OCCUPATIONAL AND ENVIRONMENTAL HEALTH

RECOGNIZING AND PREVENTING DISEASE AND INJURY

OCCUPATIONAL AND ENVIRONMENTAL HEALTH

RECOGNIZING AND PREVENTING DISEASE AND INJURY

Barry S. Levy, MD, MPH

Adjunct Professor
Department of Public Health and Family Medicine
Tufts University School of Medicine
Boston, Massachusetts

David H. Wegman, MD, MSc

Dean
School of Health and Environment
University of Massachusetts Lowell
Lowell, Massachusetts

Sherry L. Baron, MD, MPH

Coordinator, Priority Populations
National Institute for Occupational Safety and Health
Cincinnati, Ohio

Rosemary K. Sokas, MD, MOH

Professor and Director
Division of Environmental and Occupational Health Sciences
University of Illinois at Chicago School of Public Health
Chicago, Illinois

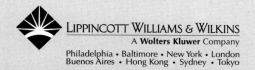

LIPPINCOTT WILLIAMS & WILKINS
A **Wolters Kluwer** Company

Philadelphia • Baltimore • New York • London
Buenos Aires • Hong Kong • Sydney • Tokyo

Acquisitions Editor: Sonya Seigafuse
Managing Editor: Nancy Winter
Developmental Editor: Molly Connors, Dovetail Content Solutions
Production Editor: Bridgett Dougherty
Senior Manufacturing Manager: Benjamin Rivera
Marketing Manager: Kathy Neely
Design coordinator: Terry Mallon
Production Services: TechBooks
Printer: Edwards Brothers

Cover photo by Earl Dotter [www.earldotter.com <http://www.earldotter.com>]

Library of Congress Cataloging-in-Publication Data

Occupational and environmental health: recognizing and preventing disease and
    injury/editors, Barry S. Levy, et al. — 5th ed.
        p. ; cm.
    Rev. ed. of: Occupational health/editors, Barry S. Levy, David H. Wegman. 4th ed.
        c2000.
    Includes bibliographical references and index.
    ISBN 0-7817-5551-4
    1. Medicine, Industrial.   I. Levy, Barry S.   II. Wegman, David H.
    III. Occupational health.
    [DNLM: 1. Occupational Diseases—prevention & control.
2. Environmental Health.   3. Occupational Exposure—prevention & control.
4. Occupational Health. WA 440 0149 2006]
RC963.022 2006
616.9′803—dc22

                                                                2005022903

Care has been taken to confirm the accuracy of the information presented and to describe generally accepted practices. However, the authors, editors, and publisher are not responsible for errors or omissions or for any consequences from application of the information in this book and make no warranty, expressed or implied, with respect to the currency, completeness, or accuracy of the contents of the publication. Application of this information in a particular situation remains the professional responsibility of the practitioner.

The authors, editors, and publisher have exerted every effort to ensure that drug selection and dosage set forth in this text are in accordance with current recommendations and practice at the time of publication. However, in view of ongoing research, changes in government regulations, and the constant flow of information relating to drug therapy and drug reactions, the reader is urged to check the package insert for each drug for any change in indications and dosage and for added warnings and precautions. This is particularly important when the recommended agent is a new or infrequently employed drug.

Some drugs and medical devices presented in this publication have Food and Drug Administration (FDA) clearance for limited use in restricted research settings. It is the responsibility of the health care providers to ascertain the FDA status of each drug or device planned for use in their clinical practice.

To purchase additional copies of this book, call our customer service department at (800) 638-3030 or fax orders to (301) 223-2320. International customers should call (301) 223-2300.

Visit Lippincott Williams & Wilkins on the Internet: at LWW.com. Lippincott Williams & Wilkins customer service representatives are available from 8:30 am to 6:00 pm, ET.

10 9 8 7 6 5 4 3 2 1

To our families for their never-ending
support and encouragement

Nancy Levy, Bernice and Jerome Levy,
Laura Levy and Ben Borowski,
and Ben Levy and Marie Knapp

Peggy, Jesse, and Marya Wegman,
Jane Dunatchik
and to the memory of
Myron, Isabel, Judy, and Betty

Dan, Traven, Reed, and Jake La Botz,
Isadora and Albert Frost,
and Henry and Ina Baron

Ahmed, Nora, Sara, and Adam Achrati
Peter Paul and Jeanne O'Toole Sokas

And to the memory of Tony Mazzocchi,
worker, advocate, labor leader, friend,
and eternal optimist, who inspired all
of us to believe in the power of workers
and people in communities to improve
the world around them.

Foreword

It is now clear that the fields of occupational health and environmental health have merged to the point that nearly all national training programs and most industrial programs include both elements. It is therefore fitting that this fifth edition of *Occupational and Environmental Health* is a fully integrated presentation of these two content areas. Indeed, now more than ever, there is a need to integrate, not only occupational and environmental health, but also health services, health promotion, and prevention in an ecological approach to inquiry, practice, and training.

The workplace and its impact on the ambient environment and the living environment of employees, family members, and their neighbors are now recognized to be much more interdependent than in the past. Workplaces of the future will be more dispersed into smaller and more rural locations. The workforce will be more diverse and include many more people with disabilities. New computer-based technologies will result in more integrated workplace designs, increased globalization, more off-site and contract work. And home-based work will become common. All of these trends will bring the workplace, the community, and the home environments closer together, making it necessary to more fully engage a variety approaches and health professionals to better understand, implement, and train those with responsibilities for workers, their family members, and the environment in which they live and work.

The challenge of the Institute of Medicine ecological model for public health—integration of broad social, economic, health, and environmental conditions; living and working conditions; social, family, and community networks; individual behavior; and innate biological traits—is to integrate employee health program elements to achieve enhanced worker protection and health more effectively, more efficiently, and more cost-effectively. This will require programs that are more performance-based, more focused on prevention and behavioral change, and more employee-centric. And it will require programs that deal with more risk factors and utilize integrated health systems.

Broader occupational and environmental health texts are therefore needed to extend these concepts beyond those traditional to occupational and environmental health. This fifth edition of *Occupational and Environmental Health,* which has been significantly expanded, provides this new perspective and meets these needs extremely well.

James A. Merchant, M.D., Dr.P.H.
Dean of The University of Iowa College of Public Health

Contents

SECTION V
An Integrated Approach to Prevention

Preface

Occupational and environmental health issues profoundly affect everyone's health and well-being. Each of us has a responsibility to address the issues that affect us as individuals, as members of families and communities, and as citizens of the world. As we prepared this fifth edition of this textbook, we directed our attention to how health professionals can recognize and prevent occupational and environmental disease and injury—at both the individual and population levels. We have, therefore, substantially revised this book to enable health professionals and students in the health professions to understand these issues and the contexts in which they occur.

In the first years of this century, dramatic changes continue to impact occupational health (ranging from the recognition of new workplace health hazards to the changing nature of work itself) and environmental health (ranging from global warming to how airborne contaminants adversely affect health). And dramatic changes continue to impact how we obtain, analyze, communicate, and use information for research, practice, and advocacy in this field. In addition, relationships between occupational health and environmental health are increasingly recognized. Occupational health hazards can affect communities. Environmental health problems often originate in workplaces. And work-related hazards, environmental degradation, poverty, and social injustice are often interrelated. This textbook aims to reflect these changes and to enable readers to prepare themselves to recognize and prevent disease and injury in a changing world.

In developing this edition, we have updated chapters from the fourth edition, emphasizing aspects of both occupational and environmental health. In addition, we have added several new chapters on environmental health issues, such as ambient air pollution, water quality, hazardous waste, and global environmental changes. We have also added a final section to the book that focuses primarily on the application and integration of occupational and environmental health principles and information. Although this book focuses primarily on occupational and environmental health in the United States, it includes several authors and many specific examples from other countries. It is designed for use by practitioners and students in health and safety professions throughout the world.

This book is divided into five sections. Section I provides an overview of occupational and environmental health—including an overview from a social perspective—as well as government regulation, legal remedies, and ethics in occupational and environmental health. Section II focuses on recognition, assessment, and prevention. Section III focuses on hazardous exposures. Section IV considers injuries and disorders by organ system, with emphasis on clinical features and prevention. Section V focuses on selected populations of workers, the roles of labor unions and nongovernmental organizations, health hazard evaluations of workplace and community exposures and illnesses, and the impact of regulation.

Information alone will not prevent occupational and environmental diseases and injuries. Prevention also depends, in part, on developing the popular and political will to support it and to implement specific preventive measures. Our society woefully undervalues the importance of prevention. Informed health and safety professionals and students, through their values, vision, and leadership, can help develop the popular and political will to ensure that occupational and environmental diseases and injuries are recognized and prevented.

The Editors
October 2005

Contributors

Henry A. Anderson, MD, MPH
Chief Medical Officer
Wisconsin Division of Public Health
Adjunct Professor
Department of Population Health
University of Wisconsin Medical School
Madison, Wisconsin
anderha@dhfs.state.wi.us

Carlos Aristeguieta, MD, MPH
Senior Service Fellow
National Institute for Occupational Safety and Health
Cincinnati, Ohio
carlos.aristeguieta@cdc.hhs.gov

Nicholas A. Ashford, PhD, JD
Professor of Technology and Policy
Director, Technology and Law Program
Center for Technology, Policy and Industrial
  Development
Massachusetts Institute of Technology
Cambridge, Massachusetts
nashford@mit.edu

David Bacon
Documentary Photographs
Berkeley, California
dbacon@igc.org

Edward L. Baker Jr., MD, MPH
Director
The North Carolina Institute for Public Health
School of Public Health
University of North Carolina at Chapel Hill
Chapel Hill, North Carolina
elbaker@email.unc.edu

Robin Baker, MPH
Director, Labor Occupational Health Program
Center for Occupational and Environmental Health
School of Public Health
University of California Berkeley
Berkeley, California
rbaker@uclink4.berkeley.edu

Elizabeth M. Barbeau, ScD, MPH
Associate Professor
Society, Human Development, and Health
Harvard School of Public Health
Researcher, Medical Oncology/Population Sciences
Dana-Farber Cancer Institute
Boston, Massachusetts
elizabeth_barbeau@dfci.harvard.edu

Sherry L. Baron, MD, MPH
Coordinator, Priority Populations
National Institute for Occupational Safety and Health
Cincinnati, Ohio
slb8@cdc.gov

Bruce P. Bernard, MD, MPH
Medical Section Chief
Hazards Evaluation and Technical Assistance
National Institute for Occupational Safety and
  Health
Cincinnati, Ohio
bpb4@cdc.gov

Leslie I. Boden, PhD
Professor of Public Health
Department of Environmental Health
Boston University School of Public Health
Boston, Massachusetts
lboden@bu.edu

Paul D. Boyce, MD, MPH
Clinical Research Fellow
Pulmonary and Critical Care Unit
Massachusetts General Hospital
MPH Candidate/Research Fellow
Occupational Health Program
Harvard School of Public Health
Boston, Massachusetts
paulboyce@post.harvard.edu

Maria J. Brunette, PhD
Wisconsin Alliance for Minority Populations
University of Wisconsin-Madison
Madison, Wisconsin
mjbrunette@engr.wisc.edu

Charles C. Caldart, JD, MPH
Research Associate/Lecturer
Department of Civil and Environmental Engineering
Massachusetts Institute of Technology
Cambridge, Massachusetts
caldart@mit.edu

John J. Cardarelli II, PhD, CIH
Health Physicist
National Decontamination Team
U.S. Environmental Protection Agency
Cincinnati, Ohio
cardarelli.john@epa.gov

Dawn N. Castillo, PhD
Chief, Surveillance and Field Investigations Branch
Division of Safety Research
National Institute for Occupational Safety and Health
Morgantown, West Virginia
dnc0@cdc.gov

Martin G. Cherniack, MD, MPH
Professor of Medicine
Director, Occupational and Environmental Medicine
    Ergonomic Technology Center
University of Connecticut Health Center
Farmington, Connecticut
cherniack@nso.uchc.edu

David C. Christiani, MD, MPH
Professor of Occupational Medicine and Epidemiology
Departments of Environmental Health and
    Epidemiology
Harvard School of Public Health
Professor of Medicine
Harvard Medical School
Boston, Massachusetts
dchris@hohp.harvard.edu

Mark R. Cullen, MD
Professor of Medicine and Public Health
Director, Occupational Health Program
Yale University School of Medicine
New Haven, Connecticut
mark.cullen@yale.edu

Denny Dobbin, MSc (OH), CIH (ret.)
President
Society for Occupational and Environmental Health
McLean, Virginia
ergo2003@hotmail.com

Joseph W. Dorsey, PhD
Assistant Professor
Environmental Science, Policy, and Geography
University of South Florida, St. Petersburg
St. Petersburg, Florida
dorseyjw@stpt.usf.edu

Earl Dotter
Photojournalist
Silver Spring, Maryland
earldotter@verizon.net

John J. Earshen, MS, FASA
Adjunct Professor
Communicative Disorders and Sciences
State University of New York
President
Angevine Acoustical Consultants, Inc.
East Aurora, New York
AngevineAc@verizon.net

Ellen A. Eisen, ScD
Professor, Department of Work Environment
University of Massachusetts Lowell
Adjunct Professor, Department of Environmental
    Health
Harvard School of Public Health
Boston, Massachusetts
eeisen@hsph.harvard.edu

Bradley Evanoff, MD, MPH
Chief, Division of General Medical Sciences
Washington University School of Medicine
St. Louis, Missouri
bevanoff@wustl.edu

Nancy L. Fiedler, PhD
Associate Professor
Environmental and Occupational Medicine
University of Medicine and Dentistry of New Jersey–
    Robert Wood Johnson Medical School
Piscataway, New Jersey
nfiedler@eohsi.rutgers.edu

Jeffrey A. Foran, PhD
President
Midwest Center for Environmental Studies and
    Public Policy
Milwaukee, Wisconsin
Adjunct Professor
Division of Environmental and Occupational
    Health Sciences, School of Public Health
University of Illinois at Chicago
Chicago, Illinois
Jforan@wi.rr.com

Linda M. Frazier, MD, MPH
Professor, Department of Preventive Medicine
    and Public Health
Adjunct Professor, Department of Obstetrics and
    Gynecology
Executive Director
University of Kansas Master in Public Health Program,
    Wichita and Kansas City
The University of Kansas School of Medicine-Wichita
Wichita, Kansas
lfrazier@kumc.edu

Deborah Barkin Fromer, MPH
Teaching Associate
Department of Preventive Medicine and
    Public Health
The University of Kansas School of Medicine-Wichita
Wichita, Kansas
dfromer@kumc.edu

Kenneth Geiser, PhD
Professor, Department of Work Environment
University of Massachusetts Lowell
Lowell, Massachusetts
Kgeiser@turi.org

Michael Gochfeld, MD, PhD
Professor, Environmental and Community Medicine
UMDNJ-Robert Wood Johnson Medical School
Environmental and Occupational Health Sciences
    Institute
Piscataway, New Jersey
gochfeld@eohsi.rutgers.edu

Gary N. Greenberg, MD, MPH
Moderator, Occupational and Environmental
    Medicine Forum
Associate Clinical Professor
Community and Family Medicine
Duke University Medical Center
Durham, North Carolina
Gary.Greenberg@Duke.edu

Simon Hales, MB BChir, MPH, PhD
Fellow
National Centre for Epidemiology and Population
    Health
The Australian National University
Senior Research Fellow
Department of Public Health
Wellington School of Medicine & Health Sciences
University of Otago
Wellington, New Zealand
simon.hales@otago.ac.nz

William E. Halperin, MD, DrPH
Professor and Chairman
Department of Preventive Medicine and Community
    Health
New Jersey Medical School
Newark, New Jersey
halperwe@umdnj.edu

John F. Halpin, MD
Undersea Medical Officer
U.S. Navy Reserve
Department of Occupational Medicine
University of Illinois at Chicago
Chicago, Illinois
halpinj36@yahoo.com

Mauricio Hernández-Ávila, MD, MPH, ScD
Director General
Instituto Nacional de Salud Pública
Cuernavaca, Morelos, Mexico
director@insp.mx

Fernando Holguin, MD
Assistant Professor
Department of Medicine
Emory University School of Medicine
Atlanta, Georgia
fholgui@sph.emory.edu

Joseph J. Hurrell Jr., PhD
Associate Director for Science
National Institute for Occupational Safety
    and Health
Cincinnati, Ohio
jjh3@cdc.gov

W. Monroe Keyserling, PhD
Professor, Department of Industrial and Operations
    Engineering and Environmental Health Science
The University of Michigan
Ann Arbor, Michigan
wmkeyser@umich.edu

Ann M. Krake, MS, REHS
LCDR, U.S. Public Health Service
El Portal, California
Ann_Krake@nps.gov

Kathleen Kreiss, MD
Chief, Field Studies Branch
Division of Respiratory Disease Studies
National Institute for Occupational Safety
    and Health
Morgantown, West Virginia
kxk2@cdc.gov

Neil T. Leifer, JD
Thornton & Naumes, L.L.P.
Boston, Massachusetts
nleifer@tenlaw.com

Barry S. Levy, MD, MPH
Adjunct Professor
Department of Public Health and Family Medicine
Tufts University School of Medicine
Boston, Massachusetts
blevy@igc.org

Jane A. Lipscomb, RN, PhD, FAAN
Associate Professor
University of Maryland School of Nursing
Baltimore, Maryland
lipscomb@son.umaryland.edu

Robyn M. Lucas, BSc, MBChB, MPH
Research Fellow
National Centre for Epidemiology and Population
    Health
The Australian National University
Canberra, Australia
robyn.lucas@anu.edu.au

Boris D. Lushniak, MD, MPH
Chief Medical Officer
Office of Counterterrorism Policy and Planning
Food and Drug Administration
Rockville, Maryland
boris.lushniak@fda.gov

Anthony J. McMichael, PhD
Director
National Centre for Epidemiology and Population
    Health
The Australian National University
Canberra, Australia
tony.mcmichael@anu.edu.au

James Melius, MD, DrPH
Administrator
New York State Laborers Health and Safety Fund
Albany, New York
melius@nysliuna.org

Donna Mergler, PhD
Professor, Department of Biological Sciences
University of Quebec at Montreal
Montreal, Quebec, Canada
mergler.donna@uqam.ca

Rick Mines
Private Research Economist
Rail Road Flat, Cailfornia
rkmines@volcano.net

Thais Catalani Morata, PhD
Research Audiologist
National Institute for Occupational Safety and Health
Cincinnati, Ohio
tcm2@cdc.gov

Rafael Moure-Eraso, PhD, CIH
Professor and Chair
Department of Work Environment
University of Massachusetts Lowell
Lowell, Massachusetts
Rafael_Moure@uml.edu

Henry Nehls-Lowe, MPH
Epidemiologist
Bureau of Environmental and Occupational Health
Wisconsin Division of Public Health
Madison, Wisconsin
nehlshl@dhfs.state.wi.us

Marie S. O'Neill, MS, PhD
Robert Wood Johnson Foundation Health and Safety
    Scholar
Center for Social Epidemiology and Population Health
University of Michigan
Ann Arbor, Michigan
marieo@umich.edu

Timothy J. Pizatella, MS
Deputy Director
Division of Safety Research
National Institute for Occupational Safety and Health
Morgantown, West Virginia
timothy.pizatella@cdc.hhs.gov

Stephanie Pollack, JD
Senior Research Associate
Center for Urban & Regional Policy
Northeastern University
Boston, Massachusetts
s.pollack@neu.edu

Margaret M. Quinn, ScD, CIH
Professor, Department of Work Environment
University of Massachusetts Lowell
Lowell, Massachusetts
Margaret_Quinn@uml.edu

Peter M. Rabinowitz, MD, MPH
Assistant Professor of Medicine
Yale Occupational and Environmental Medicine
    Program
Yale University School of Medicine
New Haven, Connecticut
peter.rabinowitz@yale.edu

Kathleen M. Rest, PhD, MPA
Executive Director
Union of Concerned Scientists
Cambridge, Massachusetts
krest@ucsusa.org

Patricia A. Roche, JD, MEd
Assistant Professor of Health Law
Department of Health Law, Bioethics, and Human
    Rights
Boston University School of Public Health
Boston, Massachusetts
pwroche@bu.edu

Bonnie Rogers, DrPH, COHN, FAAN
Director, Public Health Nursing and Occupational
    Health Nursing
University of North Carolina at Chapel Hill School
    of Public Health
Chapel Hill, North Carolina
rogersb@email.unc.edu

Isabelle Romieu, MD, MPH
Professor of Environmental Epidemiology
Salud Ambiental
Instituto Nacional de Salud Pública
Cuernavaca, Morelos, Mexico
iromieu@correo.insp.mx

Beth J. Rosenberg, MPH, ScD
Assistant Professor
Department of Public Health and Family Medicine
Tufts University School of Medicine
Boston, Massachusetts
beth.rosenberg@tufts.edu

Mark B. Russi, MD, MPH
Associate Professor of Medicine and Public Health
Yale University School of Medicine
Director, Occupational Health Services
Yale-New Haven Hospital
New Haven, Connecticut
mark.russi@ynhh.org

Thomas Schneider, MSc
Senior Scientist
National Institute of Occupational Health
Copenhagen, Denmark
ts@ami.dk

Ken Silver, SM, DSc
Assistant Professor
Department of Environmental Health
East Tennessee State University
Johnson City, Tennessee
silver@etsu.edu

Barbara Silverstein, PhD
Research Director
Safety and Health Assessment and Research for
    Prevention (SHARP)
Washington State Department of Labor and Industries
Affiliate Professor
Department of Environmental and Occupational
    Health Sciences
University of Washington School of Public Health and
    Community Medicine
Seattle, Washington
silb235@lni.wa.gov

Michael Silverstein, MD, MPH
Clinical Professor
Department of Environmental and Occupational Health
    Sciences
University of Washington School of Public Health and
    Community Medicine
Seattle, Washington
masilver@u.washington.edu

Thomas J. Smith, MPH, MS, PhD
Professor of Industrial Hygiene
Department of Environmental Health
Harvard School of Public Health
Boston, Massachusetts
tjsmith@hsph.harvard.edu

Rosemary K. Sokas, MD, MOH
Professor and Director
Division of Environmental and Occupational Health
    Sciences
University of Illinois at Chicago School of Public
    Health
Chicago, Illinois
sokas@uic.edu

Adam Spanier, MD, MPH
Clinical/Research Fellow
Division of General & Community Pediatrics
Cincinnati Children's Hospital Medical Center
Cincinnati, Ohio
Adam.Spanier@cchmc.org

Emily A. Spieler, JD
Dean and Edwin Hadley Professor of Law
Northeastern University School of Law
Boston, Massachusetts
e.spieler@neu.edu

Laura Stock, MPH
Associate Director
Labor Occupational Health Program
Center for Occupational and Environmental Health
School of Public Health
University of California Berkeley
Berkeley, California
lstock@berkeley.edu

Nancy A. Stout, EdD
Director
Division of Safety Research
National Institute for Occupational Safety
  and Health
Morgantown, West Virginia
nancy.stout@cdc.hhs.gov

David C. Strouss, JD
Thornton & Naumes, L.L.P.
Boston, Massachusetts
dstrouss@tenlaw.com

Nick Thorkelson
Graphic Designs & Illustration
Somerville, Massachusetts
nthork@cais.com

Rodney D. Turpin, MS, RPIH
Senior Science Advisor/Adjunct Assistant Professor
The New Jersey Center for Public Health Preparedness
  at UMDNJ School of Public Health
Chief National Health and Safety Advisor
Environmental Response Team
U.S. Environmental Protection Agency
Edison, New Jersey
turpin.rod@epa.gov

Gregory R. Wagner, MD
Director, Division of Respiratory Disease Studies
National Institute for Occupational Safety and Health
Morgantown, West Virginia
grw3@cdc.gov

Elizabeth M. Ward, PhD
Director, Surveillance Research
Department of Epidemiology and Surveillance
  Research
American Cancer Society
Atlanta, Georgia
elizabeth.ward@cancer.org

Michelle T. Watters, MD, PhD, MPH
Environmental Health Medical Officer
Region 5
Agency for Toxic Substances and Disease Registry
Chicago, Illinois
Watters.Michelle@epamail.epa.gov

James L. Weeks, ScD, CIH
Senior Scientist
ATL International, Inc.
Germantown, Maryland
jweeks@atlintl.com

David H. Wegman, MD, MSc
Dean, School of Health and Environment
University of Massachusetts Lowell
Lowell, Massachusetts
David_Wegman@uml.edu

Laura S. Welch, MD
Adjunct Professor
School of Public Health and Health Sciences
George Washington University
Medical Director
The Center to Protect Workers' Rights
Silver Spring, Maryland
lwelch@cpwr.com

Acknowledgments

We greatly appreciate the assistance and support of many people in the development of the fifth edition of *Occupational and Environmental Health*. We thank the many chapter authors, whose work is appropriately credited within the text. In addition, there have been many other people working behind the scenes, to whom we are deeply appreciative. We acknowledge Heather Merrell for her excellent work in preparing the manuscript and communicating with editors, authors, and the production team.

We are grateful for the outstanding work and support of Sonya Seigafuse, acquisitions editor, Nancy Winter, managing editor, and Bridgett Dougherty, project manager, of Lippincott Williams & Wilkins; Molly Connors of Dovetail Content Solutions; and John Probst.

The illustrative materials throughout the book are included to offer understanding and insights not easily gained from the text. We call special attention to the work of Earl Dotter, who provided many outstanding photographs that well illustrate occupational and environmental health issues, and Nick Thorkelson, who provided a number of creative drawings that convey concepts and perspectives that are difficult to capture in words and photographs. We are also grateful for the photographic contributions of David Bacon.

Finally, we express our appreciation to students and colleagues who, over the years, have broadened—and continue to broaden—our understanding of occupational and environmental health.

The Editors

Work, Environment, and Health

CHAPTER 1

Occupational and Environmental Health: An Overview

Barry S. Levy, David H. Wegman, Sherry L. Baron, and Rosemary K. Sokas

Occupational and environmental health is the multidisciplinary approach to the recognition, diagnosis, treatment, and prevention and control of disease, injuries, and other adverse health conditions resulting from hazardous environmental exposures in the workplace, the home, or the community. It is part of public health—what we, as a society, do collectively to assure that the conditions in which people live and work are healthy. Occupational and environmental health is an integral part of many disciplines, as illustrated by the following examples:

A 2-year-old girl, during a routine well-child checkup, is found to have an elevated blood lead level of 20 μg/dL.

A pregnant woman who works as a laboratory technician asks her obstetrician if she should change her job because of the chemicals to which she and her fetus are exposed and if it is safe to eat fish with possibly elevated levels of mercury.

A middle-aged man tells an orthopedic surgeon that he is totally disabled from chronic back pain, which he attributes to many years of heavy lifting as a construction worker.

A long-distance truck driver asks a cardiologist how soon after his recent myocardial infarction will he be able to return to work and what kinds of tasks he will be able to perform.

A chemical manufacturer, aware that a pesticide that it produces is carcinogenic and has recently been banned from sale in the United States, makes arrangements for the export of the pesticide for sale and use in developing countries.

The wife of a former asbestos worker asks her physician whether she can receive compensation for the pleural mesothelioma she has developed, presumably as a result of having washed her husband's work clothes for many years.

An oncologist observes an unusual cluster of bladder cancer cases among middle-aged women in a small town.

An elderly man with emphysema as a result of cigarette smoking asks his physician if he should curtail his activities during an air pollution alert.

Several members of a family who live adjacent to a hazardous waste site consult their physician concerning headaches, nausea, and other symptoms they note whenever they smell odors coming from the waste site.

The vice-president of a small tool and die company asks his family physician to advise his company regarding prevention of occupational disease and health promotion among his employees.

These are but a few examples of the numerous occupational and environmental health challenges facing health professionals. Virtually all health professionals need to recognize and help prevent occupational and environmental health problems.

Many hazardous exposures involve both workplaces and the general environment. Examples include:

- Chemical contamination of the air and water surrounding a factory where workers are also exposed.
- Agricultural workers' application of pesticides that may contaminate surface water and groundwater.

- Workers bringing lead, asbestos, and other hazardous materials home on their work clothes, skin, and hair.
- Exposure of workers and community residents to hazardous wastes that have been inappropriately disposed of by industrial facilities.

The biological and physical sciences that explain the pathophysiology of specific hazards in humans are the same whether the environment is a workplace, school, home, or community setting. However, the sociology and history of environmental health and of occupational health has evolved along separate tracks, with differences of focus, scale, and people involved. Hippocrates recognized the importance of air quality for health, although he was concerned with the fraction of Greeks who were citizens—not for the slaves or even for the free workers who supported them. Pliny the Elder recognized the ill effects of lead on slaves who painted ships in the first century C.E., but the use of lead in making cookware, sweetening foods, and souring vintages persisted for hundreds of years—and may have contributed to the fall of the Roman Empire. Occupational hazards were not addressed in a systematic form until the Italian physician Bernardino Ramazzini published *On the Diseases of Workers* in 1700, noting that "... we owe this to the wretched condition of the workers from whose manual toil, so necessary though sometimes so very mean and sordid, so many benefits accrue to the commonwealth of mankind." Beginning in the early 20th century, Dr. Alice Hamilton, a colleague of the great American social reformer Jane Addams, pioneered occupational health as a field of public health and preventive medicine. Rachel Carson, a popular science writer, focused public attention on the wider impact of industrial pollution in the 1960s with her widely sold book, *Silent Spring*. In the past 30 years, extraordinary changes in medical ethics, public health, and social empowerment have challenged professionals in environmental health and occupational health to work together.

Although the nature of many occupational and environmental health problems are similar, workers tend to be exposed more intensively to various hazards than community residents. As a result, the relationship between occupational exposures and adverse health effects has provided much of the information known about hazardous substances. Populations of community residents include not only workers, who are typically healthy, but also the very young and the very old and people with chronic diseases and other health conditions that may make them more vulnerable to hazardous exposures. Their exposures are often 24 hours a day, 7 days a week, although generally at lower levels of exposure. Environmental health encompasses not only hazardous substances emanating from industrial facilities but also such fundamental issues as sanitation, food and water safety, and pest control. There can be considerable overlap among occupational and environmental health issues.

Although there are many similarities and overlaps among occupational and environmental health, governmental regulatory agencies and various health and safety disciplines have evolved over time in ways that have separated occupational health and environmental health. For example, in the United States, there are separate federal regulatory agencies for occupational health (the Occupational Safety and Health Administration [OSHA]) and environmental health (the Environmental Protection Agency [EPA]). In addition, there are separate federal agencies for research in occupational health (the National Institute for Occupational Safety and Health [NIOSH] within the Centers for Disease Control and Prevention [CDC]) and environmental health (the National Institute for Environmental Health Sciences [NIEHS] within the National Institutes of Health, the Office of Research and Development of EPA, and the National Center for Environmental Health and the Agency for Toxic Substances Disease Registry within CDC). Similar separation exists within state and local government agencies, educational and research institutions, nongovernmental organizations (NGOs), professional associations, and elsewhere.

Occupational and environmental health and safety hazards can generally be classified in the following manner:

1. Safety hazards that result in injury through the uncontrolled transfer of energy to a vulnerable recipient from sources such as electrical, thermal, kinetic, chemical, or radiation energy. Examples include unsafe playground equipment, loaded firearms in the home, motor vehicle or bicycle crashes, unprotected electrical sources, working at heights without fall protection, working near unguarded moving machinery, and working in unshored trenches.
2. Health hazards that result in environmental or occupational illness, including:

a. *Chemical hazards*: These include heavy metals, such as lead and mercury; pesticides; organic solvents, such as benzene and trichloroethylene; and many other chemicals. (There are approximately 80,000 chemicals in commercial use, 15,000 of which are frequently produced or used. It is estimated that approximately 1,000 new chemicals are added to commercial use each year.)

b. *Physical hazards*: These include excessive noise, vibration, extremes of temperature and pressure, and ionizing and non-ionizing radiation.

c. *Biomechanical hazards*: These include heavy lifting and repetitive, awkward, or forceful movements that result in musculoskeletal disorders, such as carpal tunnel syndrome and many cases of low back pain syndrome.

d. *Biological hazards*: These include HIV, hepatitis B and hepatitis C viruses, the tubercle bacillus, and many other bacteria, viruses, and other microorganisms that may be transmitted through air, water, food, or direct contact.

e. *Psychosocial stress*: This includes high-stress work environments resulting from excessive work demands on workers and low control by workers as well as stress and hostility resulting from urban congestion, such as "road rage." Unemployment is a major stressor.

MAGNITUDE OF PROBLEMS

An estimated 10 million work-related injuries and 400,000 new work-related illnesses occur each year in the United States. In developing countries, occupational injury and illness rates are much higher than in the United States. Each day in the United States, an average of 9,000 workers sustain disabling injuries on the job, approximately 16 workers die from workplace injury, and an estimated 140 workers die from work-related diseases. Occupational injuries and diseases, affecting many organ systems (Table 1-1), however, are reported infrequently. Table 1-2 describes employed civilians in the United States by industry. There has been a declining percentage of workers in the United States in heavy industry (Figs. 1-1 and 1-2) and an increasing percentage in service industries (Fig. 1-3). According to the Bureau of Labor Statistics (BLS) Census of Fatal Occupational Injuries, approximately 5,700 traumatic occupational

TABLE 1-1

Major Categories of Occupational Illness, by Organ System

Musculoskeletal disorders

Respiratory disorders

Neurologic and psychiatric disorders, including hearing impairment

Skin disorders

Reproductive and developmental disorders

Cardiovascular disorders

Hematologic disorders

Hepatic disorders

Renal and urinary tract disorders

fatalities occur in the United States each year; the highest rates are in mining, construction, and agriculture/forestry/fisheries (see Chapter 32). Although these statistics provide some idea of the scope and types of occupational health problems, they grossly underestimate the role of the workplace in causing new disease and injuries and exacerbating existing ones. In addition, statistics do not represent the relative distribution of various work-related

TABLE 1-2

Employees on Nonfarm Payrolls by Major Industry Sector, Seasonally Adjusted (February 2005)

Industry	Size of Workforce (in millions)
Services	52.1
Wholesale and retail trade	20.8
Manufacturing	14.3
Finance, insurance, real estate	8.1
Transportation, warehousing, utilities	4.9
Construction	7.1
Natural resources and mining	0.6
Government	21.8
Information	3.1
Total	132.8

From the Bureau of Labor Statistics, U.S. Department of Labor. Available at: www.bls.gov. Accessed March 10, 2005.

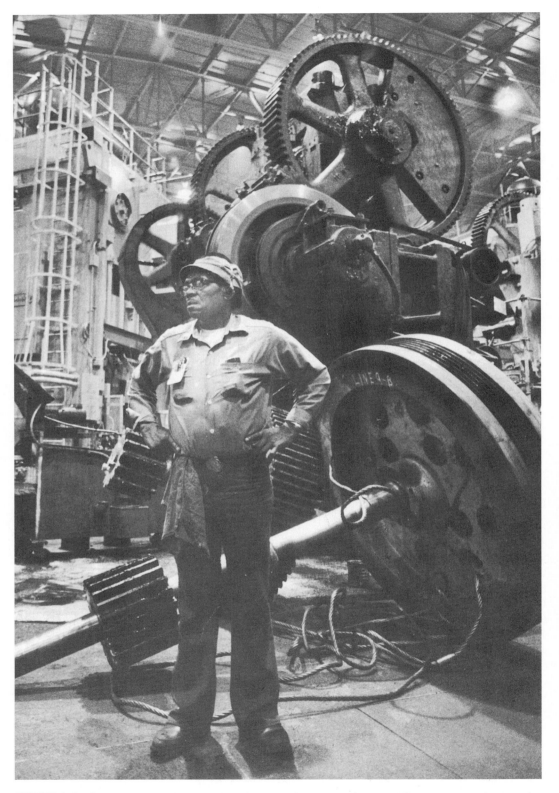

FIGURE 1-1 ● Worker at a wheel-stamping plant in Michigan. Manufacturing still represents a major part of the economy and a source of many occupational health and safety hazards. (Photograph by Earl Dotter.)

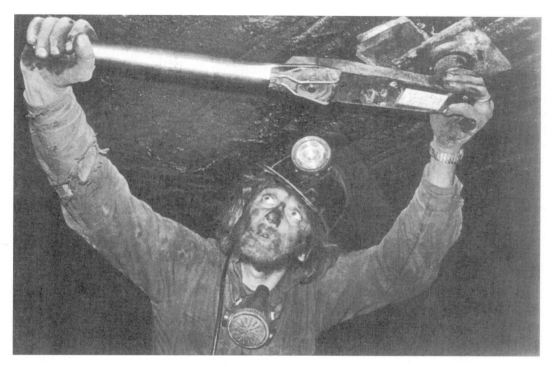

FIGURE 1-2 ● Roof bolting in coal mines is essential to prevent roofs from collapsing. Miners, like this man testing the mine roof support bolts in a Pennsylvania coal mine, face many other injury risks as well as exposure to hazardous dusts, gases, and other substances. (Photograph by Earl Dotter.)

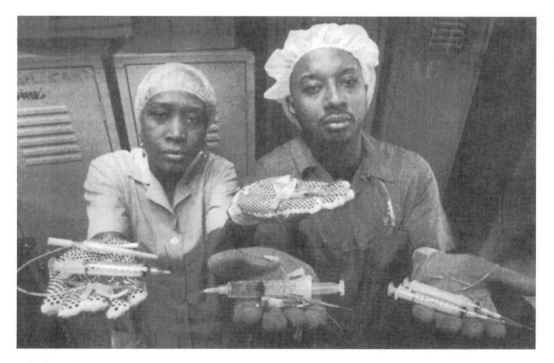

FIGURE 1-3 ● Health care workers, including these laundry workers in New York, face a number of occupational hazards, including human immunodeficiency virus, hepatitis B virus, hepatitis C virus, and other infections associated with needlestick injuries. These laundry workers found these "sharps" in soiled bed linens over the course of a year. (Photograph by Earl Dotter.)

diseases. For example, because skin disorders are easy to recognize and relate to working conditions, their representation in BLS data exaggerates their relative importance.

The scope of environmental health problems is broad (Table 1-3). Outdoor air pollution remains a widespread environmental and public health problem, causing chronic impairment of the respiratory and cardiovascular systems, cancer, and premature death (Fig. 1-4). Approximately 113 million people in the United States reside in areas designated as "nonattainment areas" by the EPA for one or more of the six air pollutants for which the federal government has promulgated health-based standards (ozone, carbon monoxide, sulfur dioxide, lead, particulates, and nitrogen dioxide). Motor vehicles and power plants account for a substantial share of ambient air pollution in the United States. Water quality continues to be a problem due to both point sources, such as industrial sites, and non-point sources, such as agricultural runoff (Fig. 1-5). Toxic and hazardous substances, in addition to posing health problems for exposed workers, may also cause health problems to people exposed where they live and play. Children are at increased risk for a number of environmental health problems, including pesticide poisoning, because of their smaller body mass and because pesticides and other toxic substances may be improperly stored or applied in areas that are easily accessible to children.

Many additional environmental factors can affect people's health in their homes and communities. These include poor indoor air quality, lead-based paint (Fig. 1-6) and lead-containing water pipes, household cleaning products, mold, radon, and electrical and fire hazards. More than 90 percent of poison exposures reported by the American Association of Poison Control Centers have occurred in the home environment.

There are fewer reliable data available for the occurrence of environmentally related diseases than for occupationally related diseases and injuries in the United States. For some disorders, such as childhood lead poisoning, there are extensive data from screening programs, which, for example, show that 2.2 percent of children ages 1 to 5 years had elevated blood lead levels (greater than 10 μg/dL) in 2000. On the other hand, data on pesticide poisoning are rather limited, and many cases go unreported because of the nonspecificity of symptoms. California, the state with the most extensive pesticide poisoning reporting system, found that

TABLE 1-3

Subjects of Environmental Health Objectives in *Healthy People 2010*, United States

Outdoor Air Quality
　Harmful air pollutants
　Alternative modes of transportation
　Cleaner alternative fuels
　Airborne toxins

Water Quality
　Safe drinking water
　Waterborne disease outbreaks
　Water conservation
　Surface water health risks
　Beach closings
　Fish contamination

Toxics and Waste
　Elevated blood lead levels in children
　Risks posed by hazardous sites
　Pesticide exposures
　Toxic pollutants
　Recycled municipal solid waste

Healthy Homes and Healthy Communities
　Indoor allergens
　Office building air quality
　Homes tested for radon
　Radon-resistant new home construction
　School policies to protect against environmental hazards
　Disaster preparedness plans and protocols
　Lead-based paint testing
　Substandard housing

Infrastructure and Surveillance
　Exposure to pesticides
　Exposure to heavy metals and other toxic chemicals
　Information systems used for environmental health
　Monitoring environmentally related diseases
　Local agencies using surveillance data for vector control

Global Environmental Health
　Global burden of disease
　Water quality in the U.S.–Mexico border region

Source: Department of Health and Human Services. Healthy people 2010 (second edition). Washington, DC: U.S. Government Printing Office, 2000. Available at: www.healthypeople.gov/document/HTML/Volume1/08Environmental.htm. Accessed March 6, 2005.

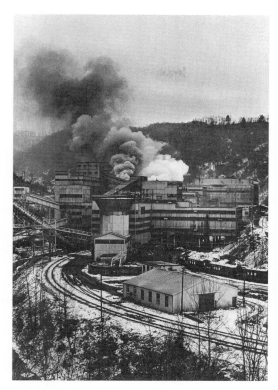

FIGURE 1-4 ● Ambient air pollution from a coal-cleaning plant in West Virginia. (Photograph by Earl Dotter.)

40 percent of the more than 1,300 reported cases were due to nonoccupational exposures. As another example, there are extensive data on acute injuries in the home, on the road, and in other settings and due to various factors, ranging from vehicles to firearms. In 2000, 29.5 million people were treated for injuries in emergency departments in the United States and more than 148,000 people hospitalized. Motor vehicle crashes are the leading cause of injury deaths, accounting for 30 percent. And while there are extensive data on ambient air pollution, there are only limited data on acute and chronic morbidity and on mortality that may be associated. The prevalence of asthma increased 74 percent from 1980 to 1996. In 1996, there were an estimated 14.6 million persons with asthma. Researchers believe that environmental factors, such as air pollution, environmental tobacco smoke, and other allergens, play an important role in the problem. Firearms account for approximately 30,000 deaths in the United States each year.

Many occupational and environmental health problems escape detection for a variety of rea-sons. The difficulty in obtaining accurate estimates of the frequency of exposure-related diseases is due to several factors, as indicated below and on Fig. 1-7:

1. Many problems do not come to the attention of health professionals, employers, and others and therefore are not included in data collection systems. A worker or community resident may not recognize a medical problem as being occupationally or environmentally related, even when the connection is known. Training workers and community residents about hazards, such as through the community and workplace right-to-know campaigns, has been helpful.

2. Many occupational and environmental medical problems that do come to the attention of physicians, employers, and others are not recognized as occupationally and environmentally related. Recognition of occupational and environmental disorders is often difficult because of the long period between initial exposure and onset of symptoms (or time of diagnosis), making cause-and-effect relationships difficult to assess. It is also difficult because of the many and varied occupational and environmental hazards to which people are exposed over many years. The training of health professionals in occupational and environmental health has begun to improve health care providers' knowledge of these factors, resulting in increased recognition of occupational and environmental diseases and injuries.

3. Some health problems recognized by health professionals, employees, or others as occupationally or environmentally related are not reported because the association with the workplace or other environments is equivocal and because reporting requirements are not strict. For example, there are only a few states where reporting of pesticide poisoning by physicians is mandatory. The initiation of occupational and environmental disease and injury surveillance activities by federal and state governments has begun to address this problem.

4. Because many occupational and environmental health problems are preventable, their very persistence implies that some individual, group, or organization is legally and economically responsible for creating or perpetuating them.

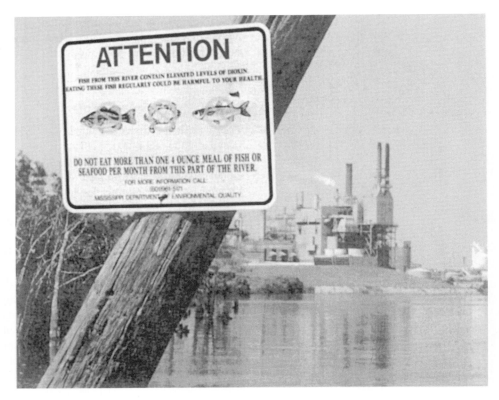

FIGURE 1-5 ●   Although non-point sources account for increasing amounts of water pollution in the United States, stationary point sources still account for a substantial amount of water pollution, such as with dioxin, a by-product of the manufacture of bleached white paper at this Mississippi plant. (Photograph by Earl Dotter.)

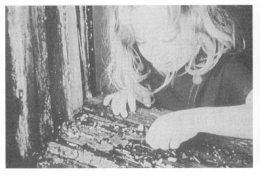
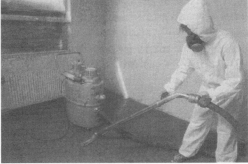

A   B

FIGURE 1-6 ●   Lead-based paint in many older homes still represents a serious health hazard to many young children. **A.** Potential child exposure to peeling lead-based paint on a windowsill, a common site for such exposure. Although the most important pathway of exposure to lead-based paint is through house dust and hand-to-mouth activity by young children, paint chips may be directly ingested, and toddlers often stand at a windowsill while chewing or sucking on the paint. **B.** Lead-abatement worker, with personal protective equipment, performs postabatement cleanup. Workers performing lead abatement must be trained and certified, and they must carefully adhere to safe practice standards. (Photographs by the California Department of Health Services.)

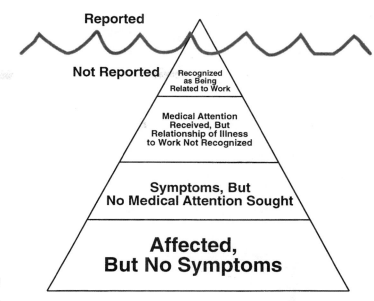

Reported

Not Reported

Recognized as Being Related to Work

Medical Attention Received, But Relationship of Illness to Work Not Recognized

Symptoms, But No Medical Attention Sought

Affected, But No Symptoms

"The Iceberg" of Occupational Disease

FIGURE 1-7 ● Most occupational disease is below the surface, as illustrated by the iceberg effect in this figure. Most environmental disease is also below the surface.

CONTEXT

Occupational and environmental health problems must be understood in social, economic, political, and historical contexts (see Chapter 2). In addition, the health and well-being of people exists in a broad ecological context (Fig. 1-8). Health and safety professionals as well as many other "actors" become involved in the detection, evaluation, and prevention and control of occupational and environmental health problems. These include workers and employers; community residents; representatives of business and industry; representatives of labor unions and environmental NGOs; officials in the executive, legislative, and judicial branches of government at the federal, state, and local levels; representatives of international organizations; educators and trainers; researchers; print and broadcast journalists and other representatives of the news media; workers in foundations that financially support programs and projects to recognize and prevent occupational and environmental problems; and people involved with other groups and organizations.

This book focuses on the recognition and prevention of these problems. Recognition focuses not only on detecting occupationally and environmentally related adverse health effects in symptomatic and asymptomatic individuals but also on applying the principles of public health surveillance for detecting individual cases and overall trends of disease

and injury occurrence in populations (see Chapter 6). Public health principles have been applied to occupational and environmental health in preventing and controlling these adverse health effects (see Chapter 7). Primary prevention focuses on diseases or injuries before they occur. Secondary prevention focuses on early identification and treatment of diseases to cure them or halt their progression. Tertiary prevention focuses on treatment and rehabilitation of individuals who have already developed diseases or injuries.

Another useful perspective on identifying opportunities for prevention and designing and implementing preventive measures is the traditional public health model of host, agent, and environment. Many preventive measures focus on the host, such as the individual worker or community resident. These measures include education and labeling, screening programs, and, where other measures cannot be implemented, use of appropriate personal protective equipment. Other preventive measures focus more on the agent, such as gasoline containing lead and insulation containing asbestos, and control measures are focused on restricting or banning production or use of the agent or on reducing human exposure to acceptable levels of risk. Some preventive measures focus on the environment; for example, designing and implementing engineering measures, such as local exhaust ventilation, can remove airborne hazards in the workplace, or installing

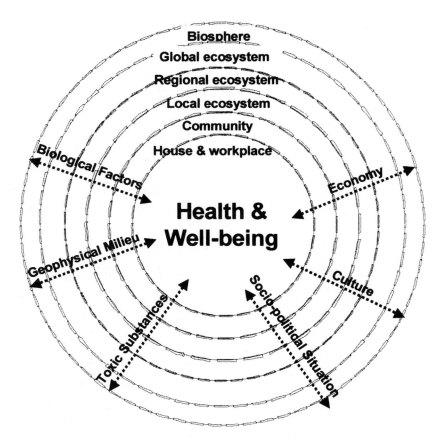

FIGURE 1-8 ● An ecosystems approach offers the opportunity to employ a wide variety of resources to achieve maximum health of individuals, groups, and communities. (Adapted from presentation by Donna Mergler, III Conference on Occupational and Environmental Health in the Americas, Alajuela, Costa Rica, February 2005.)

soundproofing materials can reduce exposure to excessive noise.

ILLUSTRATIVE OCCUPATIONAL AND ENVIRONMENTAL HEALTH ISSUES

Legislation, social activism, educational activities, and other developments have contributed to increased interest in occupational and environmental health problems in recent years. Some of these developments are summarized below.

Changing Nature of Work and of the Workforce

Enormous changes in work structure have taken place in recent decades, including mergers and, paradoxically, downsizing and outsourcing. For example, the production, packing, and distribution of meat in the United States is radically different

now than it was 30 years ago. The number of poultry, beef, and pork producers has decreased while the size of the producers has grown. Family farms have given way to concentrated animal production operations, with large-scale production and mechanization processes, which have led to concerns about animal welfare, environmental contamination from concentrated waste, and exploitation of workers. Meat packaging and poultry processing plants have relocated near to large producers, and their workforce has been transformed from relatively highly paid, unionized, mostly white workers to one that is increasingly composed of immigrant (mostly Latino) workers, who have low membership in labor unions, extremely high turnover, and low pay (Fig. 1-9). Poor working conditions remain a significant problem. In addition, one-third of those working in meat-processing plants are contingent workers who work for subcontracting agencies and perform such tasks as cleaning and maintenance.

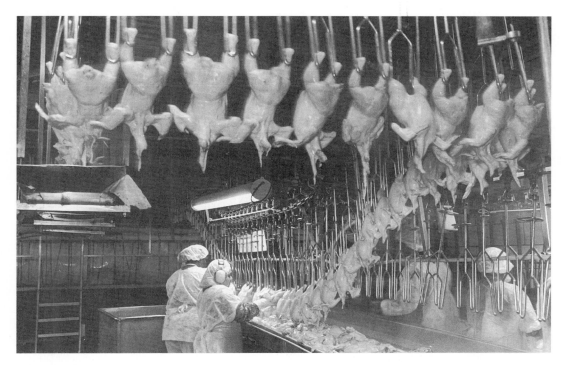

FIGURE 1-9 ● Worker processing chickens on an assembly line. Minority workers and women are overrepresented in entry-level jobs like this one, in which safety and health hazards are prevalent. Twenty-five workers in a similar chicken-processing plant died in 1991, when few workers were able to escape a fire that swept through the plant because the employer had locked most of the exit doors. (Photograph by Earl Dotter.)

Although these tasks often involve great hazard, workers' compensation and OSHA requirements often fail to adequately address these contingent workers' needs. The hazards faced by undocumented immigrant workers who find themselves in informal work arrangements or day-labor settings have resulted in mortality rates for foreign-born Hispanic workers that are one-third higher than those of native-born citizens. Reliance on contingent and outsourced labor takes place throughout the economy, from health care to manufacturing to information technology. Other changes in the workforce over the past three decades include the full integration of women into the workforce—although not in all work sectors—and the aging of the U.S. population as a whole as the "baby boom" generation ages.

Specific issues raised by these phenomena include the needs to address the integration of family health with work schedules and to accommodate workers who have significant skills but, for example, reduced physical capacity or visual acuity. In addition, advances in health care have increased the numbers of workers with severe impairments who nevertheless have the ability to contribute to society and the right to work, now recognized through the Americans with Disabilities Act. The careful development and implementation of redesigned community, home, and work spaces benefits all of us, in the same way that curb access has improved the lives of mobility-impaired individuals along with, for example, those of parents pushing strollers. All of these challenges can be met through concerted prevention activities, including development and implementation of employment policies, public health measures, engineering research, safety and health training, legislation and regulation, and the practice of clinical medicine.

Governmental Role

With the passage of the Federal Coal Mine Safety and Health Act in 1969 and legislation to establish OSHA and EPA in 1970, the federal government began taking a more active role in the creation and enforcement of standards for a safe and healthful workplace and a safe and healthy ambient environment (see Chapter 3). In addition, the 1970

Occupational Safety and Health Act also established NIOSH, which (a) has greatly expanded epidemiologic and laboratory research into the causes of occupational diseases and injuries and the methods of preventing them, and (b) has strengthened the education and training of occupational health and safety professionals. In 1969, NIEHS was established as part of the National Institutes for Health, greatly expanding the funding for environmental health research, with an initial focus on toxicologic and etiologic work, which has expanded into community-based participatory research addressing environmental justice interventions. The role of the federal government in funding scientific research, especially in the biomedical sciences, has remained strong over time. A similar sustained program to develop and implement public health measures, including surveillance tools and interventions, has never fully materialized, although interest has been rekindled in the wake of the September 11 terrorist attacks. Such a program would require strengthening of state and local government capacities through federal coordination and funding.

The roles of the federal government to set and enforce health and safety standards—for occupational or environmental contaminants, food safety, consumer protection, and a host of other public health concerns—vary and remain controversial. After the initial attempts in 1969–1970 to bring standardization to all parts of the country and to enact an initial series of environmental and occupational health laws, followed by promulgation of related standards, intense legal and political challenges slowed the setting of new standards to a crawl, and congressional budget cuts hampered enforcement of existing standards. At the present time, cooperative programs and educational outreach are prioritized. Unfortunately, increased immigration and growth in the informal workforce have occurred simultaneously, removing many financial incentives for improved safety and health at the same time that regulatory activity has dwindled. Identifying and establishing an appropriate role for government is a responsibility that all health and safety professionals share.

Occupational Safety and Health Education

A variety of factors have contributed to a recent growth in education and training opportunities for workers, employers, health professionals, and others. Unions have directed more attention to occupational health and safety through collective bargaining agreements, hiring of health professionals, workplace health and safety committees, educational programs, and support of epidemiologic studies. Worker education has been facilitated by right-to-know laws and regulations, independent coalitions for occupational safety and health (COSH groups), and employer-sponsored programs (see Box 7-3 in Chapter 7). Academic institutions concerned with occupational and environmental health have improved existing professional training opportunities and established new ones. Alerted to the critical problems associated with asbestos, lead, pesticides, ionizing radiation, and other hazards, the news media have made the public aware of many occupational and environmental health problems.

Social and Ethical Questions

Serious social and ethical problems have arisen over such subjects as the allegiance of occupational and environmental physicians who are employed by management, worker and community right-to-know about occupational and environmental hazards, confidentiality of workers' medical records kept by employers, and the restriction of female workers of childbearing age from certain jobs (see Chapters 2–5). Some of the controversies surrounding these subjects may eventually be settled by labor–management and community–company negotiations and by the deliberations of the courts, legislatures, and executive bodies of government. For example, the U.S. Supreme Court has upheld a worker's right to refuse hazardous work, stating that a worker cannot be discharged or discriminated against for exercising a right not to work under conditions reasonably believed to be very dangerous.

Environmental Justice

One of the major priorities for public health in this century is the elimination of disparities in access to health care and in disease rates for racial and ethnic minority communities. The role of disparities in environmental exposures between high- and low-income communities has been raised as one of the explanations for these health disparities. An active community-based campaign, known as the environmental justice movement, has emerged as a network of people and organizations in low-income and minority communities who are fighting against the placement in their communities of hazardous waste sites and polluting facilities. This movement has transformed the environmental movement from one supported primarily by the middle class, focused on ecological issues, into a grassroots struggle of poor and working-class communities, concerned primarily with preserving the health of their families. Many environmental health researchers now work together with teams of urban sociologists, economists, and community activists to develop multidisciplinary community-based screening and prevention programs to decrease these contributors to health disparities.

Risk Assessment

Some decision makers in business, government, and the community now expect that quantitative risk assessment will play an important role in influencing their decisions. This has increased the demand for risk-assessment models, which draw upon increasingly complex statistical analyses to provide scientific support for new standards, programs, and legislative initiatives. In occupational and environmental health, it is often difficult to compile all of the necessary health effects, exposures, and other data to support a new policy, and therefore the development of risk-assessment models that incorporate complex statistical methods to adjust for the inherent errors in measurement has become a central focus of research. In addition, policymakers and researchers now recognize the need to incorporate risk-assessment models that evaluate the complex mixtures of exposures that occur in the workplace and the community. Similarly, innovations in molecular and genetic research are providing new opportunities to identify health impacts of exposures at earlier stages in the exposure–disease chain. Molecular epidemiology deals with the potential for genetic and environmental risk factors identified at the molecular level to be used in studies to identify the etiology, distribution, and control of disease. Ideally, when risks are identified at a very early stage, interventions will be more successful in the prevention of disease.

Security and Terrorism Preparedness

The terrorist attack on the World Trade Center in 2001, followed quickly by the discovery of anthrax-tainted envelopes in Congressional offices and at media companies, resulted in major social and po-

litical changes. These events led politicians and the general public to become acutely aware of the need for a public health infrastructure that was better prepared to limit the consequences of possible future events. The emergence of public health preparedness as a key national priority highlighted the important role of occupational and environmental experts in public health. The environmental contamination from the collapse of the World Trade Center left many community residents and rescue workers with persistent respiratory problems. Twenty-three people contracted anthrax and five died as a result of their exposure to the anthrax-contaminated letters. Environmental and occupational health workers played key roles in both of these situations, in identifying and measuring contaminants and in developing screening, treatment, and prevention programs. Subsequent investigations have identified key vulnerabilities for potential future terrorist attacks, including the security of the food supply and of chemical manufacturing facilities near heavily populated areas. These concerns are likely to continue to have an impact on the training and future roles of environmental and occupational health specialists.

Liability

Some workers, barred from suing their employer under workers' compensation laws, have turned to "third-party," or product-liability, lawsuits as a means of redress for occupational disease; some community residents exposed to environmental hazards have also done so (see Chapter 4). The fear of liability suits has driven many employers to focus on preventive activities. Such lawsuits play an important role in directing attention to prevention of some diseases, although this approach can be cumbersome and the outcomes may not be equitable. In some jurisdictions, some of the most egregious health and safety offenders have been criminally prosecuted. In recent years, plaintiffs and their attorneys have found it increasingly difficult to recover damages in such lawsuits for a variety of reasons, including federal and state court decisions that have disqualified the testimonies of experts.

Advances in Technology

Advances in technology continue to facilitate identification of workplace hazards and potential hazards, including increasing use of *in vitro* assays to determine the mutagenicity of substances—and therefore their possible carcinogenicity—improvements in ways of determining the presence and measuring the levels of hazardous exposures, and new methods of monitoring concentrations of hazardous substances in body fluids and the physiologic impairments they cause (see Chapter 13). In addition, technological breakthroughs have introduced new hazards into the workplace and ambient environment (see Box 9-2 in Chapter 9).

Health Promotion

As social and behavioral sciences have expanded our understanding of the role individual factors play in health-related behaviors such as smoking or exercise, theories of personal behavior have developed that incorporate both the importance of contextual environmental factors as well as the importance of personal and community empowerment in effecting and maintaining positive change. Careful study and understanding is required to evaluate any interventions to demonstrate which aspects work and which do not. These processes are often more time-consuming and expensive than traditional approaches that might rely on a pamphlet to, for example, tell patients to eat more fruits and vegetables, but the lack of effectiveness of the pamphlet approach means this has been money wasted. Instead, through community-based participatory research approaches that identify both structural issues (the absence of stores selling fruits and vegetables in a given neighborhood) and personal and cultural factors (traditional cooking methods and tastes), projects have been developed that engage community members to develop, implement, and assess change. Similar projects addressing lead poisoning, home and community asthma triggers, and exercise recommendations in low-income neighborhoods have been studied and are being implemented. In the workplace, the relationship between frontline worker input and intervention development has been used to reduce work-related injuries, and approaches that address both personal as well as occupational hazards have been shown to improve smoking cessation success rates among blue-collar workers.

Economic Globalization

The growth of multinational corporations, reduction in trade barriers, and development of regional treaty arrangements (such as the North American Free Trade Agreement [NAFTA]) and global organizations (such as the World Trade Organization [WTO]) are having an increasing impact on occupational and environmental health, much of which is adverse to the safety, health, and well-being of workers and their families. In many developing countries, multinational corporations have exploited workers by employing them in jobs that have low wages and few benefits, offering them little or no training or upward mobility, and exposing them to serious health and safety hazards.

Additional Challenges in Developing Countries

The occupational and environmental health issues described above are important in countries throughout the world. In addition, developing countries—which comprise two-thirds of all countries and include the vast majority of people worldwide—face the following challenges.

Export of Hazards

Developed countries often export their most hazardous industries, as well as hazardous materials (such as banned or restricted pesticides) and hazardous wastes, to developing countries, where laws and regulations concerning these substances are more lax or nonexistent, and people may be less aware of these hazards (Fig. 1-10).

Inadequate Infrastructure and Human Resources

In developing countries, there are far fewer adequately trained personnel to recognize, diagnose, treat, and prevent and control occupational and environmental health problems. Governments and other sectors of society have fewer resources to devote to occupational and environmental health, and labor unions, facing other challenges such as low wages and high unemployment rates, may give little attention to occupational health.

Transnational Problems

Occupational and environmental health problems in developing countries often involve several countries in the same region, requiring transnational or regional approaches to problems, such as development and implementation of transnational standards.

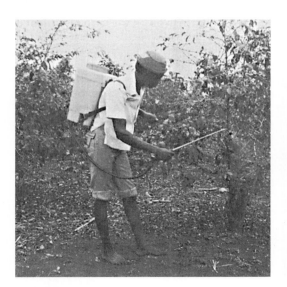

FIGURE 1-10 ● Agricultural workers in developing countries are at high risk of poisoning from pesticides, including those banned or restricted in developed countries. (Photograph by Barry S. Levy.)

Relationship Between the Workplace and the Home Environment

In developing countries, where so many people work in or near their homes, the distinction between the workplace and the home environment is often blurred. As a result, family members may often be exposed to workplace hazards.

Economic Development

In the context of economic development and accompanying rapid industrialization and urbanization, there is often pressure to overlook occupational and environmental health issues, given limited resources and the fear that attention to these issues may drive away potential investors or employers. Similarly, workers desperate for jobs in economies with high unemployment rates are unlikely to complain about occupational and environmental health and safety hazards once they are employed. In addition, many children are forced to leave school in order to work, often in hazardous jobs (Fig. 1-11).

Occupational and Environmental Health Services and Primary Health Care

Given limited resources and infrastructure, many developing countries are exploring ways to integrate occupational and environmental health services with primary medical care and with a broader range of public health services. Although some successes have been achieved with this approach, there

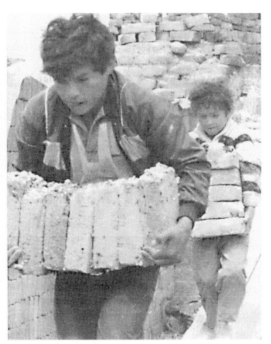

FIGURE 1-11 ● Young brick workers in Colombia. Thousands of children work as forced labor in brick kilns, rock quarries, or mines. (From the International Labor Office, Geneva, Switzerland.)

remains much untapped potential in fully achieving this kind of integration.

DISCIPLINES AND CAREERS IN OCCUPATIONAL AND ENVIRONMENTAL HEALTH SCIENCES

The identification and remediation of threats to our environment is a stewardship responsibility of us all. For those who work in health care or in public health, there are a wide range of career options that span the physical, biological, and social sciences, in addition to career options in communications, policymaking, and other fields. One of the most important challenges we face is the ability to communicate effectively across disciplines to develop the collaborative approaches needed to create safe, healthy, and sustainable environments for our children and their children's children.

Virtually everyone who enters the field of medical practice encounters environmental health issues. Primary care physicians incorporate health and safety into daily practice. Specialists and subspecialists adopt specific aspects of environmental and occupational safety and health as appropriate. So do trauma surgeons who advocate for car-seat restraints and ear-nose-and-throat specialists who treat vocalists.

In addition to the routine incorporation of prevention into the practice of medicine, the American College of Graduate Medical Education recognizes the specialty area of preventive medicine, which includes three areas of expertise: preventive medicine and public health, occupational and environmental medicine, and aerospace medicine. Physicians who choose to specialize in any of these areas may wish to become board certified by completing a postgraduate training program and passing the specialty board examinations. The American College of Occupational and Environmental Medicine is a primary professional association for physicians engaged in the practice of occupational and environmental medicine.

The field of nursing is similarly integrated with communication and prevention, key aspects of environmental and occupational health practice. For those who wish to specialize in the application of the science of occupational and environmental health in nursing practice, advanced practice degrees in nurse-practitioner programs and advanced master of science in nursing and doctoral programs are available. The American Association of Occupational Health Nurses is the primary professional association for occupational health nurses and represents nurses across the spectrum of practice.

Public health practitioners are also trained through a variety of programs, although the core public health sciences—epidemiology, biostatistics, environmental health, health services administration, and health education/behavioral sciences— form the basis for the master of public health, the core professional degree. The American Public Health Association is the main professional association for a wide range of workers in public health. A broad range of environmental health science programs are available at levels ranging from community colleges to postgraduate doctoral programs, with credentialing available for registered environmental health specialists, sanitarians, environmental health technicians, food safety professionals, hazardous substance professionals, and others, based on education, experience, and certifying examinations.

Engineering and public health programs overlap in the training of industrial hygienists, ergonomists, and environmental engineers, who provide primary prevention through a combination of exposure as-

sessment and design and implementation of interventions. Radiation physicists and biologists address a specific aspect of environmental and occupational exposure assessment and prevention. A sub-area of psychology programs includes a specialty area of industrial and organizational psychology concerned with healthy work organizations. The major professional organizations for these professions are: the American Industrial Hygiene Association, for industrial hygienists; the Human Factors and Ergonomics Society, for ergonomists; the Health Physics Society, for radiation health physicists; and the Society for Industrial and Organizational Psychology division in the American Psychological Association, for organizational psychologists.

Accreditation of training programs is rigorous. Certifying examinations are available. Safety professionals also have education in engineering disciplines, often with additional management training. Bachelor of science, master, and doctoral programs are available.

Research into any of the occupational and environmental health sciences can form the basis for a doctoral program, which focuses on advancement of scientific knowledge. These sciences include toxicology, the study of the effects of foreign substances on living organisms; epidemiology, the science of the distribution and determinants of disease in populations; environmental chemistry, concerned with the fate and transport of pollutants in the environment; systems engineering, the study of processes and their improvement; and sociology, psychology, and anthropology, critical to the understanding of human behavior in relation to the environment. Communications science, including social marketing and journalism, represents an important related area of study and practice. Environmental law, economics, policy, urban planning, and environmental management are other important areas of work. Finally, the many fields of ecology, agronomy, chemistry, physics, and geology that do not directly address human health impacts, but are nevertheless critical to our understanding of the external environment and our impact on it, provide additional career opportunities in occupational and environmental health.

CONCLUSION

Many health professionals will eventually work on occupational and environmental health and safety issues, and some will become occupational and environmental health and safety specialists. But almost all health professionals, in one way or another, will be involved with the recognition, diagnosis, treatment, or prevention and control of occupational and environmental illnesses and injuries.

BIBLIOGRAPHY

Selected Books

Ashford NA, Caldart CC. Technology, law, and the working environment. New York: Van Nostrand Reinhold, 1991.
An in-depth analysis of the technical, legal, political, and economic problems in occupational health and safety.

Burgess W. Recognition of health hazards in industry: A review of materials and processes. 2nd ed. New York: John Wiley & Sons, 1995.
An excellent summary of industrial hazards, updated, made more comprehensive, and well illustrated with photographs, drawings, and graphs in this second edition.

Fleming LE, Herzstein JA, Bunn WB III. Issues in international occupational and environmental medicine. Beverly, MA: OEM Press, 1997.
A very good, succinct primer on international issues.

Frumkin H, ed. Environmental health: From global to local. San Francisco, CA: Jossey-Bass, 2005.
An excellent new text that covers the broad field of environmental health.

Hamilton A. Exploring the dangerous trades: An autobiography. Boston: Little, Brown, 1943. (Also published by OEM Press in 1995.)
A classic historical reference.

Hathaway GJ, Proctor NH. Proctor and Hughes' chemical hazards of the workplace. 5th ed. Hoboken, NJ: John Wiley & Sons, 2004.
Brief summaries of many chemical hazards, including basics about their chemical, physical, and toxicologic characteristics; diagnostic criteria, including special tests; and treatment and medical control measures.

Harrington MM, Gill FS, Aw TC, et al. Occupational health. 4th ed. Oxford: Blackwell, 1998.

LaDou J, ed. Current occupational and environmental Medicine. 3rd ed. New York: Lange Medical Books/McGraw-Hill, 2004.
Both of these well-organized, well-written textbooks are valuable resources.

Levy BS, Wagner GR, Rest KM, Weeks JL, eds. Preventing occupational disease and injury. 2nd ed. Washington, DC: American Public Health Association, 2005.
A systematically organized handbook designed for the primary care clinician and public health worker.

Lippmann M, Cohen BS, Schlesinger RB, eds. Environmental health science: recognition, evaluation, and control of chemical and physical health hazards. New York: Oxford University Press, 2003.
A standard, widely used textbook of environmental health.

McCunney RJ, Rountree PP, eds. A practical approach to occupational and environmental medicine. 3rd ed. Philadelphia: Lippincott Williams & Wilkins, 2003.
A comprehensive practical guide on occupational medical services, occupational disorders, evaluation of hazards and the work environment, and environmental medicine.

Rom WN, ed. Environmental and occupational medicine. 3rd ed. Philadelphia: Lippincott–Raven, 1998.

Rosenstock L, Cullen MR, Brodkin CA, et al., eds. Textbook of clinical occupational and environmental medicine. 2nd ed. Philadelphia: Elsevier Saunders, 2005.

Both of these are excellent, comprehensive, in-depth references.

Stellman JM, ed. Encyclopedia of occupational health and safety. 4th ed. Geneva: International Labor Office, 1998.
A four-volume, comprehensive review of occupational hazards as well as occupational diseases and injuries.

Wald PH, Stave GM, eds. Physical and biological hazards of the workplace. 2nd ed. Hoboken, NJ: John Wiley & Sons, 2002.
A practical reference on the diagnosis, treatment, and control of these hazards.

Waldron HA, Edling C, eds. Occupational health practice. 4th ed. Oxford: Butterworth-Heinemann, 1998.
A general overview of occupational disease and health services with a non-U.S. orientation.

Wallace RB, Last JM, eds. Maxcy-Rosenau-Last public health and preventive medicine. 14th ed. Stamford, CT: Appleton & Lange (McGraw-Hill), 1998.
A standard text on preventive medicine, with chapters covering many occupational and environmental hazards.

Selected Periodical Publications

Occupational and Environmental Health

American Journal of Industrial Medicine, published monthly by Wiley-Liss, Inc., 605 Third Avenue, New York, NY 10158-0012.

American Journal of Public Health, published monthly by the American Public Health Association, 800 I Street, NW, Washington, DC 20001.

Environmental Health Perspectives, published monthly by the National Institute of Environmental Health Sciences, P.O. Box 12233, Research Triangle Park, NC, 27709-2233.

International Journal of Occupational and Environmental Health, published quarterly by Abel Publication Services, Inc., 1611 Aquinas Court, Burlington, NC, 27215.

Journal of Occupational and Environmental Medicine, published monthly by the American College of Occupational and Environmental Medicine, Lippincott Williams & Wilkins, 16522 Hunters Green Parkway, Hagerstown, MD 21740-2116.

New Solutions: A Journal of Occupational and Environmental Health Policy, published quarterly by the Baywood Publishing Company, Inc., 26 Austin Avenue, Amityville, NY 11701.

Occupational and Environmental Medicine, published monthly by the BMJ Publishing Group, BMA House, Tavistock Square, London WC1H 9JR, United Kingdom.

Scandinavian Journal of Work Environment & Health, published bimonthly by occupational health agencies and boards in Finland, Sweden, Norway, and Denmark; Topeliuksenkatu 41A, FIN-00250, Helsinki 29, Finland.

Occupational Health Nursing

American Association of Occupational Health Nurses Journal, published monthly by the American Association of Occupational Health Nurses, SLACK, 6900 Grove Road, Thorofare, NJ, 08086.

Occupational Hygiene (Industrial Hygiene)

Journal of Occupational and Environmental Hygiene, published monthly by the American Industrial Hygiene Association and the American Conference of Governmental Industrial Hygienists, Taylor & Francis, Inc., 325 Chestnut Street, Suite 800, Philadelphia, PA 19106.

The Annals of Occupational Hygiene, published eight times a year by Oxford University Press, 2001 Evans Road, Cary, NC, 27513.

Occupational Safety

Professional Safety, published monthly by the American Society of Safety Engineers, 1800 E. Oakton Street, Des Plaines, IL 60018-2187.

Safety + Health, published monthly by the National Safety Council, 1121 Spring Lake Drive, Itasca, IL 60143-3201.

Occupational Ergonomics

Applied Ergonomics, published bimonthly by Elsevier, 6277 Sea Harbor Drive, Orlando, FL, 32887-4800.

Ergonomics, published monthly by Taylor & Francis Ltd, Rankine Road, Basingstoke, Hants, RG24 8PR, United Kingdom.

Human Factors, published quarterly by The Human Factors Society, Inc., Box 1369, Santa Monica, CA 90406.

International Journal of Industrial Ergonomics, published monthly by Elsevier, 6277 Sea Harbor Drive, Orlando, FL, 32887-4800.

General News and Scientific Update Publications

BNA Occupational Safety and Health Reporter, published weekly by the Bureau of National Affairs, 1231 25th Street N.W., Washington, DC 20037.

The findings and conclusions in this chapter are those of the authors and do not necessarily represent the views of the National Institute for Occupational Safety and Health.

CHAPTER 2

The Social Context of Occupational and Environmental Health

Kenneth Geiser and Beth J. Rosenberg

Case 1

A small smelting and scrap company made the news in the early 1980s after the Occupational Safety and Health Administration (OSHA) charged the company with administering chelating drugs to employees to lower their blood lead levels (BLLs). The company, located in Massachusetts, was charged with illegally providing these lead-purging drugs to non–English-speaking, immigrant employees while they continued to work in a lead-contaminated environment. After the administration of these drugs, two employees became severely ill. One suffered from kidney failure and was ultimately diagnosed with kidney cancer. The other employee died, with lead poisoning as a significant contributing factor to his death. Although OSHA cited the company for many serious violations of standards, the fines and some of the charges were significantly re-duced after negotiation. The company agreed to clean up the plant and reduce employee lead exposures. Ten years later, however, not much had changed. One of the first reports of multiple poisonings in a single workplace listed in the state's new adult lead poisoning registry came from employees of the company. Every "shop-floor" employee was reported to the registry as having an elevated BLL, the average being 40 μg/dL—a level associated with adverse health effects in adults. After repeated violations over decades, the workers started to organize a union and contacted a worker advocacy group, the Massachusetts Coalition for Safety and Health (MassCOSH). Although a union was never formed, the workers, with the help of MassCOSH, were able to communicate, through interpreters, with the state Division of Occupational Hygiene and OSHA. The case was highly publicized in the local news media. The company's lead-generating processes were shut down, but the scrap metal recycling business remained. The lead smelting operation moved to Rhode Island.[1]

Case 2

In the 1930s, a chemical company started producing polychlorinated biphenyls (PCBs) in a community of color in Anniston, Alabama. Within 10 years, workers complained of serious chloracne and liver disease. Residents noted unexplained fish kills in local streams. In 1957, a paint made with PCBs was rejected for use by the U.S. Navy because it was too toxic for use in a submarine. The company did not warn any of its customers, its employees, or nearby residents of toxicity reports developed by the Navy. In 1960, years prior to the public's learning about the persistent nature of PCBs in the environment, the company noted that if the material is discharged to a stream, it will sink to the bottom and adversely affect the organisms there. By 1970, rates of cancer and diabetes in the nearby community were far above normal; rashes and skin disease were pervasive; and children were having more trouble than expected at school. In 1970, fish caught in a local creek contained 37,800 ppm of PCBs in their fat; the government action level in fish is 2 ppm. The company concealed its own fish tests. In 1971, the company bought hogs from a farmer that had grazed near the plant; they were found to have a PCB level of 19,000 ppm. The company told the farmer nothing, nor did it warn residents about the danger of grazing animals on polluted land. It was not until 1993 that Anniston residents were told by the Alabama Department of Public Health not to eat fish from the local creek. In 2000, community residents, through grassroots action, sued the company for contaminating their community with a known toxic substance and suspected carcinogen. In 2003, a jury found the company guilty of reckless indifference but also of "outrage"; the company's conduct "was so outrageous in character and extreme in degree" that it went "beyond all possible bounds of decency" and was thus regarded as "utterly intolerable in a civilized society."[2,3] Anniston became a rallying point for the environmental justice movement.

Case 3

In the 1950s, two companies were considering the full-scale production of an extremely effective pesticide, dibromochloropropane (DBCP), when scientists from both companies discovered that it caused testicular atrophy in rats. The companies ignored this result and mass-produced DBCP in a few plants in the United States. It was used throughout the world. In 1976, male manufacturing workers in California realized they were sterile. With their union, the Oil Chemical and Atomic Workers (OCAW), they tried to get information about the chemical composition of the pesticide they were formulating, but the company refused, stating that it had no legal obligation to provide it. Manufacturing workers in other company facilities were also found to be sterile. OSHA intervened and quickly lowered the permissible exposure limit of DBCP to such a low level that manufacturing was essentially banned. However, use of DBCP, regulated by EPA, continued. Five years later, when DBCP was polluting the groundwater of the San Joaquin Valley in California, the use of DBCP was finally prohibited in the United States, except on pineapples in Hawaii. Throughout the 1980s, remaining stocks were sold to countries in Africa and Central America as well as the Philippines, with agreements signed that freed the manufacturers from any liability. This scandal in the United States brought about right-to-know laws in a few states, which were soon preempted by the federal OSHA Hazard Communication Standard. More than 25,000 men worldwide became sterile.[4]

HEALTH AS A SOCIAL CONSTRUCT

Many diseases arise from exposures to hazards in the workplace or the community. They are typically treated through medical interventions. However, it is important to understand that occupational and environmental diseases are the result of the social, economic, and political organization of a society. Improving workplace and environmental conditions and preventing resultant illnesses and injuries requires understanding the social context that produced the hazardous conditions, the barriers to change, and opportunities for intervention.

Historically, occupational health and environmental health have been considered separate fields. By considering the two fields together, their commonalities become clear. First, the source of environmental pollution is often a workplace. The toxic chemicals used in a factory are released into the air, water, and soil outside the factory. So although exposures for workers are higher than those outside, the exposures are often the same. Not all environmental exposures originate in manufacturing, but by eliminating the use and production of toxic and hazardous chemicals inside, environmental exposures are eliminated as well.

Second, and more important, unlike malaria or smallpox, all occupational and environmental diseases and injuries are human-made. They are the result of decisions about the way we produce and use almost everything. For example, if a country chooses to heat with coal, this may result in coal workers' pneumoconiosis (black lung disease) and acid rain. Use of leaded gasoline produces lead poisoning. Assembly lines inevitably lead to repetitive strain disorders. Excess packaging of products results in either more incineration or more landfills. Poor mass transit means more cars, more smog, more traffic jams. Occupational and environmental injuries and illnesses are a direct, although unintended, result of economic activity—simply, the way we do things. But because they are the result of human decisions, they are amenable to change. This chapter describes the social context that "produces" occupational and environmental disease and injury. Improving workplace and environmental conditions requires understanding the social context of our lives, the barriers to change, and the possible points of intervention (Fig. 2-1).

The magnitude and pattern of occupational and environmental injuries and illnesses in a particular society are strongly affected by the level of economic and technological development, the societal distribution of power, and the dominant ideology of a particular social and political system. These factors bear on the way in which diseases and injuries are "produced," on the recognition and prevention of these problems, and on the extent to

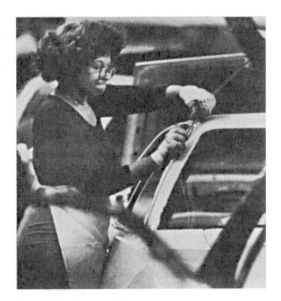

FIGURE 2-1 ● Automobile assembly line worker. (Photograph by Earl Dotter.)

which workers and the rest of the public receive compensation for them. Fully understanding occupational and environmental injuries and illnesses therefore requires an understanding of the broad context in which production takes place. This context includes the economic and technological basis of production and consumption; ideological, religious, and cultural factors determining the organization of communities and the design of work and the workplace; and the main social "actors" who determine these outcomes.

One approach to occupational and environmental health is defined by the medical/scientific model that focuses on disease and injury causation and uses scientific methods to discover, explain, and solve public health problems. By focusing on the individual (patient), this approach rarely addresses critical economic, social, and political conditions. The analysis presented here provides a different perspective, one that places control of the market by private business, the workplace, the technologies, and the labor process at the center of occupational and environmental health. This chapter focuses primarily on the United States, although parallels to other countries are drawn wherever possible. Many of the underlying issues addressed here cross national boundaries.

The organization of work, the structures of communities, and the roles played by key actors are deeply influenced by ideology—a set of beliefs,

norms, and values. Ideologies of workers, managers, government officials, scientists, and others reflect what they think about society and about themselves. Ideologies also reflect what they expect from work and from employers, government, and each other.

A capitalist, free-market economic system incorporates presumptions about human behavior that most people have come to accept: notions about individual "choice" and "rights," a belief in the primacy of private property, and the efficiency of markets. Americans, in particular, are deeply suspicious of government. It is, therefore, necessary to examine the role of ideology in order to identify the assumptions that determine power relations in the workplace and how they are reflected in the problem of occupational and environmental health and safety.

The typical workplace in the United States is organized hierarchically. In large workplaces, the model is owner or owners, leading managers, supervisors, and then workers. Smaller workplaces compress this structure. The hierarchy reflects the distribution of power: Owners and managers have complete control over investment decisions, the budget, the structure of production, what is produced, how and when production occurs, hiring and firing of workers, and, ultimately, the conditions of work.

Labor unions, considered to be a counterweight to this power, have had some success in gaining better wages and working conditions. They have usually been constrained, however, by a number of factors: the strength of the general economy, the level of unemployment, their own economic and political strength, and an ideology that supports the rights of property. Labor's achievements have also depended importantly on the level of government support for protecting and promoting the rights of workers. In Europe, although the rights of private property remain relatively sacrosanct, the power of unions and workers' parties, as well as the acceptance and expectation of government regulation of working conditions, has led to a greater ability by government to regulate private industry and working conditions than is found in the United States.

The culture of most liberal democracies, including the United States, has supported belief in the rationality and apolitical nature of science and technology—a belief that social and public health problems (indeed most societal problems) are amenable to technical solutions. Remarkably enduring has been the ideology of the "technical fix" and the notion that science can be separated from politics and issues of power and control. Before we elaborate on this framework, some historical background will reveal how we got to where we are.

A BRIEF HISTORY OF OCCUPATIONAL AND ENVIRONMENTAL HEALTH

Occupational and environmental health have rarely received much attention in most societies. Historically, the commitment to economic advancement through technology has made us blind to the toll on community and workers' health. Workers have been engaged in the more pressing task of making a living for their families to pay too much attention to widespread occupational safety and health problems, and little has been known of how environmental stresses affect human health.

In most countries, the process of industrializations, which resulted in the creation of the factory system, propelled urbanization, and generated a working class, radically changed people's lives. Forced by economic necessity into the newly created factories of the machine age, workers found themselves controlled by bosses whose sole concern was the maximization of profit. Working in large-scale plants and using the new technology of modern industry, workers confronted a whole new set of conditions: powerless and tied to the speed of the machine they served, facing the ever-present dangers of physical injury from conveyor belts and speeding looms, and exposed to a range of dyes, bleaches, and gases. The workplace became a source of injury, disease, disability, and death.

When they left their jobs at the end of the workday, many workers went home to neighborhoods that were equally polluted and dangerous. Industrial discharges fouled the air and contaminated drinking water. Food was often contaminated and easily spoiled, and housing was filled with pests and without adequate sanitation.

With the help of social reformers and professionals, people struggled to improve these conditions. In countries such as Britain and Germany in middle and late 19th century, people improved conditions somewhat through government regulation. There was an increase in laws restricting working hours and the employment of women and children and promoting protection against safety hazards and some hazardous chemical exposures. Smoke abatement programs were established, oil replaced coal in home heating, municipal sewers were constructed, and playgrounds and parks opened, providing places to relax and recreate. By the 20th century, workers, unions, and social reformers had achieved political representation in the form of labor, socialist, and social democratic parties. This gave citizens the power to demand reform and was a major factor in establishing laws to improve working and living conditions.

In the United States, the Settlement House Movement during the late 19th century provided a platform for social reformers and early public health advocates to press for municipal regulation of multifamily housing, slaughterhouses, tanneries, foundries, and landfills. As public health and sanitary engineering became increasingly professionalized, cities established garbage-collection and street-cleaning services and water-treatment plants. Congress passed the Pure Food and Drugs and Meat Inspection Act in 1906 and established the Food and Drug Administration in 1938 to inspect and regulate the food and drug industries.

In the 19th century, the Industrial Revolution brought to the United States—as it had to Europe—many safety problems and some public concern about these problems. Massachusetts created the first factory inspection department in the United States in 1867 and in subsequent years enacted the first job safety laws in the textile industry. The Knights of Labor, one of the earliest labor unions, agitated for safety laws in the 1870s and 1880s. Social reformers and growing union power, by 1900, gained minimal legislation to improve workplace health and safety in the most heavily industrialized states. However, regulations and the system of inspection were inadequate. Those states that had some legislated protections rarely enforced them and focused largely on safety issues; little was done to protect workers from exposure to the growing number of chemicals in the workplace or to clean up polluted rivers and protect air quality.

After 1900, the rising tide of industrial injuries resulted in passage of state workers' compensation laws, so that by 1920, almost all states had passed these no-fault insurance programs. In 1897, Britain passed its Workmen's Compensation Act for occupational injuries, and Germany had passed similar a similar law by 1900.

Mobilization for World War II required that the U.S. government become involved in the organization of production. Wartime production plants were built. Workers were transferred across the country and settled into new production-focused communities. Concern for the health of workers increased during this period, as a healthy workforce was considered indispensable to the war effort. However, after the war, health and safety receded from public attention. An exception to this general neglect was passage, in 1954, of the Atomic Energy Act, which included provision for workplace radiation-safety standards.

Not until the 1960s, when labor and environmental activists gained some political clout under the Democratic administrations of Presidents John Kennedy and Lyndon Johnson, did occupational and public health issues reemerge as significant. Injury rates rose 29 percent during the 1960s, prompting concern, but it was a major mine disaster in 1968 in Farmington, West Virginia, in which 78 miners were killed that captured public sympathy. In 1969, the Coal Mine Health and Safety Act was passed and, in 1970, the first comprehensive federal legislation to protect workers, the Occupational Safety and Health Act (OSHAct), was passed.

In the United States, the modern environmental movement was born in 1962, when *Silent Spring* by Rachel Carson was published. The book documented the negative consequences of pesticide use for the general public, which, until that time, was quite enchanted with technology. The overwhelmingly positive response to this book spurred organizing for the nation's first Earth Day celebration and the founding of the Environmental Protection Agency (EPA) in 1970. In a short period of time, new federal legislation—such as the National Environmental Protection Act (1969), the Clean Air Act (1970), the Clean Water Act (1972), the Safe Drinking Water Act (1974), and the Resource Conservation and Recovery Act (1976)—moved the federal government solidly into the business of protecting the environment (see Chapter 35).

This brief history illustrates only some of the dimensions of the struggle to provide workplace and community safety. Although today many countries provide regulatory protection for workers and the environment, occupational and environmental health problems persist. New chemicals in products, wastes and workplaces, limits in regulatory enforcement, and the demands of an increasingly competitive global economy exacerbate the need to maintain and improve working and living conditions.

THE GLOBAL CONTEXT
The Global Commons

Our planet has a mighty system of chemical and ecological cycles. Scientists say that the earth has a finite reserve of materials, but that its energy systems are open to the daily fluxes of the solar gain and atmospheric loss. At one time, it was possible to view the impacts of human activities on the planet as largely local and episodic. Today, with a global human population of well over 6 billion people, the impact of this one species extends throughout the world. Air pollutants released on one continent are readily transported by atmospheric currents around the world. Today, the Inuit peoples of the Arctic region carry some of the highest rates of chemical contaminants in their bodies, even though they live far from any industrial sources, because the natural air currents carry pollutants northward. Municipal wastewater discharges flow to the oceans and alter estuaries and fish-spawning areas, impacting the food patterns of the ocean. The Mississippi River washes out into the Gulf of Mexico such a volume of pollutants as to create a marine zone incapable of supporting life that is nearly the size of Delaware. Excessive releases of carbon from industrial and transportation combustion activities now threaten the chemical balance in the upper atmosphere, inhibiting the natural dissipation of global energy and gradually raising the overall temperature of the earth. As temperatures rise, viruses, pests, and other vectors expand their habitats and increase the incidence of disease and damage in large areas previously unaffected.

The unprecedented growth in human population has long been seen as a threat to the planet's resources. Although Thomas Malthus's gloomy predictions of global famine have failed to materialize because agricultural productivity and food distribution technologies have expanded, the environmental costs of food production appear likely to be an even greater threat than food scarcity. The transition from agricultural to industrial economies has had a profound effect on the ecological systems of the planet. Industrial economies consume far larger amounts of energy and generate far larger volumes of waste. Both industrial economies and "modern" pesticide- and fertilizer-intensive agricultural economies stretch the capacity of natural systems.

These problems are global in scope. The globalization of production, trade, and consumption has made occupational and environmental safety and health problems ubiquitous. Workers in developing and newly industrialized countries now face a range of workplace hazards. Stricter environmental regulations in developed countries make it attractive for companies to use developing countries in Latin America, Asia, and Africa as dumping grounds for toxic waste and as places to export highly toxic substances and hazardous industries.

Trade and Economic Development

Some of the most pressing problems in occupational and environmental health stem from the increasing integration of the world economy. In North America, the development of continental free trade has threatened the more advanced work environment standards of Canada and the United States while bringing many new hazards to Mexico. In Europe, cross-national economic integration has made the movement of capital and labor across borders much easier; as a result, industries can move to countries with less strict occupational and environmental standards. Multinational companies in developed countries invest heavily in developing countries seeking new markets and new places of production with lower wages, less regulation, and less taxation. The mobility of capital undercuts the ability of advanced industrial countries to regulate domestic industry for fear that it might cause industry to flee regulation. Developing countries, such as India, Thailand, Vietnam, China, and others in Africa and Latin America, are now the questionable beneficiaries of much of this newly mobile capital. In some cases, this intrusion has led to threats to occupational and environmental health; in others, the more advanced standards of some countries are being imposed on the less advanced. In both situations, conflict over standards has arisen. The export of hazardous technologies, hazardous products, and hazardous wastes represents increasing challenges for public health worldwide. On the one hand, our understanding of the nature of health hazards to workers and the environment has been improving; on the other hand, however, the restructuring of the world economy may undercut the political will to control these hazards.

By 1990, the global economy had undergone a fundamental realignment, with four major effects on the United States and the developed countries of Europe:

1. Their economies shifted from heavy manufacturing (of chemicals and steel) toward the service sector (banking, insurance, food, and clerical work). American businesses lost approximately 38 million manufacturing jobs during the 1970s and 1980s.[5]
2. Their economies became dominated by extremely mobile and mostly large international corporations.
3. Ownership of industry has become concentrated in a few very large firms. The frequent buying and selling of companies during the 1980s and 1990s led to the U.S. economy becoming increasingly controlled by the banking and finance sector.
4. With decreasing profitability during the 1970s, management in the United States began to (a) cut the costs of production by demanding reductions in wages or benefits and (b) fight increases in health, safety, and environment regulation. In Europe, similar economic changes ushered in a period of political conservatism, resulting in the deregulation of the market and reduction in government control over private industry.

All this had an impact on workers; for example, in the United States, real wages fell by 17 percent between 1973 and 1988. Real average wages were $9 per hour in 1973; 25 years later they were $8 per hour.[5,] Housing, education, and medical costs have all increased at a rate faster than inflation over this period. Despite more two-earner families, U.S. workers are much worse off than they had been in 1970. (The Global Sustainable Development Resolution was proposed by Congressman Bernie Sanders in 2000 to address the harmful effects of the global economy on workers.)

These transitions have also had significant impacts on community and environmental health. The U.S. economy is increasingly based on commodity consumption, resulting in a significant increase in the volume of domestic trash. Today, Americans generate nearly 208 million tons of trash per year, or about 4.3 pounds of waste per person per day. We are increasingly dependent on automobiles with commuting taking an increasing share of daytime hours. We have increased gasoline consumption, which has led to rising levels of carbon emissions. With 5 percent of the world population, the United States generates 24 percent of the planet's greenhouse gas emissions. This has led to some of the warmest years on record for the planet, with the 1990s appearing to have been the warmest decade in the past 1,000 years. Indeed, air pollution has become a major problem throughout most of the industrializing countries with the most deteriorated air now in cities like Mexico City, Sao Paulo, Beijing, and Delhi. All of this is affecting the biological diversity of the planet. Some estimate that nearly one-fourth of all species now alive may become extinct over the next 50 years.

As the 1990s drew to a close, globalization continued to be the major factor in the social and economic life of all countries. The collapse of many of the southeast Asian economies in the second half of the past decade, the rise and fall of the U.S. "dot.com economy," the chronic high levels of unemployment in Europe, and the continued economic slump in Japan place a heavy burden on workers and communities and inhibit efforts to promote environmental and health and safety policies throughout the world.

Technology Development

Technology has created a wealth of new products and services. After World War II, the rate of product innovation and availability rose rapidly. Automobiles, refrigerators, washing machines, televisions, stereos, computers, and hundreds of other products have become common throughout developed and developing countries. Because of the need to expand markets and maintain steady sales of products, many commodities were designed for rapid obsolescence and easy disposability. However, as the useful life of products has been shortened and products and packages designed to be disposed, the volume of domestic wastes has risen dramatically, with litter and waste dumps proliferating throughout the landscape, setting up new sources of pollution and chemical hazards.

Technology has also increased the speed of production, putting greater pressure on workers to perform rapid and repetitive motions that are damaging to mental and physical health. The characteristic jobs of a service-sector economy often replicate the alienating, repetitive work once associated with assembly-line production and the monotony of the modern factory. In developed countries, however, improved technology and the ubiquitousness of computers have enormously increased the potential pace of work as well as the ability of the work rate to be monitored. Technology combines with pressures for increased productivity in an increasingly competitive world economy. "Competitiveness" and the drive for productivity have enormous costs to the health and well-being of workers.

Stress and related psychological and physiologic illnesses are increasing in developed countries, as the pace of work and life increases and pressures increase to work longer hours—in order to compensate for falling wage rates and a declining standard of living.[6] In some countries, however, such as those in Europe, because of historical and cultural reasons and pressure from powerful trade unions, a shorter work week with reduced working hours has been adopted since World War II. More recently, unemployment pressures have furthered the call for a shorter work week.[7]

With speed-up has come automation. Apart from obvious physical hazards associated with use of robots, robotic systems, and highly automated machinery, automation also eliminates jobs and deskills others, leaving fewer workers responsible for complex systems. With the help of automation, one worker can do a job that may have required ten workers before. This advance, however, has been accompanied by greater stress and generally more overtime work. Under these circumstances, rather than achieving the promise that automation would replace grueling mindless labor, it has resulted in more stress, longer hours, and sometimes overwhelming responsibility at work.[7]

Another profound influence on workplace and public health has been the rapid increase in the use of chemicals, especially since World War II. There are currently 80,000 chemicals in use in the United States, with approximately 1,000 new chemicals introduced each year (Fig. 2-2).[8] A similar number of chemicals and chemical processes exist in most developed countries and increasingly so in developing countries as production is shifted to them. The vast majority of these chemicals are unregulated and their human health effects unknown. They are used in a variety of production settings to produce a wide range of products, but they are also encountered in a range of occupations not traditionally considered dangerous. Indeed, many commercial products on the market today, ranging from cleaners and paints to cosmetics and computers, contain a wide array of chemicals that create consumer and environmental exposure during production and use and long afterwards as products are disposed in landfills and burned in incinerators.

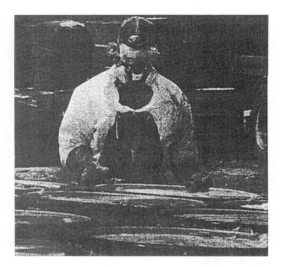

FIGURE 2-2 ● Hazardous waste worker sealing abandoned drums of waste chemicals.

THE REGIONAL AND NATIONAL CONTEXT

The Distribution of Power

The spread of new technologies, the globalization of the economy, and vast changes in the international division of labor both directly and indirectly affect not only the work environment but also the general power relations in society. Class, race, and gender are key dimensions in the political and economic power relationships in the United States that shape substantial aspects of the workplace and the general environment.

The distribution of such power and influence is another essential factor shaping workplaces, communities, and the environment. In many liberal democracies, although the stated goal is equality, power in society at large is unevenly distributed along the lines of class, race, and gender. Inequities in the distribution of power have a profound influence on work and health because power determines who does what work and under what conditions, who lives where and under what conditions, who gets exposed to various risks, and what is considered "acceptable" risk.[9]

All the cliches and pleasant notions of how the old class divisions have disappeared are exposed as hollow phrases by the simple fact that American workers must accept serious injury and even death as a part of their daily reality while the middle class does not. Imagine ... the universal outcry that would occur if every year several corporate headquarters routinely collapsed like mines, crushing sixty or seventy executives. Or suppose that all the banks were filled with an invisible noxious dust that constantly produced cancer in the managers, clerks, and tellers. Finally, try to imagine the horror ... if thousands of university professors were deafened every year or lost fingers, hands, sometimes eyes, while on their jobs.[9]

Low income threatens health at home, as well as at work. Environmentally, lower class communities bear the brunt of highway and airport expansions, landfills, toxic waste sites, incinerator and factory sitings, and other polluting activities. Dilapidated housing is associated with increased lead poisoning from lead paint and lead solder in old water pipes. Poorly maintained housing, with mold contamination from water damage, is one of the suspected causes—along with dusty old heating systems, environmental tobacco smoke, and general poor air quality—of the increased asthma rates in lower income neighborhoods.

The Impact of Race and Racism

In the workplace and in society as a whole, racism plays a role in determining where one lives, what work one does, how much he or she will be paid for it, and what alternatives are open. For most of its history, the United States has depended on minorities to do the least desirable and most dangerous work. Immigrant and minority communities have been the major sources of labor to build the railways, pick cotton and weave it in the mills, work in the foundries in the automobile industry, run coke oven operations in the steel industry, sew in the sweatshops, and provide migrant agricultural labor (Fig. 2-3). Minorities are still overrepresented in the most hazardous and least desirable occupations, such as agriculture harvesting, manual labor, and janitorial services (Fig. 2-4). The vast majority of farm laborers are Hispanic, with many coming from Mexico as illegal immigrants. Low education and fear of corporate or governmental reprisal motivates these workers to assume serious risks from pesticides and dangerous farm machinery. Some of the most flagrant corporate violations of health and safety regulations occur in the livestock and slaughtering industries, in which many minority workers work.

Minority workers may leave a hazardous work environment only to arrive home to a hazardous

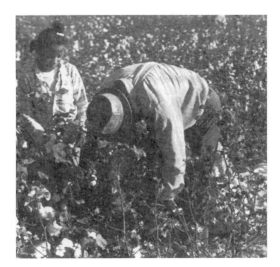

FIGURE 2-3 ● Migrant workers picking cotton. (Photograph by Earl Dotter.)

community environment. Since the early 1980s, in the United States, scientific evidence has increasingly pointed to discriminatory environmental practices of certain industries, of state and local governments, and, in some instances, of the federal government. One well-documented example is that minority communities have a disproportionate number of toxic threats to their health.[10] For example, the traditional diet for many Native American tribes relies heavily on meat and fish that is prefer-

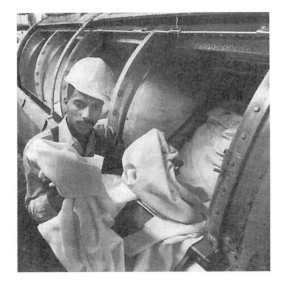

FIGURE 2-4 ● Worker in a commercial laundry. (Photograph by Earl Dotter.)

ably caught in the wild, although this food source is often so heavily tainted with persistent and bioaccumulative substances, such as mercury, that the government must issue health warnings on its consumption.

The national Environmental Justice Movement was spawned by the realization of the unfair concentration of hazardous waste sites and hazardous facilities in minority, especially African-American and Hispanic, areas. This movement that today includes hundreds of local organizations seeks to attain compensation for victims of environmental injustice and achieve remediation of the remaining contamination. The experience of Anniston, Alabama, cited at the beginning of this chapter, offers an example of the regional discrimination that locates hazardous waste sites and polluting industries in mainly minority communities. As another example, those living nearest the vast petrochemical production facilities in Louisiana's "Cancer Alley," along the Mississippi River, are predominantly African American.

The Impact of Gender and Sexism

Any discussion of power relations must include the situation of women, whose experience of work is generally different from that of men. Most obviously this is reflected in the wage differentials paid to women for comparable work. Despite a political and legal commitment to equality in the United States, as of 2004 white women were earning 87 cents to every dollar earned by white men. African-American women earn only 75 percent, and Latinas only 61 percent, of white men's pay.[11]

Even though women frequently work outside the home for as many hours as their spouses, domestic duties are rarely shared equally. Working mothers sleep less, get sick more, and have less leisure time than their husbands. One study finds that women who are employed full-time outside the home and whose youngest child is less than 5 years old spend an average of 47 hours per week on household work, while their male counterparts spend a mere 10 hours.[12] Although the situation may have improved somewhat over the past 10 to 20 years, the stress and fatigue from balancing work and home life remain a serious problem. The average working woman puts in an estimated 80 hours a week in job and household work—and up to 105 hours if she has sole responsibility for children.

Women are also the main targets of sexual harassment at work. Any unwanted verbal or physical sexual advance constitutes harassment, and this can range from sexual comments and suggestions, to pressure for sexual favors accompanied by threats concerning one's job, to physical assault, including rape. Between 40 to 60 percent of women have experienced some form of sexual harassment at work.[13] An estimated one-third of the largest 500 companies in the United States spend approximately $6.7 million per year in dealing with sexual harassment.[13]

Gender relations have political, and hence work-environment, implications. Cultural assumptions about gender can have strong impact on the distribution of power in society. A strongly patriarchal society that bars women from positions of power is also likely to have a profoundly sex-segregated labor market. As a result, sexual harassment and occupational health in female-dominated jobs like retail trade or nursing may not be considered important.

In contrast to the workplace, women have had a dominant role in a variety of environmental initiatives. The grassroots "toxics movement" in the United States has been largely led and influenced by women. Many of these women have been empowered housewives, such as Lois Gibbs, who led protests over hazardous wastes at Love Canal, New York, during the 1970s and then founded a national environmental advocacy coalition. Women have spurred and supported the organic food movement. Although small, it is the fastest growing segment of the food industry and is decreasing the amount of toxic pesticides in use somewhat in the United States—and more in Europe, where the cultural standards for quality food are higher. Finally, in urban environments, it is women who reclaim vacant lots and turn them into community gardens. This initiative not only supplies fresh produce and outdoor, communal activity to urban residents but also converts land that was often used for gang activities and/or garbage dumping into something useful and beautiful.

THE LOCAL CONTEXT

The Changing Structure of Production

The economy of the United States and many other developed countries is changing rapidly. The shift from heavy manufacturing toward the service sector affects the structure of work and the work experience for many Americans. In general, in service industries, the most rapidly growing sector of the economy, wages are lower, benefits scanty, job security limited, and unions virtually nonexistent. Much of this work is part-time or temporary.

In response to the shrinking economic pie of the 1980s, employers are increasingly using part-time and temporary workers to cut costs. The average part-time worker earns only 60 percent of a full-time worker on an hourly basis. Fewer than 25 percent of part-timers have employer-paid health insurance, compared to nearly 80 percent of full-time workers. Sixty percent of full-time workers have pensions provided by employers, whereas only 20 percent of part-time workers have this coverage.[12]

In addition to lower pay and fewer benefits, there are other negative aspects to this trend toward temporary and part-time work. Temporary workers live with the stress of not knowing when and for how long they will work. They have little or no job security. Neither part-time nor temporary workers receive equal protection under government laws and regulations, including those concerning occupational safety and health, unemployment insurance, and pensions. Few are represented by unions.[12] A case study commissioned by OSHA of contract labor in the petrochemical industry (usually small contractors of nonunion workers who are brought into a plant to do maintenance and other work) showed that contract workers get less health and safety training and have higher injury rates than do noncontract workers.[14] The consequence for occupational health and safety of an increasingly unorganized, temporary, and part-time workforce means that many people spend time unemployed.

Unemployment is more destructive to physical and mental health than all but the most dangerous jobs. Recent studies have even suggested a correlation between unemployment and mortality from heart disease, liver disease, suicide, and other stress-related ailments.[15] In the 1980s, the unemployment rate in the United States fluctuated between 6 and 11 percent. Some economists have proposed that a 5.0 percent unemployment rate be considered "full employment." In 2004, the unemployment rate was 5.6, with the threat of outsourcing increasing numbers of white-collar jobs at an all-time high.

Another increasingly common characteristic of changes in the structure of work in the United States is the rise in home-based industry. In 1949, Congress passed a law making industrial home work illegal, largely because it was almost impossible to enforce workplace regulations and labor standards (such as the minimum wage) for home work. Under the Reagan administration, Congress reversed this policy and legalized home work. The consequence was a rapid growth of home-based manufacturing and service work throughout the 1980s.[12] Many home workers are women, typically garment and clerical workers who are paid on a piece-rate system. Piece-rate payments encourage speed, increase the risks of injuries, and cause or exacerbate cumulative trauma disorders due to ergonomic problems in workplaces not designed for the work being done. Chemical exposures also pose a problem. Product manufacture at home, for example, not only exposes workers and their families to toxic substances used in the manufacturing process but also may contaminate local sewage systems.

The Changing Structure of Consumption

Changes in the economy have also profoundly changed the composition of products and the nature of consumption. A century ago, even as industrialization made steady progress, most families continued to live modestly, making many products, such as clothing, tools, and toys, at home or buying locally from small shops that offered regionally defined foods and staples. Housing for most was marginal and travel was limited with longer distances covered by train or boat. This economy began to change after World War I. The automobile significantly increased mobility, offering families weekend and vacation options unheard of before. The price of cars, kept low by automakers to increase purchases, began to offer wider settlement patterns as commuting to work became easier and cheaper.

In Europe, reliance on coal for fuel generated large amounts of coal by-products as wastes that could ingeniously be converted into a wide range of synthetic organic compounds, such as methane, ethylene, and benzene and many other aromatic compounds. In the United States, the automobile combustion engine rapidly drove the need for large amounts of petroleum-based fuels, and the residuals from oil refineries soon offered the same low-cost synthetic compounds. These innovative chemistries soon began to generate a host of new paints, dyes, solvents, adhesives, fibers, and plastics. The low cost of these synthetics undercut traditional chemicals and materials, and soon a whole new generation of inexpensive household products entered the market.

The period that followed World War II only accelerated this trend. Well-subsidized housing mortgages and new roadways greatly expanded the suburbs. At first, women stayed home to manage an increasingly sophisticated range of electronic kitchen and cleaning appliances, but access to education and new personal expectations propelled women to enter the workforce, as office and service work began demanding low-wage workers. As wages fell and families increasingly required two wage earners, even more synthetic products emerged to ease domestic needs. Prepared foods, low-cost clothing, disposable paper, and tons of packaging soon swelled the municipal waste stream. Waste dumps grew and waste incinerators appeared to treat the ever-growing waste stream.

The economy was now propelled by a continually growing flood of highly packaged commodities that were intended for short life, rapid obsolescence, and easy disposal. With prices falling, product production increasingly moved offshore to low-wage, industrializing countries in Asia and Latin America. In 2003, the United States imported more than $120 billion worth of commodities from China alone.[16] Waste and pollution have become hallmarks of commodity markets, largely inflated by artificial needs and unobtainable aspirations. The material throughput depletes the mineral, forest, and fossil-fuel supplies and congests the ecological systems expected to assimilate the residues.

KEY ACTORS

The relationships among major social actors—labor, management, and government—define rules of the work and community environment, including health and safety standards and practices as well as the boundaries within which health care providers, occupational health specialists, environmental advocates, university scientists, and health and safety advocates operate. While this web of rules sets real limits on reform, the changes in the global factors that threaten public health and the environment can also open up new possibilities to provide safe and healthful communities and workplaces.

Managers and Corporations

The production process starts at the level of the firm. Managers decide what will be produced, how it will be produced, and with what materials. All these decisions have a direct effect on occupational and environmental health. Managers are trained and rewarded to produce financial results. Most see the world through the lens of a financial record. Corporate owners, vendors, customers, and investors are critical judges of performance. The condition of workers, nearby residents, and the environment are often secondary factors, and, when challenged about the state of these other factors, managers are prone to be defensive and even dismissive. Expenditures on health and safety are often seen by management as limiting profit. As a business school textbook advises:

> In making decisions about their workplace, managers have two choices. They can remedy health and safety problems or they can provide risk compensation to workers. If reducing risk is less costly than the additional compensation, then working conditions will be improved. However, if the marginal cost of worker compensation is less than the marginal cost of safety improvements, then the firm will choose the compensation alternative. This outcome represents an efficient allocation of resources in that the firm minimizes its total costs.[17]

Unquestionably, there are many companies that seek to maintain safe and healthy work environments. They abide by environmental regulations and may even surpass them by using sustainable, clean technologies. These are frequently large, profitable companies that have relatively secure markets for their products and that have decided that their continued success depends on a well-motivated, high-quality, and healthy workforce and a reputation for environmental responsibility. Frequently, these are companies that have a commitment to collective bargaining and to negotiating industrial peace. Managers in these firms have decided that the only way that they can attract and keep highly skilled workers is to ensure the quality of working life. Other companies, concerned about product safety because of consumer concerns or the inherent risks of their technology, have attended to worker health and safety virtually as a spillover from their other essential activities. Finally, some companies have been motivated to adopt sound environmental management systems because they have paid the cost of irresponsibility through substantial insurance premiums, waste treatment or remediation costs, previous judicial judgments, or government compliance penalties.

The remarkable success of Japanese industry in reducing injury rates, as a consequence of its attention to quality in general and its abhorrence of waste, may have beneficial consequences in U.S. and European firms pursuing Japanese-style manufacturing success. Firms such as Volvo, Saab, Herman-Miller, Xerox, Interface Carpet, Ikea, Patagonia, and others that have committed themselves to missions of environmental sustainability produce annual environmental reports that serve as models for their industries. Sometimes, these company efforts may miss problems associated with low-level chemical exposures or hazards that are well "downstream" from their point of production. Nevertheless, such efforts are to be applauded.

Some small companies pay serious attention to safety and health hazards because their owners or managers came up from the ranks, know the processes well, and maintain close social contact with the employees. However, the fierce competitive economic pressures on small companies may undercut even the most responsible employer. For both small and large companies, the pressures of the market and the demands of stockholders or financial investors can be overwhelming. Technological short cuts, increased pressure on workers, deferred equipment maintenance and repair, unnoticed safety violations, reduced record-keeping, and late-night transgressions can make the difference between a positive and a negative financial quarterly performance report. In these cases, the role of government in enforcing work environment standards is particularly important.

Workers and Trade Unions

Workers are the first group of people directly influenced by decisions about the terms of production. A hundred years ago, when a cobbler woke up in the morning, the decision to make boots or shoes, to buy hides, or to take some of his wares to the neighboring town was under his control. If the cobbler acquired an allergy to a certain polish or was told that it caused cancer, he could choose not to use it. If he realized that the dyes he used were polluting the fishing stream, he could find an alternative. If he found that carving heels bothered his elbow, he could do a few every other day instead of spending a long stretch of time on a bothersome or painful task, or he could try redesigning the tools or using alternative carving methods that might be better for him. He was his own manager. He set the pace and conditions of his work.

Contrast the cobbler's situation with the working lives of most people today. These options are not open to modern-day shoemakers—or to nurses, autoworkers, bank tellers, or employees in countless other occupations. Of the 131 million American workers, approximately 92 percent work for other people. Approximately one-fourth have professional, managerial, or supervisory employment and the partial autonomy that comes with it. Most people, however, have no say about what they will make, how they will make it, what will happen to it after it is made, and under what conditions they will work. Management controls the work environment; the hours of work, the pace, the tasks, the tools, the chemicals, the conditions of the work environment, and the technologies are all determined by someone other than the worker.

In addition to the detrimental effects of lack of control, which by itself causes stress, workers' interests conflict with those of management. Management's goal is to maximize profit, labor's goal is a fair wage for a fair day's work. With increasing numbers of people working for others, the structure of work has changed, to the detriment of occupational and environmental health.

Innovations, such as word-processing technology, computerized recordkeeping, electronic mail, and computer and video monitoring have turned large offices into assembly lines. New forms of work organization have broken the close personal tie that frequently existed between secretaries and their employers, and new technology has downgraded the skills required. With these changes, clerical work becomes subject to the same kind of machine-like analysis and control as factory work. Similar situations are often found in service, retail, distributive, and other types of work. What is true for the autoworker, the word processor, and the keypunch operator is increasingly the case for the short-order cook, the checkout clerk, and the telephone operator. One young woman describes her sense of powerlessness and alienation as a grocery store cashier:

> It was extremely repetitive work. Pushing numbers all day sort of got to me. I used to have dreams, or should I say nightmares, all night long of ringing up customers' orders when it was after closing time. I have even woken up and found myself sitting up in bed talking to customers. That job ended when the whole building exploded one

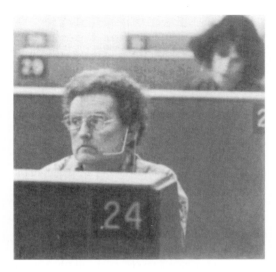

FIGURE 2-5 ● Long-distance telephone operators. Monotony characterizes many jobs. (Photograph by Earl Dotter.)

night because of some faulty electrical work. The summer of my senior year in high school I got another job as a cashier in a discount department store, doing the same thing, pushing numbers again. My nightmare of talking to customers in my sleep began again. . . . This was a job that was an extremely strict one. There was no leeway about anything. They had cameras above the registers watching us to see if we were polite, if we checked inside of containers for any hidden merchandise, checked the tags to see if they were switched, etc. If we failed to do something we were given a written warning.

> Everyone who worked there, with the exception of the management, was part-time. The schedules were made so that no one had exactly forty hours. I worked for three months, 35 to 38 hours per week. By not giving us those few extra hours, they saved themselves a lot of money by not having to give their employees benefits, insurance, etc. Of course, their hiring, firing, quitting went on week after week. There weren't too many loyal employees.[*]

A fractionated division of labor and "scientific" work discipline are ways of exerting managerial control in the interests of efficiency and profit (Fig. 2-5). The experience of alienation and powerlessness on the part of the workers, however, is not limited to workplaces where this type of organization is imposed. Many jobs in small shops—particularly

---

[*] *Miller L. Unpublished interview, Southeastern Massachusetts University, 1980.*

in the service and retail sectors, which employ the largest number of women and youth—are equally unattractive despite their lack of specialization.

Organized Labor

Unions are a way to counteract the power of management and the disempowering and disenfranchising effects of class, race, and gender. They provide workers a voice in determining the rules and conditions of work, wage rates, and benefits. They are the collective strength that provides a counterweight to management power and prerogative. Some unions have been deeply involved in health and safety issues but, for most unions, the health and safety issues are only a few among many. In the United States, given the weakness of unions and the historic antagonism to organized labor, unions have not always been able to give the necessary resources to protect their members from workplace hazards. In Europe, organized labor has been more successful in combating the prerogatives of management and, in a number of European countries, social democratic political parties that have been supported by labor movements have frequently been in power. Even in the United States, unions offer some protection against arbitrary exercise of power.

Formally, unionized workers try to regain some control over the labor process through collective bargaining—the negotiation of work rules and grievance mechanisms, the institutionalized process for adjudicating individual complaints. However, only approximately 15 percent of workers in the United States are unionized, and even where grievance mechanisms exist, they are not always respected.

Organized labor in the United States is now weaker numerically and politically than at any time since World War II. This decline began in the 1970s and continues today. From 1985 to 1995, unionization rates in the United States declined 21 percent.[18] The decline is evident across the whole range of union activity: loss of negotiating strength, decrease in membership, decline in strike activity, and a vast increase in "concessionary" collective bargaining agreements between unions and industry.

In contrast to the United States, in Great Britain 55 percent of workers are in unions, and labor governments have ruled the country. In Sweden, more than 95 percent of blue-collar workers are organized, and approximately 75 percent of white-collar employees are in unions. From the late 1980s to the late 1990s, unionization rates in Sweden increased by 8.7 percent.[18] For much of the late 20th century, Sweden had a labor government; its labor laws reflect that power.[19] In Germany, France, and many other countries, the existence of a labor party (or a social democratic party) has enabled workers to push for and defend significant legislation to control workplace hazards and provide extensive programs of social insurance and welfare.

The strength of a labor movement determines many issues that directly influence worker health. Unionized workers are more likely to be informed about the presence of health and safety hazards than are nonunion members in the same jobs.[19] In addition to union-sponsored education programs, the union provides a shield against employer discrimination. This shield is extremely important for health and safety because employers may fire a worker for raising concern about health and safety problems.

Unions in the United States and elsewhere have fought to create legislation requiring employers to clean up the workplace, to control the employment of women and children, to limit the hours of work, and to set and enforce industrial hygiene standards. In the United States, where OSHA requires that workers be informed about the hazards associated with the chemicals with which they work, unions have pushed to make sure that employers comply with these right-to-know regulations. When there was no federal right-to-know law, some unions negotiated this right, as well as the right to refuse unusually hazardous work. The strength of a labor movement determines what information is generated about workplace hazards, who has access to it, what workplace standards are set and how strictly they are enforced, and the effectiveness of workers' compensation (Fig. 2-6).

Yet, it is increasingly difficult to form a union in the United States. Unions were originally formed by workers who all came to work in the same mill or factory, at the same time; but the structure of work and production is changing. More shift work, more "temp" work, the threat of outsourcing, and the fear of unemployment make for disconnected, docile workers who cannot advocate for themselves, because regardless of how dangerous or unpleasant a job is, most people would rather have a job than be unemployed.

Nongovernmental Organizations

A range of nongovernmental organizations (NGOs) exist to protect and advocate for workers, communities, and the environment. Environmental health

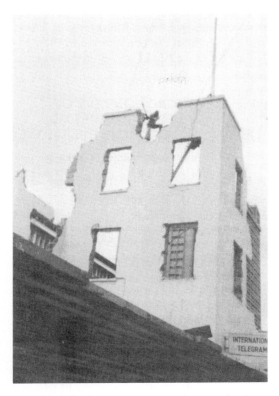

FIGURE 2-6 ● Non-union demolition worker in East Africa. (Photograph by Barry S. Levy.)

issues are most often brought to public attention by NGOs, which range from staid professional associations to strident advocacy organizations. These organizations typically rely on the breadth and character of their membership to provide legitimacy and often use scientific studies and journalistic reports to document their concerns (see Chapter 35).

The United States has thousands of such advocacy and service organizations. The large majority are local neighborhood and community advocacy associations. Some, like the Sierra Club and the American Public Health Association, work on national environmental health issues and are large organizations with state and local chapters. Others, like the Natural Resources Defense Council and Environmental Defense, use litigation to press for environmental protections. In the occupational health arena, the AFL-CIO advocates for workplace health and safety as do some 20 regional organizations called COSHs (Coalitions for Occupational Safety and Health). The COSH in Massachusetts was instrumental in cleaning up the smelter mentioned at the beginning of the chapter.

At the international level, the World Health Organization, the International Labor Organiza-

tion, the United Nations Environment Program, and other agencies of the United Nations create guidelines to improve conditions for workers and the environment. It is then up to local NGOs to pressure governments to adopt and enforce the standards. Over the past 20 years, as the U.S. government has been more reluctant to enforce environmental and labor laws, local NGOs and local branches of international NGOs, like Greenpeace, have become more active.

Citizens and advocacy groups have played significant roles in investigating disease clusters, like the cluster of childhood leukemia in Woburn, Massachusetts, in the 1980s, which was first noticed by some housewives and mothers, and the polychlorinated biphenyl (PCB) contamination of Anniston, Alabama, which was publicized by local activists. Such advocacy work is often quite confrontational because government agents tend to be reluctant to react, particularly when the potential sources of environmental contamination involve powerful business interests. Because the most effective way to raise public awareness of a potential environmental or occupational health hazard requires coverage by the news media, NGOs often find that they must be confrontational to provide the type of dramatic stories that the media will cover.

Environmental protection, inasmuch as it is seen to interfere in the control of the production process and the prerogatives of business, has been a long-standing source of controversy. Battles between environmental advocates and business are waged at all levels, including conflict over how much old forest can be logged, the relative destructiveness of strip-mining methods, the strictness of auto-emissions standards, and the use of pesticides and habitat destruction by business interests, such as sugarcane growers in the Everglades in Florida. These conflicts are inevitable, when the incentives of the economic system violate a sense of social justice and environmental integrity.

Although scientists are often quite conservative in drawing causal connections between known hazards and specific health outcomes for fear of overstating results, citizens would rather be safe than sorry. Their persistence has exposed many environmental problems that would otherwise never be known. Citizen groups also advocate for a variety of changes to remove certain toxics, such as mercury and polyvinyl chloride (PVC) and a range of pesticides, from production and use. They advocate for cleaner mass transit and stricter environmental and labor laws and their enforcement. Citizens' organizations often provide a change-seeking counterbalance to government's and industry's attachment to the status quo.

Governments

A fourth key actor in the complex of environmental health and workplace health and safety is "government" in the form of regulatory agencies, such as OSHA, the Centers for Disease Control and Prevention (CDC), and the Environmental Protection Agency (EPA). The impact of government intervention is defined by the set of institutions—legislative, executive, judicial, and civil service—that responds to needs, initiates policy, enacts laws, and promulgates and enforces regulations. In the past 100 years, social policies created by government have embraced such measures as unemployment benefits, pensions, and medical insurance and have protected consumers (such as by control of food additives and laws on advertising and product liability), preserved the environment, and promoted public health and safety.

Government regulations of the workplace are designed to protect workers, but they are infrequently enforced. This is not surprising, given that OSHA resources would allow the federal government to inspect each of 6 million workplaces once every 108 years.[20] As of 2002, EPA's budget was 23 times that of OSHA. Fines for serious OSHA violations—life-threatening conditions—average approximately $625[21] (see Chapter 3).

Why should the government in free-market economies interfere in the operation of the market to ensure the achievement of public welfare goals? What prompts the government to ascribe to itself a regulatory role? The effort to protect the health and safety of workers and the environment provides an excellent example of the contradictory forces operating on governments.

On the one hand, the government must respond to public pressures; to demands that it intervene to prevent illness, injury, and death on the job; to maintain a safe environment; and to appear to be responsible and responsive to the concerns of trade unions, workers, and the public. On the other hand, such regulation may have enormous costs for the economy as a whole and for individual firms. By controlling activities at the point of production, such direct state intervention challenges control of the workplace, and, by requiring certain levels of safety and minimum health and environmental measures,

it imposes costs on industry that may affect profitability. In addition, such intervention gives specific rights to workers, such as the right to refuse unsafe work, which threatens managerial and corporate control of the production process.

The particular ways in which government develops and implements policy are constrained by the constitutional and governing structures of a given country and by the ideological and cultural "mix" arising from history and traditions. Since the passage of the OSHAct in the United States and the creation of OSHA, the struggle for healthful and safe working conditions has raised issues of control of the workplace and organization of production. Throughout the 1970s, intense debates occurred over the role and actions of OSHA, the validity of the scientific evidence on the dangers posed by chemicals, the enforcement of standards, the extent and legitimacy of government regulation, and workers' rights to a hazard-free working environment. From the time the first draft of the OSHAct appeared before Congress, industry associations, chambers of commerce, trade unions, and government agencies all became deeply embroiled in a highly politicized and emotionally charged issue.

Scientists and Professionals

In the United States, the largest group of people working in occupational health are occupational health nurses. Environmental engineers and public health professionals make up a majority of those working on environmental health. Other professionals include physicians, industrial hygienists and industrial hygiene technicians, safety engineers, epidemiologists, ergonomists, educators, and program administrators. Ideological assumptions determine aspects of scientific investigation and research. Scientific disciplines focus attention on the technical aspects of occupational hazards and underestimate the importance of the macro and micro social, economic, and political context. In this regard, some workplaces have worker or union safety stewards and, increasingly, joint labor–management occupational safety and health committees; that is, nonprofessionals who are involved in hazard surveillance as well as injury and illness prevention. These individuals tend not to be imbued with the scientific model of research and hazard control, which, in some circumstances, may be advantageous in dealing with workplace hazards.

Where do these different types of people responsible for occupational health work? Some are blue-collar workers in factories with special assignments on health and safety. Many of the larger firms hire occupational health professionals and environmental engineers as staff. In most companies, they are part of human-resources or labor-relations departments or, more recently, part of an integrated environmental safety and health (ES&H) department that is directly responsible to top management. Rarely are these professionals given direct responsibility and authority over production; they can be influential, but basic decisions are typically made by "production" managers, even in service industries.

Small companies—where most people in the United States and the rest of the world work—rarely have environmental or health and safety professionals on the payroll. Usually, such firms rely on *ad hoc* consultations with independent professionals or simply on emergency medical services. Occasionally, there may be a relationship with specialist health clinics or services. Such consulting operations must sell their services; they are sometimes confronted with ethical difficulties because their clients are companies. Indeed, a large amount of professional time of in-house environmental health and safety staff or even the hired consultants is spent on routine paperwork and issues involved more with regulatory compliance than direct health services.

Although labor unions, such as the United Mine Workers of America, have had health and safety staff members for many years, the real growth of occupational health and safety professionals in labor unions has happened since the 1970 passage of the OSHAct. Nevertheless, the number of physicians, industrial hygienists, and other work-environment professionals employed by the labor movement remains small—and most are at the national or international level. These individuals generally provide policy assistance rather than direct services to workers. Many professionals involved with environmental health work for universities, NGOs, and medical schools and hospitals. Many environmental and occupational health professionals are members of regional and local professional groups that exchange technical information. These groups have codes of ethics (see Chapter 5) that can inspire and strengthen efforts to improve the work environment. Finally, and perhaps most important, many practitioners, including those in the full range of occupational and environmental health profes-

sions, are employed by government agencies, usually as inspectors but sometimes as technical advisers to government or industry or as educators. In the United States, practitioners are employed by such federal agencies as OSHA, EPA, the National Institute for Occupational Safety and Health (NIOSH), and other parts of CDC, the National Institute of Environmental Health Sciences, the Mine Safety and Health Administration, the Department of Energy, and state departments of labor, environmental protection, and public health.

CONCLUSION

What can be said about the importance of understanding the social context of occupational and environmental health? First, ideology shapes the way we think about problems and how to solve them. Second, the changing structure of the economy and, hence, of production and consumption has presented new problems for workers and the environment and for people involved with occupational and environmental health. Third, the direction of technological development may create new hazards and may set limits on our ability to remedy them. Finally, the distribution of power in the society can have profound impact on the attention given to worker health and safety and the environment.

The significance, then, of a social analysis of the fundamental, but often unrecognized, problem facing health care providers and others working in occupational and environmental health is that they frequently are in the difficult situation of having responsibilities for worker health and the environment while working in organizations with other priorities. Management and government organizations are influenced by economic responsibilities that may compromise the health and safety of workers and communities. Even labor organizations, with their key responsibility to rank-and-file workers, may find health and safety low down on a list of concerns and demands.

Health professionals can be successful in improving community and workplace environments, especially if they understand the social and economic context of their efforts and work toward "win–win" situations. Some have argued that environmental health and safety regulation may stimulate companies to technological innovations that might not otherwise have been considered.[22] For example, where workers' compensation costs to a company are high, it may be possible to improve the economic performance of the company and improve worker health through preventive measures. When OSHA mandated reductions in vinyl chloride exposure, the controls introduced by the companies resulted in increased profits. Environmental health and safety practitioners need to master economic, as well as humanist, arguments for change.

Sometimes, however, the economic arguments alone are not sufficiently convincing to sway management. Professionals in occupational and environmental health need to think in broader terms than usual when confronting difficult situations and recalcitrant employers. In many states, such professionals have played important roles in new coalitions of labor activists and environmentalists. Committees or coalitions for occupational safety and health have engaged in worker education and advocacy since the early 1970s and have been instrumental in focusing the attention of labor unions and the general public on health and safety issues. Likewise, broad public health and environmental advocacy organizations have led the way in promoting community and environmental health. These groups represent a grassroots movement that links professionals and concerned citizens in new ways to protect and improve the natural and work environments. It is these broad coalitions of professionals, community leaders, trade unionists, and workers that offer some of the best hopes for achieving a truly healthier and safer environment.

The authors gratefully acknowledge the contributions of Charles Levenstein and John Wooding to versions of this chapter in previous editions of this textbook.

REFERENCES

1. Levenstein C, Wooding J, Rosenberg B. Occupational health: A social perspective. In BS Levy, DH Wegman, eds. Occupational health: Recognizing and preventing work-related disease and injury. 4th ed. Philadelphia: Lippincott Williams & Wilkins, 2000:27–50.
2. McClure V. Monsanto, Solutia liable. The Birmingham News, February 23, 2002.
3. Environmental Working Group, Chemical Industry Archives, Anniston. (Available at: <www.chemicalindustryarchives.org/dirtysectrets/annistonindepth/wildlife.asp>. Accessed February 26, 2004.)
4. Rosenberg B, Levenstein C, Wooding J. Down on the farm: The agricultural extension service as a model for manufacturing? New Solutions 1998;8:3.
5. Kuhn S, Wooding J. The changing structure of work in the U.S. Part 1: The impact on income and benefits. New Solutions 1994;4:43.
6. Karasek R, Theorell T. Healthy work. New York: Basic Books, 1990.
7. Schor J. The overworked American. New York: Basic Books, 1991.
8. Rizer-Roberts E. Bioremediation of petroleum contaminated sites. Boca Raton, FL: CRC Press, 1992:4.
9. Levison A. The working class majority. New York: Coward, McGann Geohegan, 1974.
10. Bullard RD. Reviewing the EPA's draft environmental equity report. New Solutions 1993;3:78.
11. Bureau of Labor Statistics. Table 2: Median usual weekly earnings of full-time wage and salary workers by age, race, Hispanic or Latino ethnicity, and sex, fourth quarter averages, not seasonally adjusted. February 11, 2004.
12. Amott T. Caught in the crisis: Women and the U.S. economy today. New York Monthly Review Press, 1993, p. 88.
13. Spangler E. Sexual harassment: Labor relations by other means. New Solutions 1992;3:24.
14. Managing workplace safety and health. Beaumont, TX: John Gray Institute, Lamar University, 1991.
15. Leeflag RLI, Klein-Hasselink DJ, Spruit IP. Health effects of unemployment. Social Science Medicine 1992;34:351–363.
16. U.S. International Trade Commission, United States Department of Commerce US-China Business Council. Table 3. Available at: <www.uschina.org/statistics/tradetable/html>. Accessed February 18, 2005.
17. Peterson HC. Business and government 3rd ed. New York: Harper & Row, 1989:429–430.
18. International Labor Organization. World labor report 97–98. Geneva: ILO, 1998.
19. Elling R. The struggle for workers health. Farmingdale, NY: Baywood, 1986.
20. AFL-CIO. Death on the job: The toll of neglect. Washington, DC: AFL-CIO Department of Occupational Safety and Health, April 1992.
21. Armenti K, Moure-Eraso R, Slatin C, Geiser K. Joint occupational and environmental pollution prevention strategies: A model for primary prevention. New Solutions 2003,13:3.
22. Ashford NA, Heaton GR Jr. Regulation and technological innovation in the chemical industry. Law and Contemp Prob 1983;46:109–157.

BIBLIOGRAPHY

Levenstein C, Wooding J, eds. Work, health and the environment: Old problems, new solutions. New York: Guilford Press, 1997.
　Selected articles from New Solutions: A Journal of Occupational and Environmental Health Policy.
Ashford N, Caldart N. Technology, law and the working environment. Washington, DC: Island Press, 1996.
　A detailed compendium of laws and important court cases that govern the workplace in the United States.
Levenstein C, Wooding J. The point of production. New York: Guilford Press, 1999.
　A political economic framework of the work environment and occupational safety and health based on contradictions arising at the point of production.

CHAPTER 3

Government Regulation

Nicholas A. Ashford and Charles C. Caldart

The manufacturing, processing, and use of chemicals, materials, tools, machinery, and equipment in industrial, construction, mining, and agricultural workplaces are often accompanied by environmental, health, and safety hazards and risks. Occupational and environmental factors cause or exacerbate major diseases of the respiratory, cardiovascular, reproductive, and nervous system and cause systemic poisoning and some cancers and birth defects. Occupational and environmental disease and injury place heavy economic and social burdens on workers, employers, citizens, and taxpayers.

Because voluntary efforts in the unregulated market have not succeeded historically in reducing the incidence of these diseases and injuries, government intervention into the activities of the private sector has been demanded by citizens, consumers, and workers. This intervention takes the form of the regulation of environmental health and safety hazards through standard setting, enforcement, and transfer of information. This chapter addresses the major regulatory systems (or regimes) designed to protect public and worker health from chemicals discharged from sources that pollute the air, water, ground, and workplace. The setting of standards and other legal requirements in these regulatory regimes has occurred over a more than 30-year period that has seen changes in the use of scientific and technical information in regulatory initiatives and in legal doctrine, including the manner in which science, economics, and technological capability are viewed by the courts. The concepts of risk assessment, cost–benefit analysis, and technology forcing have evolved—both through the development of case law and through changes in the political environment. Often, changes in one of the regulatory regimes has affected the other regulatory regimes as well.

Several themes run through the discussion of the different regulatory systems: distinctions between performance and design/specification standards*; differences in the extent to which economics or cost are taken into account in the setting and enforcement of standards; and distinctions between interventions that encourage technological innovation and those that encourage diffusion of existing technologies.

---

*Actually, standards (what we will call direct controls) can be classified in a number of ways. A performance standard is one that specifies a particular outcome—such as a specified emission level above which it is illegal to emit a specified air pollutant—but does not specify how that outcome is to be achieved. A design or specification standard, on the other hand, specifies a particular technology—such as a catalytic converter—that must be used. In either case, the standard can be based on (a) a desired level of protection for human health or environmental quality, (b) some level of presumed technological feasibility, (c) some level of presumed economic feasibility, or (d) some balancing of social costs and social benefits. Within each of these options, there is a wide spectrum of possible approaches. A human health-based standard, for example, might choose to protect only the average member of the population, or it might choose to protect the most sensitive individual. A technology-based standard might be based on what is deemed feasible for an entire industry, or on what is deemed feasible for each firm within the industry. Moreover, some standards might be based on a combination of these factors. Many standards based on technological feasibility, for example, are also based on some concept of economic feasibility. Other requirements that could be considered "standards" include (a) information-based obligations, such as the disclosure of (and retention of, or provision of access to) exposure, toxicity, chemical content, and production data and (b) requirements to conduct testing or screening of chemical products.

In the United States, toxic substances in the workplace have been regulated primarily through three federal laws: the Mine Safety and Health Act of 1969 (Box 3-1 and Figs. 3-1 and 3-2), the Occupational Safety and Health Act (OSHAct) of 1970, and the Toxic Substances Control Act (TSCA) of 1976. These federal laws have remained essentially unchanged since their passage, although serious attempts at reform have been made from time to time. Since 1990, sudden and accidental releases of chemicals (chemical accidents), which may affect both workers and community residents, are now also regulated under the Clean Air Act.

The OSHAct established the Occupational Safety and Health Administration (OSHA) in the Department of Labor to enforce compliance with

---

BOX 3-1

Essentials of the Mine Safety and Health Administration

James L. Weeks

The Mine Safety and Health Administration (MSHA) in the U.S. Department of Labor has responsibility for writing and enforcing regulations to protect the health and safety of the approximately 200,000 miners in the United States. These miners work in underground and surface mines that produce coal, metal ore, other nonmetal commodities (such as salt and trona), and in sand, stone, and gravel quarries. Mining is one of the most dangerous industries worldwide and in the United States. There are high rates of fatal and nonfatal traumatic injuries, occupational lung disease (coal workers' pneumoconiosis, silicosis, and lung cancer), and noise-induced hearing loss. Underground miners are also exposed to high concentrations of exhaust from diesel engines.

Historically, federal government intervention in mine safety and health was the responsibility of the U.S. Bureau of Mines in the Department of the Interior. The bureau was organized in 1910 for the purpose of investigating coal mine disasters, and over the next six decades, it acquired increasing authority and responsibility to enter and inspect mines and promote mine safety, but it had limited authority to compel compliance with safety regulations. When Congress passed the Federal Coal Mine Health and Safety Act of 1969, it significantly changed the relationship between the federal government and the mining industry. This act was passed after a widespread miners strike for compensation for black lung and a spectacular and disastrous explosion that caused 78 deaths in a mine in West Virginia. Among other things, the act created an agency to perform epidemiologic research (NIOSH), an agency to continue its engineering research and development to develop safe mining practices (Bureau of Mines, since then absorbed into NIOSH), and a federal program to compensate miners totally disabled by pneumoconiosis.

The 1969 act created the federal black lung program to compensate miners totally disabled by pneumoconiosis. This program has been controversial, in part, because of the many manifestations of disease caused by inhaling coal mine dust. One innovative aspect of the program is that it allowed for decisions about eligibility when etiology was ambiguous by establishing a series of presumptions based on the miner's clinical status and work history. Originally, claims were paid out of the general treasury, but, in 1981, claims were paid by the operator who last employed the miner or, if that operator could not be found, by a disability trust fund to which operators contribute based on their tons of coal produced. The 1969 act also created the Mining Enforcement and Safety Administration (MESA), which enforced the basic structure and function of regulation as described later.

The 1969 act was amended in 1977, with passage of the Mine Safety and Health Act. The 1977 Mine Act moved MESA to the Department of Labor, changed its name to MSHA, preserved the basic structure of the 1969 act, and extended authority beyond coal mining to all other mines and quarries. The 1977 act also required that miners receive 40 hours of training in safety and health when first hired and 8 hours annually thereafter.

MSHA is structurally similar to OSHA but differs in some important ways. Both agencies write and enforce regulations, and disputes are adjudicated by administrative law review commissions with opportunities to appeal decisions to federal district courts.

(continued)

BOX 3-1

Essentials of the Mine Safety and Health Administration (Continued)

The standards-setting language in both acts is practically identical. Regulations covering toxic substances must be based on the best available evidence; must be designed to prevent material impairment of health for all miners, even if exposed for their entire working life; and standards must be feasible. Consequently, for the purpose of establishing regulations covering exposure to hazardous substances, the legal and scientific requirements of MSHA and OSHA are essentially the same.

But MSHA is significantly different from OSHA in its enforcement capabilities. Under MSHA, underground mines must be inspected four times and surface mines must be inspected twice each year. Most OSHA inspections are discretionary. Under MSHA, an inspector may, on his or her own authority, close all or part of a mine in case of imminent danger; the OSHA inspector does not have this authority and must get a court order. All mines are covered under MSHA, without exception; under OSHA, employers with 10 or fewer employees are exempt from general schedule inspection. Mine operators must submit a mine plan and have it approved before it can produce; only with confined spaces must employers under OSHA's jurisdiction obtain a permit and only then under limited conditions. Some numerical comparisons are informative. OSHA has jurisdiction over approximately 100 million workers, and MSHA has jurisdiction over less than 250,000, even though both agencies have approximately the same number of inspectors (including state plans). Thus, the number of inspectors per worker under MSHA is approximately 400 times that under OSHA.

Information about injuries and accidents in mining is more pertinent and more available. Mine-specific data on the number and rates of injuries, hours worked, and (coal) production is reported by mine operators to MSHA every quarter and some of it is available on the Internet. Surveillance data on exposure to dust, crystalline silica, other hazardous materials, and noise is also available from MSHA. Under OSHA, estimates of injury rates are available for SIC (Standard Industrial Classification) categories based on an annual survey of a sample of employers conducted by the Bureau of Labor Statistics. Employer-specific data are not available. Employers must post injury data annually, but they are not required to report it to OSHA. OSHA or workers' representatives may request it from each employer, but it is not available from a single source, as are MSHA's data. The accuracy and reliability of all surveillance data, however, is not guaranteed. Most injury and exposure data are provided by employers and passed on by either MSHA, OSHA, or the Bureau of Labor Statistics with little, if any, validation.

What has this regulatory intervention into the mining industry achieved? Before the passage of the 1969 Coal Mine Act, the fatality rate of U.S. miners was approximately 0.25 fatalities per 100 workers per year, four times that of miners in Western European coal-mining countries. For the first 10 years after the act, it declined each year to a level approximately the same as that in European mines. Since then, it has declined further, so that now, coal mines in the United States are among the safest in the world at an annual fatality rate of approximately 0.03 fatalities per 100 workers (see Fig. 3-2). Even so, the fatality rate in mining remains the highest of any major industrial group in the United States.

Trends in nonfatal injury rates are harder to measure because occurrence of these injuries varies significantly by occupation and among different age and experience cohorts. Trends in age- and experience-specific injury rates are not available. The crude rate of nonfatal injuries in coal mining has declined steadily, but this could be because very few new and inexperienced miners have been hired at the same time that the population of working miners is getting older and more experienced. This change in the age and experience distribution alone could account for the steady decline in the overall injury rate. Mine operators also must report certain accidents that do not cause injury but that signal the existence of hazards that could cause serious injury. These accidents include nonplanned roof falls, inundations with water, fires, and failure of ventilation.

(continued)

BOX 3-1

Essentials of the Mine Safety and Health Administration (Continued)

This regulatory scheme has also significantly reduced miners' exposure to respirable dust and has reduced the prevalence of coal workers' pneumoconiosis (CWP). Respirable coal mine dust was measured at 6 to 8 mg/m^3 before the 1969 act but, for the same job, declined to less than 3 mg/m^3 within 6 months and to approximately 2 mg/m^3 in another year. For continuous mining operators, the level is now regularly below 1 mg/m^3. This progress was achieved in spite of mine operators claiming, in 1969, that it was impossible to reduce exposure to the statutory limit of 2 mg/m^3. Exposure remains high at some mines and with some mining methods, such as longwall mining. Consistent with this reduction in exposure, the experience-adjusted prevalence of CWP has also been reduced since passage of the 1969 and 1977 mine acts. Problems persist, however. Noise exposure remains high, exposure to crystalline silica is also elevated, where it is known, and underground miners are exposed to high levels of diesel exhaust.

MSHA's program of surveillance and control of exposure to respirable dust and its enforcement of dust regulations is part of a more comprehensive effort to prevent the occurrence and progression of CWP. Other aspects of this plan include a federal program to compensate underground coal miners totally disabled by CWP, a prospective study of a cohort of miners, engineering research and development on methods of monitoring and controlling exposure to dust, and a program to allow miners to transfer to less dusty jobs in a mine if they have a positive chest radiograph for CWP. All these facets of the prevention effort are and have been controversial, but nevertheless they contain the essential elements for preventing occupational disease: exposure monitoring, enforcement, disease surveillance, right to transfer, epidemiologic research, and engineering research and development.

In sum, MSHA is an intensive intervention in a dangerous industry and, as such, is a laboratory on a number of issues important to worker health and safety generally. One important lesson from MSHA is that a concerted and multifaceted effort at controlling occupational hazards can succeed at reducing rates of traumatic fatalities and of pneumoconiosis. The important aspects of such an effort include sufficient resources, surveillance, exposure monitoring, worker training, epidemiologic research, and engineering research and development—all of which are supported, in one way or another, by regulatory authority.

---

the act, the National Institute for Occupational Safety and Health (NIOSH) in the Department of Health and Human Services (under the Centers for Disease Control and Prevention) to perform research and conduct health hazard evaluations, and the independent, quasijudicial Occupational Safety and Health Review Commission to hear employer contests of OSHA citations. The Office of Pollution Prevention and Toxic Substances in the Environmental Protection Agency (EPA) administers TSCA. The Office of Air, Water, and Solid Waste and the Office of Emergency Response in EPA regulate media-based pollution. The Office of Chemical Preparedness and Emergency Response in EPA is responsible for the chemical safety provisions of the Clean Air Act.

The evolution of regulatory law under the OSHAct has profoundly influenced other environmental legislation, including the regulation of air, water, and waste, but especially the evolution of TSCA.

STANDARD SETTING AND OBLIGATIONS OF THE EMPLOYER AND THE MANUFACTURER OR USER OF TOXIC SUBSTANCES

The Occupational Safety and Health Act of 1970

The OSHAct requires OSHA to (a) encourage employers and employees to reduce hazards in the workplace and to implement new or improved safety and health programs, (b) develop mandatory job safety and health standards and enforce them effectively, (c) establish "separate but dependent responsibilities and rights" for employers

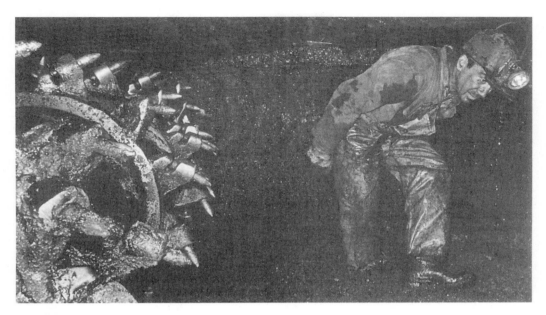

FIGURE 3-1 ● Mine hazards such as the increased dust exposure from continuous mining machines are regulated by the Mine Safety and Health Administration (MSHA). (Photograph by Earl Dotter.)

and employees for the achievement of better safety and health conditions, (d) establish reporting and record-keeping procedures to monitor job-related injuries and illnesses, and (e) encourage states to assume the fullest responsibility for establishing and administering their own occupational safety and health programs, which must be at least as effective as the federal program.

As a result of these responsibilities, OSHA inspects workplaces for violations of existing health and safety standards; establishes advisory committees; holds hearings; sets new or revised standards for control of specific substances, conditions, or use of equipment; enforces standards by assessing fines or by other legal means; and provides for consultative services for management and for employer and employee training and education. In all

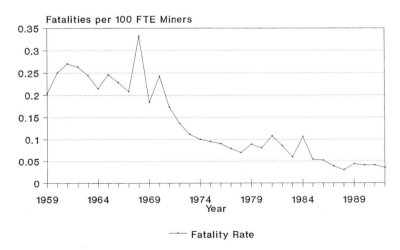

FIGURE 3-2 ● Underground bituminous coal mine fatality rates, 1959 to 1991. FTE, full-time equivalent miners. (From the Mine Safety and Health Administration.)

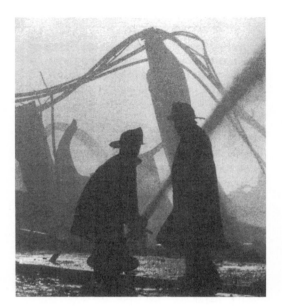

FIGURE 3-3 • The Occupational Safety and Health Administration's (OSHA's) positive impact on general industry health and safety in the United States unfortunately does not extend to municipal workers, such as firefighters. (Photograph by Marvin Lewiton.)

of its procedures, from the development of standards through their implementation and enforcement, OSHA guarantees employers and employees the right to be fully informed, to participate actively, and to appeal its decisions (although employees are limited somewhat in the latter activity).

The coverage of the OSHAct initially extended to all employers and their employees, except self-employed people; family-owned and -operated farms; state, county, and municipal workers (Fig. 3-3); and workplaces already protected by other federal agencies or other federal statutes. In 1979, however, Congress exempted from routine OSHA safety inspections approximately 1.5 million businesses with 10 or fewer employees. (Exceptions to this are allowed if workers claim there are safety violations.) Because federal agencies (except the U.S. Postal Service) are not subject to OSHA regulations and enforcement provisions, each agency is required to establish and maintain its own effective and comprehensive job safety and health program. OSHA provisions do not apply to state and local governments in their role as employers. OSHA requires, however, that any state desiring to gain OSHA support or funding for its own occupational safety and health program must provide a program to cover its state and local government

workers that is at least as effective as the OSHA program for private employees.

OSHA can begin standard-setting procedures either on its own or on petitions from other parties, including the Secretary of Health and Human Services, NIOSH, state and local governments, any nationally recognized standards-producing organization, employer or labor representatives, or any other interested person. The standard-setting process involves input from advisory committees and from NIOSH. When OSHA develops plans to propose, amend, or delete a standard, it publishes these intentions in the *Federal Register*. Subsequently, interested parties have opportunities to present arguments and pertinent evidence in writing or at public hearings. Under certain conditions, OSHA is authorized to set emergency temporary standards, which take effect immediately, but which are to be followed by the establishment of permanent standards within 6 months. To set an emergency temporary standard, OSHA must first determine that workers are in grave danger from exposure to toxic substances or new hazards and are not adequately protected by existing standards. Both emergency temporary and permanent standards can be appealed through the federal courts, but filing an appeals petition does not delay the enforcement of the standard unless a court of appeals specifically orders it. Employers may make application to OSHA for a temporary variance from a standard or regulation if they lack the means to comply readily with it, or for a permanent variance if they can prove that their facilities or methods of operation provide employee protection that is at least as effective as that required by OSHA.

OSHA requires employers of more than 10 employees to maintain records of occupational injuries and illnesses as they occur. All occupational injuries and diseases must be recorded if they result in death, one or more lost workdays, restriction of work or motion, loss of consciousness, transfer to another job, or medical treatment (other than first aid). Because this self-reported information relies on the employer determining that injuries and illness arose out of their "work-relatedness" at his or her facility, injuries, but especially illnesses, are acknowledged to be underreported.

Key OSHA Standards and Decisions

The OSHAct provides two general means of protection for workers: (a) a statutory general duty to provide a safe and healthful workplace, and (b) adherence to specific standards by employers. The act imposes on virtually every employer in the private sector a general duty "to furnish to each of his employees employment and a place of employment which are free from *recognized hazards* that are causing or are likely to cause death or serious physical harm. . . ." (emphasis added). A recognized hazard may be a substance for which the likelihood of harm has been the subject of research, giving rise to reasonable suspicion, or a substance for which an OSHA standard may or may not have been promulgated. The burden of proving that a particular substance is a recognized hazard and that industrial exposure to it results in a significant degree of exposure is placed on OSHA. Because standard setting is a slow process, protection of workers through the employer's general duty obligation could be especially important, but it is crucially dependent on the existence of reliable health effects data, as well as on the willingness of a particular OSHA administration to use this as a vehicle for protection.

The OSHAct addresses specifically the subject of toxic materials. It states, under Section 6(b)(5) of the act, that the Secretary of Labor (through OSHA), in promulgating standards dealing with toxic materials or harmful physical agents, shall set the standard that "most adequately assures, *to the extent feasible*, on the basis of the *best available evidence* that no employee will suffer material impairment of health or functional capacity, even if such employee has a regular exposure to the hazard dealt with by such standard for the period of his working life" (emphases added). These words indicate that the issue of exposure to toxic chemicals or carcinogens that have long latency periods, as well as to reproductive hazards, is covered by the act in specific terms.

In 1971, under Section 6(a) of the act, allowing for their adoption without critical review, OSHA initially adopted as standards the so-called *permissible exposure limits* (PELs): the 450 threshold limit values (TLVs) recommended by the American Conference of Governmental Industrial Hygienists (ACGIH) as guidelines for protection against the toxic effects of these materials. In the 1970s, under Section 6(b), OSHA set formal standards for asbestos, vinyl chloride, arsenic, dibromochloropropane, coke oven emissions, acrylonitrile, lead, cotton dust, and a group of 14 carcinogens. In the 1980s, OSHA regulated benzene, ethylene oxide, and formaldehyde as carcinogens and reg-

ulated asbestos more rigidly as a carcinogen at 0.2 fibers/cm^3. In the early 1990s, OSHA regulated cadmium, bloodborne pathogens, glycol ethers, and confined spaces. OSHA also lowered the PEL for formaldehyde from 1 to 0.75 parts per million (ppm; averaged over an 8-hour period) and issued a *process safety management* (PSM) rule (see later discussion). More recent rule-making activity by OSHA is discussed later in this chapter.

The burden of proving the hazardous nature of a substance is placed on OSHA, as is the requirement that the proposed controls are technologically feasible. The necessarily slow and arduous task of setting standards, substance by substance, makes it impossible to deal realistically with 13,000 toxic substances or approximately 250 suspect carcinogens on NIOSH lists. Efforts were made to streamline the process by (a) proposing generic standards for carcinogens and (b) proposing a generic standard updating the TLVs (PELs). As discussed later, neither of these efforts was successful.

The inadequacy of the 450 TLVs adopted under Section 6(a) of the act is widely known. The TLVs originated as guidelines recommended by the ACGIH to protect the *average* worker from either recognized acute effects or easily recognized chronic effects. The standards were based on animal toxicity data or the limited epidemiologic evidence available at the time (1969) of the establishment of the TLVs. They do not address sensitive populations within the workforce or those with prior exposure or existing disease, nor do they address the issues of carcinogenicity, mutagenicity, and teratogenicity. These standards were adopted en masse in 1971 as a part of the consensus standards that OSHA adopted along with those dealing primarily with safety.

As an example of the inadequacy of protection offered by the TLVs, the 1971 TLV for vinyl chloride was set at 250 ppm, whereas the later protective standard (see later) recommended no greater exposure than 1 ppm (as an average over 8 hours)—a level still recognized as unsafe, but the limit that the technology could detect. Another example is the TLV for lead, which was established at 200 μg/m^3, whereas the later lead standard was established at 50 μg/m^3, also recognizing that that level was not safe for all populations, such as pregnant women or those with prior lead exposure. In 1997, OSHA promulgated a new PEL for methylene chloride of 25 ppm, replacing the prior TLV of 500 ppm. The ACGIH updates its TLV list every 2 years. Although useful, an updated list would have little legal significance unless formally adopted by OSHA. OSHA did try, unsuccessfully, to adopt an updated and new list of PELs in its Air Contaminants Standard in 1989 (see later discussion). However, OSHA continues to maintain that it is intent on revising the list. The fact that the official OSHA TLVs are more than 30 years out of date compared with industry's own "voluntary" consensus standards is not welcomed, especially by the more modern firms in industry.

Under Section 6(b) of the OSHAct, new health standards dealing with toxic substances were to be established using the mechanism of an open hearing and subject to review by the U.S. Circuit Courts of Appeals. The evolution of case law associated with the handful of standards that OSHA promulgated through this section of the OSHAct is worth considering in detail. The courts addressed the difficult issue of what is adequate scientific information necessary to sustain the requirement that the standards be supported by "substantial evidence on the record as a whole." The cases also addressed the extent to which economic factors were permitted or required to be considered in the setting of the standards, the meaning of "feasibility," OSHA's technology-forcing authority, the question of whether a cost–benefit analysis was required or permitted, and, finally, the extent of the jurisdiction of the OSHAct in addressing different degrees of risk.

The 14 Carcinogens Standard

In an early case challenging OSHA's authority to regulate 14 carcinogens, the District of Columbia Circuit Court of Appeals first addressed the issue of substantial evidence. For 8 of the 14 carcinogens, there were no human (epidemiologic) data. Industry challenged OSHA's ability to impose controls on employers in the absence of human data. Here the court expressed its view that some facts, such as the establishment of human carcinogenic risk from animal data, were on the "frontiers of scientific knowledge" and that the requirement for standards to be supported by substantial evidence in these kinds of social policy decisions could not be subjected to the rigors of other kinds of factual determinations. Thus, OSHA was permitted to require protective action against substances known to produce cancer in animals but with no evidence of producing cancer in humans. It was not until 1980 that the U.S. Supreme Court in the benzene case (see later) placed limits on the extent of OSHA's policy determination on carcinogenic risk.

The Asbestos Standard

In the challenge to OSHA's original asbestos standard, in which asbestos was regulated as a classic lung toxin and not as a carcinogen, the Industrial Union Department of the American Federation of Labor and Congress of Industrial Organizations (AFL-CIO) unsuccessfully challenged the laxity of the standard, claiming that OSHA improperly weighed economic considerations in its determination of feasibility. OSHA indeed was permitted to consider economic factors in establishing feasibility. The District of Columbia Circuit Court of Appeals went on to state, however, that a standard might be feasible even if some employers were forced out of business, as long as the entire asbestos-using industry was not disrupted. In 1986, OSHA revised the standard from 2.0 to 0.2 fibers/cm^3, thus finally acknowledging asbestos as a carcinogen.

The Vinyl Chloride Standard

In the industry challenge to OSHA's regulation of vinyl chloride at 1 ppm, the Second Circuit Court of Appeals reiterated OSHA's ability to make policy judgments with regard to matters "on the frontiers of scientific knowledge" when it declared that there could be no safe level for a carcinogen. In addition, the court said that because 1 ppm was the lowest feasible (here meaning the lowest detectable) level, OSHA was permitted to force employers to comply even though it had performed no formal risk assessment or knew how many tumors would be prevented by the adoption of this protective level. Another noteworthy aspect of the case was the recognition that OSHA could act as a *technology forcer* and require controls not yet fully developed at the time of the setting of the standard.

The Lead Standard

Protection from lead exposure had been provided through the TLV of 200 μg/m^3. This level was long recognized as inadequate for workers who accumulated lead in their body tissues and for women (and possibly men) who intended to have children. As a result, based on the limits of technological feasibility, OSHA promulgated a new standard that permitted no exposure greater than 50 μg/m^3 averaged over an 8-hour period. In addition, because this was still unsafe for many workers, OSHA also provided that workers be removed with pay and employment security if their blood lead levels (BLLs) exceeded 50 μg/dL or if there were grounds to remove them based on risks to their reproductive system. The legality and necessity of this additional provision, known as *Medical Removal Protection* (MRP), was unsuccessfully challenged by the Lead Industries Association. OSHA specifically provided that workers in workplaces with air lead levels over an "action level" of 30 μg/m^3 have the benefit of a continuing medical surveillance program, including periodic sampling of BLLs and removal from exposure above the action level after finding a BLL in an individual worker above 50 μg/dL, with job return when the worker's BLL fell below 40 μg/dL.

Removal could also be triggered by other medical conditions deemed especially sensitive to risks associated with lead exposure, such as pregnancy. OSHA provided that workers' pay and seniority be maintained by the employer during any periods of medical removal (up to 18 months), even if such removal entailed sending the worker home. In actual practice, many employers have reduced the ambient air lead level well below 50 μg/m^3, which results in the removal of fewer workers. (In the 1980s, MRP was required in a limited way in the cotton dust and benzene standards. In 1998, medical removal requirements were added to the methylene chloride standard.)

The Benzene Standard

After the first serious successful industry challenge of an OSHA benzene standard in the Fifth Circuit Court of Appeals, the U.S. Supreme Court, in a controversial and divided majority opinion, chided OSHA for not attempting to evaluate the benefits of changing the PEL for benzene from 10 ppm (the former TLV) to 1 ppm. The Court argued that OSHA is obligated to regulate only "significant risks" and that without a risk assessment of some kind, OSHA could not know whether the proposed control addressed a significant risk. The Court was careful to state that it was not attempting to "statistically straitjacket" the agency, but that at a minimum the benefits of regulation needed to be addressed to meet the substantial evidence test. The Court did not give useful guidance concerning what constituted a significant risk. It stated that a risk of death of 1 in 1,000 was clearly significant, whereas a risk of 1 in 1 billion was clearly not so. This six-orders-of-magnitude range, of course, represents the area on which the political arguments have always been centered. The implications of the benzene decision for subsequent standards would come to reflect the political and philosophical leanings of future OSHA administrations. Unfortunately, worker protection has since gravitated to the largest permissible exposure, approximating 1 in 1,000 lifetime risk of cancer, to be contrasted with some public health protections under the Clean Air Act of 1 in 1,000,000.

There is little question that had OSHA submitted a risk assessment for benzene at the time, it could have argued that the risk it was attempting to address was actually significant. The precise requirement and nature of a risk assessment sufficient to meet the substantial evidence test remains unclear. In late 1985, OSHA again proposed to lower the PEL from 10 to 1 ppm, and, in 1987, the standard was set at that level. OSHA, however, after intervention by the Office of Management and Budget, declined to establish a short-term exposure limit.

The petroleum industry argued in the benzene case that not only must a risk assessment be performed, but a cost–benefit analysis must be done in which the risks of exposure are balanced against the benefits of the chemical. The question, however, was not decided in the benzene case but was addressed in a later case challenging OSHA's cotton dust standard. The Supreme Court not only acknowledged that cotton dust did represent a significant risk but also indicated that a cost–benefit balancing was neither required nor permitted by the OSHAct because Congress had already struck the balance heavily in favor of worker health and safety.

The Generic Carcinogen Standard

In 1980, OSHA promulgated a generic carcinogen standard by which questions of science policy, already settled as law in cases dealing with other standards, were codified in a set of principles. During the process of developing the generic carcinogen standard, OSHA and NIOSH developed lists of chemical substances that would probably be classified as suspect carcinogens. Each agency composed a list of approximately 250 substances. After revising the generic standard to reflect the need to determine if a particular carcinogenic risk was *significant*—as required by the U.S. Supreme Court in the benzene decision—OSHA declined to formally list any substance under the carcinogen standard. In setting or revising standards for formaldehyde, ethylene oxide, asbestos, and benzene, OSHA has proceeded to act as if the generic carcinogen standard did not exist, thus following the historically arduous and slow path to standard-setting.

Emergency Temporary Standards

In Section 6(c), the OSHAct authorizes OSHA to set, on publication in the *Federal Register* and without recourse to a formal hearing; *emergency temporary* (6-month) *standards* (ETSs) for toxic exposures constituting a "grave danger." Before OSHA lowered its permanent standard for asbestos from 2.0 to 0.2 fibers/cm^3, it attempted to protect workers by promulgating an ETS at 0.5 fibers/cm^3. In 1984, the Fifth Circuit Court of Appeals denied OSHA the ETS, arguing that the cost involved defeated the requirement that the ETS be "necessary" to protect workers. Attempts by OSHA to establish an ETS for hexavalent chromium likewise failed court review.

OSHA has issued nine emergency temporary standards under the OSHAct. Standards for vinyl chloride, dibromo-3-chloropropane (DBCP), and the first ETS on asbestos were not challenged in court and remained in effect until superseded by permanent standards. An ETS for acrylonitrile survived court challenge. ETSs on benzene, commercial diving, pesticides, 14 carcinogens, and asbestos were stayed or vacated by the courts.

Over the past decade, OSHA has avoided setting ETSs and instead has proceeded directly— but slowly—to establishing permanent standards for toxic substances under Section 6(b)(5). Thus, OSHA denied a 1993 request from Public Citizen for a temporary emergency hexavalent chromium standard but promised an advanced notice of rule making for 1995. After a successful court challenge, in October 2004, 9 years after OSHA's promised action, it finally issued a proposed revision of its 8-hour exposure limit, lowering the standard to 1 μg/m^3 from the previous 33-year-old standard of 52 μg/m^3, thus preventing 350 excess cancers annually. A 2001 petition requesting an ETS for beryllium was unsuccessful. However, OSHA is currently planning for a permanent standard.

Short-Term Exposure Limits

Short-term exposures to higher levels of carcinogens are in general considered more hazardous than longer exposures to lower levels. OSHA issued a new standard for exposure to ethylene oxide in 1984 but excluded a *short-term exposure limit* (STEL) that had originally been prepared, in deference to objections from the Office of Management and Budget. Ralph Nader's Health Research Group sued the Secretary of Labor in 1986 over OSHA's continuing failure to issue the STEL. In 1987, the District of Columbia Circuit Court of Appeals ordered OSHA to establish a STEL for ethylene oxide by March 1988. OSHA complied by setting a STEL of 5 ppm over a 15-minute period.

The Air Contaminants Standard

It is obvious that the slow, arduous process of promulgating individual health standards under Section 6(b)(5) of the OSHAct could never catch up with advances in scientific knowledge concerning the toxicity of chemicals. The ACGIH has updated its TLV list every 2 years, and although not as protective as workers and their unions would have liked, the recent updated lists did advance protection over the 1969 list that OSHA adopted into law in 1971. In 1989, OSHA decided to update the original list in a single rule-making effort through the 6(b) standard revision route. The agency issued more protective limits for 212 substances and established limits for 164 chemicals that were previously unregulated. Neither industry nor labor was satisfied with the standards. Industry, although giving general support, objected to the stringency of some of the PELs. Labor objected to their laxity, citing NIOSH recommendations not adopted, and generally objected to the rush-it-through process.

The Eleventh Circuit Court of Appeals vacated the standard in 1992, ruling that OSHA failed to establish that a significant risk of material health impairment existed for each regulated substance (required by the benzene decision) and that the new exposure limit for each substance was feasible for the affected industry. OSHA decided not to appeal the decision to what it perceived as a conservative Supreme Court. Thus, the original and inadequate TLV list remains in effect, and 164 new substances remain unregulated. OSHA periodically expresses its intent on updating the list through new rule making, but no new action has been forthcoming.

In the meantime, OSHA could argue that those 164 substances are "recognized hazards" and enforceable through OSHA's general duty clause, but OSHA administrations have not been willing to emphasize this approach in the case of the TLVs, although OSHA has used the general duty obligation to force compliance with good ergonomic practices in nursing homes. In 20 years, OSHA has issued only about a dozen general duty citations for substances covered by the original TLV list. Recently, OSHA's reluctance to use the general duty obligation in the case of the outdated TLVs was in part due to the many congressional attempts to pass legislation prohibiting such use.

The Toxic Substances Control Act

TSCA enables EPA to require data from industry on the production, use, and health and environmental effects of chemicals. TSCA also requires the manufacturer of new chemicals, or of existing chemicals put to a significant new use, to file a premarket notification with EPA. EPA may regulate chemicals under TSCA—by requiring labeling, setting tolerances, or banning completely and requiring repurchase or recall—where the chemicals present "an unreasonable risk of injury to human health or the environment." EPA may also order a specific change in chemical process technology. In addition, TSCA gives aggrieved parties, including consumers and workers, specific rights to sue to enforce under the act, with the possibility of awards for attorneys' fees. (This feature was missing in the OSHAct.)

Under TSCA, EPA must regulate "unreasonable risks of injury to human health or the environment." EPA has issued a regulation for worker protection from asbestos at the new OSHA limit of 0.2 fibers/cm^3, which applies to state and local government asbestos abatement workers not covered by OSHA. Although the potential for regulating workplace chemicals is there, EPA has not been aggressive in this area. Between 1977 and 1990, of the 22 regulatory actions taken on existing chemicals, 15 addressed polychlorinated biphenyls (PCBs), which EPA has a specific statutory directive to address under TSCA. Only regulations pertaining to asbestos, hexavalent chromium, and metalworking fluids had a strong occupational exposure component. Although EPA declared formaldehyde a "probable carcinogen" and the International Agency for Research on Cancer classified it as a confirmed human carcinogen, EPA chose not to take regulatory action on this substance, opting instead to defer to OSHA workplace regulations.

Used together, the OSHAct and TSCA provide potentially comprehensive and effective information-generation and standard-setting authority to protect workers. In particular, the information-generation activities under TSCA can provide the necessary data to have a substance qualify as a *recognized hazard* that, even in the absence of specific OSHA standards, must be controlled in some way by the employer to meet the general duty obligation under the OSHAct to provide a safe and healthful workplace.

The potentially powerful role of TSCA regulation was seriously challenged by the Fifth Circuit Court of Appeals in 1991, when it overturned the omnibus asbestos phase-out rule that EPA had issued in 1989. The court held that, under TSCA, EPA should not have issued a ban without having first considered alternatives that would have been less burdensome to industry. This would require the agency to perform a more comprehensive, detailed, and resource-intensive analysis. Rightly or wrongly, EPA has viewed this case (which was not appealed to the U.S. Supreme Court) as a significant impediment to future TSCA regulations, and the agency generally regards regulation of chemicals other than PCBs under TSCA to be a dead letter for now. With an unsympathetic Congress, there are no successful attempts to resurrect the regulatory authority of TSCA. However, TSCA continues to be important for its surviving authority to require the testing of chemicals and for its information reporting and retaining requirements (see the discussion later in this chapter on the *right to know*).

Control of Gradual Pollution in Air, Water, and Waste

The Clean Air Act

The modern Clean Air Act (CAA) came into being in 1970, and although significant changes were made in 1977 and 1990, the basic structure of the act has remained the same, with the addition of provisions for authority over acid rain, chlorofluorocarbons (CFCs), indoor air, and chemical safety. (The last of these is discussed later in this chapter.) The CAA regulates both stationary and mobile sources of pollution, taking into account the relative contributions of each to specific air pollution problems—and the relative capacity of different kinds of sources within each category to reduce their emissions. The recognition that sources using newer technology might be able to achieve greater emission reductions than older sources with older technology led to the act's distinction—both in the stationary and mobile source provisions—between new and existing sources. Although driven by equity considerations regarding the relative financial and technical burdens of pollution reduction, however, this approach unwittingly discouraged modernization or replacement of facilities and resulted in the operation of older (especially energy) facilities beyond their expected useful life. For new sources within each industrial sector, there was a recognition of the need for uniformity and also for encouraging technological innovation through technology-forcing inherent in stringent standards.[*] (See Chapter 17.)

The 1970 CAA directed EPA to establish primary ambient air quality standards that would protect public health with "an adequate margin of safety." [see §109(b)(1)] As interpreted by the courts and supported by congressional history, these standards were to be established without consideration of economic or technological feasibility. In addition, secondary ambient air quality standards were to be established to protect "the public welfare"..."within a reasonable time" [see §109(b)(2)].

Both federal and state government were to be involved in protecting the ambient air. Ambient air quality (concentration) standards were to be established by the federal government, and these were to be attained through (a) emission limitations placed on individual existing polluters through permits issued by state government as a part of their *State Implementation Plans* (SIPs) [§110]; (b) emission limitations for new sources, established not by the states but rather by EPA as *New Source Performance Standards* [§111]; and (c) by a combination of federal and state restrictions on mobile sources. In specifying compliance with federal emission standards, Congress expressed concern with possible *hot spots* of localized intense pollution and also with intermittent versus continuous versus sudden and accidental releases of harmful substances. Emission standards, in contrast with ambient concentration standards, are expressed as an emissions rate (mg emitted per 100 kg of product, per hour, per day, per week, per quarter, per year, per BTU, per passenger mile, or other unit of measurement).

The 1970 CAA also made a distinction between the federal control of criteria pollutants through ambient air standards and the control of *hazardous air pollutants* by means of federal emission limitations. Hazardous air pollutants were those recognized as extraordinarily toxic and eventually regarded as non- or low-threshold pollutants. Initially, these were to be regulated to protect public health with "an ample margin of safety" [§112] and, as with the standards for primary ambient air pollutants, standards were to be established without consideration of economic burden. These pollutants, Congress determined, were sufficiently dangerous

to preclude any reliance on atmospheric dispersion and mixing as a means of reducing their ambient concentrations. Because of their extraordinary toxicity, hot spots were to be avoided, and because ambient concentration air quality standards were considered impractical and of little relevance for sporadic and idiosyncratic sources, uniform federal emission standards were considered necessary. (Note, however, that California did establish an ambient standard complement to the federal emission limitation on vinyl chloride.)

In the early stages of the implementation of the stationary source provisions of the Clean Air Act (approximately 1970–1975), EPA focused on (a) the primary and secondary ambient air quality standards and (b) emission standards for both new sources of criteria pollutants and for all sources emitting seven regulated hazardous air pollutants (discussed below). Prior advisory standards for carbon monoxide (CO), sulfur dioxide (SO_2), oxides of nitrogen (NO_X), large particulate matter, and photochemical oxidants were made mandatory. In February 1979, the standard for photochemical oxidants was narrowed to cover only ground-level ozone, and the standard was relaxed from 0.08 ppm to 0.12 ppm averaged over a 1-hour period. The standard for particulate matter (PM_{10})—"inhalable" particulates up to 10 μm in diameter—was adopted in 1987. In July 1997, the ozone standard was further revised to 0.08 ppm. At the same time, the particulate standard was altered to place more stringent requirements on smaller (<2.5 μm) "respirable" particles ($PM_{2.5}$). A standard for a new criteria pollutant—airborne lead—was promulgated in October 1978. Current primary air quality standards set under Section 109 are found in Table 3-1.

In Section 112, Congress directed the administrator to set emission standards for hazardous air pollutants at a level that protects public health "with an ample margin of safety." It is likely that this phraseology reflected an early assumption that, though very dangerous, hazardous pollutants did exhibit a finite threshold (a nonzero level of exposure below which no harm would occur). As the 1970s progressed, however, there was a growing recognition that this assumption might be wrong, and that for many hazardous pollutants there was no level of exposure (at least at levels within the limits of detection) below which one could confidently predict that no harmful or irreversible effects (especially cancer or birth defects) would occur.

---

[*] *The court decisions recognizing EPA's technology-forcing authority were greatly influenced by OSHA's early technology-forcing approach to worker protection.*

TABLE 3-1

National Ambient Air Quality Standards

Carbon monoxide	Primary: 35 ppm averaged over 1 hour and 9.0 averaged over 8 hours; neither to be exceeded more than once per year. Secondary: none.
Particulate matter: PM$_{10}$	(Note that PM$_{xy}$ below refers to particles equal to or less than xy μm in diameter.) Primary: 150 μg/m^3 averaged over 24 hours, with no more than one expected exceedance per calendar year; also, 50 μg/m^3 or less for the expected annual arithmetic mean concentration. Secondary: same as primary.
PM$_{2.5}$	Additional primary: 65 μg/m^3 averaged over 24 hours; 15 μg/m^3 annual maximum.
Ozone	Prior primary: 235 μg/m^3 (0.12 ppm) averaged over 1 hour, no more than one expected exceedance per calendar year (multiple violations in a day count as one violation). Prior secondary: same as primary. Revised (current) primary: 0.08 ppm averaged over 8 hours.
Nitrogen dioxide	Primary: 100 μg/m^3 (0.053 ppm) as an annual arithmetic mean concentration. Secondary: same as primary.
Sulfur oxides	Primary: 365 μg/m^3 (0.14 ppm) averaged over 24 hours, not to be exceeded more than. once per year; 80 μg/m^3 (0.03 ppm) annual arithmetic mean. Secondary: 1,300 μg/m^3 averaged over a 3-hour period, not to be exceeded morethan once per year.
Lead	Primary: 1.5 μg/m^3 arithmetic average over a calendar quarter. Secondary: same as primary.

This presented an implementation challenge for EPA. Arguably, given its mandate to protect public health "with an ample margin of safety," the agency was required to ban the emission of several hazardous substances. This would, as a practical matter, essentially ban the use of these substances in many industries. Seeking to avoid this result, EPA adopted a policy of setting Section 112 emission standards at the level that could be achieved by technologically feasible technology.[*] Using this approach, EPA set finite (nonzero) standards for arsenic, asbestos, benzene, beryllium, coke oven emissions, mercury, vinyl chloride, and radionuclides. The standard-setting process was slow and had to be forced by litigation; it took 4 to 7 years to establish a final standard for each of these substances. Had EPA continued to set standards for

more substances, and had it used the technological feasibility approach to spur the development of cleaner technology, the environmental groups may well have been content to allow the implementation of Section 112 to proceed in this fashion. When the setting of new Section 112 standards all but stalled during the Reagan administration, however, the NRDC was determined to press the issue in court.

NRDC *v.* EPA, decided by the District of Columbia Circuit Court of Appeals, placed new limitations on EPA's approach to regulating hazardous air pollutants by requiring the EPA to determine an "acceptable" (nonzero) risk level prior to setting a hazardous air pollutant standard. In reaction to this case and to revitalize the moribund standard-setting process, Congress amended Section 112 in 1990 to use a two-tiered approach: the use of technology-based standards initially, with residual risks to be addressed (at a later date) by health-based standards. In the 1990 CAA amendments, Congress listed 189 other substances for

---

[*] *This is the approach then followed by OSHA in setting standards for exposure to workplace chemicals. In the case of carcinogens, OSHA considered no levels to be safe and established control requirements at the limit of technological feasibility.*

which *Maximum Achievable Control Technology* (MACT) technology-based standards were to be set over 10 years for major sources (defined as those emitting more than 10 tons per year of any single toxin or more than 25 tons combined). EPA was further mandated to issue a new rule, "where appropriate," adding pollutants "which present or may present . . . a threat of adverse human effects (including, but not limited to, substances which are known to be or may be reasonably anticipated to be, carcinogenic, mutagenic, teratogenic, neurotoxic, which cause reproductive dysfunction, or which are acutely or chronically toxic) or adverse environmental effects whether through ambient concentration, bioaccumulation, deposition or otherwise." In addition, for nonmajor (that is, so-called area) sources, restrictions may be less—*Generally Achievable Control Technology* (GACT) or management practices. More stringent requirements are allowed for all new sources. Emission standards established under MACT must require "the maximum degree of reduction (including a prohibition on emissions, where achievable)" but must reflect "the cost of achieving emissions reduction and any non-air and environmental impact and energy requirements." For pollutants with a health threshold, EPA could alternatively consider regulating an ample margin of safety in establishing emission levels—essentially the original mandate of the 1970 CAA. Finally, EPA was obligated to issue a report on risk, which it did in 2004. If no new legislation recommended by that report is enacted within 8 years, EPA must issue such additional regulations as are necessary to protect public health with an ample margin of safety—in general—and, specifically for carcinogens, protect against lifetime risks of one-in-a-million or more. EPA did make substantial progress on establishing MACT and GACT standards but has just begun working on risk- or health-based approaches.

Water Legislation

The two most important federal statutes regulating water pollution are the Clean Water Act (CWA) and the Safe Drinking Water Act (SDWA). The CWA regulates the discharge of pollutants into navigable surface waters (and into smaller waterways and wetlands that are hydrologically connected to navigable waters), and the SDWA regulates the level

of contaminants in public drinking-water supplies. (See Chapter 19.)

The Clean Water Act

The modern Clean Water act has its origins in the Federal Water Pollution Control Act Amendments of 1972. The basic structure of the act was established at that time, although it was refined and refocused by the Clean Water Act Amendments of 1977 (from which it also took its name) and by the Water Quality Act Amendments of 1987. The regulatory focus of the CWA is the discharge of pollutants to surface waters from "point sources," principally industrial facilities and municipal sewage treatment plants (known under the act as *publicly owned treatment works*, or POTWs). The CWA flatly prohibits any discharge of a pollutant from a point source to surface waters unless it is done in conformance with the requirements of the act, and the statute has since 1972 retained as an explicit "national goal" the elimination of all point—source discharges to surface waters by 1985. Although the "no discharge" goal may never be attainable in practical terms, it has helped focus the act's implementation on gradual—but inexorable—pollution reduction, as discharge limits are made more stringent over time.

The centerpiece of this pollution reduction scheme is the *National Pollutant Discharge Elimination System* (NPDES) permit. In theory, all point sources must have an NPDES permit before discharging pollutants to surface waters. In practice, however, many dischargers (mostly smaller ones) still do not. The NPDES permit, which is issued after public notice and an opportunity for comment, is to incorporate all of the various requirements of the act—including discharge limits—that are applicable to the point source in question. Point sources are subjected both to technology-based and water quality-based limits and to the more stringent of the two when they overlap.

The technology-based limits are established by EPA as national standards. To set these standards for industrial dischargers, EPA first divided industry into various industry categories and then established effluent limits for each category based on its assessment of what was technologically and economically feasible for the point sources within that category. Further, as required by the act, EPA set different standards within each industrial category for conventional pollutants (biochemical oxygen demand, fecal coliform, oil and grease, pH, and total suspended solids), toxic pollutants (currently a list of 129 designated chemical compounds), and nonconventional pollutants (which simply are other pollutants, such as total phenols, which are listed neither under the conventional nor the toxic designation).

In recognition of the fact that conventional pollutants usually are amenable to treatment by the types of pollution control equipment that has long been in use at conventional sewage treatment facilities, the standards for conventional pollutants are set according to what can be obtained through the use of the *Best Conventional Pollution Control Technology* (BCT), taking into account the reasonableness of the cost. The standards for toxic and nonconventional pollutants, on the other hand, are set according to EPA's determination of the level of pollution reduction that can be achieved through the application of the *Best Available Technology Economically Achievable* (BAT). Originally, Congress had directed EPA to set health-based standards for toxic pollutants, on a pollutant-by-pollutant basis, but this resulted in only a handful of standards (mostly for pesticide chemicals). The political difficulty of establishing national health-based standards for toxic chemicals led environmental groups, in a suit against EPA to compel regulation, to agree to a schedule for setting technology-based standards for a list of designated toxic pollutants. Congress formally endorsed this approach in 1977 by amending the act to require EPA to set BAT standards for all of the toxic pollutants on that list.

Under the CWA, EPA is to consider both control and process technology in setting BAT standards, which are to "result in reasonable further progress toward the national goal of eliminating the discharge of all pollutants" and are to require "the elimination of discharges of all pollutants [where] such elimination is technologically and economically achievable." An individual discharger may obtain a cost waiver from BAT standards for nonconventional pollutants if it cannot afford to comply, but no cost waiver is available from the standards for toxic pollutants. For new industrial sources within an industry category, EPA is to set standards based on *Best Available Demonstrated Technology* (BADT), which can be more stringent than BAT or BCT because of the greater technological flexibility inherent in the design and construction of a new facility. Although industry-wide costs are to be considered by EPA in establishing BADT standards, no waivers

are available to individual applicants once the standards are set.

The CWA also imposes technology-based standards on POTWs, based on the limitations that can be met through the application of secondary sewage treatment technology. In essence, this requires an 85 percent reduction in biochemical oxygen demand and total suspended solids. In addition, the act imposes limitations on discharges by industrial sources into POTWs. Such discharges are known under the act as "indirect" discharges (because the pollutants are not discharged directly to surface waters but rather are discharged indirectly to surface waters through a public sewer system). Limitations on indirect discharges are known under the act as "pretreatment" standards, because they have the effect of requiring the indirect discharger to treat its wastewater before discharging it to the POTW for further treatment. EPA has set national technology-based limitations (known as the "categorical" pretreatment standards) on indirect discharges of toxic pollutants by firms in certain industrial categories. In addition, the act requires the POTW to set such additional pretreatment limits and requirements as is necessary both to ensure the integrity of the sewage treatment process and to prevent the indirectly discharged pollutants from "passing through" the sewer system and causing a violation of the POTW's discharge permit.

For the first 15 to 20 years of the act's implementation, the primary focus was the establishment and implementation of the technology-based limits discussed above. More recently, however, considerably more attention has been given to the act's system of water quality–based limits, which is equally applicable to industrial sources and POTWs. Since 1972, the CWA has directed the states to establish, and periodically revise, ambient (in-stream) water quality standards for all of the lakes, rivers, streams, bays, and other waterways within their borders and has required EPA to set and revise these standards to the extent that a state declines to do so. Further, the act has required since 1977 that NPDES permits include such additional discharge limits—beyond the national technology-based limits—as may be necessary to meet the ambient water quality standards of the waterway in question.

To help call attention to these water quality requirements, Congress in 1987 added what became known as the "toxic hot spot" provision of the CWA, which directed EPA and the states to identify those waters that were in violation of ambient water quality standards because of toxic pollution, to identify those point sources whose discharges of toxic pollutants were contributing to those violations, and to develop an "individual control strategy" for that source (which almost always meant a revision of the source's NPDES permit to add or tighten limits on toxic pollutants). Another provision of the act that has prompted the addition or tightening of water quality–based discharge limits has been the requirement that the states (and, if they decline, the EPA) to calculate a *total maximum daily load* (TMDL) for all waters that are in violation of ambient water quality standards. For any particular body or water, the TMDL for a particular pollutant is the total amount of that pollutant that may be discharged to the water body in a day without violating the relevant ambient water quality standard. When a TMDL is set, it often leads inexorably to a tightening of the NPDES permits of those point sources whose discharges are contributing to the particular violation of water quality standards. Although the TMDL requirement has been in the act since 1972, the states and EPA have been slow to implement it. Over the past 10 years or so, however, as a result of several successful suits by environmental groups seeking to compel EPA to set TMDLs in the face of state inaction, the TMDL requirement has come considerably more to the fore. Consequently, the inclusion of water quality–based limits in NPDES permits has become considerably more commonplace.

The Safe Drinking Water Act

Although some sources of drinking water are also regulated as surface waters under the CWA, the legislation specifically designed to protect the safety of the drinking water delivered to the public from public water systems is the SDWA. Passed in 1974 after a series of well-publicized stories about the number of potential carcinogens in the Mississippi River water used as drinking water by the City of New Orleans, it contains very little that is designed to address the sources of drinking water pollution. Instead, the SDWA directs EPA to set national health-based goals—known as *maximum contaminant level goals* (MCL goals)—for various drinking water contaminants and to set *maximum contaminant levels* (MCLs) that are as close to the MCL goals as is technologically and economically feasible. All public water systems, defined as those with at least 15 service connections or that

serve at least 25 people, are required to meet the MCLs.

Over the act's first 8 years, EPA set only 23 federal drinking water standards. Dissatisfied with the pace of implementation, Congress amended the act in 1986 to spur the agency into action. It directed EPA to set standards (MCLs and MCL goals) for 83 specified contaminants within 3 years and to set standards for 25 additional contaminants every 3 years thereafter. Ten years later, with scores of MCLs and MCL goals now on the books, Congress scaled back. In a 1996 compromise endorsed by environmental groups and water suppliers alike, Congress eliminated the requirement for 25 new standards every 3 years. At the same time, it added provisions that effectively ensured both that the standards that had been set would largely be allowed to remain in place and that new standards would be far slower in coming (and likely would be—because of the addition of a cost–benefit requirement— relatively weaker).

Since then, the primary focus of the SDWA program has been bringing public water systems throughout the country into compliance with the existing standards. Although the MCLs are set at a level deemed to be technologically and economically feasible, many water systems have had difficulty affording the cost of meeting, and monitoring for, the MCLs. To attempt to ameliorate the financial burden on municipal water systems, the SDWA has periodically made federal funds available for technology upgrades and infrastructure improvements. The task, however, remains a daunting one. In 2002, EPA estimated that approximately $151 billion would be needed over the next 20 years to upgrade the nation's 55,000 community water systems.

The Regulation of Hazardous Waste

Broadly speaking, the generation, handling, and disposal of hazardous wastes are regulated by the interaction of two federal statutes. The primary federal law regulating hazardous wastes is officially known as the Solid Waste Disposal Act. In 1970, Congress amended that statute with the Resource Conservation and Recovery Act (RCRA), and the law has come to be popularly known by that name. RCRA was given regulatory "teeth" with a set of 1976 amendments under which EPA, in 1980, promulgated regulations establishing a "cradle-to-grave" system for hazardous wastes that tracks the generation, transportation, and disposal of such wastes and establishes standards for their disposal. Initially, however, EPA's disposal standards were minimal to nonexistent and did little to discourage the landfilling of chemical wastes. This led Congress, in 1984, to pass sweeping amendments to RCRA that (1) established a clear federal policy against the landfilling of hazardous wastes unless they have first been treated to reduce their toxicity and (2) gave EPA a specific timetable by which it had to either set treatment standards for various categories of waste or ban the landfilling of such waste altogether. Consequently, EPA has set treatment standards—which are commonly known as the *land disposal restrictions* (LDRs)—for hundreds of types of hazardous wastes. These standards are based on EPA's assessment of the Best Demonstrated Available Technology for treating the waste in question.

Thus, RCRA directly regulates the handling and disposal of hazardous wastes. And by establishing a set of requirements that must be followed once hazardous waste is generated, it also indirectly regulates the generation of hazardous wastes. RCRA regulations have increased the cost of disposing of most types of waste by two orders of magnitude over the past 25 years. In this sense, RCRA operates as a *de facto* tax on the generation of hazardous waste. (See Chapter 20.)

Another statute that acts as an indirect check on hazardous waste generation (and that provides additional incentive to ensure that one's waste is safely disposed) is the Comprehensive Environmental Response, Compensation, and Liability Act (CERCLA, also known as the federal Superfund law). The primary focus of this law is the remediation (cleanup) of hazardous waste contamination resulting from imprudent handling and disposal practices of the past and the recovery of remediation costs from those designated as "responsible parties" under the act. CERCLA imposes liability for the costs of remediating a hazardous waste site both on the owners and operators of the site and on those generators of hazardous waste that sent waste to the site. Because the owners and operators are often business entities that are no longer financially viable, CERCLA liability often falls most heavily on the generators. And CERCLA liability is strict liability, meaning that the exercise of reasonable care by the generator is not a defense. Further, unless the generator can establish a convincing factual basis for distinguishing its waste from all or part

of the contamination being remediated, CERCLA liability is joint and several, meaning that each responsible party is potentially liable for the full cost of remediation. As a practical matter, this means that the cost of remediation will be borne by those among the responsible parties who are financially solvent.

The prudent business entity, then, has a strong financial incentive to take such actions as will minimize the likelihood that it will face CERCLA liability in the future. As the only certain way to avoid such liability is to refrain from generating the waste in the first instance, CERCLA does provide a rationale for pollution prevention. Further, it provides firms with an incentive to meet—or perhaps to go beyond—RCRA regulations in dealing with such wastes as they do generate.

This is not to say, of course, that substantial amounts of hazardous waste are no longer generated in the United States, that all hazardous wastes are adequately treated and safely disposed, or that all instances of hazardous waste contamination are being adequately addressed (or addressed at all). RCRA and CERCLA both contain what might reasonably be called loopholes and gaps in coverage, and hazardous waste contamination remains an ongoing issue. Further, the most common treatment methodology incorporated into EPA's RCRA treatment standards is incineration, which has brought with it a release of airborne contaminants that has yet to be comprehensively addressed by regulation. There is no question, however, that the country has made considerable progress from the late 1970s, when disposal of chemical wastes in unlined landfills—at a cost of roughly $15 per ton—was the common practice.

The Chemical Safety Provisions of the Clean Air Act: Obligations Shared by EPA and OSHA

Although the first congressional response to the country's concern generated by the deadly industrial accident in Bhopal, India, was the Emergency Planning and Community Right to Know Act of 1986, the chemical safety provisions of that law are focused almost solely on mitigation and not on accident prevention. A much greater potential for a direct focus on accident prevention can be found in the 1990 amendments to the Clean Air Act, although that potential has yet to be realized by EPA and OSHA.

As amended in 1990, Section 112 of the Clean Air Act directs the EPA to develop regulations regarding the prevention and detection of accidental chemical releases and to publish a list of at least 100 chemical substances (with associated threshold quantities) to be covered by the regulations. The regulations must include requirements for the development of *risk-management plans* (RMPs) by facilities using any of the regulated substances in amounts above the relevant threshold. These RMPs must include a hazard assessment, an accident prevention program, and an emergency release program. Similarly, Section 304 of the Clean Air Amendments of 1990 directed OSHA to promulgate a *Process Safety Management (PSM) standard* under the OSHAct.

Section 112(r) of the revised Clean Air Act also imposes a "general duty" on all "owners and operators of stationary sources," regardless of the particular identity or quantity of the chemicals used on site. These parties have a duty to:

> "... *identify hazards* that may result from [accidental chemical] releases using appropriate hazard assessment techniques,
> ... *design and maintain a safe facility* taking such steps as are necessary to prevent releases, and
> ... *minimize the consequences* of accidental releases which do occur." [emphases added]

Thus, firms are now under a general duty to anticipate, prevent, and mitigate accidental releases. In defining the nature of this duty, Section 112(r) specifies that it is "a general duty in the same manner and to the same extent as" that imposed by Section 5 of the OSHAct. Because Section 112(r) specifically ties its general duty obligation to the general duty clause of the OSHAct, case law interpreting the OSHAct provision should be directly relevant. Specifically, in the General Dynamics case, the District of Columbia Circuit Court of Appeals held that standards and the general duty obligation are distinct and independent requirements and that compliance with a standard does not discharge an employer's duty to comply with the general duty obligation. Similarly, compliance with other Clean Air act chemical safety requirements should not relieve a firm's duty to comply with the act's general duty clause. Further, the requirement on owners and operators to design and maintain a safe facility would seem to extend their obligations into the area of primary prevention rather then merely hazard control.

The Clean Air Act also requires each state to establish programs to provide small business with technical assistance in addressing chemical safety. These programs could provide information on alternative technologies, process changes, products, and methods of operation that help reduce emissions to air. However, these state mandates are unfunded and may not be uniformly implemented. Where they are established, linkage with state offices of technical assistance, especially those that provide guidance on pollution prevention, could be particularly beneficial.

Finally, the 1990 amendments established an independent Chemical Safety and Hazard Investigation Board (CSHIB). The board is to investigate the causes of accidents, perform research on prevention, and make recommendations for preventive approaches, much like the Air Transportation Safety Board does with regard to airplane safety.

As required by the 1990 Clean Air Amendments, in 1992 OSHA promulgated a standard requiring chemical PSM in the workplace that became effective later that year. The PSM standard is designed to protect employees working in facilities that use "highly hazardous chemicals" and employees working in facilities with more than 10,000 pounds of flammable liquids or gases present in one location. The list of highly hazardous chemicals in the standard includes acutely toxic, highly flammable, and reactive substances. The PSM standard requires employers to compile safety information (including process flow information) on chemicals and processes used in the workplace, complete a workplace process hazard analysis every 5 years, conduct triennial compliance safety audits, develop and implement written operating procedures, conduct extensive worker training, develop and implement plans to maintain the integrity of process equipment, perform pre-startup reviews for new (and significantly modified) facilities, develop and implement written procedures to manage changes in production methods, establish an emergency action plan, and investigate accidents and near-misses at their facilities. Many aspects of chemical safety are not covered by specific workplace standards. Most that do apply to chemical safety have their origin in the consensus standards adopted under Section 6(a) of the OSHAct in 1971 and hence are greatly out of date. Arguably, the general duty obligation of the OSHAct imposes a duty to seek out technological improvements that would improve safety for workers.

In 1996, the EPA promulgated regulations setting forth requirements for the RMPs specified in the Clean Air Act. The RMP rule is modeled after the OSHA PSM standard and is estimated to affect some 66,000 facilities. The rule requires a hazard assessment (involving an offsite consequence analysis—including worst-case risk scenarios—and compilation of a 5-year accident history), a prevention program to address the hazards identified, and an emergency response program. In 2003, the Chemical Safety and Hazard Investigation Board urged OSHA to amend its 1996 regulations in order to achieve more comprehensive control of "reactive hazards" that could have catastrophic consequences and asked OSHA to define and record information on reactive chemical incidents that it investigates or is required to investigate. These recommendations have largely fallen on deaf ears. The board also expressed concern that the *material safety data sheets* (MSDSs) issued by OSHA do not adequately identify the reactive potential of chemicals. Legislation is being promoted to require OSHA to prepare or revise MSDSs for the list of chemicals in the PSM standard and generally strengthen OSHA's approach to chemical safety. Despite the fact that a memorandum of understanding between EPA and OSHA had been signed in 1996, in 2001 the U.S. General Accounting Office (GAO) issued a report indicating the need for better coordination between EPA, OSHA, the CSHIB, and other agencies.

ENFORCEMENT ACTIVITIES

Regulations and standard setting, of course, are only the beginning of the regulatory process. For a regulatory system to be effective, there must be a clear commitment to the enforcement of standards (see Chapter 37). Under OSHA, a worker can request a workplace inspection if the request is in writing and signed. Anonymity is preserved on request. When an inspector visits a workplace, a representative of the workers can accompany the inspector on the "walk-around."If specific requests for inspections are not made, OSHA makes random inspections of those workplaces with worse-than-average safety records. However, the inspection frequency is low. Furthermore, firms with significant exposures to chemicals may not be routinely inspected, simply because their record for injuries—which make up the overwhelming majority of the reported statistics—is good.

Inspections are usually conducted without advance notice, but an employer may insist that OSHA inspectors obtain a court order before entering the workplace. Federal OSHA continues to have approximately 1,000 inspectors, and state agencies have approximately another 2,000. OSHA and OSHA-approved state programs conducted approximately 97,000 annual inspections in the federal fiscal year 2002, focusing inspections on the most hazardous industries, construction and manufacturing. Clearly, not all 6 million workplaces covered by the OSHAct could be inspected on anything like a regular basis. With the relatively recent expansion of OSHA authority to cover U.S. post offices, the agency continues to be short of the resources needed to perform its statutory duties. In sharp contrast, the number of inspectors per worker is 10 times larger in British Columbia, Canada, and in many European countries.

OSHA can fine employers up to $7,000 for each violation of the act that is discovered during a workplace inspection and up to $70,000 or up to 6 months imprisonment if the violation is willful or repeated. The failure to abate hazards can result in a $7,000 fine per day. These penalties are very much less than those for violations of environmental statutes. Since Congress last adjusted OSHA's civil penalties, those fines are in effect 38 percent lower, when pegged to inflation. Management can appeal violations, amounts of fines, methods of correcting hazards, and deadlines for correcting hazards (abatement dates). Workers can appeal only deadlines. All appeals are processed through the Occupational Safety and Health Review Commission, established by the OSHAct.

The OSHAct requires OSHA to encourage states to develop and operate their own job safety and health programs. State programs, when "at least as effective" as the federal program, can take over enforcement activities. Once a state plan is approved, OSHA funds half of its operating costs. Approximately 20 state plans, which OSHA monitors, are in effect. State safety and health standards under such approved plans must keep pace with OSHA standards, and state plans must guarantee employer and employee rights, as does OSHA.

During the 1980s, OSHA inspection policy resulted in directives given to the field staff to deemphasize general duty violations. In addition, inspectors were actually evaluated by the managers of the establishments they inspected. Follow-up inspections after violations were often restricted to checks by telephone. Thus, incentives for aggressive inspection activity were not great under the Reagan and Bush administrations. Although inspection activity increased under the Clinton administration, it has retreated under the second Bush administration. Although inspections were up in numbers, in the Clinton administration, the time spent on inspections was less.

Enforcement of laws administered by the EPA is initiated by the agency under its various legislative mandates. As with OSHA, agency activity has been greatly inadequate over the past 25 years, with increased responsibilities and the lack of a corresponding increase in human resources since 1980.

WORKER AND COMMUNITY RIGHT TO KNOW

The right of workers and citizens to be apprised of the substances to which they are exposed is popularly referred to as "the right to know." This simple term actually encompasses several rights and duties that are complex and complementary. Political and legislative initiatives focusing on the right to know arose during a time when direct regulation of toxic substances was being deemphasized by the federal agencies. Historically, regulatory initiatives under the 1970 OSHAct encompassing the worker right-to-know preceded by more than 15 years the more general community right-to-know efforts embodied in the 1986 Emergency Planning and Community Right to Know Act (EPCRA), but the worker right-to-know initiatives are relevant to, and greatly influenced, the evolution of the community right-to-know.

Although the initiatives for the worker right to know and the community right to know both initially focused on "scientific" information about chemicals—(a) product ingredients and the specific composition of pollution in air, water, and waste; (b) the inherent toxicity and safety hazard of the related chemicals, materials, and industrial processes; and (c) information related to exposure of various vulnerable groups to harmful substances and processes—disseminating or providing access to other categories of information, namely technological information, and legal information[1] may be even more important for empowering workers and citizens to facilitate a transformation of hazardous industry and practices. Technological information includes (a) monitoring technologies, (b) options that control or minimize pollution, waste, and chemical accidents, and (c) available substi-

tute or alternative inputs, final products, and processes that prevent pollution, waste, and chemical accidents. Legal information refers to notification of the rights and obligations of producers, employers, consumers, workers, and the general public. Though important, legal information is not a fundamental type of information but rather the (mandated) diffusion of information about rights and duties stemming from the nature and exposure profiles of hazardous substances and processes.

Worker Right to Know

The transfer of information regarding workplace exposure to toxic substances has received considerable public attention. Workers need an accurate picture of the nature and extent of probable chemical exposures to decide whether to enter or remain in a particular workplace. Workers also need to have knowledge regarding past or current exposures to be alert to the onset of occupational disease. Regulatory agencies must have timely access to such information if they are to devise effective strategies to reduce disease and death from occupational exposures to toxic substances. Accordingly, laws designed to facilitate this flow of information have been promulgated at the federal, state, and local levels. Indeed, the right to know has become a political battleground in many states and communities and has been the subject of intensive organizing efforts by business, labor, and citizen-action groups.

In essence, the right to know embodies a democratization of the workplace. It is the mandatory sharing of information between management and labor. Through a variety of laws, manufacturers and employers are directed to disclose information regarding toxic substance exposure to workers, to unions in their capacity as worker representatives, and to governmental agencies charged with the protection of public health. The underlying rationale for these directives is the assumption that this transfer of information will prompt activity that will improve worker health.

Although the phrase *right to know* is a useful generic designation, it is an inadequate description of the legal rights and obligations that govern the transfer of workplace information on toxic substances. A person cannot have a meaningful right to information unless someone else has a corresponding duty to provide that information. Thus, a worker's right to know is secured by requiring a manufacturer or employer to disclose. The disclosure requirement can take a variety of forms, and the practical scope of that requirement may depend on the nature of the form chosen. In particular, a duty to disclose only such information as has been requested may provide a narrower flow of information than a duty to disclose all information, regardless of whether it has been requested. The various rights and obligations in the area of toxics information transfer may be grouped into three categories. Although they share a number of similarities, each category is conceptually distinct:

1. The duty to generate or retain information refers to the obligation to compile a record of certain workplace events or activities or to maintain such a record for a specified period of time if it has been compiled. An employer may, for example, be required to monitor its workers regularly for evidence of toxic exposures (biological monitoring) and to keep written records of the results of such monitoring.
2. The right of access (and the corresponding duty to disclose on request) refers to the right of a worker, a union, or an agency to request and secure access to information held by a manufacturer or employer. Such a right of access would provide workers with a means of obtaining copies of biological monitoring records pertaining to their own exposure to toxic substances.
3. Finally, the duty to inform refers to an employer's or manufacturer's obligation to disclose, without request, information pertaining to toxic substance exposures in the workplace. An employer may, for example, have a duty, independent of any worker's exercise of a right to access, to inform workers whenever biological monitoring reveals that their exposure to a toxic substance has produced bodily concentrations of that substance above a specified level.

In general, the broadest coverage is found in rights and duties emanating from the OSHAct. By its terms, that act is applicable to all private employers and thus covers the bulk of workplace exposures to toxic substances. Most private industrial workplaces are also subject to the National Labor Relations Act (NLRA). Farm workers and workers subject to the Railway Labor Act, however, are exempt from NLRA coverage. TSCA provides a generally narrower scope. Although many of the act's provisions apply broadly to both chemical manufacture and use, its information transfer requirements extend only to chemical manufacturers, processors, and importers. On the state level, the relevant coverage of the various rights and duties depends on the specifics of the particular state and local law defining them. In general, common-law rights and duties evidence much less variation than those created by state statute or local ordinance.

Under OSHA's *Hazard Communication Standard,* employers have a duty to inform workers of the identity of substances with which they work through labeling the product container and disclosing to the purchaser (the employer) using MSDSs.

Employers are under no obligation to amend inadequate, insufficient, or incorrect information provided by the manufacturer. Employers must, however, transmit certain information to their employees: (a) information on the standard and its requirements, (b) operations in their work areas where hazardous chemicals are present, and (c) the location and availability of the company's hazard communication program. The standard also requires that workers must be trained in (a) methods to detect the presence or release of the hazardous chemicals; (b) the physical and health hazards of the chemicals; (c) protective measures, such as appropriate work practices, emergency procedures, and personal protective equipment; and (d) the details of the hazard communication program developed by the employer, including an explanation of the labeling system and the MSDSs and how employees can obtain and use hazard information.

Rights and duties governing toxic information transfer in the workplace can originate from a variety of sources. Some are grounded in state common-law, whereas others arise out of specific state statutes or local ordinances. Although the states have been increasingly active in this field, the primary source of regulation is federal law. Most federal regulation in this area emanates from three statutes: the OSHAct of 1970, the Toxic Substances Control Act of 1976, and the National Labor Relations Act (NLRA), the last of which is administered by the National Labor Relations Board (NLRB).

The scope of a particular right or duty depends on many factors. The first, and perhaps most important, is the nature of the information required to be transferred. As discussed above, the main categories of information can be divided into scientific, technological, and legal information. In the context of the workplace, scientific information can be divided into three subcategories:

1. Ingredients information provides the worker with the identity of the substances to which he or she is exposed. Depending on the circumstances, this information may constitute only the generic

classifications of the various chemicals involved or may include the specific chemical identities of all chemical exposures and the specific contents of all chemical mixtures.

2. Exposure information encompasses all data regarding the amount, frequency, duration, and route of workplace exposures. This information may be of a general nature, such as the results of ambient air monitoring at a central workplace location, or may take individualized form, such as the results of personal environmental or biological monitoring of a specific worker.

3. Health effects information indicates known or potential health effects of workplace exposures. This information may be general data regarding the effects of chemical exposure, usually found in an MSDS or a published or unpublished workplace epidemiologic study, or it may be individualized data, such as worker medical records compiled as a result of medical surveillance.

The federal standard preempts state right-to-know laws in the worker notification area in a minority of jurisdictions; it would appear to be coexistent with state requirements in most jurisdictions, although its stated intent is to preempt all state efforts.

Under OSHA's Medical Access Rule, an employer may not limit or deny an employee access to his or her own medical or exposure records. The current OSHA regulation, promulgated in 1980, grants employees a general right of access to medical and exposure records kept by their employer. Furthermore, it requires the employer to preserve and maintain these records for 30 years. There appears to be some overlap in the definitions of medical and exposure records, because both may include the results of biological monitoring. Medical records, however, are in general defined as those pertaining to "the health status of an employee," whereas the exposure records are defined as those pertaining to "employee exposure to toxic substances or harmful physical agents."

The employer's duty to make these records available is a broad one. The regulations provide that on any employee request for access to a medical or exposure record, "the employer *shall* assure that access is provided in a reasonable time, place, and manner, but in no event later than 15 days after the request for access is made."

An employee's right of access to medical records is limited to records pertaining specifically to that employee. The regulations allow physicians some discretion as well in limiting employee access. The physician is permitted to "recommend" to the employee requesting access that the employee (a) review and discuss the records with the physician, (b) accept a summary rather than the records themselves, or (c) allow the records to be released instead to another physician. Furthermore, where information in a record pertains to a "specific diagnosis of a terminal illness or a psychiatric condition," the physician is authorized to direct that such information be provided only to the employee's designated representative. Although these provisions were apparently intended to respect the physician–patient relationship and do not limit the employee's ultimate right of access, they could be abused. In situations in which the physician feels loyalty to the employer rather than the employee, the physician could use these provisions to discourage the employee from seeking access to his or her records.

Similar constraints do not apply to employee access to exposure records. Not only is the employee ensured access to records of his or her own exposure to toxic substances, but the employee is also ensured access to the exposure records of other employees "with past or present job duties or working conditions related to or similar to those of the employee." In addition, the employee has access to all general exposure information pertaining to the employee's workplace or working conditions and to any workplace or working condition to which he or she is to be transferred. All information in exposure records that cannot be correlated with a particular employee's exposure is accessible.

One criticism of the OSHA regulation is that it does not require the employer to compile medical or exposure information but merely requires employee access to such information if it is compiled. The scope of the regulation, however, should not be underestimated. The term *record* is meant to be "all-encompassing," and the access requirement appears to extend to all information gathered on employee health or exposure, no matter how it is measured or recorded. Thus, if an employer embarks on any program of human monitoring, no matter how conducted, he or she must provide the subjects access to the results. This access requirement may serve as a disincentive for employers to monitor employee exposure or health if it is not clearly in the employer's interest to do so.

The regulations permit the employer to deny access to "trade secret data which discloses manufacturing processes or . . . the percentage of a chemical substance in a mixture," provided that the employer (a) notifies the party requesting access of the denial; (b) if relevant, provides alternative information sufficient to permit identification of when and where exposure occurred; and (c) provides access to all "chemical or physical agent identities including chemical names, levels of exposure, and employee health status data contained in the requested records."

The key feature of this provision is that it ensures employee access to the precise identities of chemicals and physical agents. This access is especially critical for chemical exposures. Within each "generic" class of chemicals, there are a variety of specific chemical compounds, each of which may have its own particular effect on human health. The health effects can vary widely within a particular family of chemicals. Accordingly, the medical and scientific literature on chemical properties and toxicity is indexed by specific chemical name, not by generic chemical class. To discern any meaningful correlation between a chemical exposure and a known or potential health effect, an employee must know the precise chemical identity of that exposure. Furthermore, in the case of biological monitoring, the identity of the toxic substance or its metabolite is itself the information monitored.

Particularly in light of the public health emphasis inherent in the OSHAct, disclosure of such information does not constitute an unreasonable infringement on the trade secret interests of the employer. In general, chemical health and safety data are the least valuable to an employer of all the proprietary information relevant to a particular manufacturing process.

TSCA imposes substantial requirements on chemical manufacturers and processors to develop health effects data. TSCA requires testing, premarket manufacturing notification, and reporting and retention of information. TSCA imposes no specific medical surveillance or biological monitoring requirements. However, to the extent that human monitoring is used to meet more general requirements of assessing occupational health or exposure to toxic substances, the data resulting from such monitoring are subject to an employer's recording and retention obligations.

EPA has promulgated regulations requiring general reporting on several hundred chemicals, including information related to occupational exposure. The EPA administrator may require the reporting and maintenance of those data "insofar as known"

or "insofar as reasonably ascertainable." Thus, if monitoring is undertaken, it must be reported. EPA appears to be authorized to require monitoring as a way of securing information that is "reasonably ascertainable."

In addition to the general reports required for specific chemicals listed in the regulations, EPA has promulgated rules for the submission of health and safety studies required for several hundred substances. A health and safety study includes "[a]ny data that bear on the effects of chemical substance on health." Examples are "[m]onitoring data, when they have been aggregated and analyzed to measure the exposure of humans . . . to a chemical substance or mixture." Only data that are "known" or "reasonably ascertainable" need be reported.

Records of "significant adverse reactions to [employee] health" must be retained for 30 years under Section 8(c). A rule implementing this section defines significant adverse reactions as those "that may indicate a substantial impairment of normal activities, or long-lasting or irreversible damage to health or the environment." Under the rule, human monitoring data, especially if derived from a succession of tests, would seem especially reportable. Genetic monitoring of employees, if some basis links the results with increased risk of cancer, also seems to fall within the rule.

Section 8(e) imposes a statutory duty to report "immediately . . . information which supports the conclusion that [a] substance or mixture presents a substantial risk of injury to health." In a policy statement issued in 1978, the EPA interpreted "immediately" in this context to require receipt by the agency within 15 working days after the reporter obtains the information. Substantial risk is defined exclusive of economic considerations. Evidence can be provided by either designed, controlled studies or undesigned, uncontrolled studies, including "medical and health surveys" or evidence of effects in workers. From 1978 to 2003, EPA received more than 25,000 8(e) submissions. During the years 2001 and 2002, 19 to 21 percent of these reports addressed reproductive/developmental toxicity; 7.5 to 14 percent, ecotoxicity; 9 to 11 percent, cancer; and 5 to 11 percent, mutagenicity.[2]

In the EPA's rule for Section 8(c), Section 8(e) is distinguished from Section 8(c) in that "[a] report of substantial risk of injury, unlike an allegation of a significant adverse reaction, is accompanied by information which reasonably supports the seriousness of the effect or the probability of its occurrence." Human monitoring results indicating a substantial risk of injury would thus seem reportable to EPA. Either medical surveillance or biological monitoring data would seem to qualify. Section 14(b) of TSCA gives EPA authority to disclose from health and safety studies the data pertaining to chemical identities, except for the proportion of chemicals in a mixture. In addition, EPA may disclose information, otherwise classified as a trade secret, "if the Administration determines it necessary to protect . . . against an unreasonable risk of injury to health." Monitoring data thus seem subject to full disclosure.

In addition to the access provided by OSHA regulations, individual employees may have a limited right of access to medical and exposure records under federal labor law. Logically, the right to refuse hazardous work (see later discussion), inherent in Section 7 of the NLRA and Section 502 of the Labor Management Relations Act, carries with it the right of access to the information necessary to determine whether or not a particular condition is hazardous. In the case of toxic substance exposure, this right of access may mean access to all information relevant to the health effects of the exposure and may include access to both medical and exposure records. These federal labor law provisions are clearly not adequate substitutes for OSHA access regulations, however, because there is no systematic mechanism for enforcing this right.

Collective employee access, however, is available to unionized employees through the collective bargaining process. In four cases, the NLRB has held that unions have a right of access to exposure and medical records so that they may bargain effectively with the employer regarding conditions of employment. Citing the general proposition that employers are required to bargain on health and safety conditions when requested to do so, the NLRB adopted a broad policy favoring union access: "Few matters can be of greater legitimate concern to individuals in the workplace, and thus to the bargaining agent representing them, than exposure to conditions potentially threatening their health, well-being, or their very lives."

The NLRB, however, did not grant an unlimited right of access. The union's right of access is constrained by the individual employee's right of personal privacy. Furthermore, the NLRB acknowledged an employer's interest in protecting trade secrets. Although ordering the employer in each of the four cases to disclose the chemical identities of substances to which the employer did not assert a trade secret defense, the NLRB indicated that employers are entitled to take reasonable steps to safeguard "legitimate" trade secret information. The NLRB did not delineate a specific mechanism for achieving the balance between union access and trade secret disclosure. Instead, it ordered the parties to attempt to resolve the issue through collective bargaining. Given the complexity of this issue and the potential for abuse in the name of "trade secret protection," the NLRB may find it necessary to provide further specificity before a workable industry-wide mechanism can be achieved.

The legal avenues for worker and agency access to information relevant to workplace exposures to toxic substances have been expanded substantially. Despite certain inadequacies in the current laws and despite current attempts by OSHA to narrow the scope of some of these even further, access to toxics data remains broader than it has ever been. By itself, however, this fact is of little significance. The mere existence of information transfer laws means little unless those laws are used aggressively to further the objective of the right to know: the protection of workers' health. The various rights and duties governing toxics information transfer in the workplace present workers, unions, and agencies with an important opportunity. The extent to which they seize this opportunity is a measure of their resolve to bring about meaningful improvement in the health of the American worker.

The category of technological information is not addressed in the context of worker right to know, although it has been argued that shifting the focus of debate between workers and management from the risks in the workplace to a discussion of [technological] solutions may be a much more fruitful avenue for collective bargaining.[3] In contrast, information about technology and approaches for reducing toxic substance exposure and the chances of sudden and accidental releases of chemicals (discussed below) is reflected in community right-to-know initiatives.

Community Right to Know

In 1986, Congress amended the federal hazardous waste cleanup law (commonly referred to as the Superfund statute) with the Superfund Amendment and Reauthorization Act of 1986 (known as SARA). Beyond cleanup, Congress took in SARA what may prove to be a significant step toward reducing the likelihood of new hazardous substance contamination in the future. Title III of SARA, called the Emergency Planning and Community Right to Know Act (EPCRA), now codified at 42 U.S.C. §§11001, *et seq.*, is a comprehensive federal community right-to-know program, implemented by the states under guidelines promulgated by EPA. The central feature of this federal program is broad public dissemination of information pertaining to the nature and identity of chemicals used at commercial facilities.

Although EPCRA is not a workplace right-to-know law *per se*, it does provide an alternative means through which many employees can learn about toxic substance use, not only in their own workplaces but in other workplaces in which they may wish to work.

EPCRA has four major provisions:

- Emergency planning (§§301–303)
- Emergency release notification (§304)
- Hazardous chemical storage reporting requirements (§§311–312)
- The Toxic Chemical Release Inventory (TRI) (§313)

The various requirements are summarized in Table 3-2 and are discussed below.

The implementation of EPCRA began with the creation of state and local bodies to implement this community right-to-know program. Section 301 of the act required the governor of each state to appoint a *state emergency response commission* (SERC), to be staffed by "persons who have technical expertise

TABLE 3-2

EPCRA Chemicals, Reportable Actions, and Reporting Thresholds

	Section 302	Section 304	Sections 311/312	Section 313 (TRI)
Chemicals covered	356 extremely hazardous substances	>1,000 substances	500,000 products with MSDSs[a] (required under OSHA regulations)	650 toxic chemicals and categories[b]
Reportable actions and thresholds	Threshold planning quantity 1–10,000 lb present on site at any one time requires notification of the SERC and LEPC within 60 days upon on-site production or receipt of shipment.	Reportable quantity, 1–5,000 lb, released in a 24-hour period; reportable to the SERC and LEPC.	TPQ or 500 lb for Section 302 chemicals; 10,000 lb present on site at any one time for other chemicals. Copy if requested to SERC/LEPC; annual inventory Tier I/Tier II report to SERC/LEPC/ local fire department by March 1.	25,000 lb per year manufactured or processed; 10,000 lb a year used; certain persistent bioaccumulative toxics have lower thresholds; annual report to EPA and the state by July 1.

MSDS, material safety data sheet; OSHA, Occupational Safety and Health Administration; EPA, Environmental Protection Agency; EPCRA, Emergency Planning and Community Right to Know Act; SERC, State Emergency Response Commission; LEPC, Local Emergency Planning Committee; TRI, Toxics Release Inventory; TPQ, Threshold Planning Quantity.
[a] MSDSs on hazardous chemicals are maintained by a number of universities and can be accessed through <http://www.hazard.com>.
[b] The TRI reporting requirement applies to all federal facilities that have 10 or more full-time employees and those that manufacture (including importing), process, or otherwise use a listed toxic chemical above threshold quantities and that are in one of the following sectors: Manufacturing (Standard Industrial Classification (SIC) codes 20 through 39), Metal mining (SIC code 10, except for SIC codes 1011,1081, and 1094), Coal mining (SIC code 12, except for 1241 and extraction activities), Electrical utilities that combust coal and/or oil (SIC codes 4911, 4931, and 4939), Resource Conservation and Recovery Act (RCRA), Subtitle C hazardous waste treatment and disposal facilities (SIC code 4953), Chemicals and allied products wholesale distributors (SIC code 5169), Petroleum bulk plants and terminals (SIC code 5171), and Solvent recovery services (SIC code 7389).
Source: The Community Planning and Right-to-Know Act, EPA 550-F-00-004, March 2000.

in the emergency response field." In practice, these state commissions have tended to include representatives from the various environmental and public health and safety agencies in the state. Each state commission, in turn, was required to divide the state into various *local emergency planning districts* and to appoint a *local emergency planning committee* (LEPC) for each of these districts. These state and local entities are responsible for receiving, coordinating, maintaining, and providing access to the various types of information required to be disclosed under the act.

EPCRA established four principal requirements for reporting information about hazardous chemicals. Section 304 requires all facilities that manufacture, process, use, or store certain "extremely hazardous substances" in excess of certain quantities to provide "emergency" notification to the SERC and the LEPC of an unexpected release of one of these substances. Section 311 requires facilities covered by the OSHA Hazard Communication Standard to prepare and submit to the LEPC and the local fire department MSDSs for chemicals covered by the OSHA standard. Under Section 312, many of these same firms are required to prepare and submit to the LEPC an *emergency and hazardous substance inventory form* that describes the amount and location of certain hazardous chemicals on their premises. Finally, Section 313 requires firms in the manufacturing sector to provide to EPA an annual reporting of certain routine releases of hazardous substances. These reports comprise what is known as the *Toxics Release Inventory* (TRI). In addition, Section 303 requires certain commercial facilities to cooperate with their respective LEPCs in preparing "emergency response plans" for dealing with major accidents involving hazardous chemicals. The applicability of these provisions to any particular facility depends on the amount of the designated chemicals that it uses or stores during any given year.

Taken as a whole, these requirements constitute a broad federal declaration that firms that choose to rely heavily on hazardous chemicals in their production processes may not treat information regarding their use of those chemicals as their private domain. Indeed, except for trade secrecy protections that generally parallel those available under the OSHA Hazard Communication Standard, there are no statutory restrictions on the disclosure of EPCRA information to the general public. Indeed, Section 324 of the act mandates that most of the

information subject to EPCRA reporting requirements "be made available to the general public" upon request and requires that each local emergency planning committee publicize this fact in a local newspaper. However, since the September 11 terrorist attacks, EPA is undertaking a review of the proper balance to strike between the public's right to know and the possible increased risk to disseminating information collected under the informational provisions of various legislation.

EPCRA requires certain industries to report the releases and transfers of certain chemical substances to air, water, land, or transferred off-site. The data have to be entered on a standardized form and are collected by EPA in the TRI, which is publicly available.[*] The number of chemicals that are covered is about 650—double the number required in 1987.

The TRI imposes its requirements on firms having more than 10 employees and that manufacture or process[†] More than 25,000 pounds per year, or use 10,000 pounds per year of the designated chemicals. For some six *persistent, bioaccumulative, and toxic chemicals* (PBTs), EPA lowered the reporting thresholds in 1999 to 100 lb, for 11 highly persistent and highly bioaccumulative chemicals to 10 lb, and for dioxin and dioxin-like compounds to 0.1 g. All 6,100 facilities of the manufacturing sector and several other industries including metal and coal mining, electric utilities, and commercial hazardous waste treatment, among others, are required to report. Approximately 6 to 7 percent of all chemical releases are subject to TRI reporting. In addition to the reporting requirements for chemicals releases, EPCRA now includes requirements to report pollution-prevention activities.[‡] The potential power of TRI depends on the extent to which the data represents actual releases and the quality of the data, as well as the capacity of the public to understand and interpret the data. Considering the representativeness of the data, TRI focuses only

---

[*] *The data can be found on EPA's Webpage <http://www.epa.gov/tri/>.*

[†] *The term* manufacture *means to produce, prepare, import, or compound a toxic chemical. The term* process *means the preparation of a toxic chemical, after its manufacture, for distribution in commerce. See 42 U.S.C. 11023 (b)(1)(C). See also 42 U.S.C. 11023 (a)(b)(1) and (g)(2).*

[‡] *The Pollution Prevention Act (PPA) of 1990 advocates a general shift in approach from pollution control to pollution prevention. The PPA amends EPCRA and adds further requirements to report the firms' pollution-prevention activities to EPA. These include source-reduction and waste-management practices.*

on the releases of chemicals and does not include releases that occur during the whole life cycle of a product. A reported reduction of reported chemical releases does not necessarily mean a total reduction of all releases, because there could be shifts in releases from covered to not-covered chemicals. The firms are not required to produce risk information about the covered substances but only have to report their releases, so the public may have an inadequate picture of what changes in reported releases mean in terms of reduction (or increases) in overall risk. In addition, within the covered substances, no distinction is highlighted between the different severity (health or environmental consequences) of different releases. Aside from the recent exception of reporting the specific categories of the persistent, bioaccumulative, and toxic chemicals, unless interested observers factor in differential hazardousness of different releases, they cannot make a meaningful assessment of changes in overall risk. In addition, many of the releases directly to air and water have simply been transferred to the waste stream, and it is extremely difficult to evaluate the resulting consequences for overall risk.

Although there are limitations of using the TRI data as a good environmental indicator, the publication of the data appeared to have had an enormous positive impact on the reduction of reported releases. During the 1988–2001 period, on- and off-site releases of the core chemicals were reduced by 55 percent while the production of chemicals increased. Forty percent of the decreases were already reached by 1995. However, although emissions to air and water decreased, there were corresponding large increases in hazardous waste. As a result, the success of the TRI reporting is far from clear.

The September 11 terrorist attacks have brought in a new dimension to the right to know. The Clean Air Act requires that chemical manufacturers and refineries file *start-up, shut-down, and malfunction* (SSM) plans with EPA or state air regulators. Industry has argued that public access to this information increases the vulnerability of those facilities to terrorist attacks and has requested of EPA that industry not be required to routinely submit those plans. EPA countered with a proposal that the information could be screened before dissemination. EPA has since dismantled its risk management website containing general information about emergency plans and chemicals used at 15,000 sites nationwide, allowing selective access to sensitive information contained in the Offsite Consequence Analysis—about "worst case" chemical accidents—in special reading rooms.

THE RIGHT TO REFUSE HAZARDOUS WORK

The NLRA and the OSHAct provide many employees a limited right to refuse to perform hazardous work. When properly exercised, this right protects an employee from retaliatory discharge or other discriminatory action for refusing hazardous work and incorporates a remedy providing both reinstatement and back pay. The nature of this right under the NLRA depends on the relevant collective bargaining agreement, if there is one. Nonunion employees and union employees whose collective bargaining agreements specifically exclude health and safety from a no-strike clause have the *collective* right to stage a safety walkout under Section 7 of the NLRA. If they choose to walk out based on a good-faith belief that working conditions are unsafe, they will be protected from any employer retaliation. Union employees who are subject to a comprehensive collective bargaining agreement may avail themselves of the provisions of Section 502 of the NLRA. Under this section, an employee who is faced with "abnormally dangerous conditions" has an *individual* right to leave the job site. The right may be exercised, however, only where the existence of abnormally dangerous conditions can be objectively verified. Both exposure and medical information are crucial here (see Chapter 4).

Under a 1973 OSHA regulation, the right to refuse hazardous work extends to all employees, *individually*, of private employers, regardless of the existence or nature of a collective bargaining agreement. Section 11(c) of the OSHAct protects an employee from discharge or other retaliatory action arising out of his or her "exercise" of "any right" afforded by the act. The Secretary of Labor has promulgated regulations under this section defining a right to refuse hazardous work in certain circumstances: where an employee reasonably believes there is a "real danger of death or serious injury," there is insufficient time to eliminate that danger through normal administrative channels, and the employer has failed to comply with an employee request to correct the situation.

Under the federal Mine Safety and Health Act, miners also have rights to transfer from unhealthy work areas if there is exposure to toxic substances or harmful physical agents or if there is medical evidence of pneumoconiosis.

ANALYSIS OF OSHA'S PERFORMANCE AND COMMENTARY ON NEW INITIATIVES

In the 1980s, OSHA turned to negotiated rule-making allowed by the revisions to the Administrative Procedure Act. However, negotiation for the benzene standard failed, and, in 1983, OSHA issued a standard essentially the same as had been remanded by the U.S. Supreme Court, but with the required scientific/risk-assessment justification. OSHA then promulgated formally negotiated standards for formaldehyde in 1992 and methylenedianiline in 1992 and used an informal negotiation process for the butadiene standard issued in 1996, but they were neither as protective as the law would have allowed nor as technology-forcing.[4]

Although OSHA standard-setting efforts continued in the latter part of the 1990s, its early commitment to worker protection has been further seriously compromised by both procedural requirements imposed by new legislation and by the chilling effect that this legislation has had on agency willingness to set stringent standards. This legislation—the Regulatory Flexibility Act, the Paperwork Reduction Act, the Unfunded Mandates Reform Act, the Small Business Regulatory Enforcement Fairness Act, and the National Technology Transfer and Advancement Act—has placed time-consuming burdens on the agency, contributing to a serious slowdown and resource intensiveness in the development of standards, compounding the effects of executive (presidential) orders requiring the Office of Management and Budget to review OSHA's assessment of costs and benefits for major rules, defined as those having more than $100 million in costs per year.

Equally disturbing is the inadequacy of protection offered by some of the new health standards. The standard for the carcinogen methylene chloride was finally promulgated in 1997—after 13 years of delay. The United Autoworkers Union (UAW) first petitioned OSHA in 1987 for a reduction of the permissible 8-hour exposure allowed by the prior PEL of 500 to 10 ppm. OSHA promulgated a standard of 25 ppm, without medical removal protection. That level was argued to present a lifetime cancer risk of 1 in 1,000 for the average exposed worker (and ensured that 95 percent of the workers were exposed to no lifetime risk higher than 3.6 in 1,000), a risk considerably greater than that allowed in prior standards for individual carcinogens, such as vinyl chloride and benzene (but in line with the lax formaldehyde standard), and in sharp contrast to the level of 1 in 1 million required by the Clean Air Act of 1990 for environmental ambient air exposures to carcinogens. Originally challenging the standard in court as being too lax, the UAW negotiated a legal settlement with the opposing industry for a revision of the standard, retaining the 25 ppm level but adding medical surveillance and removal requirements. Legislation introduced in Congress to veto the standard was unsuccessful.

As discussed earlier, OSHA has to make findings of fact with regard to both the significance of the risk and the feasibility of a proposed standard. Unfortunately, OSHA has pulled back from its historically protective determinations of these factors by (a) being content to regulate near the 1 per 1,000 lifetime risk, which was the *lower* bound of significance suggested by the U.S. Supreme Court in its benzene decision; and (b) finding gratuitously that a proposed standard is feasible, rather than protecting workers to the extent feasible—that is, to the limits of feasibility, using its technology-forcing authority. A study undertaken by the now-defunct Congressional Office of Technology Assessment (OTA) examined the postpromulgation costs of past OSHA standards (including vinyl chloride, ethylene oxide, lead, cotton dust, and formaldehyde) and, in general, found them to be a fraction of the prepromulgation estimates. The OTA concluded:

> OSHA's current economic and technological feasibility analyses devote little attention to the potential of advanced or emerging technologies to yield technically and economically superior methods for achieving reductions in workplace hazards. . . . Opportunities are missed to harness leading-edge or innovative production technologies (including input substitution, process redesign, or product reformulation) to society's collective advantage, and to achieve greater worker protection with technologically and economically superior means.
>
> [I]ntelligently directed effort can yield hazard control options—attributes that would, no doubt, enhance the "win-win" (for regulated industries and their workforces) character of OSHA's compliance requirements in many cases and support the achievement of greater hazard reduction.

Thus, OSHA in no way seems to be pushing regulation to its limits of technology.[5]

OSHA ran into tremendous industry resistance to a proposed ergonomics standard. Congress actually repealed the standard under recently new congressional authority, and OSHA ultimately withdrew the standard. However, OSHA has made it clear the employer has obligations to protect workers from ergonomic hazards under the general duty clause and that enforcement activity will be applied in appropriate situations. The Review Commission upheld OSHA's authority to use the general duty clause in these circumstances. OSHA also experienced political difficulty in establishing standards for secondary tobacco smoke (environmental tobacco smoke) as part of its concern for indoor air quality. OSHA issued a proposed rule in 1994, but action is yet to be taken.

The Clinton administration's record on worker protection was not impressive. No new health standards for chemicals had been issued. The two standards that were issued for 1,3-butadiene and methylene chloride had actually been proposed in the Bush administration prior to Clinton's. In the first George W. Bush administration, OSHA not only withdrew the proposed ergonomic standard, it also withdrew its plans for issuing a rule on metal-working fluids. OSHA does plan the promulgation of some new standards and the review/reconsideration of standards more than 10 years old as required by the Regulatory Flexibility Act. After a successful court challenge, in 2004, OSHA finally issued a proposed revision of its 8-hour exposure limit for hexavalent chromium, lowering the standard to $1\mu g/m^3$ from the previous 33-year-old standard of $52\ \mu g/m^3$, thus preventing 350 excess cancers annually. A peer review for a risk assessment for silica exposure was scheduled for February 2005, but, as of mid-2005, a proposed rule was not yet scheduled. Initial action on beryllium was scheduled for early 2005, but no action has yet been taken. In addition, a rule was planned for requirements for employers to pay for personal protective equipment. Four older standards are also being reviewed: lock-out/tag-out, ethylene oxide, cotton dust, and grain-handling facilities. Also under consideration for revision is a rule for the Process Safety Management of Highly Hazardous Chemicals, to add other reactive chemicals to the rule and to bring it more in line with the EPA's Risk Management Plan. As provided by the Small Business Regulatory Enforcement Fairness Act, the effects of revisited standards on small business must be assessed, and that assessment is now reviewable by the circuit courts of appeals.

With only enough inspectors to inspect 2 percent of the 6 million worksites covered by the OSHAct each year, OSHA has historically used a variety of targeting schemes to decide which sites get inspected. Nearly half of the inspections are reserved to respond to worker complaints, referrals from other agencies, or reports of major or fatal incidents. Begun in mid-2003, OSHA's Site-Specific Targeting (SST) Inspection program selects workplaces with high lost-workday injury and illness rates for inspections from self-reported survey data of about 80,000 employers (mainly mid-sized or larger employers with the lower cutoff at about 40 employees). Lost-workday injury and illness rates are dominated by injuries, and workplace exposures to harmful substances are acknowledged to be grossly underreported, thus biasing the strategy. Out of the approximately 35,000 inspections OSHA conducts each year, about 3,000 are SST-based. Further, based on the 2003 survey of recorded injuries and illnesses, OSHA contacted about 13,000 high-hazard sites, notifying them that their injury rates are above average (usually greater than twice the average) and advising them to seek safety consultations and that they would be targeted for random inspections. Those with four times the national average would be targeted for "wall-to-wall inspections." These 13,000 worksites contribute approximately 20 percent of the 3 million (reported) lost-workday cases annually. In addition to the national targeting strategy, special emphasis programs for specific hazards in selected industrial sectors are conducted at the regional level.

In the current antiregulatory climate, OSHA has, as have other regulatory agencies, shifted toward more voluntary initiatives, including the use of expert advisors, outreach, compliance assistance, consultation, and partnering with industry, trade unions, and workers. OSHA has designated Special Emphasis Programs and Initiatives on silicosis, mechanical power press injuries, lead in construction, nursing home accidents, and workplace violence. These programs and initiatives target a specific occupational hazard or industry and combine outreach and education with enforcement. OSHA has issued to its field staff a Directive on Strategic

TABLE 3-3

Summary of OSHA's Four Voluntary Compliance Programs

Program and Year Established	Target Participants	Program Description	OSHA Oversight
State Consultation Program, 1975	Small businesses in high-hazard industries.	Free, usually confidential reviews of employers' worksites to identify hazards and abatement techniques.	Program operates in all states and is run by state governments, but funded mainly by OSHA.
Voluntary Protection Programs, 1982	Single worksites typically with injury and illness rates below average for their industry sector.	Recognizes worksites that have safety and health programs with specific features that exceed OSHA standards.	Employers must pass a weeklong on-site worksite review by OSHA personnel. Participants complete yearly self-evaluations. OSHA recertifies worksites every 1 to 5 years.
Strategic Partnership Program,[a] 1998	Priority for participation is given to groups of employers and employees in high-hazard workplaces, with a focus on employers working at multiple worksites.	Flexible agreements between OSHA and partners to address a specific safety and health problem.	OSHA conducts verification inspections for a percentage of partner worksites to ensure compliance with the partnership agreement.
Alliance Program, 2002	Trade and professional organizations, employers, labor unions, governmental organizations.	Agreements with organizations that focus on training, outreach, and promoting the consciousness of safety and health issues.	OSHA meets quarterly with participants to ensure progress toward alliance goals is being met.

[a] Although the Occupational health and Safety Administration (OSHA) had partnership agreements prior to 1998, the Strategic Partnership Program was not formalized until that year.
Source: General Accounting Office (GAO) analysis.

Partnerships for Worker Safety and Health. OSHA Strategic Partnerships are intended to establish co-operative efforts at improving health and safety. However, OSHA continues to favor the more voluntary initiatives of *voluntary protection programs*— which it intends to expand tenfold—and alliances discussed below. All in all, the United States stands out in its slow, if not reluctant, approach to protect workers sufficiently with all the tools at its disposal.

The GAO recently reviewed OSHA's four voluntary initiatives and concluded that OSHA had not collected the data necessary to evaluate their effectives. GAO describes the four voluntary compliance programs as follows (Table 3-3):

(Through) the Voluntary Protection Programs (VPP), the State Consultation Program, the Strategic Partnership Program, and the Alliance Program,[*] OSHA has extended its reach to a growing number of employers. While worksites directly involved in these programs represent a small fraction of the 7 million sites over which OSHA has authority, their numbers suggest an expansion in the number of employers the agency

---

[*] *The State Consultation and the Strategic Partnership programs are sometimes referred to by slightly different names. The State Consultation Program is also known as the Onsite Consultation Program and the Consultation Program and the Strategic Partnership Program is also known as OSHA Strategic Partnerships for Worker Safety and Health.*

is able to reach through enforcement. OSHA's four voluntary compliance programs have involved employers both directly and indirectly through trade and professional associations. These programs represent a mix of strategies designed to reach different types of employers, including those that recognize employers with exemplary safety and health practices and programs designed to address serious hazards in workplaces. The State Consultation Program—a state run, but largely OSHA-funded, program—provides consultations, usually confidentially, to small businesses in high-hazard industries and exempts worksites that meet certain standards from routine inspections. Almost 29,000 consultation visits were made in 2003 as a part of this program. The VPP recognizes employers with exemplary safety records and practices by exempting them from routine inspections. The VPP has grown substantially over the past decade and currently includes over 1,000 worksites. The Strategic Partnership Program encourages employers in hazardous industries to develop measures for eliminating serious hazards. To date, there are more than 200 partnerships. In the Alliance Program, OSHA has collaborated with more than 160 organizations, such as trade and professional associations, to promote better safety and health practices for their members. To support all of its voluntary compliance strategies, OSHA has increased the proportion of resources dedicated to them from about 20 percent of its total budget in fiscal year 1996 to about 28 percent in 2003. The agency also plans to expand its voluntary compliance programs in the future, although national and regional OSHA officials we interviewed acknowledged that doing so would be difficult given the agency's current resources. For example, OSHA plans an eightfold increase in the number of worksites for the VPP, from 1,000 to 8,000. OSHA's voluntary compliance programs have reduced injuries and illnesses and yielded other benefits, according to participants, OSHA officials, and occupational safety and health specialists, but the lack of comprehensive data makes it difficult to fully assess the effectiveness of these programs. Participants we interviewed in the three states and nine worksites we visited told us they have considerably reduced their rates of injury and illness. They also attributed better working relationships with OSHA, improved productivity, and decreased worker compensation costs to their involvement in the voluntary compliance programs. However, much of the information on program success was anecdotal, and OSHA's own evaluation of program activities and impact has been limited to date. OSHA currently does not collect complete, comparable data that would enable a full evaluation of the effectiveness of its voluntary compliance programs. For example, OSHA requires participants in the Strategic Partnership Program to file annual reports but does not collect consistent information about each partnership. The agency has begun planning but has yet to develop performance measures to use in evaluating the programs and a strategic framework that will allow it to set priorities and effectively allocate its resources.

In addition to these formal programs, OSHA conducts other compliance assistance activities, such as outreach and training activities, to aid employers in complying with OSHA standards and to educate employers on what constitutes a safe and healthy work environment.

ANALYSIS OF EPA'S PERFORMANCE AND COMMENTARY ON NEW INITIATIVES

As with OSHA, EPA has underperformed in its effort to implement the legislation under its authority.[6] TSCA is internally regarded as a "dead letter" when it comes to the regulation of toxics and continues to move slowly on the testing of chemicals. As of mid-2005, the number of significant final rules promulgated by EPA under all the legislation under its authority during the two George W. Bush administrations was 11, compared to 31 and 40 in the two Clinton administrations and 31 in the George H. W. Bush administration. In 2004, EPA withdrew 25 items from its regulatory agenda, 12 of them coming from Clean Water Act items. During the first administration of George W. Bush, there have been 90 withdrawals as of September 2004: 39 from Clean Air Act planned action. 16 from Clean Water Act actions, and 12 from RCRA actions. EPA is resource-strapped but also without determined leadership. As of June 2004, EPA failed to achieve fully 73 percent of the benchmarks announced in its December 2003 agenda.

Like OSHA, EPA has invested its efforts in voluntary and conciliatory overtures to industry. What is euphemistically called regulatory reinvention was begun (at least under that name) in the Clinton administration and continues today in evolving forms. The most prominent early example was EPA's Common Sense Initiative (CSI), wherein the agency assembled groups of interested parties to focus on regulatory issues concerning a particular industry sector, such as automobile manufacturing, with an eye toward developing "cleaner, cheaper, smarter" ways of reducing or preventing pollution. In contrast, EPA's Project XL focused on negotiations with individual firms. Both programs have now been phased out, and the Bush administration's National Environmental Performance Track program is now occupying center stage in regulatory reinvention. This program focuses on creating partnerships with individual firms in which the firms agree to exceed regulatory requirements, implement environmental management systems, work closely with their communities, and set 3-year goals to improve continuously their environmental performance in exchange for reduced priority status for inspections, reduced regulatory, administrative, and reporting requirements, and positive public recognition.[*] The program is too new to evaluate for inclusion in this writing.

OCCUPATIONAL HEALTH AND SAFETY IN BRITISH COLUMBIA

The discussion in this chapter has focused on occupational health and safety in the United States. The system in British Columbia, Canada, is very different and provides another useful perspective. (The following is based on a 1997 analysis of that system.)

Profile of British Columbia

British Columbia is Canada's third-largest province, with 1.4 million workers of a total population of 3 million people. Thirty-seven percent of the workers are unionized, compared with approximately 15 percent in the United States. Ninety-five percent of the firms have 50 or fewer workers, and 75 percent have five or fewer workers.

Administrative Structure

In British Columbia, the occupational safety and health regulation and enforcement activities and the workers' compensation system are part of the same administrative public corporation, the Workers' Compensation Board (WCB), and both are funded by assessed premiums on employers (see Box 4-2). The WCB is administered by a panel of administrators appointed by the Minister of Labour.

The Prevention Division (formerly the Occupational Safety and Health Division) employs approximately 400 people, which would translate into 28,000 for the United States (compared with the actual number of approximately 2,000). The annual division budget would be equivalent to a U.S. $1.5 billion budget for OSHA, five times larger than the amount actually allocated in the United States.

Legal/Structural Basis

Two provincial pieces of legislation—the Workers' Compensation Act (see Chapter 4) and the Workplace Act—provide the basis for the WCB's standard-setting authority. The federal Workplace Hazardous Materials Information System serves as the basis for provincial right-to-know activities. The Panel of Administrators adopts regulations, with the assistance of a tripartite Regulation Advisory Committee, including professionals from the division, which was responsible for developing new regulations and revising older ones during the last extensive regulation review process. A Policy Bureau in the division provides advice to the Panel of Administrators concerning the final regulations. Thereafter, there is no legal mechanism to challenge the regulations in the British Columbia system. Thus, the development of regulatory policy by the courts discussed for the U.S. system does not exist in British Columbia, for all practical purposes.

Enforcement

Historically, British Columbia standards have not been technology forcing. For example, until 1993 the lead standard permitted exposures up to 150 $\mu g/m^3$, compared with the U.S. standard of 50 $\mu g/m^3$. First-instance citations (mandatory citations on discovery of violations) exist only for a few, mostly safety, violations. There is pressure to include specific chemical exposures and failure of the employer to provide an adequate health and safety program/health and safety committee in the list of violations requiring first-instance citations. The Prevention Division can and does impose penalty assessments; criminal penalties are rarely issued. Labor participates in the WCB's enforcement and appellate process in a significant way.

Inspection activity is targeted by a combination of industry hazard classification, payroll, compensation claims, and inspector experience through a rational targeting system called WorkSafe. The

---

[*] Approximately 350 firms have joined the program from a diverse cross-section of the economy. In contrast to Project XL, regulatory flexibility seems to relate to discretionary activities of agency inspection and reporting policies rather than to extensive exclusion of individual firms from mandatory regulatory provisions. See <http://www.epa.gov/performancetrack>.

construction and logging industries are targeted for special attention because of their high-hazard nature and poor claims experience. The Prevention Division places serious emphasis on its data collection and analysis activities, which appear to be more useful than those of OSHA and the Bureau of Labor Statistics. Accident reporting, which is being computerized, increasingly provides the information needed to focus prevention activities, such as the cause of the accident, rather the cause of the injury. The Prevention Division is implementing the Diamond Project, which, like OSHA's Cooperative Compliance Program, is based on the Maine 200 Program, and seeks to shift responsibility to firms and workers when justified by a good record of occupational injuries (and diseases).

Consultation

Most inspection activity results in warnings and corrective orders rather than monetary penalties on the employer. Some consultation and technical assistance is usually rendered by the inspector at the time of the inspection or closing conference. The division provides engineering guidance and advice to employers in the form of technical bulletins and on-site consultation. The WCB also has an active first-aid certification program for workplace-based first-aid attendants, which is required by law. The WCB does not charge a fee for consulting advice or laboratory assistance/analysis.

Worker Participation

Workplace safety and health programs are required to be provided by all employers with a workforce of 50 or more employees (5 percent of the firms). For especially hazardous industries, the programs are required for employers with a workforce of 20 or more employees. Joint workplace safety and health committees are considered an essential part of these programs. There is pressure to expand the number of firms required to have such a program. Workers complain that they need more authority in the functions of the safety and health committees. They also complain of the inadequacy of the antidiscrimination provisions of the current law/structure, such as in relation to the right to refuse hazardous work.

Comment

Features of the British Columbia system suggest possible U.S. OSHA reforms, such as mandatory health and safety programs and committees, greater recognition of occupational disease, a streamlined standard-setting process, and a linkage of compensation and prevention activities. The period since 1970 has revealed both the strengths and weaknesses of the U.S. system, including the need to strengthen the connection between OSHA and the EPA through the OSHAct, TSCA, and the safety provisions of the Clean Air Amendments.

OCCUPATIONAL HEALTH AND SAFETY IN THE EUROPEAN COMMUNITY

Occupational health and safety legislation in individual European countries is in a great deal of flux after the formation of the European Community (EC), now the European Union (EU). (The following is based on a 1998 analysis.) The Single European Act establishing the EC was enacted in 1987. Article 118A of the act addresses employment, working conditions, and occupational health and safety and provides a streamlined legislative process for the development of health and safety directives and minimum health and safety standards affecting approximately 150 million people. The EC directives have the force of law and set down general principles for the protection of workers. However, individual countries are obligated to adopt national legislation implementing these principles, with important technical details concerning enforcement and administration left to the EC member states. Thus, programs may be expected to differ considerably among countries in the near future, although these differences may narrow as European integration becomes a reality. Therefore, it may be some time before innovations in health and safety regulatory approaches can be evaluated and serve as models for OSHA reform in the United States. Nevertheless, the EC experience may be important for the United States because (a) with the formation of a North American Free Trade Zone, the problems of harmonization of legislation may be similar; (b) the EC will be an important force in occupational safety and health; and (c) the EC will be a major trade competitor. The recent agreement between the EC and the European Free Trade Association countries to set up a free trade area means that the EC safety and health legislation is applicable in 19 countries in Europe.

Legal and Structural Basis

Regulatory activity within the EC can include regulations, decisions, directives, resolutions, and recommendations, varying from commitments in principle to legally enforceable mandates on the Member States. The European Commission, aided by expert groups, makes formal proposals to the EC Council of Ministers. The council, in consultation with the Economic and Social Committee and the European Parliament, adopts, rejects, or modifies the proposals and issues directives by a qualified majority vote of 54 of a total of 76. Individual member states can maintain or introduce more stringent measures for the protection of working conditions than those contained in the directives.

Until 1988, EC directives, such as those dealing with occupational exposure limits for vinyl chloride, lead, asbestos, and benzene, were very detailed and prescriptive. STELs were also specified. After Article 118A was enacted, a more general Framework Directive 89/391/EEC "on the introduction of measures to encourage improvements in the safety and health of workers at work" was issued. This directive is the centerpiece of EC health and safety policy and establishes the guiding principles on which more specific directives are issued. There are now seven so-called daughter directives to the Framework Directive. Directive 90/394/EEC addresses carcinogens at work. Directive 88/642/EEC addresses risks related to exposure to chemicals and physical and biological agents at work and has led to some 27 indicative limit values (ILVs), which are advisory only. The enforcement of those limits is left to the individual regulatory systems and styles of the various member states. Nevertheless, there is a preferred hierarchy of control for "dangerous substances and products." In order of preference, these are substitution of dangerous substances by safe or less dangerous ones, the use of closed systems or processes, local extractive ventilation, general workplace ventilation, and personal protective equipment.

Other EC directives address biological agents, asbestos, video display terminals, work equipment, personal protective equipment, and handling of loads. In 1988, the European Parliament adopted a Resolution on Indoor Air Quality, which is receiving attention for development into a directive.

All commission proposals are submitted to the Advisory Committee on Safety, Hygiene and Health Protection at Work, composed of representatives of employers, workers, and governments. Initially, an expert scientific group evaluates all scientific data relevant to protecting workers from a particular substance. The commission makes a proposal and solicits Advisory Committee

opinion. The Technical Progress Committee votes on the proposal. The limit values may be adopted as indicative values by commission directive. If the exposure limits are mandatory, they are adopted by the Council of Ministers as directives pursuant to Article 118A. Compared with the United States, relatively few health standards have been established, reflecting the slowness of the tripartite process of participatory standard setting envisioned by the EC.

The Framework Directive applies to all sectors of employment activity, both public and private. However, it excludes the self-employed and domestic workers. Employers have a general "duty to ensure the safety and health of workers in every aspect related to the work" (Article 5.1). Among the employer's specific duties are (a) to evaluate risks in the choice of work equipment, chemicals, and design of the workplace; (b) to integrate prevention into the company's operations at all levels; (c) to inform workers or their representatives of risks and preventive measures taken; (d) to consult workers or their representatives on all health and safety matters; (e) to train workers on workplace hazards; (f) to provide appropriate health surveillance; (g) to protect especially sensitive risk groups; and (h) to keep records of accidents and injuries.

Enforcement

Labor inspectorates in each member state have the responsibility to ensure employer compliance with health and safety requirements. However, beyond broad principles and duties, the EC directives are often advisory, and not many specific requirements are enforceable through EC channels. Attempts to place binding obligations on national governments to establish the necessary institutional elements to support proper implementation of safety and health regulations, such as health and safety technical centers, have been unsuccessful. The commission established a Committee of Senior Labor Inspectors in 1982 to facilitate information exchange to encourage coordination of policy. The commission also established the European Agency for Safety and Health at Work in Bilbao, Spain.

The commission does have the authority to bring action against a member state for failure to adhere to EC directives, but the commission does not yet have the institutional capacity to monitor compliance effectively. Action against a member state has never been brought, however, even though some countries have not adopted national legislation to conform with specific mandatory exposure limits, such as for noise. No uniform policy on enforcement of standards, such as first-instance citations or penalty levels, exists, and it is likely that intercountry variations will be allowed.

Worker Participation

The Framework Directive calls for "the informing, consultation, balanced participation . . . and training of workers and their representatives" to improve health and safety at the workplace (Article 1.2). The directive gives workers the rights to consult in advance with their employers on health/safety matters, to be paid for safety activities, to communicate with labor inspectors, and to exercise the right to refuse dangerous work. Safety committees are not explicitly addressed by the directive, although many European countries have required them in transposing the directive into national law. Similarly, joint decision-making is not mandated but may occur in practice.

Comment

The health and safety policy of the EC is evolving. Although the general principles declared in EC legislation and specific directives are laudable, it remains to be seen what course implementation will take and how much variation will continue to exist among the different member states. European regulatory systems tend to be more advisory. On the other hand, they are also more participatory, inviting decision making on a tripartite basis.

REFERENCES

1. Ashford NA, Caldart CC. Technology, law and the working environment. Second ed. Washington, DC: Island Press, 1996:311.
2. Karstadt ML. The Toxic Substances Control Act Section 8(e) Database: A rich source of data for studies of occupational carcinogenesis. Eur J Ocol 2003;8:159–64.
3. Ashford N, Ayers C. Changes and opportunities in the environment for technology bargaining. Notre Dame Law Rev 1987;62:810–58. Available at: <http://hdl.handle.net/1721.1/1546>.
4. Caldart CC, Ashford NA. Negotiation as a means of developing and implementing environmental and occupational health and safety policy. Harvard Environ Law Rev 1999;23:141–202.
5. U.S. Congress, Office of Technology Assessment. Gauging control technology and regulatory impacts in occupational safety and health: An appraisal of OSHA's analytic approach. Publication no. OTA-ENV-635. Washington, DC: U.S. Congress, Office of Technology Assessment, 1995.
6. The Bush regulatory record: A pattern of failure. Washington, DC: OMB Watch, 2004.

BIBLIOGRAPHY

Ashford NA. Promoting technological changes in the workplace: Public and private initiatives. In: Brown M, Froines J, eds. Technological change in the workplace: Health impacts for workers. Los Angeles: UCLA Institute of Industrial Relations, 1993:23–36.
A series of essays on the effects of technological change on workers and suggestions for improvement of workers' health and safety.

Ashford NA. The economic and social context of special populations. In: Frumkin H, Pransky G, eds. *Special populations in occupational health.* Occup Med 1999;14: 485–93.
Introductory chapter on changes in the nature of technology, work, and labor markets and their impact on different worker populations at risk.

Ashford NA, Caldart CC. *Technology, law and the working environment.* Washington, DC: Island Press, 1996.
A textbook of law and policy related to the workplace, with court cases, law review articles, and policy analysis.

Ashford NA, Caldart CC. Environmental law, policy, and economics. 2006.
A textbook of law, policy, and economics related to the general environment, with court cases, law review articles, and policy analysis.

Caldart CC, Ashford NA. Negotiation as a means of developing and implementing environmental and occupational health and safety policy. Harvard Environ Law Rev 1999;23:141–202.
A major review of negotiated rule making in both OSHA and EPA, assessing the strengths and weaknesses of regulatory negotiation.

Commission of the European Community. Social Europe: Health and safety at work in the European Community. Brussels: Commission of the European Community, February 1990.
Text and explanation of EC directives and legislation pertaining to occupational safety and health.

Hecker S. Part 1: Early initiatives through the Single European Act. New Solutions 1993;3:59–69; Part 2: The Framework Directive: Whither harmonization? New Solutions 1993;4:57–67.
A critical look at health and safety policy in the European Union.

Rest KM, Ashford NA. *Occupational safety and health in British Columbia: An administrative inventory of the WCB Prevention Division.* Cambridge, MA: Ashford Associates, 1997.
A review of the Occupational Health and Safety Administration in British Columbia.

U.S. Congress, Office of Technology Assessment. Preventing illness and injury in the workplace. Washington, DC: U.S. Government Printing Office, 1985.
A comprehensive assessment of earlier political problems faced in preventing occupational disease and injury.

U.S. Congress, Office of Technology Assessment. Gauging control technology and regulatory impacts in occupational safety and health: An appraisal of OSHA's analytic approach. Publication no. OTA-ENV-635. Washington, DC: U.S. Congress, Office of Technology Assessment, 1995.
An analysis of the differences between preregulatory estimates of cost and postregulatory costs of OSHA regulation, focusing on the importance of taking technological change into account.

CHAPTER 4

Legal Remedies

Leslie I. Boden, Neil T. Leifer, David C. Strouss,
and Emily A. Spieler

Physicians often express anxiety or confusion about the treatment of patients with occupational and environmental health problems. The anxiety occurs, in part, because questions may arise about the legal responsibility for the consequences of occupational and environmental health problems. Disputes about who carries this burden—employer or worker, manufacturer or consumer, polluter or community member—often involve the physician in providing input about causation or extent of injury. This role, in turn, can interfere with the trust and openness needed to ensure the best health outcome for the patient.

The provision of occupational health services presents particular problems for the treating physician. When treating a patient for a minor illness or injury incurred at home, the physician can deal directly with the patient—both the cause of the problem and its treatment will, in many cases, be within the patient's control. Health problems caused at work present greater legal, economic, and social complexities. Neither the patient nor the physician can ignore the external forces that will influence the patient's progress and prognosis. Neither the patient nor the physician has control over the workplace design and the hazards that cause the medical problem. The employer's attitudes and policies regarding workplace hazards and workplace-induced disabilities, the extent of job security that the employer offers during periods of disability, and the availability of monetary benefits all influence the course of the patient's recovery. Ultimately, any successful attempt to deliver health services to working people must consider the roles played by the employer, the employer's representatives (including employer-retained attorneys and physicians), the employer's insurer, the job security and job mobility of the patient, and the economic prospects for the patient.

As a result, many others—employers, attorneys, insurers, various state and federal health and safety and compensation agencies—will be looking over the shoulder of the treating physician when a patient's medical problem is due to work. The interests of these others cause the special legal problems associated with occupational injuries and illnesses.

Environmentally induced illnesses do not cause as wide a range of outside forces to intrude on the physician–patient relationship. Still, treating physicians may play a critical role in determining how their patients fare in the legal system. Physicians are often uncomfortable with the responsibility for preparing medical-legal reports about work-relatedness, degree of disability, work restrictions, readiness to return to work. These are tasks for which they have often been poorly prepared.

These patients' economic and employment status may depend on whether physicians are willing to provide documentation regarding the occupational causation or the degree of impairment resulting from the health problem. The patient may need assistance from the physician in order to be excused from work and to return to work— and to obtain compensation or disability benefits and medical insurance coverage during the course

---

Leslie I. Boden is the overall chapter editor and is primarily responsible for the workers' compensation section. Neil T. Leifer and David C. Strouss are primarily responsible for the section on toxic tort litigation. Emily A. Spieler is primarily responsible for the section on job security.

of treatment. Patients' trust in their physicians—and, therefore, their degree of compliance with medical instructions—will be influenced by the physicians' understanding of the pertinent legal issues and their willingness to provide assistance to the patient. Ignorance of the patients' situation and the legal rules surrounding them may lead to serious adverse consequences for patients, including discharge from employment.

Physicians' primary ethical and legal obligations are to their patients. The economic interests of other people and entities, including those of the patients' employers, are well protected by the legal system. Physicians who treat individuals with occupationally induced health problems and are concerned about the long-term health of their patients must become familiar with the various legal rules that govern requests for (a) information that will be made by others and (b) assistance that will come from their patients.

This chapter provides an understanding of the legal and institutional environment in which people with occupational or environmental health conditions are treated. It describes the ways in which actions by treating physicians can affect their patients' legal rights to financial recovery and how physicians may interact directly with the legal system. The chapter is divided into four parts: (1) workers' compensation insurance and Social Security programs for the disabled; (2) the role of personal injury litigation in providing access to compensation for people with occupational and environmental health conditions; (3) laws that protect workers' job security; and (4) privacy rights of workers and potential conflicts with the information needs of the employers of injured workers.

WORKERS' COMPENSATION

Workers' compensation is a legal system that shifts some of the costs of occupational injury and illness from workers to employers. Workers' compensation laws generally require employers or their insurance companies to reimburse part of injured workers' lost wages and all of their medical and rehabilitation expenses.

Historical Background

Before passage of the first workers' compensation act in 1911, workers generally bore the costs of their work-related injuries. Injured workers and their families were forced to cope with lost wages and medical care and rehabilitation costs. Under the *common law,*[*] workers had to prove in a court of law that their injuries were caused by employer negligence in order to recover these costs.

For several reasons, it was extremely difficult for workers to win such negligence suits. Injured workers had the burden of proof and had to show that their employers were negligent, that there were work-related injuries, and that negligence caused these injuries. To sustain this burden of proof, workers had to hire lawyers (which was costly) and often had to rely on the testimony of fellow workers (who, along with suing workers, might be fired for their part in suits). All of this was enough to deter most workers from bringing suit.

In addition, employers had three very strong common-law defenses that usually protected them from losing negligence suits when they were brought:

Doctrine of contributory negligence: If judges found that employees had contributed in any way to their injuries, they were barred from winning.
Fellow-servant rule: If judges found that fellow employees' actions had caused the injuries, employers were not considered responsible.
Assumption of risk: If judges found that injuries were caused by common hazards or by unusual hazards of which workers were aware, they could not recover damages.

In the late 19th century, these defenses were widely used, and less than one-third of all employees who brought such negligence suits won any award. In one case, a New York woman lost her arm when it was caught between the unguarded gears of the machine she had been cleaning. Unguarded gears were in violation of New York State laws then, and before the accident she had complained to her employer about this hazard. Still, her employer refused to guard the machine. After the accident, the worker sued her employer, but the court held that she could not be compensated; she had obviously known about the hazard and, of her own free will, had continued to work. This evidence showed that she had "assumed the risk" and that her employer was not responsible for the consequences.

---

[*] *The common law is a body of legal principles developed by judicial decisions rather than by legislation. Statutory law can override these judge-made laws.*

The inability to hold employers responsible for their negligent actions persisted in the face of the high and increasing toll of occupational death and disability at the beginning of the 20th century. After a disabling injury, workers and their families were left largely to their own resources and to assistance from relatives, friends, and charities.

By 1920, some efforts had been made to provide better means of compensation to injured workers and their families. Some of the larger corporations had established private compensation schemes, and several states and the federal government had enacted employers' liability acts. These laws retained the basic common-law liability scheme but reduced the role of the three common-law defenses.

Most injured workers, however, were not able to take advantage of these changes. There was growing support for a major change in the law from the social reformers of the Progressive Era and from major corporations. These pressures gave rise to the passage of the first workers' compensation law in New York State. Many other states rapidly followed suit, and by 1920 all but eight states had passed similar laws, although most did not cover occupational disease. Mississippi, in 1948, was the last state to establish a workers' compensation system.

Description of Workers' Compensation

Workers' compensation provides income benefits, medical payments, and rehabilitation payments to workers injured on the job as well as benefits to survivors of fatally injured workers. There are 50 state and 3 federal workers' compensation jurisdictions, each with its own statute and regulations.

Although state and federal systems are different in numerous ways, they have several characteristics in common. Benefit formulas are prescribed by law. Generally, medical care and rehabilitation expenses are fully covered, but lost wages are only partially reimbursed. Employers are legally responsible for paying benefits to injured workers. Some large employers pay these benefits themselves, but most pay yearly premiums to insurers, which process all claims and pay compensation to injured workers. Workers' compensation is a no-fault system. Injured workers do not need to prove that their injuries were caused by employer negligence. In fact, employers are generally required to pay benefits even if the injury is entirely the worker's fault.

The change to a no-fault system was established to minimize litigation. For a worker to qualify for workers' compensation benefits, only three conditions must be met: (1) there must be an injury or illness, (2) it must "arise out of and in the course of employment," and (3) there must be medical costs, rehabilitation costs, lost wages, or disfigurement.

Clearly, these conditions are much easier for the injured worker to demonstrate than employer negligence. For example, if a worker falls at work and breaks a leg, all three conditions are easily met. Unusual cases sometimes arise in which the question of the relationship of an injury to employment is difficult to resolve, and there may be questions about when a worker is ready to return to work. Such issues may result in litigation, but they are the exception, not the rule. In most cases, a worker files a claim for compensation with the employer, and the claim is accepted and paid either directly by the employer or by the workers' compensation insurance carrier of the employer.

The following case is typical of the events that follow many minor claims for workers' compensation:

> Mr. Fisher developed a painful muscle strain while lifting a heavy object at work on Monday afternoon. He went to the plant nurse and described the injury. He was sent home and was unable to return to work until the following Friday morning. On Tuesday, the nurse sent an industrial accident report to the workers' compensation carrier and a copy to the state workers' compensation agency. Three weeks after he returned to work, Mr. Fisher received a check from the insurance company covering part of his lost wages—as mandated by state statute—and all of his out-of-pocket medical expenses related to the muscle strain.

Workers' compensation provides wider coverage than the common-law system did. Under workers' compensation, workplace injuries and illnesses are compensable—even if they are only, in part, work-related. Generally, injuries and illnesses are considered eligible for compensation if occupational exposure is the sole cause of the disease, is one of several causes of the disease, was aggravated by or aggravates a nonoccupational exposure, or hastens the onset of disability (Table 4-1). Suppose, for example, a worker with preexisting chronic low back pain becomes permanently disabled as a result of lifting a heavy object at work. In this case, the

TABLE 4-1

Likelihood of Compensation, by Source of Preexisting Condition and Source of Ultimate Disability

	Source of Preexisting Condition	
Source of Ultimate Disability	Work Related	Nonwork Related
Work related	Compensable	Generally compensable
Nonwork related	Generally compensable	Not compensable

Adapted from Barth PS, Hunt HA. Workers' compensation and work-related illnesses. Cambridge, MA: MIT Press, 1980.

workers' preexisting condition might just as easily have been aggravated by carrying out the garbage at home, but the fact that the disabling event occurred at work is generally sufficient for compensation to be awarded.

Cases in which an occupational injury or illness becomes disabling as a result of nonwork exposures are similar in principle. For example, a worker with nondisabling silicosis may leave a granite quarry job for warehouse work. Without further exposure, the silicosis will probably never become disabling. However, the worker may begin to smoke cigarettes and lose lung function until partial disability results. In most states, this worker should receive compensation from the owner of the granite quarry if the work relationship can be demonstrated.

During the 1990s, nine states passed laws that undermined the long-standing principle of workers' compensation that workers are eligible for benefits even if their disabilities are in part caused by nonwork factors. These laws (a) require that work be a major or predominant cause of the disability or (b) eliminate compensation for the aggravation of a preexisting condition or for a condition related to the aging process.[1]

Several states, including California and Florida, allow disability to be apportioned between occupational and nonoccupational causes. Although at first this may seem like a sensible approach, apportionment creates some difficult decisions for workers' compensation administrators. Many disabilities are not additively caused by two separable exposures. With silica exposure or cigarette exposure alone, the worker in the above example would probably not have become disabled. Often, as in the case of lung cancer caused by asbestos exposure and smoking, the contribution to disability or death of two factors is many times greater than that of one alone. Such issues make the apportionment of disability very difficult, if not impossible.

When workers' compensation was introduced, workers gained a swifter, more certain, and less litigious system than existed before. In return, however, covered workers waived their right to sue employers through common law. (See Box 4-1 for situations in which workers with occupational injuries and illnesses can sue.) They also accepted lower awards than those given by juries in negligence suits: Workers' compensation provides no payments for "pain and suffering" as there might be in a common-law settlement. In addition, disability payments under workers' compensation are often much less than lost income, especially for more severe injuries.

The United States does not have a unified workers' compensation law. Each state has its own system with its own standards and idiosyncrasies. In addition, federal systems cover federal employees, longshoremen and harbor workers, and workers employed in the District of Columbia. Except for Texas, all states require employers either to purchase insurance or to demonstrate that they are able to pay any claims that might be made by their employees. In most states, private insurers underwrite workers' compensation insurance paid for by premiums from individual employers. In some states, a nonprofit state workers' compensation fund has been established; the state government therefore acts as an insurance carrier, collecting premiums and disbursing benefits. State funds seem to be very effective in delivering benefits: They disburse a higher percentage of premiums in the form of benefits than do private insurance carriers.

BOX 4-1

When Employers Are Subject to Lawsuits for Workplace Injuries and Illnesses

Generally speaking, workers are barred from suing their employers for injuries covered by workers' compensation laws. However, in most states, injured workers can sue their employer:

- If the employer has not properly purchased workers' compensation insurance coverage.
- If the particular injury or illness is not compensable under the state's workers' compensation law: For example, if a state specifically excludes coverage for a specific occupational diagnosis such as stress-related mental illness or cumulative trauma disorders, the employer is not shielded from lawsuit. To be successful, the worker must, however, prove that the employer was negligent; the no-fault principles of workers' compensation do not apply.
- If the claim is related to a specific employment law: Until relatively recently, employers of occupationally injured employees could pay workers' compensation benefits and discharge the workers, without adverse legal consequences. This practice is often no longer legal. Actions brought by employees alleging violation of various state

and federal employment laws are not affected by workers' compensation rules—generally, including situations where the workers allege mental injury as a result of illegal discrimination or retaliation.

In addition, when an injury is the result of intentional—not merely negligent—conduct by the employer, some states will allow the worker to bring a common-law action against the employer. Most states still preclude these actions or require the worker to prove that the employer specifically intended to injure the worker—the *specific intent* standard. Under this standard, even employers who intentionally violate health and safety rules or are reckless in their approach to occupational safety are protected by workers' compensation immunity. In contrast, a growing minority of states now allow workers to bring common-law actions against an employer when the employer knowingly allows hazardous conditions to exist that are "substantially certain" to result in serious injury. In these states, an employer's knowledge that conditions were extremely hazardous is relevant to determining whether the employer will be held liable for damages above those provided by workers' compensation.

The Role of the Physician in Workers' Compensation

Workers' compensation is basically a legal system, not a medical system. The decision points for claims in this complex system are shown in Fig. 4-1. If a claim is rejected by the workers' compensation carrier or self-insured employer, it will generally be necessary for the injured worker to hire a lawyer. The worker's lawyer may then bargain with the lawyers for the insurance carrier in an attempt to settle the dispute informally. If this bargaining does not result in agreement, the claim must either be dropped or taken before an administrative board—a quasijudicial body established by state statute—for a hearing. To the worker or to a physician who may be called to testify in such a hearing, such a proceeding may be indistinguishable from a formal trial: Witnesses are sworn,

rules of evidence are followed, and testimony is recorded.

As a part of this legal proceeding, medical questions are often raised. There may be disagreement about the degree of disability of a worker, when an injured worker is ready to return to work, or whether a particular injury or illness is work-related. In order to settle these disputes, physicians may be called on to give their medical opinions about employees' disabilities. Most often, physicians provide written opinions, but sometimes they may be called upon to testify. Many physicians do not like to testify, and most are not prepared by their training or experience to assume this role. Their expertise may be challenged; moreover, they may be confused by the different meanings of legal and medical terminology.

In workers' compensation, decisions are based on legal definitions, and the legal distinction between disability and impairment is often unclear to

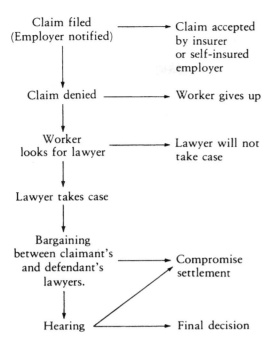

FIGURE 4-1 ● Decision points for workers' compensation claims.

physicians. A physician called in to testify about whether or not a worker is permanently and totally disabled may understand total disability as a state of physical helplessness and may therefore testify that the injured worker is not totally helpless. However, this standard is not what a workers' compensation board would apply. The term *disability,* as used in workers' compensation proceedings, means that wages have been lost, whereas *total disability* means that the injured worker loses wages as a result of not being able to perform gainful employment. A relatively small impairment could result in a substantial disability. For example, airline pilots might be barred from working because of a level of visual impairment that might minimally interfere with other aspects of their lives. On the other hand, a worker who has been exposed to silica at work may have substantially reduced pulmonary function and therefore impairment. However, if the worker continues to work at the same job, no wages have been lost, and therefore no disability payment is made. Many states, however, offer specified payments for disfigurement or losses of sight, hearing, or limbs, with compensation based on impairment and not on disability (Table 4-2).

Although physicians may feel that they have not been trained adequately for their role in workers'

compensation, workers do need their support in this area. A lack of assistance may mean unnecessary financial hardship for the victim of an occupational injury or disease. The best way a physician can help identify a work-related disease or injury is by taking an occupational history (see Chapter 6). If the physician suspects a work-related disease or injury, the patient should be informed of the right to receive workers' compensation and the time limits on such claims. (The period for filing a claim generally begins when the patient is informed that the disease is work-related.) Physicians should also suggest the possibility of seeking legal counsel, and they can provide direct help by completing any required reports, including descriptions of the illness or injury and why it is believed to be work-related. The extent of probable disability should also be noted. In most states, none of these steps requires testimony before a workers' compensation judge, most workers' compensation claims are either paid without contest or settled without a hearing.

A primary care physician may be the only person willing and able to provide documentation for an employee wishing to file a workers' compensation claim. Support for valid compensation claims not only assists injured workers but also helps to ensure that employers and their insurance carriers will appropriately shoulder the costs that result from workplace hazards. If these costs are not paid under workers' compensation, they will be borne by workers and their families or by all of us through our share of the costs of third-party medical payments, welfare, Social Security, and other public support programs.

The Adequacy of Workers' Compensation for Occupational Injuries

The fundamental problems of the common-law scheme were that litigation was a necessary element of compensation and that it was very difficult for workers to win suits against their employers. Even when workers won negligence suits, payments were made long after they were injured, and one-third or more of each settlement was diverted for legal fees and expenses. Today, workers with minor injuries covered by workers' compensation generally can expect to receive payments promptly and without a contest. In fact, fewer than 10 percent of all claims for occupational injuries—as opposed to occupational diseases—are contested.

TABLE 4-2

Income Benefits for Scheduled Injuries in Selected Jurisdictions (As of January 1, 2003)[a]

Jurisdiction	Arm at Shoulder ($)	Hand ($)	Foot ($)	Eye ($)	Hearing: Both Ears ($)
Alabama	48,840	37,400	30,580	27,280	35,860
Connecticut	142,896	115,416	85,875	107,859	71,448
Delaware	122,892	108,145	78,651	98,314	86,024
District of Columbia	239,148	187,026	157,388	122,640	153,300
Georgia	90,000	64,000	55,000	60,000	60,000
Illinois	299,436	189,643	1540709	159,699	108,434
Mississippi	68,212	49,659	41,382	33,106	49,659
New York	124,800	97,600	82,000	64,000	60,000
North Carolina	161,760	134,800	97,056	80,880	101,100
Washington	89,469	80,522	89,469	61,050	47,952
Wisconsin	111,000	88,600	111,000	61,050	47,952
Federal employees	498,071	389,517	459,757	255,421	319,276
U.S. longshore	310,920	243,155	287,005	159,446	199,308

[a] Amounts in table reflect maximum potential entitlement.
Source: U.S. Department of Labor, Employment Standards Administration, Office of Workers' Compensation Programs. Available at:
<http://www.dol.gov/esa/regs/statutes/owcp/stwclaw/tables-pdf/table-9a.pdf>. Accessed July 20, 2004.

Under workers' compensation, insurance carriers or self-insured employers have the right to contest a claim. A claim may be contested because the injury is not considered work-related, for example, or because the claim is for a larger amount than the insurer is willing to pay. However, in most injury cases, the employer or insurance carrier has little incentive to contest because proof of eligibility is easy, and the potential gain to the insurer of postponing or eliminating small payments is not enough to offset the legal costs of pursuing a claim.

For expensive injury claims, such as permanent total disability and death claims, insurance companies are much more likely to contest. More than 80 percent of all compensation claims for chronic occupational diseases (Table 4-3) and almost 50 percent of all injury claims for permanent total disability or death are contested, leading to delays of a year or more in settling workers' compensation claims (Table 4-4). Even if they do not win, a contest enables insurers to keep the settlement money temporarily, invest it, and receive investment income until the case is closed and the injured worker paid. Because a contest delays the date of payment, this investment income is an incentive to

TABLE 4-3

Percentage of Alleged Occupational Disease Cases Controverted (Contested) by Category of Disease

Category	Percentage
Dust disease	88
Disorders due to repeated trauma	86
Respiratory conditions due to toxic agents	79
Cancers and tumors	46
Poisoning	37
Skin diseases	14
Disorders due to physical agents	10
Other	54
All diseases	63[a]

[a] In contrast, the percentage for all injuries is 10%. Adapted from Barth PS, Hunt HA. Workers' compensation and work-related illnesses. Cambridge, MA: MIT Press, 1980.

Delays in Compensation for Occupational Disease by Category of Disease

Category	Mean Number of Days from Notice to Insurer to First Payment
Skin diseases	59
Dust diseases	390
Respiratory conditions due to toxic agents	389
Poisoning	111
Disorders due to physical agents	79
Disorders due to repeated trauma	362
Cancers and tumors	260
Other illnesses	180[a]

[a] In contrast, the mean delay for all injuries is 43 days.
Adapted from Barth PS, Hunt HA. Workers' compensation and work-related illnesses. Cambridge, MA: MIT Press, 1980.

contest even those cases that the insurer is likely to lose. The higher the potential settlement, the stronger is the incentive to contest. Claims for permanent disability and death are contested 5 to 10 times more frequently than are claims for temporary disability.

Long delays caused by contests may put great financial pressure on injured workers, who may have high medical costs and substantial lost earnings. This can lead workers to accept settlements that leave them seriously undercompensated. Also, legal fees, commonly 15 to 20 percent of cash benefits paid, must be paid by the injured worker. Among injured workers represented by attorneys in Wisconsin who were injured in 1989 or 1990, workers paid their attorneys an average of $3,200 of $20,900 in income benefits.

Aside from the incentives to contest major claims, several other important problems can be cited in the more than 50 workers' compensation systems in the United States. In theory, workers' compensation should cover all employees; however, some states exempt agricultural employees, household workers, and/or state and municipal employees.

The maximal weekly benefit provided varies widely among the jurisdictions: The highest, on January 1, 2003, was for federal employees ($1,596) and the lowest was for Mississippi workers ($331) (Table 4-5). Some jurisdictions do not provide for cost-of-living adjustments; a person injured 30 years ago and still disabled may receive total disability payments of only $10 to $20 a week. Benefits also do not account for the increased wages that would have been earned if the employee had continued to work.

Recent studies have raised substantial concerns about the adequacy of workers' compensation benefits. Several suggest that a substantial number of workers with occupational injuries never enter the workers' compensation system and, as a result, never receive benefits.[2] Other recent studies in five states (California, New Mexico, Oregon, Washington, and Wisconsin) show that many workers receive workers' compensation income benefits that are less than one-half their lost earnings, especially when injuries have long-term impacts.[3] Workers with long-term disabilities who do not receive permanent disability benefits do the worst—often receiving benefits that are less than 20 percent of their injury-related losses.[4]

Workers' Compensation Medical Costs

Figure 4-2 shows that, during the 1980s, the annual rate of growth of workers' compensation medical costs was consistently above the growth of medical costs outside workers' compensation. From 1980 to 1990, there was a 265 percent increase in workers' compensation medical costs, compared to a 183 percent increase in medical costs outside workers' compensation. Between 1990 and 1992, there was no clear pattern. However, from 1992 to 1997 workers' compensation medical costs have grown more slowly than other medical costs, actually falling by 3 percent, compared to the 32 percent increase in medical costs outside workers' compensation during the same period. Since 1997, the two systems have been growing at about the same rate. Studies in Minnesota[5] and California[6] suggest that medical costs for similar injuries may be higher in workers' compensation than in general medical practice.

Causes of Higher Workers' Compensation Medical Costs

Factors specific to workers' compensation may have caused its medical costs to accelerate. Certain

TABLE 4-5

Maximum Weekly Benefits for Total Disability Provided by Workers' Compensation Statues of Selected States (As of January 1, 2003)

Jurisdiction	Fraction of Worker's Wage	Maximum Weekly Benefit (to Nearest Dollar)
Alabama	2/3	569 (SAWW)
Alaska	4/5 of worker's spendable earnings	814
California	2/3	602
District of Columbia	2/3 up to 4/5 of worker's spendable earnings	1,022 (SAWW)
Florida	2/3	608 (SAWW)
Iowa	4/5 of worker's spendable earnings	1,103 (200% of SAWW)
Massachusetts	3/5	882 (SAWW)
Michigan	4/5 of worker's spendable earnings	653 (90% of SAWW)
Mississippi	2/3	331 (66% of SAWW)
New Hampshire	3/5	1,018 (150% of SAWW)
New York	2/3	400
North Carolina	2/3	674 (110% of SAWW)
Pennsylvania	2/3	675 (SAWW)
Rhode Island	3/4 of worker's spendable earnings	702 (110% of SAWW)
Texas	7/10	537 (SAWW)
West Virginia	2/3	526 (SAWW)
Federal employees	2/3 or 3/4[a]	1,596 (66% or 75% of GS-15)[a]
U.S. longshore	2/3	997 (200% of NAWW)

SAWW, state's average weekly wage; NAWW, national average weekly wage.
[a] Maximum is 3/4 if one dependent or more.
Source: U.S. Department of Labor, Employment Standards Administration, Office of Workers' Compensation Programs. Available at:
<http://www.dol.gov/esa/regs/statutes/owcp/stwclaw/tables-pdf/table-6.pdf>. Accessed July 20, 2004.

cost-control techniques are absent in workers' compensation, and others are more difficult to perform. For example, copayments and deductibles are used regularly outside workers' compensation to reduce the demand for medical care and, thus, its cost. Yet workers' compensation systems traditionally have paid all medical costs resulting from covered injuries and illnesses.

Workers' compensation insurers or self-insured companies may find discounts for medical care difficult to negotiate for two reasons: (1) workers' compensation has only a small share of the medical care market (about 2 percent) and therefore has less bargaining power, and (2) workers have the legal right to choose a treating physician in about half the states, making it more difficult for employers to direct them to lower cost providers. Evidence about the impact on costs of who chooses the treating physician is equivocal, with studies suggesting that employer choice does not reduce, and may even raise, costs.[7]

Because workers' compensation payers pay for both medical care and a portion of lost wages, they may be willing to pay for more intensive medical treatment in the belief that the worker will return to work more quickly. The increase in medical costs would then be offset by a decline in income benefits.

Litigation also increases the medical costs of workers' compensation beyond those that might be incurred in other settings. Litigation can interfere with the trust that is essential to the doctor–patient relationship, possibly prolonging the duration of medical treatment paid for by workers' compensation. In addition, most states allocate the expense of medical evaluations used to resolve legal disputes, which are often substantial, as medical costs.

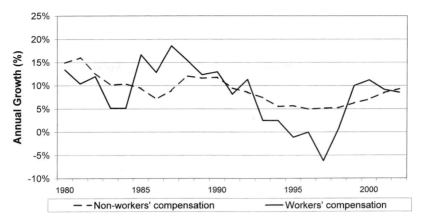

FIGURE 4-2 ● Annual U.S. medical care cost growth: Workers' compensation versus non–workers' compensation. (Sources: For 1980–1993, workers' compensation data are from Schmulowitz J. Workers' compensation: Coverage, benefits, and costs, 1992–93, Social Security Bull 1955;58(2)51–7. For 1994 and 1995 workers' compensation data: National Academy of Social Insurance. Workers' compensation: Benefits, coverage, and costs, 1994–95: New estimates. Washington, DC: National Academy of Social Insurance, 1997. For non–workers' compensation medical costs: Centers for Medicare and Medicaid Services. Available at: <http://www.cms.hhs.gov/statistics/nhe/historical/tables.pdf> (filenhe02.zip).

Workers' Compensation Medical Cost Control

Rapidly increasing medical costs have driven many states to place controls on medical costs. The most common of these are

- Fee schedules that list maximum reimbursement levels for health care services or products;
- Limited employee initial choice of medical care provider, or limitations on changing medical care providers;
- Mandatory bill review for proper charges, generally tied to a fee schedule;
- Mandatory utilization review of the necessity and appropriateness of admissions and procedures, length of hospitalization, and consultations by specialists before, during, or after an inpatient admission;
- Managed care programs that seek to reduce the price and utilization of medical care (for example, health maintenance or preferred provider organizations); and
- Treatment guidelines designed to reduce the provision of ineffective or harmful medical care.

In the 1990s, many states adopted one or more of these methods of containing medical costs. From 1991 to 1997, 13 states added medical fee schedules, and 14 states added hospital payment regulation. In addition, six employee-choice states gave employers and insurers the right to provide managed care, where none had done so before 1991.

The importance of these changes goes beyond their impact on medical costs. When they choose the medical provider or managed care organization, employers and insurers have a greater say about the medical treatment but also about the provider's behavior in litigated cases. In many workers' compensation systems, treating providers furnish information about when a worker is ready to return to work (and when temporary disability benefits may be terminated) or the worker's level of impairment (affecting permanent disability benefits). Because provider choice can affect income benefits, it would be in contention even if everybody agreed it did not affect medical costs.

Medicolegal Roadblocks to Compensation for Occupational Diseases

The burden of proving that occupational injuries "arose out of and in the course of employment" is usually straightforward. However, workers with occupational illnesses face a different situation (Table 4-6). The workers' compensation system expects a physician to say whether or not a worker's illness was caused by or aggravated by work. Physicians are asked, "Was this illness caused by workplace

TABLE 4-6

Roadblocks to Compensation for Occupational Disease

Limitations of Medical Science	Statutory Limitations	Other Limitations
Difficulty of differential diagnosis	Time limits	Lack of exposure records
Lack of epidemiologic and	Burden of proof	(duration and intensity)
toxicologic studies	Restrictive definitions of disease	
Multiple causal pathways		
Limitations of physicial training		

conditions?" This is a question for which medical science often does not have a simple answer.

Many aspects of occupational diseases make the disabled worker's burden of proof difficult to sustain. Physicians may not realize that their patients may have become ill as a result of workplace exposures. Many physicians are not able to identify occupational diseases because their medical training in this area has been inadequate—many have not even been trained in taking occupational histories. Furthermore, the signs and symptoms of most occupational diseases are not uniquely related to an occupational exposure. Medical and epidemiologic knowledge may be insufficient to distinguish clearly a disease of occupational origin from one of nonoccupational origin. For example, shortness of breath, an important symptom of occupational lung disease, is also associated with other chronic lung diseases (Fig. 4-3).

Another complicating factor is that a disease may have multiple causes, only one of which is occupational exposure. A worker who smokes and is exposed to ionizing radiation at work may develop lung cancer. Because both cigarette smoke and ionizing radiation are well-established risk factors for lung cancer, it may be impossible to say which of these two factors "caused" the disease. In many cases, occupational disease may develop many years after exposure began and perhaps many years after exposure ceased. Consequently, memories of events and exposures may be unclear, and records of employment may not be available.

Some occupational injuries occur as a result of extended exposure to a hazard. These are cumulative trauma disorders, such as carpal tunnel syndrome, noise-induced hearing loss, and chronic low back pain. As with chronic occupational diseases,

it may be difficult to prove the work-relatedness of these injuries. Moreover, records of exposure to occupational hazards are not often kept, so that even when a worker knows the type and duration of exposure, no written evidence of this can be presented.

These aspects of occupational disease mean that many victims do not even suspect that their disease is job-related. For those who do and wish to make a claim, the causal relationship between

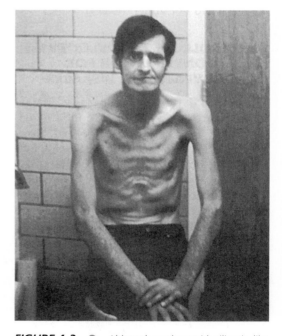

FIGURE 4-3 ● Although workers with silicosis, like this rock driller, qualify for workers' compensation, most workers with chronic occupational diseases often find their claims denied. (Reprinted from Banks DE, Bauer MA, Castellan RM, et al. Silicosis in surface coal mine drillers. Thorax 1983;30:275.)

disease and workplace exposures may be very difficult to establish. These are major reasons why so few claims for compensation for occupational disease are filed. A study of occupational disease in California and Washington revealed that, of the 51 probable cases of occupational respiratory conditions, only one was reported as a workers' compensation claim.

When claims for chronic occupational disease are filed, many are contested by the insurance carrier or self-insured employer (see Table 4-3). Therefore, payments to disabled workers are delayed and uncertain (see Table 4-4). Workers with chronic occupational diseases wait more than a year, on average, to receive compensation payments. In addition, administrative and legal costs absorb many of the resources devoted to compensating workers for their occupational diseases.

Establishing Work-Relatedness for Compensation

The burden of proving that disease is occupational in origin lies with workers. They must find physicians who are convinced that their illnesses are occupational in origin or that their illnesses were aggravated or hastened by occupational exposures. Physicians must then be able to convince judges who hear the cases that the diseases are indeed work-related.

The burden of proof might at first seem to be impossible for those diseases that are not uniquely occupational in origin. For example, lung cancer may be caused by smoking, air pollution (although not definitely established), occupational or nonoccupational radiation exposure, or all of these factors.

Suppose that a worker with lung cancer has smoked cigarettes, has had diagnostic x-rays, and has also been occupationally exposed to ionizing radiation in a uranium mine. Because occupational lung cancer does not have distinctive clinical features, an expert medical witness, using clinical judgment, cannot say that the disease is, without question, occupational in origin—although he or she may be able to say that, more likely than not, it is a cause of the lung cancer. In this case, the legal standard is that there must be a *preponderance of evidence* that the disease is occupational in origin, or the case is unlikely to be settled in favor of the disabled worker. A *preponderance of evidence* means that it is more likely than not (probability greater than 50 percent) that the illness in question was caused by, aggravated by, or hastened by workplace exposure.

In some cases, workers' compensation laws have been written so that payment of a claim may be denied even though convincing evidence is presented that the illness was caused by or aggravated by the worker's employment. Some states require that a disease not be "an ordinary disease of life." In other words, diseases such as emphysema and hearing loss may not be compensable because they often occur among people with no occupational exposure. More than 20 states have a related requirement that diseases are only compensable if they are "peculiar to" or "characteristic of" a worker's occupation.

All jurisdictions have a statute of limitations (often 1 or 2 years) for workers' compensation claims. A 2-year statute of limitation means that the worker must file the claim within 2 years of a given event. A time limit of 2 years after the worker has learned that a disease is work-related imposes no particular hardship on occupational disease victims. In some states, however, the time period begins when the disease becomes symptomatic, even if this takes place before the disease is diagnosed or determined to be work-related. The latter policy for starting the statute of limitations may be a special problem if the worker's physician is not familiar with the occupational disease. The most burdensome statutes require that a claim be filed 1 or 2 years after exposure. Because chronic occupational diseases commonly do not manifest themselves until 5, 10, 20, or more years after exposure, such rules effectively eliminate the possibility of compensation for workers with these illnesses. Time limits in some states for filing workers' compensation claims are described in Table 4-7.

The Problem of Compromise Settlements

A workers' compensation claim that is denied by the employer or insurer does not automatically go to a hearing. The injured worker must first find a lawyer who will take the case. The lawyer's fee is often based on the portion of the award attributed to lost wages, which means that the lawyer's fee will be small in a small award and that the lawyer will receive nothing if the claim is denied. Thus, it is difficult for injured or ill workers to find lawyers to represent them when claims are small or success is unlikely.

TABLE 4-7

Time Limits on Filing Occupational Disease Claims in Selected Jurisdictions (As of January 1, 2003)

Jurisdiction	Time Limit on Claim Filing
Alabama	Within 2 years after injury, death, or last payment. Radiation: within 2 years after disability or death and claimant knows or should know relation to employment. Radiation or pneumoconiosis: exposure during at least 12 months over 5 years prior to last exposure.
California	Disability: within 1 year from injury or last payment. Death: within 1 year after death (for death within 1 year after injury), 1 year after last medical payment, or 1 year after death if no compensation paid and in no case more than 240 weeks after injury, except for asbestos-related disease claims. Date of injury is defined as when claimant is disabled and knows or should know of relation to employment.
Massachusetts	Within 4 years of diagnosis or knowledge of relation to employment.
Michigan	Within 2 years after the claimant knows or should know relation to employment.
New York	Within 2 years after disability or death, and within 2 years after the claimant knows or should know relation to employment
North Carolina	Within 2 years after final disability determination or death. Within 6 years after death from an occupational disease.
Oregon	Within 1 year of the latest of worker's discovery of the disease, onset of disability, physician diagnosis, or beneficiaries' discovery that death was caused by occupational disease.
Utah	Within 6 years after cause of action arose but no later than 1 year after death. Notification must be given to employer or Industrial Commission within 180 days of this date.
Virginia	Within 2 years after diagnosis is first communicated to worker or within 5 years after exposure, whichever is first; within 3 years after death, occurring during a period of disability.
Federal employees	Within 3 years after injury, death, or disability and claimant knows or should know relation to employment; delay excusable.
U.S. longshore	Within 2 years of knowledge of relation to employment or 1 year after last payment.

Source: 2003 Analysis of workers' compensation laws, prepared and published by the U.S. Chamber of Commerce. (The full report may be ordered at 1-800-638-6582.) Reprinted with permission.

A settlement reached outside the courtroom is called a compromise settlement because the amount paid to the injured worker generally is a compromise between the maximum and minimum amounts that the worker could receive in a court decision.

In the face of protracted litigation with uncertain results, a compromise settlement may seem very attractive to an injured worker who may have no wage income for a considerable period and may be facing large medical bills. The injured worker may therefore prefer a small settlement paid immediately to a much larger, but uncertain, settlement that would not be available for 1 or 2 years. Especially where the worker does not foresee a quick return to work, a settlement may be accepted that might seem quite small to an outside observer. Insurers may use their

knowledge of the financial pressures on the injured worker to obtain a small settlement; they will thus contest, delaying the time when the case is closed in the hope of obtaining a small compromise settlement.

The compromise settlement will usually be paid in a lump sum to the injured worker and the attorney. This lump-sum settlement will take the place of future payments for lost earnings and medical and rehabilitation costs. Many compromise settlements also release the insurer from future liability: If the worker's condition should change at a later date or if future medical needs or increased costs were inadequately estimated, the insurer would not incur the costs of any increased disability or medical or rehabilitation expenses. The injured worker who has accepted a *compromise and release* settlement may later need additional medical care but not have the resources to pay for that care.

For example, a worker with a back injury was denied compensation by his employer, who claimed that the injury was not work-related. He then took action that led to his being offered a lump-sum settlement:

> I went to my union representative and filled out the forms for the industrial accident board, and about 3 weeks later they sent me an award which was about $600 . . . and I wouldn't take it. But then I applied for an attorney and talked to my attorney, and then filed suit. They turned around and told my attorney that they would consider [the injury] an industrial accident. So, I never did go to court. All they did was talk to my lawyer. They settled out of court. My lawyer told me while I was in the hospital that they wanted to settle it for $7,500. The fee for him [would be] $2,500.*

If the settlement of $7,500 was the result of a compromise and release agreement, the insurer or employer will not be liable for any future disability or medical costs resulting from this injury.

Recommendations of the National Commission

As part of the Occupational Safety and Health Act of 1970, Congress established the National Commission on State Workmen's Compensation Laws to "undertake a comprehensive study and evaluation of state workmen's compensation laws in order to determine if such laws provide an adequate, prompt, and equitable system of compensation." In 1972, the commission released its report, which described many problems of workers' compensation and made recommendations for improving state workers' compensation systems. This report, still relevant today, included these seven "essential" recommendations:

1. Compulsory coverage: Employees could not lose coverage by agreeing to waive their rights to benefits.
2. No occupational or numerical exemptions to coverage: All workers, including agricultural and domestic workers, should be covered, and all employers, even if they have only one employee, should be covered.

3. Full coverage of work-related diseases: Elimination of arbitrary barriers to coverage, such as highly restrictive time limits, occupational disease schedules, and exclusion of "ordinary diseases of life."
4. Full medical and physical rehabilitation services without arbitrary limits.
5. Employees' choice of jurisdiction for filing interstate claims.
6. Adequate weekly cash benefits for temporary total disability, permanent total disability, and fatal cases.
7. No arbitrary limits on duration or sum of benefits.

When this report was issued, some federal legislators threatened to establish federal minimum standards for state workers' compensation programs or to supersede them with a national program. In the 1970s and 1980s, many states changed their statutes to follow some or all of the recommendations of the National Commission. By increasing coverage and raising benefits, they substantially improved the value of workers' compensation to injured employees. However, this trend ended in the 1990s, and, in fact, some states have moved backwards during the 1990s,[1] Moreover, general changes in coverage have done little to discourage the litigation of occupational disease claims and costly occupational injury claims.

Alternatives to U.S. Workers' Compensation Systems

Other countries have workers' compensation systems with considerably less controversy surrounding compensation for occupational diseases (Box 4-2). These countries have social programs that provide medical benefits and disability benefits that are substantially greater than those provided to many American workers. Thus, a worker who does not receive workers' compensation still can pay for needed medical care and continue to help support the family through disability payments. Countries with national health systems, such as Great Britain and Sweden, provide universal medical care whether or not illnesses are occupational; Belgium and Denmark have excellent social insurance and disability programs, providing a significant amount of wage replacement for disabled workers, whether or not disability is work-related.

Adapted from Subcommittee on Labor, Committee on Labor, and Public Welfare, U.S. Senate. Hearings on the National Workers' Compensation Standards Act, 1974. Statement of Lawrence Barefield.

BOX 4-2

Another North American System: Workers' Compensation in British Columbia*

Canadian workers' compensation systems are administered at the provincial level, just as most workers' compensation systems in the United States are state systems. The workers' compensation system in British Columbia is similar to U.S. systems in states with exclusive state funds. The Workers' Compensation Board (WCB) of British Columbia is the only organization allowed to offer workers' compensation insurance to employers in that province.

The British Columbia workers' compensation system offers the same types of benefits to injured workers as systems in the United States: temporary and permanent disability benefits, fatality benefits for survivors, medical benefits, and vocational rehabilitation benefits. Benefits to replace lost wages are high compared with most U.S. jurisdictions. This is, in part, because maximum benefits are high. Also, British Columbia has no waiting period for wage-replacement benefits; in contrast, U.S. jurisdictions have waiting periods ranging from 3 to 7 days. Therefore, more workers are paid wage-replacement benefits in British Columbia than in the United States.

British Columbia provides payments through its Medical Services Plan to cover health care for all its citizens. Yet the workers' compensation system pays the medical expenses of injured workers. Providers are paid fees that are 10 percent higher than those in the private sector, to cover the additional paperwork required by the workers' compensation system.

Four separate organizations within the Ministry of Labour and Consumer Services administer the workers' compensation act. The WCB provides insurance and administers the payment of claims. The Workers' Compensation Review Board (WCRB) adjudicates disputed claims, as do workers' compensation commissions and industrial

accident boards in the United States. Two other agencies provide services that generally have no parallel in U.S. systems. (Oddly, the Appeals Division of the WCB can review decisions of the WCRB.) The Workers' Advisers Office (WAO) helps workers to bring claims and may represent them before the WCB or WCRB. The WAO also trains union personnel to represent their members in disputed claims. The Employers' Advisers Office (EAO) provides similar services to employers. An ombudsman in the WCB responds to complaints. In addition, outside the Ministry of Labour and Consumer Services, the Ombudsman of British Columbia responds to complaints and provides oversight of other agencies.

The WAO, the EAO, and the Ombudsman of British Columbia have no counterpart in U.S. workers' compensation jurisdictions, although some workers' compensation agencies in the United States do provide information about the law to workers and employers. These agencies reflect a less litigious approach to workers' compensation, an approach that makes British Columbia's appeals rate similar to those in the least litigious U.S. states. Compared with U.S. jurisdictions, British Columbia has many fewer appealed claims. In 1994, workers or employers appealed only 4 percent of new claims filed, or 11 percent of claims with lost wages in British Columbia. In Wisconsin, a low-litigation state, 10 percent of claims with lost wages involve a request for hearing. This rate is 10 percent in North Carolina, 19 percent in Pennsylvania, 25 percent in Georgia, 42 percent in California, and 43 percent in Missouri.

In 1994, 74 percent of workers in appealed claims were represented, primarily by the WAO or union. It is likely that most of the unrepresented workers had consulted with their unions, the WAO, or somebody else prior to their hearings. Virtually all U.S. workers with appealed claims hire attorneys. This difference between the British Columbia system and the U.S. systems is probably produced in part by the availability of assistance from the WAO and the EAO. A study of the British Columbia system suggests that another reason is "the strong posture in the Act and by the WCB that it should administer the law in an inquiry, rather than an adversarial, manner."

Unless otherwise noted, the source of the information presented here is Hunt HA, Barth PS, Leahy MJ. The workers' compensation system of British Columbia: Still in transition. Kalamazoo: W.E. Upjohn Institute for Employment Research, 1996.

(continued)

BOX 4-2

Another North American System: Workers' Compensation in British Columbia (Continued)

Another interesting feature of the British Columbia workers' compensation system is the Medical Review Panel (MRP). When a medical issue is in dispute, a worker or employer can appeal that issue to an MRP. The provincial government (with advice from the British Columbia College of Physicians and Surgeons) appoints and keeps a list of private physicians who can chair panels. Chairs are chosen sequentially from this list. When a physician's name comes up, that physician is chosen to head a panel. The chair then sends the worker and employer a list of specialists in relevant disciplines from which they can each choose one. This panel of three physicians sees the worker, reads relevant records, and can order additional medical testing. The decision of the panel on medical issues is binding; it cannot be appealed. This feature probably would not survive a legal challenge in the United States. A Massachusetts law that established medical referees that could issue binding opinions was overturned in the Massachusetts state court because it limited the parties' access to appeals and therefore to due process (Meunier's Case, 319 Mass. 421, 66 N.E. 2d 198 [1946]).

Medical payments are much lower in the British Columbia workers' compensation system than in U.S. systems. In 1994, medical payments were 39 percent of all workers' compensation benefits in the United States[1]; in that year, they were 28 percent of all benefits paid in British Columbia. The reason for this is not clear. It may reflect generally lower Canadian medical costs. Perhaps higher litigation rates in the United States lead to more medical care or reduce the effectiveness of medical care, thus leading to greater use. Also, this ratio may be lower in British Columbia because wage-replacement benefits are higher there.

In British Columbia, unlike U.S. jurisdictions, the workers' compensation agency has authority to develop and enforce workplace safety and health regulations. WCB inspectors can require correction of hazards, recommend penalties, or issue 24-hour closure orders where imminent dangers exist. For firms above a certain size and hazard level, the law in British Columbia requires occupational health and safety programs, including labor–management health and safety committees. WCB inspectors review these programs, decide whether they are adequate, and provide advice on improving them.[2]

REFERENCES

1. National Academy of Social Insurance. Workers' compensation: Benefits, coverage, and costs, 1994–95: New estimates. Washington, DC: NASI, 1997.
2. Rest KM, Ashford NA. Occupational health and safety in British Columbia: An administrative inventory of the prevention activities of the Workers' Compensation Board. Cambridge, Mass.: Ashford Associates, 1997.

Because national medical care systems in these countries cover costs that might otherwise be paid by workers' compensation, they provide a medical "safety net" for victims of occupational disease. Still, in these countries, workers' compensation may not provide benefits for many occupational disease claims. As in the United States, physicians do not identify occupational diseases, workers are unaware of their exposures to workplace hazards, and, when they are, they find that exposures are difficult to document. Also, legislation and regulation may be restrictive in covering occupational diseases.[8]

SOCIAL SECURITY DISABILITY INSURANCE AND SUPPLEMENTAL SECURITY INSURANCE

Social Security Disability Insurance (SSDI) is a federal insurance program: workers contribute to it through a payroll tax, and their benefit amount will be based on the amount they contribute. Disabled workers may also apply for and receive SSDI benefits during the same period in which they receive workers' compensation benefits.*

---

* *The Social Security laws provide that a worker cannot receive more than 80 percent of his or her preinjury earnings, including workers' compensation benefits.*

To be eligible for workers' compensation benefits, the worker must:

- be under 65 years of age,
- have worked in covered Social Security employment for an adequate amount of time, and
- currently have a qualifying disability (or, if the worker has recovered, the period of disability must have lasted at least 12 months and ended less than 12 months before he or she applied for benefits).

To establish eligibility for benefits, a worker must obtain medical certification of disability. Particular weight is given to the opinion of the treating physician in the Social Security program, especially when the opinion is supported by medically acceptable diagnostic techniques and is not in conflict with other evidence. Primary care physicians who are knowledgeable about the process may therefore have important impact on the outcome for the patient.

For the purposes of the SSDI program, disability means that the worker is unable to engage in substantial gainful activity as a result of severe, medically determinable physical or mental impairment that has lasted or can be expected to last for at least 1 year or that will result in death. The worker must be unable to do not only his or her previous job but also any other substantial gainful activity that is available in the national economy. Individuals with severe impairments who have only marginal education and have worked exclusively in jobs involving unskilled physical labor will almost always be considered disabled for the purposes of this program. A person who is currently employed is obviously not eligible for benefits. The extent of disability that is required for eligibility for SSDI benefits is considerably more severe, therefore, than the extent required for eligibility for temporary total or permanent partial disability benefits from workers' compensation programs.

Physicians may determine disability by relying on the patient's history and description of symptoms, including pain. Ultimately, a designated state agency will make the eligibility determination, including an evaluation as to whether the patient's description of symptoms are consistent with the medical signs and laboratory and other diagnostic findings.

The Social Security Administration has documents on the Internet that describe the disability determination process and how disability evaluations are done. Several of these can be found at <http://www.ssa.gov/disability/professionals/publications.htm>. One publication, "Disability Evaluation Under Social Security," also known as the "Blue Book," describes the disability evaluation process and provides information about the information needed in medical reports to establish the degree of disability. It also lists specific impairments, by organ system, that are considered severe enough to lead to a determination of total disability. An individual lacking such impairments may, however, still be eligible for SSDI benefits because that person has other totally disabling problems. Some people with less severe impairments may still qualify for SSDI benefits because their impairments combined with their age, education, and labor market experience combine to make them unable to engage in substantial gainful activity. For example, a physical impairment that might allow a physician to continue working might be much more disabling for a 60-year-old manual laborer with a fourth-grade education.

SSDI is considerably different from workers' compensation programs. Eligibility for SSDI benefits does not require that any impairment be caused by the patient's work. Eligibility may be based on the patient's total disability resulting from a combination of impairments; physicians therefore should document all health problems of the patient, not just those that are job-related. This creates a record-keeping problem for those patients who have filed simultaneous claims for workers' compensation and SSDI, as only the occupational injury–related records should be made available in any litigation over workers' compensation eligibility.

Disabled people who are very poor may qualify for Supplemental Security Income (SSI) benefits. The determination of disability status is the same as for the SSDI program. However, eligibility is not based on payment of Social Security. Instead, SSI is a need-based program based on demonstration of both poverty and disability. Most workers who are severely disabled from occupational injury or disease will meet the requirements of the SSDI program and will not need to meet the need-based requirements of the SSI program.

ENVIRONMENTAL AND OCCUPATIONAL TOXIC TORT LITIGATION

The Industrial Revolution that began in the 19th century was a revolution in mass production. Much of this involved the manufacture and sale of products containing hazardous materials with little or no investigation into the risks they posed to the health and safety of workers, consumers, or others who might be exposed to these products. Concurrent with this industrialization was the growth of the chemical industry and the innovation of synthetics. There was use of lead in many products, including paint and gasoline; widespread use of asbestos, and incorporation of many chemicals into manufacturing processes and end products. As a result, there has been significant dispersion of toxic chemicals into the workplace, ambient, and home environments.

The Development of Environmental and Toxic Tort Litigation

Environmental litigation for personal injuries was largely unknown for most of the 20th century. This was due in large part because general legal assumptions about injury and causation did not fit the circumstances of environmental and toxic injuries. In the mid to late 1960s, advances in medical knowledge about the effects of exposure to toxins changed the courts' understanding of these kinds of injuries and allowed for the development of environmental and toxic tort litigation.

Prior to this time, there were multiple legal barriers to lawsuits for environmental and toxic tort injuries. First, under the common law, the courts generally required that there be a *privity relationship* (a direct connection) between the defendant (the party allegedly causing injury) and the injured party. Because injuries from environmental exposures rarely arose in such contexts, claims for these injuries were barred for lack of privity. In addition, the *statute of limitations* (the period of time in which an injured party must initiate a civil action), as it then existed, did not anticipate these kinds of injuries. It generally began at the time of exposure, which was then considered to be the time of injury. However, unlike traumatic injury, in which impact and injury occur simultaneously, exposures to environmental toxins often do not manifest injury until years after exposure. Thus, claims for injuries from environmental exposure were often time-barred long before the injury had become manifest. Finally, the concept of legal causation, as it then existed, did not allow for these kinds of claims. During this period, an injured party often was required to prove that the toxic exposure was the sole cause of the injury. However, unlike traumatic injury, in which an injury arose from a solitary event, such as a broken

leg from an automobile crash, proof of injury from chemical or toxic exposure was not so obvious. Often, these environmental injuries resulted from prolonged exposure to a variety of products or other circumstances, any one of which could be sufficient to cause the injury, leaving a worker or bystander incapable of proving which actually caused the injury. Thus, claims for injuries from environmental exposure were uncompensated because defendants argued that injured parties could not prove that their products were the cause in fact of injuries, or alternatively could not prove how much of each injury was caused by that defendant.

Advances in medicine during this period, including a better understanding of the long-term and synergistic effects of exposure to environmental and occupational toxins, led to modifications and adaptations of these barriers to recovery. The most notable development occurred in the context of asbestos exposure and disease. Asbestos, a naturally occurring mineral that is incombustible, was widely used for many years in insulation and fireproofing materials in many workplaces. Asbestos is also a potent carcinogen with a long latency period between exposure and the onset of disease. The asbestos industry knew for decades of its hazardous properties but chose not to warn the public, thus exposing millions of people. The seminal case confronting the environmental effects of asbestos and the illogical legal barriers to recovery was decided in Texas in 1973 (Borel v. Fibreboard, 493 F.2d 1076, 5th Cir. 1973). In the wake of this and other cases decided at about this time, the barriers of access to the courts largely fell and the standards for prosecution of such cases were established. Privity was abolished. The statute of limitations was reinterpreted to begin, not at the date of exposure, but when the injured person knew or should have known of the injury or disease. Finally, injured parties no longer had to prove that a toxic exposure was the sole cause of the injury or disease; rather, they only had to show that the exposure was a substantial contributing cause of the injury or disease.

The Elements of Proof in Environmental and Toxic Tort Claims

The basis for liability in any environmental or toxic tort case will depend on the circumstances of the case. In cases in which exposure occurs because of a product, the theories of liability known as *products liability* generally apply. In cases in which exposure occurs because of contamination of the environment, such as the contamination of groundwater, soil, or air, the theories of liability in environmental law generally apply.

Products-Liability Claims

Environmental or toxic tort injuries litigated in the products-liability setting usually arise when someone is exposed to and injured by a pollutant or hazardous substance that is contained in, or is part of, a manufactured product.

In an environmental or toxic tort claim for products liability, an injured person may proceed under a theory of negligence or under a theory of strict products liability. In the case of negligence, the injured person must prove that:

- The manufacturer or seller of the product owed a duty to exercise reasonable care;
- The manufacturer breached that duty (failed to exercise reasonable care);
- The person was exposed to and injured by the product as a result of the manufacturer's or seller's failure to exercise reasonable care; and
- The person has suffered damages as a result of that exposure and injury.

In the case of strict products liability, the first two elements of the negligence claim are essentially satisfied by proof that the product was "unreasonably dangerous." In other words, the focus of the strict products liability case is less on the manufacturer or seller's conduct and more on the condition of the product. However, the distinction becomes somewhat semantic because both require proof of what dangers inherent in a product, such as toxins, were known or knowable by the industry at the time of sale.

The role of physicians and scientists is essential in environmental and toxic tort cases. Often, these cases can only be proved by reference to the scientific literature and the testimony of treating physicians and expert witnesses. These cases are very different from traumatic injury cases, in which cause and effect occur simultaneously and can be readily observed. Injury from environmental and toxic exposures is usually far more insidious and complicated. Causation in toxic cases is often less obvious because there frequently is a long latency period between start of exposure and manifestation of disease. Moreover, with a few no-

table exceptions, such as asbestosis and mesothelioma, most diseases from toxic exposure are not *pathognomonic*—the presence of the disease does not definitely point to cause. Thus, medical judgments must not only be made concerning the diagnosis but also concerning causation.

Effective proof in an environmental or toxic tort case will therefore often require the participation of a variety of medical and scientific professionals, frequently including treating physicians, pathologists, toxicologists, specialists in occupational or environmental medicine, epidemiologists, and those in allied fields. The need for and role of these professionals is required because medical and scientific issues tend to permeate every aspect of these cases. For example, in a case of exposure to hazardous fumes in a work environment, the plaintiff may have to prove that:

- Hazardous nature of the product was known or knowable at the time of exposure;
- Dose and duration of the plaintiff's exposure was sufficient to cause disease;
- The plaintiff has the type of disease associated with exposure to that substance;
- Even after consideration of other factors in his or her history, the exposure probably contributed to the development of the disease; and
- The plaintiff has some impairment or loss as a result of the disease.

One can observe that an occupational medicine physician might be needed to establish general knowledge about the toxicity of the product, an industrial hygienist might be needed to measure or model exposure, an epidemiologist might be needed to testify about the causal association between a specific exposure and a specific disease, and the treating physician might be needed to apply this general knowledge to the specific medical history of the worker.

Environmental Injuries and Tort Claims

Environmental and toxic tort claims also arise in settings that do not involve products. They are typically circumstances in which person or property has been damaged because of the presence of hazardous or toxic substances in the immediate environment. In the late 1960s, the effects of decades of industrial waste disposal practices began to emerge in the form of groundwater contamination. As residential growth crossed paths with industrialization, contamination of water supply sources became a major public heath issue. Ironically, resort to civil action in the courtrooms was triggered not by well-known dumping practices or reporting of contaminants by the EPA but often by unusual patterns or clustering of serious illness. The most well-known case of this type involved the alleged poisoning of children from tainted groundwater in Woburn, Massachusetts.

In 1982, 16 families from Woburn filed a lawsuit alleging that cases of leukemia and other illnesses resulted from contamination of drinking water wells. Plaintiffs further alleged that two major defendants disposed of toxic chemicals, including trichloroethylene (TCE) and tetrachloroethylene, that ultimately reached potable water supplies consumed by the families. The challenge to the families in the Woburn case was to present to lay jury members the scientific evidence of groundwater contamination and its adverse health effects in terms that they could understand.

Perhaps the most important lesson from the Woburn case was the enormous difficulty and complexity in proving a groundwater contamination case. The families had to show that the two companies negligently dumped TCE and other toxic solvents that eventually entered groundwater, migrated to city wells, and caused childhood leukemia. Although the jury found that one of the companies had negligently contaminated the drinking water wells, it also found that the contamination occurred after some of the children developed leukemia. Before the trial continued to the question of medical causation, the parties settled with this company, motivated largely by the uncertainty of establishing causation in light of the jury's prior findings. The partial trial lasted months, cost the families millions of dollars, and involved the testimony of numerous witnesses.

The Woburn case is not unique. Similar lawsuits across the United States include (a) the contamination of Anniston, Alabama, where more than 22,000 people brought suit for damages caused by 40 years of dumping polychlorinated biphenyls (PCBs) by a chemical manufacturer; and (b) widespread contamination of groundwater caused by methyl *tert*-butyl ether (MTBE) that leaked from underground storage tanks in gas stations and elsewhere.

Medical and scientific experts play key roles in these cases, such as in assessing the concentration and duration of exposure. As the Woburn case demonstrated, these experts must also establish the pathways of such exposures. These experts often perform complex modeling and health assessment of the potentially affected community. Ultimately, experts render opinions, based on review of exposure, health effects, and other data.

Lawsuits Against "Third Parties"

Although workers' compensation systems bar workers from suing their employers at common law for negligently caused injuries (those caused by a breach of the duty to use reasonable care), there is no such bar applicable to suits against third parties. Not surprisingly, workers and their lawyers have sought substantial additional damages from a variety of third parties—entities other than the employer. Most commonly, people involved in automobile crashes at work have sued the drivers of the other vehicles. In addition, people have frequently sued manufacturers of equipment or substances that contributed to or caused their injuries. For example, workers injured by faulty machinery at work have sued manufacturers of the machinery. Similarly, workers whose lung disease or cancer is related to workplace exposure to asbestos have successfully sued asbestos manufacturers.

These lawsuits always require that the worker show that the third party was negligent—the mere fact of the injury is never enough. In the case of third-party manufacturers of equipment, this negligence is tied to the failure to warn the users of the product (including the injured worker and, in some cases, his or her employer) regarding the safe handling or use of the dangerous machinery or substances. Other third parties who have sometimes been found liable to workers for events surrounding workplace injuries range from workers' compensation insurance carriers (for bad faith dealings regarding the handling of claims or for negligent safety inspections of the workplace) to the Occupational Safety and Health Administration (OSHA; for failing to cite a flagrant workplace safety hazard). Employers have also sometimes been sued—with varying success—by workers who claimed that their employers were not wearing the "employer hat" when the injury occurred. These lawsuits have involved a wide variety of situations, including when employers made or substantially altered the equipment causing the injury or when employers have negligently provided medical services to employees.

Differences Between Lawsuits and Workers' Compensation Claims

It is not surprising that workers attempt to pursue common-law litigation instead of, or in addition to, workers' compensation claims. Although workers' compensation covers medical care and vocational rehabilitation costs and a fraction of lost earnings, a successful lawsuit will provide full recovery of lost earnings, cover medical care and rehabilitation, pay an additional amount for "pain and suffering," and may pay other benefits as well, including in some instances punitive damages. A successful lawsuit can provide benefits that are many times those of a successful workers' compensation claim. Moreover, filing a workers' compensation claim does not preclude filing a lawsuit against a third party.

But the barriers to successful litigation of lawsuits are also high. Injured workers must prove in most cases that the defendant was negligent; the no-fault rules of workers' compensation do not apply. Lawsuits are tried in the regular civil courts rather than in specialized workers' compensation administrative courts. Trials in the civil courts are conducted under much more stringent rules of evidence, and proceedings tend to be much longer and require much more work by attorneys. Unlike workers' compensation claims, these cases cannot be pursued without a lawyer.

Challenges to Expert Testimony in Environmental and Toxic Tort Cases

Physicians and research scientists are essential witnesses to show causality (that the chemical in question actually caused the disease) in environmental and toxic tort cases. For example, a patient who believes that contaminated groundwater caused his or her cancer must be able to prove with medical and scientific evidence that the contamination caused or significantly contributed to the cause of the cancer, even after accounting for genetics, lifestyle, and bad luck. In order to prove causation, treating physicians and research scientists provide their expert opinions about the cause of the patient's disease.

Expert opinions of physicians and scientists often are decisive in these kinds of cases and, as such, the admissibility of those opinions is often strongly contested. Until 1993, judges relied on a simple standard to determine the admissibility of medical and scientific testimony: whether the evidence was relevant and whether the science itself, including methods, theories, and the scientist's training, was "generally accepted" by the scientific community (Frye *v*. United States, 293 F. 1013 [1923]). The requirement that science be "generally accepted" had the effect of preventing new scientific methods or new facts about the causes of human disease from being used in the courtroom.

In 1993, the U.S Supreme Court changed the manner in which judges decide whether scientific evidence and expert testimony can be used in court. In a case called Daubert *v*. Merrell Dow Pharmaceuticals, Inc., two children with birth defects and their parents sued the manufacturer of the drug Bendectin alleging that the antinausea medication used during pregnancy caused the children's birth defects. The scientific literature indicated that the drug was safe for maternal use. The plaintiffs' experts, however, examined *in vitro* studies, animal studies, and reanalyzed and recalculated the published data on Bendectin and found that Bendectin did, in fact, cause birth defects. The trial court rejected the plaintiffs' experts' opinions because they were not "generally accepted" scientific methods under the Frye standard. In Daubert, the U.S Supreme Court replaced the "generally accepted" standard with a much more flexible analysis of whether the medical opinion and scientific evidence are based on a reliable scientific methodology.

Under the Daubert approach, a physician's opinion may be admitted as evidence if it is based on a reliable scientific methodology. The determination takes into account: (1) whether the subject matter of the science can be, and has been, tested; (2) whether the science has been subjected to peer review and publication; (3) whether there is a known or potential rate of error and the existence of standards controlling a technique's operation; and (4) whether the theory or technique is widely accepted in the field. These are factors for the judge to consider, but the standard is not meant to be used as a checklist. The rationale for such a standard is to allow the judge more flexibility to keep out unreliable science but to allow for new medical and scientific theories into evidence, which may be reliable and well founded but not yet published or widely recognized.

Today in toxic tort cases, industry defendants attempt to discredit the plaintiff's scientific evidence before the trial by arguing that it does not meet the Daubert standard. This is known as a Daubert challenge. Typically, industry defendants challenge the medical and scientific evidence by arguing that the differential diagnosis was unreliable and cannot be proved, the physician was not up-to-date on current literature, the test or study design was flawed, the statistics were bad, and the experts were not well qualified. The challenge takes place during pretrial motions, briefs, and a hearing where the parties argue extensively about whether the science meets the Daubert criteria.

Physician or research scientists whose opinions are challenged under Daubert must be able to explain to the court the scientific methods that they employed to reach their opinion. They may be based on some type of instrument, test, examination, clinical observation, or other generally reliable method of analysis.

The trial judge's role in the Daubert challenge is not to determine whether the jury should believe the expert testimony but rather to determine if the expert testimony is reliable science that will assist the jury in deciding questions of fact at the trial. The judge's discretion as to which medical and scientific evidence is "good enough" for the jury has made challenges to the admissibility of scientific evidence much more common and has made it more difficult for injured people to have their day in court. The judge's rejection of medical opinions frequently ends the litigation, as it is virtually impossible for plaintiffs to proceed if the judge decides the necessary medical or scientific evidence cannot be used at trial.

JOB SECURITY FOR WORKERS

When workers become injured or sick, they confront three important challenges. First, those who cannot work need to find a source of income to replace the temporary or permanent loss of wages. Second, injured workers need health care and assistance in paying for that care. Third, injured workers need protection of their legal rights to jobs—the focus of this section.

This is a complicated arena. People without severe health impairments generally want to continue working or, if their work was interrupted, to return to work. An injured worker may or may not be physically capable of returning to the preinjury job or the job may have been filled and no longer be available. If the old job is unavailable, he or she may seek a different job with the same employer or a new job with a new employer. Social and private insurance benefits may be limited in both quantity and duration. Keeping or finding a job is critical to the patient's economic and physical well-being.

Physicians become key players in this process. Employers, insurers, and workers look to physicians to determine eligibility for benefits, as well as a worker's ability to return to work and what work he or she can perform. Employers may informally rely on physicians to assess the ability of an employee to perform a job. In addition, a wide range of critical employment laws rely on physicians as gatekeepers—in ways that may be contrary to the traditional physician–patient relationship.

Under these laws, the physician is called upon to assess the capability of the individual to work and the risks of certifying the individual for work. These decisions can be complex. For example, if a physician certifies an individual's ability to work, this may result in the termination of workers' compensation or other wage replacement benefits. Has a job been offered? Is the individual going to be able to perform the job? If not, the patient may be left without benefits and without wage income.

Despite the laws that provide job protection for disabled workers, many working people are vulnerable to employer retaliation and discrimination. Individuals with health impairments have difficulty both in keeping their old jobs and finding new ones.

Basic Regulation of Employment

Patients are often deeply aware of the practices of the employers with whom they are dealing. Workers' own sense of job security will affect the ways in which they, as patients, will act regarding issues that affect the physician–patient relationship:

- Whether they will raise concerns to an employer regarding hazards;
- Whether they will tell an employer that they suffer from health impairments;
- Whether they will file for workers' compensation benefits;
- Whether they will seek (or avoid) a return to work, either at a regular or light duty job; and
- Whether they will authorize release of medical information to their employers.

The *employment-at-will* doctrine is at the core of the U.S. legal code governing private-sector employment. Under this doctrine, employers may discharge or discipline an employee without articulating a reason—and an employee can quit without notice. This is most often described as the right of an employer to discharge someone for a good reason, a bad reason, or no reason at all. As a practical matter, this also means that an employer may change the specific elements of the bargain with a worker without notice: if the employee continues to work, he or she is generally deemed to have accepted the new terms.

In the pure application of the doctrine (as it existed in the early 20th century), an employer could legally discharge an employee because of any stigma or prejudice or because the employee was unproductive, too old, disabled, African American, an immigrant, a woman, or simply because the employer disliked the employee. This is no longer true. The terms of this at-will "agreement" can be, and have been, modified by legislation, judicial decisions, individual and union contracts, and public-sector employment rules. Nevertheless, the at-will doctrine remains the default rule for private employment in almost every American jurisdiction. If there is no specific applicable exception to the rule, then the default rule applies and the employee is legally unprotected.

In addition to this basic private-sector employment rule, a patient's general legal rights at work are affected by three key factors.

First, does he or she work in the private or the public sector? By and large, public-sector employees (comprising about 21,800,000 U.S. workers in early 2005, 16.4 percent of the nonfarm workforce) are protected by civil service and other rules that may provide legal protections. These protections, which generally provide a broader range of rights to employees than those available under the at-will doctrine, range from specific entitlements under insurance programs to general protections against discharge.

Second, is his or her workplace unionized? Workers who are covered by collective bargaining agreements have two advantages: (a) They can rely on the union to assist them in evaluating work hazards and actions of an employers; and (b) These agreements almost always provide for protections that are unavailable to private-sector workers who are not covered by union contracts. Collective bargaining agreements set wages and benefits (includ-ing health insurance), establish progressive disciplinary procedures, require employers to have "just cause" to discipline or terminate an employee, and establish rights to job allocation and retention based, at least in part, on seniority.

Third, where does the patient live and work? Basic employment protections and the health of the general labor market, both of which vary from state to state, affect attitudes of patients and employers.

Employees have differing views regarding their job security, which will also affect their behavior. They may know the past behavior of their employers with regard to other employees who have been in similar situations. They may trust—or distrust—their own employers, irrespective of the relevant legal rules. In fact, employees have been found to overstate their general level of legal protection at work.[9,10]

Moreover, workers may have difficulty enforcing legal rights that do exist, and efforts to enforce their rights may put them in jeopardy due to inappropriate or illegal retaliation by employers. Legal rights are not self-executing. Enforcement of rights can be costly, time-consuming, and cumbersome and can require medical and other forms of proof. Physicians should be aware that this complex set of legal rules and attitudes justifiably influences the behaviors of their patients.

Specific Legal Protections for Disabled Workers

Eligibility for job protection under an employer-specific disability program or under any of the following disability-based laws will depend on the assessment of the physician as to whether the patient is capable of performing the work in question. In order to provide useful information to workers, employers, and agencies, physicians must understand the specific rules relevant to each wage-replacement program or disability-based law. Definitions of disability and the implications of a finding of disability or impairment vary tremendously from one program to another. Physicians must also realize that a finding that an individual is not capable of performing a particular job or particular job functions may result in adverse employment consequences for the patient.

Given the extraordinary power in the hands of physicians, more than one opinion will often be sought. For example, if the physician is the individual's treating physician, a determination regarding whether an individual is able to work may only provide the patient with a "foot in the door." Others will still have the opportunity to develop and submit alternative medical data. This adversarial process means, however, that physicians may be called upon to defend their conclusions; in order to do so, it is essential for physicians to understand the particular legal rules associated with any given program. A failure to understand the relevant rules can result in medical reports and testimony that fail to accomplish what the physician intends.

Disability Discrimination

Discrimination and exclusion from the workforce due to disabilities is a continuing problem in the U.S. labor market. Disabled workers face barriers that rest both on their special needs and on prejudice or stigma.

The Americans with Disabilities Act (ADA) and similar state laws were specifically intended to encourage employers to employ disabled workers and to provide enforceable employment rights to workers who were subjected to discrimination based on disability. Hailed as the great civil-rights advance of the late 20th century, these laws forbid discrimination by employers against individuals who currently have disabilities, are incorrectly perceived as being disabled, or have a record of disability.

To qualify for protection under these laws, people with disabilities must have "a physical or mental impairment that substantially limits one or more major life activities of an individual, as, for example, walking, talking, seeing, hearing, or caring for oneself" (42 U.S.C. 12102(2)). If the life activity at issue is the individual's ability to work, he or she must be unable to perform a class of jobs or a broad range of jobs; the inability to perform a specific job does not qualify for protection under the ADA. Temporary health problems, such as strains and sprains from workplace injuries, were never intended to qualify as disabilities under the ADA. An employer is prohibited under the ADA from refusing to hire or rehire an employee because of the worker's history of injuries or because the employer fears that the worker may manifest problems in the future, unless the future risk is more than speculative.

A qualified individual with a disability cannot be excluded from work if he or she can perform the essential functions of the job in question, with or without reasonable accommodation. Essential job functions include only the fundamental duties of the job. Employers are expected to analyze jobs in order to determine which duties are in fact essential. The fact that a job has historically included certain peripheral duties does not mean that the employer can insist that it continue to include those duties. A disabled employee may not be able to perform these essential functions without some form of accommodation. The ADA requires that employers provide "reasonable accommodation" to qualified disabled employees. The definition of reasonable accommodation is quite broad:

> (a) making existing facilities used by employees readily accessible to and usable by individuals with disabilities; and (b) job restructuring, part-time or modified work schedules, reassignment to a vacant position, acquisition or modification of equipment or devices, appropriate adjustment or modifications of examinations, training materials or policies, the provision of qualified readers or interpreters, and other similar accommodations for individuals with disabilities.

Reasonable accommodation may include modification to the work environment or to the manner in which a job is performed, elimination of nonessential tasks from a job, or transfer of the disabled worker to another vacant job that he or she can perform. The determination of the need for, and the scope of, reasonable accommodation was intended to be made through a flexible, interactive process that involves both the employer and the disabled worker. This process requires the individual assessment of the particular job and the specific limitations of the individual.

The employer can legally refuse to employ disabled persons who qualified under these definitions only if (a) the necessary accommodation would pose an "undue hardship" on the employer, or (b) the persons pose a "direct threat" to their own health and safety or that of their co-workers.

This definitional structure gave disability rights activists hope that the courts would intervene to expand the rights of disabled employees. But a series of court cases have narrowed the possibilities for legal protection for these workers.

Most importantly, individuals with impairments have found it difficult to persuade the courts that they suffer from a qualifying disability. After an initial ruling that found HIV-positive individuals to be disabled within the meaning of the Act (Bragdon *v.* Abbott, 524 U.S. 624 [1998]), the court has rejected one claim after another. For example, the U.S. Supreme Court concluded that "a person whose physical or mental impairment is corrected by medication or other measures does not have an impairment that presently 'substantially limits' a major life activity" (Sutton *v.* United Airlines, 527 U.S. 471 [1999]; Murphy *v.* United Parcel Service, 527 U.S. 516 [1999]). The result of this determination is that people with chronic diseases that are controlled with medication, such as hypertension, diabetes, and epilepsy, are not part of the class of people who qualify for protection under the ADA.

In 2002, the Supreme Court further restricted the reach of the ADA, holding that the definitional terms in the ADA "need to be interpreted strictly to create a demanding standard for qualifying as disabled" (Toyota Motor Mfg, Kentucky, Inc. *v.* Williams, 534 U.S. 184 [2002]). This case involved an individual with occupationally-related musculoskeletal impairments who claimed that she was substantially limited in performing manual tasks, housework, gardening, playing with her children, lifting, and working due to musculoskeletal injuries sustained at work. In order to qualify for protection under the ADA, the Court noted that "an individual must have an impairment that prevents or severely restricts the individual from doing activities that are of central importance to most people's daily lives" and concluded that repetitive work with hands and arms extended at or above shoulder levels for extended periods of time did not qualify automatically for protection. The decision goes even further, to suggest that an individual's impairments must be of "central importance in most people's daily lives." In this case, it was insufficient that the plaintiff's impairments "caused her to avoid sweeping, to quit dancing, to occasionally seek help dressing, and to reduce how often she plays with her children, gardens, and drive long distances."

In litigated ADA cases in the lower federal courts, judges have tended to dismiss ADA cases at a very high rate because people have been unable to prove that they are "disabled" in a legal sense.[11,12] Individuals with common occupationally caused disabilities, such as those due to musculoskeletal injuries or respiratory disorders, have faced particular resistance in the courts.[13] However, state courts in several states, including Massachusetts, California, and West Virginia, have rejected the federal interpretation of the ADA and interpret state disability laws more favorably for disabled workers. This is one illustration of employment laws varying from state to state.

Individuals who cannot meet the court's strict interpretation of the meaning of "disability" are not entitled to any protection under the ADA and may therefore be "at-will" employees with no protections at all. The result of the court cases has been to create difficult barriers for individuals with disabilities: They must show that they are sufficiently disabled to be entitled to protection while still being able to do the job. Individuals who suffer from qualifying disabilities must also be able to demonstrate that they are able perform the "essential functions" of the job, with or without "reasonable accommodation." This has frequently been characterized as the "Catch 22" of disability law: If the person is sufficiently disabled to be a member of the protected class, he or she may be viewed as too disabled to perform the job.

In addition, employers can refuse to employ a qualifying individual if he or she poses a "direct threat" to safety. Again, the regulatory language is broad, stating that the assessment must be based on individualized, objective evidence and involve a high probability of imminent and significant risk of substantial harm to the worker or to others. In determining whether to exclude a qualified individual from a job, the employer must consider the duration of the risk, the nature and severity of the potential harm, the likelihood the harm will occur, and the imminence of the potential harm. Future speculative risk, such as an underlying back condition that might worsen over a period of years, would not be sufficient to justify an individual's exclusion from a job. Employers have successfully argued, however, that there is a tension between the legal obligation to continue the employment of employees who are disabled and the obligation to provide a safe workplace for all employees, as mandated by the Occupational Safety and Health Act (OSHAct) (see Chapter 3). In Chevron U.S.A. Inc. *v.* Echazabal, 536 U.S. 73 (2002), a case involving an individual with hepatitis C who sought work in an oil refinery, the U.S. Supreme Court relied on the provisions of the OSHAct to uphold the employer's exclusion of the worker. The court noted:

> The text of OSHA itself says its point is 'to assure so far as possible every working man and woman in the Nation safe and healthful working conditions,' and Congress specifically obligated an employer to 'furnish to each of his employees employment and a place of employment which are free from recognized hazards that are causing or are likely to cause death or serious physical harm

to his employees." Although there may be an open question whether an employer would actually be liable under OSHA for hiring an individual who knowingly consented to the particular dangers the job would pose to him. . ., there is no denying that the employer would be asking for trouble: his decision to hire would put Congress's policy in the ADA, a disabled individual's right to operate on equal terms within the workplace, at loggerheads with the competing policy of OSHA, to ensure the safety of "each" and "every" worker.

Although this decision endorses the general principle that employers have an obligation to provide a safe and healthy working environment for each and every worker, it also underscores the fact that public policy does not guarantee job security to individual workers with disabilities who are at risk at work. If a worker poses substantial safety risks to self or others, and the employer does not have an open job to which the disabled worker can be reassigned, the employer may terminate the employee.

The disability discrimination statutes initially appeared to create very broad requirements for employers to accommodate the needs of disabled workers through job redesign or reassignment. Despite the narrow reading of the ADA by the courts, some disability advocates maintain that the changing treatment of disabled employees may simply not be mirrored in the visible litigation of claims but rather is lodged in changing norms that encourage employers to accommodate workers. This position is challenged by current research that strongly suggests that employment of people reporting disabilities that affect their ability to work did not rise during the economic boom of the 1990s.[14] Disability discrimination has, in fact, proved to be a remarkably intractable form of labor-market exclusion.

When these interventions are effective, the ability of disabled workers to remain in the workforce is substantially enhanced. Job accommodation has unquestionably been shown to successfully extend a worker's working life for a period of years.[15–17] To the extent that a physician can assist an employer and a worker to reach a reasonable accommodation of a patient's disability, the likelihood that the individual will continue a productive life is considerably enhanced.

Because employee rights under the ADA are rooted in analyses of the employee's health impairments and functional capacity, physicians play critical roles in determining whether an employee may be entitled to legal protection. Employees and employers call on physicians to determine whether an individual has a qualifying disability, to assess an individual's functional abilities and limitations in relation to job functions, and to evaluate whether the individual's impairment poses a direct threat to health and safety.

Workers with disabilities may be required by their employers to provide medical documentation about their disability and their ability to work. In writing a written report, the physician should be as specific as possible and should be attentive to both the patient's functional capacities and to the functional requirements of the job and the possible hazards. Physicians who treat employees will want to discuss the issues of future injury carefully with patients before supporting a patient's application to return to work.

The ADA explicitly forbids an employer from making employment decisions based on medical problems that are unrelated to the applicant's ability to perform the job in question. Preplacement physicals can only be performed after the employer has made a conditional offer of employment. An employer can require "fitness for duty" medical examinations before returning employees to work after an injury, but these examinations must be limited to job-related inquiries. If, based on medical examination, the patient/worker cannot perform the essential functions of the job, with or without reasonable accommodation, or if the patient poses a "direct threat" to self or others, then the employer may refuse to hire or rehire that individual.

Work Injuries and Job Security

If employees are not "disabled" within the meaning of the disability discrimination laws, they may have remarkably little guaranteed job security if they have been injured on the job. Many employers and employees are able to work together to reach reasonable decisions regarding when, and if, a worker should be away from work, and when he or she should return. Some employers, of course, will voluntarily provide transfers to workers who would prefer to keep working. But employers are never required to provide light- or modified-duty programs for employees with temporary disabilities.

These situations raise complex issues if there is not an agreement between the employer and employee. When injured, workers are not legally entitled to a temporary or permanent job transfer in order to accommodate a partial or temporary disability.* This means that an employee who would prefer to continue to work may be forced to seek nonwage benefits.

If the employee does leave work, the return-to-work process can be complex and confusing for the worker, the employer, and physicians. Sometimes, the individual worker wants to return, but the employer does not offer a job. In other situations, an employer may offer a job that the worker and his or her physician believe does not adequately accommodate the worker's continuing impairments. In general, workers' compensation laws make it illegal for an employer to discharge an injured worker in retaliation for filing for compensation benefits but do not provide broad protection against discharge for lengthy absences, even if the absence is the result of a compensation-related injury. Most states will require workers who are receiving temporary total disability workers' compensation benefits to return to work or lose their benefits if the employer offers them a light-duty job. The extent to which there is assurance that the job appropriately accommodates any continuing impairments varies. This can put both the worker and his or her physician in a difficult position. The refusal to take the offered position may result in termination of workers' compensation benefits; a decision to take it does not guarantee that any continuing impairments will be appropriately addressed through job accommodations.

There are a few state systems, as well as the Federal Employees' Compensation Act, in which people who receive workers' compensation benefits have a legal right to return to work after an absence for a compensable injury. In most of these states, a physician must certify that the patient is fit to return to work. Again, the physician and patient are confronted with a dilemma. If a physician notes serious functional limitations, this may ensure that

the employee will receive appropriate job accommodation. On the other hand, noting these limitations may lead to the opposite result: The lack of availability of light-duty jobs—or the refusal to provide one—may leave the patient without a job. If the patient does not qualify for protection under the disability discrimination laws, then he or she has no recourse in this situation. And even if he or she is a "qualified person with a disability," employers are not required to create light-duty jobs in order to meet their obligation to provide accommodation.

The goal, in general, is to ensure that a disabled worker continues to have an income stream, either through nonwage benefits or appropriate accommodation at work. Because of the interplay between the various laws and systems, workers can be left without either source of income, through no fault of their own.

Leaves of Absence for Employees

Workers may need to be absent from work, sometimes for extended periods, as a result of health problems that are caused by or exacerbated by their work. Larger employers often have their own disability programs, including light duty as well as short- and long-term disability insurance. In situations in which these voluntary benefits are not available, employees have some clear, albeit limited, rights to time off from work.

First, under the disability discrimination laws, a leave of absence can be considered a reasonable accommodation if the individual has a qualifying disability. This will depend on the specifics of an individual's situation. The person must have a qualifying disability and be able to perform the essential functions of the job; time away from work must not interfere with these principles. Not surprisingly, courts have held that someone who is chronically absent is not protected by the ADA because he or she cannot perform the essential functions of the job. See Moore *v.* Payless Shoe Source, Inc., 139 F.3d 1210, 1213 (8th Cir. 1998); Rogers *v.* Int'l Marine Terminals, Inc., 87 F.3d 755, 759 (5th Cir. 1996): "Because [the plaintiff] could not attend work, he [was] not a 'qualified individual with a disability' under the ADA"; coming to work regularly was an "essential function" (Carr *v.* Reno, 23 F.3d 525, 530 [D.C. Cir. 1994]).

Second, the Family and Medical Leave Act (FMLA) provides that employees who meet minimum work duration requirements and whose employers employ more than 50 employees are

---

There are exceptions to this statement. Under the Americans with Disabilities Act, qualified workers may in certain circumstances be entitled to job reassignment to a vacant position. Under the Mine Safety and Health Act, coal miners with medical evidence of pneumoconiosis may transfer to a job with guaranteed exposure to less than 1 mg of coal dust per cubic meter. Since 1977, the Mine Safety and Health Administration has had broad rights (which have not been implemented) to establish other job transfer programs for miners exposed to toxic substances or harmful physical agents. Federal regulations governing specific hazards under the Occupational Safety and Health Act require temporary (but not permanent) job reassignment. For example, the regulation governing occupational exposure to lead provides that workers with elevated blood lead levels may be entitled to a temporary transfer until their lead levels are reduced.

entitled to take 12 weeks of unpaid leave in each calendar year; the leave can be continuous or intermittent. Leave is granted if the employee needs to care for a family member with a serious health condition or if the employee needs time off because of his or her own serious health condition. The employer must guarantee reinstatement to the prior job at the end of the leave, unless the employee is a high-level manager.

Notably, the definition of a qualifying health condition under the FMLA is very different from the requirements for a qualifying disability under the ADA. A "serious health condition" requires either inpatient care or continuing treatment by a health care provider and can include conditions that are work-related. Department of Labor regulations require, when inpatient care is not involved, that the absence from work be for a period of more than 3 days in addition to requiring the continuing treatment of a health care provider. The FMLA can provide guaranteed job security for workers who are temporarily disabled by occupational injuries. This protection is separate from any benefits a worker may receive through workers' compensation and is also distinct from the prohibitions against discrimination under the ADA. Instead of providing cash benefits or extending protection against discrimination solely to those with substantial impairments, the FMLA simply guarantees that eligible employees will be guaranteed the right to return to work after an absence. Employers covered by the law are required, once the leave period is concluded, to reinstate the employee to the same or an equivalent job—that is, one in which the pay, benefits, and other terms and conditions of employment are equivalent. They are also required to maintain any preexisting health insurance coverage during the leave period.

To be eligible for a leave under the FMLA, employees must have medical certification from a health care provider that they are either unable to work at all or are unable to perform "any of the essential functions" of the position. Leave may be taken by the employee whenever "medically necessary." The employee need not, however, be so incapacitated that he or she is unable to work at all. An employee may also request intermittent leave, or a reduced work schedule, in order to accommodate planned medical treatment; the health care provider must then certify that this type of leave is medically necessary and the expected duration and schedule of the leave. Employers who want a health care provider to review an employee's ability to per-

form his or her essential job functions will have the option of describing these functions in a position description provided to the health care provider for this purpose. Failure of the patient to obtain medical certification for the leave may result in denial of the leave and, in some situations, discharge of the employee.

When Can Employees Fight Retaliatory Actions by Employers?

Not all adverse actions taken against employees are the result of employees' functional impairments or disabilities. Sometimes, workers assert that they have been retaliated against because they raised concerns about health and safety or other matters of significant concern. The procedure for challenging retaliation under the Occupational Safety and Health Act (see Chapter 3) is weak: Time limits are short, the procedure is cumbersome and controlled by the agency, and the remedy is quite limited. In keeping with the continuing viability of the employment-at-will doctrine, there is no general federal law that prohibits retaliatory discharge. In part in reaction to this vacuum, many state courts have developed remedies for individuals who assert that they have been discharged "against public policy." The exact meaning of this concept varies tremendously from one state to another. Some states have extended this concept to include situations in which workers have been discharged for activism around health and safety concerns.

The fact that a worker may have a valid legal claim against an employer's retaliatory actions does not, however, guarantee success or reinstatement to a job. It can be quite difficult to enforce these rights. Moreover, employers are rarely ordered to employ an individual, even after a lawsuit. The remedy commonly provided in successful retaliatory discharge claims is monetary compensation, not a job. In general, this monetary compensation fails to pay for the full loss of income of the worker. In fact, reinstatement to jobs is rarely ordered in any kind of employment litigation, including successful claims under the ADA.

ISSUES OF CONFIDENTIALITY AND PRIVACY

In connection with all the issues described in this chapter, physicians and other health professionals need to understand their obligations with regard to confidentiality and privacy (Box 4-3).

BOX 4-3

Patient Rights to Confidentiality

Patricia A. Roche

No single law in the United States governs every aspect of privacy including the privacy of medical information. Physicians who strive to understand their legal obligations regarding patient information are advised to consult people who know the applicable state laws, are familiar with federal laws that govern medical information, and understand the relationship between such state and federal laws. Physicians should also recognize that such knowledge, although necessary for achieving compliance with the law, would not satisfactorily resolve all legal questions and ethical dilemmas that arise over information in clinical practice. For example, some laws may permit—but not require—physicians to disclose some information to certain third parties without the patient's authorization, thus leaving it up to physicians to decide whether or not to disclose. Medical ethics, rather than the law, will guide such decisions. This box identifies some laws that apply to some of the questions that arise when physicians have patients who are involved in workers' compensation claims and third parties request information on these patients.

Duty of Confidentiality

The physician's duty to maintain the confidences of patients is well established as a legal obligation that derives from case law and state statutes. In general, the duty requires that the physician not disclose private information obtained from the patient to anyone who is not directly involved in the patient's treatment without first obtaining the patient's authorization.[1] It does not matter whether the disclosure is made verbally or in writing, but for the duty to apply, a physician–patient relationship must be established.*

Case law and state statutes have also established exceptions to this general rule. For example, all states have mandatory reporting statutes that not only permit, but require physicians to report certain diseases or

---

The law does not ordinarily view the relationship between an employee and a physician retained to conduct physical examinations on behalf of an employer as one of patient and physician.

conditions to designated public authorities without patient authorization and typically provide immunity from breach of confidentiality suits in relation to such reporting.[1] Depending on the state, additional exceptions may permit disclosures to employers, without patient authorization when the patient presents a serious danger to self or others or go so far as to mandate such disclosures.

A physician may have a statutory obligation to obtain patient authorization in writing before disclosing medical information. And depending on the specific medical information involved, the process for obtaining valid consent for disclosure as well as the form and content of the written authorization may be dictated by a state statute or regulation.

Caution should also be exercised when a physician is presented with a subpoena or similar legal process to compel attendance in a judicial proceeding or production of medical records. Consultation with a lawyer may be necessary to determine if the subpoena has been validly issued, whether grounds exist to ask the court to "quash" the subpoena, whether any testimonial privilege applies to the provider and the information sought, and the legal consequences for failure to obey a (valid) subpoena.

Confidentiality, Federal Privacy Laws, and Workers' Compensation Claims

When workers' compensation is involved, how much information may be disclosed without obtaining patient consent is sometimes spelled out in the applicable state statue or relevant court decisions. Where it is not and the physician is unsure of what information may be disclosed without risking breach of confidentiality, the guiding principle should be to provide the minimum information necessary to achieve the purpose of the disclosure. Specifically, the physician should take care to release only information directly relevant to the workers' compensation case, unless the patient has requested and authorized that additional information be released. The physician should out of concern for the patient's best interests consult with the patient before releasing data, even in states where a signed claim for workers' compensation or occupational disease benefits

(continued)

BOX 4-3
Patient Rights to Confidentiality (Continued)

operates as an authorization for disclosure of information by a health care provider to the relevant insurer. The physician should recognize that not only is the patient's privacy at issue but that disclosure may affect employment, access to workers' compensation benefits, or the outcome of a lawsuit.

Physicians hired by an insurer or employer to evaluate the worker's readiness to return to work, degree of disability, or other nontreatment issues are not considered *treating physicians* under the law. If the examining physician has findings outside the purpose of the evaluation, the physician should respect the privacy of the person being examined by disclosing only the required information.

This *minimum necessary* principle is incorporated into several privacy laws, including federal rules under the Health Insurance Portability and Accountability Act (HIPAA) that went into effect in 2003, which regulates how physicians, health plans, pharmacies, hospitals, and other "covered entities" can use and disclose patients' personal medical information. (Most practicing physicians will fit the definition of a "covered entity" used in the regulations and therefore will be governed by them.) Under these rules, covered entities are required to limit the amount of individually identifiable information that is disclosed without patient

authorization. The regulations also explicitly address disclosures of health information regarding workers' compensation claims and permit disclosures without the individual's authorization to the extent necessary to comply with laws relating to programs providing benefits for work-related injuries or illnesses. In addition, these regulations permit physicians to rely on a public official's representation that the information requested is the minimum necessary for the intended purpose of the disclosure.

The HIPAA privacy rules set a floor rather than a ceiling for protecting the privacy of medical information. Consequently, when other federal or state laws on medical information provide more protection than the HIPAA rules, the more protective federal or state law governs. For this reason, it is imperative that physicians become familiar with and understand applicable state laws on confidentiality and medical information. Most importantly, physicians' legal and ethical obligations to their patients require physicians to limit disclosure of patient information (other than to the patient) to the minimum necessary to comply with applicable laws and regulations.

REFERENCE

1. Annas GJ. The rights of patients. Carbondale, Ill.: So. Illinois University Press, 2004:246–54.

REFERENCE

1. Burton JF, Speiler EA. Workers' compensation and older workers. In: Hunt HA, ed. Ensuring health and income security for an aging workforce. Washington DC National Academy of Social Insurance, 2001:41–84.
2. Azaroff LS, Levenstein C, Wegman DH. Occupational injury and illness surveillance: Conceptual filters explain underreporting. Am J Public Health 2002;92:1421–9.
3. Reville RT, Boden LI, Biddle J, et al. New Mexico workers' compensation permanent partial disability and return-to-work: An evaluation. Santa Monica, Calif.: RAND, 2001.
4. Boden LI, Galizzi M. Economic Consequences of workplace injuries and illnesses: Lost earnings and benefit adequacy. Am J Industrial Med 1999;36:487–503.
5. Thornquist L. Health care costs and cost containment in Minnesota's workers' compensation program. John Burton's Workers' Compensation Monitor 1990;3: 3–26.
6. Johnson WG, Baldwin ML, Burton JF Jr. Why is the treatment of work-related injuries so costly? New evidence from California. Inquiry 1996;33:53–65.
7. Pozzebon S. Medical cost containment under workers' compensation. Industrial Labor Relations Rev 1994;48:153–67.
8. Mony AT. Compensation of occupational illnesses in France. New Solutions 1993;4:57–61.
9. Kim P. Bargaining with imperfect information: A study of worker perceptions of legal protection in an at-will world. Cornell Law Rev 1997;83:105–60.
10. Kim P. Norms, learning, and law: Exploring the influences of workers' legal knowledge. University of Illinois Law Rev 1999;447–515.
11. Colker R. The Americans with Disabilities Act: A windfall for defendants. Harvard Civil Rights Civil Liberties Law Rev 1999;34:99–162.
12. Colker R. Winning and losing under the Americans with Disabilities Act. Ohio State Law J 2001;62:239–79.
13. Rabinowitz RS. The Americans with Disabilities Act and the Family and Medical Leave Act. In:

Occupational safety and health law. 2nd ed. Washington, DC: BNA, Inc, 2002:845–910.

14. Burkhauser RV, Daly MC, Houtenville AJ. How working-age people with disabilities fared over the 1990s business cycle. In: Budetti PP, et al., eds. Ensuring health and income security for an aging workforce. Kalamazoo: W.E. Upjohn Institute for Employment Security, 2001:291–346.

15. Burkhauser RV, Butler JS, Kim YW, et al. The importance of accommodation on the timing of male disability insurance application: Results from the survey of disability and work and the health and retirement study. J Human Resources 1999;34:589–611.

16. Daly MC, Bound J. Worker adaptation and employer accommodation following the onset of a health impairment. J. Gerontol B Psychol Sci Soc Sci 1996;51:S53–S60.

17. Strunin L, Boden LI . Paths of reentry: Employment experiences of injured workers. Am J Industrial Med 2000;38:373–84.

BIBLIOGRAPHY

Barth PS, Hunt HA. Workers' compensation and work-related illnesses. Cambridge, Mass.: MIT Press, 1980.
Even though it is two decades old, this remains the most complete description available of how workers' compensation programs handle occupational diseases. Describes how different states compensate occupational diseases and gives an overview of litigation and settlement of workers' compensation disease claims in the United States. Also reviews workers' compensation in other countries.

Boden LI. Workers' compensation in the United States: High costs, low benefits. Annu Rev Public Health. 1995;16:189–218
A review of workers' compensation programs in the United States, focusing on safety, medical costs, litigation, and benefit adequacy.

Burton JF Jr. John Burton's Workers' Compensation Resources. Available at: <http://www.workers compresources. com/>.
Information about workers' compensation maintained by an academic expert. Links to other Internet resources as well.

Harr J. A civil action. New York: Vintage Books, 1996.
A gripping book describing the legal battle between eight families of leukemia victims and companies that polluted their water supply. Winner of the National Book Critics Circle Award.

National Academy of Social Insurance. Workers' compensation: Benefits, coverage, and costs, annual. Washington, DC: NASI. Also available at: <http://www.nasi.org/search_site2710/search_site_list.htm?attrib_id=2758>.
An annual summary of workers' compensation benefits, coverage, and cost.

National Commission on State Workmen's Compensation Laws. Report and compendium on workmen's compensation. Washington, DC: U.S. Government Printing Office, 1972 and 1973.
The national commission was created by the Occupational Safety and Health Act of 1970 to evaluate the status of workers' compensation. It undertook a 2-year study. The compendium is a descriptive report on workers' compensation in 1973, and the report makes recommendations to upgrade workers' compensation programs. Available at: <http://www.workerscompresources.com/National_Commission_Report/national_commission_report.htm>.

Scientific evidence and public policy. Am J Pub Health 2005; 95 (Suppl 1): S1-S150.
A recent comprehensive compendium of articles on this subject.

Social Security Administration, Office of Disability Programs. Disability evaluation under social security. Available at: <http://www.ssa.gov/disability/professionals/publications.htm>.
This publication provides information from the Social Security Administration (SSA) for physicians regarding the disability programs administered by the SSA. It explains how each program works and the kinds of information a physician should provide to ensure appropriate decisions on disability claims.

Spieler EA. Perpetuating risk? Workers' compensation and the persistence of occupational injuries. Houston Law Rev 1994;31:119–264.
A legal and political analysis of the most important public policy debates concerning workers' compensation. Critical of efforts to contain costs that focus on reducing benefits instead of reducing hazards.

CHAPTER 5

Ethics in Occupational and Environmental Health

Kathleen M. Rest

Case 1

A team of university scientists (epidemiologists, physicians, industrial hygienists, toxicologists, and statisticians) is funded to conduct a large industry-sponsored epidemiologic study. The team wants to establish an independent advisory board to oversee the design and conduct of the study, as well as the data analyses and reporting and dissemination of study findings. The industry is reluctant to agree.

Case 2

A large industry is sponsoring a study of a community's exposure to two carcinogenic chemicals in its air emissions over the past 15 years, as well as a study of cancer incidence. Although the community is concerned about cancer, residents are much more concerned about birth defects and childhood respiratory illnesses, which they believe may be associated with many of the chemicals emitted from the plant.

Case 3

Hazardous wastes from industrial operations have contaminated the soil and water supply of a poor neighborhood with a large minority population. The government and responsible industrial parties have decided to incinerate the waste on site. Their contractor performs a risk assessment that indicates no health risk to the community. The residents want the waste removed from the neighborhood. They have used Environmental Protection Agency (EPA) funding to obtain their own technical advisor, who presents a risk assessment suggesting that

incineration on-site will indeed pose health risks to community residents.

Case 4

On petition from a labor union, the Occupational Safety and Health Administration (OSHA) is considering whether to lower the permissible workplace exposure limit of a chemical, because recently completed epidemiologic studies suggest neurotoxic effects at the current exposure level. The epidemiologists who conducted the studies are reluctant to get involved in the policy debate, but other experts from industry, labor, and academia are asked to comment about the need for such action. They present conflicting interpretations of the studies, different views about the findings from previous studies, and widely divergent opinions on the need for more stringent regulation.

Case 5

A U.S. company decides to move its pesticide manufacturing operations to another country because labor costs are cheaper there and because the other country's environmental and occupational regulations are less stringent and virtually unenforced. The other country's ministry of commerce and development welcomes the company.

Case 6

A hospital-based occupational health program has a contract to provide clinical and consultation services to a local furniture manufacturer. The company has many ergonomic problems, and many workers have experienced musculoskeletal and repetitive strain injuries. The company physician, nurse, and safety engineer have recommended ergonomic changes in the work environment many times, but the company has taken no action. Instead, the company has asked the nurse to institute a weight reduction program and a class on safe lifting techniques for the workers.

Case 7

An occupational medicine resident conducts an "independent medical evaluation" of a person who has been out of work for 6 months with a work-related injury. The workers' compensation insurer requested the evaluation. The resident tells her preceptor that she cannot understand why the patient seems uncooperative and even hostile during the medical evaluation.

Case 8

A company contracted with a local family physician to perform preplacement physical examinations, periodic screening examinations, and fitness-for-duty and return-to-work evaluations. The company told the physician what it wanted to include in the preplacement and screening examinations. The physician has never visited the plant and has little information about workplace conditions and job demands. During the first 6 months of the contract, the physician is called many times by the company's human resource manager and asked for what she considers to be confidential medical information about specific employees' fitness for duty and return-to-work issues.

These cases typify the range of issues and types of ethical and moral questions that occupational and environmental health professionals, researchers, regulators, and others can expect to encounter. Literature from the United States and elsewhere frequently reflects on the ethical problems encountered by occupational and environmental health professionals in their work. Because the environments in which these health and safety professionals function can be characterized as having competing goals and interests and differential power structures, thorny ethical issues are common.

As a field of study, ethics is a complex discipline that attempts to analyze, define, and defend the moral basis of human action. For our purposes, we can use the term *ethics* to refer to the rightness

and wrongness of human behavior. Ethics entails a sense of "ought"; that is, ethics helps us decide how we ought to act or what ought to be done. Ethics is not law, social custom, personal preference, or consensus of opinion, although any of these may derive from or inform ethical considerations. Rather, ethics is both an approach to moral reasoning and a collection of principles and rules to help guide judgment and action. Ethics can facilitate reflection that leads to consistent, informed, and justifiable decisions that can withstand close moral scrutiny.

In the field of occupational and environmental health, conflict and disagreement occur at many levels—from actions taken or not taken by regulatory and other governmental agencies in matters of public policy to decisions made by researchers and occupational and environmental health professionals in the context of their daily work. Difficult questions abound: Should a substance or condition in the workplace be regulated? At what level? How safe is safe enough? How clean is clean enough? What research should be done? Who should decide? Should medical screening or epidemiologic surveillance (or both) be instituted for a group of workers or residents of a contaminated community? When and how should information or concern about actual or potential health risks associated with present or past exposures be disclosed—to those exposed, to appropriate authorities, and to peers in the scientific community? How much information about their workers are employers entitled to have? How should trade-offs among health, productivity, jobs, environmental protection, and economic development be made? Not all aspects of these conflicts and decisions are ethical in nature; some may reflect simple disagreements about facts, methods, processes, or desired outcomes. Many of the disagreements, however, have some underlying moral dimension, even when the arguments are framed in technical or economic terms.

The moral issues encountered in occupational and environmental health are socially constructed and therefore may vary temporally and geographically. These issues cannot be considered fully outside the social, cultural, institutional, political, and, increasingly, economic contexts from which they arise.[1] In the workplace and in many environmentally contaminated communities, an important contextual dimension is the power imbalance between employer and worker, polluter and resident, government, and citizen. These power imbalances are reflected in the significant differences in economic and technical resources, decision-making authority, access to powerful institutions, and distribution of risks and benefits among the stakeholders. A second important contextual dimension is the scientific uncertainty that attends many of the problems and issues encountered. Other contextual dimensions include the powerful economic forces generated by market competition and world trade and the very nature of the employer–employee relationship.

This chapter provides a brief and basic discussion of the ethical dimensions of common occupational and environmental health issues in public policy, scientific research, and practice. It also presents an array of principles, processes, and guidelines that have been suggested as aids to problem solving and decision making in situations that pose ethical dilemmas, conflicts, or problems. Probing the ethical dimensions of these situations can make a unique contribution to improved decision making and action.

REVIEW OF ETHICAL PRINCIPLES, PROCESSES, AND GUIDELINES

A lengthy and comprehensive discussion of moral philosophy and ethics is neither possible nor warranted in a textbook such as this. Yet it is important that the reader appreciate some of the concepts and constructs that are commonly applied when assessing or analyzing ethical problems. The literature of ethics and bioethics is replete with discussions of moral rights and their attendant moral obligations and duties; character traits and virtues of moral persons; moral principles against which actions can be judged; and necessary or established procedural and behavioral guidelines, such as ethical codes. This chapter considers a set of principles that has been prominent historically in bioethics, along with additional concepts that may further enrich ethical inquiry.

In 1994, Beauchamp and Childress provided a standard approach to bioethical issues with their focus on the principles of *autonomy* (which has come to mean individual self-determination but is also defined as respect for persons), *nonmaleficence* (the duty to do no harm), *beneficence* (the duty to do or promote good), and *justice* (the duty to be fair). The principle of justice may be further refined to include the distribution of risks, costs, and benefits. Although these principles remain central, important, and helpful in moral reasoning, they have been criticized, as has the general approach of applying abstract moral principles to complex problems. It is suggested that they do not help in the most difficult of situations (when principles conflict); that they suggest application devoid of context; and that they are preoccupied with individual rights and removed from larger social and collective concerns.[2] Additional guidance is offered by other scholars. Some emphasize the concept of moral responsibility, which arises from interpersonal relationships or from the special knowledge that one person has in relation to another person's welfare.[3] Others suggest inquiry into the social construction of the moral issue—the vested interests and social, cultural, and institutional contexts that give rise to the problem.[1]

ETHICAL ISSUES IN RESEARCH

Although science, in its pursuit of truth, is often held to be "objective," it is now generally acknowledged that individual, social, and cultural values influence scientists in many aspects of their work. These values may influence what researchers decide to study, how they frame research questions and design studies, what data they collect, how they analyze and interpret data, how they report study results, and how they participate in policy debates that involve the use of their findings. It is helpful when researchers are honest with themselves and with the public about the influence of their own values and conflicts of interest, or those of relevant interest groups—including their funders and collaborators—on their activities and pronouncements, because it adds an important dimension to public and private decision making. There have been cases in which science and scientists have been bought (directly or indirectly) to serve political or ideological interests under the guise of "objectivity."[4] Concerned about bias and conflict of interest, many journals are signatories to the 2001 uniform requirements for manuscripts submitted to biomedical journals developed by the International Committee of Medical Journal Editors <http://www.icmje.org>, and some have adopted even stiffer policies.[5] Recent reports of close ties between government agencies and the pharmaceutical and biotechnology industries have surfaced in the press, resulting in public hearings, new ethics regulations for government scientists, and questions about public trust in government pronouncements.[6,7] The corporate sector's growing influence on the academy is also generating concern, raising real questions about the long-term effects on science and innovation, academic freedom, and the erosion of the academy's role in serving the public interest.[8]

In occupational health research, there are additional complexities. Because the workplace is the primary subject of the research, industry will always have an interest in the outcome, even if it does not fund the research. Powerful institutions may also have a strong interest in the conduct and results of environmental health research.

An often-discussed area of conflict in the research process is the reporting of results and dissemination of findings. There are both historic and current examples of situations in which occupational health professionals have failed to report relevant research findings or have experienced adverse personal and professional consequences after doing so.[9,10] Questions relevant to this part of the research process include the following: How much control does the research sponsor have—over the research question(s), study design and methods, data analyses, and reporting of results? Does the author have full access to all the data in the study? Can the sponsor delay or even prevent presentation, publication, or dissemination of a study's findings? Are publications or presentations subject to approval of the sponsor? Can the sponsor edit, change, delete, or add to any manuscript prepared for publication?

These questions suggest consideration of the researcher's autonomy and integrity. Because research findings can have serious consequences for the interest groups involved, they may seek to influence the researcher and the work. In the past, industry sponsors have tried to influence the design, conduct, and interpretation of research and the dissemination and publication of results. For this reason, it would behoove independent researchers to institute structural safeguards before conducting a study sponsored by an industry or other interest group. Case 1 illustrates how one research team sought to protect the integrity and independence of their industry-sponsored research project. The sponsor's reluctance should signal the need for careful examination of the potential for interference or influence.

The questions listed also suggest consideration of the researcher's professional responsibility. In many studies, researchers establish a direct or implied relationship with their subjects, from whom they obtain personal and medical information and, perhaps, biological specimens. This special relationship confers a responsibility on researchers to at least respect and refrain from harming their sub-jects, whose welfare may be affected by inappropriate disclosure of personal information or by the researchers' failure to communicate the results of the study. Protection and promotion of worker and public health (beneficence) and fairness and justice for research subjects also merit deliberation.

A more subtle influence may be found in the way researchers themselves choose to interpret and report their findings. Will they refer to contradictory evidence and fairly discuss the significance of their own findings in this light? Will they fully discuss the limitations of their study—perhaps with reference to the study's statistical power? Although honesty and integrity demand attention to these matters, the researcher may be influenced by sources of previous, present, and potential future funding when findings are presented, interpreted, and discussed. Self-censorship can have a potent influence on the research process; it can affect any aspect, from the questions the researcher seeks to answer to the ways in which results are interpreted and reported.

The initial framing of the research question is also subject to influence. For example, a corporation concerned about the frequency of musculoskeletal injuries in its workforce may be willing to sponsor research on a device or method to identify susceptible workers, whereas the ergonomics researcher might prefer to study etiology or potential process, work practice, or product interventions. Industrial sponsors may directly influence toxicologists' or epidemiologists' decisions about which chemicals to study and which end points to investigate (see Case 2). Researchers concerned with the costs of workers' compensation may limit the focus of their studies to medical care cost-containment strategies, effectively precluding research on the prevention of workplace injury—perhaps because the sponsors view the problem solely in this light. Certainly, framing the research question is partly a function of the researcher's professional interests and abilities, but external factors and pressures can play a role during this phase of the research process. Important questions include the following: Who has defined the research question: the investigator, the sponsor, or both? If funding were not an issue, would this be the right question, the right issue, the right problem? Whose interests are being served by the way in which the question is framed?

Of course, the conduct of the study also poses ethical challenges. The concept of informed consent (justified by an appeal to autonomy and respect for persons) is especially important. Research subjects should be informed of the risks and benefits of their voluntary participation in any study. In occupational and environmental health research, there may be additional requirements. For example, subjects should be informed about the reasons for the study, the sponsors of the study, the timetable for completion of the study, and how the results will be used.[11] Study subjects should also be informed about possible economic risks of participation, both for themselves and for their employers. Box 5-1 provides some ethical guidance for medical research on workers. Informed consent also has bearing on the conduct of medical examinations and screening and surveillance activities, performed by occupational and environmental health professionals, that are often carried out at the behest of third parties. This is discussed in a later section.

ETHICAL ISSUES IN SCIENCE POLICY

In the field of occupational and environmental health, most debates of science and public policy focus on the regulation and control of health and safety hazards. Beneath the technical and economic arguments regarding the basis, process, and content of regulation lie clear differences in values and in the deference given to widely held moral principles.

Several cases mentioned at the beginning of this chapter illustrate common ethical issues in science policy. In these cases, scientists and experts have differing opinions about what a study means or which risk assessment reveals "the truth." These views may involve honest disagreements about methodology, but they may also reflect different understandings about the duties imposed by widely held moral principles, such as beneficence and autonomy, as well as differences in personal preferences, political ideology, and disciplinary biases.

In deciding whether to incinerate or remove the waste from a poor community (Case 3), whether to lower the permissible exposure limit of a potential workplace neurotoxin (Case 4), or whether to move a hazardous operation to a country with less stringent environmental controls (Case 5), scientists, regulators, government officials, and employers are dealing with concepts of nonmaleficence, beneficence, autonomy, justice, fairness, responsibility. Consideration of these moral concepts are particularly important in decisions involving health and safety issues and environmental regulations, which to a large extent transfer choice about "acceptable" risk from individuals to other entities, such as governments or corporations.

Although there is debate about the extent to which individuals are morally obligated to take positive action to contribute to the welfare of others, there is little disagreement that they should refrain from doing harm and, in some cases, take positive action to prevent harm from occurring. If the waste is incinerated, the health and well-being of community members may be harmed; if a chemical is not regulated more stringently, the health of workers may be endangered; if a hazardous facility is moved abroad, residents and workers in the new host country may be harmed. On the other hand, it could be argued that trucking the waste out of the community would create potential risks to others; that more stringent regulation of a chemical would adversely affect the financial resources of some manufacturers and might even cause some workers to lose their jobs; or that the economy of the other country would be improved by the migration of the potentially hazardous industry. How should these trade-offs be made?

Many disagreements are likely to revolve around issues of scientific and technological uncertainty, in many ways an inherent element of occupational and environmental health research, policy, and practice. The effectiveness of technologies to clean up hazardous waste may be unknown. Risk assessments vary by orders of magnitude, depending on the models and assumptions made by the investigators. Most epidemiologic studies show association, not causation, and reported mortality risks are bounded by confidence intervals of varying widths. Furthermore, the models chosen, the assumptions made, and the designs employed may reflect the investigator's values or the values and interests of the study sponsors.

The comments of scientists and the decisions of policymakers often reflect their value-laden approaches to issues of uncertainty. What level of proof is needed to trigger action, and who bears the burden of proof? Should we wait for certain evidence of harm before we take action, or is a reasonable suspicion enough? Should consumers or workers be responsible for showing that a product is dangerous, or should the manufacturer or employer be required to show that the product is safe before it is allowed into the market or workplace?

BOX 5-1

Ethical Guidelines for Medical Research on Workers

All sets of ethical guidelines for medical research on workers should advance the three basic ethical precepts underlying all research on human subjects, as stated in the *Common Rule,* which refers to the regulations for the protection of human subjects of research as promulgated by the U.S. Department of Health and Human Services and the Food and Drug Administration and which are applicable to all federal agencies sponsoring biomedical research. These ethical principles are

1. Respect for persons, which includes autonomy and informed consent;
2. Beneficence, which includes nonmaleficence (not inflicting harm); and
3. Justice, which involves the fair allocation of the benefits and burdens of research.

The following guidelines are intended to supplement the requirements of the Common Rule and should be followed in all instances of medical research on workers.

1. If possible, the research should be performed by a party other than the employer, such as a university, medical institution, nongovernmental organization, or government agency.
2. Employers and employees (including union representatives) should be involved from the beginning in developing all aspects of the study, including study design, recruitment practices, criteria for inclusion and exclusion, informed consent process, confidentiality rules, and dissemination of findings.
3. The sponsor of the research must be indicated to potential participants, and investigators must disclose any financial interests in the research.
4. Individuals with supervisory authority over potential research participants should not be involved in the recruitment process, and lists of research participants should not be shared with supervisors.
5. No inducements should be offered for participation in the research.
6. In the informed consent process, it must be made clear to potential participants that there will be no adverse employment consequences for declining to participate or withdrawing from the research; potential participants also should be informed whether treatment or compensation for injuries will be provided.
7. Research should be conducted, and results should be disclosed, in the least identifiable form consistent with sound scientific methodology.
8. If the investigators believe that the findings will be of sufficient scientific validity and clinical utility to warrant offering participants the opportunity to obtain their individual results, the participants should be advised of all the potential risks of disclosure, including any psychological, social, or economic risks.

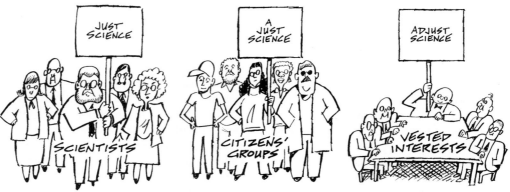

Different groups sometimes have different perspectives on science. (Drawing by Nick Thorkelson.)

(continued)

BOX 5-1

Ethical Guidelines for Medical Research on Workers *(Continued)*

9. Reasonable steps should be taken to ensure the confidentiality of participant-specific information generated by the research, including storing the information in secure locations separate from other employment records, destroying biological samples that are no longer needed, destroying linking codes when no longer needed, and applying

for a certificate of confidentiality from the Department of Health and Human Services when appropriate.

10. Investigators should take special precautions at all stages of study if the research has the potential to adversely affect groups of individuals on the basis of race, ethnicity, gender, age, or similar factors.

Source: Rothstein MA. Ethical guidelines for medical research on workers. J Occup Environ Med 2000;42:1166–1171.

Although science may contribute information and even define the parameters of the debate, the answers to these questions reflect policy judgments that invariably are influenced by values. Some scientists, regulators, and members of the public prefer to wait for additional evidence and accept the risk of future harm rather than expend potentially unnecessary resources to impose costly regulations now. These persons are likely to frame their arguments in economic terms and to focus their critiques on the design flaws and technical limitations of individual studies bearing on the question.

Others prefer to err on the side of caution in protecting the health of workers and the public and seek to impose regulations or deny siting permits, even at the risk of being found wrong at some future date. Their arguments focus on human health or environmental impacts and are more likely to synthesize the available data, overlook the design flaws of individual studies, and give weight to the aggregate suggestive evidence. They employ the *precautionary principle*. To what extent are these determinations "scientific" and to what extent are they driven by different views of one's duty to prevent harm, do good, or fulfill one's responsibility toward others in a personal or fiduciary relationship?

Cases 3 and 5 also illustrate an especially important dimension of justice. Many policy decisions reflect a utilitarian approach to policymaking; that is, decisions are made to maximize benefit or to confer the greatest good on the greatest number. This approach, deeply rooted in ethical theory, often has salutary effects and can justify actions that harm a few while helping many. However, this approach often fails to consider issues of distribution.

Distributive justice relates to fairness in the distribution of risks, costs, and benefits. Who benefits? Who bears the risks or costs? Who gets to make the decision? What is the relationship between those who bear the costs, those who reap the benefits, and those who make the decisions?

The environmental justice movement has provided evidence of environmental inequity, whereby economically disadvantaged and minority communities have borne more than their fair share of landfills, hazardous waste facilities, polluting industries, and environmentally related health problems, such as lead and pesticide poisoning.[12,13] In these cases, it seems that the most vulnerable members of society are asked to bear a disproportionate share of environmental pollution and associated health risks. Distributive justice requires us to examine and justify the allocation of risks, costs, and benefits.

Applications in Public Policy

The application of ethical principles to occupational and environmental health policy is more than just the fodder for interesting debate. We can see their reflection in many of the regulatory decisions taken by governmental agencies.

For example, the OSHA lead standard addresses issues of autonomy, justice, nonmaleficence, and beneficence. The regulatory debate on lead included scientific questions about safe airborne levels and the merits of using blood lead concentrations as the primary measure of compliance with the standard. An interesting part of the debate centered on the establishment of medical removal protection, with (hourly) rate retention for workers found to have elevated blood lead concentrations. There was little argument about the wisdom of removing such workers from exposure. Rather, the conflict arose over a proposal that obligated employers to maintain workers' hourly rates and seniority rights during the period of removal. The Lead Industries Association argued against this proposal on legal grounds. Workers' representatives focused on issues of autonomy and fairness, noting that workers would choose not to participate in a blood lead screening program that might threaten their livelihoods. Although medical removal was in the best interest of the workers' health, their representatives argued that it was unfair to penalize them by putting their wages and seniority benefits at risk in an exposure situation over which they have little, if any, control. The courts ruled in favor of the policy of medical removal with rate retention, but the ethical issues surrounding the regulation of lead did not abate. (Somewhat more recently, OSHA's failure to include a medical removal protection requirement in its revised methylene chloride standard prompted the United Auto Workers union to sue the agency. The Halogenated Solvents Industry Alliance also sued, but on economic grounds involving the costs of compliance. After the lawsuits were filed, the opposing parties worked together and proposed a settlement, which OSHA adopted in 1998. The final rule addressed some concerns for both parties. It included provisions for medical removal protection and extended compliance dates for certain employers to implement requirements for engineering controls and respiratory protection.)

Recognizing the effects of lead on reproduction, some employers began to institute *fetal protection* policies. Such policies ostensibly sought to protect actual and potential fetuses of pregnant women or women of reproductive capacity. These policies involved the principles of beneficence and nonmaleficence, which in this case clashed with the principles of autonomy and justice. In weighing their options, employers who adopted such policies placed a higher value on protecting the fetus from harm (and themselves from future liability) than on providing autonomous choices to female workers, who could take steps to control their fertility. In addition, because lead is known to have toxic effects on both men and women, one could question the fairness of differentially protecting female and male employees.

The U.S. Supreme Court ruled against the use of fetal protection policies on the basis of sex discrimination (fairness), upholding the autonomy of women workers, in United Auto Workers *v.* Johnson Controls, U.S. 111 Sup. Ct. 1196 (1991). The Court stated that such policies force female workers "to choose between having a child and having a job" and that "it is no more appropriate for the courts than it is for individual employers to decide whether a woman's reproductive role is more important to herself and her family than her economic role." Rather, the Court found that "Congress has left this choice to the woman as hers to make." Thus, the Court gave overriding weight to the woman's autonomy.

Freedom and noninterference are tightly guarded and highly cherished rights in the United States. In occupational and environmental health, these concepts are reflected in right-to-know laws and regulations (see Chapter 3). In this context, autonomy suggests that individuals have a right to know about their workplace or environmental exposures so that they can make decisions and take individual or organized action. Such decision making requires information—in this case, information about the exposures, their potential health effects, methods of protection, and, ideally, possible substitutes or alternatives.

In the United States, the concept of right-to-know has been embodied in both occupational and environmental legislation. The OSHA Medical Access Rule provides workers with access to their own medical records and to records pertaining to their exposures to toxic substances to the extent that the employer compiles such records. Under this rule, information is provided on request. The OSHA Hazard Communication Standard obliges employers to educate and train workers about the hazardous chemicals in the workplace. Employers must provide this information as a matter of course, even without a request. Congress extended the right to know about toxic hazards to communities in 1986 with the enactment of the Emergency Planning and Community Right-to-Know Act. Its many provisions provide local citizens with access to information about the location, use, and release of toxic chemicals in their communities.

In promulgating these right-to-know laws and regulations, the government recognized workers' and citizens' needs for information about toxic substances in their workplaces and communities, granted them a right to such information, and conferred on manufacturers and employers the duty to provide it. However, provisions were also enacted to balance these needs with the needs of employers and manufacturers to protect their trade secrets. The existing power imbalances in workplaces and communities have called into question the adequacy of these right-to-know provisions. It is argued that, in addition to the right to know, workers and citizens need the right to act.

In enacting the Occupational Safety and Health Act of 1970, U.S. legislators recognized the potential harm that might befall workers who take action to protect their health and safety, for example by refusing hazardous work, calling unsafe conditions to the attention of their employers or fellow workers, or alerting authorities about health and safety problems at work. Section 11(c) of the Act seeks to protect workers in the exercise of these rights from retaliation and discrimination by their employers. A 1997 report issued by the Inspector General of the Department of Labor criticized the adequacy of OSHA's 11(c) program. Workers who invoke this statutory right often do so at great personal risk. It is critical that the agency vigorously enforce this provision to provide workers with the protection and justice they need when they take action to secure their health and safety on the job.

Applications in Corporate Policy

Public policy and regulation can go only so far in protecting workers and communities from occupational and environmental hazards. Corporate and business policies and decisions have the most immediate impact on health, safety, and the environment. They can promote good (beneficence) or result in significant harm. Although many employers have excellent health, safety, and environmental programs and function as responsible corporate citizens, there have been too many cases of business policies and practices that demonstrate wanton disregard for worker and community health.[14,15]

The public is well aware of and disillusioned by these corporate failures. Surveys indicate that the public considers industry the least trusted (but most knowledgeable) source of information about chemical risk.[16] A 2004 global poll of citizens in 20 countries found very low levels of public trust in global companies.[17] Recognizing the impact of this public perception, private industry has developed a variety of initiatives and policies to upgrade its practices and reassure a skeptical public. For exam-

ple, the American Chemistry Council (formerly the Chemical Manufacturers Association) instituted a voluntary program (Responsible Care) for its member companies, which provides management practices, performance measures, a risk-based security management system, and guidelines for community and employee outreach activities. New program enhancements are now a condition of membership. Some companies participate in OSHA's Voluntary Protection Program, taking steps to enhance their own internal responsibility for worker health and safety. Others participate in OSHA's more recently established cooperative Alliance and Strategic Partnership programs. Independently, some individual employers also have refined their policies and practices to improve their health, safety, and environmental programs; facilitated right-to-know programs and worker training; and eliminated discriminatory practices against their workers. Business schools have instituted courses in business ethics.

Obviously, the employer community plays a significant part in creating ethical problems relating to occupational and environmental health. Employers need opportunities and incentives to enhance their abilities to recognize, understand, and respond to their ethical obligations and responsibilities and to respect the ethical duties and responsibilities of others. They must also obey the law.

Workers and their representatives, including organized labor, also have ethical duties and responsibilities to prevent harm, do good, be fair, and tell the truth. However, most workers in the United States and other countries are not in a position to enact and enforce policies and programs in the workplace. The conduct of individual workers, like that of everyone else, should be guided by moral considerations both on and off the job. Although individual workers (and labor organizations) can and sometimes do create ethical dilemmas for occupational health professionals, in most cases they are not a powerful and organized group, and they are not treated as such in this chapter.

OCCUPATIONAL HEALTH AND SAFETY PRACTICE

Most occupational and environmental health professionals routinely encounter conflicts and ethical problems that challenge their values as well as their professionalism. Those who provide occupational and environmental health services directly, such as occupational physicians, nurses, industrial hygienists, safety professionals, and occupational ergonomists, have clear professional and moral responsibilities that derive from their special knowledge of occupational and environmental health and safety and from the special relationships they develop with workers, employers, and communities. This section examines the ethical dimensions of activities commonly conducted or encountered by these professionals. Problem areas relate to dual agency, conflict of interest, confidentiality, professional competence, taking action in the face of scientific uncertainty or opposition, and responsibility for others.

In exploring these issues, it is important to appreciate the very real and personal consequences that these individuals may experience as a result of their work. Their actions can enhance their own reputation, status, and esteem or incur the wrath and distrust of employers, patients, and colleagues. Their decisions can affect their income, their employability, their standing in the professional community, and their respectability in the eyes of persons for and to whom they are responsible. Courageous and unpopular decisions may take a personal and emotional toll on these professionals and their families. The difficulty of "doing the right thing" in such situations should not be underestimated.

Working for Companies

Health and safety professionals who work for companies, whether full-time, part-time, contractually, or on a fee-for-service basis, frequently face a host of ethical issues that call their allegiance and values into question. Their goals, interests, and values may differ significantly from those of both employers and workers. The company's primary purpose and interest is to profitably manufacture a product or provide a service and to stay in business. The workers are primarily interested in earning a living, providing for their families, and finding some personal satisfaction in their work—without damage to their health. When the health and safety professional and the worker share the same employer, and the interests of the employer and worker diverge, what is the role of the health care provider? Whose interests take precedence: those of the worker/patient or those of the employer/client?

Within this complicated structure, the practice of occupational medicine, nursing, safety, or industrial hygiene is inherently difficult and challenging. Employers may expect physicians and nurses to function as agents of social control, making determinations about when, where, and whether a person can work. A company's satisfaction with the services of these health care professionals may depend in large measure on their ability to get injured workers back to work quickly. Employers may limit the ability of their health and safety professionals to take preventive action regarding workplace hazards. At the same time, workers may expect occupational health professionals to protect their interests and function as their advocates when problems arise. The worker and the health professional may not always agree on issues related to return-to-work directives or job restrictions. When the employer/client's interests differ from those of the worker/patient, it is not surprising that skepticism, distrust, and hostility arise on all fronts. The occupational medicine resident in Case 7 has probably failed to appreciate the significant economic and psychosocial factors, as well as the power dynamics, that often come into play when a worker is injured on the job and issues of compensation or return-to-work are raised.

The issue of confidentiality is perhaps the most frequently discussed ethical problem in the occupational health literature—and for good reason. Consider, for example, the almost unbelievable case of an employer installing hidden video equipment in a nurse's examining room—and then firing the nurses when they discovered and complained about it.[18]

How much personal and medical information obtained by the health care provider is the company entitled to? This question frequently arises in the context of preplacement medical examinations, diagnosis and treatment of work-related injuries or illnesses, medical surveillance examinations, and fitness-for-work evaluations. Should employers be informed that a job applicant has diabetes or a history of back injury? Should the employer be told that the executive being considered for promotion has cardiac disease or is seeing a psychiatrist? What about liver abnormalities related to alcohol use discovered in a hazardous waste worker participating in a medical surveillance program?

As in Case 8, physicians and nurses may encounter direct or indirect pressure to disclose or release this type of information, which the company believes will help protect its legitimate business interests. However, such disclosures invade workers' privacy and may threaten their job status. How should the health care provider reconcile these competing interests? Clarification of legal requirements and restrictions (especially in light of the Americans with Disabilities Act) may be a helpful first step. Reflection on the widely held professional ethic of maintaining patient confidentiality is also in order. In most cases, the employer does not need diagnostic or medical data but merely information about the employee's ability to work and the need for job modifications or work restrictions.

A larger and even more difficult problem relates to the extent to which occupational health and safety professionals are obligated to take action regarding suspected or known problems. The physician, nurse, and safety engineer in Case 6 have expressed their concern about the company's ergonomic problems and have made numerous recommendations for correcting them. The company has taken no action. Having expressed their concern (perhaps even in writing), do these professionals have any further obligation to follow up on these problems? Do the principles of nonmaleficence and beneficence impose an ethical duty to do more than make recommendations? Workers have already been injured, and there is every reason to believe that injuries will continue to occur. Should the physician, nurse, or safety officer notify OSHA? Try to organize the workers to take action? Quit? How far should the company-employed health and safety professional go to protect the workers? Similarly, if the company's environmental engineer is aware that the company has violated federal or state regulations on waste disposal, should he or she notify the appropriate authorities if the company continues to break the law?

The situation becomes even more complex when it is attended by uncertainty. Suppose, for example, that a hospital-based occupational health physician discovers several cases of serious disease (such as interstitial lung disease) among a group of workers (such as workers in the nylon flock industry), and that he suspects the disease may be related to unidentified exposures in the workplace. The physician commences an investigation, with the consent of the company. The physician wants to report his findings and suspicions about a new occupational disease to his colleagues at a professional meeting. If the flock manufacturer objects, citing a confidentiality agreement with the physician not to release trade secrets, and even the physician's hospital and affiliated university medical school object, what should the physician do? Continue to gather more scientific evidence? Provide the information to colleagues on an informal and *ad hoc* basis? Alert the workers and advise them to take action on their own? Take the personal and professional risk and report the findings anyway? (To find out what can happen in the real world of occupational medicine, see refs. 10, 19, 20, and 21.)

Worker Screening and Medical Examinations for Third Parties

Employers frequently ask physicians and nurses to perform medical examinations as part of various worker screening programs, for both predictive and preventive purposes. Preplacement examinations and medical surveillance programs are two examples—the latter possibly offered to comply with specific OSHA standards. Employers and insurers may also request examinations to assess work-relatedness, measure impairment or functional capacity, determine fitness for work, and make recommendations on return-to-work and job accommodation needs. Physicians have insisted and courts have agreed that no physician–patient relationship exists when a person is being examined on behalf of an employer or for another third party.[22] This lack of a physician–patient relationship dilutes the legal duty of care a physician has for the patient and may relieve the physician of other traditional legal obligations in medical practice. In this situation, attention to the ethical aspects of these activities is of special importance.

Issues of privacy, confidentiality, fairness, informed consent or refusal, and professional competence and responsibility pervade almost every form of worker screening, as well as medical examinations required by third parties for other reasons. Ethical concerns may relate to the purpose and content of examination or screening programs or to the use of the results generated by these activities.

It is helpful to ascertain why the employer wants the workers screened or examined: To help ensure that the worker can do the job without injury to self or others? To comply with government regulations? To help evaluate the effectiveness of workplace controls? (For example, the employer may want to know whether the ventilation and respiratory protection programs are adequately protecting workers from chemical exposure.) Does the employer want to weed out applicants who may pose a future liability risk? Or to find medical reasons to justify the removal of a troublemaker or a frequently absent employee? Who is the intended beneficiary of the medical examination or screening program?

Decisions about what the screening program or examination should include can also be problematic. Sometimes these examinations and their content are mandated by OSHA regulations; sometimes the company has its own ideas about what the examination should include, such as back x-ray studies, strength testing, and drug screening. Although it is certainly within the employer's rights to require preplacement, random, or for-cause drug testing, ideally it is the health care provider who defines the clinical content of the medical examination, based on knowledge of the job requirements, workplace exposures, conditions, and risks and the diagnostic and preventive value of medical testing. Many worker screening programs are ill-conceived from both a scientific and an ethical point of view. Problems with test validity (sensitivity and specificity) and predictive value may weaken any appeal to beneficence. For example, with their low predictive value in forecasting future back injury, the use of lumbosacral x-ray studies to screen out persons with back problems provides no real benefit to the company and exposes the worker to unnecessary radiation, as well as the risk of job loss. The use of cardiovascular stress testing for healthy young adults applying for jobs in the hazardous waste industry is another questionable practice.

In all cases, the physician or nurse should be aware that a worker's participation in a screening program or consent to a medical examination does not necessarily reflect an autonomous and voluntary decision. Individuals may consent to these examinations simply because they need a job. During the examination, they may knowingly or unknowingly (through testing) divulge highly personal and sensitive information to the health care provider. They may not know how or even whether such information will be passed on to others and used to their benefit or detriment.

In Case 8, the employer wants to dictate the contents of the preplacement and other periodic screening evaluations to a community physician, who has agreed to provide these services although she has never visited the plant. Can physicians exercise their professional and ethical responsibility to practice competently when, in making judgments about a worker's ability to perform a job, they have neither seen the job nor are well acquainted with its demands? Even if the physician understands the nature of the job, how will she balance fairness to the employer with protection of the prospective or current employee? Will the workers be in-

formed that the results of the medical evaluation may adversely affect their employability, remuneration, or advancement in the company? Will they be informed of their test results, counseled about their meaning, or referred elsewhere for this type of follow-up? Will the results of medical evaluations be used to help improve workplace conditions or simply to weed out "unfit" employees? If the screening program is the employer's sole approach to controlling workplace illness and injury, health care providers should weigh their involvement very carefully.

These factors place stringent ethical obligations on physicians and nurses who participate in worker screening programs. They must decide whether the purpose and content of the proposed screening program is medically reasonable and ethically justifiable. They must decide how much information employers need and are entitled to. The concepts of nonmaleficence, beneficence, fairness, and professional competence and responsibility must also be considered in decisions about the use of screening information and the need for follow-up action. Any action or inaction may adversely affect the employer, the worker, and, possibly, the provider's own standing with the company.

In considering these and other issues related to worker screening, one group of authors suggested that such testing should be used only if (a) it is an appropriate preventive tool that addresses a specific workplace problem; (b) it is used in conjunction with environmental monitoring; (c) it is not used to divert attention and resources from reducing worker exposure to toxic substances and improving workplace conditions; (d) the tests are accurate, reliable, and have a high predictive value in the population screened; and (e) medical removal protection for earnings and job security is provided.[23]

More recently, a bill of rights for persons who are subject to medical examinations at the direction of their employers has been proposed.[22] This proposal suggests that each examinee should have the right (a) to be told the purpose and scope of the examination; (b) to be told for whom the physician works; (c) to provide informed consent for all procedures; (d) to be told how results will be conveyed to the employer; (e) to be told about confidentiality protection; (f) to be told how to obtain access to the medical information in the worker's file; and (g) to be referred for medical follow-up, if necessary.

Because workers involved in medical screening or medical examinations at the behest of third parties have few legal protections, occupational health professionals must take special care when engaging in these activities.

Workplace Health Promotion

This country's economic engine depends on both a healthy workplace and a healthy workforce, and there is resurging interest in workplace health promotion. Employers have always been attracted to wellness programs because of rising health care cost and concerns about productivity and competitiveness. In many ways, the workplace is an ideal site for such intervention programs. It is a place where large numbers of relatively healthy people spend a significant amount of time. It is a potential locus for encouraging, delivering, or providing access to recommended screening exams and for distributing information about health and community-based health services. Worksites also offer the potential for social and peer supports and organizational interventions that could influence personal behavior, such as smoking, diet, and exercise. In this sense, workplace health promotion programs are buttressed by the principle of beneficence. Yet, occupational health professionals and workers often have viewed these programs with suspicion and outright distrust. Indeed, the historically narrow focus of these programs on the personal health behaviors of workers has created the potential for misuse and presented ethical challenges to the unwary health professional.[24,25]

The primary issue has been concern that a focus on individual lifestyle risks diverts attention away from workplace risks that are under the direct control of the employer and that certainly affect worker health. This appears to be happening in Case 6; the employer has ignored recommendations for ergonomic changes in the workplace and has decided to institute weight-reduction and safe lifting classes for the workers instead—essentially shifting the entire prevention burden onto the worker. Is this the best way of preventing musculoskeletal injury in this workplace? Doesn't the employer have some responsibility for the back injuries that occur in the workplace? Is it fair to place the sole burden on the workers? Should the nurse agree to conduct these health promotion programs in the absence of workplace ergonomic changes? Should the nurse encourage workers to participate in these wellness programs without also informing them of their substantial job-related risks and the actions the employer could take to reduce or eliminate them?

The debate has been framed as one between health promotion and health protection—or between the behavioral approach and the environmental approach to public health. The priority and emphasis given these approaches by occupational health professionals may reveal something of their primary allegiance or, perhaps, their biases, comfort level, or philosophy of health. It is encouraging that efforts are underway to encourage the coordination and integration of worksite health promotion and occupational health and safety programs and to bridge the gap between the professionals who design and deliver these programs. (See the NIOSH Website http://www.cdc-gov/niosh/steps/ for information about its Steps to a Healthier U.S. Workforce Initiative.) However, in the absence of effective health and safety programs focused on workplace hazards and risks, worksite wellness programs will continue to pose ethical challenges.

The Business of Providing Occupational Health Services

The United States lags behind in requiring or providing occupational health services for its workers. Most European countries have legal requirements for the provision of these services. Of growing concern, however, is the increasingly competitive environment within which occupational health services must be delivered. Competition for contracts and business among external, community-based occupational health services and competition for resources within companies have raised challenges associated with business ethics for health care providers.[26] These include issues relating to advertising and marketing; provider expertise, competence, and qualifications; commitment beyond contract periods; handing over records and responsibilities to new contractors; complying with regulations; and supervising trainees who help provide services. It has been suggested that there has been a shift from a professional ethic to a business orientation in the provision of medical care and that tension between the forces of business and professional practice gives rise to serious ethical conflicts. One study found widespread agreement on the need for a code of business ethics for occupational health services.[26] (see Chapter 12).

A popular axiom for how to succeed in a competitive business environment is to provide client-focused, customer-friendly products and services that are responsive to customer needs. This approach may be problematic for the ethical provision of occupational health services in several ways. The customer (most often an employer) may have no appreciation for what is needed or what an occupational health service can provide. Activities and actions that are necessary to keep the company happy and retain its business may conflict with a provider's ethical duties or even the customer's (or provider's) legal obligations (such as recording or reporting cases of work-related injury or illness). The status of workers or patients and the provider's relationship and responsibility to them is murky, at best. Competition on the basis of price or cost may limit the array or dilute the intensity of services that are needed to prevent work-related illness and injury. The movement of managed care organizations and techniques into the arena of workers' compensation medical care in the United States is another area that may present ethical challenges worthy of attention.

PROBLEM SOLVING AND DECISION MAKING: GUIDELINES, CODES, AND CONSULTATION

Codes of ethics are vehicles for articulating core values, establishing standards of ethical care and practice, and providing guidelines for conduct. Professional organizations of occupational and environmental health specialists have acknowledged the need for guidance in the face of ethical problems and have produced codes of ethics for their disciplines and members. In the United States, codes have been developed and adopted by the American College of Occupational and Environmental Medicine (ACOEM); the American Association of Occupational Health Nurses (AAOHN); four industrial hygiene associations (the American Conference of Governmental Industrial Hygienists, the American Board of Industrial Hygiene, the American Industrial Hygiene Association, and the American Academy of Industrial Hygiene); and the American Society of Safety Engineers (see Appendix to this chapter). Professional groups in other countries have done the same. For example, in the United Kingdom, the Faculty of Occupational Medicine has issued *Guidance on Ethics for Occupational Physicians*. The International Commission on Occupational Health has adopted an international and interdisciplinary code of ethics for oc-

cupational health professionals. One U.S. group, the Association of Occupational and Environmental Clinics, has expressed its clear preference for the international code over the code promulgated by the largest professional organization of occupational and environmental medicine physicians in the United States. There is no paucity of written guidance or debate on the subject (see Bibliography).

Although these ethical codes address many of the same issues and problems, their articulation of principles varies in clarity, depth, emphasis, strength, and directness. The codes vary, for example, in what they say about the professional's primary purpose and what should be done when the needs, demands, or expectations of employers and workers conflict. The ACOEM code for occupational physicians directs them to "*accord the highest priority to the health and safety of individuals* in both the workplace and the environment." The hygiene code advises hygienists to "practice their profession following recognized scientific principles with the realization that the lives, health and well-being of people may depend on their professional judgment and that they are obligated *to protect the health and well-being of people*." The nursing code enjoins nurses to "provide health care in the work environment with regard to human dignity and client rights . . . and promote collaboration with other health professionals and community health agencies in order *to meet the health needs of the client*." The safety engineering code indicates a duty to "*protect people and property and the environment*." The international code is perhaps the most straightforward; it states that "*the primary aim of occupational health practice is to safeguard the health of workers and to promote a safe and healthy working environment*." (Italics were added for emphasis in all instances.) A comparison of the provisions of various codes can be found in refs. 27 and 28.

Although they often are vague, these codes can be helpful. They could be appended to any contract or agreement that an occupational or environmental health professional enters into with a company or other organization. Ethical codes, however, cannot solve the moral dilemmas that arise in the day-to-day practice of occupational and environmental health. Studies suggest that occupational health professionals are often unaware of published guidelines and codes, or, if aware, seldom consult them.[29,30] Further, the codes and guidelines do not provide the protection that health professionals may need when they take action that is contrary to the wishes of their employer or other powerful interests. In the final analysis, these professionals must make their own decisions and live with the consequences.

Beyond codes, there are other concepts and methods that may help occupational health professionals in approaching ethical dilemmas. Light and McGee suggested that insights can be gained from an examination of the social construction of the moral or ethical issue at hand, as well as consideration of the vested interests; the type of action involved (starting, stopping, continuing, or abstaining); the social, political, economic, and institutional contexts; the degree of volition; and the potential for various types of harms[1]. For Philipp and colleagues, the tenets of professionalism are closely linked to ethics and can help guide conduct.[26] These tenets include competence, a sense of dedication and purpose, responsibility, autonomy, accountability, a willingness to collaborate and work effectively with others, adherence to an ethical code, and conducting one's practice with personal integrity and for the public health. Weed urges public health professionals to examine and proclaim their own philosophic commitments or values in the interest of making better choices.[31] At the same time, he acknowledged that the examination and disclosure of economic interests, political ideologies, and other social forces may also be needed.

A clarification of legal responsibilities may be a helpful first step in trying to resolve ethical problems, but compliance with legal obligations alone may be insufficient. In many cases, consultation and deliberation with others can help clarify the underlying ethical dimensions of the conflict, help define a basis for decision making, suggest or help weigh ethical criteria and justifications for various courses of action, and share the moral responsibility for decision making. Questions that may stimulate reflection and discussion include the following: What makes this an ethical problem? Why does the health professional see it that way? Who will benefit or be harmed by each alternative? Who is the least advantaged or most affected person or group in this situation? Are the needs and preferences of this party known, and have they been given the appropriate weight? What are the consequences of each action? What will happen if a particular action is not taken? What does the professional stand to lose or gain from each possible alternative? Does the professional feel pressured, or can independent judgment be exercised? Would the professional make a

different decision or determination if the issue arose while practicing in another setting? How would the professional like to be treated–or have a family member treated–in this situation?

CONCLUSION

The fields of occupational and environmental health are charged with ethical problems and dilemmas that are not easy to resolve. Consideration of widely held moral principles—such as autonomy, respect for persons, nonmaleficence, beneficence, justice, responsibility, and the integrity of personal and fiduciary relationships—can help guide decision making. Honest and careful assessment of the social, economic, political, and institutional contexts of the problem may provide insight, as may meaningful deliberation and discussion with others. Although these steps can help point the way, they do not necessarily make hard choices any easier in the practical sense. Advances in medicine, science, and technology presage a growing number of complex ethical problems, as does the increasingly competitive market for health care, including occupational health services. The need for structural safeguards for occupational and environmental health professionals has never been more clear. Unless these professionals can somehow be insulated from personal and economic reprisals, it will remain difficult for them to make the bold decisions needed to ensure worker and community environmental health. The development of structural safeguards will require creativity and, most likely, legislative action. Constructive solutions also demand honest dialogue and a clear understanding by all parties of how their actions and expectations can contribute to both the creation and the resolution of ethical issues in occupational and environmental health.

APPENDIX

Selected Codes of Ethical Conduct for Occupational Health and Safety Professionals.

AMERICAN COLLEGE OF OCCUPATIONAL AND ENVIRONMENTAL MEDICINE CODE OF ETHICAL CONDUCT

Adopted October 25, 1993 by the Board of Directors of the American College of Occupational and Environmental Medicine (ACOEM).

This code establishes standards of professional ethical conduct with which each member of the ACOEM is expected to comply. These standards are intended to guide occupational and environmental medicine physicians in their relationships with the individuals they serve; employers and workers representatives; colleagues in the health professions; the public; and all levels of government, including the judiciary.

Physicians should:

1. Accord the highest priority to the health and safety of individuals in both the workplace and the environment.
2. Practice on a scientific basis with integrity, and strive to acquire and maintain adequate knowledge and expertise on which to render professional service.
3. Relate honestly and ethically in all professional relationships.
4. Strive to expand and disseminate medical knowledge and participate in ethical research efforts as appropriate.
5. Keep confidential all individual medical information, releasing such information only when required by law or overriding public health considerations, or to other physicians according to accepted medical practice, or to others at the request of the individual.
6. Recognize that employers may be entitled to counsel about an individual's medical work fitness but not to diagnoses or specific details, except in compliance with laws and regulations.
7. Communicate to individuals and/or safety groups any significant observations and recommendations concerning their health and safety.
8. Recognize those medical impairments in oneself and others, including chemical dependency and abusive personal practices, which interfere with one's ability to follow the above principles, and take appropriate measures.

From Teichman R, Wester MS. The new ACOEM code of ethical conduct. J Occup Environ Med 1994;36:27–30.

AMERICAN ASSOCIATION OF OCCUPATIONAL HEALTH NURSES CODE OF ETHICS (INTERPRETIVE STATEMENTS NOT INCLUDED)

The AAOHN Code of Ethics has been developed in response to the nursing profession's acceptance of its goals and values, and the trust conferred on it by society to guide the conduct and practices of the profession. As a professional, the occupational health nurse accepts the responsibility and inherent obligation to uphold these values.

1. Occupational and environmental health nurses provide healthcare in the work environment with regard for human dignity and client rights, unrestricted by considerations of social or economic status, personal attributes or the nature of the health status.
2. Occupational and environmental health nurses promote interdisciplinary collaboration with other professionals and community health agencies in order to meet the health needs of the client.
3. Occupational and environmental health nurses strive to safeguard employees' right to privacy by protecting confidential information and releasing information only upon written consent of the employee or as required or permitted by law.
4. Occupational and environmental health nurses, through the provision of care, strive to safeguard clients from unethical and illegal actions.
5. Occupational and environmental health nurses, licensed to provide health care services, accept obligations to society as a professional and responsible member of the community.
6. Occupational and environmental health nurses maintain individual competence in nursing practice based on scientific knowledge, and recognize and accept responsibility for individual judgments and actions, while complying with appropriate laws and regulations that impact the delivery of occupational and environmental health services.
7. Occupational and environmental health nurses participate in activities that contribute to the ongoing development of the profession's body of knowledge while protecting the rights of subjects.

From <www.aaohn.org/practice/ethics.cfm>.

CODE OF ETHICS FOR THE PRACTICE OF INDUSTRIAL HYGIENE (INTERPRETATIVE GUIDELINES NOT INCLUDED)

Objective

These canons provide standards of ethical conduct for industrial hygienists as they practice their profession and exercise their primary mission, to protect the health and well-being of working people and the public from chemical, microbiological and physical health hazards present at, or emanating from, the workplace.

Industrial Hygienists shall:

1. Practice their profession following recognized scientific principles with the realization that the lives, health and well-being of people may depend on their professional judgment and that they are obligated to protect the health and well-being of people.
2. Counsel affected parties factually regarding potential health risks and precautions necessary to avoid adverse health effects.
3. Keep confidential personal and business information obtained during the exercise of industrial hygiene activities, except when required by law or overriding health and safety considerations.
4. Avoid circumstances where a compromise of professional judgment or conflict of interest may arise.
5. Perform services only in the areas of their competence.
6. Act responsibly to uphold the integrity of the profession.

Developed jointly in 1995 by the American Industrial Hygiene Association, the American Conference of Governmental Industrial Hygienists, the American Board of Industrial Hygiene, and the American Academy of Industrial Hygiene. From: <http://www.aiha.org/about AIHA/html/codeofethics.htm>.

AMERICAN SOCIETY OF SAFETY ENGINEERS CODE OF PROFESSIONAL CONDUCT

Membership in the American Society of Safety Engineers evokes a duty to serve and protect people, property and the environment. This duty is to be exercised with integrity, honor and dignity. Members are accountable for the following Code of Professional Conduct.

Fundamental Principles

1. Protect people, property, and the environment through the application of state-of-the-art knowledge.
2. Serve the public, employees, employers, clients, and the Society with fidelity, honesty, and impartiality.
3. Achieve and maintain competency in the practice of the profession.

4. Avoid conflicts of interest and compromise of professional conduct.
5. Maintain confidentiality of privileged information.

Fundamental Canons

In the fulfillment of my duties as a safety professional and as a member of the Society, I shall:

1. Inform the public, employers, employees, clients, and appropriate authorities when professional judgment indicates that there is an unacceptable level of risk.
2. Improve knowledge and skills through training, education, and networking.
3. Perform professional services only in the area of competence.
4. Issue public statements in a truthful manner, and only within the parameters of authority granted.
5. Serve as an agent and trustee, avoiding any appearance of conflict of interest.
6. Assure equal opportunity to all.

Approved by the House of Delegates June 9, 2002.

From the American Society of Safety Engineers Web site. Available at: <http://www.asse.org/hcode.htm>.

INTERNATIONAL COMMISSION ON OCCUPATIONAL HEALTH INTERNATIONAL CODE OF ETHICS FOR OCCUPATIONAL HEALTH PROFESSIONALS (EXCERPTS)

Basic Principles

The three following paragraphs summarize the principles of ethics on which is based the International Code of Ethics for Occupational Health Professionals, prepared by the International Commission on Occupational Health.

The purpose of occupational health is to serve the health and social well-being of the workers, individually and collectively. Occupational health practice must be performed according to the highest professionl standards and ethical principles. Occupational health professionals must contribute to environmental and community health.

The duties of occupational health professionals include protecting the life and the health of the worker, respecting human dignity and promoting the highest ethical principles in occupational health policies and programmes. Integrity in professional conduct, impartiality, and the protection of the confidentiality of health data and of the privacy of workers are part of these obligations.

Occupational health professionals are experts who must enjoy full professional independence in the execution of their functions. They must acquire and maintain the competence necessary for their duties and require conditions which allow them to carry out their tasks according to good practice and professional ethics.

Duties and Obligations of Occupational Health Professionals

1. The primary aim of occupational health practice is to safeguard and promote the health of workers, to promote a safe and healthy working environment, to protect the working capacity of workers and their access to employment. In pursuing this aim, occupational health professionals must use validated methods of risk evaluations, propose efficient preventive measures, and follow up their implementation. . . .

2. Occupational health professionals must continuously strive to be familiar with the work and the working environment as well as to improve their competence and to remain well informed in scientific and technical knowledge, occupational hazards and the most efficient means to eliminate or minimise the relevant risks. . . .

4. Special consideration should be given to rapid application of simple preventive measures which are technically sound and easily implemented. Further evaluation must check whether these measures are effective or if a more complete solution must be sought. When doubts exist about the severity of an occupational hazard, prudent precautionary action must be considered immediately and taken as appropriate. . . .

5. In the case of refusal or of unwillingness to take adequate steps to remove an undue risk or to remedy a situation which presents evidence of danger to health or safety, the occupational health professionals must make, as rapidly as possible, their concern clear, in writing, to the appropriate senior management executive, stressing the need for taking into account scientific knowledge and for applying relevant health protection standards, including exposure limits, and recalling the obligation of the employer to apply laws and regulations and to protect the health of workers in their employment. The workers concerned and their representatives in the enterprise should be informed and the competent authority should be contacted, whenever necessary.

6. Occupational health professionals must contribute to the information of workers on occupational hazards to which they may be exposed in an objective and understandable manner which does not conceal any fact and emphasizes the preventive measures. . . .

8. The occupational health objectives, methods, and procedures of health surveillance must be clearly defined with priority given to adaptation of workplaces to workers who must receive information in this respect. The relevance and validity of these methods and procedures must be assessed. The surveillance must be carried out with the informed consent of the worker. The potentially positive and negative consequences of participation in screening and health surveillance programs should be discussed as part of the consent process. . . .

9. The results of examinations carried out within the framework of health surveillance must be explained to the worker concerned. The determination of fitness for a given job, when required, must be based on a good knowledge of the job demands and of the work-site and on the assessment of the health of the worker. . . .

10. The results of the examinations prescribed by national laws or regulations must only be conveyed to management in terms of fitness for the envisaged work or of limitations necessary from a medical point of view in the assignment of tasks or in the exposure to occupational hazards. . . .

14. Occupational professionals must be aware of their role in relation to the protection of the community and of the environment. . . .

Conditions of Execution of the Functions of Occupational Health Professionals

16. Occupational health professionals must always act, as a matter of prime concern, in the interest of the health and safety of the workers. . . .

17. Occupational health professionals must seek and maintain full professional independence and observe the rules of confidentiality in the execution of their functions. . . .

18. The occupational health professionals must build a relationship of trust, confidence, and equity with the people to whom they provide occupational health services. All workers should be treated in an equitable manner, without any form of discrimination. . . . Occupational health professionals must establish and maintain clear channels of communication among themselves, the senior management responsible for decisions at the highest level about the conditions and the organisation of work and the working environment in the undertaking, and with the workers' representatives.

19. Occupational health professionals must request that a clause on ethics be incorporated into their contract of employment. . . .

20. Individual medical data and the results of medical investigations must be recorded in confidential medical files which must be kept secured under the responsibility of the occupational health physician or the occupational health nurse. Access to medical files, their transmission, and their release are governed by national laws or regulations on medical data where they exist and relevant national codes of ethics for health professionals and medical practitioners. The information contained in these files must only be used for occupational health purposes.

From the International Commission on Occupational Health. <http://www.icoh.org.sg/core_docs/core_ethics_eng.pdf>.

INTERNATIONAL CODE OF CONDUCT (ETHICS) FOR OCCUPATIONAL HEALTH AND SAFETY PROFESSIONALS

This International Code of Conduct (Ethics) for Occupatonal Health and Safety Professionals was developed, in part, to address the inadequacies of the ICOH International Code of Ethics for Occupational Health Professionals, excerpts of which are printed above. The International Code of Conduct (Ethics) is the product of deliberations of leading occupational health and safety professionals from many countries. Most of the participants were Fellows of the Collegium Ramazzini, and many represented the World Health Organization and the International Labor Organization. This International Code of Conduct (Ethics) goes far beyond all existing codes. In that regard, it challenges organi-

zations and professionals to upgrade their commitments to ethical conduct.

The International Code of Conduct (Ethics) is intended to assist occupational health and safety professionals to make and support decisions that protect the interests of the worker and the needs of society. The Code requires occupational health and safety professionals to disclose the perspective from which they approach their analysis of specific issues. The Code is intended to guide professionals when confronted with conflicts of interest, and to encourage disclosure of affiliations so that potential bias can be discussed openly. Unarticulated, such affiliations threaten to undermine the objectivity of all occupational health and safety professionals and jeopardize the validity and ultimate significance of their work. The Code's important provision of a Declaration of Conflict of Interest is currently being considered by the Collegium Ramazzini and other international organizations.

I. Purposes and Goals

International occupational safety and health organizations do by consensus hereby state the following purposes and goals for the ethical professional conduct of Health and Safety Professionals:

1. Health and safety in the workplace is a right of all workers, regardless of gender, age, national or ethnic origin, religion, or race.

2. Occupational health and safety professionals have an ethical responsibility to accord priority to health and safety in the workplace. Occupational health and safety professionals shall take every practical measure to protect workers from any unreasonable risk of harm.

3. It is the responsibility of occupational health and safety professionals to promote a consistent and dependable level of health and safety regulation and enforcement for the protection of every worker in every country.

4. Occupational health and safety professionals must be trained in their own field and in relevant related disciplines, and must remain current with advances in their field in order to participate with other professionals to design, develop, implement, and safeguard policies and programs that achieve optimal health and safety for the workplace.

5. Occupational health and safety professionals should support the consideration of any

environmental impact of industrial activities, related employer policies, and governmental public health policies.

II. Definitions

This Code incorporates International Labor Office (ILO)-based definitions, as they appear in relevant international conventions, for the terms Safety, Work, Workplace, Employer, Employee Standards, Professional Responsibility, Ethics, Government Programs, Occupational Safety and Health Professional, Risk, Unreasonable Risk of Harm, and Declaration of Conflict of Interest.

III. Responsibilities

Occupational health and safety professionals have an obligation to bring to the attention of employers any health and safety policy deficiencies and any risks to the health and safety of workers. All occupational health and safety professionals have an obligation to support each other in the face of conflict of interest between the obligations to employees and the employer's economic interests.

If the occupational safety and health professional reasonably believes within the discretion of sound professional judgment and expert opinion that a given employer does not act responsibly to reduce risk, modify the impact of unavoidable harms, or prevent specific avoidable health or safety problems, the occupational health and safety professional has an obligation to notify the employer in writing of the specific health and safety risks to specific categories of workers and the likelihood of health and safety impacts from the employer's failure to correct such problems.

It is the responsibility of every occupational health and safety professional to be familiar with government agency regulations, and the occupational health and safety laws applicable to that occupational health and safety professional's workplace. Every effort should be made to remain aware of current developments in the law, emerging issues in occupational safety and health policy, and impacts of new technologies through continuing professional education in law, medicine, safety, economics, and other sciences in order to provide appropriate and effective preventive measures and interventions.

IV. Right to Know

- Workers are to be informed of any medical findings on fitness examinations and preventive

medical (surveillance) reviews where knowledge of such findings by the worker may affect the worker's future well-being.
- All medical records are confidential. They can be released to a party other than the worker only when permitted by law, required by overriding public health considerations, or at the request of the worker. It is the right of the worker to designate a representative who may receive the worker's medical, safety, and industrial hygiene records, on his or her behalf.
- Employers may be entitled to information about a worker's work fitness, but employers are not entitled to disclosure of diagnoses or to specific medical details unnecessary to the employer's responsibility to protect the worker from harm in the workplace. Employers and insurance companies are not entitled to any genetic information on workers.
- Workers are entitled to all occupational health and safety information that relates to their workplace. The worker's right to health and safety information is of greater concern than the employer's wish to protect trade secrets.
- Occupational health and safety professionals must present and explain health and safety information so that all workers are adequately informed about the level of risk.

V. Reports and Declaration of Conflict of Interest

Occupational health and safety professionals must disseminate health and safety knowledge and support research efforts. They have a responsibility to identify occupational illnesses and to publish their findings. They have a responsibility to participate in expert advisory committees, and to participate in the reviews of regulations and other public policies. When occupational health and safety professionals conduct studies, write research reports, publish in scientific journals, and appear as experts in various proceedings, they must make a Declaration of Conflict of Interest by completing and signing the attached Declaration. All sources of support, including governments, foundations, unions, and law firms should be declared.

Occupational health and safety professionals must be aware of all "conflict of interest" where their professional decisions may also provide them with incidental personal benefit. Occupational health and safety professionals should not allow personal benefit to determine or to substantially influence their professional decisions. Where such influence cannot be avoided, the occupational health and safety professional should refer the matter to another occupational health professional who is competent to make the decision and who has no such conflict of interest.

VI. Compliance Programs

It is the further responsibility of every occupational health and safety professional to comply with laws and to assist employers to comply with those laws to the greatest extent practical. Where inadequate resources or employer disagreement with the law prevent the occupational health and safety professional from fully complying with the law, that occupational health and safety professional shall nevertheless take every practical measure to protect workers from any unreasonable risk of harm.

VII. Transparency Policy

When occupational health and safety professionals participate in or are represented by a professional organization, a Transparency Policy must be adopted and enforced by the organization. "Transparency" refers to the administration of an organization in an open and above-board fashion, where leaders, members, and outsiders, are all given full opportunity to observe the administration of the organization.

The professional organization will conduct all its activities so that members are fully informed, and non-members can be informed without impediment. Meetings of the professional organization will be open to all members. Non-members may attend meetings of the officers and board without impediment. The minutes of a professional organization's meetings will be placed on a homepage and made available to non-members without impediment. All letters between officers and board members will be put into electronic format and copied to the members of the professional organization. All financial statements of the professional organization will be sent to members. Financial statements will be available on a homepage for non-members.

VIII. Enforcement Provisions

Organizations that adopt the International Code of Conduct limit membership in the organization to those who agree to abide by the provisions of the Code of Conduct.

Source: Ladou J, Tennenhouse DJ, Feitshans IL. Codes of ethics (conduct). Occup Med: State of the Art Rev 2002;17:559–585.

Declaration of Conflict of Interest

I am committed to objectivity in the collection, interpretation, and presentation of research data and information for educational purposes. I recognize the pervasive and destructive effects of conflicts of interest and appearances of conflicts of interest, and I recognize that full disclosure is the appropriate remedy for real or apparent conflicts of interest. Therefore, my signature on this Declaration signifies that during the past three years I have not engaged in any practice, or received anything of significant value, that might compromise or appear to compromise my objectivity in my areas of professional expertise or activity except as disclosed below.

a) I have neither received nor been promised anything of significant value, including but not limited to salary or wages, payment for consultancies or expert testimony, patient referrals, participation in industry advisory boards, other business relationships, honoraria, stock or stock options, cash, any travel allowance, gifts, services, or awards, from government, foundations, unions, law firms, trade associations, corporations, business, or other commercial entities with a financial interest in my areas of professional expertise or activity, including payment through all sources of support, or other person or organization representing such an entity.

b) I do not own and have no current plans to purchase stock, stock options, or any other interest with significant economic value in any corporation, business, or commercial entity with a financial interest in my areas of professional expertise or activity.

c) I have received no research support, not have my students or persons working for me received such support, from any corporation, business, or other commercial entity with a financial interest in my areas of professional expertise or activity.

d) Neither my family members, nor my students, nor my colleagues, nor my business partners or associates, nor my institution has received anything of significant value from any corporation, business, or other commercial entity in recognition of my professional activity.

e) I have received no honors, awards, or other formal recognition from any commercial corporation, business, or other entity with a financial interest in my work.

Exceptions and (optional) explanations:
____ There are no exceptions
____ There are exceptions that are described below.

_____

_____

_____

_____

_____

_____

None of the exceptions listed here in any way compromise my professional objectivity or conduct. I recognize that no printed form can adequately explore all matters that may create, or appear to create, a conflict of interest, and I will endeavor to avoid or promptly disclose any other such real or apparent conflicts of interest if they have arisen or do arise.

_____   _____

Signature   Date

REFERENCES

1. Light D, McGee G. On the social embeddedness of bioethics. In: DeVries R, Subedi J, eds. *Bioethics and society: Constructing the ethical enterprise. 4th ed.* Upper Saddle River, NJ: Prentice Hall, 1998:1–15.
2. Wolpe P. The triumph of autonomy in American bioethics: A sociological view. In: DeVries R, Subedi J, eds. *Bioethics and society: Constructing the ethical enterprise. 4th ed.* Upper Saddle River, NJ: Prentice Hall, 1998:38–59.
3. Ladd J. The task of ethics. In: Reich WT, ed. *Encyclopedia of bioethics*. New York: The Free Press, 1978.
4. Soskolne CL. Epidemiology: Questions of science, ethics, morality, and law. Am J Epidemiol 1989; 129:1–18.
5. James A, Horton R, Collingridge D, McConnell J, Butcher J. The Lancet's policy on conflicts of interest–2004. Lancet 2004;363:2–3(9402).
6. Kaiser J. NIH chief clamps down on consulting and stock ownership. Science 2005;307:824–5.
7. Harris G, Berenson A. 10 voters on panel backing pain pills had industry ties. New York Times, February 25, 2005.A1
8. Washburn J. University, Inc.: The corporate corruption of American higher education. 2005. New York: Basic Books
9. Egilman DS, Hom C. Corruption of the medical literature: A second visit. Am J Ind Med 1998;34:401–4.
10. Shuchman M. Secrecy in science: The flock worker's lung investigation. Ann Intern Med 1998;129:341–4.
11. Ozonoff D, Boden L. Truth and consequences: Health agency responses to environmental health problems. Sci Technol Hum Values 1987;12:70–7.
12. Bullard R. *Dumping in Dixie: Race, class and environmental quality.* Boulder, CO: Westview Press, 1990.
13. Bryant B, (ed). Environmental justice: Issues, policies, and solutions. Washington, DC: Island Press, 1995.
14. Fagin D, Lavelle M (Center for Public Integrity). *Toxic deception: How the chemical industry manipulates science, bends the law, and endangers your health. 2nd ed.* Monroe, ME: Common Courage Press, 1999.
15. Robinson JC. *Toil and toxics: Workplace struggles and political strategies for occupational health.* Berkeley: University of California Press, 1991.
16. McCallum DB, Covello VT. What the public thinks about environmental data. EPA J 1990;113:467–73.
17. World Economic Forum. Global survery on trust: Update 2004. http://www. weforum.org/site/homepublic.nsf
18. Larsen S. Hidden camera triggers suit: IBP nurses fired after finding video equipment. The Dispatch and The Rock Island Argus. November 27, 1997:A1–A2.
19. Kern D, Crausman RS, Durand KTH, et al. Flock worker's lung: Chronic interstitial lung disease in the nylon flocking industry. Ann Intern Med 1998;129:261–72.
20. Kern D. The unexpected result of an investigation of an outbreak of occupational lung disease. Int J Occup Med Environ Health 1998;4:19–32.
21. Davidoff F. New disease, old story. Ann Intern Med 1998;129:327–38.
22. Rothstein MA. Legal and medical aspects of medical screening. Occup Med State of the Art Rev 1996;11: 31–9.
23. Ashford NA, Spadafor CJ, Hattis DB, et al. *Monitoring the worker for exposure and disease: Scientific, legal, and ethical considerations in the use of biomarkers.* Baltimore: Johns Hopkins Press, 1990.
24. Walsh DC, Jennings SE, Mangione T, et al. Health promotion versus health protection: Employees' perceptions and concerns. J Public Health Policy 1991;12:148–64.
25. Allegrante JR, Sloan RP. Ethical dilemmas in workplace health promotion. Prev Med 1986;15:313–20.
26. Philipp R, Goodman G, Harling K, et al. Study of business ethics in occupational medicine. Occup Environ Med 1997;54:351–6.
27. Brodkin CA, Frumkin H, Kirkland KH, et al. AOEC position paper on the organizational code for ethical conduct. J Occup Environ Med 1996;38:869–81.
28. Rothstein MA. A proposed revision of the ACOEM code of ethics. J Occup Environ Med 1997;39:616–22.
29. Aw TC. Ethical issues in occupational medicine practice: Knowledge and attitudes of occupational physicians. Occup Med 1997;47:371–6.
30. Martimo KP, Antti-Poika M, Leino T, et al. Ethical issues among Finnish occupational physicians and nurses. Occup Med 1998;48:375–80.
31. Weed D. Toward a philosophy of public health. J Epidemiol Community Health 1999;53:99–104.

BIBLIOGRAPHY

ACOEM Committee on Ethical Practice in Occupational Medicine. Commentaries on the code of ethical conduct: I. J Occup Environ Med 1995;37:201–6.

Brodkin CA, Frumkin H, Kirkland KH, et al. AOEC position paper on the organizational code for ethical conduct. J Occup Environ Med 1996;38:869–81.

Brodkin CA, Frumkin H, Kirkland KH, et al. Choosing a professional code of ethical conduct in occupational and environmental medicine. J Occup Environ Med 1998;40:840–2.

Goodman KW. Codes of ethics in occupational and environmental health. J Occup Environ Med 1996;38:882–3.

Rothstein MA. A proposed revision of the ACOEM code of ethics. J Occup Environ Med 1997;39:616–22.

Teichman R, Wester MS. The new ACOEM code of ethical conduct. J Occup Environ Med 1994;36:27–30.

Teichman RF. ACOEM code of ethical conduct. J Occup Environ Med 1997;39:614–15.

The above seven articles cover the debate about the ACOEM code of ethics for occupational health physicians.

Ashford NA, Spadafor CJ, Hattis DB, et al. *Monitoring the worker for exposure and disease:scientific,legal,and ethical considerations in the use of biomarkers.* Baltimore:Johns Hopkins Press, 1990.

Koh D, Jeyaratnam J. Biomarkers, screening and ethics. Occup Med 1998;48:27–30.

Rothstein MA. Legal and medical aspects of medical screening. Occup Med 1996;11:31–9.

The above three sources provide information on ethical issues in worker screening, genetic and otherwise.

Beauchamp TL, Childress JF. *Principles of biomedical ethics.* New York: Oxford University Press, 1994.

DeVries R, Subedi J. *Bioethics and society: Constructing the ethical enterprise.* Upper Saddle River, NJ: Prentice Hall, 1998.

The above two texts provide a general discussion of bioethics.

Bullard R. *Dumping in Dixie: Race, class and environmental quality.* Boulder, CO: Westview Press, 1990.

Fagin D, Lavelle M (Center for Public Integrity). *Toxic deception: How the chemical industry manipulates science, bends the law, and endangers your health. 2nd ed.* Monroe, ME: Common Courage Press, 1999.

Robinson JC. *Toil and toxics: Workplace struggles and political strategies for occupational health.* Berkeley: University of California Press, 1991.

The above three books present accounts of historical failures described in this chapter.

Kern D, Crausman RS, Durand KTH, et al. Flock worker's lung: chronic interstitial lung disease in the nylon flocking industry. Ann Intern Med 1998;129:261–72.

Kern D. The unexpected result of an investigation of an outbreak of occupational lung disease. Int J Occup Med Environ Health 1998;4:19–32.

Shuchman M. Secrecy in science: The flock worker's lung investigation. Ann Intern Med 1998;129:341–4.

Davidoff F. New disease, old story. Ann Intern Med 1998;129:327–8.

The above four articles describe a real-world example of ethical issues in occupational health.

McCunney RJ. Preserving confidentiality in occupational medical practice. Am Fam Physician 1996;53:1751–6.

Rischitelli DG. Licensing, practice, and malpractice in occupational medicine. Occup Med 1996;11:121–35.

Rothstein MA. Legal and medical aspects of medical screening. Occup Med 1996;11:31–9.

Tilton SH. Right to privacy and confidentiality of medical records. Occup Med 1996;11:17–29.

The above four articles provide information about legal and ethical aspects of confidentiality of medical records in occupational health.

Westerholm P, Nilstun T, Ovretveit J (eds). *Practical ethics in occupational health.* Oxford: Radcliffe Medical Press, 2004.

London L, Kisting S. Ethical concerns in international occupational health and safety. Occup Med State of the Art Rev 2002;17:587–600.

Good sources for an international perspective on ethical issues in occupational health.

Recognition, Assessment, and Prevention

TABLE 6-2

Outline of a Detailed Environmental History

Components	Specific Questions and Issues
Present and prior home locations	Information on all places that a person has lived. In particular, one should ask about living hear to: (a) an industrial facility that may be polluting the air, surface water, groundwater, or the soil; (b) a hazardous waste site; and (c) a farm where pesticides or herbicides may have been applied.
Jobs of household members	Workers may bring home contaminants, such as lead. Children may be inappropriately brought to a worksite, such as a farm where pesticides have been used.
Environmental tobacco smoke	Smokers in home and other environments.
Lead exposure	Is a child living in a home built before 1978?
	Does a child have a sibling or playmate with a history of lead poisoning?
	Is lead present in water pipes?
	Is there imported pottery in the home?
	Are ethnic folk remedies used?
	Do household members work in lead-related industries or have hobbies in which they are exposed to lead?
Home insulating, heating, and cooking	What types of insulation are present?
	Are furnaces and stoves properly vented?
Household building materials	What types have been used? For example, formaldehyde-containing materials may cause irritative and respiratory symptoms. Has there been recent renovation or remodeling?
Home cleaning agents and other household products	What types have been used? Many household products contain toxic, allergenic, or irritant chemicals.
Presence of pests, mold, pets, and dust in the home	Asthmatic and other atopic individuals may be allergic to cockroaches, molds, animal dander, or dust mites. Is there a damp basement or recent flooding that might be conducive to mold growth? Are there pillows and stuffed animals, which can be a reservoir for house dust mites? Are there shag carpets, which can be a reservoir for allergens?
Pesticide usage	What types have been used and where? Do not overlook flea collars and flea treatments of pets.
Water supply	What is the source of water? People on small water systems or with private wells are especially at risk. Bottled water may not be safer than municipal water. If people are using a private well, when was it last tested?
Diet	Obtain information on diet, including dietary supplements. If there has been a possible foodborne illness, what food was eaten and what was its source during the time of likely exposure? Was lead-glazed pottery used for food preparation?
Hobbies	Hobbies such as painting, sculpting, welding, woodworking, piloting, auto maintenance and repair, ceramics, and gardening may bring chemicals into the home environment.
Safety issues	Seatbelt use, and home and recreational safety
Travel history	Obtain information on recent travel.

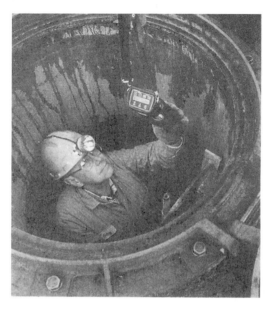

FIGURE 6-1 ● Many jobs require work in confined spaces. (Photograph by Earl Dotter.)

major past occupations of patients and key information on residential and other environmental exposures. The extent of detail depends largely on the clinician's level of suspicion that occupational or environmental factors may have caused or contributed to the patient's illness. The history should always be recorded with great care and precision.

Some hospitals and clinics have standardized forms for occupational and environmental histories, which can expedite the taking and recording of this

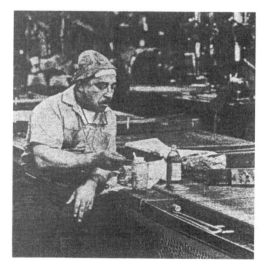

FIGURE 6-2 ● Workers eating in the workplace may ingest toxic substances. (Photograph by Earl Dotter.)

information and make gathering this information feasible for those providing comprehensive primary care. Ideally, such forms should include (a) a grid with column headings for job, employer, industry, major job tasks, dates of starting and stopping the job, and major work exposures (Fig. 6-3); and (b) a series of questions on environmental exposures. It may be helpful to ask questions from a list prepared in advance about whether the patient has had any exposures to hazardous substances or physical factors, such as noise or radiation. Further elaboration on each of the key parts of the occupational and environmental histories may be helpful, especially when (a) the patient raises concerns about potential exposures, (b) the clinician needs to further evaluate exposures of concern, (c) organ systems that are commonly associated with exposure are adversely affected, or (d) the diagnosis remains unclear.

Sometimes there is an additive or synergistic relationship between occupational and environmental factors in causing disease. The clinician should ask whether the patient smokes cigarettes, is exposed to environmental tobacco smoke, or drinks alcohol; if so, amount and duration should be quantified. For skin problems, questions should be asked regarding recent exposure to new soaps, cosmetics, or clothes.

Other information that the clinician obtains may supplement the history. It is useful to know whether the patient has had preplacement or periodic physical and laboratory examinations at work. For example, preplacement audiograms or pulmonary function test results may be helpful in determining whether hearing impairment or respiratory symptoms are work–related. Because Occupational Safety Health Administration (OSHA) regulations mandate periodic screening of workers with certain exposures, such as asbestos or coke oven emissions, and because many employers voluntarily provide health screening in the workplace, it is increasingly likely that such information may be available to a clinician, if the worker approves its release.

Finally, it is often useful to ask the patient whether there is some reason to suspect that the symptoms may be related to external exposures.

When to Take Complete Occupational and Environmental Histories

In the following situations, the clinician should have a strong suspicion of occupational and environmental factors or influences on the development of the

1. Please provide the following information on your work history.

Job	Employer	Industry	Major job tasks	Dates of starting stopping		Major work exposures*
CUSTODIAN	City of Boston	Day Care	Repair, cleaning	10/91	→	Flu, kid's infections, asbestos, cleaners
GRINDER	Hudson Engine	Engine Mfg.	metal machining	10/86	10/91	Oil mist,
LATHE OPER.	Nash Engine	Engine mfg.	metal machining	10/76	10/86	Noise,
BORE MACHINE OPERATOR	Kaiser	Die Making	Cutting metals	10/70	10/76	Lifting/Twisting
VOLUNTARY FIREFIGHTER	Town of Salem	—	Fighting House fires	10/68	10/79	Fumes, gases
STUDENT	—	—	mechanic Student	6/68	9/70	Noise, oils
Military? YES	US Air Force	Helicopter Mech.	motor. Repair	1/67	1/68	Noise, Stress
Part-time work?	Town General Store	Retail Food	Checkout Clerk	1/64	1/67	Repetitive motion

2. Have you had any possibly hazardous exposures outside of work? _Yes_ If yes, complete the following.

Major exposures	Associated activity	Location	Dates of starting stopping	
Wood dust	Cabinet making	Home	~1971	→

3. Have you ever smoked cigarettes? _Yes_ If yes, please answer the following questions.
   How old were you when you started smoking? _18_
   On average, how many packs have you smoked a day? _½_
   Do you currently smoke? _No_ If no, how old were you when you stopped smoking? _31_

*Such as chemicals, fumes, dusts, vapors, gases, noise, and radiation.

FIGURE 6-3 ● Sample occupational history form. (From Levy BS, Wegman DH. The occupational history in medical practice: what questions to ask and when to ask them. Postgrad Med 1986;79:301.)

problem and take detailed occupational and environmental histories. Many symptoms appear to be nonspecific but may have their origin in occupational and environmental exposures.

Respiratory Disease

Virtually any respiratory symptoms can be related to occupational and environmental factors. It is all too easy to diagnose acute respiratory symptoms as acute tracheobronchitis or viral infection when the actual diagnosis is occupational asthma or to attribute chronic respiratory symptoms as chronic obstructive pulmonary disease when the actual diagnosis is asbestosis. Viruses and cigarettes are too often assumed to be the sole agents responsible for respiratory disease. Adult-onset asthma is frequently work-related but often not recognized as such. In addition, patients with preexisting asthma may have exacerbations of their otherwise quiescent condition when exposed to workplace sensitizers. Less commonly, pulmonary edema can be caused by workplace chemicals such as phosgene or oxides of nitrogen; a detailed work history should be

obtained for anyone with acute pulmonary edema when no likely nonoccupational cause can be identified (see Chapter 25).

Skin Disorders

Many skin disorders are nonspecific in nature, bothersome but not life-threatening, and self-limited. Diagnoses often are nonspecific, and physicians all too often fail to take a brief occupational and environmental history that might identify the offending irritant, sensitizer, or other factor. Contact dermatitis, which accounts for about 90 percent of all work-related cases and many other cases of skin disease, does not have a characteristic appearance. Determination of the cause depends on carefully obtained occupational and environmental histories (see Chapter 28).

Hearing Impairment

Many cases of hearing impairment are falsely attributed to aging (presbycusis). Millions of American workers have been exposed to hazardous noise at work, at home, at rock concerts, or elsewhere. For this reason, detailed occupational and environmental histories should be obtained from anyone with hearing impairment. Recommendations for the prevention of future hearing loss should also be made (see Chapters 14A and 27).

Back and Joint Symptoms

Back pain is often partially work-related, but there are no tests or other procedures that can differentiate work-related from non–work-related back problems; its relationship to work depends on the occupational history. A surprising number of cases of arthritis and tenosynovitis are caused by rapid, forceful, awkward, and/or repetitive movements associated with work tasks. *Ergonomics*, the study of the complex interactions among workers, their workplace environments, job demands, and work methods, can help prevent some of these problems (see Chapters 11 and 23).

Cancer

A significant percentage of cancer cases are caused by occupational and environmental exposures, and, as time goes by, more occupational and environmental carcinogens are discovered. Often, the initial suspicion that a substance may be carcinogenic comes from individual clinicians' reports. This effort would be facilitated if occupational and environmental histories were obtained from all patients with cancer. Of importance in considering occupational and environmental cancer is that exposure to the carcinogen may have begun many years before diagnosis of the disease and that the exposure need not have been continued over the entire time interval (see Chapter 24).

Exacerbation of Coronary Artery Disease Symptoms

Exposure to stress (see Chapter 16) and to carbon monoxide and other chemicals in the workplace (see Chapter 13) may increase the frequency or severity of symptoms of coronary artery disease (see Chapter 30).

Liver Disease

As with respiratory disease, it is all too easy to give liver ailments common diagnoses such as viral hepatitis or alcoholic cirrhosis rather than the less common diagnosis of toxic hepatitis. It is always important to take a occupational and environmental histories from a patient with liver disease. Hepatotoxins encountered in the workplace and the general environment are discussed in Chapter 30.

Neuropsychiatric Problems

The possible relation of neuropsychiatric problems to occupational and environmental factors is often overlooked. Peripheral neuropathies are more frequently attributed to diabetes, alcohol abuse, or "unknown etiology"; CNS dysfunction to substance abuse or psychiatric problems; and behavioral abnormalities (which may be the first sign of work-related stress or, less frequently, a neurotoxic problem) to psychosis or personality disorder. More than 100 chemicals (including virtually all solvents) can cause CNS dysfunction, and several neurotoxins (including arsenic, lead, mercury, and methyl n-butyl ketone) can produce peripheral neuropathy. Carbon disulfide exposure can cause symptoms that mimic a psychosis (see Chapter 26).

Illnesses of Unknown Cause

Detailed, complete occupational and environmental histories are essential in all cases in which the cause of illness is unknown or uncertain (such as fever of unknown origin) or the diagnosis is obscure. The need to search carefully for an occupational and environmental source in such illnesses results from the increasing awareness of low-level environmental exposures as a cause of symptoms or disease. Such exposures may be related to hazardous wastes (see Chapter 20) or indoor air quality (see Chapter 18).

A key principle in toxicology and occupational and environmental health is that the biological response to a chemical or physical agent is primarily a function of dose. Although health effects from high levels of exposure typically are more frequent and more severe than those caused by low levels, more people are subject to low levels of exposure in the workplace and in the ambient environment. Health professionals who are approached by patients with symptoms they think are related to low levels of exposure to chemical substances should develop a caring and careful approach to addressing these concerns.

Symptoms associated with low-level exposures are often difficult to evaluate because of difficulty in documenting the exposure and because the symptom pattern is much less specific than that of a well-established disorder. Human variability is such that even a normal distribution of responses includes a few individuals who respond at very low doses. True allergic responses, unusual exposures, and new technologies may all present diagnostic challenges, and it is critically important that clinicians not arrive at premature closure or fail to listen to their patients—a process that requires thoughtful evaluation of personal, home, and other life stressors. On the one hand, symptoms as obscure as difficulty in initiating urination have been caused by very specific neurotoxins introduced into the workplace. On the other hand, patients have had needless trauma and disability imposed on them through unnecessary testing and invasive procedures.

The history is still central in the final determination of how to care for these patients as indicated below, although laboratory investigation of the syndromes represented in these individuals may predominate.

1. If the problem is related to classic allergy, it may be possible to identify patterns of response of those who are severely atopic that explain the nonspecific stimuli associated with lower symptom severity between allergic attacks.
2. Some disorders may be associated with chemical or other environmental stimuli resulting in symptoms interpreted as being caused by the environment. A careful medical history should identify the need to have such patients evaluated by a specialist, especially because the relevant diagnoses may be ones of exclusion.
3. Building-related illnesses and multiple chemical sensitivity often present as diagnostic challenges (see Chapter 18).

SURVEILLANCE

Public health surveillance is the systematic and ongoing collection, analysis, and dissemination of information on disease, injury, or hazard for the prevention of morbidity and mortality. Surveillance as it applies to populations, also sometimes called public health tracking, should be differentiated from medical monitoring of individuals. *Medical monitoring*, sometimes refered to as *periodic medical screening*, is focused on the interview, examination, and/or testing of individuals. Public health surveillance is focused on populations. Although the overriding goal of medical monitoring and public health surveillance are the same (that is, prevention), the specific goals are different.

There are five goals of public health surveillance as it is applied to occupational and environmental disease:

1. *To identify illnesses, injuries, and hazards that represent new opportunities for prevention*: New opportunities can arise from new problems, such as might occur with the introduction of a new hazardous machine, from belated identification of a long-standing but ignored problem, or the recurrence of a problem previously controlled.
2. *To define the magnitude and distribution of the problem in the workplace and the general environment:* Information on magnitude and distribution is useful for planning intervention programs. Although no hazard is acceptable, the more common and severe problems deserve more immediate attention.
3. *To track trends:* Tracking trends of the magnitude of a problem is a rudimentary method of assessing the effectiveness (or lack of effectiveness) of prevention efforts. Epidemics can be tracked on their rise or their decline.
4. *To set priorities:* To identify categories of occupations, industries, and specific workplaces and environmental sites that require attention in the form of consultation, education, or inspection for compliance with established regulations.
5. *To publicly disseminate information:* This can facilitate appropriate personal and societal decisions.

There is a continuum of outcomes that could be monitored. The continuum may range from the presence of an exposure or hazard, to early and subclinical health effects of that hazard, to morbidity and associated medical care and disability, and finally to mortality (Fig. 6-4). The choice of an appropriate exposure or health outcome for surveillance should depend on the goal of the surveillance. Other considerations should include (a) an assessment of whether the proposed reporting entity, such as physician or employer, will report the occurrence; (b) the accuracy of the system in detecting real problems and minimizing false-positive leads; (c) the timeliness of the system in producing useful information; and (d) the cost of the system in relation to other systems that could be supported instead.

There are two approaches to surveillance: one based on cases and the other based on rates. *Case-based surveillance* relies on the intensive investigation of individual cases or clusters of cases. *Rate-based surveillance* is embedded in epidemiologic methods that determine the distribution or rate of disease, injury, or hazard in a population. Like communicable disease surveillance, which relies heavily on physician and laboratory reporting of cases

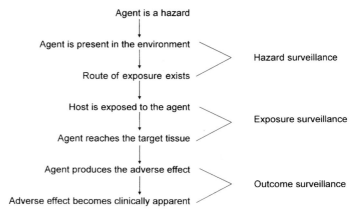

FIGURE 6-4 ● The continuum of environmental and occupational health surveillance (Adapted from: Thacker SB, Stroup DF, Parrish RG, et al. Surveillance in environmental public health: issues, systems, and sources. American Journal of Public Health 1996;86:633–638.)

of disease, occupational and environmental health practitioners often rely on surveillance of sentinel health events, which may lead to their conducting intensive investigations of unusual cases of disease or disease clusters. *Sentinel health events* are defined as cases of disease, injuries, or exposures that represent failures of the system for prevention.[1] Some examples include the discovery of lead contamination in imported candy through the investigation of a cluster of cases of lead poisoning in children, and the identification of occupational asthma in workers using solvents to remove graffiti from public spaces.

Rate-based surveillance is embedded in epidemiologic methods that determine the rate of occurrence of disease, injury, or hazard in a population, track this rate over time, or compare it with rates in other populations. Surveillance differs from *epidemiologic research* in that it is an ongoing activity with goals directly related to the functioning of the public health system; in contrast, epidemiologic research assesses possible associations between exposures and adverse health effects. Epidemiologic research also involves intensive collection of data during a limited time period, rather than the ongoing collection and assessment of data that comprise surveillance. In reality, the distinctions between surveillance and research often blur.

Surveillance can be used to monitor the occurrence of disease at each point within the exposure–disease continuum (Fig. 6-4). *Hazard surveillance* is used to determine the distribution of agents that could potentially lead to disease. Examples of hazard surveillance include the number and geographic distribution within a community of homes that contain lead-based paint or the types and quantity of pesticides used in an agricultural area. *Exposure surveillance* is used to document the frequency and distribution of indicators that the host has been exposed to the hazard, and it has reached the host's target tissues. Examples of exposure surveillance include elevated blood lead levels and depressions of cholinesterase levels in workers or community members exposed to organophosphate pesticides. *Health-outcome surveillance* measures the frequency and distribution of disease resulting from such exposure. Examples include measurement of cases of cognitive impairment in lead-exposed workers or children and of neuropathy after pesticide exposure.

The development of well-defined occupational and environmental health indicators has been extremely useful in promoting rate-based surveillance, as it allows the direct comparison of rates across different populations. *Indicators* are defined as specific health outcomes or factors associated with a health outcome, such as exposure to a hazard or an intervention to prevent a hazardous exposure. Recently, public health practitioners have developed occupational and environmental health indicators. (Tables 6-3 and 6-4).

Examples of Occupational Health Surveillance Programs

Although hazard and exposure surveillance is preferable to health-outcome surveillance, as it ideally leads to interventions before disease has occurred, hazard and exposure surveillance is often difficult and expensive to implement. Therefore, many occupational health surveillance programs have focused on health outcomes, based on sources described below.

TABLE 6-3

Types and Examples of Occupational Health Indicators

Occupational injuries and illnesses (combined)
  Nonfatal occupational injuries or illnesses reported by employers
  Work-related hospitalizations

Acute and cumulative occupational injuries
  Fatal work-related injuries
  Work-related amputations with days away from work reported by employers
  Work-related amputations with reports filed with the workers' compensation system
  Hospitalizations from work-related burns
  Work-related musculoskeletal disorders with days away from work reported by employers
  Carpal tunnel syndrome cases filed with the workers' compensation system

Occupational illnesses
  Hospitalizations due to or with pneumoconiosis
  Deaths due to or with pneumoconiosis
  Acute work-related pesticide-associated illnesses or injuries reported to poison control centers
  New cases of mesothelioma

Occupational exposures
  Elevated blood lead levels in adults

Occupational hazards
  Percentages of workers employed in industries at high risk for occupational morbidity
  Percentages of workers employed in occupations at high risk for occupational morbidity
  Percentages of workers employed in both industries and occupations at high risk for occupational mortality

Intervention resources for occupational health
  Occupational safety and health professionals
  OSHA enforcement activities

Socioeconomic impact of occupational injuries and illnesses
  Workers' compensation awards

Source: Council of State and Territorial Epidemiologists. Occupational Health Indicators: A Guide for Tracking Occupational Health Conditions and their Determinants. Atlanta, GA: CSTE, 2004. Available at <www.cste.org>. Accessed July 29, 2005.

TABLE 6-4

Types and Examples of Environmental Health Indicators

Hazard indicators (potential for exposure to contaminants or hazardous conditions)
  Criteria pollutants in ambient air
  Hazardous or toxic substances released in ambient air
  Residence in nonattainment areas (for criteria air pollutants)
  Motor vehicle emissions
  Tobacco smoke in homes with children
  Residence in a flood plain
  Pesticide use and patterns of use
  Residual pesticide or toxic contaminants in foods
  Ultraviolet light
  Chemical spills
  Monitored contaminants in ambient and drinking water
  Point-source discharges into ambient water
  Contaminants in shellfish and sport and commercial fish

Exposure indicators (biomarkers of exposure)
  Blood lead level (in children)

Health effect indicators
  Carbon monoxide poisoning
  Deaths attributed to extremes in ambient temperature
  Lead-induced adverse health effects (in children)
  Noise-induced hearing loss (nonoccupational)
  Pesticide-related poisoning and illness
  Illness or condition with suspected or confirmed environmental contribution (a case or an unusual pattern)
  Melanoma
  Possible child poisoning (resulting in consultation or emergency department visit)
  Outbreaks attributed to fish and shellfish
  Outbreaks attributed to ambient or drinking water contaminants

Intervention indicators (programs or official policies addressing environmental hazards)
  Programs that address motor vehicle emissions
  Alternate fuel use in registered motor vehicles
  Availability of mass transit
  Policies that address indoor air hazards in schools
  Laws pertaining to smoke-free indoor air
    Indoor air inspections

(continued)

TABLE 6-4 (Continued)

Types and Examples of Environmental Health Indicators

Emergency preparedness, response, and mitigation training programs, plans, and protocols

Compliance with pesticide application standards (among pesticide workers)

Health-based activity restrictions in bodies of water

Implementation of sanitary surveys

Compliance with operation and maintenance standards for drinking water systems

Advisories to boil water

Source: National Center for Environmental Health. Environmental Public Health Indicators. Atlanta, GA: NCEH, 2005. Available at <www.cdc.gov/nceh/indicators/>. Accessed July 29, 2005.

Death Certificates

The National Occupational Mortality Surveillance (NOMS) system of the National Institute for Occupational Safety and Health (NIOSH) collects and codes mortality and occupational information from about 500,000 death certificates annually from 23 states in the United States. This allows analysis of differential mortality patterns among occupations and industries and comparison of the distributions of industries and occupations among diseases.

Employer Records

An annual survey of a large sample of employers is performed by the Bureau of Labor Statistics (BLS) of the U.S. Department of Labor. Using information from the required "OSHA 300" log of injuries and illnesses, these data provide broad estimates of work-related disease and injury. However, the survey is limited by the absence of specific criteria for determining the work-relatedness of disease, the limited sensitivity of the OSHA 300 log for detecting cases, and the assurance of confidentiality, which limits the usefulness of the survey for identifying cases or workplaces for in-depth follow-up investigations.

Workers' Compensation Records

Although readily available in most states, workers' compensation data are limited because they include only those who file (generally workers with the more severe injuries and illnesses), they exclude most cases of chronic work-related disease, and they are limited by adjudication procedures and di-

agnostic criteria that vary from state to state (see Chapter 4). However, these data have been very useful in identifying new problems, such as violence toward women workers, and in providing estimates of the magnitude of newly identified problems, such as disability from knee disease in carpet installers.

Cancer Registries

Hospital-based, regional, or statewide cancer incidence registers can be useful sources of surveillance data on cancer but often provide only limited, if any, information on occupation.

Physician Reporting

In locations such as Alberta (Canada), Great Britain, Germany, and some states in the United States, the law requires physicians to report all work-related diseases and injuries or certain specified ("scheduled") conditions. Where this is effectively enforced, the scheduled diseases can be tracked and epidemics identified early.

Laboratory-Based Reporting

A state-based national system, the Adult Blood Lead Epidemiology and Surveillance (ABLES), collects information from U.S. states that require laboratories to report cases of excessive lead levels. This information has proved useful in making national estimates of lead poisoning, tracking trends, identifying underserved occupations and industries, and targeting specific worksites with excessive cases. The limitations of laboratory-based reporting include the limited number of conditions for which laboratories can be involved; an irony is that those workers with the most inadequate resources for assistance are also the least likely to be monitored for lead.

Sentinel Event Approaches

Examples of sentinel event approaches exist in both Great Britain and the United States. In Great Britain, the SWORD (Surveillance of Work-related and Occupational Respiratory Disease) system was developed to identify new and conduct surveillance on known types of occupational respiratory disease, using reports from thoracic and occupational physicians.[2] Preliminary success has led to efforts to replicate the model for occupational dermatitis. In the United States, NIOSH is working with states to develop state-based systems for surveillance of occupational disease and injury. Very successful programs have been established, for example to track cases of pesticide poisoning and occupational respiratory diseases such as silicosis and asthma.

Examples of Environmental Health Surveillance Programs

In contrast to occupational health surveillance, environmental health surveillance has traditionally focused on measuring environmental hazards and exposures rather than health outcomes. A number of factors make the surveillance of environmental health outcomes especially challenging. First, in many instances it is difficult to link health outcomes to specific environmental exposures. This difficulty may result from (a) the long latencies between exposure and some diseases, such as cancer; or (b) many diseases, such as asthma, being caused by both environmental and nonenvironmental factors. Second, many records, such as medical records, may not contain the information needed to link a disease to environmental exposures, for a number of reasons including an inadequate environmental history. Third, there are not yet biomarkers for many important environmental exposures that might allow clinicians to more definitively establish the role of a presumed environmental exposure in causing the disease of a patient.

Exposure Databases of EPA

The Environmental Protection Agency (EPA) has programs that track the levels of air and water pollution in communities throughout the United States. For example, the National Water Quality Inventory collects information on the quality of water used for drinking, swimming, and fishing, which is reported every other year by states, territories, and other jurisdictions. EPA also has an extensive national system for collecting measurements of the levels of the six criteria air pollutants (sulfur dioxide, nitrogen dioxide, ozone, lead, carbon monoxide, and particulate matter). (See Chapter 17.) The Toxic Release Inventory collects information on chemical releases and waste management reported by major industrial facilities throughout the country. These and other exposures have been organized into a national database by Environmental Defense, a nongovernmental organization, allowing individual communities to obtain a "scorecard" on local pollution levels.

Childhood Blood Lead Surveillance

The measurement of environmental lead exposure is a major public health priority, especially in young children who are especially vulnerable to its central nervous system toxicity. Since the 1970s, the Centers for Disease Control and Prevention (CDC) has been collecting data on blood lead levels from a sample of the U.S. population aged 1 to 5 through the National Health and Nutrition Examination Survey (NHANES). In 1997, CDC established a national data system to aggregate data on elevated blood lead levels in children under age 6 from state-based laboratory reporting programs. Although the threshold blood lead level that must be reported is variable and established by each individual state, CDC, in conjunction with the states, has established a standardized set of data that are collected each time a child is tested.

The CDC National Report on Human Exposure to Environmental Chemicals

CDC performs an ongoing assessment of the exposure of U.S. population to environmental chemicals using biomonitoring from blood and urine specimens. This program's first report, released in 2001, included 27 substances; the second, released in 2003, was expanded to 116 chemicals; the third, released in 2005, was expanded to 148 chemicals. The program is scheduled to continued issuing new reports every 2 years. These data allow physicians, scientists, and public health practitioners to know the "background" concentrations of certain chemicals in the general U.S. population in order to determine whether a specific population may have experienced higher exposures. These data also allow public health practitioners to focus investigations and interventions in those communities or populations with the highest exposure levels.

The Environmental Public Health Tracking Network

In 2001, the Pew Environmental Health Commission, established by the Pew Charitable Trust, concluded that there was no integrated system for tracking environmental health in the United States. Based on this commission's recommendations, the National Center for Environmental Health (NCEH) at CDC, in conjunction with governmental and nongovernmental partners, established a new environmental public health network. Central to this initiative was the creation of the environmental health indicators list shown in Table 6-4. A network of state and city health departments and a number of academic centers of excellence were funded to develop programs for capacity building and infrastructure development based on the collection of data on these indicators.

With time, it is likely that improved surveillance of occupational and environmental disease will yield additional useful information. In evaluating occupational and environmental surveillance programs, it is most important to clearly understand the goals of the specific surveillance system and to recognize that not every system will meet every goal.

More information on surveillance of occupational and environmental disease and injury can be obtained from (a) NIOSH, NCEH and the Agency for Toxic Substances and Disease Registry (ATSDR)—all at CDC; (b) workers' compensation system agencies in most states; (c) the BLS of the U.S. Department of Labor in Washington, D.C.; (d) EPA; and (e) the environmental and occupational disease and injury epidemiologists within health or labor departments in most states.

SCREENING FOR DISEASE

Screening is the search for previously unrecognized diseases or physiologic conditions in individuals who could benefit in some way from the detection of the condition, such as by removal from exposure or through treatment. It may be part of an individual clinician's evaluation of a patient's health or part of a large-scale prevention program of an employer, union, or other organization for a group of individuals, but the goal is always to improve the health of the persons screened. Screening methods can include questionnaires seeking suggestive symptoms or exposures, examinations and laboratory tests, or other procedures. To be widely used, the methods should be simple, noninvasive, safe, rapid, and relatively inexpensive. Screening is one technique in a continuum for the prevention of occupational and environmental disease. Screening only presumptively identifies those individuals who are likely (and those who are unlikely) to have a particular disease. Further diagnostic tests are almost always necessary to confirm the diagnosis or assess the severity of the condition.

Although screening data may eventually lead to more effective primary prevention measures, the purpose of screening is the identification of conditions already in existence at a stage when their progression may be slowed, halted, or even reversed. Screening is therefore a secondary prevention measure. Primary prevention measures that reduce workers' exposure to occupational and environmental hazards are, in general, more likely to

improve health and prevent disease (see Chapters 7, 9, 10, and 11).

The main goal of screening is early detection and treatment of disease. Clearly, screening data, in addition to their clinical use for the protection of the individual screened, may be analyzed epidemiologically for the protection of the population of people similarly exposed.[3]

The employees at a particular workplace are a logical target for screening for occupational disease because they have some risk factors in common (their workplace exposures) and a clear opportunity for prevention in common (reduction or elimination of those exposures). In addition, a workplace can provide excellent opportunities for screening for treatable nonoccupational diseases, such as hypertension. To be effective, screening programs for occupational disease must meet the following five criteria:

1. Screening must be selective, applying only the appropriate tests to the population at risk for development of a specific disease, given exposures, demographic features, and other factors. A "shotgun" approach, involving a battery of tests, such as a "chemistry profile," applied indiscriminately without regard to the diseases for which the population is at risk, is generally not effective. The natural history of the exposure–disease relationship should be considered in the application of screening tests. For example, screening of workers exposed to asbestos during the first few years after the start of exposure may lead to a false sense of security, because there has not been sufficient time for the disease process to become detectable on screening examination.

2. Identification of the disease in its latent stage, instead of after symptoms appear, must lead to treatment that may impede progression of the disease in a given patient or to measures that prevent additional cases (Fig. 6-5). The major justification for screening for a disease for which there is no therapy is to allow an opportunity to control exposure and prevent disease in others similarly exposed.

3. Adequate follow-up is critical, and further diagnostic tests and effective management of the disease must be available, accessible, and acceptable both to examiner and worker. Lack of follow-up is a frequent deficiency in screening programs for occupational disease. Workers who have been screened should receive test

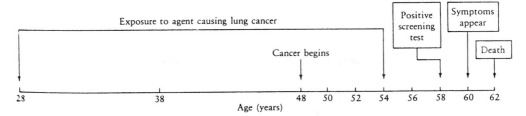

FIGURE 6-5 ● Phases of cancer development. If the course of the disease cannot be positively influenced by early detection and effective treatment, there is no advantage to screening an individual for early detection of the disease.

reports along with interpretation of test results and, if possible, summary data for the entire group tested. (OSHA requires that records of medical monitoring be made available to affected employees. These records may be transmitted to third parties only with the written consent of the worker.) Follow-up also entails action to reduce or eliminate the hazard. An example is job transfer for the ill worker combined with improvements in the ventilation systems of the workplace; job transfer without action to control the underlying problem may result in exposure of another worker to the same hazard.

4. The screening test must have good reliability and validity. *Reliability* reflects the reproducibility of the test. *Validity* reflects the ability of the test to identify correctly which individuals have the disease and which do not. Validity is evaluated by examining sensitivity and specificity. *Sensitivity* is the proportion of those with the disease that the test identifies correctly; *specificity* is the proportion of those without the disease that the test identifies correctly. Another measure of a screening test is the *predictive value positive*, which is often more useful clinically than either sensitivity or specificity; it indicates the proportion of those with a positive screening test who actually have the disease (Table 6-5). The prevalence of the disease affects the predictive value positive. The predictive value positive rises as prevalence rises, even as the sensitivity and specificity of the test remain the same.

5. The benefits of the screening program should outweigh the costs. Benefits consist primarily of improved quality and/or length of life – that is, reduced morbidity and mortality. Costs include both economic costs (the expenses of performing the screening tests and further diagnostic tests and of managing the disease in affected work-

ers) and human costs (the risks, inconvenience, discomfort, and anxiety of screening and of diagnostic workups for those with false-positive results). Screening tests in the community must be inexpensive because they compete with other public health resources, such as immunization. It should not be assumed that effective screening tests for occupational disease must be inexpensive, because they do not compete for the same resources, although the human costs to screening may be significant and should be carefully weighed in all settings. The cost–benefit equation is often difficult to determine and relies on tenuous assumptions, and workers and other patients may decline screening procedures based on their own risk–benefit assumptions. Strict financial analysis should not be allowed to obscure the primary objective of screening: early identification of work-related disease. Advocates of

TABLE 6-5

Hypothetical data: Screening of 100,000 workers for colon cancer[a]

Test Outcome	Colon Cancer Present		
	Yes	No	Total
Positive	150	300	450
Negative	50	99,500	99,550
Total	200	99,800	100,000

[a] These data assume the following:
Sensitivity = 150/200 = 75%. The test was (correctly) positive for 75% of actual cancer cases, but 25% of the actual cases were not detected.
Specificity = 99,500/99,800 = 99%. The test was (correctly) negative for 99% of those who actually did not have colon cancer.
Predictive value positive = 150/450 = 33%. Of those with a positive test, 33% actually had colon cancer.

screening should be cautious, because increased survival in those determined to have the disease by screening, compared with those detected after they become symptomatic, may be a result of lead-time bias or length bias. In *lead-time bias*, the apparently increased survival time results from adding part of the preclinical detection period to the postdiagnosis survival time and not from altering the actual duration of survival after the disease is contracted. In *length bias*, an apparently increased survival time results from the greater probability of detecting indolent, more benign disease than quickly developing disease, which is less likely to be detected because it is present for a shorter period.

Medical ethics demand that the patient encounter be conducted in the best interests of the patient (see Chapter 5). However, to the extent that screening programs are run for surveillance purposes or are otherwise required by public health or occupational health mandates, the interface between the clinician and the individual worker becomes more complex. These situations are fraught with potential ethical challenges that require care and thoughtful planning to address. There must be mutual trust among the individuals who have requested or authorized the screening program, the health professionals who are administering it, and the workers being screened. Without such trust, workers may be reluctant to be screened. This trust is developed, in part, by management personnel and health professionals assuring that screening data will be kept strictly confidential, will be used only for the stated purpose of the screening program, and will not adversely affect the worker's salary or other benefits. In addition, for any screening program to be effective, it cannot be used as a tool to discriminate—sexually, racially, or otherwise—against a specific group of workers.

Screening approaches for specific categories of work-related disease are covered in several chapters of Part IV of this book. The general industry

TABLE 6-6

Illustrative Components of Medical Monitoring in Selected OSHA Standards

Exposure	History	Physical Examination	Other Test/Procedures
Airborne asbestos	Especially respiratory symptoms	Especially chest examination	Chest x-ray, FVC*, and FEV_1*
Vinyl chloride	Especially alcohol use, history of hepatitis, transfusions	Especially liver, spleen, kidneys, respiratory system, skin, and connective tissue	Liver function tests
Inorganic arsenic	Especially respiratory symptoms	Especially nasal and skin examinations	Chest x-ray
Benzene	Including alcohol use and medications	If respirator used frequently, specific attention to cardiopulmonary exam	Complete blood count, including differential white cell count and red cell indices
Cadmium	Including respiratory, cardiovascular, and renal symptoms	Especially blood pressure, respiratory and genitourinary system	Urine cadmium, blood cadmium, β-2 microglobulin in urine
Methylene chloride	Including neurological symptoms and heart, liver, and blood disease	Particular attention to lungs, cardiovascular system, liver, skin, and neurological system	Based on medical and work history

*FVC = Forced vital capacity; FEV_1 = Forced expiratory volume in the first second.
Source: OSHA. Code of Federal Regulations (CFR) Title 29: General industry.

standards for specific hazardous exposures, published by OSHA, specify requirements for medical monitoring of exposed workers.[4] These may include preplacement and periodic screening histories, examinations, and tests. Table 6-6 illustrates some of the specific screening tests required by OSHA. OSHA also requires employers to keep records of this surveillance and to make these records available to affected employees. The records can also be made available to physicians or other third parties on specific written request.

In conclusion, as the theme of a conference on screening stated: "Screening and monitoring, in and of themselves, prevent nothing; only the appropriate intervention, in response to results of these tests, can prevent."[5]

REFERENCES

1. Rutstein D, Mullen R, Frazier T, et al. The sentinel health event (occupational): a framework for occupational health surveillance and education. Am J Public Health 1983;73:1054–1062.
2. Ross DJ. Ten years of the SWORD project: Surveillance of work-related and occupational respiratory disease. Clin Exp Allergy 1999;29:750–3.
3. Halperin WE, Ratcliffe J, Frazier TM, et al. Medical screening in the workplace: proposed principles. J Occup Med 1986;28:547–552.
4. OSHA. General industry: OSHA safety and health standards (29 CFR 1910). Washington, DC: U.S. Government Printing Office, 1978.
5. Millar JD. Screening and monitoring: tools for prevention. J Occup Med 1986;28:544–546.

BIBLIOGRAPHY

History

Goldman RH, Peters JM. The occupational and environmental health history. JAMA 1981;246:2831–6.
An excellent article with more detail on the occupational history.

Medical Monitoring/Screening

Halperin WE, Schulte PA, Greathouse DG (eds, Part I) and Mason TJ, Prorok PC, Costlow RD (eds, Part II). Conference on medical screening and biological monitoring for the effects of exposure in the workplace. J Occup Med 1986;28:543–788, 901–1126.
An in-depth, comprehensive review on screening in the workplace.

Halperin WE, Ratcliffe J, Frazier TM, et al. Medical screening in the workplace: Proposed principles. J Occup Med 1986;28:547–52.
Questions the adequacy of current recommendations on screening in the workplace and proposes a revised set of principles for such screening.
Hathaway GJ, Proctor NH. Proctor & Hughes' chemical hazards of the workplace, 5th ed. New York: Wiley-Interscience, 2004.
Includes recommended screening examinations and tests for workers exposed to some of the more than 600 substances covered in this book.
Lauwerys RR. Industrial chemical exposure: guidelines for biological monitoring, 2nd ed. Davis CA: Biomedical Publications, 1993.
Presents concepts of biologic monitoring and reviews current knowledge on numerous specific agents.
Morrison AS. Screening in chronic disease. Monographs in epidemiology and biostatistics, Vol 7, 2nd ed. New York: Oxford University Press, 1992.
An excellent text on the epidemiology of screening.
Silverstein M. Analysis of medical screening and surveillance in 21 OSHA standards: Support of a generic medical surveillance standard. Am J Ind Med 1994;26:283–95.
An excellent review article.

Surveillance

Ashford NA, Spadafor CJ, Hattis DB, Caldart CC. Monitoring the worker for exposure and disease: scientific, legal, and ethical considerations in the use of biomarkers. Baltimore: Johns Hopkins Press, 1990.
The considerations given to both screening and surveillance issues in this monograph raise a number of important questions concerning the objectives of efforts to evaluate biological materials from workers, how these measurements are used effectively, and how they can be of little or no use for the objectives identified.
Teutsch SM, Churchill RE, eds. Principles and practice of public health surveillance 2nd ed. New York: Oxford University Press, 2000.
A standard text in this field on the principles of surveillance and their application.
Maizlish NA, ed. Workplace health surveillance: An action-oriented approach. New York: Oxford University Press, 2000.
This book provides an excellent step-by-step approach to establishing or improving surveillance systems.
Mullan RJ, Murthy LI. Occupational sentinel health events: An updated list for physician recognition and public health surveillance. Am J Ind Med 1991;19:775–99.
Adaptation of the general concept of sentinel health events to occupational disease.

The findings and conclusions in this chapter are those of the authors and do not necessarily represent the views of the National Institute for Occupational Safety and Health.

CHAPTER 7

Preventing Occupational and Environmental Disease and Injury

Rosemary K. Sokas, Barry S. Levy, David H. Wegman, and Sherry L. Baron

P revention is the goal of occupational and environmental health and safety. It requires a systematic approach, effective communication, and constant feedback. Prevention generally involves a sequence of steps, including (a) gathering information about exposures and outcomes; (b) identifying problems; (c) developing, communicating, and implementing strategies for prevention; and (d) evaluating the outcome of these strategies.

All societal activities require vision, planning, and implementation—erecting buildings; establishing water, sewage, and transportation systems; developing sources of and distributing energy; growing, packaging, and distributing food; and planning entire cities. Occupational and environmental injuries and illnesses are, in one way or another, the result of these same activities. With enough care, resources, and commitment, we can prevent problems ranging from the adverse effects of air pollution and hazardous wastes to workplace illnesses and injuries. And we can continuously and sustainably shape our environment to reduce and eliminate health and safety hazards.

Whereas a coordinated, problem-solving approach is needed to reduce occupational and environmental hazards and prevent the illnesses and injuries they cause, most problems unfortunately occur where the system is either broken or does not exist, and most people affected encounter fragmented sources of assistance. The following situations demonstrate how health care providers, other health and safety professionals, and public health workers have missed opportunities for prevention and highlight common themes, such as the need for improved communication and enhanced feedback.

In the town of Libby, Montana, occupational health investigations conducted in the 1980s revealed asbestos-related diseases and deaths among workers who mined and processed asbestos-containing vermiculite ore. These workplace deaths were not seen as sentinel events. Vermiculite waste was not controlled until deaths from mesothelioma were reported in community residents in the 1990s.

Orders for leaded chemical products in an Indiana factory increased when a Pennsylvania competitor went out of business. As production increased, physicians monitoring workers for lead exposure found an increased number with high blood lead levels (BLLs). Physicians removed the workers with elevated BLLs from direct exposure to lead using the medical removal protection provision of the Occupational Safety and Health Administration (OSHA) lead standard, and returned them to work when their BLLs declined. Several workers went through this cycle repeatedly. Some of the occupational medicine records documented concerns workers had voiced about elevated BLLs among their children who had been routinely tested by their pediatricians. An OSHA inspection finally revealed that lead inadvertently brought home by workers caused the elevated BLLs in their children.

In the same factory, in response to an earlier OSHA inspection, an overhead exhaust hood was installed in the room where workers opened bags of inorganic lead to feed into a hopper to be mixed into a final product. The purpose of the hood was to provide local exhaust ventilation to capture and remove lead dust from the workers' breathing zones. The workers had been using a table to hold the bags before opening them and dumping them; with the new hood, there was no room for the table, and bags were instead placed on and lifted from the floor. The number of back injuries resulting in lost work time increased.

A Maryland woman complaining of headache and vomiting was diagnosed with a viral syndrome and treated symptomatically. She and her family members returned the following night reporting the same symptoms and this time were diagnosed with carbon monoxide poisoning. Inspection of their home revealed a faulty furnace.

In these examples, opportunities for prevention are easily identified in retrospect. The manufacturer has the responsibility to identify hazards, both within the factory and in the waste stream, and control them and communicate the nature of the hazard to workers and to community members. Physicians conducting OSHA-mandated surveillance can communicate with factory managers and raise appropriate concerns. They should expect meaningful communication with safety officers until specific problems are identified and remediated. Frontline workers should be included in remediation discussions, and alternate strategies should be explored, such as use of bags that do not need to be opened because they dissolve in the mixing process. Finally, opportunities for enhanced communication among physicians, other health care providers, and public health practitioners abound. Joint approaches to primary prevention, ranging from information about smoke detectors and carbon monoxide monitors to awareness about lead exposure (Fig. 7-1), might also involve fire departments, schools, and community-based nongovernmental organizations.

The themes that emerge reinforce the need for effective communication, sharing of data, and systematic follow-up evaluation to confirm that improvement has been achieved. Information-sharing that empowers individuals to identify hazards and take appropriate steps for intervention produces critical improvements in activities. Examples include hazard prevention and control (a) by individuals, such as seatbelt use and smoking cessation; (b) by communities, such as construction of safe bi-

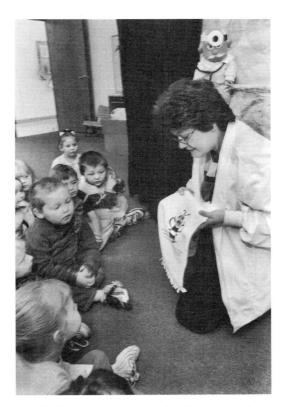

FIGURE 7-1 ● Bee Lead Safe educational project for Head Start Program children and their parents. (Photograph by Earl Dotter.)

cycle paths and speed bumps; and (c) by workplace safety and health teams. Successful programs have been shown to reduce patient assaults on nursing home workers, back injuries among hospital-based nursing assistants and orderlies, dermatitis among printing workers, needlesticks among health care workers, ambient lead levels following conversion to lead-free gasoline, and fatalities after introduction of air bags into cars.[1–3]

Systems approaches can guide comprehensive safety and health programs. In these approaches, it is often recognized that no injuries are acceptable. Comprehensive safety and health programs developed by federal OSHA for voluntary use have been required by several state-plan OSHA programs. These programs, which include a "plan–do–check–act" cycle, engage frontline workers in systems approaches. They rely on management commitment, employee participation, hazard identification and control, training, medical monitoring, and program evaluation. These programs have been successful to the extent they empower workers to identify needs and participate to bring about change. However, many of these programs have failed to share resources or genuinely empower workers, engendering suspicion and limiting program implementation and effectiveness. Similar comprehensive approaches have been developed to reduce environmental hazards. The EPA's Pollution Prevention Initiative (Box 7-1) identifies alternatives that reduce the production of pollutants. The International Standards Organization (ISO 14000) management standard can help management to reduce environmental pollution from industry. To be effective, these programs require external verification and constant engagement of vigilant civic groups and nongovernmental organizations that empower community members.

It often takes the concerted effort of professionals in health care, general public health, and occupational and environmental safety and health working together with patients, employers, representatives of community organizations, and government officials to address complex problems. However, each member of this team has the ability to initiate improvements. We are each responsible for ensuring that change happens, while at the same time we are only able to bring about positive change if we communicate effectively and engage others.

The following three examples of major improvements show how communication, focus, and persistence at the individual level and in the public health policy arena can reduce exposure and improve lives—although in each of these examples, much work remains to be done.

Lead Exposure

Lead has been widely used in plumbing and manufacturing, and its toxic effects have been recognized for centuries. Yet it continues to cause adverse health effects in some workers, young children exposed to lead-based paint, and others. One of the most significant population-based exposures in the 20th century occurred when organic lead was added to gasoline as an antiknock agent that made combustion engines more efficient and contributed to the ascent of the automobile as the dominant mode of transportation. Thousands of tons of lead oxide were exhausted from tailpipes, contaminating ambient air and settling in dust and on crops. By the mid-1970s, the geometric mean BLL for the U.S. population as a whole approached 16 μg/dL, a level now known to cause adverse neurologic ef-

fects. Based on the research of scientists and the advocacy of environmental nongovernmental organizations and associations of health professionals, EPA regulated the removal of lead from gasoline. Over the nearly three decades since, BLLs in the U.S. population have declined, with the geometric mean BLL now below 2 μg/dL. Additional efforts to ban lead as a pigment in paint, in water-carrying pipes, and in solders used for canned foods have also had a positive impact, although problem areas persist, especially in areas with older houses. With the decline of BLLs among children aged 1 to 5, only about 2 percent of them have BLLs over 10 μg/dL—the CDC level of concern.[4]

Environmental Tobacco Smoke

Since the Surgeon General's seminal report in 1964 on the hazards of cigarette smoking, the tobacco industry has fought back, such as by attacking the science that demonstrated the adverse health effects of environmental tobacco smoke on nonsmokers. Smoking cessation programs, one-on-one counseling by primary care physicians, educational and advocacy projects by nonprofit organizations, legislation restricting smoking, and individual and state lawsuits have increased public awareness and reduced the percentage of smokers in the United States. As a result, among nonsmokers, levels of cotinine (a biomarker for environmental tobacco smoke), declined 58 percent during the 1990s for children, 55 percent for adolescents, and 78 percent for adults.[4]

Mining Fatalities

Mining remains the industry with the highest rate of fatal traumatic injury, although this rate declined 92 percent from 1911 to 1997. Public outcry in response to horrific disasters led to a series of federal responses, including the establishment of agencies to conduct research in and to regulate mining. The reduction of fire, explosion, collapse, asphyxiation, and other hazards has been the result of improvements in technology, training, and enforcement. Lessons learned from improvements in this industry may help improve safety in other high-hazard industries, such as construction and agriculture.

APPROACHES TO PREVENTION

Primary prevention identifies a hazard and either (a) prevents susceptible individuals from becoming

BOX 7-1

Avoiding the Transfer of Risk: Pollution Prevention and Occupational Health

Rafael Moure-Eraso

The growing national concern with environmental pollution became acute in the past decade because of the increase in waste-generating activities by industry. The U.S. Congress responded to this concern by enacting the Pollution Prevention Act of 1990. Congress reflected the consensus of the scientific community that waste management and control alone will not resolve environmental problems in the long run and that a change of approach—a *paradigm shift*—from pollution control to pollution prevention was necessary. Source reduction is the strategy of choice to achieve pollution prevention. Only to the degree that this cannot be achieved is it appropriate to turn to pollution control activities such as treatment, disposal, and remediation.

Pollution prevention has begun to take hold. It provides, for the first time, a coordinated effort of primary prevention, eliminating the possibility of pollution-related health effects and superseding *end-of-pipe* interventions. Thousands of companies in the United States have established pollution prevention programs.

These developments have critical implications for occupational health. The important conceptual change from control of environmental exposures to their prevention through source reduction and changes in process methods allows the workplace to be seen as a separate source of pollution when undertaking a comprehensive and systematic pollution source evaluation. When industries that use chemicals as raw materials begin to look at changing materials and processes as an environmental health strategy, the opportunity exists to incorporate workplace pollution exposures into the equation and prevent the choice of substitute materials without consideration for the impacts of any proposed changes on the exposures within the plant. Consequently, the working population and work environment can be given equal footing with the general population when pollution prevention strategies are planned.

The establishment of this understanding as the foundation for pollution prevention activities requires a change in both environmental health and occupational hygiene practice. Just as previous environmental health activities did not consider root causes and their prevention, traditional workplace-based exposure control activities have been end-of-pipe interventions designed to control exposure without systematically examining root causes. Consequently, it was not recognized that a preferred engineering control such as local exhaust ventilation tended to shift the burden from the workplace to the ambient environment in the form of air pollution or solid hazardous waste (via contaminated filters or other pollution collection media). Unless source reduction or process modifications are examined comprehensively, occupational hygienists may be equally responsible for shortsightedness. So, work environment scientists must join environmental health scientists in a unified effort to avoid simply shifting risk among different media (Table 7-1).

For this conceptual potential to be realized, the occupational health professional must be at the table during discussion of pollution prevention strategies. The six general pollution prevention (source reduction) strategies that most directly affect occupational health are raw material substitution or reduced use, closed-loop recycling, process or equipment modification, improvement of maintenance, reformulation of products, and improvement of housekeeping and training.

Some examples of pollution prevention interventions that incorporate concern for reduction or elimination of work exposures are the following:

1. In industrial textile dry-cleaning operations, water-based solvents have been successfully substituted for perchloroethylene. This change eliminates exposures to a potential human carcinogen, but also leads to reduced volatile organic compounds in ambient air, improved dry-cleaning job organization, and decreased ergonomic risk factors.
2. In the offset lithography industry, the solvent with the lowest concentration of aliphatic organic chemicals has been successfully substituted for regular organic solvents to clean printing ink from metal surfaces. Products with high organic chemical content were found to perform no better than those with lowest.

(continued)

BOX 7-1

Avoiding the Transfer of Risk:
Pollution Prevention and Occupational
Health (Continued)

3. In painting of small metal parts, the introduction of an electrostatically delivered coating was successful in replacing a resin-based epoxide paint. Not only were the respiratory and skin hazards from epoxide exposures eliminated, but the paint dispenser was made substantially lighter, avoiding an ergonomic hazard.

Occupational hygiene should strive to change its most common practice from secondary to primary prevention by addressing workplace problems as an aspect of the comprehensive production system, which has impacts both inside and outside the point of production (see Table 7-1). Neither work environment problems nor worker and community concerns can be compartmentalized.

Bibliography

Ellenbecker MJ. Engineering controls as an intervention to reduce worker exposure. Am J Ind Med 1996;29:303–307.
Broadens the definition of substitution to include process changes and presents field examples of interventions. Also describes the general methods of pollution prevention (toxic use reduction).
Goldschmidt G. An analytical approach for reducing workplace health hazards through substitution. Am Ind Hyg Assoc J 1993;54:36–43.

Describes a systematic approach involving analysis of health characteristics of raw materials (162 examples from Denmark are summarized) for the purpose of choosing as alternatives more environmentally and occupationally benign materials.
Lempert R, Norling P, Pernin C, et al. Next generation environmental technologies: benefits and barriers. Santa Monica, CA: The RAND Corp., 2003.
This study of the benefits and barriers of next-generation environmental technologies in a number of U.S. industries concluded that, although in its infancy, green chemistry technologies provide significant benefits for occupational health, environmental health, and economic security.
Quinn MM, Kriebel D, Geiser K, et al. Sustainable production: A proposed strategy for the work environment. Am J Ind Med 1998;34: 297–304.
This paper calls for expansion of the role of the occupational health professional to include evaluation and redesign of production processes. It also calls for new research to develop these activities as the scientific and public health policy basis of sustainable production.
Roelofs CR, Moure-Eraso R, Ellenbecker MJ. Pollution prevention and the work environment: The Massachusetts experience. Appl Occup Environ Hyg J 2000;15:843–850.
This paper evaluates the impact on occupational health practices in 35 Massachusetts firms where the state promoted cleaner production alternatives. The study concluded that toxics use reduction activities improved the work environment, but that such improvements were neither systematically planned nor incorporated into their activities. Information about superior technologies regarding existing options to protect both workers and the environment were also missing.

---

exposed to it (usually through engineering interventions or substitution), or (b) strengthens the individual, such as through immunization. Secondary prevention identifies early evidence of a disease (usually by screening) at a stage where intervention (such as by medical treatment) can cure or prevent further progression of the disease. Tertiary prevention attempts to reduce the impact of illness or injury and associated disability, such as through medical care, rehabilitation, or environmental or workplace adjustments. All of these approaches require effective communication and information-sharing among a wide range of professionals, including some combination of physicians, nurses, physician assistants, occupational hygienists, epidemiologists, other health workers, engineers,

planners, community members, workers, managers, and others.

Primary Prevention at the Public Health Level

The Centers for Disease Control and Prevention (CDC), in partnership with a wide variety of stakeholders, has developed a nationwide goal of transforming the current patchwork of environmental health programs and services into a system of public health resources that would enable each state to provide comprehensive, updated environmental services that would adequately address traditional problems, such as water purity and food sanitation,

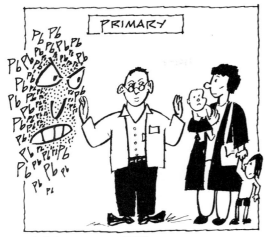

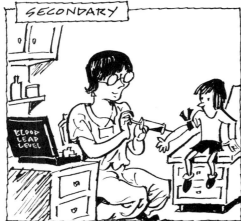

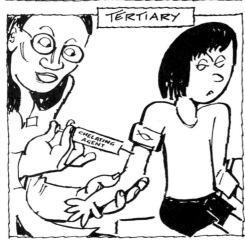

Examples of primary, secondary, and tertiary prevention. (Drawing by Nick Thorkelson.)

as well as emerging environmental health threats. This approach is similar to an occupational health systems approach, but on a larger scale. The following is an outline of 10 essential environmental health services needed for prevention:

1. Monitoring health status to identify community environmental health problems;
2. Diagnosing and investigating environmental health problems and health hazards in the community;
3. Enforcing laws and regulations that protect health and ensure safety;
4. Linking people to needed environmental health services and assuring the provision of environmental health services when otherwise unavailable;
5. Assuring a competent environmental health workforce;
6. Evaluating the effectiveness, accessibility, and quality of personal and population-based environmental health services;
7. Developing policies and plans that support individual and community environmental health efforts;
8. Mobilizing community partnerships to identify and solve environmental health problems;
9. Informing, educating, and empowering people about environmental health issues; and
10. Conducting research for new insights and innovative solutions to environmental health problems and issues.[5]

In most situations, a public health approach to prevention aims to "move upstream" to address the primary sources of a health problem (Fig. 7-2).

Primary Prevention at an Organizational Level

Substitution of a Less Hazardous Process for a More Hazardous One

Examples of process substitution may be on a large or small scale. Train, bus, and subway travel cause fewer deaths and disabling injuries due to crashes and emit fewer pollutants than automobile travel. Transdermal patches and oral medications, where effective, reduce the need for sharps exposures in health care. The use of wind or solar energy reduces pollution from fossil-fuel utilities and reduces reliance on nuclear-power plants, with attendant concerns about reactor safety and nuclear

TABLE 7-1

Pollution Prevention and Occupational Health: Occupational Hygiene as an Instrument for Primary Prevention

Occupational Hygiene Approaches	Primary Prevention	Secondary Prevention
Anticipation	*Hazard surveillance*	—
Identification	*Hazard identification*	*Medical surveillance*
Evaluation	*Exposure assessment*	—
Controls	*Exposure prevention*	*Control of generated exposures*
	Comprehensive	End-of-pipe
	Source reduction	Engineering controls
	Materials changes	Enclosure
	Substitution	Local exhaust
	Process changes	Wet methods
	Physical conditions	General ventilation
	Machinery	Administrative controls
	Operations	Personal protective equipment
	Work organization	*Early therapeutic intervention*

waste transportation and disposal. In all of these examples, residual risks remain, which require continued tracking of adverse health effects and development of additional process improvement, which relies on engineering and also requires planning, training, communication, and evaluation to be effective.

Substitution of a Less Hazardous Substance for a More Hazardous One

An example of this type of action is the substitution of synthetic vitreous fibers, such as fibrous glass, for asbestos. Substitution carries certain risks, because substitute materials often have not been adequately tested for health effects and may, in fact,

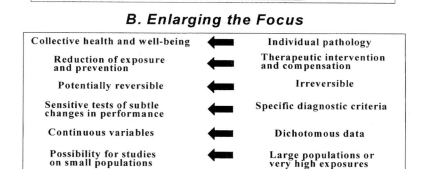

FIGURE 7-2 ● Moving upstream: Understanding the relationships of exposure to clinical illness offers the opportunity, in many different ways, to seek the earliest possible evidence of effects in order to prevent the chain of events and identify reversible changes. (Courtesy of Donna Mergler.)

be hazardous. For example, years ago fire protection was enhanced by replacing flammable cleaning solvents with carbon tetrachloride. Increased use of carbon tetrachloride led to identification of its hepatotoxicity and its subsequent replacement by less toxic chlorinated hydrocarbons. Now there is concern that use of chlorinated hydrocarbons should be reduced to better protect the general environment. The lesson in this evolution is not that substitution is hopeless, but that the introduction of a substituted material should be considered only a first step and that the impact of the substitution must always be monitored to determine whether initially unrecognized problems develop after increased use of the new material. The substitution approach is embodied in the broader concept of pollution prevention, described in Box 7-1.

Installation of Engineering Controls and Devices

These approaches are more often available than substitution and cover a wide range of effective options to reduce hazards, such as:

- Installing airbags in automobiles;
- Installing ventilation exhaust systems that remove hazardous dusts (Fig. 7-3);
- Using jigs or fixtures to reduce static muscle contractions while holding parts or tools;
- Applying appropriately designed sound-proofing materials to reduce loud noises that cannot be engineered out of a work process. (Sound barrier walls along highways help shield neighborhoods from noise using this same principle.)
- Installing tools on overhead balancers to eliminate torque and vibration transmitted to the hand;
- Constructing enclosures to isolate hazardous processes;
- Installing hoists to eliminate manual lifting of containers or parts;
- Carefully maintaining process equipment to reduce or eliminate (a) fugitive emissions from processes designed as closed systems, or (b) the development of unwanted vibrations as equipment ages;
- Using scrubbers or other mechanisms to reduce airborne pollutant emissions;
- Maximizing fuel use through cogeneration of hot water from the heat exhaust produced as a by-product of generating electricity; and
- Treating waste-water effluent before discharge.

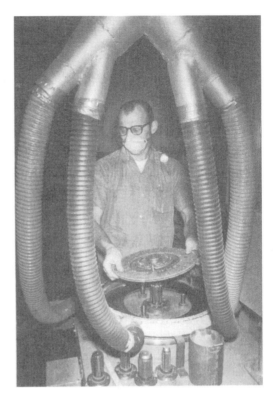

FIGURE 7-3 ● Local exhaust ventilation used to protect a worker from asbestos dust generated in working with clutch plates. (Photograph by Earl Dotter.)

Although installation of these engineering controls can involve a substantial initial capital expenditure, they often save money by reducing materials use, reducing toxic and other material wastes, and reducing costs of disease, injury, and absenteeism. Often, such approaches are not considered or implemented because of lack of awareness that such solutions are available and cost-effective.

Job Redesign, Work Organization Changes, and Work Practice Alternatives

A number of changes can be introduced that take advantage of methods that directly reduce or eliminate various types of risks in work processes. These include job redesign, changes in work organization, and alternative work practices. Job redesign, which often combines engineering and administrative aspects, typically seeks several related objectives: to increase job content, to make the physical work less redundant or repetitive, and to improve workers' opportunity to exercise individual or collective autonomy in decision making (see Chapter 16).

Changes in work organization, often closely integrated with individual job redesign, are directed at elimination of undesirable features in the structure of work processes. For example, a change from piece-rate work (with incentive wages) to hourly-rate work removes inappropriate pressure and tension—both physical and mental—on affected workers. Piece-rate work has been associated with higher rates of musculoskeletal problems in a variety of work settings. Another example is the elimination of machine pacing, which tends to enforce repetitive and mind-numbing work.

Work practice alternatives can, through relatively limited changes, lead to important improvements in the work environment. For example, dust exposures in a variety of settings can be significantly reduced by the introduction of vacuum cleaning in place of compressed air to clean dusty surfaces and wet mopping in place of dry sweeping wherever possible.

As a rule, these preventive measures are more effective than methods that primarily affect the worker. The measures that follow potentially reduce the damage that may result from workplace hazards without actually removing the source of the problem.

Primary Prevention at an Individual Level

The following sections address opportunities for primary prevention. Primary prevention in the workplace offers the opportunity for health promotion (Box 7-2).

Education

Education concerning specific environmental and occupational hazards is an essential aspect of safety and health. This is an aspect of information-sharing that is important on a number of levels: basic information about adverse effects of specific exposures conveyed in a manner that the individual is able to use is a form of empowerment. Health educators have developed and evaluated a variety of different theories in order to describe the various steps individuals use to understand a specific hazard, to assess their potential to impact that hazard, and then to decide to act. Much scientific evidence supports specific approaches to encouraging healthy behaviors, such as using seat belts and bicycle helmets,

checking home smoke detectors, and quitting smoking. Different approaches are needed for different activities.

The Environmental Protection Agency (EPA) has developed rules for effective risk communication for environmental hazards that clearly distinguish, for example, risks over which the individual has perceived control, such as automobile crashes—regardless of the extent to which individual control is actually the determining factor. Information that reintroduces some aspect of control—even if it is just information about where to obtain additional information or how to register and follow up on a complaint—is an important aspect of education and training. Workers should always be given full information about workplace hazards and means of reducing their risk (Fig. 7-4). Many safety measures necessitate changed behavior by workers, which also requires education or training. Workers who are not aware of job hazards will not take the health and safety precautions necessary to protect themselves and their co-workers. (See Box 7-3, Fig. 7-5, and information on the OSHA Hazard Communication Standard in Chapter 3.) Although training itself will not replace needed equipment, the equipment may be rendered useless or worse in the absence of effective training. Effective training that builds on life experiences and empowers the individual to address and solve problems is a cornerstone for all health and safety prevention.

Personal Protective Equipment

Use of personal protective equipment (PPE), such as respirators, earplugs, gloves, and protective clothing (Fig. 7-6), or safety devices, such as helmets, seat belts, and child restraint systems, will continue to be necessary in some workplace settings, where it is the only available protective measure, and for most transportation safety. However, this approach to controlling a hazard often has important limitations; for example, workers often resist wearing such protection because it is cumbersome or causes other difficulties. The effectiveness of PPE should be evaluated in actual use where the experimentally determined effectiveness claimed by its manufacturer may not apply. OSHA has developed lists of acceptable PPE that can be helpful in proper selection and use of this equipment. OSHA and other authorities have also emphasized the need for and importance of developing a complete program for PPE, not only a requirement for its use. Adequate programs include requirements

BOX 7-2

Health Promotion in the Workplace

Gregory R. Wagner

The protection, preservation, and improvement of the health of people who work are goals shared by workers, their families, and their employers. Ill health and injury, whether caused by work or nonwork activities, reduces income, quality of life, and opportunity, not only for the directly affected individuals but also for those dependent on them. Nevertheless, in the public health and employment communities, there has been a long-standing separation between those interested in control of health risks and hazards from work and those focused on individual and community health risk reduction outside the workplace.

Some occupational health specialists have been concerned that worksite health promotion and disease prevention programs may draw needed resources from occupational health protection programs and, at worst, may amount to victim-blaming, distracting attention from the occupational health needs of workers. There is concern that a narrow focus on health promotion could deflect employers from their legal responsibilities to provide workplaces free of recognizable hazards. Health promotion/disease prevention specialists often see the workplace as a convenient and valuable venue to provide important health improvement services to a priority population, without attention to work-related risk. These distinct perspectives are reflected in the separate training of occupational health practitioners and researchers and those focused on health promotion and health education.

The systems of payment in the United States for the medical costs of disease and injury have also contributed to this dichotomy. Conditions caused or significantly exacerbated by workplace conditions and exposures are supposed to be covered through workers' compensation insurance programs that are separate from any health insurance benefits paying for care for—or, in rare instances, prevention of—diseases and injuries "of everyday life." Any cost savings that result from improved health of workers may not be sufficiently clear or timely to be attributed to successful programs.

There is a limited, but growing, body of evidence and opinion that the separation of focus on at-work and off-the-job risks is artificial and is not optimally serving either workers or their employers. Certain health-risk behaviors, such as smoking, are nonrandomly distributed through the working population: blue-collar workers are more likely to smoke—and are less likely to quit successfully—than white-collar workers. Exposure to specific workplace conditions may increase risk for chronic diseases, such as chronic obstructive pulmonary disease (COPD), depression, and cardiovascular disease—otherwise characterized as "diseases of everyday life." Workers may inadvertently transport toxins home, putting themselves and family members at risk. Concurrent interventions at work to reduce adverse workplace hazards and to promote reduction of tobacco use in blue-collar manufacturing workers have been more successful than those focused solely on tobacco cessation.

A number of employers, with the support of the workers they employ, have implemented integrated programs to protect, preserve, and, at times, improve the health of the workers by focusing broadly on the diversity of factors—work-related and personal—that contribute to health and disease. Successful programs appear to have the following elements in common:

- Active communication among all interested parties;
- A true commitment to identification and intervention in problems of concern to the workforce;
- A commitment to health-supportive work policies (on sickness leave, tobacco use, health insurance, employee assistance programs, and other issues);
- Reasonable incentives for worker participation;
- Attention to identification and control of workplace stressors;
- A high level of coordination or integration among all program elements;
- Well-designed interventions; and
- Ongoing evaluation and program adjustment based on both process data and health and risk factor outcomes.

(continued)

BOX 7-2

Health Promotion in the Workplace (Continued)

There are a number of barriers to the adoption of integrated programs for health protection and promotion. Economic benefits may be difficult to measure, except for a few interventions, such as influenza vaccination. With chronic disease prevention strategies, economic benefits may only be realized after a significant time lag. Where employment relationships are strained and trust is low, workers may be reluctant to participate in voluntary programs. Even in stable positive work environments, many workers may feel that personal health issues are private and their employers should be uninvolved. Zealous efforts to promote health, such as through exclusive employment of nonusers of tobacco, may be seen as an unwarranted intrusion on personal autonomy.

Because of the constantly changing workplace and the nature of the workforce, some of the highest-hazard workplaces, such as in construction and mining, present unique challenges. Commercially available health promotion programs may be inadequately flexible to incorporate the particular needs of a given workforce, and small- and medium-sized

employers may not have the resources to develop their own programs. Economically marginal employers may be unable to afford to design and offer programs. Workers at highest health risk—those in low-wage work—may work multiple jobs, have lengthy commutes to work, and face language or cultural barriers to participation.

Nonetheless, there is growing awareness of the importance of a healthy workforce for the overall economic health of an enterprise and, conversely, the substantial costs of ill health through absenteeism, lost productivity, and health care expenditures. This recognition is likely to increase efforts to protect, preserve, and improve worker health through workplace-specific programs that integrate occupational safety and health with overall health promotion and health management.

Bibliography

National Institute for Occupational Safety and Health. Steps to a Healthier U.S. Workforce. Available at: <http://www.cdc.gov/niosh/steps/2004/whitepapers.html>.

U.S. Preventive Services Task Force. The Guide to Clinical Preventive Services. McLean, VA: International Medical Publishing, Inc., 2002.

for proper fitting of the equipment (especially with respirators), education about proper use, and a plan for maintenance, cleaning, and replacement of equipment or parts. The costs of an effective PPE program are significant, making it particularly important to recognize that use of such equipment should be accepted only when no alternative control is present.

Administrative Measures

Organizational measures taken by the employer may offer some protection. For example, exposure can be reduced somewhat by implementing work schedules such that workers spend carefully limited amounts of time in areas with potential exposure. Such measures require good environmental monitoring data to design appropriate schedules. Care must be taken that the result is not simply to distribute more widely the exposure to substances that can be controlled by engineering approaches.

Another preventive administrative measure is preplacement examination to avoid assigning workers to jobs in which individual risk factors place them at higher risk for specific diseases or injuries. The requirements of the Americans with Disabilities Act in the United States place a special responsibility on those performing preplacement examinations. At a community level, zoning ordinances that restrict types of industry in residential areas or that set hours for noise restriction offer important protections.

Secondary Prevention

Screening and Surveillance

Screening and surveillance, either separately or together, may lead to the identification of need for control measures to prevent further hazardous exposure to workers (see Chapter 6). Unlike the methods described previously, which are designed to

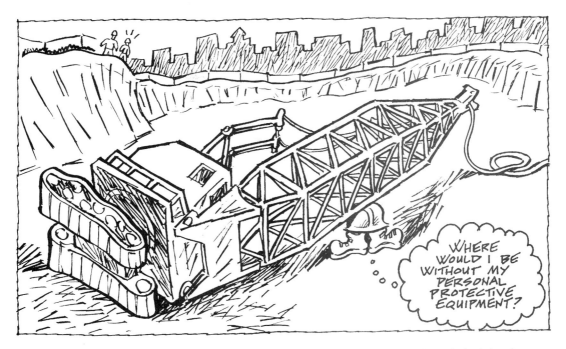

Personal protective equipment is generally not the best approach to prevention. (Drawing by Nick Thorkelson.)

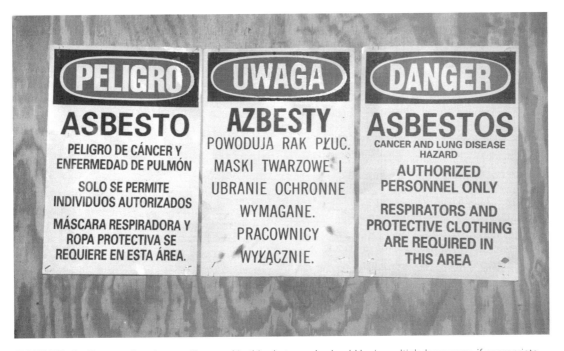

FIGURE 7-4 ● Warning signs, as illustrated in this photograph, should be in multiple languages, if appropriate. (Photograph by Earl Dotter.)

BOX 7-3

Effectively Educating Workers and Communities

Margaret Quinn and Nancy Lessin

A prerequisite to effective health and safety programs is education. The most effective approach to teaching health and safety acknowledges that the worker or community member is the one most familiar with his or her job, home, and community. Workers can identify hazards, both apparent and hidden, that may be associated with their work. Community members understand the specific cultural and political characteristics that will affect the success of a program. Community and worker involvement in prioritizing educational needs and in designing and presenting training are major ingredients in making programs meaningful and useful. They should also be involved in developing and implementing solutions to health and safety problems. Education regarding solutions should include a discussion of the traditional industrial hygiene hierarchy of hazard controls, which emphasizes hazard elimination, and should not be limited to training on the use of personal protective equipment. In addition to worker and community involvement with needs assessment and program design, additional guidelines for successful educational programs include the following:

1. Develop an educational program in the trainee's literal and technical language. The educator should also understand the social context and psychosocial factors of a workplace or community environment that may affect a person's ability to participate in an educational program or to perform certain practices in response to a potential hazard.
2. Define specific and clearly stated goals for each session based on a needs assessment that has involved representatives of the workforce or community to be trained. Begin each program with a concise overview, and reinforce the key issues that come up during the session.
3. Build an evaluation mechanism that can easily be adapted to each program. The evaluation process should be designed to judge the effectiveness of the educational

program in attaining goals set by both the trainer and trainees.
4. Use participatory teaching methods, which draw on the experience that workers and community member already have, in place of a traditional lecture approach.

Participatory, or learner-centered, teaching methods are designed to foster maximum worker participation and interaction. They constitute an approach to education that is based on the understanding that adults bring an enormous amount of experience to the classroom and that this experience should be used in the training program. In addition, adults learn more effectively by doing rather than listening passively. Learners' experiences are incorporated into the course material and are used to expand their grasp of new concepts and skills. Basing new knowledge on prior practical experience helps the learner solve problems and develop safe solutions to unforeseen hazards. Instructors offer specialized knowledge; workers have direct experience. It is the combination of these that leads to effective, long-lasting solutions to health and safety problems.

Participatory learning generally requires more trainer–trainee interaction than lecture-style presentations. Groups should be limited to approximately 20 participants, and these may be broken down into groups of 3 to 6 for small-group exercises. Participatory teaching methods may include use of the following techniques:

1. *Speakouts (large-group discussions)*: The participants share their experiences in relation to a particular hazard or situation.
2. *Brainstorming sessions*: The instructor poses a particular question or problem; the participants call out their ideas. The ideas are recorded on a flipchart so that they become a collective work. In this activity, the trainer elicits information from the participants rather than presenting it in a didactic manner.
3. *Buzz groups (small-group discussions or exercises)*: Each group of three to six participants discusses a particular problem, situation, or question and records the answers or views of the group.

(continued)

BOX 7-3

Effectively Educating Workers and Communities (Continued)

4. *Case studies (small-group exercises)*: Participants apply new knowledge and skills in the exploration of solutions to a particular problem or situation.
5. *Discovery exercises*: Participants go back into the workplace or community to obtain certain items, such as OSHA 300 logs or records of local levels of ambient air contaminants, or perform activities, such as interviewing co-workers regarding a particular hazard; this information is brought back into the classroom for discussion.
6. *Hands-on training*: The participants practice skills such as testing respirator fit, simulating asbestos removal or hazardous waste clean-up (see Fig. 7-5), taking soil samples to measure levels of contaminants calculating lost-workday injury rates from OSHA 300 logs, or handling and learning the uses and limitations of industrial hygiene or environmental monitoring equipment.
7. *Report-back sessions*: After buzz groups, the class reconvenes as a larger group, and a spokesperson for each buzz group reports the group's answers or views; similarities and differences among groups are noted, and patterns may be discovered.

Participatory, or learner-centered, techniques are well-established methods practiced in labor education programs, schools of education, labor unions, and Committees for Occupational Safety and Health (COSH groups) and community-based environmental groups. These groups have demonstrated that it is possible to use participatory methods even for educational programs that require conveyance of specific, technical knowledge. For example, the OSHA Hazard Communication Standard has worker training requirements for use of material safety data sheets (MSDSs), which are forms that contain brief information regarding chemical and physical hazards, adverse health effects, and proper handling, storage, and personal protection for a particular substance. Training on MSDSs should cover how to obtain and interpret them, and their uses and limitations; it should give the participants practice in each of

these areas. Rather than presenting the MSDS in a lecture-style format, the information can be taught more effectively with a participatory exercise, such as the one that follows.

In the first part of the exercise, workers go back into their work areas, find a labeled chemical container, and seek an MSDS for that substance. This requires workers to become familiar with where MSDSs are located in their workplace and the process required to find them. It also serves to identify problems in the system that can be corrected, such as unlabeled containers, missing MSDSs, or locked file cabinets to which no one on the shift has a key. In the second part of the exercise, the class is divided into small groups; the groups review sample MSDSs and collectively answer questions such as, "Is the substance flammable?" "What are the health effects associated with it?" "Does it require wearing of gloves?" and "What ventilation is required?" During the report-back session, the instructor asks for the answers from all of the groups and reviews how to read and interpret MSDSs in general. In the final part of the exercise, participants look up the chemicals covered in the sample MSDSs in other sources, such as the *NIOSH Pocket Guide to Chemical Hazards*. In some situations, more hazards, especially health hazards, are discovered when other sources are consulted. In this way, students learn about the uses and limitations of MSDSs and get practice in using additional sources.

Participatory or learner-centered approaches not only make learning active, but also give participants the skills and support necessary to recognize hazards and to improve health and safety conditions. These approaches broaden the objectives of worker training curricula to include learning of knowledge, attitudes, skills, and behaviors, as well as problem-solving, critical-thinking, and social-action skills.

Bibliography

Auerbach E, Wallerstein N. *ESL for action: problem-posing at work: teachers guide and student manual*. Reading, MA: Addison-Wesley, 1987.

Briggs D, Cameron B, Johnson H, et al. The evolution of worker training methods at Boeing commercial airplane group. New Solutions 1997;7:31–6.

(continued)

BOX 7-3

Effectively Educating Workers and Communities (continued)

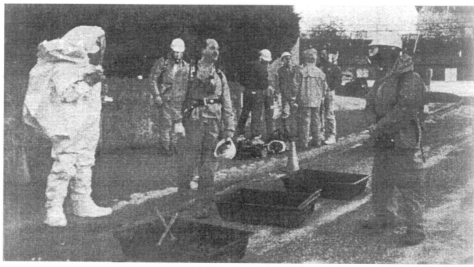

FIGURE 7-5 ● Hands-on field training for hazardous waste workers.

Cary M, Van Belle G, Morris SI, et al. The role of worker participation in effective training. New Solutions 1997;7:23–30.

Colligan M. (Ed.). Occupational safety and health training. Occup Med: State of Art Rev 1994;9(2):127–361.

Hecker S. Education and training. In: JM Stellman, ed. ILO encyclopaedia of occupational health and safety. Geneva: International Labor Organization, 1998:18.1–18.32.

McQuiston T, Coleman P, Wallerstein N, et al. Hazardous waste worker education. J Occup Med 1994;36:1310–23.

Massachusetts Coalition for Occupational Safety and Health. English as a second language health and safety curriculum for working people. Boston: Mass-COSH, 1993.

National Clearinghouse for Worker Safety and Health Training for Hazardous Materials, Waste Operations and Emergency Response, National Institute of Environmental Health Sciences (NIEHS), 5107 Benton Avenue, Bethesda, MD 20814 (telephone 301-571-4226). Materials available from all NIEHS regional training centers, including *Chemical and radioactive hazardous material workbook* (Oil, Chemical and Atomic Workers/Labor Institute, New York, 1993) and *Hazardous waste workers health and safety training manual, version 3.1* (The New England Consortium, University of Massachusetts Lowell, Lowell, MA, 1997).

Slatin C, ed. Health and safety training [special section]. New Solutions 1995;5(2):4–38.

The Labor Institute. Sexual harassment at work: a training workbook for working people. New York: The Labor Institute, 1994.

Wallerstein N, Pillar C, Baker R. Labor educator's health and safety manual. Berkeley, CA: Labor Occupational Health Program, Center for Labor Research and Education, Institute of Industrial Relations, University of California, 1981.

Wallerstein N, Rubenstein H. Teaching about job hazards: a guide for workers and their health providers. Washington, DC: American Public Health Association, 1993.

Wallerstein N, Weinger M, eds. Empowerment education [special issue]. Am J Ind Med 1992;22(5):619–784.

prevent occurrence of occupational disease or injury by primary prevention, screening and surveillance activities are part of secondary prevention. Both screening and surveillance are directed toward identification of health events or documentation of early evidence for adverse health effects that have already occurred. *Screening* is a clinical activity that seeks to identify adverse health effects in an individual before they are symptomatic and when intervention can reduce the probability the individual will develop an adverse health outcome. Specific guidelines for appropriate screening include considerations of risks and benefits to the individual. (See Chapters 6 and 12.) Screening may identify individuals who need primary workplace intervention or who need specific treatment or other therapeutic intervention. *Surveillance* is the systematic gathering, analysis, and dissemination of data. It implies watching out or watching over and may consist of watching out for single events (*sentinel events*) that signal a breakdown in prevention or may consist of reviewing grouped or aggregate data for subtle trends that may be significant across a population but not meaningful for a specific individual (such as increases in liver enzymes that do not exceed population norms). Surveillance can lead to primary prevention measures by identifying inadequate control measures, allowing them to be corrected.

By recognizing potential or existing work-related disease or injury, health professionals can initiate activities leading to one or more of these methods of prevention. They can play an active role in education by informing the community about potentially hazardous workplace exposures and ways of minimizing them. They can advise appropriate use of respirators or other PPE. They can also develop appropriate screening programs targeting high-risk workers or community members. Consultation with specialists in occupational medicine, occupational hygiene, toxicology, safety, or ergonomics may be necessary to facilitate these activities.

Roles in Environmental Health

Roles for professionals in environmental health have been developed by CDC in collaboration with stakeholders at state and local levels and are intended to guide the development of the public health workforce.[5] They can be categorized as follows:

Assessment

Research. Identifying and compiling relevant information to solve a problem and obtaining the relevant information.

Data Analysis and Interpretation. Analyzing data, recognizing meaningful test results, interpreting results, and presenting the results in a meaningful way to different types of audiences

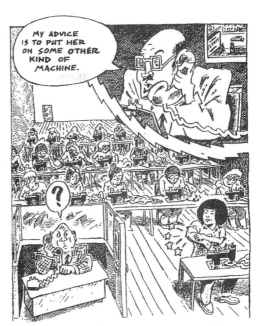

Advice to employees and employers should be practical. (Drawing by Nick Thorkelson.)

Evaluation. Evaluating the effectiveness or performance of procedures, interventions, and programs.

Management

Problem-solving. Understanding and solving problems.

Economic and Political Issues. Understanding and appropriately using information about the economic and political implications of decisions.

Organizational Knowledge and Behavior. Functioning effectively within the culture of organizations and be an effective team player.

Program and Project Management. Planning, implementing, and maintaining fiscally responsible programs and projects using skills and prioritizing projects across the employee's entire workload.

Computer Use/Information Technology. Using information technology as needed to produce work products.

Reporting, Documentation, and Recordkeeping. Producing reports to document actions, keep records, and inform appropriate parties.

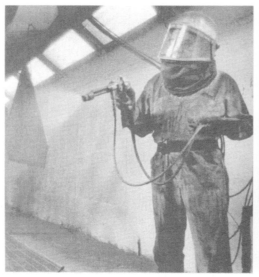 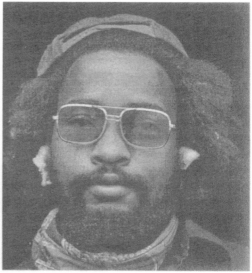

FIGURE 7-6 ● **(A)** Spray painter with respiratory protection. **(B)** Makeshift PPE. Cotton plugs are not effective as PPE; only adequately fitting earplugs or earmuffs are effective. (Photographs by Earl Dotter.)

Collaboration. Forming partnerships and alliances with other individuals and organizations to enhance performance on the job.

Communication

Education. Using environmental health practitioners' frontline role to effectively educate the public on environmental health issues.

Communication. Effectively communicating risk and exchanging information with colleagues, practitioners, clients, policymakers, interest groups, the news media, and the public through public speaking, print and electronic media, and interpersonal relations.

Conflict Resolution. Facilitating resolution of conflicts within an agency, in the community, and with regulated parties.

Marketing. Articulating basic concepts of environmental health and public health and conveying an understanding of their value and importance to clients and the public.

Roles of the Clinician

Once a clinician has identified a probable case of occupational or environmental disease or injury, it is crucial to take preventive action while also providing appropriate treatment and rehabilitation services. Failure to consider the prevention opportunities along with the necessary therapeutic measures may lead to recurrence or worsening of the disease or injury in the affected worker and the continuation or new occurrence of similar cases among workers in similar jobs, either at the same workplace or at other workplaces. A clinician has at least the following five opportunities for preventive action after identifying a case of work-related disease or injury:

- Advise the patient
- Contact the patient's union or other labor organization
- Contact the patient's employer
- Inform the appropriate government authority, and
- Contact an appropriate research or expert group.

Often, some combination of these approaches is undertaken.

Advise the Patient

The clinician should always advise the patient concerning the nature and prognosis of the condition; the possibility that there may be appropriate engineering controls to remove the hazard, such as removing lead-based paint in the home; the need, even if only temporarily, for PPE at work; or, in extreme circumstances, the necessity to change jobs or to move to a different home. The clinician should alert the patient to the need to file a workers' compensation report to protect the worker's rights to income replacement and both medical and rehabilitation services (see Chapter 4). These reports also trigger the employer to consider listing the health event as a reportable injury or illness and may lead the insurance carrier to provide consultative services to the employer to assess the problem area and consider appropriate control measures.

At times, the clinician may be called on to provide advice to the patient concerning legal remedies should a health problem result in a contested workers' compensation claim or the need for registering a complaint with an appropriate government agency (see below). Options may be limited; the worker may not wish to file a claim or register a complaint, fearing job loss or other punitive action, or a family may not have the resources to move to a better home. However, it is essential to inform the patient of potential hazards. It is not appropriate to withhold this information because of the possibility of upsetting the patient. A clinician cannot assume that even a large and relatively sophisticated employer has adequately educated its workers about workplace hazards. Once a patient is informed of the work-relatedness of a disease in writing, this may start the time clock on notification procedures and statutes of limitations for workers' compensation (see Chapter 4).

Contact the Patient's Union or Other Labor Organization

If it is agreeable to the affected worker, the health professional should inform the appropriate labor organization of the health hazards suspected to exist in the workplace. The provision of this information may help to alert other workers to a potential workplace hazard, facilitate investigation of the problem, identify additional similar cases, and eventually facilitate implementation of any necessary control measures. (Keep in mind, however, that fewer than 15 percent of workers in the United States belong to a union.)

Contact the Patient's Employer

The clinician, again only with the patient's consent, should report the problem to the employer. This can be effective in initiating preventive action. Many employers do not have the staff to deal with reported problems adequately, but they can obtain assistance from insurance carriers, government agencies, academic institutions, or private firms. In addition to triggering workplace-based prevention activity, discussions with the employer may lead to

obtaining useful information concerning exposures and the possibility of similar cases among other workers. Depending on the circumstance, it can be particularly helpful to the health professional to arrange with an employer to visit a patient's work area. This presents the opportunity to observe the possibly hazardous environment firsthand and to establish the necessary rapport with managers to involve them in prevention.

Although the law prohibits employers from firing workers for making complaints to OSHA, it does not prohibit them from firing workers who have a potentially work-related diagnosis. In the United States, only the OSHA lead and cotton dust standards mandate removal of workers from jobs that are making them sick. The medical removal protection section of the OSHA lead standard provides temporary medical removal for workers at risk of health impairment from continued lead exposure, as well as temporary economic protection for workers so removed. It states, "During the period of removal, the employer must maintain the worker's earnings, seniority and other employment rights and benefits as though the worker had not been removed." (See Chapters 13, 26, and 30 for more information on lead.) The cotton dust standard does not offer such protection.

Important is close cooperation between labor and management, such as that demonstrated by health and safety committees (Box 7-4).

Inform the Appropriate Governmental Regulatory Agency

If a case of occupational or environmental disease or injury appears to be serious or may be affecting other workers in the same workplace, company, or industry or individuals in the same community, it is wise for the patient or the health professional to consider filing a complaint with the appropriate governmental agency, such as OSHA, EPA, or the state or local health department. (See Chapter 3.) State and local health departments depend on clinicians to identify new clusters of disease, such as foodborne illness, so they can investigate and control these outbreaks.

The health professional should always inform the patient in advance of notifying federal or state governmental agencies. Although regulations of OSHA and the Mine Safety and Health Administration (MSHA) protect U.S. workers who file health and safety complaints against resultant discrimination by the employer (loss of job, earnings, or

BOX 7-4

Labor–Management Health and Safety Committees

The benefits that accrue from seeking the participation of labor unions and workers in the development and implementation of occupational health and safety programs and research can be substantial. As a consequence of their experience and intimate knowledge of the actual work processes, workers and their unions often can add significantly to the understanding of a health or safety problem and determine the best approach to prevention of risks. Their participation also aids in understanding and explaining the nature and importance of programs and research efforts and in interpreting the impact and meaning of such work to individual workers (Fig. 7-7).

One effective means for including workers and their labor unions in the development and improvement of approaches to prevention is joint labor–management health and safety committees in the workplace. These committees consist of representatives of workers and managers. They meet periodically to systematically review workplace health and safety hazards and their control and to respond to specific complaints concerning workplace health and safety. For these committees to function effectively, labor representatives must be truly representative of workers and not simply appointed by management.

Joint labor–management health and safety committees have been legally authorized and are more generally active in some countries, such as Canada. In the United States, they are less common and usually are established through collectively bargained agreements. Proposed OSHA reform legislation in the United States would require operation of health and safety committees in many more workplaces than at present.

Studies in Canada, where joint health and safety committees have been mandated, suggest that this particular form of involvement can be unusually effective. Reduction in work injuries and resolution of health and safety problems without the need for governmental intervention have been documented. Effective committees tend to have cochairs and equal representation, readily available training and information, and well-established procedures. An important feature of successful committees is sufficient authority for action, either as a committee or on the part of the management representatives.

Typically, labor–management health and safety committees meet on a monthly basis for 1 to 2 hours. They review, evaluate, and respond to worker and manager complaints and concerns about working conditions and workplace hazards. They periodically walk through the workplace to observe and assess working conditions and possible health and safety hazards. In addition, they systematically evaluate work practices and procedures and materials used in the workplace in regard to their impacts on workplace health and safety.

As effective as labor–management health and safety committees can be, they are most effective when seen as one component of a more general prevention program that also relies on the development and enforcement of government regulations.

---

benefits), this protection is difficult to enforce, and workers' fears are not unfounded. Health professionals should familiarize themselves with pertinent laws and regulations. For example, if the worker does not file an "11(c)" (antidiscrimination) complaint within 30 days of a discriminatory act, the worker's rights are lost. In the United States, health professionals and workers (or their union, if one exists) have the right, guaranteed by the Freedom of Information Act, to obtain the results of an OSHA inspection.

Help to Create New Knowledge

Occasionally, the health professional who is reporting a work-related or environmentally-mediated medical problem may undertake or assist in a research investigation of this problem. No matter who conducts the research, investigation of the workplace and identification and analysis of additional cases often lead to new information. Publication of epidemiologic studies or case reports alerts others to newly discovered hazards and ways of controlling them. The health professional may also assist

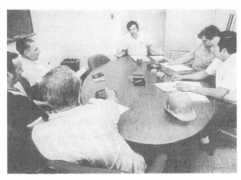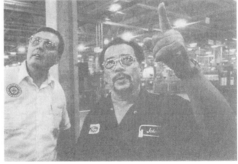

A   B

FIGURE 7-7 ● Joint labor–management health and safety committees are increasingly important in ongoing workplace prevention activity. **(A)** Medical monitoring, screening programs, and a wide variety of other occupational health issues are discussed by committee. **(B)** A worker points out a faulty oil line in a grinder to the union health and safety representative (man in white shirt). (Photograph by Earl Dotter.)

with research to evaluate the effectiveness of preventive approaches, such as the impact of OSHA regulations.

Other Available Resources

Additional resources may be available through federal, state, and local governmental agencies, as well as academic centers and professional organizations. There is a wealth of information on the Web sites of many of the following groups, but it is helpful to know the focus of each as well as their relative strengths and limitations and to be clear to individuals or community groups about the potential costs as well as benefits of engaging each.

The Association of Occupational and Environmental Clinics (AOEC)

A nonprofit association of 60 clinics and more than 250 occupational and environmental health professionals that are dedicated to improving the provision of occupational and environmental health care through information sharing and research, this is one of the most useful resources. AOEC has entered into cooperative agreements with both NIOSH and ATSDR (below) and funds members to participate in specific activities, such as providing services to populations near specific hazardous sites or developing learning materials that can be downloaded and presented for courses and education programs. Member clinics, which are often based in large academic medical centers, must provide access to industrial hygiene and other preventive services. Through AOEC, one can often identify physicians or other health care professionals with specific clin-

ical or research expertise, either for patient referral or for consultation by telephone with the treating physician. (It is in the best interest of the patient to have a therapeutic relationship with a health care provider—a relationship that cannot be established over the telephone.)

The National Center for Environmental Health (NCEH) and the Agency for Toxic Substances Disease Registry (ATSDR)

NCEH and ATSDR have recently been administratively merged at CDC. ATSDR was created by congressional mandate to address health concerns arising from chemical pollution at Superfund sites. Its mission is to assess and mitigate the effect on public health of hazardous substances in the environment. It provides public health assessments of waste sites, health consultations concerning specific hazardous substances, health surveillance and registries, response to emergency releases of hazardous substances, applied research in support of public health assessments, information development and dissemination, and education and training concerning hazardous substances. ATSDR does not conduct formal surveillance or screening, but under unusual circumstances (such as in Libby, Montana), it may contract with AOEC member clinics or other health care providers. ATSDR has also evaluated neurologic and other outcomes among occupants of a building converted from industrial use that was subsequently found to be heavily contaminated with metallic mercury, conducted investigations of unlicensed pesticide applicators using methyl parathion illegally for indoor pest control, and done preliminary studies into complaints arising from low-frequency noise exposure. ATSDR is obligated to formally respond to written citizen requests. Information about the complaint process is available on its Web site, <www.atsdr.gov>.

NCEH provides technical assistance at the request of state or local health departments. It helps to prevent or control diseases or deaths resulting from interactions between people and their environment, including but not limited to those due to chemicals. For example, it also addresses hazards and impediments to walking and bicycling introduced by poor urban planning. Its divisions and offices:

- Provide national and international leadership for coordinating, delivering, and evaluating emergency and environmental public health services;
- Focus on air pollution and respiratory health, environmental surveillance, health studies of disasters and emerging threats, and radiologic hazards;
- Respond to requests from state and local public health departments, such as by helping to evaluate the health impact of a chemical spill on the surrounding community;
- Develop and measure biomarkers for environmental exposures;
- Issue periodic reports with information on the distribution and amount of chemicals in urine and blood in a sample of the U.S. population, such as lead and cotinine, and phthalates;
- Coordinate research and provide information on human genomic discoveries that may be applied to disease prevention; and
- Provide research and technical assistance to reduce the burden of environmental hazards internationally.

The OSHA Small Business Consultation Program

In addition to developing and enforcing standards, OSHA funds a system of consultation programs throughout the United States, based in agencies and universities that provide, on request, free occupational safety and health consultation primarily to businesses with fewer than 250 employees. These programs provide workplace walkthrough surveys, obtain industrial hygiene measurements, and provide recommendations. Although these programs do not impose OSHA fines or citations, if serious hazards are encountered in the course of an evaluation, the program is obligated to inform the local OSHA office (similar to the responsibilities of

the NIOSH Health Hazard Evaluation program, described below and in Chapter 33). This program is designed to assist small businesses that do not have the resources to provide sophisticated health and safety services—although it does not reduce the employer's responsibilities. The program is most effective for those hazards that are well understood and for which OSHA standards exist, such as noise, asbestos, and general safety. In general, these programs are small. There may be a significant wait before the evaluation takes place and a longer one before it is completed. If there are serious, immediate hazards at a workplace, the best approach is still to contact the local OSHA office. However, if a health care provider is treating a patient who works for a small business where the employer is trying to do the right thing, this can be a valuable resource.

The National Institute for Occupational Safety and Health (NIOSH)

Although the Occupational Safety and Health Act of 1970 created them both, NIOSH and OSHA are distinct agencies with separate responsibilities. OSHA is part of the U.S. Department of Labor and is responsible for creating and enforcing workplace safety and health regulations. NIOSH, which is part of the CDC in the Department of Health and Human Services, is responsible for conducting and supporting research to improve workplace safety and health, promoting and supporting training in occupational safety and health, providing technical assistance to employers and employees (often in the form of health hazard evaluations), and developing the scientific basis for standards or other policies aimed at improving workplace safety and health.

NIOSH responds to requests for investigations of workplace hazards through its Health Hazard Evaluation (HHE) program (see Chapter 33). An HHE is a worksite study designed to evaluate potential workplace health hazards. HHEs can be requested by a management official, three current employees, or any officer of a labor union representing the employee. However, with the employee's consent, a health care professional can also contact NIOSH and speak with members of the HHE program. Although there are specific regulations that guide the HHE program itself, NIOSH places a high priority on identifying and preventing emerging threats. HHEs are often able to develop the state of the science, such as identifying outdoor sources of fatal carbon monoxide poisoning; establishing, identifying probable causes, and documenting successful interventions for exposures causing corneal edema; or evaluating fixed small airways disease in a popcorn packaging plant. NIOSH HHEs also result in new exposure assessment methods; for example, they developed the first validated measure of aerosolized pentamidine in clinical settings and established the limitations of dry cotton swabs in measuring environmental anthrax contamination. Because of limited resources, the NIOSH HHE program will not conduct evaluations for known hazards, such as noise or indoor air quality problems, but will instead typically provide written information to the requestor. When an evaluation is conducted, NIOSH reports the results to the workers, the employer, and the U.S. Department of Labor and makes recommendations for reduction or removal of the hazard. Although the HHE program serves as a useful surveillance tool for keeping NIOSH abreast of emerging workplace concerns, NIOSH conducts a wide range of additional surveillance activities to determine the number of workers exposed to specific hazards and which industries and occupations are at risk.

NIOSH supports research through (a) intramural programs that it conducts, (b) cooperative agreements that it initiates and in which it participates, and (c) research grants that extramural investigators initiate and conduct. In 1996, NIOSH established the National Occupational Research Agenda (NORA), a framework to guide occupational safety and health research—not only for NIOSH, but for the occupational health and safety community at large.

To disseminate research findings, NIOSH publishes a variety of reports and other materials. NIOSH publications are designed to inform workers, employers, and occupational safety and health professionals of hazards and how to avoid them.

NIOSH has headquarters in Washington, DC, with administrative offices in Atlanta and with six working divisions and one office located in Morgantown and Cincinnati, two laboratories in Pittsburgh, one laboratory in Spokane, and field stations in Denver and in Anchorage. These major units are

The Division of Applied Research and Technology (DART), which conducts research in toxicology, neurologic and behavioral science, and ergonomics. Responsibilities include laboratory and field studies of biomechanical, psychological, neurobehavioral, and physiologic effects of physical, psychological, biomechanical, and selected chemical stressors. It also develops biological monitoring and diagnostic procedures to improve worker health and conducts research to develop procedures and equipment for the measurement of occupational safety and health hazards and for the development of effective engineering controls and work practices. It also maintains a quality control reference program for industrial hygiene laboratories.

The Division of Respiratory Disease Studies (DRDS), which conducts epidemiologic, environmental, clinical, and laboratory research focusing on all aspects of occupational respiratory disease. It also has specific responsibilities from the Mine Safety and Health Act (the National Coal Workers X-ray Surveillance and the National Coal Workers Autopsy Study, certification of x-ray facilities, mine plan approvals, and B-reader examinations).

The Division of Safety Research (DSR), which conducts research on occupational injury prevention through studies of risk factors and the effectiveness of prevention efforts. It conducts research to provide criteria for improving personal protective equipment and devices.

The Education and Information Division (EID), which has responsibility for development of NIOSH policy and recommendations, with special attention to new occupational health and safety standards. It publishes *Current Intelligence Bulletins* to disseminate new scientific information and *Alerts* to identify opportunities for preventative interventions. It also undertakes quantitative risk assessment efforts to prioritize issues for regulatory attention. It provides library services and technical information services, maintains the NIOSH archives, and operates a toll-free telephone information line.

The Division of Surveillance, Hazard Evaluations and Field Studies (DSHEFS), which has responsibility for surveillance of the extent of hazards and occupational illnesses. It conducts legislatively mandated health hazard evaluations at the request of employees or employers. It also conducts a broad range of industrywide epidemiologic and industrial hygiene research programs, with wide responsibility for occupational illnesses not included in DART or DRDS. It is also responsible for energy-related health research related to workers at U.S. Department of Energy facilities.

The Health Effects Laboratory Division (HELD), which conducts basic, applied, and preventive laboratory research, develops intervention programs, and designs and implements methods for health communications in the area of occupational injury and disease. HELD collaborates with researchers throughout NIOSH and in other public and private institutions to apply the latest scientific research to workplace health problems

The National Personal Protective Technology Laboratory (NPPTL), which focuses expertise from many scientific disciplines to advance federal research on respirators and other personal protective technologies for workers.

The Pittsburgh Research Laboratory and the Spokane Research Laboratory, which conduct surveillance, research, intervention development, technology transfer and training methods development aimed at reducing illness and injuries in the mining industry.

The Office of Compensation Analysis and Support, which conducts activities to assist claimants and support the role of the Secretary of Health and Human Services under the Energy Employees Occupational Illness Compensation Program Act of 2000.

To further assist professionals and the public, NIOSH provides a toll-free information system. It can be accessed by telephone at 1-800-35-NIOSH (1-800-356-4674). NIOSH specialists provide technical advice and information on subjects in occupational safety and health.

State and Local Resources

In addition to those states where there is a state OSHA plan, each state has a state public health department, as do many counties and many large cities. Basic functions of public health departments include disease surveillance, environmental assessment, and preventive services, although the scope of these varies widely according to state history and funding. Public health departments nationally suffered neglect and decay of human resources and infrastructure as a victim of their own successes in allowing Americans to take clean water and safe food supplies for granted. Even the renewed attention to infectious diseases that took place in the wake of the AIDS pandemic and the advent of multiple drug resistant tuberculosis sparked more of a medical response, with some increased attention paid to services for sexually transmitted diseases

and public health messages. Since the September 11 terrorist attacks and the subsequent anthrax outbreak, renewed attention has been given to improving disaster preparedness in the public health system, recognizing the depleted public health infrastructure.

Public health departments generally include some aspects of environmental control or sanitation, and many have programs specifically directed toward childhood lead screening programs. Some include other housing needs, such as radon detection, window safety, and water incursion, although in some locations these programs are located in a department of housing. Control of vectors, including rats, mosquitoes, and other pests, is an additional responsibility of many health departments. State departments of environmental health or environmental resources are tasked with many of the enforcement responsibilities required by specific EPA regulations, although there is growing recognition of the need for regional collaboration among states for many of these responsibilities. These state-level departments or the EPA, for example, may provide information about certified laboratories for specific environmental testing programs. Some state health departments, such as Massachusetts, New Jersey, Wisconsin, and California, have very strong components addressing occupational safety and health. Major cities, such as Chicago, New York, Washington, D.C., and Los Angeles, have strong environmental health units within their public health departments. State, county, and municipal Web sites are useful sources of information. Governmental services are also listed in the blue pages of the telephone book.

Education and Research Centers, Environmental Health Sciences Centers, and Outreach and Training Programs

NIOSH currently funds 16 comprehensive Education and Research Centers (ERCs) that focus on occupational safety and health professional training but that also provide continuing education and research training. They are a useful source of academic expertise and may be able to fund small pilot research projects to permit a preliminary investigation into a new or emerging hazard. The National Institute of Environmental Health Sciences is part of the National Institutes of Health and funds research and training in environmental health, including 20 university-based Environmental Health Sciences Centers, all of which have community outreach and educational components, as do five Marine and Freshwater Biomedical Sciences Centers and one Developmental Center. Although attempting to identify faculty research expertise that meets a local community need is usually hit or miss, at a minimum the effort provides insight into the nearby academic expertise. NIEHS also funds worker education programs related to hazardous materials and K–12 environmental health education science curricula.

The Environmental Protection Agency

Although EPA is primarily a regulatory agency, it also has research and laboratory facilities, training and outreach programs, and environmental justice initiatives that may provide expertise and technical assistance.

RESOURCES ON THE WEB

The CDC Web site includes information on environmental and occupational health, injury prevention, and other aspects of public health. Issues of the *Morbidity and Mortality Weekly Report* are available online and cover major public health issues as well as current investigations (see <http://www.cdc.gov/node.do/id/0900f3ec8000e044>).

Environmental Health Perspectives, a print journal that is fully available online, is published monthly by the National Institute of Environmental Health Sciences, part of the NIH (see <http://ehp.niehs.nih.gov/>).

The EPA Web site includes tools to identify contaminant sources at the neighborhood level ("Enviromapper"), Toxic Release Inventory information, and real-time air pollution mapping, among other resources (see <http://www.epa.gov/>).

The NIOSH site is especially useful for educational and research materials, as well as information about Health Hazard Evaluations (see <http://www.cdc.gov/niosh/homepage.html>).

The OSHA home page includes exceptionally helpful links to technical topics, as well as information on state programs, standards, and enforcement (see <http://www.osha.gov/>).

REFERENCES

1. Held E, Mygind K, Wolff C, et al. Prevention of work related skin problems: An intervention study in wet work employees. Occup Environ Med 2002;59:556–61.
2. Evanoff BA, Bohr PC, Wold LD. Effects of a participatory ergonomics team among hospital orderlies. Am J Industr Med 1999;35:358–65.
3. Carayon P, Smith M. Work organization and ergonomics. Appl Ergon 2000;31:649–62.
4. Centers for Disease Control and Prevention. Third national report on human exposure to environmental chemicals. Atlanta, GA: CDC, 2005. Available at: <http://www.cdc.gov/exposurereport>.
5. Centers for Disease Control and Prevention. A national strategy to revitalize environmental public health services. Available at: <http://www.cdc.gov/nceh/ehs/Docs/NationalStrategy2003.pdf>.

The findings and conclusions in this chapter are those of the authors and do not necessarily represent the views of the National Institute for Occupational Safety and Health.

CHAPTER 8

Epidemiology

Ellen A. Eisen, David H. Wegman, and Marie S. O'Neill

The epidemiologic study of populations complements the clinical focus on individuals in addressing occupational and environmental health problems. *Environmental epidemiology* is the study of the health consequences of involuntary exposures to hazards in the air, water, soil, or diet that occur in the general environment—outdoor or indoor. The related field of *occupational epidemiology* is concerned with hazardous exposures in the workplace. In contrast with most other specialty areas of epidemiology, both environmental epidemiology and occupational epidemiology are defined by potential exposure and both require the construction and refinement of biologically relevant exposure measures. Exposure assessment must characterize the level of exposure while accounting for temporal and spatial variation specific to the setting.

Occupational epidemiology studies are based on a workforce that is generally healthy, whereas environmental epidemiology studies are based on the general population, which may include infants and older people as well as working-age adults in poorer health than those in the workforce. Study designs and analytic methods need to take account of these features.

cupational or environmental hazard can be a challenge because people move and exposure patterns change over time. In an occupational setting, new workers are hired and others leave the workforce. Exposures vary over time because of job transfers, changes in technology or production processes, use of different materials, and other factors. The levels of pollution, noise, and green space in a residential neighborhood can change dramatically over a short period of time, and these changes may have important health implications for those who live there. Susceptibility and activity patterns and behaviors that affect exposure, such as cigarette smoking, typically change over the life course.

Exposure can be characterized by intensity (concentration) and the duration over which it occurs. Current exposures are measured for studies of short-term, or acute, health responses; in contrast, long-term exposures are needed to examine chronic disease or to evaluate the potential impact of cumulative exposure on an acute health event. In some static situations, current exposure may be a reasonable surrogate for past exposure. In more dynamic situations, patterns of exposure over time need to be accounted for to estimate dose to an organ or tissue. There are several degrees of refinement for estimating dose.

MEASURING EXPOSURE

There are a variety of ways to estimate both current and past exposures. An accurate measurement of exposure is equally as important as an accurate measurement of health outcome in arriving at an unbiased and precise estimate of the exposure–outcome relationship. Assigning exposure to an oc-

Potential for Exposure

The most commonly available measure of exposure is documented employment in a specific industry or a specific job or residence in a particular geographic area. Although the potential for exposure is a crude surrogate for exposure, if the relation between exposure and outcome is sufficiently strong, an association can be determined in spite of measurement error. For example, lung cancer was associated with asbestos in a study of shipyard workers, despite the fact that fewer than half of the shipyard workers had asbestos exposure.[1] Nevertheless, the estimate of risk associated with exposure to a specific agent is greatly diluted with use of such a surrogate measure. For example, a study of diesel exposure among railroad workers was largely negative, but only 7 percent of workers had been exposed to diesel fumes.

Quantity of Exposure

Measures of exposure should ideally include both intensity and duration. Because data on duration of employment or distance from a toxic waste site may be more easily and accurately determined than intensity of exposure, duration of exposure or distance from a source of exposure are frequently used as exposure surrogates. It is often possible to document the number of years employed from payroll records or from union seniority records. Sometimes length of employment is unknown, but data such as pension-plan eligibility may provide at least a dichotomous measure of duration—such as more than or less than 10 years of employment.

Exposure estimates are improved when occupational or environmental exposure assessment input is available, based on either judgments of potential exposure or as measurements of actual exposure. Variation in exposure may occur over time as a result of change in the environment or changes in a subject's activities between days and within any given day. In the workplace, differences in work habits or tasks, seasonal changes in ventilation patterns, and use of personal protective equipment may also affect personal exposures.

Current exposure estimates alone can be used to study acute health effects, but for the study of chronic effects such estimates must be integrated with past exposures to develop a measure of cumulative exposure. In the work setting, a complete work history ideally includes documentation of time spent in specific jobs together with information on gaps in employment, such as prolonged sick leaves, periods of layoff, or military leaves (see Chapter 6). Estimates of cumulative workplace exposure ideally rely on compilation of current and historical industrial hygiene data and interviews of workers about the history of changes, such as in the production process and exposure controls. Es-

timates can be made of past exposures by reconstructing and testing old work environments. For example, in studies of pulmonary function in the Vermont granite industry, there was a need to account for past exposures, but no measurements were available. An old granite shed was reopened and operated without modern exhaust ventilation controls to arrive at appropriate estimates of the historical exposures.[2]

To compute cumulative exposure to an occupational hazard, estimated exposure levels are weighted by the number of years in successive jobs and summed over all jobs held by each worker. An implicit assumption in the computation of cumulative exposure is that 1 year of exposure to 20 fibers/cc of asbestos is equivalent to 10 years of exposure to 2 fibers/cc. Furthermore, exposure that occurred years ago is assumed to be biologically equivalent to the exposure last year. More complex weighting schemes are possible, but they should be based on specific biological hypotheses about the relative importance of different exposure patterns. For example, exposures in the distant past can be weighted more heavily than those in the recent past for diseases such as silicosis, in which irreversible changes are believed to accumulate gradually over years.

In contrast with workplace-based studies, cumulative exposure is rarely estimated in community-based studies because the necessary records are rarely available. Assigning long-term exposure to an environmental pollutant, such as particles in the ambient air or disinfection by-products in drinking water, requires knowledge of residential history and/or consumption habits over a long period of time. This information would need to be obtained through surveys or questionnaires or through public records of vital statistics, water supply practices, or environmental monitoring

Biological Monitoring

Biological markers (biomarkers) are indicators of an exposure, a response to exposure, an early pathologic change, or susceptibility. They include toxic agents (or their metabolites) that are measured directly in blood, urine, bone, or exhaled air. Biological markers can provide refined measures of dose* or early physiologic response. One

---

Dose is the quantity of a substance or radiation absorbed at a given point or in a given period of time.

advantage of biological markers is that they account for exposures from multiple routes of absorption, including inhalation, skin absorption, and ingestion. For example, blood lead level has been used in epidemiologic studies of workers and urban children because it integrates recent absorption through respiration and ingestion. Another advantage of biological markers is that they may reflect exposure over specific time intervals. For example, in studies of the health effects of chronic lead exposure, x-ray fluorescence (XRF) of bone provides a more relevant biomarker of exposure than blood lead level because it estimates the accumulated body burden of lead, reflecting long-term exposure. Although no biological monitoring tests currently exist for a substantial number of hazardous substances, biological monitoring is receiving more attention today, and new measures of the body burden of toxic agents can be expected.

COMMON MEASURES OF DISEASE FREQUENCY

Clusters are aggregations of disease in a specific population defined by time or space. If a disease is extremely rare, the occurrence of even a few cases in a workplace or neighborhood can prompt further investigation of a possible hazard. For example, three cases of angiosarcoma diagnosed during a 3-year period among a group of workers exposed to vinyl chloride were sufficient to make a plant physician suspect that the chemical was a carcinogen.[3] When the disease is more common, however, disease frequency can be interpreted only in relation to the size of the population at risk. To determine if a high disease frequency is beyond random variation, the epidemiologist uses one of these two measures of disease frequency: prevalence and incidence.

Prevalence

The simplest quantity, known as *point prevalence*, is the ratio between the number of cases present and the size of the population at risk at a single point in time:

$$\text{Point prevalence} = \frac{\text{Number of cases}}{\text{Population at risk}}$$

To interpret the public health significance of 68 cases of peripheral neuropathy reported in a coated fabrics plant,[4] one needs a denominator. The total plant population was 1,157. Therefore, the point prevalence was

$$\frac{68}{1,157} = 5.9 \text{ percent}$$

To determine whether this prevalence was excessive, the prevalence in the plant had to be compared with the prevalence in the general population or some other appropriate comparison group. A limitation of point prevalence is that it does not distinguish between old and new cases.

Incidence Rate

In contrast, incidence measures the occurrence of new cases. The *incidence rate* is based on the number of new cases occurring during a specified period of time:

$$\text{Incidence rate} = \frac{\text{Number of new cases}}{\substack{\text{Toal population at risk during} \\ \text{the specified period}}}$$

In the coated fabrics plant, only 50 affected workers had onset of the disease within the past year; 18 of the 68 prevalent cases occurred more than 1 year ago. Therefore, the population at risk for development of a new case within the past year was: 1,157 − 18 = 1,139. Because the number of new cases in that period was 50, the plant-wide annual incidence rate was

$$\frac{50}{1,139} = 4.4 \text{ per } 100 \text{ workers}$$

The incidence rate can also be refined to reflect monitoring of individuals for varying lengths of time. The appropriate denominator incorporates the concept of *person-time*, usually expressed in units of person-years. This denominator takes into account not only the number of at-risk persons but also the length of time during which they were at risk for development of the specific disease. An example of how to calculate the contribution of a single worker to a person-years denominator is illustrated in Fig. 8-1.

COMPARISONS OF RATES

To understand whether an incidence rate in an exposed population is excessive, it is necessary to compare it with the rate in an unexposed population. The two most common comparisons, or estimates of risk, are relative risk (the ratio of rates) and attributable risk (the difference between rates).

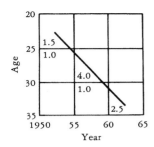

Time Period	Age Group	Person-years
1950 – 1954	20 – 24	1.5
	25 – 29	1.0
1955 – 1959	25 – 29	4.0
	30 – 34	1.0
1960 – 1964	30 – 34	2.5
		10.0

FIGURE 8-1 ● Person-years experienced by a worker entering a follow-up program at age 23 years 6 months in mid-1952 and leaving in mid-1962. (Adapted from Monson RR. Occupational epidemiology. 2nd ed. Boca Raton, FL: CRC Press, 1989.)

Relative Risk

The *relative risk*, or rate ratio, is designed to communicate the relative importance of an exposure by comparing the rate from an exposed population with that from an otherwise comparable nonexposed population. In its simplest form, it is the ratio of two rates (Table 8-1). In the case of the fabrics plant, the suspect neurotoxin was in the print department, so it was possible to create a within-plant comparison. Of the 1,139 disease-free workers in the plant, 169 worked in the print department and 34 of these workers had onset of peripheral neuropathy in the past year, resulting in an annual incidence rate of:

$$\frac{34}{169} = 20.1 \text{ per 100 workers}$$

Among the remaining 970 workers, there were 16 new cases, resulting in an annual incidence rate of:

$$\frac{16}{970} = 1.6 \text{ per 100 workers}$$

TABLE 8-1

Derivation of Relative Risk and Attributable Risk[a]

Disease	Exposure		Total
	Present	Absent	
Present	a	c	a + c
Absent	b	d	b + d
Total	a + b	c + d	a + b + c + d

[a] Calculations:
  Exposed disease rate = a/(a + b)
  Nonexposed disease rate = c/(c + d)
  Relative risk = a/(a + b) ÷ c/(c + d)
  Attributable risk = a/(a + b) − c/(c + d)

Therefore, the relative risk (or incidence rate ratio) was

$$\frac{20.1}{1.6} = 12.6$$

When examining different diseases or the effects of different hazards, relative risks can be compared directly. For example, the relative risk of lung cancer in heavy smokers compared with nonsmokers is very large (32.4), whereas that for cardiovascular disease is small (1.4). This suggests that smoking is more potent as a lung carcinogen than as a cardiotoxic agent.

Attributable Risk

Whereas the relative risk is a measure of the potency of the hazard, *attributable risk* measures the magnitude of the disease burden in the population that is ascribed to the exposure under study. This concept is particularly useful in studies of an occupational or environmental health hazard because such an exposure is generally only one of several possible causes of any specific disease. The attributable risk is calculated by subtracting the rate of the particular disease in the nonexposed population from that in the exposed population (Table 8-1). This risk difference is attributed to the exposure. In the example in the coated fabrics plant, the annual incidence rate per 100 workers in the unexposed population (1.6) is subtracted from the rate in the exposed population (20.1), yielding an attributable risk of 18.5 per 100 workers per year.

Concerning the impact of cigarette smoking on health, Table 8-2 shows that the smoking-attributable risk for lung cancer (2.20 per 1,000) is smaller than the smoking-attributable risk for cardiovascular disease (2.61 per 1,000). The attributable risk takes account of both the potency of the disease-causing factor and the magnitude of the disease in the population. Despite the lower *relative risk* of cardiovascular disease due to smoking,

> ### TABLE 8-2
>
> ### Relative and Attributable Risk of Death Among British Male Physicians from Selected Causes Associated with Heavy Cigarette Smoking
>
> | Cause of Death | Death Rate[a] | | Relative Risk | Attributable Risk |
> |---|---|---|---|---|
> | | Nonsmokers | Heavy Smokers[b] | | |
> | Lung cancer | 0.07 | 2.27 | 32.4 | 2.20 |
> | Other cancers | 1.91 | 2.59 | 1.4 | 0.68 |
> | Chronic bronchitis | 0.05 | 1.06 | 21.2 | 1.01 |
> | Cardiovascular disease | 7.32 | 9.93 | 1.4 | 2.61 |
> | All causes | 12.06 | 19.67 | 1.6 | 7.61 |
>
> [a] Number of deaths per 1,000 per year.
> [b] Smokers of ≥25 cigarettes per day
> Adapted from Doll R, Hill AB. Mortality in relation to smoking: Ten years' observations of British doctors. Br Med J 1964;1:1399.

the larger *attributable risk* indicates that in a population, reduction of smoking has a greater impact on cardiovascular disease than on lung cancer.

Relative risks are commonly presented in epidemiologic studies as a measure of association between an exposure and a disease outcome. In contrast, attributable risks are useful in setting priorities for public health interventions or control.

INTERPRETING RATES

Crude Rates

When rates are calculated without consideration of factors such as age or calendar year, they are referred to as *crude rates*. Crude rates can be misleading. For example, if the exposed group includes a high proportion of older people and disease incidence increases with age, then observed differences in crude rates may only reflect differences in age.

Specific Rates

Specific rates are rates estimated for homogeneous subgroups of a population defined by specific levels of a factor, such as age-specific rates. Sometimes, an elevated disease risk exists only in one subgroup.

Adjusted Rates

Although specific rates can sometimes provide valuable information, it is cumbersome to compare many specific rates. Methods have been developed for estimating a single summary rate that takes account of differences in the distribution of population characteristics, such as age. Such rates are known as *adjusted*, or *standardized*, *rates*. Two types of adjustment are commonly used: *direct adjustment* (rates in the study population are weighted by person-time in a reference population) and *indirect adjustment* (rates in a reference population are weighted by person-time in the study population). These methods can be illustrated with examples of adjustment for age (Table 8-3). For a description of these types of adjustment, see the Appendix at the end of the chapter.

TYPES OF EPIDEMIOLOGIC STUDY DESIGNS

Epidemiologic studies can be categorized into three general types: *cohort, case-control,* and *cross-sectional*. The population in a cohort study is defined on the basis of exposure status. An occupational cohort often represents a complete enumeration of both current employees and past workers. The cohort is monitored over time, and the incidence of symptoms, functional abnormalities,

TABLE 8-3

Age Effect on Incidence of Myocardial Infarction[a]

	Workers < 45 Years			Workers ≥ 45 Years			All Workers			
Location	Cases	Population at Risk	Age-Specific Incidence Rate	Cases	Population at Risk	Age-Specific Incidence Rate	Cases	Population at Risk	Crude Incidence Rate	Age-Adjusted Incidence Rate[b]
Factory 1	4	400	10.0	18	600	30.0	22	1,000	22.0	18.0
Factory 2	10	800	12.5	10	200	50.0	20	1,000	20.0	27.5

[a] The incidence rate is expressed as new myocardial infarctions occurring in a 10-year period of observation per 1,000 population.
[b] Based on age distribution summed for Factory 1 and Factory 2.

disease, or death is observed. By contrast, subjects in a case-control study are selected on the basis of health status (Figure 8-2), and exposures are compared between subjects with and without disease. The cross-sectional design typically focuses on a study population at a single point in time, collecting both exposure and health information simultaneously.

In addition to these three classic study designs, other types of studies are commonly used in environmental epidemiology because environmental exposure data are often available for groups or areas, rather than for individuals. To meet the challenges and opportunities of available data, epidemiologists use ecologic study designs and do cluster investigations. All study designs should consider including risk factors that act through populations along with those that act through individuals. In this regard, work in social epidemiology is instructive (Box 8-1).

Cross-Sectional Studies

The cross-sectional approach is commonly used in field investigations because it is the simplest study design to execute. The study population includes all subjects in the population of interest who are present at the time of data collection. Either the prevalence of disease is compared between subgroups defined by exposure status, or exposure is compared between subgroups defined by disease status. Exposure can be classified (a) dichotomously, such as exposed versus nonexposed; (b) categorically, as low, medium, and high; or (c) as

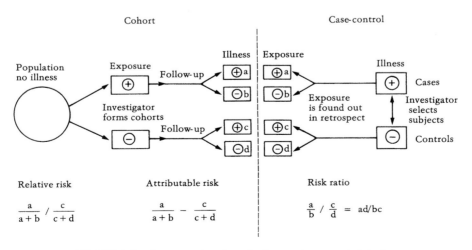

FIGURE 8-2 ● General outline of cohort and case-control studies.

BOX 8-1

Social Epidemiology
Elizabeth M. Barbeau

Social epidemiology is the branch of epidemiology concerned with the social distribution and social determinants of health.[1] The field is distinguished by its focus on social determinants as the central objects of causal analysis rather than as background characteristics to be adjusted for in the examination of biomedical phenomena.[2] If we consider social determinants, such as socioeconomic deprivation and inequality, social networks, and discrimination, to be *social exposures*, then social epidemiology can be viewed within the framework of environmental epidemiology.

Social epidemiology studies have added to our understanding about how the social context might contribute to shaping individual health behaviors. For example, these studies consider multiple levels—individual, interpersonal, and environmental—at which social conditions could impact health. Lessons learned inform approaches to intervention, calling attention to the importance of targeting systems and institutions—not just individuals—to improve health behaviors. Among the lessons learned from these approaches are that social factors can create a vulnerability or susceptibility to poor health in general and not just to one specific disorder.

The social determinants of cigarette smoking and success in quitting were recently explored in a study based on data from the 2000 National Health Interview Survey, a nationally representative sample of adults.[3] The social exposures considered as determinants of smoking habits were the commonly studied aspects of social position, including income, education, race/ethnicity, gender, and occupation.

Overall, the results indicated a socioeconomic gradient with prevalence of current smoking greatest among persons in working-class occupations, those with low education level, and those with low income. Attempts to quit, however, showed no socioeconomic gradient; however, success in quitting was highest among those with most socioeconomic resources.

These patterns held in most, but not all, race/ethnicity-gender groups, calling attention to the potential importance of tailoring public health approaches to the varying socioeconomic gradients observed in different racial/ethnic and gender groups. In addition, smoking patterns were associated with occupational class in multivariate models that also included income and education, suggesting that these measures of social class contain independent information and are not redundant.

As discussed elsewhere in this chapter, traditional methods for epidemiology are either ecologic or based on individuals. Neither design is adequate for a multilevel analysis of the impact of the social context on health. The problems with ecologic analyses have been addressed. Models based on individuals will be invalid if individuals are clustered within workplaces or neighborhoods, violating the independence assumption. Subjects who work in the same hazardous job or live in the same polluted neighborhood may share traits and experiences that make their probabilities of disease not entirely independent. *Multilevel modeling* is a recently developed approach for analyzing data that have a nested hierarchical structure, in which individuals (lower level) are nested within one or more higher order spatial or organizational units (higher levels). Social epidemiologists have pioneered the use of multilevel analyses that examine how social conditions that operate at the individual, group, and environment levels can impact health.

In a study of determinants of tobacco consumption (smoking and chewing) in India, the national family health survey provided data that could be grouped at several potentially important levels.[4] Sex, marital status, and educational attainment were available on individuals in addition to social caste, religion, and a living index (available at the household level). Households were also grouped by location in large or medium cities, towns, or villages. Using multilevel modeling, smoking and chewing tobacco were found to be associated with socioeconomic markers at the individual level (no education), household level (low living standard), and caste level (marginal caste groups). Interestingly, when these variables were accounted for in models that included state, district, and village, differences in tobacco consumption remained, with state accounting for most of the variation. The authors concluded, "The distribution of tobacco consumption is likely to maintain, and perhaps

(continued)

BOX 8-1

Social Epidemiology (Continued)

increase, the current considerable socioeconomic differentials in health in India. Interventions aimed at influencing change in tobacco consumption should consider the socioeconomic and geographical determinants of people's susceptibility to consume tobacco."

References

1. Berkman LF, Kawachi I, eds. Social epidemiology. New York: Oxford University Press, 2000.

2. Krieger N. Epidemiology and social sciences: Towards a critical reengagement in the 21st century. Epidemiol Rev 2000;11:155–63.
3. Barbeau EM, Krieger N, Soobader M. Working class matters: Socioeconomic disadvantage, race/ethnicity, gender and smoking in the National Health Interview Survey, 2000. Am J Public Health 2004;94:269–78.
4. Subramanian SV, Nandy S, Kelly M, et al. Patterns and distribution of tobacco consumption in India: cross sectional multilevel evidence from the 1998-9 national family health survey. Br Med J 2004;328:801–6.

---

a continuous measurement. Exposure classification can be based on either current or lifetime exposure. The following is an example of a cross-sectional study.

The association between environmental lead exposure and blood pressure was investigated in a cross-sectional study based on data from the second National Health and Nutrition Examination Survey (NHANES II). NHANES II was a general health survey administered to a representative sample of the U.S. population. The study population was restricted to the high-risk group of white males between the ages of 40 and 59. Treating both the outcomes and exposure as continuous variables, subjects with higher blood lead levels were found to have higher systolic and diastolic blood pressure. These associations were significant in linear regression models after adjusting for other known risk factors, including age, body mass index, nutritional factors, and blood chemistry.[5]

Cohort Studies

In a cohort study design, a potentially exposed group is identified and monitored forward in time to measure the occurrence of adverse health outcomes. The incidence is observed in the study group and compared with that in a nonexposed reference group. Cohort studies are described as either *retrospective* (the cohort is defined at some point in the past and monitored to the present) or *prospective* (the cohort is defined at the present and monitored into the future).

Cohort Mortality Studies

Although the cohort design can be used to examine nonfatal outcomes, most occupational cohort studies examine mortality from specific causes. The most common of type of cohort study is the standardized mortality study, in which the cause-specific mortality rate of the exposed cohort is compared with that of the general population (assumed to be nonexposed). This comparison results in an approximation of relative risk, known as the *standardized mortality ratio* (SMR). If the number of deaths observed in the exposed cohort is equal to the number expected based on death rates in the standard population, the SMR equals 1.0, which indicates neither an excess nor a deficit of risk. If the SMR is greater than 1.0, the data suggest an increased risk in the exposed population.

To conduct an SMR study, the following information must be obtained for each member of the cohort: date of birth, date of entry into cohort, date of leaving cohort, vital status (alive or dead), and cause of death for those who died. With these data, one can determine person-years at risk, which take into consideration times when workers entered or left during the study period. This permits a calculation of person-years at risk, adjusting for length of time since entry into the study and for age. This type of study requires personnel records with accurate employment data; if such data on the total population at risk are lacking, the mortality experience can be evaluated by proportional mortality analysis. The following is an example of a retrospective cohort mortality study.

A cohort of autoworkers was studied to examine the relation between exposure to metalworking fluids and specific causes of death.[6] All workers who had ever been employed in one of three Midwestern automobile manufacturing plants for at least 3 years prior to 1984 were included. Subjects were followed for vital status from 1941, the year Social Security records became available, through 1994. By the end of the follow-up period, almost 25 percent of the 46,400 subjects had died. When the observed number of deaths due to all causes combined was compared to the expected number, there was no obvious excess among white males (SMR = 1.0) and a slight deficit among African-American males (SMR = 0.9). When observed deaths due to specific cancers were compared to expected, slight excesses of between 1.2 and 1.4 were found for cancers of the esophagus, larynx, stomach, liver, and lung as well as leukemia among white males and for several of these same cancers, as well as pancreatic cancer, among African-American males (Table 8-4). When lifetime exposure to metalworking fluids was evaluated as a predictor in regression models for deaths due to specific cancers, increasing risk was associated with increasing exposure for cancers of the esophagus, larynx, liver, skin, brain, and prostate.

Cohort Morbidity Studies

Increasingly, the cohort design is being used to study risks associated with a variety of nonfatal health outcomes. Retrospective studies can be conducted if information on past health status is available, such as in medical records or collected in health surveys. More often, morbidity studies require prospective study designs so that the health information can be collected directly by administering medical examinations, physiologic tests, or surveys of current health status. Studies that examine episodic health events, such as recurrent symptoms or changes in pulmonary function, are referred to as *longitudinal studies*, and the change in health status over time becomes the *outcome of interest*. The following is an example of a retrospective cohort morbidity study.

A cohort of approximately 1,000 hospital nurses was studied to examine possible reproductive effects associated with use of sterilizing agents.[7] Questionnaires and medical records were used to collect information retrospectively about both exposure and pregnancy history as far back as 30 years. The frequency of spontaneous abortion among nurses currently using the sterilizing agents was only slightly higher than that for currently nonexposed nurses. A more striking difference was observed when results were stratified according to whether exposure to sterilizing agents had occurred during a past pregnancy. Among those exposed, the rate of spontaneous abortion was 16 percent, compared with 6 percent among the nonexposed. Of the three specific sterilizing agents considered, ethylene oxide showed the strongest association with spontaneous abortion.

The following is an example of a prospective cohort morbidity study.

A cohort of 1,022 infants born in the Faroe Islands* was followed forward in time to investigate the possible neurobehavioral effects of prenatal exposure to methyl mercury. The source of exposure was dietary and derived mostly from eating whale meat, a custom in this Nordic community. Batteries of neurophysiologic and neuropsychologic tests were administered to school children at approximately age 7. The exposure variables were both biomarkers: the mercury concentration in cord blood and maternal hair. Mercury concentration in the hair of the subjects at 12 months of age was also measured. Neurophysiologic and neuropsychologic testing did not reveal any mercury-related abnormalities; however, deficits in language, attention, and memory were related to prenatal exposure.[8]

Case-Control Studies

In the case-control, or case-referent, study design, the investigator compares the frequency of exposure between groups with and without the disease

---

*The Faroe Islands, part of the Kingdom of Denmark, are located between the Norwegian Sea and the North Atlantic Ocean.

TABLE 8-4

Standardized Mortality Ratios for Selected Cancers among White and African-American Male Autoworkers

Cause of Cancer Death	White Males		African-American Males	
	Observed	SMR (95% CI)	Observed	SMR (95% CI)
All cancers	2,983	1.05 (1.01–1.09)	460	0.95 (0.86–1.04)
Esophageal	83	1.22 (0.97–1.51)	21	0.76 (0.47–1.16)
Stomach	151	1.16 (0.98–1.36)	28	0.96 (0.63–1.38)
Pancreas	143	0.99 (0.83–1.16)	36	1.50 (1.05–2.07)
Liver	78	1.42 (1.12–1.77)	16	1.31 (0.75–2.13)
Larynx	44	1.16 (0.85–1.56)	11	1.26 (0.63–2.25)
Lung	1,002	1.08 (1.02–1.15)	153	0.95 (0.80–1.11)
Prostate	261	1.06 (0.94–1.20)	55	0.98 (0.74–1.28)

SMR, standardized mentality ratio; 95% CI, 95% confidence interval.

Adapted from Eisen EA, Bardin J, Gore R, et al. Exposure-response models based on extended follow-up of a cohort mortality study in the automobile industry. Scand J Work Environ Health 2001;27:240–9.

of interest (see Fig. 8-2). The case-control design is particularly well suited to study diseases that occur infrequently; a cohort study would have to be very large, and therefore prohibitively expensive, to generate enough cases to study.

There are three types of case-control studies: (a) studies nested within occupational cohorts, (b) population-based case-control studies, and (c) registry-based case-control studies. In *nested case-control studies*, all cases of the selected disease are identified from the cohort, and controls are sampled from among those without the disease. In a mortality study, disease status may be determined at death from a particular disease; in a morbidity study, disease status may be determined by disease incidence based on diagnosis. In a *population-based case-control study*, all cases occurring in residents of a defined geographic area are included, and controls are selected from the same defined population. In a *registry-based case-control study*, cases of disease that are reported to the registry with onset during a defined time period are identified, and controls are selected from the same registry base. Because registries are not necessarily population-based, such as a hospital cancer registry, the selection of controls may require identification of patients with other diseases from the same source as the cases, such as from the same hospital.

The measure of relative risk typically calculated in a case-control study is the *odds ratio* (OR), which is a ratio of the odds of exposure among the cases compared with the odds of exposure among the controls. In Table 8-1, it can be seen that a/b is the odds of exposure among the cases, and c/d is the odds of exposure among the controls. ORs approximate the incidence rate ratios that are obtained in cohort studies. Their interpretations are similar: when OR = 1, there is no excess or deficit of risk.

A case-control study need not include all the cases within a defined population. Valid results may still be obtained when the case group includes only a sample of all cases. The major requirement for a valid case-control study is that the selected controls be comparable to the population from which cases were identified and that both cases and controls be selected without prior knowledge of past exposure history. The following is an example of a population-based case-control study:

Non-Hodgkin lymphoma has been associated with agricultural pesticide use in men, but little is known about risks in women. To address this lack of knowledge, National Cancer Institute investigators conducted a population-based case-control study in

TABLE 8-5

Non-Hodgkin Lymphoma According to Insecticide Use Among Women in Eastern Nebraska

Insecticide Class	Used on Farms			Personally Handled		
	Cases	OR	95% CI	Cases	OR	95% CI
Any insecticide	56	0.8	0.5–1.3	22	1.3	0.7–2.3
Chlorinated hydrocarbons	20	1.6	0.8–3.1	5	1.7	0.5–5.8
Organophosphates	14	1.2	0.6–2.5	6	4.5	1.1–17.9
Metals	3	1.6	0.3–7.5	0	—	—

OR: odds ratio; 95% CI: 95% confidence interval.
Adapted from Zahm SH, Weisenburger DD, Saal RC, et al. The role of agricultural pesticide use in the development of non-Hodgkin's lymphoma in women. Arch Environ Health 1993;48:353–8.

which cases were defined as incident cases of non-Hodgkin lymphoma among women residing in 66 counties in eastern Nebraska, diagnosed between 1983 and 1986 in all area hospitals.[9] Controls were selected from female residents in the same counties using random-digit dialing. No risk was found to be related to living or working on a farm. Small risks were observed for women who personally handled insecticides (OR = 1.3) or herbicides (OR = 1.2), and women who personally handled organophosphate insecticides had a 4.5-fold increased risk (Table 8-5). Because non-Hodgkin lymphoma is a rare disease with a long latency, the case-control design was more feasible than a cohort study. Because exposures occur on farms, each of which employs a small number of workers, a community-based study was more practical than a workplace-based study.

The following is an example of a nested case-control study.

The carcinogenic risk of pulsed electromagnetic fields was studied in a series of case-control studies nested in a cohort of electric utility workers.[10] Case groups were defined as all diagnosed cases of selected cancers that occurred at any time after entry into the cohort until the end of follow-up in 1988. Controls were chosen at random from sets of cohort members matched to each case who had survived to the date of diagnosis of the case. Cumulative exposures were estimated up to the date of diagnosis of the case. Smoking information was obtained from company medical records. No associations were found between exposure to pulsed electromagnetic fields and cancers previously suspected of being associated with magnetic fields. However, the investigators reported a clear association between cumulative exposure to pulsed electromagnetic fields and lung cancer (after adjusting for cigarette smoking history), with an OR of 3.1 in the highest exposure category.

Ecologic Studies

In an *ecologic study*, the group is the unit of analysis, rather than the individual. Such studies require that information is available about disease and exposure that characterize the group as a whole, be it a school class, a community, a state, or a nation. Disease rates and average exposures are compared either between groups in different places at the same point in time using spatial mapping techniques or within a group over time. For example, one study in Spain used census data on cancer mortality and information on water source by municipality to assess associations between drinking water chlorination and stomach and bladder cancer.[11]

Cluster Investigations

A cluster is a small number of disease cases occurring in a population, narrowly defined over time and/or space, that attracts public concern. A cluster investigation begins with an assessment of how unusual, in a statistical sense, the disease cluster actually is. This assessment is based on verified cases and relies on judgments about how narrowly to define the affected neighborhood and time period, as well as assumptions about the probability model appropriate to describe the disease.

SELECTION OF TYPE OF STUDY

The choice of study design is based on a variety of factors, including the particular health end points and nature of exposure as well as available sources of data and other resources.

Cross-Sectional Studies

Cross-sectional studies have certain advantages over cohort studies or case-control studies. Because the subjects are all alive at the time of the study, it is possible to directly measure health and administer questionnaires to collect information on symptoms, exposure, and personal characteristics, such as smoking, diet, and health history, which are potential confounders. Also, because both disease prevalence and exposure data are collected at one point in time, cross-sectional studies usually require less time to complete than cohort or case-control studies. This explains why cross-sectional studies are common when studying risks in the workplace and the general environment.

These studies also have important limitations. They are less appropriate for investigating causal relations because they are based on prevalent rather than incident cases of disease. Prevalence is a poor proxy for incidence, especially for conditions of short duration. A related limitation in working populations is that cross-sectional studies oversample workers with long duration of employment and undersample workers with short duration of employment. Moreover, it may be difficult to determine that the exposure preceded the adverse health outcome, as information on both are obtained at the same point in time. In addition, occupational cross-sectional studies based on currently active workers do not include the workers who have left work, some of whom may be in poor health. The absence of such workers may result in an underestimate of the association of interest due to the *healthy worker effect* (see below).

Cohort Studies

The cohort study has several advantages. First, the study population includes all subjects at risk, rather than a cross-sectional sample. Second, because the population is observed over time (prospectively or retrospectively), the timing of the exposure relative to the outcome is known. Third, because the ascertainment of exposure precedes the ascertainment of outcome, there is less opportunity for subject recall bias. Thus, cohort studies can provide the strongest evidence for a causal relationship. The design is efficient for studying relatively common chronic

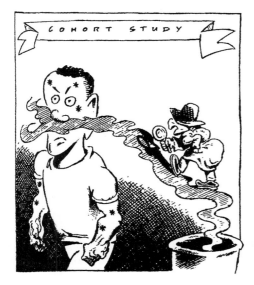

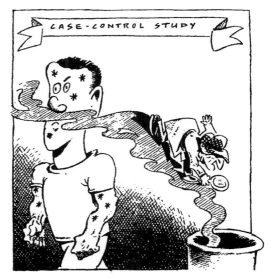

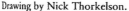

Drawing by Nick Thorkelson.

diseases. Several specific causes of death or disease can be studied in the same cohort study. However, retrospective cohort studies typically rely on outcomes recorded for other purposes, such as disease diagnosis or cause of death, and thus the end point is unlikely to be an early marker of disease.

Case-Control Studies

The principal advantage of the case-control study is its relative simplicity and relatively low cost of studying rare diseases. Case-control studies are valuable when multiple exposures are being explored in the etiology of a disease. If the investigator wishes to examine a spectrum of diseases associated with an exposure, such as lead, a cohort study is desirable; but if the interest is in the causes of a specific disease, such as bladder cancer, then the case-control study is more suitable.

Case-control studies are slightly more susceptible to biases than cohort studies (see below). For example, if exposure information depends on self-report, it may be recalled differently by subjects with and without disease. Moreover, the need to identify a control group from the same population that generated the cases often presents a challenge.

Ecologic Studies

Use of ecologic variables is common in environmental epidemiology because high-quality data often exist for a region but are unavailable for the individual subject. For example, air pollution measured at city or county monitors (an ecologic measure) may be assigned to all individuals living in the local area and associated with individual level health outcomes, as was done in a study of daily mortality and ozone in Mexico City.[12] In a recent validation study, it was found that outdoor particle measurements correlated reasonably well with personal particle exposure over time, supporting their use in longitudinal studies of air pollution and health.[13]

Studies using ecologic variables for both exposure and outcome may be more prone to a bias known as the *ecologic fallacy*. This term refers to the inappropriate inference of a causal effect at the individual level from data that is aggregated across individuals. In a famous example, it was observed that suicide rates were higher in predominantly Catholic countries than in predominantly Protestant countries, suggesting that Catholics had higher suicide rates.[14] Although possibly true, it is also plausible that being Protestant in a predominantly Catholic country could explain this observation. In addition, some other variable unrelated to religion, such as unemployment, might also be the causal agent.

Ecologic data are properly interpreted as representing a contextual effect; for example, the effect of living in a neighborhood with little green space or one with high literacy rates. Although one needs to interpret such studies with caution, there are some applications where ecologic studies are totally appropriate, such as in developing hypotheses for further study or evaluating the effectiveness of an intervention by comparing disease rates in the target population before and after the intervention.

Cluster Studies

When a scientist in a public health agency is faced with community concerns about a local source of pollution or an unexplained series of health problems, a cluster investigation may be warranted. Investigations of environmental causes of statistically significant clusters are unlikely to be conclusive, however, because the number of cases is generally small and exposure poorly characterized (see also Chapter 36). The challenges for a cluster investigation are particularly daunting when the health outcome is a chronic disease with a long latency period.

PROBLEMS RELATED TO VALIDITY

Because epidemiologic studies are observational studies rather than randomized experiments, they are prone to biases, some of which are unavoidable. Careful consideration needs to be given to a study's validity (lack of bias). *Bias* is defined as a distortion of the measure of association between exposure and health outcome, such as an SMR or an OR. The degree to which the inferences drawn from a study are warranted is determined largely by the absence of bias.

Reports of epidemiologic studies should provide sufficient information for the reader to understand what potential sources of bias were present and how these biases were addressed. There are three sources of bias: selection, misclassification of exposure, and confounding.

Selection Bias

Selection bias results from the inappropriate inclusion or exclusion of subjects in the study population. For example, in the past it was customary in studies of pulmonary function to exclude subjects who did not perform reproducible pulmonary function tests. It was subsequently discovered that subjects who had difficulty performing a reproducible forced expiratory maneuver had compromised respiratory health.[15] The exclusion of such subjects could result in an overestimation of the respiratory health of a working population and possibly the underestimation of a dose–response association, if one exists.

Most types of selection bias, such as exclusion of short-term workers from the study population, cannot easily be corrected or controlled for in the analysis; they can only be prevented. To prevent selection bias in a cohort study, investigators should be kept unaware (*blinded*) of cohort members' outcome status. Similarly, in case-control studies, investigators should be blinded as to the exposure status of cases and controls. Furthermore, selection of subjects should not be influenced by prior knowledge or suspicion of health outcome in a cohort study or of exposure status in a case-control study.

The most common type of selection bias in occupational epidemiologic studies is the *healthy worker effect* (HWE). This bias results from workers' selecting themselves out of the study groups rather than investigator error or oversight. For example, as described earlier, cross-sectional studies may result in an underestimate of the dose–response association if the occupational exposure causes disease that, in turn, causes workers to leave the workforce.

Another example of the HWE, common to cohort mortality studies, occurs because employed people are healthier than the general population, which includes the aged, the chronically ill, and those who are otherwise unfit to obtain and maintain employment.

As a result of the HWE, studies of illness or death among working populations often show lower rates of chronic diseases, such as cardiovascular diseases, than in the general population. In the mortality study of autoworkers described previously, the overall SMR, expected to be 1.00, was only 0.82 when the mortality rates of the surrounding county were used for comparison.

It is rare that an appropriate alternative comparison group of sufficient size is available. When possible, HWE bias is minimized by using a nonexposed comparison group drawn from within the study population. The HWE is reduced, although not necessarily eliminated, when analyses are based on this sort of "internal" comparison between exposed and nonexposed workers.

Misclassification

Misclassification (information bias) refers to an investigator's inadvertent placement of a worker into an incorrect category or group. (When exposure is a continuous variable, mismeasurement is referred to as *measurement error*). There are two types of misclassification: nondifferential and differential.

Exposure misclassification that is *nondifferential* is random misassignment of exposure that occurs regardless of disease status. Nondifferential misclassification is common in environmental studies, in which there is often little information on subjects' exposures, and subjects cannot be well classified into exposure categories. The problem is generally worse in retrospective studies, because adequate documentation of historical exposures is more difficult. The usual effect is to reduce estimates of the exposure–disease associations, although under certain circumstances the bias is in the opposite direction. The larger concern related to nondifferential misclassification, however, is that an existing occupational hazard may go unrecognized.

Bias of a different sort is presented by *differential* misclassification, in which the likelihood of misassignment of exposure is related to disease status. This type of bias can result in either a stronger or a weaker association than truly exists. In cohort studies, differential misclassification is commonly prevented by keeping the investigators blind to exposure status during collection of outcome information. In this manner, any errors in collection should be randomly distributed among both exposed and nonexposed groups. In case-control studies, control of differential bias is much more complicated; it is difficult for the investigator, and usually impossible for the subject, to be unaware of the disease status when exposure information is being obtained. Prevention of differential misclassification depends on collecting data as objectively as possible.

Confounding

Confounding is present when two study groups, such as those exposed and those nonexposed, are not comparable with respect to a characteristic that is also a risk factor for the disease. For example, in a study comparing stomach cancer in coal miners and iron miners, chewing tobacco was considered to be a potential confounder because (a) it is used more commonly by coal miners, who are prohibited from smoking in coal mines, and (b) it may be an independent risk factor for stomach cancer.

Confounding can be controlled either in the design of the study or in the analysis of the data. In case-control studies, matching of study subjects on potential confounders in the design phase can facilitate control of confounding in the analysis. To control confounding in the example of the stomach cancer study, subjects could be matched on tobacco-chewing habits so that the proportion of tobacco chewers is the same among cases and controls.

Stratification is the major approach to control of confounding in the analysis phase of cross-sectional, cohort, and case-control studies. A confounder, such as age, is used to define strata, such as 10-year age groups. The exposure–response association is then estimated in each stratum. Stratification, however, becomes problematic as the number of confounders increases, because the strata become too small to allow stable measures of risk. For example, if age, smoking, race, and gender must be controlled for simultaneously, there may be no nonsmoking 40- to 49-year-old white females in the study population. In this case, stratification becomes an inadequate method of controlling confounding, and mathematical modeling must be used to control confounding statistically.

Multivariate models make distributional assumptions about the outcome variable and impose particular mathematical forms on the dose–response relations, such as a linear or exponential form. By restricting the data to a specific structure, the model allows one to interpolate between sparse data strata defined by categories of the exposure and confounders.

INTERPRETATION OF EPIDEMIOLOGIC STUDIES

The interpretation of epidemiologic studies depends on the strength of the association, the validity of the observed association, and supporting evidence for causality (Box 8-2). The strength of an association usually is measured by the size of the relative risk in studies of discrete health outcomes, such as cancer, or by the magnitude of the difference between groups in studies of physiologic parameters, such as the forced expiratory volume in one second (FEV_1). Further evidence of the strength of an effect is provided by dose–response trends, in which the effect estimate rises over increasing categories of exposure.

When an association appears to be present, the validity of the association must be evaluated. This can be done in studies that provide adequate detail on design and results. The internal validity should be evaluated by examining for selection bias, misclassification, and confounding. All studies suffer to some degree from problems with validity, so a judgment must be made concerning the importance of the biases. The important biases are those that could explain the findings; that is, biases large in magnitude and operating in the direction of the finding (away from the null in positive studies, toward the null in negative studies).

Finally, the consistency of the association—that is, the repeated demonstration of a particular association in different populations and by different investigators—is valuable supporting evidence that the association truly exists. Toxicology data and reasonable consistency with a postulated biological mechanism may also assist in determining causal associations.

Results of statistical tests of significance, probability values (p-values), and/or confidence intervals, are usually presented along with estimates of the relative risk. These results contribute to interpretation of studies by providing a measure of stability of the associations reported.

Statistical tests enable investigators to decide whether or not to reject a null hypothesis. They are based on a prespecified significance level, which, in turn, is based on a probability that the observed association could have occurred by chance alone (assuming that no effect is expected *a priori*). For example, a p-value of 0.07 indicates that the likelihood of observing an effect at least as large as the one actually observed is 7 percent, given that no association truly exists. Some investigators use a significance level of $p < 0.05$ or $p < 0.01$ as the decision rule for rejecting the null hypothesis; however, a more useful way to interpret a p-value is as a measure of stability on a continuous scale. Confidence intervals provide more information than

---

BOX 8-2

Guide for Evaluating Epidemiologic Studies

To assist health professionals in reading, understanding, and critically evaluating epidemiologic studies, the following questions, adapted from Monson's *Occupational Epidemiology*, should serve as a useful guide.

Collection of Data

1. What were the objectives of the study? What was the association of interest?
2. What was the primary outcome of interest? Was it accurately measured?
3. What was the primary exposure of interest? Was it accurately measured?
4. What type of study was conducted?
5. What was the study base? Consider the process of subject selection and sample size.
6. Selection bias: Was subject selection based on the outcome or the exposure of interest? Could the selection have differed with respect to other factors of interest? Were these likely to have introduced a substantial bias?
7. Misclassification: Was subject assignment to exposure or disease categories accurate? Were possible misassignments equally likely for all groups? Were these likely to have introduced a substantial bias?

8. Confounding: What provisions, such as study design and subject restrictions, were made to minimize the influence of external factors before analysis of the data?

Analysis of the Data

9. What methods were used to control for confounding bias?
10. What measure of association was reported in the study? Was this appropriate?
11. How was the stability of the measure of association reported in the study?

Interpretation of Data

12. What was the major result of the study?
13. How was the interpretation of this result affected by the previously noted biases?
14. How was the interpretation affected by any nondifferential misclassification?
15. To what larger population may the results of this study be generalized?
16. Did the discussion section adequately address the limitations of the study? Was the final conclusion of the paper a balanced summary of the study findings?

Adapted from Monson RR. Occupational epidemiology. 2nd ed. Boca Raton, FL: CRC Press, 1989.

---

probability values alone because they provide the range in the magnitude of association consistent with the observed data as well as the stability of the estimate.

The statistical power of a study to detect a true effect depends on the background prevalence of the disease or exposure, the size of the group studied, the length of follow-up, and the level of statistical significance required. Monitoring of a small cohort for a brief period can yield a falsely negative result. For this reason, it is important, when interpreting a negative study, to examine whether the design itself precluded a positive finding. For example, a retrospective cohort study of formaldehyde exposure had only 80 percent power to detect a fourfold risk in nasal cancer mortality, despite having 600,000 person-years of observation.[16] The power

was low because nasal cancer has a very low background prevalence. Formulas for calculating the statistical power associated with a given sample size are available in standard biostatistics and epidemiology texts.

REFERENCES

1. Blot WJ, Harrington JM, Toledo A, et al. Lung cancer after employment in shipyards during World War II. N Engl J Med 1978;299:620–4.
2. Ayer HE, Dement JM, Busch KA, et al. A monumental study: reconstruction of a 1920 granite shed. Am Industrial Hygiene Assoc J 1973;34:206–11.
3. Creech JL, Johnson MN. Angiosarcoma of liver in the manufacture of polyvinyl chloride. J Occup Med 1974;16:150–51.
4. Billmaier D, Yee HT, Allen N, et al. Peripheral neuropathy in a coated fabrics plant. J Occup Med 1974;16:668–71.

5. Pirkle JL, Schwartz J, Landis JR, et al. The relationship between blood lead levels and blood pressure and its cardiovascular risk implications. Am J Epidemiol 1985;121:246–58.

6. Eisen EA, Bardin J, Gore R, et al. Exposure-response models based on extended follow-up of a cohort mortality study in the automobile industry. Scand J Work Environ Health 2001;27:240–9.

7. Hemminki K, Mutanen P, Saloniemi I, et al. Spontaneous abortions in hospital staff engaged in sterilizing instruments with chemical agents. Br Med J 1982;285:1461–3.

8. Grandjean P, Weihe P, White RF, et al. Cognitive deficit in 7-year-old children with prenatal exposure to methylmercury. Neurotoxicol Teratol 1997;19:417–28.

9. Zahm SH, Weisenburger DD, Saal RC, et al. The role of agricultural pesticide use in the development of non-Hodgkin's lymphoma in women. Arch Environ Health 1993;48:353–8.

10. Armstrong B, Theriault G, Guenel P, et al. Association between exposure to pulsed electromagnetic fields and cancer in electric utility workers in Quebec, Canada and France. Am J Epidemiol 1994;140:805–20.

11. Morales Suarez-Varela MM, Llopis Gonzalez A, Tejerizo Perez ML, et al. Chlorination of drinking water and cancer incidence. J Environ Pathol Toxicol Oncol 1994;13:39–41.

12. O'Neill MS, Loomis D, Borja-Aburto VH. Ozone, area social conditions, and mortality in Mexico City. Environ Res 2004;94:234–42.

13. Janssen NA, Hoek G, Brunekreef B, et al. Personal sampling of particles in adults: Relation among personal, indoor, and outdoor air concentrations. Am J Epidemiol 1998;147:537–47.

14. Durkheim E. Le suicide. Paris: F. Alcan, 1897. English translation by Spalding JA. Toronto, Canada: Free Press, Collier-MacMillan, 1951.

15. Eisen EA, Robins JM, Greaves IA, et al. Selection effects of repeatability criteria applied to lung spirometry. Am J Epidemiol 1984;120:734–42.

16. Blair A, Stewart P, O'Berg M, et al. Mortality among industrial workers exposed to formaldehyde. J Natl Cancer Inst 1986;76:1071–84.

BIBLIOGRAPHY

Beaglehole R, Bonita R, Kjellstrøm T. Basic epidemiology. Geneva: World Health Organization, 1993.
An introductory texts on the core ideas underlying general epidemiologic research and useful starting points for more advanced reading. Available worldwide (through WHO), and a teacher's guide can be obtained for use with the text.

Checkoway H, Pearce NE, Kriebel D. Research methods in occupational epidemiology. 2nd ed. New York: Oxford University Press, 2004.
Very readable full text on epidemiologic approaches specific to occupational studies. Numerous examples are provided to guide the reader in understanding both the simple and the complex issues that must be addressed.

Hernberg S. Introduction to occupational epidemiology. Chelsea, MI: Lewis Publishers, 1992.
An excellent introductory text that is well written and illustrated. Aimed at the reader new to occupational epidemiology but somewhat familiar with principles of epidemiology.

Olsen J, Merletti R, Snashall D, et al. Searching for causes of work-related diseases: An introduction to epidemiology at the work site. Oxford: Oxford Medical Publications, 1991.

A practical introduction to epidemiology for health professionals with no formal training in the discipline. It is written to assist professionals to better plan and carry out investigation of worksite health problems.

Pagano M, Gauvreau K. Principles of biostatistics. Belmont, CA: Duxbury Press, 1993.
Basic statistics text written in a reasonable fashion with a functional index. Good general reference for statistics.

Rothman KJ, Greenland S. Modern epidemiology. 2nd ed. Philadelphia: Lippincott-Raven, 1998.
Probably the best general text on epidemiologic methods designed both for the novice and the expert. Provides principles of epidemiology in substantial detail as well as the quantitative basis for the research methods. Particularly useful as a reference. Good chapters on ecologic studies (Morgenstern) and on environmental epidemiology (Hertz-Picciotto).

Steenland K. Case studies in occupational epidemiology. New York: Oxford University Press, 1993.
Provides the reader the opportunity to explore further many of the questions discussed in this chapter through practical and detailed presentation of case studies of various types of epidemiologic studies.

Steenland K, Savitz DA. Topics in environmental epidemiology. New York: Oxford University Press, 1997.
A survey of environmental health issues associated with different environmental media. While examining a number of different problems, the text provides an overview of important methodologic concerns, particularly exposure assessment and statistical methods.

APPENDIX:
ADJUSTMENT OF RATES

For purposes of illustration, adjusting for differences in age is examined in detail. Table 8-3 presents a hypothetical problem involving the myocardial infarction experience in two viscose rayon factories. To compare the incidence of myocardial infarction, a summary rate is calculated for each factory. If crude rates were calculated, it would appear that workers in Factory 2 have a slightly greater risk. Comparison of these rates, however, ignores the rather striking difference in age distribution of the populations in the two factories. These can be taken into account by adjusting for age differences by either the direct method or the indirect method.

Direct Adjustment

The principle of *direct adjustment* is to apply the age-specific rates determined in the study groups to a set of common age weights, such as a standard age distribution. The selection of the standard is somewhat arbitrary, but often the sum of the specific age groups for the study groups is chosen. In Table 8-3, the standard population includes 1,200 persons younger than 45 years and 800 persons 45 years or older. The specific rates are applied to this set of weights and then added to create an adjusted rate:

$$\text{Factory 1} = \frac{(0.010 \times 1,200) + (0.030 \times 800)}{2,000}$$

$$= 0.018$$

$$\text{Factory 2} = \frac{(0.0125 \times 1,200) + (0.050 \times 800)}{2,000}$$

$$= 0.275$$

Not only is the magnitude of the rate of myocardial infarction affected by the adjustment procedure, but the rank order is reversed. Note that, if another age distribution had been selected as the standard, the standardized rates would change. For example, for 1,500 persons younger than 45 years and 500 age 45 or older, the rate for Factory 1 would become 0.015 and that for factory 2 would become 0.022. Although the absolute magnitudes of the two adjusted rates have no inherent meaning, the relative magnitudes do. Although the size of the ratio will change slightly, it will be closely duplicated regardless of the weights. In these two examples of weighting, the ratios of the adjusted rates are 1.53 and 1.47.

Indirect Adjustment

In *indirect adjustment*, standard rates are applied to the observed weights or the distribution of specific characteristics, such as age, sex, or race, in the study populations. This provides a value for the number of cases (events) that would be expected if the standard rates were operating. The expected number of cases can be compared with the number actually observed for each study group in the form of a ratio. In Table 8-3, assume a national standard rate for myocardial infarction of 1 in 1,000 (0.001) for those younger than 45 years of age and 2 in 1,000 (0.002) for those

45 years or older. The expected number of cases in the two factories would then be as follows:

Factory 1 $= (0.001 \times 400) + (0.002 \times 600) = 1.6$

Factory 2 $= (0.001 \times 800) + (0.002 \times 200) = 1.2$

These expected values are compared with the observed values to calculate a standardized morbidity ratio, as follows:

$$\text{Factory 1 SMR} = \frac{22}{1.6} = 13.8$$

$$\text{Factory 2 SMR} = \frac{20}{1.2} = 16.7$$

It is tempting to compare the two SMRs and calculate a ratio similar to that calculated for the directly standardized rates. However, a drawback of indirect standardization is that SMRs cannot be compared. Because the age distributions and age-specific rates are significantly different for the two factories, the resulting comparison of the two SMRs would not distinguish differences caused by a different disease incidence rate from differences caused by a different age distribution.

It is reasonable, then, to ask why indirectly standardized rates are used. One reason is that often, only one population is being studied, so comparison with the general population experience is convenient and possibly the only reasonable comparison available. Probably of greater importance is the instability of observed rates. In the example presented here, if five rather than two age groups were used and it was also necessary to adjust for both race and sex, then the total number of subdivisions necessary would be $5 \times 2 \times 2 = 20$. With a maximum of 22 cases in either factory, several of the subdivisions would contain no cases and therefore have no reliable rate estimate. Even in the illustration provided, one case more or one case less among the group of younger workers in Factory 1 would have changed the age-specific incidence rate to 12.5 or 7.5, respectively—a very large difference.

CHAPTER 9

Occupational and Environmental Hygiene

Thomas J. Smith and Thomas Schneider

Occupational hygiene (industrial hygiene) is the environmental science of anticipating, recognizing, evaluating, and controlling health hazards in the working environment with the objectives of protecting workers' health and well-being and safeguarding the community at large. It encompasses the prevention of chronic and acute conditions emanating from hazards posed by physical agents, chemical agents, biological agents, and stressors in the occupational environment as well as concern for the outdoor environment. For example, an occupational hygienist determines the composition and concentrations of air contaminants in a workplace where there have been complaints of eye, nose, and throat irritation and determines if the contaminant exposures exceeded Occupational Safety and Health Administration[1] (OSHA) permissible exposure limits or other national limits. If the problem is new and appears to be the result of airborne materials, which might be determined in consultation with a physician or an epidemiologist, then the hygienist would be responsible for selecting (a) the techniques used to reduce or eliminate the exposure, such as installing exhaust ventilation around the source of the air contaminants and isolating it from the general work area, and (b) performing follow-up sampling to verify that the controls were effective.

Most occupational hygienists have earned either a bachelor's degree in science or engineering or a master of science degree in industrial hygiene. Occupational hygienists tend to specialize in specific technical areas because the scope of the field has so greatly expanded. Occupational hygienists must work with physicians to develop comprehensive occupational health programs and with epidemiologists to perform research on adverse health effects. It has been traditional to separate occupational hygiene and occupational safety, but the recent trend has been to broaden the training for each discipline to include that of the other. This has led to the specialty of risk management for evaluating and controlling all types of workplace hazards. At present, occupational hygienists generally do not deal with mechanical hazards or job activities that can cause physical injuries; these are the responsibility of safety specialists (see Chapter 10). However, it is not uncommon for private companies to have a single individual responsible for both occupational hygiene and safety who has no formal training in either area.

Most occupational hygienists work for large companies or governmental agencies. A small, but growing number, work for labor unions. For whomever they work, occupational hygienists unfortunately are often located in organizational units where they have little organizational power to bring about necessary changes. Hygienists who work for labor unions may be restricted in their access to the workplace for sampling and exposure measurements, which can limit their ability to assess and control hazards.

The closeness of working relationships between occupational hygienists and occupational physicians varies. Some have close collaborative activities with an extensive exchange of information, whereas others operate with nearly complete independence and have little more than formal contact. A physician who is familiar with the workplace, job activities, and health status of workers in all parts of the process may be very helpful in guiding the occupational hygienist in assessing environmental hazards, and vice versa. Within a framework of multidisciplinary approaches, occupational hygienists and physicians should collaborate with safety specialists, workers in production units, staff members in personnel departments, worker representatives, and delegates of the health and safety committees. Where contact among these groups is minimal, many opportunities are lost for improving the effectiveness of health hazard control and the prevention of adverse effects.

The integration of occupational hygiene into an overall program for occupational health is an important issue, without which the effectiveness of intervention strategies may be limited. An effective hygiene program must have good working relationships with the production, personnel, and health and safety departments and strong support by upper management. Core activities of hazard anticipation, recognition, evaluation, and control must be well integrated with the day-to-day activities of the enterprise. There is no single organizational structure that is optimal.

ANTICIPATION, RECOGNITION, EVALUATION, AND CONTROL OF HAZARDS

Formal strategies for workplace assessment have not been well developed. The American Conference of Governmental Industrial Hygienists (ACGIH) monograph on exposure assessment, *A Strategy for Occupational Exposure Assessment*[2] (see Bibliography) is focused on sampling and does not address program management issues. European Union (EU) regulations now require workplace assessment to identify occupational hazards. However, no formal mechanism has been established or validated to demonstrate its consistency. It is expected that EU regulations, when fully implemented, will be beneficial to small- and medium-sized enterprises because they will create awareness and an expectation of controlling the problems identified.

Anticipation

Anticipation of hazards has become an important responsibility of the occupational hygienist. *Anticipation* refers to the application and mastery of knowledge that permits the occupational hygienist to foresee the potential for disease and injury. The

occupational hygienist should thus be involved at an early stage in planning of technology, process development, and workplace design.

An electronics company was developing a new process for making microcomputer chips. The process involved dissolving a photographic masking agent in toluene and then spraying the mask on a large surface covered with chips. The company's hygienist noted that this would expose the workers to potentially high airborne levels of toluene. She suggested they substitute xylene, which has a lower vapor pressure, and modify the process to use smaller amounts of solvent, which would reduce the amount of hazardous waste generated by the process.

It is common that process engineers or industrial researchers will propose using hazardous materials or will not consider the interaction of the worker and the process or machine. Consequently, hygienists can prevent many problems that will be expensive to fix after installation by reviewing early plans and findings of pilot-plant experiments.

Identification of hazards may be most easily accomplished using an overview of the production process that describes the complete flow from raw material to final product. Production can be subdivided into its component unit processes. In this stepwise fashion, the processes with hazards can be recognized, worker exposures evaluated, and exposures in nearby areas assessed. Examples of some common unit processes and their hazards are shown in Table 9-1. This general approach and the hazards of a wide range of common industrial processes are discussed in more detail in Burgess' *Recognition of Health Hazards in Industry: A Review of Materials and Processes* (see Bibliography).

This approach can be illustrated by considering a small company that manufactures toolboxes from sheets of steel by a six-step process: (1) sheets of steel are cut into the specified shape; (2) sharp edges and burrs are removed by grinding; (3) sheets are formed into boxes with a sheet metal bender; (4) box joints are spot welded; (5) boxes are cleaned in a vapor degreaser in preparation for painting; and (6) boxes are painted in a spray booth. Production steps 2, 4, 5, and 6 use unit processes with known sources of airborne emissions, and their hazards, which are listed in Table 9-1, should be evaluated. Exposures of workers involved with steps 1 and 3 may need to be evaluated because they may be

TABLE 9-1

Common Unit Processes and Associated Hazards by Route of Entry[a]

Unit Process	Route of Entry and Hazard
Abrasive blasting (surface treatment with high velocity materials, such as sand, steel shot, pecan shells, glass, or aluminum oxide)	Inhalation: silica, metal, and paint dust Noise
Acid/alkali treatments (dipping metal parts in open baths to remove oxides, grease, oil, and dirt)	
Acid pickling (with HCl, HNO_3, H_2SO_4, H_2CrO_4, HNO_3/HF)	Inhalation: acid mist with dissolved metals Skin contact: burns and corrosion, HF toxicity
Acid bright dips (with HNO_3/H_2SO_4)	Inhalation: NO_2, acid mists
Molten caustic descaling bath (high temperature)	Inhalation: smoke and vapors Skin contact: burns
Blending and mixing (powders and/or liquid are mixed to form products, or undergo reactions)	Inhalation: dusts and mists of toxic materials Skin contact: toxic materials
Cleaning (application of cleansers, solvents and strong detergents to clean surfaces and articles; and operation of devices to aid cleaning such as floor washers, waxers, polishers and vacuums)	Inhalation: dust, vapors Skin contact: defatting agents, solvents, strong bases
Crushing and sizing (mechanically reducing the particle size of solids and sorting larger from smaller with screens or cyclones)	Inhalation: dusts and mists of toxic materials Noise
Degreasing (removing grease, oil, and dirt from metal and plastic with solvents and cleaners)	
Cold solvent washing (clean parts with ketones, cellosolves, and aliphatic, aromatic, and stoddard solvents)	Inhalation: vapors Skin contact: dermatitis and absorption Fire and explosion (if flammable) Metabolic: carbon monoxide formed from methylene chloride
Vapor degreasers (with trichloroethylene, methyl chloroform, ethylene dichloride, and certain fluorocarbon compounds)	Inhalation: vapors; thermal degradation may form phosgene, hydrogen chloride, and chlorine gases Skin contact: dermatitis and absorption
Electroplating (coating metals, plastics, and rubber with thin layers of metals, such as copper, chromium, cadmium, gold, or silver)	Inhalation: acid mists, HCN, alkali mists, chromium, nickel, cadmium mists Skin contact: acids, alkalis Ingestion: cyanide compounds
Forging (deforming hot or cold metal by presses or hammering)	Inhalation: hydrocarbons in smokes (hot processes), including polyaromatic hydrocarbons, SO_2, CO, NO_x, and other metals sprayed on dies (for example, lead and molybdenum) Heat stress Noise
Furnace operations (melting and refining metals; boilers for steam generation)	Inhalation: metal fumes, combustion gases (for example, SO_2 and CO) Noise from burners Heat stress Infrared radiation, cataracts in eyes

(continued)

TABLE 9-1 (Continued)

Common Unit Processes and Associated Hazards by Route of Entry[a]

Unit Process	Route of Entry and Hazard
Grinding, polishing, and buffing (an abrasive is used to remove or shape metal or other material)	Inhalation: toxic dusts from both metals and abrasives Vibration from hand tools Noise
Industrial radiography (x-ray or gamma ray sources used to examine parts of equipment)	Radiation exposure
Machining (metals, plastics, or wood are worked or shaped with lathes, drills, planers, or milling machines)	Inhalation: airborne particles, cutting oil mists, toxic metals, nitrosamines formed in some water-based cutting oils, endotoxin Skin contact: cutting oils, solvents, sharp chips Noise
Materials handling and storage (conveyors, forklift trucks are used to move materials to/from storage)	Inhalation: CO, exhaust particulate, dusts from conveyors, emissions from spills or broken containers
Mining (drilling, blasting, mucking to remove loose material, and material transport)	Inhalation: silica dust, NO_2 from blasting, gases from the mine Vibration stress Heat stress Noise
Painting and spraying (applications of liquids to surfaces; for example, paints, pesticides, coatings)	Inhalation: solvents as mists and vapors, toxic materials Skin contact: solvents, toxic materials
Repair and maintenance (servicing malfunctioning equipment; cleaning production equipment and control systems)	Inhalation: dusts, vapors, and gases from the operation Skin contact: grease, oil, solvents
Quality control (collection of production samples, performance of test procedures that produce emissions)	Inhalation: dusts, vapors and gases Skin contact: solvents
Soldering (joining metals with molten lead or silver alloys)	Inhalation: lead or cadmium particulate (fumes) and flux fumes
Welding and metal cutting (joining or cutting metals by heating them to molten or semimolten state) Arc or resistance welding Flame cutting and welding Brazing	Inhalation: metal fumes, toxic gases and materials, flux particulate, and other substances Noise: from burner Eye and skin damage from infrared and ultraviolet radiation

[a] The health hazards may also depend on the toxicity and physical form(s) of the materials used. For further information, see Burgess WA. Recognition of health hazards in industry: A review of materials and processes. 2nd ed. New York: John Wiley & Sons, 1995.

located near enough to the operations with hazards to have significant exposure.

The design of job tasks and an individual's work habits can both have an important influence on exposures. For example, a furnace tender's exposure to metal fumes will depend on the length of tools used to scrape slag away from the tapping hole in the furnace and on the instructions for performing the task. Lack of adequate tools or sufficient oper-ating instructions may cause excessive exposure to fumes emitted by molten materials. Similarly, the furnace tender, who is positioned close to the slag as it runs out of the furnace, may receive a much higher exposure to fume than a co-worker who stands farther away from the molten slag. Therefore, an important part of an evaluation is the observation of work practices used in hazardous unit processes.

Recognition

Recognition of problems in a new or unfamiliar workplace generally requires that the occupational hygienist engage in collection of background information on production layout, processes, and raw materials.

Visits to the workplace to become familiar with the production processes and their hazards are crucial for detecting unique aspects of the workplace that may strongly affect exposures. Information is collected on:

- Types, composition, and quantities of substances and materials, including raw materials, intermediate products, and additives;
- Design of work processes and tasks;
- Emission sources; and
- Design and capacity of ventilation systems or other control measures.

Flow visualization with smoke tubes (glass tubes with a packing that produces dense white smoke when air is forced through it) can give information on effectiveness of local exhausts or process ventilation. Work practices, worker position relative to sources, and task duration can be recorded. Information can be collected on cleaning routines and performance as well as tidiness, which are important determinants of exposure.

Farm workers were experiencing episodes of depressed blood cholinesterase levels from organophosphate exposure despite the fact that they were observing the required waiting times before reentry into sprayed fields and wearing long-sleeved shirts and gloves to prevent skin contact. The pesticide had a very low vapor pressure so there was no significant inhalation exposure. However, it was known that environmental moisture decomposes this type of pesticide. Because the weather was very dry during these episodes, there was concern that the pesticide was not decomposing as rapidly as expected. Consequently, despite the skin protection, there could still be sufficient skin absorption of the pesticide to depress cholinesterase levels. Skin sampling with patches showed that fine dust was sifting through the cloth of the shirt sleeves and depositing pesticide on workers' arms in large amounts. The problem was solved by extending the standard reentry times.

If the initial appraisal cannot definitely rule out a hazard, a basic survey has to be performed to provide quantitative information about exposure of workers. Particular account has to be taken of tasks with high exposure. Sources of information are:

- Earlier measurements;
- Measurements from comparable installations or work processes;
- Reliable calibrations or modeling based on relevant quantitative data; and
- Air-sampling measurements to determine the range of exposures.

Sampling may show that sensory impressions underestimate or overestimate exposures; for example, the odor threshold for most solvents is well below the level at which they present a toxic exposure hazard.

If this information is insufficient to enable valid comparisons to be made with the limit values, a full-scale survey must be performed. The full-scale survey examines all phases of workplace activities—both normal activities and abnormal or infrequent ones, such as maintenance, reactor cleaning, or simulation of malfunctions. The survey activities may take several weeks or months in a complex manufacturing or chemical plant.

Evaluation

The evaluation of recognized or suspected hazards by the hygienist uses techniques based on the nature of the hazards, emission sources, and the routes of environmental contact with the worker. For example, air sampling can show the concentration of toxic particulates, gases, and vapors that workers may inhale; skin wipes can be used to measure the degree of skin contact with toxic materials that may penetrate the skin; biological samples (blood or urine) can provide data where there are multiple routes of entry; and noise dosimeters record and electronically integrate workplace noise levels to determine total daily exposure. Both acute and chronic exposures should be considered in the evaluation because they may be associated with different types of adverse health effects.

The workplace is not a static environment: Exposures may change by orders of magnitude over short distances from exposure sources, such as welding, and over short time intervals because of intermittent source output or incomplete mixing of air contaminants. In addition, operations and materials used or produced commonly change, as do job titles and definitions. The nature of these changes and their possible effects must be recognized and taken into consideration by the occupational hygienist.

All monitoring programs for both long-term and acute problems should be structured with a clear focus on the individual's sources of exposures and the ultimate objective to estimate dose. Monitoring organized solely around compliance with today's standards will probably be unable to answer tomorrow's questions about hazards associated with personal exposures. The effects of environmental controls, such as ventilation and personal protective equipment, that intervene between the emission source and the worker must also be considered.

The hygienist's decision on whether a hazard is present is based on three sources of information:

1. Scientific literature and various exposure limit guidelines, such as (a) the threshold limit values (TLVs) of the ACCIH*—a set of consensus standards developed by occupational hygienists, toxicologists, and physicians from governmental agencies and academic institutions, or (b) the World Health Organization (WHO) recommendations.†
2. The legal requirements of OSHA (in some cases, these are less stringent than the TLVs because the TLVs have been updated) or regulatory agencies of other countries.[1]
3. Interactions with other health professionals who have examined the exposed workers and evaluated their health status.

In cases where health effects are present but exposures do not exceed the TLVs, WHO recommendations, or OSHA (or other national) requirements, prudent hygienists will conclude that there is a relationship between adverse health effects and workplace exposures if it is consistent with the facts. Exposure limits are designed to prevent adverse effects in most exposed workers but are not absolute levels below which effects cannot occur. The supporting data for many of these exposure limits are sometimes viewed as insufficient, out of date, or based too much on evidence of acute toxic effects and not enough on recent evidence of carcinogenicity, mutagenicity, or teratogenicity.

Once a hazard is identified and the extent of the problem evaluated, the hygienist's next step is to design a control strategy or plan to reduce exposure to an acceptable level. Such controls may have two phases, an immediate response with personal protective equipment to quickly reduce the hazard and an engineering follow up to more effectively control the problem, including:

1. Changing the industrial process or the materials used to eliminate the source of the hazard, such as changing to clean technologies.
2. Isolating the source and installing engineering controls such as ventilation systems.
3. Using administrative directives to limit the duration of exposure a worker receives, or, as a final resort, requiring the development of a formal program for the prolonged use of personal protective equipment.

The controls in the last of these three approaches are less reliable because they depend on enforcement by managers and conscientious application by the workers, both of which can fail. In designing control strategies, account should also be taken of the environmental impact of emissions, waste, accidents, storage, spills, and leaks. Action can be taken at the process, materials, component, system, and workplace levels. Education of both workers and supervisors is an important part of any control strategy; both must understand the nature of the hazards and support the efforts taken to control or eliminate them. Implementation of control measures should be supervised and their efficacy evaluated.

Automobile manufacturers have been very concerned about the hazards of coolants used in machining and grinding operations. Workers complain of skin and inhalation problems associated with exposures to liquids splashed on their skin and mists in the air. In the recent past, controls were installed based on hypotheses about the causal factors but without an investigation of the specific causes for exposures. As is often the case, some hypotheses were later found to be incorrect and it was determined that incomplete control had been achieved despite substantial expenditures. It was shown that inhalation exposures had been only partially controlled by local exhaust ventilation and enclosure of processes, but a relationship was still found between symptoms and reduced pulmonary function associated with exposures at levels below the current allowable exposure. Analysis of the coolants also revealed that material safety data sheets (MSDSs) were inaccurate, and more hazardous materials were being used than were known to the machining

---

*Can be obtained from ACGIH, 6500 Glenway Avenue, Building D-5, Cincinnati, OH 45211.
†Can be obtained from WHO, Avenue Appia 20, 1211 Geneva 27, Switzerland.

department. Investigations are now being planned to determine what engineering controls will be needed to further reduce the exposures. Substitution of alternate types of coolant components and better control of microbial contaminants are part of the planned investigations.

This example indicates that controlling hazards in large, complex manufacturing operations is very frequently a stepwise process. Control strategies are most effective when based on complete knowledge of the nature of problems.

After hazards are controlled, the hygienist may recommend a routine hazard surveillance program to ensure that controls remain adequate. This type of surveillance is most effective when done in close association with a medical surveillance program designed to detect subtle effects that may occur at low levels of exposure.

The following sections indicate how assessment and control techniques are used. The approach for toxic materials is used as a paradigm, which can also be used for other environmental hazards, including noise, vibration, ionizing and nonionizing radiation, temperature extremes, poor lighting, and infectious agents.

TOXIC MATERIALS

Exposure Pathways

The hazard of a given exposure to a toxic material depends on the toxicity of the substance and on the duration and intensity of contact with the substance. Thus, adverse effects can result from chronic low-level exposure to a substance or from a short-term exposure to a dangerously high concentration of it. However, the pharmacologic mechanisms by which effects are caused may differ for acute and chronic effects. Occupational hygienists are concerned with both long-term, low-level exposures and brief acute exposures.

In assessing a given hazardous material, the hygienist determines the route of exposure by which workers contact it and by which it may enter their bodies. There are four major routes of exposure: (1) direct contact with skin or eyes; (2) inhalation, with deposition in the respiratory tract; (3) inhalation, with deposition in the upper respiratory tract and subsequent transport to the throat and ingestion; and (4) direct ingestion with gastrointestinal uptake from food or drink. In the workplace, sev-

eral concurrent routes of exposure may occur for a single toxic substance.

Inhalation of airborne particulates, vapors, or gases is, by far, the most common route of exposure and therefore occupies much of a hygienist's assessment and control activities. Skin absorption may be important if the substance is lipid soluble or the skin's barrier is damaged or otherwise compromised. Ingestion of contaminated food and drink is a problem, especially for particulate and liquid materials, whose degree of risk may depend on the worker's level of awareness of the hazard and personal hygiene habits and on the availability of adequate facilities for washing and eating at the workplace. Contamination of cigarettes with toxic materials and their subsequent inhalation is also a problem for some substances.

For example, workers handling lead ingots are exposed to a low-level hazard from ingesting small amounts of lead by eating contaminated food or by inhaling small amounts of lead fumes from contaminated cigarettes. However, workers refining lead at temperatures above 800°F are exposed to a serious hazard from inhaling large amounts of lead fume if they work close to unventilated refining kettles for several hours daily. Workers handling liquid nitric acid are exposed to the hazard of direct contact with the liquid on their skin, but they may also be exposed to a respiratory hazard from inhaling acid mist generated by an electroplating process using the nitric acid. In these examples, the toxic materials cause different types and magnitudes of hazards because their physical forms vary: solid material versus small-diameter airborne particulates, and liquid material versus airborne droplets.

Anticipation and Recognition

The first problem the hygienist faces in evaluating an unfamiliar workplace for toxic hazards is the identification of toxic materials. In many cases, such as a lead smelter or pesticide-manufacturing process, the emission sources for toxic materials are clearly evident. But even in these examples, some hazards may not be evident without a careful examination of an inventory of the chemicals to be used or in use in the facility, including raw materials, by-products, products, wastes, solvents, cleaners, and special-use materials. Lead smelter workers are also exposed to carbon monoxide and sometimes to arsenic and cadmium; pesticide workers are subjected to solvent exposures. Relatively nontoxic chemicals may be contaminated with highly toxic ones; for example, low-toxicity chlorinated hydrocarbons used in weed killers, such as 2,4-D may contain dioxin, which is highly toxic, and technical-grade toluene may contain significant amounts of highly toxic benzene. In some cases, toxic materials may not be hazards because there are no emissions into the workplace and only small amounts are handled, such as in a chemical lab.

Material safety data sheets (MSDSs), which list the composition of commercial products, are available from manufacturers and can be useful, but they are sometimes too general or out of date. Toxicity data on specific substances can be obtained by literature searches or by searches of toxicity data indices.

Because exposure to toxic substances can occur by contamination of food, drink, or cigarettes, the hygienist determines if eating and drinking facilities are physically separated from the work area, if facilities for washing are close to eating areas, and if sufficient time is permitted for workers to use these facilities. Protective clothing and facilities for showering after a work shift should also be provided. Workers' understanding of hazards from the toxic materials that they are using must also be assessed. Finally, the hygienist determines the existence and enforcement of rules prohibiting eating, drinking, and smoking in areas with toxic substances.

Evaluation

Measurement Techniques

Two types of environmental sampling techniques are available.

Direct-reading instruments have sensors that detect the instantaneous air concentration and may produce a reading on a dial or store a complete 8-hour time profile for later retrieval. Some are expensive, and all require careful calibration and maintenance to obtain accurate data. The detector tube is another type of direct-reading instrument of considerable use in determining approximate concentrations of air contaminants. This simple device uses a small hand pump to draw air through a bed of reagent in a glass tube that changes color or develops a length of stain that is dependent on the concentration of a given gaseous air contaminant. The conventional tube is suitable for short-term sampling, such as for 10 minutes, but short-term samples can misrepresent long-term average exposures. Tubes

with 8-hour collection times are also available that are capable of measuring *time-weighted average* (TWA) exposure levels. Detector tubes are available that have been manufactured under strict quality control, and their degree of measurement uncertainty is specified. Consideration must always be given to interference from other substances (cross-sensitivity), which usually is specified on the tube's data sheets.

Sample collectors that remove substances from the air for analysis in a laboratory may be a less expensive alternative to direct-reading instruments. *Personal sampling* is a common approach used by the occupational hygienist to obtain accurate and precise measurements of workers' exposures. Particulate contaminants are collected with filters, and gases and vapors are collected by solid adsorbents or liquid bubblers. The sampling apparatus is generally quite simple, consisting of a small air pump usually worn on a worker's belt, connected by tubing to the collector and attached to the worker's shirt at the neck (Fig. 9-1). (Some gas and vapor collectors are passive, using diffusion instead of an air pump to move the contaminant into the sampler.) With the appropriate selection of a gas or particulate collector or both combined in a sampling train, it is possible to measure the average concentration of an air contaminant in the worker's breathing zone during an 8-hour work shift.

Collection devices for toxic particulates may capture either *inhalable dust* (that is, particles that can enter the nose and mouth, less than about 10 μm) or only the *respirable dust* (that is, only particles that can penetrate the terminal airways and alveolar spaces [less than 4 μm]). Total particulate samples are collected if the toxic substance causes systemic health problems, as lead and pesticides do. Respirable dust samples are collected if the particulate causes chronic pulmonary disease, such as pneumoconiosis. There is some controversy about the size of particles that cause chronic bronchitis and, therefore, which type of sample to collect. The type of sampler should be matched to the route of entry, type of effect, and target tissue.

Charcoal and other sorbent packed into tubes have been the most common absorption collectors for gases and vapors; a small amount of charcoal inside a small glass tube acts as an activated surface that will retain nonpolar materials, such as benzene. These collectors are commonly used to measure inhalation exposures to solvents, such as vapor exposures of printers. The specific methods

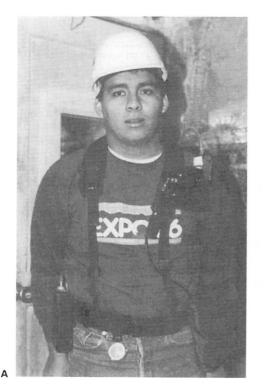
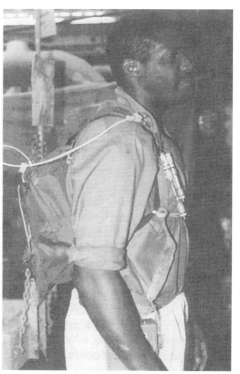

A   B

FIGURE 9-1 ● Monitoring equipment can be used to collect samples for measurement of personal exposure on the job. (**A**) Particulate sampler is connected to portable pump located on worker's right hip. Here, more sophisticated sampling is being accomplished by adding a real-time direct-reading aerosol sampler and logging device (black box on chest and package on left hip). (**B**) Vapor sampling tubes on worker's chest usually collect a time-weighted sample to measure chemical exposure. Here, a direct-reading aerosol measurement system has been added (in the backpack) to permit collection of real-time data in a logging device. (Photographs by Susan Woskie.)

for chemicals are discussed in detail in the *OSHA Analytic Methods Manual* (see Bibliography).

Passive or badge-type samplers are much more convenient to use for gas and vapor sampling than the collectors requiring air pumps, are relatively inexpensive, and have better worker acceptance because many workers do not like the weight of the pumps. At the start of sampling, the face of the badge is uncovered to allow diffusion into the badge, and at the end of the sampling period, the cover is replaced on the badge and it is sent to a laboratory for analysis. Several passive samplers have well-documented sampling rates. They may surpass active samplers in accuracy, if contamination from liquid splashes during use can be avoided.

Sampling Strategy

The hygienist must design a sampling strategy that takes into account the types of hazards, variations in exposure, routes of exposure, and the uses for the data, such as risk assessment or source evaluation and control. The approach should enable most efficient use of resources. Personal measurements are designed to reflect the accumulation of exposure from a variety of sources that a worker may encounter during a work shift. In some cases, exposure may occur only during certain operations. Worst-case sampling is the approach used when it is clear that high emissions from certain activities or sources will occur and it is decided that sampling will only be done during the period of highest exposure. Workers in adjacent areas not directly involved with the air contaminant of interest are frequently found to have significant exposures because the air contaminant drifts into their work areas.

Variability in exposure levels can be large due to day-to-day variation in work pattern, production rate, and differences in the process. Differences in personal work habits, wind velocity, and direction also cause variation. The exposed populations should be subdivided into smaller, well-defined groups of workers performing identical or similar tasks. Properly selecting subgroups reduces within-group variability so that measurement resources can be concentrated on the highest exposed groups, although these may be difficult to identify *a priori*. Single samples are generally avoided, because it is difficult to know what the sample value represents. Additionally, because workers have different work habits and techniques, there may be differences in average exposures among workers.[2] Several replicate samples on workers may indicate how important these differences are and how much the assumption of uniform mean exposure within groups is violated.

In addition to personal sampling, the occupational hygienist also uses *fixed-location sampling*. In this strategy, the sampler is set at a given location that has some useful relationship to a source of exposure. This type of sampling is advantageous because it can enable determination of features of the exposure that would be difficult with personal samples. For example, a large sampler can be used to determine the particle size distribution of airborne dust in a work area or to provide sufficient airborne material for detailed chemical analysis if the composition of the contaminants is not known. These samplers can be very useful for identifying and characterizing sources of exposure and assessing the effectiveness of engineering controls. As with personal sampling, in order to get the most out of the effort, it is very important to select carefully the sampling location and strategy for fixed-location sampling. In some cases, a combination of personal and fixed-location samples is used to describe a given problem completely. For example, personal samples are used to describe the highly variable exposures of steel workers tending a blast furnace, while stationary samples measure exposures to the uniform, well-mixed air levels they experience while waiting in the lunchroom for their next job assignment (for 2 to 4 hours per work shift).

Many large plants use continuous multipoint sampling of gases and vapors with central analysis. Instant action can be taken if concentrations exceed specified limits. Continuous monitoring at stationary sites should be part of the total quality management process.

In some occupational settings, the most important route of exposure is skin contact. Skin contact is difficult to evaluate with environmental sampling because even if the amount of skin contamination can be determined at a point in time it is not possible to know how much of the contaminant has already entered the body or would enter, given sufficient time. Two principal sampling approaches are employed. First, cloth patches can be used to cover given locations of skin, such as the forehead, back of the neck, back of the hands, and forearms, to measure the amount of contamination per unit area that resulted during a period of exposure. The second approach is to use wipe sampling in which an area of skin is washed with an appropriate, nontoxic solvent to determine the quantity of contamination.

Both of these techniques have been used to estimate pesticide exposures of agricultural workers. Addition of a fluorescent whitening agent to the pesticide as a tracer allows visualization of contamination. Additionally, wipe sampling on surfaces can be used as a method to detect and control the indiscriminate distribution of toxic materials throughout the workplace environment with which workers may come in contact. This type of sampling is also useful in estimating the risk of one person relative to another or of one area relative to another. It is, however, difficult to know in absolute terms the quantity of contaminant that may actually penetrate the skin and become a health problem. Biological monitoring is probably the best method for determining the intensity of skin exposures to a substance for which such a monitoring test is available (see Chapter 6).

Some nonpolar substances, such as pesticides and solvents, may enter the body both via the respiratory tract and through skin contact. In these cases, both skin contact and air exposure must be evaluated to completely assess the risk. Biological sampling that integrates these two routes of intake may be a practical necessity. However, two important theoretical problems are associated with biological monitoring. Some types of tests may represent detection of adverse effects, such as monitoring red blood cell cholinesterase in pesticide-exposed workers. As a result, they detect excessive exposures only after the effects have occurred. Tissue levels of environmental contaminants represent a dynamic interaction because the exposure is rarely constant. As a result, there is a complex relationship between exposures and levels of compounds and metabolites in blood, urine, exhaled breath, and other biological media. This relationship is controlled by toxicokinetics of the particular agents.[3] Consequently, proper interpretation of findings from biological monitoring for a given worker requires some knowledge of the temporal variations in the worker's exposure. In many situations, biological monitoring should only be used to verify that exposures have been controlled. Its use in detecting high exposures should be limited, such as when absorption is primarily through the skin.

It is almost never possible to evaluate ingestion as a route of exposure with sampling. Occasionally, samples of food and drink may be collected to assess the level of contamination; however, this sort of exposure is likely to be extremely variable and episodic in nature, so that environmental sampling is usually an ineffective way of assessing exposure.

Exposure measurements on workers performing the same job under similar conditions commonly show substantial variation in mean exposure between workers. These differences are the primary limitation to what can be achieved with exposure controls. There are many reasons why differences might occur. First, individuals have differences in skill, training, and experience, which may lead them to perform a job with differences in techniques that affect personal exposure. Second, they may have differences in their level of concern about the hazards of the job and take more or fewer precautions to avoid exposure through the use of personal protective equipment or engineering controls. Differences among workers on these factors are generally assigned to "work practices" and dismissed. As a result, there has been little systematic investigation of the nature of these differences, especially the behavioral components and effective ways for intervening to reduce the exposures.

Controls

Substitution

Substances and materials that pose risks to impair health and safety should not be used if they can be substituted. Substitution is part of the concept of toxics use reduction and waste management. Potential benefits to health and safety have to be balanced against technological and economic consequences. This balance should include product properties, production process, environment, and reliability of supply. For example, less-toxic toluene may be an adequate replacement for benzene. Regular auditing of use of substances and materials provides inspiration for substitution and keeps the substitution process active.

Limitation of Release and of Build-up of Contamination

If substitution is not possible, then the next step is to attempt to control or limit releases and prevent the buildup of toxic materials in the worker's environment. Local exhaust ventilation combined with source isolation will control process emissions. General room ventilation is used to prevent the build-up of hazardous concentrations in the work area from contaminants escaping local exhaust, from spills, or from fugitive emissions (from seals, valves, or pumps). An example of these two ventilation approaches is shown in Fig. 9-2.

Local exhaust systems surround the point of emission with a partial or complete enclosure and attempt to capture and remove the emissions before they are released into the worker's breathing zone. Figures 9-3 and 9-4 show examples of local ventilation systems; various types with differing degrees of effectiveness are available. Unfortunately, it is not possible before installation to determine precisely the effectiveness of a particular system, although this is an area of active research. As a result, it is important to measure exposures and evaluate

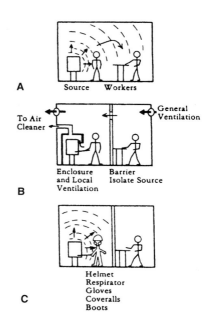

FIGURE 9-2 ● Examples of controls for airborne exposures. (**A**) Workers with primary and secondary exposure to source emissions. (**B**) Ventilation and source isolation to control exposures. (**C**) Personal protection and source isolation to control exposures. (Diagrams prepared by T. J. Smith, Harvard School of Public Health, Boston, Massachusetts.)

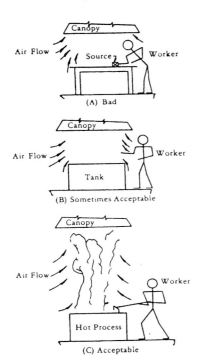

FIGURE 9-3 ● The proper use of a canopy hood, which does not allow the air contaminants to be drawn through the worker's breathing zone. The worker's location is crucial. (From National Institute for Occupational Safety and Health. The industrial environment: Its evaluation and control. Washington, DC: NIOSH, 1973:599.)

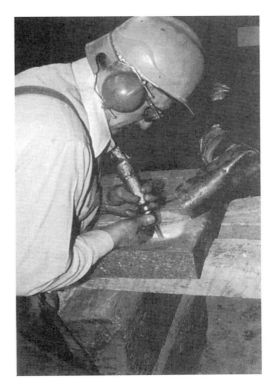

FIGURE 9-4 ● Local exhaust ventilation successfully captures dust produced by stone cutting. (From W. A. Burgess, Harvard School of Public Health, Boston, Massachusetts.)

how much control has been achieved after a system is installed. Unless contaminant sources are totally enclosed, collection will only capture a fraction of the total emission. Release of smoke from smoke tubes at the point of contaminant generation is a useful technique for visualizing the flow of air toward the exhaust. It may reveal if the distance to the exhaust is too large, if there are cross-drafts or strong air disturbances, or if the worker creates wakes, all of which greatly reduce the collection efficiency. A good system may collect 80 to 99 percent, but a poor system may capture only 50 percent or less. Careful maintenance must be performed on the system to maintain efficiency. Poor maintenance is probably most responsible for system failures.

The increasing cost of energy has made the practice of ventilating work areas with outside fresh air an increasingly expensive process; considerable effort is being directed to the design of systems that can recirculate decontaminated air or use heat exchangers so the heat value is not lost.

Limitation of Contact

The third important approach to controlling exposures to toxic materials is to limit worker contact by (a) automating processes, (b) isolating processes using toxic materials from the remainder of the work area so that the potential for contact with these materials is limited, or (c) by furnishing workers with personal protective equipment, such as dust or gas masks (respirators) or hoods or suits with externally supplied air for controlling inhalation of toxic materials. Many people mistakenly think that the use of respirators is a simple and inexpensive way to control exposure to toxic airborne materials. However, there is discomfort in wearing these masks, poor worker acceptance, and variable levels of protection achieved. There are extensive OSHA requirements for an adequate respirator program to ensure that the quality of the devices is maintained and that workers are receiving adequate protection. It should be noted that the annual cost of a good respirator program for lead dust exposures is reported to be approximately $1,000 per worker or more. Fitting of respirators is extremely important but is often neglected; a poorly fitting respirator provides substantially less protection than expected because, even if the filters are highly efficient, air leaks around the edges of the face mask.

The use of rubber gloves and protective clothing does not automatically ensure that workers are protected adequately. Toluene and other aromatic solvents readily penetrate rubber gloves; thus, glove composition must be matched to the chemical nature of the substance. Similarly, long-sleeved shirts or coveralls may not prevent skin contact with toxic dusts because small dust particles can sift through the openings between threads in woven cloth. A study of orchard workers showed the effects of pesticide exposures even though they had been wearing dust masks to prevent inhalation of the dust and long-sleeved shirts to prevent skin exposure. Special testing indicated that, despite their wearing the shirts, their arms were covered with dust that contained pesticide. Tests with fluorescent dusts showed similar findings, which indicated that even impermeable protective suits are difficult to seal to prevent migration of dust past cuffs and the neck opening.

An important part of limiting contact with hazardous substances is the requirement that protective clothing be changed each day and not worn outside the work area. This effort is also facilitated by the requirement for showers after the work shift.

Some reduction in exposure can be obtained by administrative controls, such as scheduling workers to spend limited amounts of time in areas with potential exposure, which may reduce their cumulative exposure below recommended guidelines. Although this approach may be effective in certain situations, (a) it requires good exposure data to demonstrate its effectiveness and the careful attention of supervisory personnel, (b) it may be an inefficient use of workers, and (c) it may be inappropriate for controlling exposures to carcinogens.

Ideally, all the control approaches described should be used together to develop an overall control strategy that will deal with all aspects of toxic material exposure in a particular workplace. Short-term measures, such as extensive use of personal protective equipment, may be adopted immediately after a problem is recognized to allow time for developing engineering controls or process modifications that will provide more long-term control. In spite of their undesirable aspects, respirators may be the only effective control device for some exposures, such as those faced by maintenance or clean-up workers. (OSHA policy is to use them only as a last resort.)

NOISE PROBLEMS

Occupational exposure to excessive noise is an important problem that is evaluated and controlled in part by occupational hygienists (see also Chapters 14 and 27). Hygienists are trained to measure the intensity and quality of noise, assess its potential for producing damage, and devise means to control noise exposures. Two principal types of workplace noise, continuous and impact, require somewhat different techniques of evaluation and control. *Continuous noise* is produced by high-velocity air flow in compressors, fans, gas burners, and motors. Crushing, drilling, and grinding are important sources of continuous noise because a large amount of energy is used in a small space. *Impact noise* results from sharp or explosive inputs of energy into some object or process, such as hammering or pounding on metal or stone, dropping heavy objects, or materials handling.

During the evaluation of a workplace, a hygienist looks for sources of excessive noise, determines which workers are exposed, and then selects an evaluation strategy to clarify the nature and extent of the exposures. If the noise is continuous or almost continuous, a hand-held noise survey meter may be used to determine the noise levels at the worker's location. If the exposure involves impact noises, an electronic instrument that records and averages the high-intensity, but short-duration, pulses is used to characterize the source and exposures.

Typically, workers spend variable amounts of time exposed to noise sources, and they may work at different distances from the sources, which will alter their exposures. Exposures may also vary because the output of noise sources may change over time. Therefore, the average (time-weighted) exposure may not be easy to estimate, even though the sources may present clear potential for overexposure. This problem has been solved by the use of small noise dosimeters worn by workers that electronically record sound levels and indicate average noise levels during work shifts. Dosimeters are very useful for describing average exposures. Some dosimeters store 8-hour time profiles, where they can be displayed and linked to records of worker activities. A typical noise evaluation will include both source noise level and dosimeter measurements.

National requirements and TLV guidelines are used by the hygienist to evaluate noise data and decide if a hazard is present. In addition to the hazard to hearing, noise affects verbal communication, which may create a hazard by masking verbal communication or warning sounds, and worker detection of safety hazards, such as moving equipment. The current OSHA standard for continuous noise for 8 hours is 90 dBA.* Higher levels are permitted for shorter periods of time.[4] The OSHA standard allows levels of noise exposure that will protect some, but not all workers, from the adverse effects of workplace noise. The TLV for an 8-hour exposure to noise is 85 dBA, which is significantly lower than the 90 dBA OSHA standard for (continuous) noise.

Although techniques exist to obtain an overall time-weighted average (TWA) of noise exposures received in several different work settings, no techniques exist for assessing the hearing risks of combined exposure to both continuous and impulse noise. Many workers are exposed to both continuous and impulse noise, such as brass-foundry workers who are exposed to continuous noise from gas burners and to impulse noise from brass ingots dropping into metal bins from conveyors.

The strategies for controlling noise are similar to those used for toxic material control and are discussed below.

Substitute

Use another process or piece of equipment. For example, electrically heated pots for melting metal can be used instead of gas-heated pots to eliminate burner noise.

Prevent or Reduce Release of Noise

Modify the source to reduce its output, enclose and soundproof the operation, or install mufflers or baffles. For example, noisy air compressors can be fitted with mufflers and placed in soundproofed rooms to control their noise; impact-absorbing materials can be installed to eliminate impulse noise from ingots dropping into a metal bin.

Prevent Excessive Worker Contact

Provide personal protective equipment, such as earplugs or earmuffs, or provide a control booth. As with toxic materials, the overall strategy to control exposures usually involves separate approaches for various aspects of the problem. It may be necessary to consult an acoustical engineer with advanced evaluation and engineering expertise for dealing with complex noise problems. If engineering controls are not completely effective or are impractical, ear protectors may be required; however, the effectiveness of these devices is limited because sound may also reach the ear by bone conduction. A full-shift exposure above 120 dBA cannot be controlled adequately using earplugs or muffs (see Chapter 14).

RADIATION PROBLEMS

Radiation hazards are commonly first identified by occupational hygienists, but the responsibility for their evaluation and control overlaps among the occupational hygienist, the health physicist, and the radiation protection officer (see Chapter 14).

Exposure to ionizing radiation can be external (from x-ray machines or radioactive materials) or internal (from radioactive substances in the body). External exposures can be monitored instrumentally by several methods; the type of detector system chosen for a given problem depends on the nature of the ionizing radiation. Personal monitoring is commonly performed with badges of photographic emulsions, thermal luminescent materials, or induced radiation materials that will indicate the cumulative dose during the period worn. Data from these measurement systems can be used to construct relatively accurate estimates of tissue exposure. If there are also detailed supporting data on worker activities, sources of exposure and points of intervention can also be identified.

Nonionizing radiation is also an external exposure problem. This type of radiation includes a variety of electromagnetic waves, ranging from short-wavelength ultraviolet, to visible and infrared, to long-wavelength microwaves and radiowaves. Exposures to ultraviolet, visible, and infrared radiation are measured with photometers of various types. Microwaves and radiowaves can also be measured by several standardized techniques, but there is some controversy over the exposure intensities required to produce adverse health effects.

---

*The unit dBA denotes decibels on the "A" scale, which is related to the human ear's response to sound.

Exposures to radioactive materials can be evaluated with similar methodology to that used for toxic substances. Personal air sampling, surface sampling, and skin contamination measurement can be used to quantify exposures by their route of contact or entry into the body. For example, personal air sampling in uranium mines can measure the miners' exposure to respirable radioactive particles that will be deposited in their respiratory tracts. Internal levels of some radionuclides can be detected outside the body and measured directly if they emit sufficient penetrating radiation, such as gamma rays emitted from radioactive cobalt. However, most cannot be detected externally; the quantities of radioactive substances reaching sensitive tissues usually must be estimated by determining the worker's external exposures and making assumptions about the amount entering the body and being transported to the site(s) of adverse effects.

The Nuclear Regulatory Commission (NRC) has set standards for allowable ionizing radiation exposures for both external and internal sources. These exposure limits can be used, like TLVs, to decide if a given exposure presents a health risk. Radiation protection programs have strict requirements about techniques for handling radioactive materials and working with radiation sources and also require extensive routine exposure monitoring and medical monitoring.

Exposure limits for nonionizing radiation have been set by OSHA, based on published scientific data, the TLVs developed by the ACGIH, and standards developed by the American National Standards Institute (ANSI). Equivalent limits have been developed by WHO and several countries (see Bibliography). The eyes and the skin are the critical organs to be protected, and the standards are set for the most susceptible areas. There is concern about reproductive hazards for these agents. Standards also have been developed for lasers based on ophthalmoscopic data and irreversible functional changes in visual responses. As with other types of standards, the numerical limits cannot be treated as absolute, and the margin of safety for many is uncertain.

Control of external ionizing and nonionizing radiation exposures is achieved by minimizing the amounts of radiation used, isolating the processes, shielding the sources, using warning devices, interlocking door and trigger mechanisms to prevent accidental exposures, educating workers and supervisors about the hazards, and, if necessary, requiring use of personal protective equipment.

For example, an industrial x-ray machine used to check castings for flaws is placed in a separate room with extensive lead shielding, and the x-ray machine cannot be triggered when the door is open. The room also has signs warning of the hazard. A red warning light inside the room is lit for 30 seconds before the x-rays are released so that a worker inside the room when the door is closed could activate an emergency override switch to prevent operation of the x-ray machine. All personnel working around the x-ray operation are required to wear film badges to monitor their accumulated x-ray exposure.

Control of internal radiation exposures from radioactive materials is very similar to controls for toxic materials. The objectives are to use minimal amounts of radioactive materials; isolate the work areas; enclose any operations likely to produce airborne emissions; use work procedures that prevent or minimize worker contact with contaminated air or materials; have workers wear personal protective equipment to prevent skin contact, eye exposure, or inhalation of materials; monitor environmental contamination levels; and educate workers about the hazards. Careful supervision of work activities and monitoring of program implementation are required to provide adequate protection.

CONCERNS FOR THE FUTURE

Traditional work environments, such as factories and other workplaces in heavy industry, have been long-term concerns of hygienists. These are now a growing concern in developing countries that seek to balance the economic benefits of industry against the health costs of insufficient worker protection. In some developed countries, there has been a growing concern about the office environment and the health effects associated with energy-efficient, tightly sealed buildings. The scientific basis for occupational hygiene practice has been eroding because of limited research funding and a small number of researchers. Examination of the scientific literature in occupational hygiene shows it to be narrowly focused on limited issues. Internal research funded by companies is often not published because it may aid competitors or it may raise liability concerns. Gaining access to workplaces for academic studies has also become more difficult. There is a reluctance of industries to examine the hazards of their operations because of concerns about the costs of additional government regulation and legal liability for health claims from previously unrecognized hazards. As a result of this, there is little development and refinement of exposure assessment methods, control technology, or intervention strategies. This has occurred despite the extensive worldwide development of new materials, production technologies, biomedical and drug manufacturing, and other advances. Occupational hygiene has not kept up with this development. A number of occupational hygienists in North America and other parts of the world are very concerned about this situation. They have begun working to strengthen local research and to develop more collaborative international research programs. Joint labor and management research programs supported by company funds have also become increasingly important sources of workplace access and research funding, such as the joint health and safety research programs of the United Auto Workers with the Daimler Chrysler Corporation and with the General Motors Corporation.

ENVIRONMENTAL HYGIENE

Environmental hygiene has much in common with occupational hygiene. There is considerable overlap in basic concepts and approaches for hazard recognition, exposure assessment, and source controls, especially for air pollution. The major difference is the occupational hygienist is dealing with a prescribed setting and generally a healthy adult population. In contrast, the environmental hygienist covers the whole environment, and all of its population, including the young, elderly, and ill, in addition to healthy adults. Exposures tend to be higher in occupational settings but are not always higher. Environmental transport of contaminants is usually more extensive in the outdoor environment than the workplace setting, which allows more time for reactions, transformations, and removal processes that selectively modify what is present. Residents of an area will have exposure to general environmental conditions in addition to those inside their homes and public buildings.

Source–Transport–Receptor Model

There is a simple but powerful representation of environmental exposures that has been widely used by environmental scientists. This representation is known as the *source–transport–receptor model.*

The *source* produces and releases emissions into the environment, such as airborne emissions from a power plant or toxic organic solvents released into groundwater by a waste dump. The source defines the composition and release rate of the emissions. Source sampling is very useful when it can be accomplished. Sometimes, there are many small sources that are dispersed, such as individual vehicles in traffic and heating units in homes. Given knowledge about the source, we can identify what types of hazards might be present and what to measure. Environmental processes during *transport* of emissions are important in many ways; these include dispersion and dilution, photochemical reactions with sunlight, and removal by rain, adsorption to soil particles, and sedimentation. Our primary concern is the concentration and composition reaching the *receptor*—the exposed person.

Major Problems

Air and water emissions from traffic, power plants, industrial operations (especially chemical and mining), food sanitation, municipal and agricultural wastes, sewage, and solid waste are all major problems. Some characteristics of these major sources are listed in Table 9-2. In most cases, it is necessary to investigate in detail the characteristics of a given source to fully understand the hazards it presents. There is no simple summary that can adequately indicate the complexity and variety of source releases. It is also important to consider the natural sources that may affect the background levels of an environmental contaminant.

EXPOSURE CHARACTERIZATION

As with occupational hygiene, there is a set of common and/or dangerous exposures for which well-characterized methods have been developed that are used by the EPA and other regulatory agencies. These methods are based on (a) sample collection and analysis, and (b) more commonly, direct-reading instruments. The most important part of an evaluation is the sampling strategy, which specifies how, when, and where samples will be obtained and measurements performed. The goal is to define the magnitude of exposures. Exposures can be highly variable among individuals, across time, and across space. Thus, a series of measurements must be made to define the distribution of exposures that may be received. For environmental problems, we are

TABLE 9.2		

Major Sources of Environmental Emissions and Releases

Major Sources	Emissions and Contaminated Media	Route of Entry
Natural processes • Erosion • Vegetation and microbes • Volcanoes • Geothermal springs • Forest and grass fires • Storm runoff and floods • Sea spray • Radon	Airborne dusts, pollen, terpenes, ammonia, methane, sulfur dioxide, hydrogen sulfide; Waterborne particles, dissolved carbon and metals, hydrogen sulfide, arsenic Soil contamination with metals, radon	Inhalation and ingestion
Power plants	Airborne ash, nitrogen oxides, metals; sulfur oxides, arsenic from coal; sulfur oxides, vanadium from oil Radionuclides in air and water from nuclear power	Inhalation and ingestion
Vehicle emissions • Traffic: cars, trucks, buses • Off-road: trains, mining • Boats and ships	Airborne unburned fuel, nitrogen oxides, polycyclic aromatic hydrocarbons (PAHs), particles, lead Secondary photochemical smog Waterborne hydrocarbons, lead in street runoff water Soil contamination with hydrocarbons, lead Ship ballast water releases of oil, organisms	Inhalation
Home-heating emissions	Particles, hydrocarbons, sulfur oxides, metals	Inhalation
Sewage systems • Human wastes • Small business wastes	Waterborne pathogens, nutrients, toxic chemicals, solvents, metals	Ingestion
Industrial activities • chemical releases	Airborne contaminants (depend on the specific industry) Waste-water contaminants (depend on the specific industry)	Inhalation and ingestion

interested in contamination of air, water, food, and soil. There are also evaluation techniques for noise and radiation hazards.

Sampling Strategy

One of the most challenging aspects of environmental sampling is ensuring that the samples are representative of exposure because there are so many different sources of variation. For example, there can be important temporal variations on the scale of minutes, hours, days, weeks, months, seasons, and years; and spatial variations on the scale of feet, yards, hundreds of yards, miles, and more. Wells, streams, rivers, and lakes can vary dramatically. So

can individual and batches of food items. As a result, we need to be clear about the exposure distribution we are attempting to characterize: for adults, children, the elderly, or the ill, for homes along a busy street, for a neighborhood, for a particular time period, or for a certain activity? Do we need to collect personal samples or will fixed-location area samples be acceptable? If we wish to define the mean and standard deviation of an exposure, fewer samples are required than if we are trying to define the range or the probability of the highest values (the upper tail of the exposure distribution). If we are looking for exposures that exceed a legal limit, it may be necessary to use a strategy and methods defined by law or regulation. Therefore, it is critical that the hygienist have a well-developed set of questions to answer and a sampling strategy that will obtain the answers as efficiently as possible.

Sample Collection

Each exposure media has different collection approaches, as indicated in Table 9-3. Airborne particles may be collected on filters, impacted on surfaces, or electrostatically collected. Nonreactive gases can be collected in bags and bottles. Reactive gases may be collected in liquids using bubblers, or treated substrates, such as filters or adsorbents. Vapors, such as gasoline vapors, are gaseous, but they will readily condense to a liquid or solid state. Consequently, they will readily condense on surfaces like the inside of bags. The preferred method for sampling these materials is with special

TABLE 9.3

Examples of Environmental Sampling and Analysis Methods for Common Contaminants

Media and Contaminant	Collection Method Examples	Analytical Method
Air: Metals (lead, cadmium)	Total metals: Membrane filter (0.2 -μm pore size) and pump (4 Lpm) Respirable particles: use cyclone or impactor precollector before filter Direct analysis[a] by specific light scattering instrument	Acid digestion of filter and sample, atomic absorption (AA) measurement
Air: Organic vapors	Hydrocarbon vapors: charcoal in canister; Pesticides: Tenax or XAD or other suitable resin	Strip vapors with solvent and gas chromatography (GC) analysis
Air: Reactive gases (ozone, ammonia, sulfur dioxide)	Collect on treated substrate; selective for gas Direct analysis by specific electrochemical instrument Direct analysis by specific colorimetric detector tubes	Specific reaction products; ion chromatography analysis
Air: Carbon monoxide	Collect in bag Direct analysis by specific electrochemical instrument	Gas sample injected for direct analysis by GC
Water: Metals (lead)	Collect sample[b] with acid-cleaned polyethylene bottle (1 L)	Free Pb: Acidify water and AA analysis; Total Pb: perchlorate digestion then AA
Water: Microorganisms	Collect water in sterile bottle	Filter water; culture organisms on filter or directly culture water; digest filtered organisms and polymerase chain reaction (PCR) analysis
Food and soil: Pesticides	Collect food or soil sample[c] in chemically clean container	Macerate and prepare[d] food and soil; extract preparation with solvent; GC analysis

[a] Direct analysis is a real-time measurement with a very short averaging time, usually 1 minute or less.
[b] A variety of components may need to be characterized to accurately represent a water contamination problem, such as organisms, suspended materials, or sediments.
[c] Because food and soil are very heterogeneous, careful sampling strategies are needed to collect representative samples that indicate human exposures.
[d] Food and soil are complex matrices and may require extensive preparation to prepare them for analysis.

materials in small holders, such as charcoal in tubes or reactants impregnated on papers or fibrous glass. The collection process may be either active, using a pump to draw air through the collector, or passive, using diffusion to bring the gaseous materials into the collector. Badge-type passive collectors are better accepted by subjects for personal sampling. Automated collectors may be used to collect a long series of air or water samples in a chosen location or drifting with balloons or floating devices.

Sample Analysis

Sampling media or containers are sent to a laboratory with experience performing the desired analyses; accredited labs are best. Analyses for all regulated substances must follow the method given in regulations if the data are to be used for determining compliance or legal proceedings. If the measurements are to be used for a research project, where there is no accepted method for the substances of interest, then the investigator must work closely with the lab to ensure the validity of the data. Developing new methods to measure an environmental contaminant is a major undertaking, even for highly skilled environmental chemists. It is not unusual for the development and validation process to take several years.

In all cases, there must be detailed quality-control and quality-assurance plans, which should include lab and field blank samples, analysis of standards with each batch of samples, duplicate field samples, replicate analyses, and sometimes spiked blanks or spiked samples to verify that there were no problems in the field collection or lab analyses. More information about quality-assurance programs can be found in standard texts on environmental monitoring or in publications by regulatory agencies.

DEFINING A HAZARD

Complaints

It is common for residents of an area to complain about odors, dust, and damage to materials from air pollutants. Likewise, they may complain about the odors, color, and opacity of water in ponds, lakes, streams, and rivers, and all of these problems in addition to the taste of drinking water. Any of these may indicate a potential problem. In some cases, the problem is one of esthetics, and in others it is

a health risk. If the source of the poor quality can be identified, such as a chemical plant upwind or a sewage treatment plant upriver, then it may be possible to identify what might be contaminating the environment. Often the source is not known, but the odor or other characteristics may be identified. For example, in the past many private wells were contaminated with gasoline leaking from underground storage tanks, and the gasoline odor from the water was notable. Spills or accidental releases are most often noted by people living or passing nearby, and they may be the most at risk.

Exposure Assessment Study

Where the resources are present, an exposure study may be conducted to define what contaminants are present and determine if they exceed allowable exposure standards developed by the EPA, WHO, or other organizations. However, one of the most difficult exposure analysis problems is to determine what unknown agents are present in a sample media. Unfortunately there are no general, broad-spectrum methods that can readily determine the components of the black gunk scraped off the bottom of the pond, material obtained from an abandoned barrel left at a waste site, or a substance causing an unpleasant odor in air, water, or food. In general, one must tell the laboratory what to measure, so it can choose the appropriate methods. If a suitable, sample collection strategy is used, then exposure levels can be compared to exposure standards. When measured levels are less than the standard, it may mean that there is no hazard; however, if there are health complaints related to the exposure, the findings may also mean that the exposure standard has been set too high.

Epidemiologic Study

If there are local health complaints, such as by neighbors of a local industry, then a small study may be conducted by the local health department. A larger, full-scale epidemiological study may also be warranted in some cases. The water contamination problems from the Woburn, Massachusetts, waste dump represent a good example. Excess leukemia in children was found to be associated with residence near the dump. Other community studies have been launched to examine apparent unusual clusters of cases of disease.

CONTROL OF HAZARDS

The same processes used to control industrial exposures and waste emissions are also used in environmental controls. Elimination of the source is the only completely successful control approach. Sometimes it is possible to change the source or limit its output. Personal exposure controls are less successful for general environmental hazards than they are for occupational hazards. Respirators and protective clothing are impractical and unreasonable for the general public. Although there is an active market for home and personal air cleaners, the amount of protection they can provide is limited; in addition, some of them will expose people to ozone, which is not recommended. Therefore, emission controls at the source are the most common and effective way to deal with emissions from large or numerous sources.

EXAMPLES OF MAJOR PROBLEMS

In this section, we consider some of the major types of environmental problems, their sources, transport phenomena, and characterization of exposures at the receptors.

Air Pollution

In recent years, airborne particulate matter less than 10 or 2.5 μm in diameter (PM_{10} or $PM_{2.5}$) has received much attention because daily variation in concentrations are well correlated with daily fluctuations in mortality, especially from respiratory and cardiovascular diseases. This has been seen in many cities worldwide. Because these effects occur at low concentrations (20 to 200 μg/m^3), public health officials are concerned. Part of this effect is associated with premature mortality, but part is also associated with increased mortality of people with preexisting diseases that would not have otherwise been fatal.

Environmental hygienists have been challenged to better define the air pollution exposures associated with general-population health effects. Time-activity studies have followed the daily lives of children, adults, the elderly, and the ill, while monitoring their exposures. Surprisingly, aside from children playing outdoors and people engaged in outdoor sports, most people spend limited time outdoors exposed to urban air pollution. Indoor exposures account for a much larger fraction of their time. When it was found that exposures to some general categories of air contaminants can be higher inside people's homes than outdoors, there was considerable concern. However, there are several reasons why that may not be as inconsistent with the health findings as it first might seem (Box 9-1).

Indoor and outdoor exposures are qualitatively and quantitatively different because the emission sources are different. Air contaminants generated inside the home come from cooking, pets, combustion sources, home and personal care products, paints, furnishings, hobbies, pesticides, vapors in water from bathing and showering, and other materials. $PM_{2.5}$ indoors comes from reentrainment of dust and dirt tracked into the house or from vacuuming and sweeping, whereas outdoor $PM_{2.5}$ comes from combustion sources and atmospheric reaction products (smog). Importantly, some outdoor air contaminants can readily penetrate indoors, such as small-diameter particles in $PM_{2.5}$, and some gases. However, highly reactive ozone in smog is found at lower concentrations indoors than outside.

Once materials are released to the environment, there are a number of processes that operate to modify and remove them—processes that differ for particles and gases. Combustion processes can produce dense clouds of very small particles (0.01 to 0.1 μm), sometimes visible as smoke (Box 9-2). These rapidly agglomerate into larger particles ($\sim$1 μm). As the particles become larger, they settle out of the air or are removed by impaction on surfaces of buildings and trees. During periods of high humidity, water-soluble particles will absorb water and may grow large enough to be removed by sedimentation and impaction. Particles can also be removed by precipitation—by nucleating raindrops and washout. Semivolatile vapors of polynuclear aromatic hydrocarbons (PAHs), tars, and greases condense on the particles as hot combustion gases cool. Gaseous emissions can also undergo atmospheric reactions. Sulfur dioxide from burning materials containing sulfur, such as coal and fuel oil, can react with water to form sulfuric acid, which absorbs water to form tiny droplets. Atmospheric ammonia reacts with the sulfuric acid to form ammonium sulfate. Some hydrocarbons will be oxidized to peroxides, aldehydes, and organic acids by ozone and other strong oxidants.

The hydrocarbons and nitrogen oxides released by vehicles in the summer can be photochemically converted to intense eye and upper respiratory

---

BOX 9-1

Assessing Indoor Air Pollution

In many cases, indoor problems cannot be characterized by a generally uniform clinical picture and a specific cause (see Chapter 18). These problems must be considered as being a result of complex interactions between several factors, including air contaminants (including their odor), temperature, ventilation, air movement, illumination, noise, ergonomics, and psychological and social factors. Emerging complaints about indoor environment quality should be dealt with immediately, assessing and controlling the problems while making it clear that management cares. The latter is important to set a positive social context. Actions taken could follow a cost-effective stepwise approach as indicated below:

1. Check whether operational conditions are normal, such as for the HVAC system. Instruct those who complain about the possibilities for individual control of the HVAC system.
2. Determine type and extent of problem by using a standardized "sick building" questionnaire or, if there are few employees, structured interviews.

3. Perform a technical survey to assess risk factors inherent in the building or its use and operation.
4. Assess the building and its construction materials and furniture, quality of cleaning, moisture damage and mold growth, temperature, air movement using smoke tubes, and carbon dioxide concentration. Estimate degree of recirculation of air and possible contamination of intake air.
5. Measure ventilation efficiencies with tracer gas studies.
6. Make a detailed assessment of contaminant sources and concentrations.
7. Perform clinical examination of affected persons and additional occupational hygiene investigations, such as detailed chemical analyses of complex mixtures, or assessment of individualized work habits to guide training interventions.

This approach is recommended because buildings are now recognized as a possible source of hazardous exposure to emissions from building materials, such as formaldehyde, and to biological agents and their toxins (see Chapter 18). All of these problems are of interest to the occupational hygienist.

---

irritants, especially highly reactive oxidants including ozone, under the action of ultraviolet radiation from the sun. The classic time pattern is as follows: vehicle emissions during the morning rush hours are converted to afternoon smog, as occurs in Los Angeles, Denver, and Houston. Although emission controls on cars, improved engines and fuel, and catalytic mufflers have dramatically reduced the emissions per car over the past three decades, the number of cars has increased over that same time period. As a result, the number of smog alerts has decreased, but not proportionally to individual vehicle-emission reductions.

Common Personal Sources

Although many personal items, such as cars, home heating units, barbeques, and power mowers, are minor sources by themselves, when taken together in large numbers in a city or in locations with poor local ventilation, such as valleys, they can cause

major generalized air pollution. Vehicle traffic, predominantly cars and trucks, is one of the largest sources of emissions in urban and suburban areas. These emissions include particulates containing elemental carbon, oils, grease, unburned fuel, and PAHs, as well as gases containing carbon monoxide, carbon dioxide, oxides of nitrogen, benzene, toluene, xylene, aldehydes, organic acids, and other volatile organic compounds (VOCs).

Biological Sources

Biological hazards include airborne molds, pollens, and infectious agents. Seasonal allergies are a consequence of pollens released by plants. Less familiar are the releases of terpenes by pine trees (chemicals found in terpentine, a paint solvent). The haze in the Smoky Mountains in North Carolina is produced by the photochemical reaction of sunlight with the summertime releases of terpenes. This is supplemented by sulfuric acid aerosol from power

BOX 9-2

Occupational and Environmental Particle Exposure, with Special Focus on Ultrafine Particles and Nanotechnologies

Margaret Quinn

For many occupational exposures, inhalation is the major route of entry into the body. The primary target organ for pathogenic effects is the respiratory system; however, submicrometer particles can translocate to other organs where they may cause disease. For example, asbestos can penetrate the alveolar lining and migrate not only to the pleura but also to the peritoneum to cause mesothelioma. The respiratory system of a normal adult processes 1,000 to 2,500 L of air a day. The surface area for gas exchange is about 75 m² —half the size of a singles tennis court. This area is perfused with more than 2,000 km (about 1,240 miles) of capillaries.

The human respiratory system is typically described as being composed of three major regions: nasopharyngeal, tracheobronchial (or thoracic), and alveolar (or pulmonary). The likelihood that an inhaled particle will deposit in one of these regions depends on three main factors: (a) the particle's physicochemical properties, including size, density, shape, and hygroscopic or hydrophobic character; (b) the geometry of the respiratory tract, including the diameter of the airways and their branching angles; and (c) airflow patterns in the respiratory tract, such as those resulting from heavy (as opposed to shallow) or mouth (as opposed to nose) breathing.

A high fraction of coarse particles (with diameters more than 4 μm) is deposited within the nasopharyngeal region, whereas fine particles (with diameters less than 4 μm) are deposited more efficiently in the tracheobronchial and alveolar regions (Fig. 9-5A). The distribution of particle sizes generated in most occupational and environmental settings is usually quite broad; it is common to find differences of several orders of magnitude between the smallest and largest particle diameters. Figure 9-5B shows typical particle diameter size ranges for common occupational and environmental exposures. In general, dusts, ground material, and pollen are

in the micrometer size range or larger, and fumes and smokes are submicrometer. The smallest aerosol particles approach the size of large gas molecules and have many of the same properties. These particles—called *ultrafine particles* (especially in the environmental literature) or *nanoparticles* (especially in the occupational literature)—range from approximately 1 to 100 nm in size.

In the past, exposure to ultrafine particles or nanoparticles was measured for occupational and environmental studies in units of mass, such as milligrams of particles per cubic meter of air (mg/m³). However, results of occupational studies of asbestos and human-made mineral (synthetic vitreous) fibers and environmental studies of ultrafine particles indicate that it is the number of particles, and perhaps even more importantly the surface area of particles, that may be most relevant for studies of adverse health effects in humans. Evidence from occupational and environmental epidemiologic studies indicate that exposure to these particles is associated with increases in overall mortality and in adverse effects on the respiratory, cardiovascular, neurologic, and immune systems. When particles get smaller, their number and surface area increase many orders of magnitude per unit mass; that is, the same material in ultrafine or nanoparticle form can be more toxic than in the form of larger, still respirable, particles.

A new field called *nanotechnology* is beginning to emerge and will likely be a dominant technology of this century. It is based on the principle of building particles and devices, with chemistry and biology, one atom at a time. The evolution of nanoparticles and nanotechnologies can be described in three phases, representing their level of structural complexity:

1. Some nanoparticles are naturally occurring or human-made and are part of exposures that have existed for years, including diesel exhaust, flour dust, welding fume, silica flour, asbestos, some human-made mineral fibers, and combustion products, such as asphalt fume and ultrafine air pollution. Other types of nanoparticles are made by applying new processes to conventional

(continued)

BOX 9-2

Occupational and Environmental Particle Exposure, with Special Focus on Ultrafine Particles and Nanotechnologies (Continued)

materials, including nanoscale metals, such as iron, beryllium, chromium, lead, cadmium, manganese, zirconium, titanium, gold, silver, and aluminum.

2. Engineered nanoparticles or nanodevices have more structural complexity than those described above. The most common examples are nanotubes, microspheres, and fullerenes (buckyballs, geodesic-dome-like particles named after Buckminster Fuller), all with engineered surfaces and hollow interiors. Carbon-60 nanotubes are used commercially to form harder, more-flexible composite materials, including plastics. In more advanced applications, the surface chemistry of fullerenes or nanotubes can be changed, such as by attaching an antibody, or they can be used to encase other nanomaterials and then applied as, for example, targeted drug delivery devices.

3. Engineered devices and systems on the nanoscale are being developed to collect data, monitor chemical and biological systems, and provide communications and computing. Many of these devices and systems are still in the research and development phase.

Nanotechnology has the potential to radically change the study of basic biological mechanisms, and to significantly improve the prevention, detection, diagnosis, and treatment of diseases and other medical conditions. It operates at the same scale as biological processes, offering a unique perspective from which to view and manipulate fundamental biological pathways and processes. Nanotechnology may offer ways to study how individual molecules work inside an organism, with potential benefits and hazards. For example, it has been proposed that nanotechnologies could be used to develop effective screening tools for Alzheimer disease; however, there is also evidence suggesting that exposure to nanoparticles may cause this disease.

Although full evaluations of the health, safety, and environmental impacts of nanotechnology have not been conducted, toxicologists have postulated potential effects to guide future research. They hypothesize that nanoparticles may not be detected by normal phagocytic defenses. Because very small nanoparticles are smaller than some molecules, they could act like haptens to modify protein structures, either altering their function or rendering them antigenic, thus raising the potential for immune effects. Of special concern is the apparent ability of nanoparticles to redistribute from their site of deposition. For example, after inhalation exposure, nanoparticles have been reported to (a) travel via the olfactory nerve to the brain, as has been described for polio virus; and (b) enter the bloodstream and, in turn, the brain and other organs.

In 2002, an estimated 2 million U.S. workers were exposed to nanometer-diameter particles on a regular basis. It has been estimated that an additional 2 million workers globally will be required to work in nanotechnology industries in order to meet predicted demand for products over the next decade.

Bibliography

Department of Health and Human Services, National Institutes of Health. Statement for the record on nanotechnology before the Senate Committee on Commerce, Science, and Transportation, May 1, 2003.

Donaldson K, Stone V, Tran CL, et al. Nanotoxicology. Occup Environ Med 2004;61:727–8.

European Commission Community Health and Consumer Protection. Nanotechnologies: A preliminary risk analysis. Brussels: European Commission. 2004.

Hinds WC. Aerosol technology: Properties, behavior, and measurement of airborne particles. Second ed. New York: John Wiley & Sons, 1999.

Hood E, Nanotechnology: Looking as we leap. Environ Health Persp 2004;112:A740-A749.

IEEE Technology and Society Magazine. Nanotechnology [special issue]. 2004; Winter.

Kreyling WG, Semmler M, Moller W. Dosimetry and toxicology of ultrafine particles. J Aerosol Med 2004;17:140-152.

National Nanotechnology Initiative (NNI). Available at: <www.nano.gov>.

Quinn MM, Smith TJ, Schneider T, et al. Determinants of airborne fiber size in the glass fiber manufacturing industry. Occup Environ Hygiene 2005;2:19–28.

Royal Academy of Engineering and The Royal Society (UK). Nanoscience and nanotechnologies: Opportunities and uncertainties. Available at: <http://www.nanotec.org.uk/finalReport.htm>.

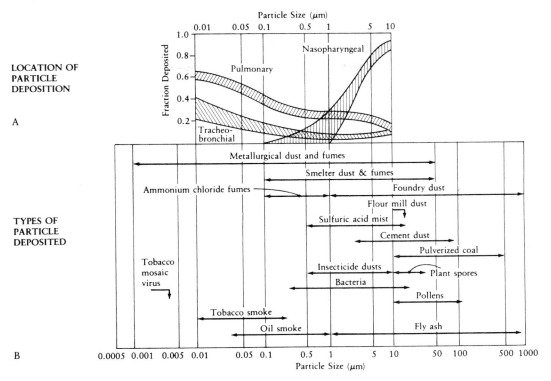

FIGURE 9-5 ● **A.** Fractional deposition plotted against particle size (effective aerodynamic diameter) for three functional parts of the respiratory tree, based on the model of the International Committee on Radiation Protection. The broad bands reflect large standard deviations. **B.** Examples of inhaled particles, classified by size. By comparing (**A**) and (**B**), approximate predictions of the deposition pattern for each particle can be generated. (Adapted from Brain JD, Valberg PA. Aerosol deposition on the respiratory tract. Am Rev Respir Dis 1979;120:1,325–73.)

plants in the Midwest burning high sulfur coal. Natural decomposition of vegetation and animals by microorganisms produces a number of common air contaminants. Proteins are reduced to ammonia, nitrates, hydrogen sulfide, and sulfates. Organic carbon is ultimately reduced to methane under anaerobic conditions and carbon dioxide when there is sufficient oxygen; both are greenhouse gases produced in large amounts by natural sources.

Natural Sources

Forest and grass fires, volcanoes, erosion, and sea spray produce large amounts of air contaminants across broad areas. Natural fires are dangerous from both their direct destruction and from the large amounts of smoke they produce. Outdoor fires release many of the same combustion products that are found in emissions from cars, trucks, and other human-made sources. Volcanoes release inorganic particles of ash and sulfur dioxide and produce hazardous conditions in broad areas downwind. The rare catastrophic eruptions, such as of Mount

Pinatuba in the Philippines, can inject thousands of tons of ash and sulfur high into the stratosphere, which can remain in the air for a year or more and enhance sunsets worldwide. Erosion produces soil particles that can be entrained into the air if the soil is dry and dusty. Dust storms scour tons of dust into the air, leading to very high dust exposures of populations. Coastal areas receive constant inputs of sea salt aerosol from breaking waves and bursting bubbles on the ocean.

Industrial Sources

Generally, these are point sources associated with local operations, such as power plants, chemical manufacturers, and petroleum refineries. Most of these are required to meet local and central governmental regulations on emissions. The specific emissions from these operations depend on the specific industry, which can be determined from reference texts and information collected by governmental agencies. This is effective for recognized hazards, such as the criteria pollutants defined by EPA and WHO. However, with the continuous development of new chemicals and materials, this strategy will not protect against new hazards. Public health agencies must maintain surveillance to verify that controls are effective and to detect when they are not.

Power plants are one of the most common industrial sources of airborne materials. They burn coal or oil, and some can also burn natural gas and switch between different fuels. They are major sources of carbon dioxide and nitrogen oxides, and, depending on their fuel, they may also release major amounts of sulfur oxides (coal and oil with sulfur), and fine particles of ash that contain metals (mercury, lead, and cadmium in coal, and vanadium in oil). Exposures will depend on wind direction and weather conditions.

Industrial operations run as designed most of the time. Unfortunately, there can be acute situations that result in large emissions. Spills of chemicals, fires, breakdowns of processing equipment, accidents, and failures of control systems can all produce massive emissions. In cases where the failure of a key part of the operation, such as a cooling system, will result in an explosion or chemical releases, a special system is usually in place to deal with a potential breakdown. One of the best examples of this is a nuclear power plant, which has back-up systems to maintain the flow of cooling water and control rods to limit the nuclear reaction. The few cases of malfunctions are well-known. One lesson from the Three Mile Island reactor accident in 1979 is that despite "fail-safe" engineering, unforeseen failures can still occur. Catastrophic breakdowns and accidents do occur, and community planning to minimize their effects is critical.

Emission Controls

Thereare well-developed emission controls for nearly all of the common industrial processes that produce airborne waste products. Particles can be collected by filters, cyclone separators, electrostatic precipitators, and gases and can be removed by scrubbers and other specialized devices. Collection efficiency is never 100 percent. As a result, even if the percent collection is 98 percent, as it is in some power-plant electrostatic precipitators, if the amount of particles produced is very large, then the amount that escapes collection can be large. Engineering controls used to minimize emissions must be well designed and carefully maintained to operate effectively. Assessment of these systems must

be done by specialists. In general, elimination of waste production is a much more effective control strategy than removal of waste. Changes in processes and raw materials can sometimes eliminate problematic wastes; for example, residual amounts of sulfur can be reduced in fuels, such as coal and oil.

Water Pollution

Problems with water pollution tend to be more localized that air pollution, although contamination of large watersheds can affect large populations. Water contaminants can take several forms: dissolved substances, such as salts and gases; suspended particles, such as clay and organic matter, which will settle out of the water; colloids—stable suspensions of very small particles that will not settle out; and floating substances, such as oils and grease. Oxygen content is one of the critical dimensions of water quality because it is necessary to sustain plants and animals in the water and sediments. Solubility of oxygen varies inversely with temperature; cold water holds more oxygen than warm water. The exchange of oxygen with the atmosphere is relatively slow, so conditions that either block the surface uptake or rapidly use up dissolved oxygen can create anaerobic conditions. Oil slicks block oxygen uptake. Large amounts of biological debris and organic carbon, such as from bacterial decay of vegetation, can deplete water of its oxygen. Then decay becomes anaerobic, which limits what can grow and creates odor and other problems.

Bioaccumulation

Accumulation and concentration of toxic chemical contaminants in the food chain is a serious problem for stable materials with long-term storage, such as lipid-soluble materials with very low water solubility that are not broken down by natural biochemical processes or organisms in the environment. Biological transport into and out of organisms requires some water solubility, and phase II metabolism of toxic materials increases their water solubility. The classic example of a substance that accumulates in biological systems is DDT. Because DDT has a low order of human toxicity, it was extensively sprayed to control mosquitoes and other insect pests in the 1940s and 1950s. Then during the 1960s, it was found that, in addition to many birds directly killed by pesticides, avian predators, such as fish-eating ospreys and eagles, were rapidly declining because of high losses of bird eggs—the shells had become very fragile and easily broken. Rachel Carson brought the story of the losses of birds and useful insects to national attention in 1962 with her book *Silent Spring*. Researchers had found that trace concentrations of DDT in natural waters accumulated in the lipids of tiny plants. Small aquatic animals that ate those plants effectively collected the lipids from many plants and concentrated DDT into their own body fats. Small fish ate relatively large amounts of those small animals, further concentrating DDT in their fat. Medium-sized fish ate the small fish, and large fish ate the medium-sized fish. This concentrating process progressed up the food chain, with DDT becoming more concentrated at each step—as much as 10,000-fold relative to the starting concentration in the plants. Finally, at the top of the food chain, the ospreys and eagles ate the large fish, whose fat now contained toxic levels of DDT. A high degree of chemical stability is a critical requirement for bioaccumulation. The stability of DDT and some other chemicals has allowed them to spread throughout the world so that even in the most remote places one can find DDT in the body fat of "top predators." Bioaccumulation also occurs for methyl mercury, which is formed in aquatic sediments by bacterial methylation of inorganic mercury. Tuna and swordfish accumulate methyl mercury, and when people eat these fishes they accumulate mercury in body fat, including in neurological tissues with high lipid content. Polychlorinated biphenyls (PCBs) and some radioactive materials, such as strontium-90, also bioaccumulate.

Common Sources

The major sources of water pollution in developed countries are storm runoff and sanitary waste water from cities, wastes from industries, and runoff from agriculture where fertilizers and pesticides are used and from concentrated animal feeding operations. Large industrialized animal-feeding operations can produce as much fecal and urinary waste as a small city. Fertilizers as well as animal and human wastes are major stimulants of plant growth in the receiving waters, leading to algal blooms. The bacterial decay of large amounts of organic wastes can strip the oxygen from the water, producing anaerobic conditions that kill fish and aquatic vegetation and lead to the growth of fungi, slug worms, and bacteria.

Although large oil spills are catastrophic when they occur, they are rare. A larger problem is the discharging of contaminated ballast and bilge water from ship tanks. After a ship unloads its cargo, the ballast tanks must be refilled with water to stabilize the ship. When the ship prepares to take on another cargo, it must pump out the ballast water. This procedure is a common way that aquatic species are transferred from one area to another, where they may not be native.

Industrial-waste releases have historically resulted in water-quality problems, from spills and accidental releases as well as routine releases. Specific hazards depend on the industry. Reference works on water pollution and toxic chemicals can help one identify which materials a given industry may commonly release and the problems they cause. Governmental regulations have greatly reduced the problems in areas where they are enforced. However, new industrial processes can produce wastes with unrecognized hazards.

There are natural cleaning processes that can lead to recovery in polluted waterways. Given sufficient time without further pollution, natural processes will remove the organic oxygen demand and lead to the return of plants and organisms that prefer clean, well-oxygenated conditions. Acidic and alkaline wastes will be neutralized. Toxic metal ions will be removed by complexation and formation of insoluble complexes and sedimentation. The bottom sediments will remain toxic, but without much effect if they remain undisturbed.

Water Treatment

Drinking water treatment is directed toward removing floating particle contaminants and killing pathogens. Surface waters with minimal contamination are purified by (a) addition of chemicals, such as alum or ferric sulfate, that will cause any particles to stick together (*flocculation*); then (b) sedimentation to allow the big particles to deposit on the bottom of large tanks; and then (c) filtration through beds of sand, which removes the fine particles. After filtration, water is disinfected by adding chlorine, chloramines, or other bactericides until there is free bactericide in the water flowing to the customer. The free bactericide provides some residual protection against pathogens introduced through breaks or problems in the distribution system. In places where there are mineral contaminants in the source water, such as iron or hydrogen sulfide, or hardness, additional chemical treatments can be used.

Drinking water treatment is directed toward bacterial contamination, which may not be effective for viruses or toxic chemicals. Chlorination creates carcinogens by oxidizing some trace organic chemicals found in surface water. However, we believe that the risk from bacterial diseases far outweighs the added cancer risk. Some alternative treatment methods do not have this risk but are more expensive. There is little routine water-quality monitoring for chemical hazards. There are small expensive devices using reverse osmosis that can be used to purify personal drinking water, but they are impractical for wide use in areas where local drinking-water supplies are contaminated.

Sanitary wastewater treatment is also focused on the presence of pathogenic bacteria and on the large amount of particulate organic matter that requires oxygen in order to decompose. Biological oxidation in standard sewage-treatment plants is the current method of choice. Typically, raw sewage is filtered with coarse screens and passed through settling tanks to remove large particles, which form sludge on the bottom of the tanks. The water phase is then aerated, which produces more particles and sludge. The bacteria are mostly collected in the sludge. The sludge is passed to an anaerobic digester, where more of the oxygen demand is removed and many of the bacteria are killed. The water continues to a trickle filter while a bacterial biofilm (slime) on a solid phase removes much of the remaining organic waste, followed by a sand filter. In some cases, there is a final disinfection tank to minimize releases of viable organisms. These steps constitute tertiary treatment, which can remove almost 100 percent of suspended solids and approximately 99 percent of biological oxygen demand. Additional steps, such as pH control, addition of complexing agents, and air stripping, can remove inorganic and volatile hydrocarbons. Many areas in developing countries do not have any sewage treatment or only primary treatment to remove suspended solids.

The bacteria in digesters are vulnerable to releases of chemical wastes. For example, a chrome-plating shop dumped its acid bath directly into a sanitary sewer and shut down the Salem, Massachusetts, municipal treatment plant, with considerable hazard to workers. The strong acid and toxic metals killed the bacteria and produced a major release of hydrogen sulfide from the sludge and the anaerobic sludge digester. Fortunately, the plant workers escaped without harm when they were warned by alarms from sensors detecting high concentrations of hydrogen sulfide. Several weeks were needed to clean out the system and restart the treatment process, during which raw sewage went into Salem Harbor.

Food Contamination and Sanitation

Food animals and plants can become contaminated by ingestion or absorption of hazardous materials. They can also be contaminated externally by contact with contaminants. Bioaccumulation of aquatic contaminants can be a hazard to humans as well as other animals. Plants can absorb metals, such as lead and cadmium, from the soil. Pesticides can contaminate the surface of food. Many pesticides are biodegradable, but sufficient time and appropriate environmental conditions must occur to reduce pesticide residues to safe levels. Food crops are tested routinely for pesticide levels and other contaminants; there are strict requirements for allowable application levels.

Animal carcasses are visually inspected for quality by government inspectors in many countries. However, the frequency and extent of chemical testing of food items is limited. When testing is done, it is focused on detecting extensive contamination, so limited and localized contamination can easily pass undetected. This situation was highlighted by the testing for mad cow disease in the United States in 2003, when only a few thousand animals were tested out of the millions processed into meat. Testing is expensive and adds to the complexity of the food distribution system for producers. Unless testing is performed by government agencies, it is likely to be very limited.

Contamination of food items by biological agents, such as bacteria and molds, is common and well recognized as a hazard. Most do not produce disease, but some infectious agents may be transmitted by food. Similarly, it is extremely difficult to prevent contamination of food by materials from rodents and insects. Consumers routinely reject food that has visible contamination or has been exposed to insects. Handling and preparing food under sanitary conditions can minimize contamination and subsequent adverse health effects. Many texts extensively discuss foodborne illness and its prevention.

Solid Waste and Land Pollution

The disposal of wastes in landfills ("dumps") has been a widespread and ancient practice of human societies, which includes human wastes, discarded broken implements, and food wastes. Archeologists have developed a set of research tools to gather information from these remnants about how people have lived. As the human population has grown, especially in large cities, the quantity of these wastes has become overwhelming, sparking recycling programs for paper products, plastics, metals, and petroleum products. As our consumer culture has expanded the range of items available to purchase and discard, the complexity and composition of materials in landfills has also expanded. Today's new home computer will be tomorrow's toxic waste because of its guaranteed obsolescence and the exotic toxic materials it contains. Developing societies are experiencing these problems too.

Surface water and groundwater have been contaminated by runoff and leakage from improperly discarded wastes. Although the problem with pathogens from sanitary wastes has been well recognized, the hazard from small amounts of toxic materials in homes, such as mercury and cadmium in batteries, waste paint solvents, home and garden pesticides, and chemical cleaners, has not been recognized. It is easier to recognize the problems from industrial wastes from large producers. In developed countries, there generally are strong regulations to control and limit industrial releases. Most large industries have actively sought to recycle and reclaim wastes. However, that has not been as effective for small businesses because they lack both knowledge about the hazards and resources to control them.

REFERENCES

1. Occupational Safety and Health Administration, U.S. Department of Labor. General industry: OSHA safety and health standards (29 CFR 1910). Washington, DC: U.S. Government Printing Office, 1984.
2. Hawkins NC, Norwood SK, Rock JC. A strategy for occupational exposure assessment. Fairfax, VA: American Industrial Hygiene Association, 1991.
3. Fiserova-Bergerova V. Modeling of inhalation exposure to vapors: Uptake, distribution, and elimination. Boca Raton, FL: CRC Press, 1983.
4. Rappaport SM. Assessment of long-term exposures to toxic substances in air [review]. Ann Occup Hygiene 1991;35:61–121.

BIBLIOGRAPHY

Bingham E, Cohrssen B, Powell CH, Harris RL, eds. Patty's industrial hygiene and toxicology, Fifth edition (13-volume set). New York: Wiley, 2001.

DiNardi S, ed. The industrial environment—Its evaluation and control. Fairfax, VA: American Industrial Hygiene Association (AIHA), 1993.
Two useful and comprehensive general references on industrial hygiene. Patty's, although somewhat unwieldy, is the professional's reference work. A The AIHA volume is very comprehensive but is somewhat uneven in quality.

American Conference of Governmental Industrial Hygienists. Industrial ventilation. 23th ed. Cincinnati: ACGIH, 1999.

Colton CB, Birkner LR, Brosseau L. Respiratory protection—A manual and guideline. Akron: AIHA 1991.

Schwope AD, Costas PP, Jackson JO. Guidelines for selection of chemical protective clothing. Cincinnati: ACGIH, 1987.
Manuals containing recommendations for the design and operation of ventilation systems to control air contaminants, along with other protective approaches.

Burgess WA. Recognition of health hazards in industry: A review of materials and processes. 2nd ed. New York: John Wiley & Sons, 1995.
The source of much of the data in Table 9-1 and a highly recommended reference for all occupational health professionals.

Considine DM. Chemical and process technology encyclopedia. New York: McGraw-Hill, 1974.
Although out-of-date for newer technologies, such as semiconductors or biotechnology, it is a good technical source for gathering background information on basic industries and industrial processes.

Hawkins NC, Norwood SK, Rock JC, eds. A strategy for occupational exposure assessment. Akron: AIHA, 1991.

Rappaport SM. Assessment of long-term exposures to toxic substances in air [review]. Ann Occup Hyg 1991;35: 61–121.
Although these two works contain much useful information, they are difficult to follow in places and require a strong background in statistics. They are important because they lay out the rationale for sampling strategies to determine compliance with OSHA's permissible exposure limits.

OSHA analytical methods manual, part I—Organic substances, Vols. 1–3 (1990); Part 2—Inorganic substances, Vols. 1–2 (1991). Washington, DC: OSHA, U.S. Department of Labor.
Designed for the laboratory chemist and industrial hygienist. New methods are continuously being added and all can be found at the OSHA Web site: www.osha.gov.

World Health Organization, Occupational Hygiene in Europe. Development of the profession. European occupational health series no. 3. Copenhagen, Denmark: WHO Regional Office for Europe, 1992.

Harvey B, Crockford G, Silk S, eds. Handbook of occupational hygiene. Vols. 1–3. London: Crone Publications Ltd, 1992.
These references contain relevant material about exposure standards in Europe and a number of other countries.

Lippmann M, Cohen BS, Schlesinger RB. Environmental health science. New York: Oxford University Press, 2003.

Manahan S. Environmental chemistry. Boca Raton: Lewis Publishers, 1994.
These are two general references on environmental problems with good sections on air, water, and soil pollution and control techniques. The Lippmann book is less technical and more suitable for the nonspecialist.

CHAPTER 10

Safety

Maria J. Brunette

The interaction of the various and complex elements of the work environment exposes workers to situations that might cause them to suffer injuries at work. Safety deals with this interacting relationship and its effects on workers' health and well-being. The evolving and dynamic nature of the work environment and the continuous introduction of new technologies demand that professionals from several disciplines, such as engineering, epidemiology, medicine, sociology, and psychology, work together in promoting safe workplaces for all. This interdisciplinary nature of occupational safety represents an advantage when the goal is to protect workers from harm while making the workplace more efficient and productive.

Preventing fatal and disabling injuries that result from work-related events is one of the major goals in the field of occupational safety. Occupational injuries are acute effects of work-related hazards that occur in real-time. They are caused by the release of, or the contact with, some sort of energy, with observable outcomes. In most of the cases, the sequence of events leading to these injuries can easily be reconstructed, allowing a better understanding of the injury causation process. Sprains, cuts, fractures, and amputations are typical examples of these injuries. (See Box 10-1 for examples of actual occupational incidents leading to fatal and nonfatal injuries.) Considering that injuries are highly preventable, strategic measures should be planned and implemented to manage and control workplace safety hazards and, ultimately, save workers' lives.

Lack of injuries does not necessarily mean working in a safe environment. Safety is more than merely a "noninjury" situation.[1] It needs to be considered proactively, with an approach that goes beyond injury prevention. However, to identify, evaluate, and control the most hazardous work situations, data on injuries provide a clear understanding of the outcomes of these situations.

Injury data can be based on the nature of the injury, such as cut or laceration; the part of the body affected, such as back or finger; or the event or exposure by which the injury occurred, such as a fall from a ladder. In addition, injuries can be categorized as fatal and nonfatal.

Tables 10-1, 10-2, and 10-3 provide information on fatal and nonfatal occupational injuries for 2001 and 2002 (see also Chapter 22). Approximately 25 percent of fatal injuries occurred in the construction sector, where dangerous work is usually performed (Fig. 10-1). In contrast to the striking differences in fatality rates among industrial sectors, there are relatively smaller differences in nonfatal or disabling injuries among industrial sectors. For both fatal and disabling injuries, construction and agriculture are among the three most dangerous sectors.

Many environmental safety hazards exist outside work—at home, in the community, and on the road. Work-related fatalities were only 5 percent of all fatal injuries in the United States in 2001. On average, each hour in the United States, there are 12 unintentional injury deaths per hour: 5 related to motor vehicles, 1 related to work, 4 at home, and 2 in public (Table 10-4).[2]

BOX 10-1

Selected Occupational Incidents

Case 1

Six people were killed by gunfire in an auto parts warehouse after a man described as a disgruntled former employee opened fire with a semiautomatic pistol. The shooter was later killed in a shoot-out with police.[1]

Case 2

A mechanic was working in the grease pit in a repair shop. Due to the cold weather, the doors and windows were closed. A nearby vehicle was left with the engine running. The mechanic was overcome by carbon monoxide, a gas that interferes with the blood's ability to transfer oxygen.[2]

Case 3

An electrician was working on a high-voltage machine while it was "hot" to save time. The screwdriver slipped and shorted between two contact points. The resulting explosion severely burned the electrician, damaged the control box, and shut down part of the manufacturing process.[2]

Case 4

A 22-year-old man was reversing his truck when his brake pedal snapped. His truck continued moving and trapped his left foot against a pillar. He sustained a 4-inch (10-cm) laceration and degloving injury to the sole of his foot, with associated neurological injury. He was treated with cleaning and primary closure of his wound.[3]

Case 5

A 16-year-old was working on a forklift truck unsupervised. He was standing on a pallet supported by the forks, unloading fibrous glass balls. The forks moved upward and he was trapped against the ceiling and suffered asphyxiation due to crushing. He required ventilation for 48 hours to reverse effects of hypoxia, including cerebral edema.[3]

Case 6

A maintenance worker descended alone into a machine pit. Downsizing had ended the practice of entering pits with a partner. His sleeve snagged in an unguarded conveyor belt; he struggled desperately to free himself. It was nearly 3 hours before his screams were heard. The friction from the belt had sanded his arm away, so that even his elbow joint was worn smooth and flat. His arm had to be amputated.[4]

Case 7

Two employees were riding a load, which was tied onto the forks of a forklift. The load was being lifted additionally with the aid of a crane. The men were standing on the load as it was lifted about 23 feet in the air, above packed dirt. The load shifted and slipped off the forks, propelling the two men off the load. One man was seriously injured, but survived; the other died of his injuries.[5]

Case 8

An inventory control person was standing on a step of a portable stairway stand placed against and parallel to a rack containing rolls of carpeting. Another employee was operating a forklift with a pole attached to the front on which had been placed a roll of carpeting. When the forklift operator turned a corner from one aisle to another, the roll caught the rear leg of the stairway stand. This jostled the inventory control worker and he fell 3 feet to the concrete floor, landing on his back, and then his head was injured as it struck the floor. He died 20 days later.[5]

References

1. Disaster News Network. Workplace shooting stuns IL. Available at: <http://www.disasternews.net>.
2. Bird FE, Germain GL. Practical Loss Control Leadership. Loganville, GA: International Loss Control Institute, Inc., 1990.
3. Darcy CM, Lovell ME, Metcalfe JW. Injuries from forklift trucks. Injury 1995;26:285.
4. Death on the Job. PBS online. Available at: <http://www.pbs.org/wgbh/pages/frontline/shows/workplace/mcwane/>.
5. Summaries of selected forklift fatalities investigated by OSHA. Available at: <http://www.osha.gov/dcsp/ote/trng-materials/pit/fatalities_sum.pdf>.

TABLE 10-1

Fatal and Disabling Injuries at Work, Excluding Homicides and Suicides, by Industry Sector, United States, 2001

Industry Sector	Fatal Injuries			Disabling Injuries		
	Number	Rate[a]	Percent	Number	Rate[a]	Percent
Mining/oil and gas extraction	180	31.8	3	20,000	3.5	1
Agriculture/forestry/fishing	700	21.3	13	130,000	4.1	3
Construction	1,210	13.3	23	470,000	5.2	12
Transportation/public utilities	930	11.4	18	410,000	5.0	11
Manufacturing	630	3.3	12	600,000	3.2	15
Government	490	2.4	9	580,000	2.9	15
Wholesale and retail trade	470	1.7	9	740,000	2.7	19
Finance, insurance, real estate	690	1.4	13	950,000	2.0	24
Total	5,300	3.9	100	3,900,000	2.9	100

[a] Rate per 100,000 workers.
From National Safety Council. Injury facts®. Itasca, IL: NSC, 2002.

SOCIAL AND ECONOMIC COSTS OF INJURIES

Measuring the cost of work injuries is complex. Although there is no generally accepted methodology to do so, it has been estimated that occupational injuries are responsible for more lost time from work and more lost work productivity than any other threats to health, including cancer and cardiovascular disease. The economic costs of both fatal and nonfatal injuries include both direct and indirect costs. Lost wages, medical expenses, and workers' compensation premiums and other insurance costs are examples of direct costs. Indirect costs, often difficult to define, make work-related injuries more expensive. These include the costs to train and compensate replacement workers, repair damaged property, investigate accidents, implement corrective action, and maintain insurance coverage. Other indirect costs are related to schedule delays, added administrative time, lower morale, increased absenteeism, higher turnover, and poorer customer relations. Work-related injuries have many consequences to those injured, their family members, their employers, and the economy (Fig. 10-2).[3] Although there are research methods and techniques for calculating economic costs, there are few to explore the indirect costs of work-related injuries and their social impact. Integrated research in this area is in its infancy.

WHY INCIDENTS HAPPEN: CAUSATION THEORIES

Occupational injuries result from multiple causes. In the past, many theories about the causes of occupational incidents focused on the worker. However, it is now recognized that the interaction of various personal and workplace factors produces hazardous situations and resultant incidents and injuries. Any strategy for control and prevention should consider these factors and their interaction. Workplace factors that might contribute to traumatic injuries include hazardous exposures, workplace and process design, work organization and environment, and economics. Among the theories describing the relationship between these factors are the domino theory, the energy-transfer theory, the accident/incident theory, the systems theory, and the behavioral theory—although no one prediction theory of accident causation has been universally accepted.

Domino Theory

Herbert W. Heinrich proposed, in the 1920s, that the sequence of events leading up to an accident include five factors represented in a series of aligned toppling dominos: (a) a person's social environment, where character traits are developed; (b) undesirable traits, such as recklessness, nervousness,

TABLE 10-2

Fatal Workplace Injuries, by Event or Exposure, United States, 2002

Event or Exposure	Number	Percent
Transportation incidents	2,381	43
Highway	1,372	25
Nonhighway (farm and industrial)	322	6
Aircraft	192	3
Worker struck by a vehicle	356	6
Water vehicle	71	1
Rail vehicle	64	1
Assaults and violent acts	840	15
Homicides	609	11
Self-inflicted injuries	199	2
Contact with objects and equipment	873	16
Struck by object	506	9
Caught in or compressed by equipment or objects	231	4
Caught in or crushed in collapsing materials	116	2
Falls	714	13
Fall to lower level	634	11
Fall on same level	63	1
Exposure to harmful substances or environments	538	10
Contact with electrical current	289	5
Contact with temperature extremes	60	1
Exposure to caustic, noxious, or allergenic substances	98	2
Oxygen deficiency	90	2
Fires and explosion	165	3
Other events or exposures	13	
Total	5,524*	100*

*Total represents sum of major categories of events/exposures.
From Bureau of Labor Statistics. National census of fatal occupational injuries in 2002. Washington, DC: Bureau of Labor Statistics, 2003.

violent temper, or lack of safety knowledge; (c) unsafe acts of workers or hazardous conditions at work, such as those due to mechanical or physical hazards; (d) the accident; and (e) the injury. The domino theory proposed that removal or control of these contributing factors, especially unsafe acts or hazardous conditions, could prevent accidents and injuries.

Energy-Transfer Theory

In 1970, William Haddon, Jr., proposed an accident causation theory that proposed that accidents and injuries involve the transfer of energy. Haddon suggested that the kind and severity of injuries are directly related to their corresponding quantities of energy, means of energy transfer, and rates of energy transfer. This theory, also known as the *energy-release theory*, proposes an accident prevention scheme in which measures to prevent accidents should be established simultaneously at the source of energy (engineering controls to eliminate the source), the path (enclosure of the path, such as with machine guarding), and the receiver (appropriate use of personal protective equipment). This parallel approach of accident prevention differs from the series approach, previously suggested by Heinrich.[4]

TABLE 10-3

Nonfatal Occupational Injuries Involving Days Away from Work, by Nature of Injury and Frequent Occupations, United States, 2000

Nature of Injury	Nonfatal Cases	Percent	Frequent Occupations
Sprain, strains	728,202	44	Materials handlers, miners, baggage handlers, mail handlers, construction workers
Fractures	116,713	7	Materials handlers, miners, construction workers
Cuts, lacerations, punctures	141,649	9	Sheet-metal workers, butchers, press operators, sawyers, fabric cutters
Bruises, contusions	151,680	9	Materials handlers, any workers exposed to low-energy impacts
Heat (thermal) burns	24,298	1	Foundry workers, smelter workers, welders, glass workers, laundry workers
Chemical burns	9,395	1	Masons, process workers, hazardous-waste workers
Amputations	9,658	1	Press operators, butchers, machine operators
Other nonfatal injuries[a]	482,423	29	
Total	1,664,018	101*	

*Because of rounding of component categories, sum of percents is 101.
[a] Includes carpal tunnel syndrome, tendonitis, soreness/pain, and multiple injuries.
From National Safety Council. Injury facts®. Itasca, IL: NSC, 2002; and Jovanovic J, Arandelovic M, Jovanovic M. Multidisciplinary aspects of occupational accidents and injuries. Working and Living Environmental Protection 2004;2:325–33.

Accident/Incident Theory

This theory, also known as the *Petersen accident/incident theory*, establishes that accidents and injuries are caused by two major components: human error and systems failure. Three broad factors leading to human error are:

- *Overload*: Too much pressure, physical and mental fatigue, lack of motivation.
- *Ergonomic traps*: Incompatible workstation or extreme physical workload.
- *Decision to err*: "It won't happen to me" syndrome.

An important contribution of this theory is the inclusion of the systems failure factors—policy, responsibility, training, inspection, and standards—in the causal path of accidents, as it makes clear the role that management has in injury prevention.[5]

Systems Theory (The Balance Theory)

The balance theory, proposed by Michael J. Smith and Pascale Carayon-Sainfort, is used to analyze different elements of the work system and their interrelations and outcomes.[6] This theory analyzes the work system and its five subsystems: (a) organization, (b) tasks, (c) tools and technologies, (d) physical environment, and (e) the person. Each one of these factors has specific characteristics than can influence exposure to hazards and injury potential.[7] The balance theory states that an element in the system will influence any other element, originating a continuous interplay among elements (*systems-balance principle*). At the same time, interactive effects can cause or mitigate exposures, so "positive" aspects of the system could compensate for "negative" aspects (*compensatory balance principle*). For example, having a good relationship with one's supervisor, considered as a positive element in the system, could be used to overcome some adverse aspects perceived by workers, such as inflexible working schedules.

Behavioral Theory

This theory, also known as *behavior-based safety* (BBS), applies behavioral theories from psychology to occupational safety. It promotes the idea that the behavior of workers is the most important determinant for their safety, and consequently positive reinforcement, such as incentives and rewards, could be used to promote the desired (safe)

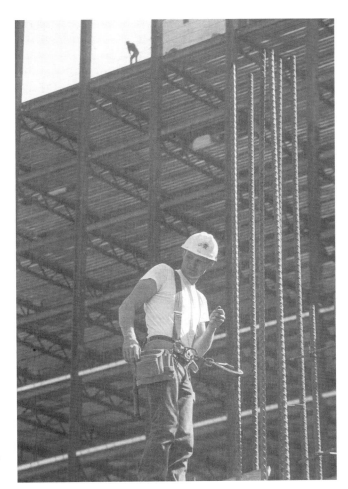

FIGURE 10-1 ● Construction is one of the most dangerous industries and accounts for 20 percent of all work-related deaths in the United States. (Photo: Construction worker in Chicago. Used with permission from ILO, ® International Labour Organization/Jacques Maillar.)

TABLE 10-4

Principal Classes of Unintentional-Injury Deaths, 2001

Class	Number	Rate[a]
Motor vehicle	42,900	15.4
Work	5,300	1.9
Home	33,200	12.0
Public nonmotor vehicle	19,000	6.8
Total[b]	98,000	35.3

[a] Per 100,000 population.
[b] Excludes duplications among motor vehicle, work, and home deaths.
From National Safety Council. Injury facts®. Itasca, IL: NSC, 2002.

behaviors and to discourage undesirable (unsafe) behaviors.[5] Major criticism of this theory is that behavior alone cannot make a dangerous job safe. Incentives aimed at enhancing employee awareness and motivation, such as annual safety awards dinners and annual safety contests, are not very effective in influencing worker "safe" behavior or company safety performance. The relationship between these incentives to actual safety hazards and considerations is unclear to the extent that workers are not able to translate the reward to specific actions that need to be taken.[7]

OCCUPATIONAL SAFETY HAZARDS

This section describes exposures to safety hazards at work and measures to prevent them. These hazards include those caused by walking and

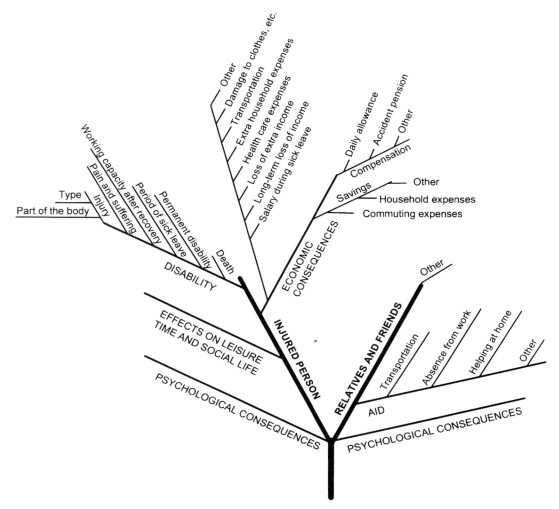

FIGURE 10-2 ● The accident consequence tree: Consequence of injuries to individuals. (From Aaltonen MVP, Uusi-Rauva E, Saari J, et al. The accident consequence tree method and its application by real-time data collection in the Finnish furniture industry. Safety Sci 1996;23:11–26.)

working surfaces; mechanical hazards; materials handling; electrical hazards; confined space hazards; and workplace violence.

Walking and Working Surfaces Hazards

A *walking and working surface* is "any surface, whether horizontal or vertical, on which an employee walks or works, including but not limited to floors, roofs, ramps, bridges, runways, formwork, and concrete-reinforcing steel. It does not include ladders, vehicles, or trailers on which employees must be located to perform their work duties."[8] Standing, walking, working, and climbing

at work are associated with slips, trips, and fall-related events—accounting for a substantial portion of occupational injuries and deaths. In 2002, for example, 13 percent of all the fatalities at work were related to falls. Although many fall-related cases are fatal, nonfatal falls often lead to extremely severe injuries. The problem is greater in specific industries. In construction, for example, falls from heights are the leading cause of deaths accounting for 31 percent of deaths.[9] Two fall-related incidents described in Box 10-2 indicate the severity of the problem for a residential construction contractor and a carpenter.

Trips occur when workers encounter unseen foreign objects in their path that interrupts the motion

---

BOX 10-2

Fall-Related Fatal Incidents

Self-Employed Residential Contractor Dies in 10-Foot Fall Through Floor Opening on Construction Site

A 39-year-old male self-employed residential construction contractor was fatally injured when he fell 10 feet through a floor opening and strock his head on the concrete chimney footing below. The victim was working with a co-worker to true up the gable end of the second floor of a single family home under construction. The victim was holding a level to the gable end wall when he apparently stepped backwards into the opening in the floor intended for a chimney. Two laborers were on the second-floor level with the victim: one went to assist the victim while the other laborer went to call for emergency assistance. The victim was transported to a local hospital, where he was pronounced dead.[1]

Carpenter Dies in Fall Through Wall Opening in Factory Renovation Site

A 33-year-old male carpenter was fatally injured when he fell through the open side of the third floor of a structure being renovated from a factory into an office building. The victim was working with two co-workers to place a 300-lb wooden box beam onto the roof 8.5 feet above the floor using a manual hoist. The hoist mechanism let go, allowing the beam to fall, striking the victim and pushing him out the opening. He fell approximately 22.5 feet to the ground below, sustaining severe head injuries. The victim was transported to a nearby hospital where he never regained consciousness and died 2 days later of his injuries.[2]

References

1. OSHA Regional News Release. Conveyor hazards at Worcester, Massachusetts, CVS Pharmacy leads to nearly $62,000 in OSHA fines. January 7, 2003.
2. OSHA Regional News Release. Amputation of worker's arm by unguarded conveyor at Milan, N.H. lumber mill leads to $49,000 OSHA fine. June 9, 2003.

---

of their feet. Slips occur when workers' feet unexpectedly slide on a surface. Slips can cause strains to muscles and joints, even if a fall does not occur. If the expected resistance between the floor (or another surface) and the worker' shoes is not present or sufficient, then a slip might occur. The resistance of one surface, such as a shoe, against another, such as a floor, is measured by the coefficient of friction (μ). A coefficient of 0.5 defines a safe level of shoe/floor resistance. Whereas a higher value is considered slip-resistant, lower values are related to different levels of slippery surfaces. There is also an increased chance for slipping when changes in floor conditions occur, such as moving from a dry surface to a wet one. Basic measures that can make walking and working surfaces safe include:

- Good housekeeping, such as by keeping surfaces clean and dry especially around machinery and equipment where spills may occur
- Use of warning signs, such as by marking areas being mopped
- Proper selection of shoe, such as by use of nonskid footwear

- Surface materials and floor finishes, such as abrasive coatings
- Proper illumination, such as by additional lights on stairs
- Effective use of painting in hazardous locations
- Use of safety mats and abrasive strips.

Many falls that occur on floors at the same level do not have fatal consequences, but they often cause injury. When a worker falls to a lower level, such as from ladders, scaffolds, elevated structures, a severe or fatal injury will likely occur. Falls from as little as 4 to 6 feet above the floor or ground can cause serious lost-time incidents and even deaths. The number of fatal injuries due to falls to a lower level in the United States is more than 10 times higher than the ones on the same level.[10] Fall prevention is critical among some industries, such as construction, where almost all the falls occurring to a lower level result in fatalities (98 percent).

Fall protection is needed in walkways and ramps, open sides and edges, roofs, wall openings, floor holes, concrete forms and rebar, excavations, and bricklaying. Table 10-5 provides information

TABLE 10-5

Preventing Falls and Injuries: Objectives and Methods

Objective	Method
To prevent falls of people	Remove tripping and slipping hazards
	Protect edges and openings
	Provide barriers (such as guardrails, covers, and cages)
	Provide visual and auditory warnings
	Provide grab bars, handrails, and handholds
	Provide fall-limiting equipment
To prevent objects from falling on people	Housekeeping (remove objects that could fall)
	Barriers (such as toe boards, guardrails, and covers)
	Proper stacking and placement
	Fall zone
	Overhead protection
To reduce energy levels	Reduce fall distances
	Reduce weight of falling objects
To reduce injuries from falls and impact	Increase area of impact force
	Increase energy absorption distance

From Brauer RL. Safety and health for engineers. New York: Van Nostrand Reinhold, 1990.

on the basic objectives to prevent falls at work and corresponding methods for prevention. The most common methods for preventing people from falling are barriers (such as guardrails), fall-limiting devices (such as safety nets), and personal fall arrest systems. These fall protection systems must be in place before work starts. Workers should be trained to recognize hazards of falling and to follow procedures to minimize these hazards. Other important hazards from walking and working surfaces are those related to the use of stairs, ramps, ladders, and scaffolds. Proper design, adequate housekeeping, good lighting, provision of handrails, and frequent inspection could help decrease potential for falls.

Mechanical Hazards

Exposure to mechanical hazards derived from any machine part, function, or process might cause serious injuries. Safeguarding machines is essential for protecting workers from exposure to these hazards. The basic goal of machine guarding is to prevent machines from doing to a worker what they are supposed to do to materials—cut, tear, shear, puncture, and crush—and to prevent machine–operator contact. Even though innovative technology to guard machines has been developed, mechanical haz-

ards remain a major concern. In the United States, workers who operate and maintain machinery suffer approximately 18,000 amputations, lacerations, crushing injuries, and abrasions every year. Eight hundred deaths occur annually, and many of the nonfatal injuries result in permanent disability. Unfortunately, machine guarding and related machinery violations continue to rank among the most frequent Occupational Safety and Health Administration (OSHA) citations (Box 10-3). Mechanical hazards are found at the machine point of operation—the point where work is performed on the material, such as cutting; any machinery part that moves, such as flywheels, pulleys, belts, couplings, chains, and gears; feeding mechanisms and auxiliary parts; in-running nip points; and flying objects. Moving and rotating parts, such as belts and pulleys, are generally easier to guard than the point of operation, and their access is usually limited to maintenance operations. In-running (or ongoing) nip points, which are pinch points created by the rotation of machine parts toward each other or toward a fixed component, can cause injury by catching loose clothing and pulling a worker into the machine (Box 10-3). Mechanical hazards from flying objects relate to chips or sparks thrown from the area of the point of operation and to the

---

BOX 10-3

Unguarded Machinery, Workers' Injuries, and Willful Violations

A conveyor belt used to move product between the basement and a first-floor storage area lacked guarding to prevent employees from coming in contact with its pinch points, resulting in more than $60,000 in fines from OSHA. Having workers exposed to possible fractures and crushing injuries due to unguarded conveyor belts was not a first-time event. It was found that the company, cited for an alleged willful violation, had two workers injured by unguarded machinery in previous months. In addition, workers did not receive training in how to prevent accidental start-up of the conveyor belt while clearing product jams, and there were no written instructions for doing so. OSHA cited the company for an

alleged willful violation and fined it more than $60,000.[1]

A material-handling conveyor that was not properly guarded caused the amputation of a worker's arm at a lumber mill when his shirt became caught between the unguarded drive chain and sprocket wheels of the operating conveyor and he was pulled into the machinery. The company had previously been cited for unguarded chains and sprockets on other machinery. OSHA cited the company for an alleged willful violation and fined it $49,000.[2]

References

1. NIOSH. Fatality Assessment and Control Evaluation (FACE) report 1999–22. Morgantown, WV: NIOSH, 2004.
2. NIOSH. Fatality Assessment and Control Evaluation (FACE) State Program: Massachusetts Report 1997-050-01. Morgantown, WV: NIOSH, 2004.

---

potential breaking of machine parts or products being manufactured that could fall on or be thrown at the operator.

Machines can be made safe by guards and devices. Guards prevent access of the worker's hands, fingers, or other body parts to the danger zone during machine operation. They also protect against falling objects by shielding the moving parts of machines from falling objects. Where possible, guards should be a permanent part of the machine or equipment while not interfering with operation. Safe guards should also be durable and strong enough to resist the anticipated wear and tear. Their design should allow for safe inspection and maintenance activities, such as lubrication, adjustment, and repair, to be performed without removing the guard. Provision of machine guards must not create additional hazards, such as new pinch points.

Some types of devices restrain worker's hands, fingers, or other body parts from inadvertently reaching into the point of operation, and others prevent machine operation by breaking or shutting it down so the machine does not cycle. Two types of devices are illustrated in Fig. 10-3. A two-hand control device keeps operator hands at a predetermined safe location—on control buttons—far enough from the danger area while the machine completes its closing cycle. A self-feeding device

also ensures proper distance between the worker and the hazards at the point of operation. Major disadvantages of these devices are

- The possibility of being easily rendered or blocked by the workers, such as in a two-hand control button device where a worker could hold one button with an arm;
- Potential obstruction of the workspace around the worker (Fig. 10-3B); and
- The need for frequent inspection and regular maintenance.

Accidental or inadvertent energizing of a machine or equipment while performing service or maintenance tasks is one of the main causes of machine-related incidents. In order to prevent injury to workers, lockout/tagout procedures disable machines by an energy-isolated device that prevents unexpected energization, start up, or release of stored (and hazardous) energy. Energy-isolating devices are mechanical devices that physically prevent the transmission or release of energy, including manually operated electrical circuit breakers, disconnect switches, line valves, and blocks. Lockout/tagout procedures ensure that the machine or equipment being controlled does not operate until the lockout or tagout device is removed (Fig. 10-4). A lockout procedure involves the placement of a

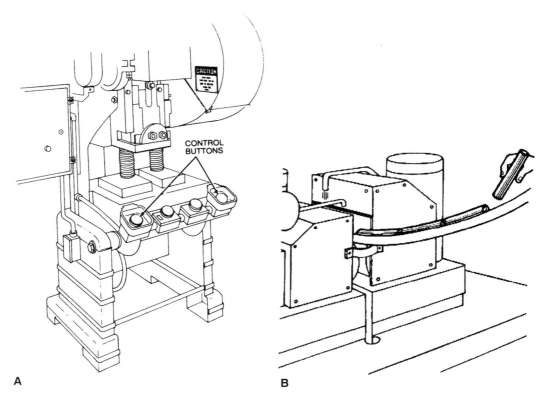

A   **B**

FIGURE 10-3 ● Machine safeguarding: (**A**) Two-hand control buttons ensure that the operator's hands are at a safe location (on control buttons) and at a safe distance from the danger area before the machine cycle is started (From Occupational Safety and Health Administration. Concepts and techniques of machine safeguarding. Publication No. OSHA 3067. Washington, DC: U.S. Department of Labor, Occupational Safety and Health Administration, 1992 revised). (**B**) A machine with self-feeding device keeps the operator's hands away from dangerous parts of the machinery. (From International Labor Organization and the International Ergonomics Association. Ergonomics checkpoints: Practical and easy to implement solutions for improving safety, health and working conditions. Geneva: International Labor Office, 1999.)

lockout device, such as a padlock, on an energy-isolating device. A tagout procedure establishes the placement of a warning device, such as a tag, that is securely fastened to an energy-isolating device and indicates that the machine or equipment must not be operated. Lockout/tagout devices should be

- *Durable*: The means of attachment must be sturdy enough to prevent inadvertent removal.
- *Standardized*: Devices must have the same color, shape, or size and the format of tags should be standardized.
- *Identifiable*: Tags must identify the worker who applies them and must warn against hazardous conditions if the machine is energized.

Effective initial training and periodic training are critical to ensure workers understand lockout/tagout procedures.

Safety responsibilities regarding machine guarding and lockout/tagout need to be shared by managers, supervisors, and workers. Managers must ensure that all machinery and equipment is properly guarded. Supervisors must train workers on specific machine guarding rules in their work areas, ensure that guards remain in place and are properly working, and, when needed, immediately correct any deficiencies. Workers should not remove guards unless machines are properly locked and tagged, should not operate equipment unless guards are in place, and should immediately report machine guarding problems to supervisors.

Materials-Handling Hazards

Materials handling is the movement of raw materials, semifinished products, and finished products

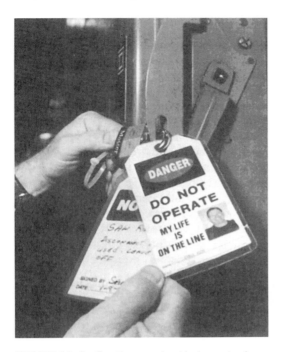

FIGURE 10-4 ● Three workers' locks are in place on this machine power switch. All must remove their locks before the machine can be started. (From Occupational Safety and Health Administration. Concepts and techniques of machine guarding. Publication No. OSHA 3067. Washington, DC: Occupational Safety and Health Administration, 1980:60.)

within a plant. Industry moves about 50 tons of material for each ton of product. Lifting, the most basic material handling activity, can be performed manually or assisted by mechanical aids, such as industrial trucks, tractors, or cranes. Although manual material handling has been replaced increasingly more often by the use of mechanized lifting and transport equipment, manual handling operations are performed in most industrial plants.

Hazards derived from materials handling activities include sprains and muscle strains from improper manual lifting. Objects and loads may fall and pinch, fracture, sever, or crush workers' hands, feet, and legs. A moving part of a processing machine can strike a worker, resulting in a severe injury. Speed and mass of the materials and equipment may also contribute to serious injuries. Workers may injure themselves and others by operating equipment too quickly. Workers may be run over by powered vehicles. Failure of lifting equipment, such as a chain of a lifting device, may also lead to injuries.

Measures to prevent materials handling injuries vary and depend on the type of lifting and carrying activity, the machine or equipment being used, and the characteristics of the materials or load, such as weight, size, and shape. In general, they include:

- The reduction, or elimination if possible, of manual material-handling steps (mechanical handling is preferred).
- Selection of appropriate equipment, such as adequate loading capacity in a vehicle.
- Proper and safe use of equipment and tools, such as proper steering of a vehicle.
- Adequate worker training on the recognition of hazards derived from the equipment, such as learning to judge the stability of a vehicle.
- Control of environment factors, such as housekeeping, poor lighting, visibility problems, weather changes, and surface conditions. A proper design of the work area will provide a better access to the load being moved, with aisles clear of obstacles and signs posted where needed (Fig. 10-5).

Powered industrial trucks (PITs) are power-propelled trucks used to carry, push, pull, lift, stack, or tier materials. Known as forklifts, pallet trucks, rider trucks, or lift trucks, they are very commonly used for lifting and transporting materials in manufacturing plants, warehouses, and freight-handling terminals. Forklift trucks, the most common type of PIT, cause more than 90 deaths and an estimated 90,000 nonfatal incidents in the United States each year. Forklift hazards include pedestrian traffic, poor workstation design, slippery surfaces, vehicle overloading and stability, excessive driving speed, steering problems, lack of knowledge and training of the driver, visibility problems, and vehicle condition (see Cases 5, 7, and 8 in Box 10-1). Basic guidelines for the safe use of forklifts include proper training of the forklift operator, correct loading and unloading procedures, routine checks, never leaving a forklift unattended, repairs and maintenance, watching for pedestrians, care on ramps, and keeping the work area organized and clean (see Fig. 10-5).

Electrical Hazards

Electrical incidents cause nearly one fatality every day in the United States and more than half of these deaths are in the construction industry. Electricity is the flow of energy (electrons) from one place to

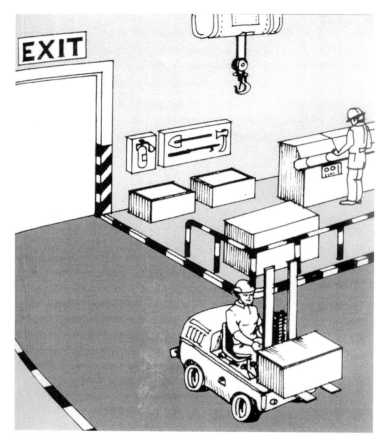

FIGURE 10-5 ● Materials handling. (From International Labor Organization and the International Ergonomics Association. Ergonomics checkpoints: Practical and easy to implement solutions for improving safety, health and working conditions. Geneva: International Labor Office, 1999.)

another that travels in a closed circuit via an electrically conductive material. Most electrical injuries are attributed to electrocution, electrical shocks, and electrical burns. Electrical shocks and burns do not occur as frequently as many other types of occupational injuries, but they are disproportionately fatal. Electrical shocks occur when the human body becomes part of the path through which current flows, such as by touching a live wire and an electrical ground. Electrocution can be the direct result of an electrical shock. It takes very little electricity to cause harm. The severity of the electric shock depends on the path, amount, and duration of the shocking current through the body. While a current as little as 3 mA (milliamperes) will cause a painful shock, a fatal shock might occur with currents between 100 mA and 4 A (amperes). More than 4 A will cause severe burns and cardiac arrest. Burns, the most common shock-related injury, occur when a person touches electrical wiring or equipment that is improperly used or maintained. Typically, burns occur on hands causing serious injury that demands immediate attention. Workers in elevated work surfaces who receive an electric shock may fall, suffering additional serious or fatal injury. Electricity is also a common cause of fires and explosions. The most frequent electrical hazards found at the workplace include contact with power lines, lack of ground-fault protection, the path to ground missing or being discontinuous, equipment not being used in the manner prescribed (including inadvertent activation of equipment), improper use of extension and flexible cords, and ignition of combustible materials. Most fatal electrical incidents are (a) installation and maintenance not involving power lines; (b) incidental contact of an overhead power line with a handheld object; (c) incidental contact of an overhead power line through mobile equipment; (d) incidental contact with energized circuits other than overhead or buried power lines; and (e) installation and maintenance work on power lines.[11]

Grounding and bonding can prevent electrical injuries. Grounding allows one or more charged bodies to have a conductor between them and connect to an electrical ground. It ensures a path to the earth from the flow of excess current. Bonding is the process where two bodies have a conductor between them and the charge between them is equalized. Other basic controls include:

- Proper use of cords including three wire cords (a hot wire, a neutral wire [grounded conductor], and a ground wire [grounding conductor]) and cords marked for hard or extrahard usage.
- Isolating electrical parts (such as with electrical panels) by using guards or barriers to prevent passage through areas of exposed energized equipment.
- Recognizing and using proper lockout and tagout procedures.
- Avoiding wet conditions and overhead power lines.
- Use and placement of adequate warning signs.

- Implementing training procedures in working with electric equipment and safe work practices.
- Use of appropriate protective equipment, such as proper foot protection, rubber insulating gloves and hoods, and insulated-nonconductive hard hats.

Confined Space Hazards

Confined spaces are enclosed areas that have limited or restricted means of entry or exit. These spaces are not designed for permanent occupancy and require special procedures to ensure that the workers are safe while entering and working in them. Typical confined spaces include tanks, manholes, boilers, silos, vaults, trenches and pits (Box 10-4). Work in confined or enclosed spaces is dangerous. It is not unusual for an untrained worker to use inadequate

---

BOX 10-4

Typical Confined Spaces in the Construction Industry

Condenser Pits

A common confined space found in the construction of nuclear power plants is the condenser pit, which is often overloaded because of its large size. This below-grade area creates a large containment area for the accumulation of toxic fumes and gases, or for the creation of oxygen-deficient atmospheres when purging with argon, freon, and other inert gases. Additional hazards may be created by workers above dropping equipment, tools, and materials into the pit.

Containment Cavities

These large below-grade areas are characterized by little or no air movement. Ventilation is always a problem. In addition, there is a possibility of oxygen deficiency. Welding and other gases may easily collect in these areas, creating toxic atmospheres. As these structures near completion, more confined spaces will exist as rooms are built off the existing structure.

Heat Sinks

These larger pit areas hold cooling water in the event that there is a problem with the pumps located at the water supply to the plant—normally a river or lake, which would prevent cooling water from reaching the reactor core. When in the pits, workers are exposed to welding fumes and electrical hazards, particularly because water accumulates in the bottom of the sink. Generally, it is difficult to communicate with workers in the heat sink, because the rebar in the walls of the structure deadens radio signals.

Manholes

Throughout the construction site, manholes are a necessary means of entry into and exit from vaults, tanks, and pits. However, these confined spaces may present serious hazards that could cause injuries and fatalities. A manhole could be a dangerous trap into which the worker could fall; often, covers are not provided or are removed and not replaced.

Pipe Assemblies

Piping of 16 to 32 in. in diameter is commonly used for a variety of purposes. For any number

(continued)

BOX 10-4

Typical Confined Spaces in the Construction Industry (Continued)

of reasons, workers enter this piping. Once inside, they are faced with potential oxygen-deficient atmospheres, often caused by purging with argon or another inert gas. Welding fumes generated by workers in the pipe, or by other workers operating outside the pipe at either end, subject the worker to toxic atmospheres. The generally restricted dimensions of the pipe provide little room for the workers to move about and gain any degree of comfort while performing their tasks. Once inside the pipe, communication is extremely difficult. In situations where the pipe bends, communication and extrication become even more difficult. Electrical shock is another potential hazard, due to ungrounded tools and equipment or inadequate line cords. Heat within the pipe run may cause the worker to suffer heat prostration.

Sumps

Sumps are used as collection places for water and other liquids. Workers entering sumps may encounter an oxygen-deficient atmosphere. Because of the wet nature of the sump, electrical shock represents a hazard when power tools are used inside. Sumps are often poorly illuminated. Inadequate lighting may create a safety hazard.

Tanks

Tanks are used for many purposes, including the storage of water and chemicals. Tanks require entry for cleaning and repairs. Ventilation is always a problem. Oxygen-deficient

atmospheres, along with toxic and explosive atmospheres created by the substances stored in the tanks, present hazards to workers. Heat, another problem in tanks, may cause heat prostration, particularly on a hot day. Because electrical line cords are often taken into the tank, electrical shock is always a potential hazard. The nature of the tank's structure often dictates that workers must climb ladders to reach high places on the walls of the tank.

Vaults

A variety of vaults are found on the construction site. Workers often enter these vaults to perform a number of tasks. The restricted nature of vaults and their frequently below-grade location can create a variety of safety and health problems.

Ventilation Ducts

Ventilation ducts are sheet-metal enclosures that create a complex network that moves heated and cooled air and exhaust fumes to desired locations in the workplace. Ventilation ducts may require that workers enter them to cut out access holes, install essential parts of the duct, and so forth. Depending on where these ducts are located, oxygen deficiency could exist. The ducts usually possess many bends, which create difficult entry and exit and which also make it difficult for workers inside the duct to communicate with those outside it. Electrical shock hazards and heat stress are other problems associated with work inside ventilation ducts.

From OSHA. Anatomy of confined spaces in construction. Washington, DC: Construction Safety and Health Outreach Program, 1996.

equipment to attempt to rescue a co-worker from a confined space; when the impulsive rescue attempt fails, both workers become trapped and die. More than half of the deaths in confined spaces are of attempted rescuers.

In confined spaces, oxygen-deficient atmospheres (with oxygen concentrations lower than 19.5 percent) may lead to loss of consciousness and death; oxygen-enriched atmospheres (with oxygen concentrations greater than 23 percent) may cause

flammable and combustible materials to ignite very quickly and burn. Presence of combustible gases and liquids, such as methane, hydrogen, acetylene, propane, and gasoline fumes, and of toxic materials, such as hydrogen sulfide, carbon monoxide, and welding fumes, is also considered a problem associated with confined spaces. Other hazards include pressurized atmospheres that might cause injury if opened, mechanical hazards from related equipment such as mixers and crushers, hazards derived from electrical equipment, and engulfment hazards where workers could die from asphyxia or by being crushed by sand, grain, or other granular materials.

Hazards can be first avoided by evaluating the hazards of the confined space prior to entry. Workers might accomplish this by checking the atmosphere inside the confined space by appropriate devices and continually monitoring it during work; by providing proper and continuous ventilation, either natural or mechanical; by properly purging toxic vapors and other toxic substances; and by checking that access and exit equipment such as ladders and steps are in good working conditions. Workers should also be provided and properly trained in the use of personal protective equipment

(Fig. 10-6) and should have a contingency plan including provisions for appropriate equipment and backup assistance. This plan should be developed by the workers, and rescuers should be briefed before the job begins.

Workplace Violence

Workplace violence—violent acts, including physical assaults and threats of assault, directed toward persons at work or on duty—has been recently recognized as a major problem nationwide (Box 10-5). Every year in the United States, more than 2 million workers suffer from nonfatal assaults. Police officers, taxi drivers, and health care,

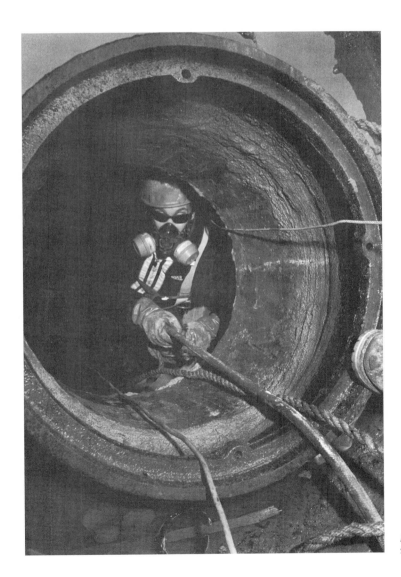

FIGURE 10-6 ● Confined space. (Photograph by Earl Dotter.)

BOX 10-5

Violence in the Workplace: Types and Vulnerable Occupations

Type I: Criminal Intent

The perpetrator has no legitimate relationship to the business or its employees and is usually committing a crime in conjunction with the violence, such as robbery, shoplifting, and trespassing. The vast majority of workplace homicides (85 percent) fall into this category. Convenience store clerks, taxi drivers, security guards, and proprietors of "mom-and-pop" stores are all examples of the kind of workers who are at higher risk for Type I workplace violence.

Type II: Customer/Client

The perpetrator has a legitimate relationship with the business and becomes violent while being served by the business—during the course of a normal transaction. This category includes customers, clients, patients, students, inmates, and any other individuals for which the business provides services. Many customer/client incidents occur in health care, in settings such as nursing homes or psychiatric facilities; the victims are often patient caregivers. Police officers, prison staff members, flight attendants, and teachers are some other examples of types of workers who may be exposed to this kind of workplace violence.

Type III: Worker-on-Worker

The perpetrator is an employee or past employee of the business who attacks or threatens another employee(s) or past employee(s) in the workplace. In some cases, these incidents occur after a series of increasingly hostile behaviors from the perpetrator. Worker-on-worker assault is often the first type of workplace violence that comes to mind for many people, possibly because some of these incidents receive extensive media coverage, leading the public to assume that most workplace violence falls into this category. Worker-on-worker fatalities account for approximately 7 percent of all workplace violence homicides. There do not appear to be any kinds of occupations or industries that are more or less prone to Type III violence. Some of these incidents appear to be motivated by disputes.

Type IV: Personal Relationship

The perpetrator usually does not have a relationship with the business but has a personal relationship with the intended victim—almost always a female. This category includes victims of domestic violence who are assaulted or threatened while at work. (Occasionally, the abuser—who usually has no working relationship to the victim's employer—will appear at the workplace to engage in hostile behavior.) There are many adverse effects of domestic violence perpetrated in the workplace.

From Lovelace L, ed. Workplace violence: A report to the nation, 2001. Iowa City, IA: University of Iowa Injury Prevention Research Center, 2001.

---

community services, and retail workers are among the most vulnerable occupations (Table 10-6). In addition to injuries and homicide, violence at the workplace can lead to a wide range of negative effects, including anxiety, fears, depression, psychosomatic complaints, and an overall climate of distrust.

One of the first widely reported cases of workplace violence took place in Oklahoma in 1986, when a part-time letter carrier with a troubled work history and facing possible dismissal walked into the post office where he worked and shot 14 people to death before killing himself. Since then, workplace violence has markedly increased. In 2002, for example, assaults and violent acts accounted for 15 percent of occupational fatalities, ranking it as the third most prevalent cause of work-related deaths, after motor vehicle crashes and machine-related injuries.[12] Recent major workplace homicides in the United States have included four co-workers killed by a 66-year-old former forklift driver (Chicago, 2001); three killed by an insurance executive (New York City, 2002); three killed by a plant worker at a manufacturing plant

TABLE 10-6

Violent Victimization in the Workplace, by High-Risk Occupation, United States, 1993–1999

Occupation	Number	Average Annual Rate[a]
Police officer	1,380,400	260.8
Corrections officer	277,100	155.7
Taxi-cab driver	84,400	128.3
Private security officer	369,300	86.6
Bartender	170,600	81.6
Mental health custodian	60,400	69.0
Special education teacher	102,000	68.4
Gas station worker	86,900	68.3
Mental health professional	290,000	68.2
Junior high teacher	321,300	54.2
Convenience store worker	336,800	53.9

[a] Per 1,000 workers.
From Bureau of Justice Statistics. Violence in the workplace, 1993–1999. Washington, DC: BJS, 2001.

(Missouri, 2003); and six killed by a plant worker at an aircraft plant (Mississippi, 2003).[13] Although these cases reveal how severe the problem might be (Fig. 10-7), they represent only a very small fraction of workplace assaults that occur daily. Violence in the workplace includes not only assaults but also domestic violence, stalking, threats, harassment, bullying, and physical and emotional abuse—the magnitude of which is difficult to assess due to underreporting and other factors.

More research on and prevention of workplace violence are needed. A proactive approach to minimize the effects of this problem needs to be developed and validated. Basic strategies for prevention of workplace violence include (a) environmental and engineering controls, such as improved lighting, security hardware, and placement of physical barriers; (b) organizational and administrative controls, including development of programs, policies, and work practices; and (c) behavioral and interpersonal controls, including training staff to anticipate, recognize, and respond to unexpected conflicts and assaults, as well as communication and reporting techniques for violent, inappropriate, disruptive, or threatening behaviors.[14] A workplace vi-

olence prevention program should engage all employees. It should (a) ensure that they understand that all claims of workplace violence will be investigated and remedied promptly, (b) provide safety education, (c) introduce a "buddy system," (d) develop policies and procedures for home visits, and (e) conduct periodic inspections.[15]

A HOLISTIC APPROACH TO SAFETY AT WORK

Many people work in hazardous and unsafe environments. All people have a right to healthy and safe work and to work environments that enable them to live socially and economically productive lives.[1] We should commit not only to preventing injuries but also to a broader concept of safety that engages a sustainable way of being healthy and safe at, and outside of, work—a holistic approach that supports workplaces where workers' well-being, health, and satisfaction are given high priority. This holistic approach must be multidisciplinary, integrated, and systemic. For better identification, prediction, and control of safety problems at work, there needs to be multidisciplinary involvement of experts in engineering, manufacturing processes, technical equipment, health sciences, management, finance, insurance, behavioral sciences, and other areas. An integrated approach implies that everyone in the organization is responsible for safety, with efforts structured and coordinated within each area of the organization and the safety department having responsibility for overall planning and implementation. Finally, a systemic approach includes each element of the work system and their interaction. Elements of the work system include tasks, technology and tools, environment, organizational aspects, and individual factors.[6] A systemic approach relies on two basic principles: (1) the systems-balance principle, in which an element in the system will influence any other element, resulting in a continuous interplay among them; and (2) the compensatory-balance principle, in which positive aspects of the work system may counterbalance its negative effects.

Environmental Safety

We must adopt appropriate approaches to establish a sustainable way of being healthy and safe at and outside of work. Environmental safety concerns beyond work include safety on the road, at home, and

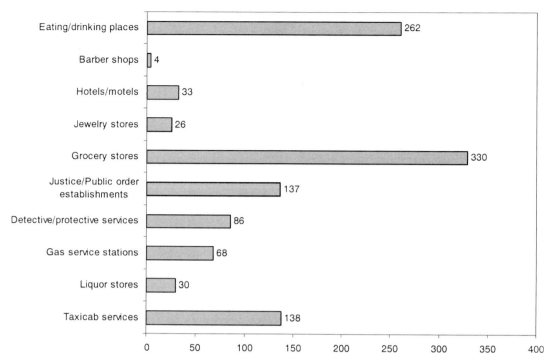

FIGURE 10-7 ● Workplace homicides in high-risk industries, United States, 1990–1992. (From NIOSH. Violence in the workplace: Risk factors and prevention strategies [Bulletin 57, Publication No. 96-100]. Washington, DC: NIOSH, 1996.)

in the community. The magnitude of environmental safety problems is demonstrated by data on fatal injuries in the United States in 2002: 5 percent occurred at work, while 43 percent were related to motor-vehicles crashes, 33 percent occurred in the home, and 19 percent occurred in the community.[2] Road traffic injuries accounted for more than 42,000 deaths and almost 3 million nonfatal injuries. They are the leading cause of death for people aged 1 to 34. While the United States has the most motor vehicles per capita of any country in the world (765 motor vehicles per 1,000 population), its 16 percent decline in motor vehicle–related deaths since 1979 has been less than in Canada (50 percent), Australia (48 percent), and Great Britain (46 percent).[16] Risk factors contributing to motor-vehicle fatalities are lack of seat belt use, especially among teenage drivers; driving under the influence of alcohol; and lack of proper occupant protection, such as use of appropriate safety seats for children and use of helmets by motorcyclists.[17]

Poisoning, falls, suffocation by ingested objects, and fires are the major causes of fatal injuries at home. Four out of five of the falls are suffered by people over the age of 65. Prevention and control

of safety hazards in the home requires cooperation among the public, government agencies, and the research community. Development and application of successful interventions for promoting safe workplaces can be adapted to the home environment

TABLE 10-7

Percentages of Types of Unintentional-Injury Deaths in the Community, United States, 2001

Falls	24
Poisoning	15
Drowning	12
Suffocation by ingestion	11
Air transport	3
Rail transport	3
Water transport	2
Mechanical suffocation	2
Other	28

From National Safety Council. Injury facts®. Itasca, IL: NSC, 2002.

and evaluated for their effectiveness. Disseminating home-safety information at the workplace can improve safety at home.

Community safety aims to prevent injuries occurring in public places, such as sports and recreation facilities. The leading causes of fatal injuries in the community are falls, poisoning, drowning, and suffocation by ingestion (Table 10-7). Appropriate interventions need to consider culture, language, and socioeconomic aspects of the community. Community safety can also be promoted by workplace programs that disseminate information.

REFERENCES

1. World Health Organization. Global strategy on occupational health for all. Geneva: WHO, 1995.
2. National Safety Council. Injury facts. Itasca, IL: National Safety Council, 2002.
3. Aaltonen MVP, Uusi-Rauva E, Saari J, et al. The accident consequence tree method and its application by real-time data collection in the Finnish furniture industry. Safety Sci 1996;23:11–26.
4. Brauer RL. Safety and health for engineers. New York: Van Nostrand Reinhold, 1990.
5. Goetsch DL. Occupational safety and health for technologists, engineers, and managers. 5th ed. Upper Saddle River, NJ: Prentice-Hall, 2004.
6. Smith MJ, Carayon-Sainfort P. A balance theory of job design for stress reduction. Int J Ind Ergon 1989;4:67–9.
7. Smith MJ. Design for health and safety. In: Salvendy G, ed. Handbook of industrial engineering. 2nd ed. New York: John Wiley & Sons, 1990.
8. OSHA. Fall protection in construction. Washington, DC: OSHA, 1998.
9. The Center to Protect Workers' Rights. The construction chart book: The U.S. construction industry and its workers. 3rd ed. Silver Spring, MD: Center to Protect Worker's Rights, 2002.
10. United States Bureau of Labor Statistics. National census of fatal occupational injuries in 2002. Washington, DC: BLS, 2003.
11. Cawley JC, Homce GT. Occupational electrical injuries in the United States, 1992–1998, and recommendations for safety research. J Safety Res 2003;34:241–8.
12. United States Bureau of Labor Statistics. Workplace injuries and illnesses in 2002. Washington, DC: BLS, 2003.
13. National Center for the Analysis of Violent Crime. Workplace violence: Issues in response. Quantico, Virginia: United States Department of Justice, 2004.
14. Lovelace L, ed. Workplace violence: A report to the nation, 2001. Iowa City, IA: University of Iowa Injury Prevention Research Center, 2001.
15. OSHA. Workplace violence. OSHA Fact Sheet. Washington DC: OSHA, 2003.
16. Binder S, Runge JW. Road safety and public health: A U.S. perspective and the global challenge. Injury Prevention 2004;10:68–9.
17. World Health Organization. World report on road traffic injury prevention. Geneva: WHO, 2004.

BIBLIOGRAPHY

Asfahl CR. Industrial safety and health management. Fifth ed. Upper Saddle River, NJ: Pearson Prentice-Hall, 2003.
Practical textbook that is targeted to the safety and health professional. Coverage of workplace hazards include walking and working surfaces, materials handling and storage, machine guarding, welding, electrical hazards, flammable and explosive materials, personal protection and first aid, and fire protection. An entire chapter covers hazards unique to the construction industry. Numerous case studies provide good examples of how to control and prevent safety hazards at the workplace.

Brauer RL. Safety and health for engineers. New York: Van Nostrand Reinhold, 1990.
A comprehensive text that is significantly more quantitative and engineering oriented than most contemporary books on safety and health. This book covers a broad range of topics of problems faced by engineers and other safety and health professionals and places major emphasis on the description of occupational hazards and their control. Numerous illustrations, sample problems, and reference citations enhance the presentation of technical topics.

Goetsch DL. Occupational safety and health for technologists, engineers, and managers. Fifth ed. Upper Saddle River, NJ: Prentice-Hall, 2004.
A useful reference or instructional text that covers both engineering and management aspects of occupational safety. Chapters are organized by generic hazard types and include machine guarding, falls, vision, temperature extremes, electrical, fire, pressure, radiation and noise, vibration, and workplace violence hazards. Ergonomics and stress hazards are also covered.

International Labor Organization and the International Ergonomics Association. Ergonomics checkpoints: Practical and easy to implement solutions for improving safety, health and working conditions. Geneva: International Labor Office, 1999.
A very easy-to-read reference that covers a broad range of the hazards encountered at the workplace. Each topic includes several illustrations that provide good examples of how hazards can be prevented and controlled.

CHAPTER 11

Occupational Ergonomics: Promoting Safety and Health Through Work Design

W. Monroe Keyserling

Ergonomics is the study of humans at work to understand the complex interrelationships among people, their work environment (such as facilities, equipment, and tools), job demands, and work methods. A basic principle of ergonomics is that all work activities place some level of physical, mental, and psychosocial demands on the worker. If these demands are kept within reasonable limits, work performance should be satisfactory, and the worker's health and well-being should be maintained. If demands are excessive, however, undesirable outcomes may occur in the form of errors, accidents, injuries, and/or a decrement in physical or mental health.*

Ergonomists evaluate work demands and the corresponding abilities of people to react and cope. The goal of an occupational ergonomics program is to maintain a safe work environment by designing facilities, furniture, machines, tools, and job demands to be compatible with workers' attributes, such as size, strength, aerobic capacity, information-processing capacity, and expectations. A successful ergonomics program should simultaneously improve health and enhance productivity.

The following examples call attention to ergonomic issues that may affect health and safety in the contemporary workplace.

ACCIDENT PREVENTION

- Designing a machine guard that allows a worker to operate equipment with smooth, comfortable, time-efficient motions. This reduces inconveniences introduced by the guard and decreases the likelihood that it will be bypassed or removed, thus exposing the worker to mechanical hazards. A well-designed guard may also eliminate awkward postures that lead to musculoskeletal disorders in vulnerable body parts, such as the lower back, shoulder, and upper extremity.

- Evaluating the mechanics of human gait to determine forces acting between the floor surface and the sole of the shoe. This information is used to determine friction required to reduce the risk of a slip or fall. Falls can also be prevented by eliminating slip and trip hazards, such as puddles of oil on the floor, uneven floor surfaces, and changes in floor elevation. The ability of workers to perceive and react to these hazards can be enhanced by providing good lighting and contrasting surface colors.

- Designing warning signs for hazardous equipment and work locations so that workers take appropriate actions to avoid accidents. Warnings are particularly important for visitors, inexperienced

---

*An accident *is defined as an unanticipated, sudden event that results in an undesired outcome, such as property damage, injuries, and/or death. An* injury *is defined as damage to body tissues. Injuries can be associated with accidents but can also result from normal stresses in the environment.*

workers, and contract workers, or if the hazards are hidden or subtle.

PREVENTING EXCESSIVE FATIGUE AND DISCOMFORT

- Designing a computer work station (equipment and furniture) and associated tasks so that an operator can use a monitor, mouse, and keyboard for extended periods without experiencing visual fatigue or musculoskeletal discomfort. Discomfort in the back, neck, or upper extremities may be a precursor of potentially disabling problems, such as tendonitis or carpal tunnel syndrome.
- Evaluating the metabolic demands of a job performed in a hot, humid environment to develop a work-rest regimen that prevents heat stress.
- Establishing maximum work times for transportation workers, such as truck drivers and airline pilots, to reduce the risk of drowsiness, performance errors, and accidents caused by sleep deprivation.

PREVENTING MUSCULOSKELETAL DISORDERS CAUSED BY OVEREXERTION OR OVERUSE

- Evaluating lifting tasks to determine biomechanical strain on the lower back, and designing lifting tasks to prevent back disorders.
- Evaluating work-station layouts to discover causes of postural stress (such as torso bending and twisting and/or overhead work with the arms and hands) and implementing changes to eliminate awkward work postures associated with the development of musculoskeletal disorders in the trunk and shoulders. Eliminating awkward postures may also reduce fatigue and enhance performance.
- Evaluating highly repetitive manual assembly-line jobs and developing alternative hand tools and work methods to reduce the risk of cumulative trauma disorders of the upper extremities, such as tendonitis, epicondylitis, tenosynovitis, and carpal tunnel syndrome.

ACCOMMODATION OF PERSONS WITH DISABILITIES

The previous examples focused primarily on preventing situations and workplace exposures that could cause death, injury, discomfort, or fatigue. Ergonomic methods and principles can be used to assist workers with disabilities who may need special accommodations to work safely, effectively, and comfortably. For example:

- Fire alarms with strobe lights are needed to warn the hearing disabled.
- Computers equipped with voice-recognition hardware and software can accommodate persons who have lost the use of their hands or where traditional data-entry devices (keyboards and mice) cause or aggravate upper extremity musculoskeletal disorders.
- Older workers may also require accommodations because many human capabilities, such as vision, hearing, balance, aerobic endurance, reaction time, and strength, begin to slowly decline starting at about age 40. The aging of the workforce in North America and Western Europe will present increasing accommodation challenges in the future. When designing work, ergonomists must consider the capabilities and needs of older workers.

Ergonomists involved in designing and implementing workplace modifications to accommodate individuals with disabilities work as members of multidisciplinary teams, with physiatrists, psychologists, physical/occupational therapists, rehabilitation engineers, and others, to establish a work environment and job demands that are matched to the specific capabilities of the worker, allowing him or her to return to work.

The remainder of this chapter describes several subdisciplines of ergonomics concerned with occupational safety and health.

COGNITIVE ERGONOMICS

Cognitive ergonomics—sometimes referred to as *human factors engineering* or *engineering psychology*—is concerned with the perceptual, information processing, and psychomotor aspects of work. Engineering psychologists design displays, controls, procedures, software, equipment, warning signs, alarms, and the general work environment to improve work performance and to reduce accidents caused by human error. Common causes of work accidents due to human error include:

1. *Failure to perceive or recognize a hazardous condition or situation*: In order to react to a dangerous situation, a worker must first perceive that danger exists. Many workplace hazards, such as excessive pressure inside a boiler, a fork truck

or automatic guided vehicle (AGV) approaching from behind in a noisy factory, uneven flooring in a poorly lit room, or the sudden release of an odorless, colorless toxic gas, are not easily perceived through human sensory channels. These situations require special informational displays. The boiler should be equipped with a gauge that displays internal pressure, coupled with an audible alarm that activates when the pressure exceeds safe limits. Fork trucks and AGVs should have beepers and flashing lights that operate when the vehicle moves. Good lighting is required near trip hazards, and alarm systems should sound if toxic gases are released. Warning signs at locations with concealed hazards, such as confined space entry points, enhance awareness and help to prevent accidents.

2. *Failure in information-processing and/or decision-making processes*: Decision-making involves combining new information with existing knowledge to provide a basis for action. Errors can occur at this stage if information is misleading or if the information-processing load is excessive. For example, during the Three Mile Island nuclear power plant accident in 1979, operators were required to react to multiple alarms and interpret a complex array of informational displays, making it difficult to prioritize actions required to stabilize the reactor. Decision-making errors can also occur if critical information is unavailable or misleading or if previous training was incorrect or inappropriate for handling a specific situation. As a result of the terrorist attacks on the World Trade Center, changes were made to communication systems to enhance the information flow among different groups of emergency responders (fire, police, and emergency medical technicians). In addition, established procedures for evacuating high-rise buildings and performing rescue operations after catastrophic events have been changed to enhance the safety of building occupants and rescue personnel.

3. *Failures in motor actions after correct decisions*: After a decision, it is frequently necessary for a worker to perform a motor action, such as flipping a switch or adjusting a knob, to control the status of a system or machine. Problems can occur if required actions exceed motor abilities. For example, the force required to adjust a control valve in a chemical plant should not exceed a worker's strength. Errors can occur if

controls are not clearly labeled or if manipulation of the control causes an unexpected response. Switches that start potentially dangerous machinery or equipment should be guarded to prevent accidental activation. This is accomplished by covering the switch, locking it in the "off" position, or placing it in a location where it cannot be accidentally touched.

WORK PHYSIOLOGY

Physical work (such as walking, carrying, lifting, and gripping) occurs as the result of muscular contractions. *Work physiology* is the branch of ergonomics concerned with the metabolic conversion of stored biochemical energy sources to physical work. If work demands exceed metabolic capacities, the worker will experience fatigue. Fatigue may be localized to a relatively small number of muscles or may affect the entire body.

Static Work and Local Muscle Fatigue

Static work occurs when a muscle remains in a contracted state for an extended period. Static work may be caused by sustained awkward posture, such as when an automobile mechanic flexes the trunk while working in the engine compartment, or when an electrician elevates the shoulders for prolonged periods when reaching overhead to install wires. In other instances, static work may involve short-duration, forceful exertions, such as using a tire iron to unfreeze a rusted lug nut when changing a tire.

When a muscle contracts, internal blood vessels are compressed. Because vascular resistance increases with the level of muscle tension, the blood supply to the working muscle decreases. Without periodic relaxation, the demand for metabolic nutrients and oxygen exceeds the supply, and metabolic wastes accumulate. The short-term effects of this condition may include ischemic pain, tremor, and a reduced capacity to produce tension; long-term exposure may cause injury.[1] Figure 11-1 shows the relationship between the intensity and duration of a static exertion.[2] A contraction of maximum intensity can be held for only about 6 seconds. At 50 percent of maximum intensity, the limit is approximately 1 minute. To sustain a static contraction indefinitely, muscle tension must be kept below 15 percent of maximum strength. The endurance curve shown in Fig. 11-1 reflects time to exhaustion.

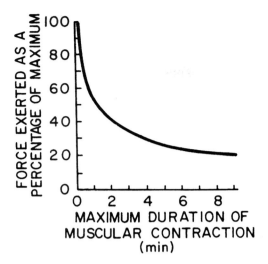

FIGURE 11-1 ● Maximum duration of a static muscle contraction for various levels of muscular contraction. (Source: Keyserling WM, Armstrong TJ. Ergonomics. In: Last JM, ed. Maxcy-Rosenau public health and preventive medicine. 12th ed. Norwalk, CT: Appleton, Century, Crofts, 1986:734–50.)

It is not desirable for workers to exert themselves to the point of exhaustion; therefore, static work demands should stay below the curve. One study used electromyography and measurements of blood lactate levels to document residual fatigue in muscles 24 hours after sustained handgrip exertions at only 10 percent of maximum strength.[3] Work activities should be designed so that static exertions are of limited duration and that adequate recovery time is built into the job. Dynamic activities involving cyclical contraction and relaxation of working muscle are generally preferable to static work.

Dynamic Work and Whole-Body Fatigue

Whole-body dynamic work occurs when large skeletal muscle groups repeatedly contract and relax while performing a task. Common examples of dynamic work include walking on a level surface, pedaling a bicycle, climbing stairs, shoveling snow, and carrying a load.

The intensity of whole-body dynamic work is limited by the capacity of the pulmonary and cardiovascular systems to deliver adequate supplies of oxygen and glucose to the working muscles and to remove the products of metabolism. Whole-body fatigue occurs when the collective metabolic demands of working muscles throughout the body exceed this capacity. Symptoms of whole-body fa-

tigue include shortness of breath, weakness in working muscles, and a general feeling of tiredness. These symptoms continue and may increase until the work activity is stopped or decreased in intensity.

For extremely short durations of whole-body dynamic activity (typically 4 minutes or less), a person can work at an intensity equal to his or her aerobic capacity before a rest break is required. As the duration of work increases, the intensity must decrease. For a 1-hour work period, the average energy expenditure should not exceed 50 percent of the worker's aerobic capacity. Over an 8-hour shift, the average energy expenditure should not exceed 33 percent of the worker's aerobic capacity.[4]

Aerobic capacity varies considerably within the population. Table 11-1 presents mean aerobic capacities for untrained males and females (nonathletes) of various ages. Aerobic capacity peaks in the third decade (20 to 29 years) for both men and women. At age 50, average aerobic capacity decreases to about 90 percent of the peak value; by age 65, it falls to about 70 percent of the peak.[5] Note that these are average values for each age–sex stratum and do not reflect the full range of variability among the adult population. This variability is an important consideration when evaluating ergonomic stress; a job that is relatively easy for a person with high aerobic capacity can be extremely fatiguing for a person with low capacity.

The prevention of whole-body fatigue is accomplished through good work design. The energy demands of a job should be sufficiently low

TABLE 11-1

Average Aerobic Capacities (kcal/min) of Untrained Males and Females for Various Ages

Age	Males	Females
20	15.0	11.0
30	15.0	9.5
40	13.0	8.5
50	12.0	8.0
60	10.5	7.5
70	9.0	6.5

Source: Stegemann J. Exercise physiology: Physiologic bases of work and sport. Chicago: Yearbook Medical Publishers, 1981.

to accommodate the adult working population, including persons with limited aerobic capacity. This can be accomplished by designing the workplace to minimize unnecessary body movements (excessive walking or climbing) and providing mechanical assists, such as hoists or conveyors for handling heavy materials. If these approaches are not feasible, it may be necessary to provide additional rest allowances to prevent excessive fatigue. This is particularly true in hot, humid work environments due to the metabolic contribution to heat stress (see Chapter 14).

In establishing metabolic criteria for jobs that involve repetitive manual lifting, the National Institute for Occupational Safety and Health (NIOSH) recommends that the average energy expenditure during an 8-hour work shift should not exceed 3.5 kcal/min.[6-8] Applying the "33 percent" rule to the values in Table 11-1, the NIOSH rate would be acceptable to most of the adult population. Caution should be practiced when placing persons with low levels of physical fitness on metabolically strenuous jobs.*

To assess the potential for whole-body fatigue, it is necessary to determine the energy expenditure rate for a specific job. This is usually done in one of three ways:

1. *Table reference*: Extensive tables of the energy costs of various work activities have been developed and can be looked up. (The text by McArdle, Katch, and Katch cited in the Bibliography provides tables describing the energy cost of many work tasks.)
2. *Indirect calorimetry*: Energy expenditure can be estimated for a specific job by measuring a worker's oxygen uptake while performing the job.[5-9]
3. *Modeling*: The job is analyzed and broken down into fundamental tasks such as walking, carrying, and lifting. Parameters describing each task are inserted into equations to predict energy expenditure.[10]

There is no "best" method for determining energy expenditure. The selection of a method is often a trade-off between the availability of published tables or prediction equations for the specific work activities of interest versus the time and expenses associated with data collection for indirect calorimetry. Indirect calorimetry is indicated when a precise measure of energy expenditure is required.

BIOMECHANICS

Biomechanics is concerned with the mechanical properties of human tissue and the response of tissue to mechanical stresses. Some injury-causing mechanical stresses in the work environment are associated with overt accidents, such as crushed bones in the feet caused by the impact of a dropped object. The hazards that produce these injuries can usually be controlled through safety engineering techniques (see Chapter 10). Other mechanical stresses are more subtle and frequently do not cause immediately perceptible injury. Work-related overexertion disorders (also called *cumulative trauma disorders,* or CTDs) are frequently seen in the lower back, neck, shoulders, and/or upper extremities and include a variety of injury and disease entities, such as sprains, strains, tendonitis, bursitis, and carpal tunnel syndrome.[11-14] Because these disorders impair mobility, strength, tactile capabilities, and/or motor control, affected workers may be unable to perform their jobs. In many industries, overexertion is the leading cause of workers' compensation expenditures. Adding in indirect costs, the annual economic burden of these disorders is conservatively estimated to be approximately $50 billion in the United States.[14] (For additional information on musculoskeletal disorders and related overexertion syndromes, see Chapter 23.)

Ergonomists and other health professionals are often called on to perform job analyses to identify and control exposures to risk factors that may cause overexertion injuries and disorders. Primary risk factors include the following categories:[11-15]

- Forceful exertions
- Awkward postures
- Localized mechanical contact stresses
- Vibration
- Temperature extremes.

All of these risk factors are modified by the temporal factors:

- Repetition (frequency of exposure to primary risk factors)
- Duration (total time of exposure to primary risk factors).

---

*Aerobic capacity can be determined by measuring oxygen uptake and carbon dioxide production during a stress test. For additional information on measuring or estimating aerobic capacity, see the texts by McArdle, Katch, and Katch and by Rodahl (reference 9).

In addition to identifying the presence of these risk factors, ergonomic job analysis evaluates specific job attributes, such as work-station layout, production standards, incentive systems, work organization, and/or work methods, that affect the magnitude, frequency, and duration of worker exposure. This information must be obtained in order effectively design and implement job modifications.

FORCEFUL EXERTIONS

Whole-body exertions such as strenuous lifting, pushing, and pulling can cause back pain and other injuries and disorders (Fig. 11-2). Because the lifting and handling of heavy weights are the most commonly cited activities associated with occupational low-back pain, NIOSH has issued guidelines for the evaluation and design of jobs that require manual lifting.[6-8] These guidelines consider task factors, such as lift frequency, work duration, workplace geometry, and posture, to establish the amount of weight that a person can safely lift. Factors other than object weight play a significant role in the amount of force that workers can safely exert during lifting and other manual transfer tasks. Due to the effect of long moment arms, handling relatively light loads can stress muscles in the back and shoulder if the load is held at a long horizontal distance in front or to the side of the body (Fig. 11-3).

One or more of the following approaches may prove useful in reducing the magnitude of forces exerted during whole-body exertions:

1. Reduce the weight of the object by decreasing the size of a unit load, such as by placing fewer parts in a tote bin or purchasing smaller bags of powdered or granular materials.
2. Reduce extended reach postures by removing obstructions that prevent the worker from getting close to the lifted object.
3. Use mechanical aids, such as conveyors, hoists, conveyors, or articulating arms, to assist the worker and/or eliminate the manual exertion (Fig. 11-4).

Forceful exertions of the hands, such as cutting with knives or scissors, tightening screws, "snapping" together electrical connectors, and using the hands or fingers to sand or buff parts, can cause upper extremity disorders such as tendonitis or carpal tunnel syndrome.[11-14] Pinch grips, heavy tools, poorly balanced tools, poorly maintained tools (such as dull knives or scissors), or low friction between the hand and tool handle increase the forces exerted by the finger flexor and extensor muscles and tendons. Gloves may increase force requirements of some jobs due to reduced tactile feedback, reduced friction, or resistance of the glove itself to stretching or compression. Environmental conditions may also increase force requirements as some rubber and plastic materials lose their flexibility when cold and become more difficult to shape or manipulate. One or more of the following approaches may prove useful in reducing the forcefulness of hand exertions:

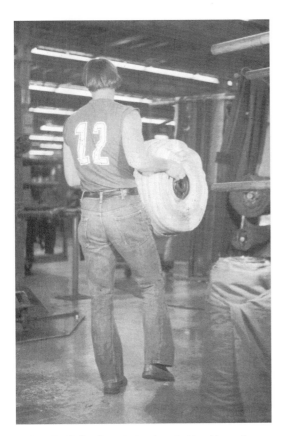

FIGURE 11-2 ● The load carried by this worker exceeds 50 kg (110 lb). A mechanical-assist device such as an overhead hoist would reduce the risk of back injuries on this job.

1. Substitute power tools for manual tools. If a power tool is infeasible, redesign the manual tool to increase mechanical advantage or otherwise decrease required hand forces.

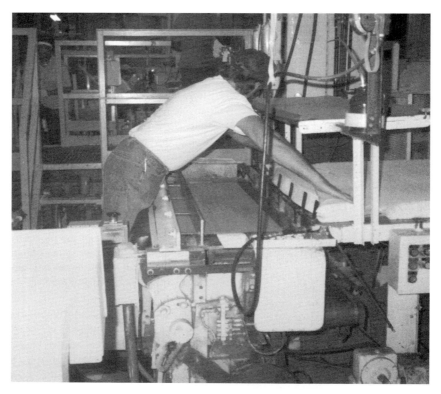

FIGURE 11-3 ● Although the lifted load is relatively light (approximately 8 kg), the combination of forward bending and lifting place a high load on the spine, increasing the risk of a back injury.

2. Suspend heavy tools with "zero-gravity" balance devices.
3. Treat slippery handles with friction-enhancing coatings to minimize slippage and reduce hand force.
4. Move the handle of an off-balance tool closer to the center of gravity or suspend the tool in a way that minimizes off-balance characteristics.
5. Use torque control devices (such as reaction arms or automatic shut-off) on power tools such

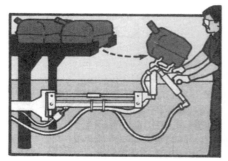
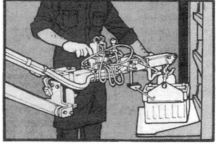

FIGURE 11-4 ● Mechanical-assist devices can reduce or eliminate forceful exertions during manual materials handling activities such as lifting or carrying. (Courtesy of The University of Michigan and the UAW/Ford Joint National Committee on Health Safety. Source: The University of Michigan Center for Ergonomics. Fitting jobs to people: An ergonomics process. Ann Arbor, MI: The Regents of the University of Michigan, 1991.)

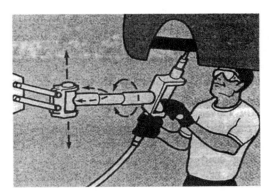

FIGURE 11-5 ● Torque-control devices can substantially reduce the amount of force exerted when using air wrenches and similar tools. Note that the weight of the tool is also borne by the device, further reducing the force exerted by the worker. (Courtesy of The University of Michigan and the UAW/Ford Joint National Committee on Health Safety. Source: The University of Michigan Center for Ergonomics. Fitting jobs to people: An ergonomics process, Ann Arbor, MI: The Regents of the University of Michigan, 1991.)

as air wrenches, nut runners, or screwdrivers (Fig. 11-5).

6. If high force is required to engage tightly fitting parts, improve quality control to achieve a better fit and/or use a lubricant to reduce force.

7. Prewarm rubber and plastic components if these become cold and unmalleable during storage.

Awkward Posture

Awkward posture at any joint may cause transient discomfort and fatigue. Prolonged awkward postures may contribute to disabling injuries and disorders of musculoskeletal tissue and/or peripheral nerves. Awkward trunk postures such as those shown in Figs. 11-3 and 11-6 increase the risk of back injuries.[12,14,16] Raising the elbow above shoulder height or reaching behind the torso can increase the likelihood of musculoskeletal problems in the neck and shoulders. The worker shown in Fig. 11-7 must position his arms in an extended forward reach due to poor work-station layout.

Most awkward postures of the trunk and shoulder result from excessive reach distances, such as bending into bins to place or retrieve parts, reaching overhead to high shelves and conveyors, or reaching overhead or in front of the body to activate machine controls. These postures can be eliminated through improved work-station layout. In general, workers should not reach below knee height or above shoulder height for prolonged periods. Routine forward reaches should be performed with the trunk upright and the upper arms nearly parallel to the trunk. Where possible, work stations and equipment should offer adjustability to accommodate workers of different body sizes. Anthropometry is the branch of ergonomics concerned with designing facilities and equipment to accommodate work populations of varying body dimensions. A detailed presentation of anthropometry is beyond the scope of this chapter. For additional information, refer to the textbook by Pheasant in the Bibliography.

Allowing workers to sit while working reduces fatigue and discomfort in the legs and feet and can increase stability of the upper body. (A high level of body stability is essential for precision manual tasks.) However, prolonged sitting may be a factor in the development of back pain. A well-designed work seat, such as one with a good lumbar support and adjustability of the seat pan and backrest, enhances comfort and can reduce the risk of health problems. Layouts that allow workers to alternate between standing and sitting postures are also desirable.

Awkward upper extremity postures can occur at the shoulder, elbow, or wrist. It is important to avoid frequent or prolonged activities that require a worker to bend the wrist. Jobs that involve precise manipulation to align and position handled parts and materials frequently require substantial wrist deviations (Fig. 11-8). Hand-tool features, such as the shape and orientation of handles, in combination with work-station layout (location and orientation of work surfaces) play an important role in determining wrist postures.

Localized Contact Stresses

Local mechanical stresses result from concentrated pressure during contact between body tissues and an object or tool. *Hand hammering* (using the palm as a striking tool) is used in some manufacturing and maintenance tasks as a method for joining two parts. This activity, which can irritate nerves and other tissues in the palm, can be avoided by using a mallet. Hand tools with hard, sharp, or small-diameter handles, such as knives, pliers, and scissors, can irritate nerves and tendons in the palm and/or fingers. This problem can be controlled by padding and/or by increasing the radius-of-curvature of handles. In some bench-assembly activities and office jobs, contact stresses result from resting the forearms or wrists

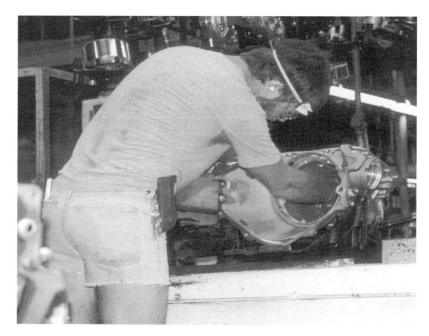

FIGURE 11-6 ● This assembly-line worker must twist and laterally bend his back in order to see his hands to install a part.

against a sharp, unpadded workbench edge. This problem can usually be controlled by either rounding or padding the edge or by providing a support for the forearm and wrist.

Seated work stations that produce localized pressure on the posterior knee and thigh can impair circulation causing swelling and discomfort in the lower legs, ankles, or feet. A common cause of this condition is a work seat that is too high, allowing the lower legs to dangle, producing concentrated compressive forces on tissues where the thighs contact the front edge of the seatpan. Solutions to this problem include adjustable seats and/or providing a footrest to partially support the weight of the lower extremities.

Vibration

Exposure to whole-body vibration that occurs while driving or riding in motor vehicles (including fork trucks and off-road vehicles) may be a factor that

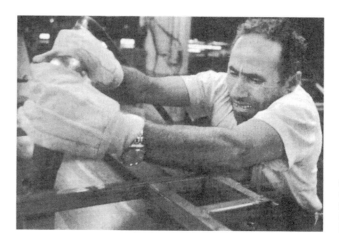

FIGURE 11-7 ● This job requires exerting high hand force with elevated shoulders, increasing the risk of shoulder and upper extremity injuries. (Photograph by Earl Dotter.)

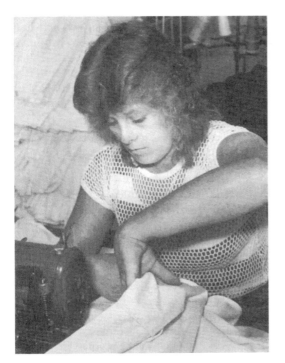

FIGURE 11-8 ● Garment workers must repetitively use awkward wrist and shoulder postures when operating sewing machines. (Photograph by Earl Dotter.)

increases the risk of back pain.[12,14] Because driving tasks are usually performed in a seated posture, most drivers are exposed to two back-pain risk factors. Driving over rough surfaces for prolonged periods while sitting in a poorly suspended seat can increase vibration exposure.

Localized vibration of the upper extremity (also called *segmental vibration*) can occur when using powered hand tools, such as screwdrivers, nut runners, grinders, jackhammers, grinders, or chippers. Segmental vibration may contribute to the development of hand–arm vibration syndromes, such as vibration white finger.[12,14] Proper tool selection can help in reducing exposure. For example, an air wrench that uses an automatic shut-off system produces less vibration exposure than a slip-clutch mechanism. Many manufacturers offer a variety of low-vibration hand tools (see Chapter 14).

Temperature Extremes

Exposure to unusually hot or cold ambient temperatures can produce a variety of adverse health effects, as discussed in Chapter 14. In addition to considering the general thermal characteristics of the workroom (air temperature, air movement, and relative humidity), it is also necessary to look at temperature extremes that affect the hands. For example, handling extremely hot or cold parts may require the use of special gloves that increase the force requirements of the job. In jobs that involve the use of pneumatic tools, air from high-pressure lines and tool exhaust ports may be directed onto the hands, causing local chilling and reducing manual dexterity and tactile sensitivity. This exposure can be controlled by eliminating leaks and/or by directing exhaust air away from the hands.

Repetitive and Prolonged Activities

The biomechanical and physiological strain experienced by a worker is related to the cumulative exposure to all the risk factors discussed above.[11–14] Because ergonomic risk factors are often related to specific work tasks, jobs that involve high repetition and/or duration, such as driving 5,000 screws a day on an assembly line or continuous word processing in an office, typically involve higher exposures than nonrepetitive jobs, such as inspection tasks in a factory or a supervisory position in an office. Repetitiveness is not a risk factor limited to upper extremity problems. Frequent lifting and repetitive/prolonged use of awkward trunk postures increase the risk of back pain.

Repetitiveness can often be measured or estimated using industrial engineering records and other work standards. For example, on an assembly line, repetitiveness is a function of the line speed or the time allowed to complete one unit of work. For a clerk in a bank or insurance office, repetitiveness can be a function of the number of forms processed a day. For a supermarket checker, repetitiveness is a function of the number of items scanned over the course of a work shift. Repetitiveness can also be measured using an observational technique where the rapidity and intensity of hand motions are compared against benchmarks or a scale with verbal anchors.[17] An ordinal scale for describing the repetitiveness of hand-intensive work is presented in Fig. 11-9. This scale has been incorporated into an American Conference of Governmental Industrial Hygienists (ACGIH) threshold limit value (TLV) for evaluating worker exposure to repetitive hand activities.[18]

Resolving problems of repetition and prolonged exertions can be a major challenge. Two possible approaches are job enrichment and job

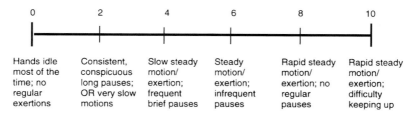

FIGURE 11-9 • Visual analog scale for rating repetition/hand activity with verbal anchors. (Source: Latko WA, Armstrong TJ, Foulke JA, et al. Development and evaluation of an observational method for assessing repetition in hand tasks. Am Ind Hyg Assoc J 1997;58:278–85.)

rotation. The premise behind these approaches is to increase the overall variety of activities performed by a worker to reduce the repetitiveness of any specific stressful activity. Although good in theory, these approaches may be very difficult to implement. Job enrichment and job rotation will not prove feasible in work locations where there are no "low-repetition" jobs to combine with the "high-repetition" jobs. Even in situations with a good mix of low- and high-repetition jobs, there may be other factors, such as increased learning time and seniority restrictions, that present significant barriers. In these instances, it may be necessary to establish a participative ergonomics program and to educate management and workers before attempting these interventions.

COMPONENTS OF AN ERGONOMICS PROGRAM

An effective ergonomics program starts with the commitment and involvement of management to provide the organizational resources and motivation to control ergonomic hazards in the workplace. Management must also perform regular reviews and evaluations of the program to assure program goals are met in a deliberate and timely manner. Because ergonomic programs focus on improving the complex interrelationships among workers and their jobs, employee involvement is essential to assuring the success of the program.[19]

An effective program should include the following components:

- Reviews of health and safety records to identify patterns of overexertion injuries and illnesses. In some instances, these records are incomplete, so it is difficult to establish direct links between outcomes and specific work exposures. When this occurs, it is necessary to supplement review of

archival records with plant walk-throughs and interviews of workers, supervisors, and/or ergonomic teams to identify specific work locations with excessive exposure to ergonomic risk factors.[20] In addition, record-keeping should be enhanced so that future overexertion injuries and disorders can be linked to specific jobs and work stations.

- Training of managers, engineers, and workers in the recognition and control of ergonomic risk factors.
- Job analysis to identify worker exposures to risk factors that cause overexertion injuries and illnesses.
- Job design, and redesign if necessary, to reduce or eliminate ergonomic risk factors.
- Medical management of injured workers to improve the chances for a speedy return to work.

Limited resources must be directed at those jobs with the greatest ergonomic problems. One approach for identifying high-hazard jobs is to analyze available medical, insurance, and safety records, such as workers' compensation payments and Occupational Safety and Health Administration (OSHA) logs, for evidence of high rates of overexertion disorders in certain departments, job classifications, or work stations. This approach is called *passive surveillance* because it relies on previously collected information. Passive surveillance may underestimate the true level of cumulative trauma problems. (For example, at small plants that do not have in-plant medical services, a worker may seek treatment from his or her personal physician. Unless the worker requests coverage under the workers' compensation system, the complaint and associated treatment may not appear in any company records.) Active surveillance involves a more aggressive approach to identifying potential problems. Active surveillance may include employee surveys to identify jobs associated with elevated rates of discomfort in the back, neck, shoulders, and upper extremities. Active surveillance may also include interviews with supervisors and personnel managers to identify jobs with high turnover. If other employment opportunities are available, workers often seek relief by leaving jobs with unusually high physical stresses before a cumulative trauma injury develops (see Chapter 6).

Once the high-risk jobs have been identified, the next step is to determine the specific causes of exposure so that corrective actions can be taken. This activity involves job analysis to identify the various risk factors discussed above and the development of engineering and/or administrative controls to reduce or eliminate exposures. The appropriateness of an intervention to reduce ergonomic stress will vary among and within facilities. Changes that are practical at one work station may not be appropriate for other work stations. Alternatives must be evaluated to determine the best strategy for resolving each ergonomic problem. It is also important to recognize that most solutions will require some degree of "fine tuning" to assure that they are acceptable to workers and accomplish the intended reductions in ergonomic stress. Follow-up job analyses should be performed to assure that the solution is working effectively and that no new stresses have been introduced. Follow-up health surveillance is also recommended to detect any changes in the pattern of injuries, illnesses, or employee complaints.

REFERENCES

1. Lieber RL, Frieden J. Skeletal muscle metabolism, fatigue, and injury. In: Gordon SL, Blair SJ, Fine LJ, eds. Repetitive motion disorders of the upper extremity. Rosemont, IL: American Academy of Orthopedic Surgeons, 1995.
2. Rohmert W. Statische Haltearbeit des Menchen, Special issue of REFA-Nachrichten, 1960; cited in Kroemer KHE, Grandjean E. Fitting the task to the human—A textbook of occupational ergonomics. London: Taylor and Francis, 1997.
3. Bystrom S, Fransson-Hall C. Acceptability of intermittent handgrip contractions based on physiologic response. Human Factors 1994;36:158–71.
4. Eastman Kodak Company. Work-rest cycles. In: Ergonomic design for people at work. Vol. 2. New York: Van Nostrand Reinhold, 1989:207–29.
5. McArdle WD, Katch FI, Katch VL. Exercise physiology: Energy, nutrition, and human performance. 4th ed. Baltimore: Williams and Wilkins, 1996.
6. National Institute for Occupational Safety and Health. Work practices guide for manual lifting. NIOSH Publication No. 81-122. Cincinnati: NIOSH, 1981.
7. Waters TR, Putz-Anderson V, Garg A, et al. Revised NIOSH lifting equation for the design and evaluation of manual lifting tasks. Ergonomics 1993;36:749–76.
8. National Institute for Occupational Safety and Health. Applications manual for the revised NIOSH lifting equation. NIOSH Publication No. 94–110. Cincinnati: NIOSH, 1994.
9. Rodahl K. The physiology of work. London: Taylor and Francis, 1989.
10. Garg A, Chaffin DB, Herrin GD. Prediction of metabolic rates for manual materials handling jobs. Am Ind Hyg Assoc J 1978;39:661–74.
11. Kuorinka I, Forcier L, eds. Work-related musculoskeletal disorders (WMSDs): A reference book for prevention. London: Taylor and Francis, 1995.
12. National Institute for Occupational Safety and Health. Musculoskeletal disorders and workplace factors—A critical review of epidemiologic evidence for work-related musculoskeletal disorders of the neck, upper extremity, and low back. NIOSH Publication No. 97–141. Cincinnati: NIOSH, 1997.
13. Violante F, Armstrong T, Kilbom A. Occupational ergonomics: Work related musculoskeletal disorders of the upper limb and back. London: Taylor and Francis, 2000.
14. National Research Council. Musculoskeletal disorders in the workplace: Low back and upper extremities. Washington, DC: National Academy Press, 2001.
15. Keyserling WM, Armstrong TJ, Punnett L. Ergonomic job analysis: A structured approach for identifying risk factors associated with overexertion injuries and disorders. Appl Occup Environ Hyg 1991;6:353–63.
16. Punnett L, Fine, LJ, Keyserling WM, et al. A case-referent study of back disorders in automobile assembly workers: The health effects of non-neutral trunk postures. Scand J. Work Environ Health 1991;17:337–46.
17. Latko WA, Armstrong TJ, Foulke JA, et al. Development and evaluation of an observational method for assessing repetition in hand tasks. Am Ind Hyg Assoc J 1997;58:278–85.
18. American Conference of Governmental Industrial Hygienists. 2003 TLVs® and BEIs®. Cincinnati: ACGIH Worldwide, 2003.
19. Cohen AL, Gjessing CC, Fine LJ, et al. Elements of ergonomics programs: A primer based on workplace evaluations of musculoskeletal disorders. NIOSH Publication No. 97–117. Cincinnati: NIOSH, 1997.
20. Keyserling WM, Ulin SS, Lincoln AE, et al. Using multiple information sources to identify opportunities for ergonomic interventions in automotive parts distribution—A case study. Am Ind Hyg Assoc J 2003;64:690–8.

BIBLIOGRAPHY

Chaffin DB, Andersson GBJ, Martin BJ. Occupational ergonomics. 3rd ed. New York: Wiley-Interscience, 1999.
This text discusses in detail the biomechanical basis of many occupational injuries and disorders, with special coverage of the lower back and upper extremities. Quantitative methods of job analysis are presented with numerous examples of ergonomic approaches to equipment, tool, and work-station design.

Cohen AL, Gjessing CC, Fine LJ, et al. Elements of ergonomics programs: A primer based on workplace evaluations of musculoskeletal disorders. NIOSH Publication No. 97–117. Cincinnati: National Institute for Occupational Safety and Health, 1997.
This document presents general guidance for establishing and managing worksite-based ergonomic programs.

Topics include organizational elements of effective ergonomics programs, training for managers and workers, health surveillance, job analysis, engineering interventions to reduce exposure to ergonomic stress, and medical management. Text includes many illustrations, examples, and references.

Kroemer KHE, Grandjean E. Fitting the task to the human— A textbook of occupational ergonomics. 5th ed. London: Taylor and Francis, 1997.

A well-written survey text that covers all aspects of ergonomics. Chapters on fatigue, work physiology, anthropometry, biomechanics, and cognitive ergonomics provide an excellent introduction to these topics.

Kuorinka I, Forcier L, eds. Work related musculoskeletal disorders (WMSDs): A reference book for prevention. London: Taylor and Francis, 1995.

Written by a multidisciplinary team of international experts in occupational health and ergonomics, this book provides comprehensive and sophisticated coverage of musculoskeletal diseases and disorders resulting from repeated trauma. Topics include a conceptual model that describes the development of WMSDs, a review of the clinical and epidemiological literature, evaluation of workplace risk factors, and medical management of affected workers. Although this is an excellent reference book, it should be noted that occupational low-back pain is not covered.

McArdle WD, Katch FI, Katch VL. Exercise physiology: Energy, nutrition, and human performance. 4th ed. Baltimore: Williams and Wilkins, 1996.

This comprehensive textbook covers a wide range of issues in work and exercise physiology. Early chapters cover basic exercise physiology (nutrition, energy conversion during exercise, structure and function of the pulmonary, cardiovascular, and neuromuscular systems), and advanced chapters cover applied topics such as measurement of human energy expenditure, training for muscle strength and aerobic power, and rehabilitation training programs. Appendices include comprehensive tables of energy expenditure costs of common household, occupational, and recreational activities.

National Institute for Occupational Safety and Health. Applications manual for the revised NIOSH lifting equation.

NIOSH Publication No. 94–110. Cincinnati: National Institute for Occupational Safety and Health, 1994.

A "hands-on" users' guide for evaluating work activities that require manual lifting. Numerous examples demonstrate application of the 1991 Revised NIOSH Lifting Equation in a variety of work environments. The guide includes a brief summary of the scientific basis of the 1991 Lifting Equation with references to biomechanical, physiological, psychophysical, and epidemiological research. The text is supplemented with numerous illustrations and examples.

National Research Council. Musculoskeletal disorders in the workplace: Low back and upper extremities. Washington, DC: National Academy Press, 2001.

A comprehensive review of the scientific literature on the relationship between work and musculoskeletal disorders of the low back and upper extremities. Major sections include discussions of epidemiology, tissue pathology, biomechanics, and interventions. Summary tables provide descriptive synopses of key studies, and the list of references is extensive.

Pheasant S. Bodyspace: Anthropometry, ergonomics, and the design of work. London: Taylor and Francis, 1996.

This textbook provides comprehensive coverage of the anthropometric aspects of ergonomics. Introductory chapters describe methodologies for measuring and statistically summarizing human body dimensions. This is followed by an excellent presentation of how anthropometric principles are used to design furniture, equipment, and work stations in the home, office, and factory environment. Numerous examples, illustrations, and anthropometric tables make this text an indispensable reference book for both novice ergonomists and experienced ergonomic designers.

Wickens CD, Lee JD, Liu Y, et al. An introduction to human factors engineering. 2nd ed. Upper Saddle River, NJ: Pearson Prentice Hall, 2004.

This textbook provides a good introduction to all aspects of ergonomics with special emphasis on cognitive ergonomics. Introductory chapters cover human sensory mechanisms, displays, cognition, decision making, and design of controls. Advanced chapters cover a variety of topics, including human–computer interaction, human factors in transportation, usability testing, stress and work performance, and the role of human error in accidents.

CHAPTER 12

Clinical Occupational and Environmental Health Practice

Gary N. Greenberg and Bonnie Rogers

Occupational and environmental health programs can range from those that are very comprehensive and offer a large array of services for the worker population to those that provide services to meet mandatory regulatory requirements. Although each organization needs to determine the types of programs and services that best meet the needs of the employees, the central tenets are the following:

- To protect employees from work-related health hazards;
- To foster health promotion and prevention strategies;
- To facilitate worker job placement and to monitor ongoing work compatibility within the context of physical and mental health capabilities;
- To provide for health care and rehabilitation for work-related injuries and illnesses and to provide case management;
- To assess and monitor the work environment for health hazards and to provide strategic recommendations for prevention and risk control;
- To enhance interdisciplinary collaboration for occupational health care and services; and
- To engage in decision making to help resolve ethical issues in occupational and environmental health.

By applying occupational health principles to the workplace, all employees, including those who are disabled, are placed in jobs according to their abilities to perform the work. This approach also promotes continuing health care and rehabilitation of occupationally ill and injured workers. The achievement of these objectives benefits both employees and employers by improving health, morale, and productivity.

THE MULTIDISCIPLINARY APPROACH

Essential to the success of an effective occupational health and safety program is (a) a thorough assessment of the work and work environment to determine potential and actual work-related exposures and (b) continuous monitoring to prevent and control workplace hazards. This is a complex process that requires the knowledge and skills of many disciplines.[1] A multidisciplinary approach to occupational health care is necessary and requires occupational medicine physicians, nurses, safety specialists, industrial hygienists, ergonomists, and others with experience related to the problem at hand to collaborate in recognizing, treating, and preventing occupational illness and injury.[1] There is great diversity among providers of occupational and environmental health services. Physicians are one source of providing occupational and environmental health services, and their training and backgrounds vary. Some physicians who designate their practice as occupational medicine were specifically trained in occupational medicine residencies; however, most occupational medicine physicians are trained in other specialties. About 20 percent are board-certified in occupational medicine.[2]

Industry has traditionally provided the most employment in clinical occupational medicine. Physicians who work at the upper management level are more involved in questions of policy, whereas those at the worksite level are more involved in clinical duties. Physicians also work for governmental agencies at the federal and state levels. Opportunities to practice occupational medicine can also be found in clinical settings in the community. In some cases, occupational medicine clinics exist as independent contractors that sell services to client companies. Some clinical occupational medicine units exist as parts of hospital staffs, usually within departments of medicine or family practice. Physicians may perform complex illness/injury management, evaluate patients for insurance companies (such as for disability impairment ratings), and participate in health/medical surveillance programs on a consultative basis and subcontract with industrial hygiene and clinical laboratory facilities when appropriate.[1]

Many physicians in other specialties also see patients with occupational illnesses and injuries. For example, patients with work-related injuries and musculoskeletal disorders may be cared for by orthopedic surgeons or specialists in physical medicine and rehabilitation; patients with occupational asthma may be referred to pulmonologists or allergists. Most cases of work-related injury or illness are seen in the offices of primary care/family practice physicians or in emergency departments; however, the association between disease and work-related causes may not always be recognized.

Occupational health care is also provided by occupational health nurses. Although not all nurses working in occupational health are specialty-trained, available training curricula include a master's degree in occupational health nursing. Certified occupational health nurses have completed requisite work experience and educational training and have passed a certification examination.[3]

The nurse practicing in the clinical setting needs to be familiar with occupational and environmental diseases and injuries within the contexts of nursing practice and the processes and exposures affecting the workforce population served. For example, a major cause of occupational illnesses among production workers is exposure to toxic chemicals, such as solvents, acids, and those chemicals found in soaps, petroleum fractions, paints, plastics, and resins. Additional problems occur from exposure to dusts, gases, and metals. The occupational and environmental health nurse will need to be able to assess the problem and provide treatment and/or refer the injured or ill worker to the appropriate health care provider when necessary. Nurses are often the

only licensed professionals at the worksite and thus manage the functions of an occupational health clinic, refer employees needing medical management to consulting physicians, or serve as case managers in managed care organizations and insurance companies.

Industrial (occupational) hygiene is the environmental science of anticipating, recognizing, evaluating, and controlling health hazards in the work environment with the objectives of protecting workers' health and well-being and safeguarding the community at large.[4] It encompasses the study of chronic and acute conditions emanating from hazards posed by physical agents, chemical agents, biological agents, and stress in the workplace as well as concern for the outdoor environment. However, all members of the occupational health and safety team play an integral role in identifying and managing workplace exposures and hazards.

Hazard recognition requires skill in assessing the work and work environment and investigating conditions that may be contributory to health risks. A full-scale worksite assessment and walk-through survey is a major component of the hazard recognition process, which should be done using a multidisciplinary context.

Safety in the workplace is everyone's responsibility, and awareness of safety and health issues is key to accident prevention. The principal responsibility of the safety professional is to design, implement, and evaluate strategies aimed at preventing and controlling workplace exposures that result in unnecessary injuries and deaths and to emphasize training and education of workers about job safety. An effective safety program requires a multidisciplinary effort. The emphasis on and commitment to safety starts with top management and extends, by example, throughout the organization to managers and all employees.

The establishment of a workplace safety (and health) committee is vital to transforming safety ideas into prevention and protection strategies in terms of policy, procedure, program development, and training and education about safety in the workplace. The safety committee should include representatives of various levels of management and of the employees, the physician, the occupational and environmental health nurse, the safety manager, other appropriate health care professionals, and, if applicable, union representatives. The safety and health plan with specific goals and objectives should be established within the context of the committee with input from employees and all levels of management.

Although ergonomics is concerned with matching work and job design to fit the capabilities of most people by adapting the product to fit the user rather than vice versa, the design of the work environment should be flexible enough to consider the need for individual variation.[5,6] For example, two people with the same height and weight may have a different arm reach or strength, and accommodations for those differences should be available.[1] An effective ergonomic health and medical program should encompass a multidisciplinary approach and include early identification, evaluation, treatment, follow-up, rehabilitation, and recording of signs and symptoms by health care providers knowledgeable in these areas and with respect to the company's operations, work practices, and light-duty job options. The ergonomist or other qualified person should analyze the physical procedures used in the performance of each job, including lifting requirements, postures, hand grips, and frequency of repetitive motion. Resolution of ergonomic problems is best accomplished through a team problem-solving approach.

A comprehensive occupational health and safety program is one that looks beyond the specific requirements of the law in addressing general and specific workplace hazards. Doing so requires substantial knowledge in the occupational health sciences as well as an interdisciplinary approach to recognizing and understanding work-related risks and hazards so that effective occupational health and safety services can be delivered.

WORKPLACE VISITS AND WALK-THROUGHS

An important and practical aspect of occupational and environmental health is the clinician's awareness of work processes and related demands and potential hazards. Because many occupational health evaluations address specific permissions, clinicians need to know the health parameters of concern and to detect health-related situations of potential risk or prior harm.

To provide a well-informed and reality-based judgment regarding the fitness of workers to perform specific tasks, clinicians should routinely visit workplaces and assess work processes. Such visits provide clinicians with a huge advantage in determining work limitations and endorsements. Beginning with providing a useful vocabulary specific to the work being performed, workplace visits also instill insight into the pace, protection, and demands of individual assignments and hazards.

From a preventive perspective, experienced clinicians can often identify job elements of specific danger that require protections not yet in place. Ethical worker protection involves a hierarchy of control measures: first, primary prevention strategies, such as substitution and engineering control measures, and clinical actions only infrequently for difficult hazards for which control is not immediately achievable by other preventive measures. Use of personal protective equipment, such as respirators, should be a backup method to protect employees only when more effective measures are not available (see Chapter 7).

Clinically triggered actions, such as medical evaluation and monitoring, are secondary prevention and can be late-onset interventions for worker protection. Whether the intention is to select workers for special capability to withstand hazards (such as with pre-employment exams for heavy lifting), to tolerate burdensome personal protective gear (such as with respirator exams), or to identify and remove workers harmed by prior exposures (such as with hearing protection programs), clinical and individual interventions are intrinsically less protective than more widespread and anticipatory programs, where exposures are eliminated or distanced from workers.

Clinicians' questions that provide important recognition of potential hazards include using basic concepts in industrial hygiene and safety. Health care providers need to be knowledgeable about the work situation and its dangers. The insight to perform these critical workplace assessments is central to industrial hygiene expertise. Repeated visits make for even greater awareness.

Questions need to be posed about speed and volume of work, the purpose of personal protective equipment, precautions used for workers who bypass safety measures, and the chemical nature of materials in use. Important vocabulary is acquired by asking about job titles and team definitions. Useful topics are ventilation, noise measures, weather stressors, spill management, and break rooms and associated personal hygiene topics, such as handwashing and laundering of work clothes. Inquiry into routine cleaning operations, the roles of contract laborers (who often face greater hazards and are poorly supervised), and product packaging (a frequent source of ergonomic problems) are necessary. Managers often expect clinicians visiting the workplace to discuss first-aid preparations and smoking cessation programs, but these subjects should not dominate the visit. Workers' interactions with their jobs require the closest scrutiny and insight.

OCCUPATIONAL HEALTH CLINICAL VISITS

The clinical service provided to workers and employers varies greatly in the occupational clinic. For each visit type, the focus is unique. Examples discussed here are the most common and include preplacement evaluations, drug-testing evaluations, specific work approvals, and biological agent–exposure evaluations.

Preplacement Evaluations

Preplacement evaluations, which were formerly termed *pre-employment physicals*, were renamed with the enactment of the Americans with Disabilities Act (ADA) in 1990, which prohibits use of medical screenings before employment is offered. Now, these evaluations yield clinical approvals for particular jobs or recommendations for specific work accommodations. The ADA limits which restrictions can be considered disqualifying and which must be accommodated. An important principle is whether a specific prohibited task is an "essential function of the job," and whether accommodating the restriction would involve "undue hardship" to the employer. (See Chapter 4.)

Experienced clinicians recognize that nearly all pertinent health and medical information required for clinical assessment is derived from the patient's narrative. Most illness is not apparent by physical exam and requires the patient's candor to reveal such pertinent diagnoses as asthma, coronary artery disease, low back pain, carpal tunnel syndrome, and epilepsy. Established and reliable confidentiality rules are required. In addition, workers should be informed by management that later discovery of intentional concealment of medical information in this process will have administrative consequences.

Because the patient is not yet a company employee, clinicians should expect a more rigorous and inflexible management response against proposed restrictions. The ADA rules protect workers who would once have been disqualified for having a "tarnished" work approval. When restrictions apply to "nonessential" job aspects, current rules prohibit management from barring individuals from employment, because minimal work modifications may be all that is required to include otherwise well workers into employment.

Drug-Testing Evaluation

The exception to the restricted duty nature of the occupational health report is the evaluation of preemployment drug-testing results, usually involving forensic urinary measurement of metabolites from illicit "recreational" drugs. Here, an unexcused positive result requires a report to management that the candidate—not yet an employee—"does not meet the employer's standards for employment." Such a judgment does not involve a diagnosis of addiction, intoxication, or documented safety risk. It is simply an assessment of whether the urinary metabolites are present and whether they can be considered forgivable, based on confidential review of authorized prescriptions or reasonable dietary constituents.

This unusual evaluation is called a *medical review officer* (MRO) assessment and involves explicitly designated physician training and certification, especially for specific federally designated programs, such as those of the U.S. Department of Transportation (DOT). Forensic skills are additional aspects of this process, including assessment of the documentation of the chain of custody for a urine sample, the worker's proof of authorized medications, and assessment of the specimen's biological validity.

The social policy that established drug testing is also intended to create a deterrent against recreational drug abuse, in addition to screening abusers from safety-sensitive positions. Although a clinical license is required, this process is ultimately quite remote from the collaborative development of medical care plans in nonoccupational clinical settings and even distinct from the usual protective assessments for occupational and environmental medicine. These activities are unique in medical practice, because the patient's narrative is considered suspect, and external documentation is required to confirm any assertion.

Other occasions for drug testing are similarly accusatory and nonclinical, including mandated randomly timed testing programs for safety-sensitive positions and postinjury assessment. In some states, this last program allows employers' insurers to assume that metabolites of intoxicating materials are proof of impairment and thus to remove workers' compensation coverage for both indemnity and clinical care. No documentation of neurological, behavioral, or judgment impairment is required or sought.

Specific Work Approvals

Many work assignments require focused clinician assessment to permit a single activity. The most common of these evaluations are respirator exams and commercial driver certification examinations, both of which are covered by specific federal guidelines and evaluation criteria.

Required medical record management for occupational and environmental medicine evaluations is unique and specific. The Occupational Safety and Health Administration (OSHA) regulation specifies that medical records for employees be preserved and maintained for at least 30 years beyond the duration of employment. With rare exception, job-related evaluations are maintained by the employer (or designated clinical contractor) in permanently available files. Explicit arrangements for both written and radiological records must distinguish occupational health from other clinical documentation, for essentially permanent availability.

Respirator evaluations are narrowly directed at whether the device would itself pose a health hazard to the worker. Employees with underlying pulmonary disease may be unable to cope with the supplemental inspiratory or expiratory demands of the respirator's filter. Some severely claustrophobic employees are unable to withstand the perceived confinement of the face mask's opacity or compression. Clinicians should also determine the nature of the potential hazard for which respirators are needed and recognize that individuals with highly reactive airways who are exposed to even a minor irritant leak may develop serious bronchospasm, resulting in panicky removal of an otherwise protective device.

Although universally performed in the past, spirometry is not required for approval for most respirator users. Based on illness and the respiratory dangers of potential exposures, selective pulmonary flow and volume testing is still more frequent than in most clinical settings and helps to provide objective criteria for workers at additional risk for respiratory disease or incapacity for respirator use.

Even facial hair (a healthy advantage for patients who would otherwise suffer pseudofolliculi-

tis barbae) needs to be recognized as a reason that a negative-pressure mask would be inadequate protection from airborne hazards. Facial deformities may also prevent proper respirator sealing and warrant comment about individualized fit-testing to be performed by safety personnel. Powered air-purifying respirators are often required for individuals in the categories described above but represent an increased cost to management over negative-pressure filtering respirators.

Department of Transportation requirements for truck drivers of interstate or hazardous loads represent a special set of considerations, governed explicitly by regulatory language and by evolving agency guidelines. Special concerns regarding any medical condition associated with interrupted or reduced operator vigilance, such as coronary artery disease, sleep disorders, cardiac arrhythmias, diabetes, or seizures, dominate the critical but arcane debates over such workers. Special training is available and published texts* are helpful. Also, many evaluators share opinions in national electronic forums on occupational medicine, such as Occ-Env-Med-L,[†] which represents an evolving clinical database.

Exposure-specific assessment may be the entire focus for a clinical encounter in an occupational health setting based simply on the worker's employment category. These extremely narrow assessments include mandated evaluations[‡] for injury from specific situations. The clinician's findings on a worksite walk-through may suggest other circumstances, such as ergonomic stress, where medical monitoring can provide early data for potential harm. Examples below represent a tiny fraction of the selective reasons for clinical monitoring for exposure-attributable harm. Please consult other publications and OSHA regulations for more comprehensive protocols on such monitoring.

- Noise-exposed workers are monitored annually for personal compliance with hearing protection and for impaired hearing. An OSHA-defined *standard threshold shift* is a specific reportable degree of deterioration. Regulatory-required response to such changes is minimal, but

---

*The *DOT Medical Examination: A Guide to Commercial Drivers' Medical Certification.* 3rd ed. Edited by Natalie Hartenbaum, MD., OEM Press, Beverly Farms, MA, 2003.

[†] Available at: <http://archives.occhealthnews.net>.

[‡] Available at: <http://www.osha.gov/SLTC/medicalsurveillance/hazardspecific.html>.

investigations regarding workplace policies and protections are often worthwhile for the individual and workforce as a whole.

- Lead-exposed workers are required to be monitored for exposure (with blood lead levels) and for metabolic effects (with erythrocyte protoporphyrin levels). Peripheral neuropathy and renal abnormalities are often markers for other toxic harm. Because significant exposure can result from accidental ingestion, worksite personal hygiene (lunchroom handwashing, cigarette contamination) merits discussion. The OSHA Lead Standard offers specific regulatory requirements to remove workers from this exposure when findings show increased lead exposure.

- Asbestos-exposed workers are routinely provided extensive personal protective gear (clothing, respirators, closed environments), and so the most immediate clinical agenda is to monitor their ability to tolerate these devices (which may cause heat stress and increased respiratory workload). Because health risks from asbestos usually occur after a long latency, the required health monitoring for toxic injury is usually premature (and clinical monitoring regulatory requirements ironically end when exposure does). Nonetheless, pulmonary radiographs and spirometry for restrictive disease are required. Because the various dangers of asbestos exposure are greatly amplified by smoking, clinical encounters should routinely include time spent on tobacco cessation counseling.

- Cadmium exposure (determined by environmental sampling exceeding a regulatory *action level*) requires clinical monitoring for absorbed exposure levels and renal harm. Blood and urine cadmium levels and urinary β_2-microglobulin (reported per gram of excreted creatinine) are indicators of potential disease. Obviously, serum creatinine assessment and questions about other renal dangers are additionally important.

Biological Agent Exposure Evaluation

Each year, an estimated 600,000 to 800,000 health care workers experience a needlestick injury, making them at risk to acquire hepatitis B (HBV), hepatitis C (HCV), human immunodeficiency virus (HIV), and other virulent pathogens. Unfortunately, many health care workers still lack knowledge about exposure risk, the availability of immediate treatment, and the urgent need for action. Occu-

pational health clinicians are in a key position to educate health care workers about the risks and prevalence of bloodborne pathogen exposures in the workplace and about steps to take immediately after an exposure.[7] Consider the following examples of cases with exposure to bloodborne pathogens as a result of needlestick injury. (See Chapter 15.)

Case 1

A hospitalized patient with AIDS became agitated and tried to remove the intravenous (IV) catheters in his arm. Several hospital staff members struggled to restrain the patient. During the struggle, an IV infusion line was pulled, exposing the connector needle that was inserted into the access port of the IV catheter. A nurse at the scene recovered the connector needle at the end of the IV line and was attempting to reinsert it when the patient kicked her arm, pushing the needle into the hand of a second nurse. The nurse who sustained the needlestick injury tested negative for HIV that day, but she tested HIV positive several months later.[8]

Case 2

A physician was drawing blood from a patient in an examination room of an HIV clinic. Because the room had no sharps disposal container, she recapped the needle using the one-handed technique. During clean-up, the cap fell off the phlebotomy needle, which subsequently penetrated her right index finger. The physician's baseline HIV test was negative. She began postexposure prophylaxis with zidovudine but discontinued it after 10 days because of adverse side effects. Approximately 2 weeks after the needlestick, the physician developed flu-like symptoms consistent with HIV infection. She was found to be seropositive for HIV when tested 3 months after the needlestick exposure.[8]

In determining intervention, prevention, and control strategies, the health care provider will need to determine several issues: if an exposure occurred and what were the exposure circumstances; how best to treat and educate the health care worker; and what follow-up is important.

HBV, HCV, and HIV are all biological agents of concern. The health care provider needs to obtain an accurate and detailed health history and occupational history including the events surrounding the exposure. This will include determining the serostatus of the source person, recognizing issues of informed consent and confidentiality. Testing the exposed individual with appropriate markers/antibody tests for HBV, HCV, and HIV should be done according to recommended (Centers for Disease Control and Prevention; CDC) interval schedules. Prophylaxis and treatment should then be offered and given according to U.S. Public Health Service guidelines. For example, for HIV, antiretroviral agents are available for both prophylaxis and treatment. Prophylaxis for HIV exposure has been formally available since 1996 when the CDC first issued provisional guidelines. The CDC (1996) based its decision on studies showing prophylaxis with antiretrovirals may reduce the risk of transmission of HIV in both occupational and maternal–child exposures. A case-control study focusing on exposed health care workers showed the use of zidovudine (AZT) reduced the risk of HIV infection by 79 percent.[9] Studies of mothers infected with HIV found the administration of AZT during pregnancy, labor, and delivery decreased the risk of HIV in infants by 67 percent. Early postexposure prophylaxis is thought to inhibit HIV replication. Studies have shown systemic infection does not occur immediately, and, therefore, a brief window of opportunity exists to prevent viral replication.[10] Three classes of antiretroviral medications are available for the prophylaxis and treatment of HIV:

- Nucleoside reverse transcriptase inhibitors (NRTIs).
- Nonnucleoside reverse transcriptase inhibitors (NNRTIs).
- Protease inhibitors (PIs).

Those at risk of exposure must have a clear understanding of the nature of the risk, how best to prevent exposure, important risk factors, modes of transmission, and the need for continued follow-up and treatment. In addition, management must put in place systems and strategies to eliminate or mitigate the risk. The health care provider must work with multidisciplinary teams including management to determine the most effective approaches to risk reduction.

Reports to Workers and to Management

Just as for all clinical evaluations, workers must be told (in explanatory and direct fashion) the results and meaning of their exposure and effect monitor-

ing. Findings requiring clinical management and follow-up (for example, high blood pressure, or alcohol-related transaminase elevations) are to be expected. The occupational health clinician should expect to hold the responsibility for full disclosure of any measurements, as well as for customized supportive recommendations for personal and ongoing clinical care.

Management's approach to medical surveillance is at a minimum to mandate regulatory compliance that screening occurred satisfactorily. Regulatory compliance falls to the employer, and the clinic's operation needs to provide adequate documentation that these standards are being followed. Individual clinical reports should reflect simply that each worker was evaluated according to these requirements (see the example "Health Recommendation Form" on page 258). Usually, individual results are suppressed unless a work-related health consequence was found, and then rules regarding workers' compensation findings apply (see below).

An aggregate report should also be created, combining results from similar workers to demonstrate and document the number of workers screened, the proportion with health findings of significance, and to enumerate those evaluations that required either worker removal or exposure modification. Statistical reports regarding the distribution of numerical results (usually biological exposure indices), comparison with prior years, and explanatory efforts regarding any changes show the clinic's programmatic efforts to improve the overall success of the occupational safety program. These aggregate reports are not confidential and should be discussed with employers' hygiene and safety professionals and also made available to workers and their representatives.

Work-Related Care and Workers' Compensation

The care of recognized work-related injuries and illnesses is influenced by state-specific workers' compensation laws and regulations (see Chapter 4). This care is affected by whether the worker or the employer selected the site of care. When workers are allowed to choose the site of care, it is usually in the same site as for their personal illness—usually because of comfort, confidence, and convenience. When employers choose the site of care, it is much more likely to be provided in a designated occupational medicine practice by health professionals

DUKE UNIVERSITY MEDICAL CENTER

Division of Occupational & Environmental Medicine
Department of Community & Family Medicine

HEALTH RECOMMENDATION FORM

Employee Name	Social Security Number
Employer	Report Date

Examination Date	**Y / N** Work-Related Illness / Injury	This clinical evaluation was designed to meet the regulatory requirements for:
Position / Title	Date Follow-up Required	☐ Arsenic Work Ethylene Oxide ☐ ☐ Asbestos Work Fluoride Work ☐ ☐ BCG Work Formaldehyde Exposure ☐ ☐ Benzene Exposure Hazardous Waste ☐
Examining Clinician	Other Specialist Involved	☐ Cadmium Work Lead Exposure ☐ ☐ Cotton Dust Methylene Chloride Work☐
Visit Type	Restrictions expire	☐ D.O.T. certification Noise Exposure ☐ Respirator Wear ☐

Based on my evaluation, there is (**no**) detected medical condition which would place the examinee or fellow workers at increased risk of physical impairment from his/her work duties.

Recommended work / duty modifications:

1.

Clinician's Signature: _____

BOX 3886, DUKE UNIVERSITY MEDICAL CENTER, Durham, NC 27710
Appointments & Messages: 684-6721 **Fax** 684-8975

● (Displayed as an example by permission of the Duke Occupational Health Service.)

known to management and familiar with the workplace and its activities and policies.

In workers' compensation care, confidentiality rules are suspended. Once an employee files a claim, whether for lost wages or for medical care, the employer or the workers' compensation insurer is permitted direct involvement in the review of decisions regarding clinical management, attribution, and specialty referrals. Release of personal health information, even for prior and unrelated illness, is permitted. Reports to management are not required to conceal diagnosis or medical details, and health care providers can choose to abandon the customary confidential restricted-duty reports in favor of simple photocopies of the clinical record. Where permitted by management, reports that voluntarily respect the worker's privacy are preferred but are no longer required by regulation.

Often, even when the patient's care involves clinical specialists apart from the occupational health situation, employers will use their customary physicians and nurses to monitor the care and its consequences. Occupational health specialists review determinations of work absences and work restrictions, including those that enable workers to return to specially modified duty.

Tertiary Consultations in Occupational and Environmental Health

Occupational and environmental health physicians also consult to other specialists and attorneys on attribution and causation, sometimes on diseases that have resolved or patients already deceased. In legal situations, opposing experts' opinions can be expected. Most of these tertiary consultations regard questions about work-related illnesses rather than work-related injuries. In these situations, the specialist's knowledge and experience in exposure assessment, toxicology, and regulatory matters can be useful.

The following guidelines may be helpful in developing a consultation:

- Identify the source of all cited information.
- Consider and report every aspect of the employee's work experience. Exposure histories require an entirely open narrative style, in which much collected information is synthesized and condensed into a smooth, but highly detailed, description of the exposure situation.

- Maintain a textual tone of open impartiality. Make sure that conclusions do not contaminate statements of facts and objective findings. All collected information should be stated in a factual, nonjudgmental tone. Consultations can never include all potentially significant information, so the expert must leave open the opportunity to change opinions if new information, such as correction of misstatements or objective measures of prior estimates, comes to light after the consultation report is filed.
- Disclose the scientific basis for an expert opinion, such as from:

    Textbooks of occupational and environmental medicine;

    Clinical textbooks related to the specific organ system of concern;

    Medical and scientific journals, many of which can be accessed through the National Library of Medicine (MedLine and ToxLine);

    The National Institute for Occupational Safety and Health (NIOSH) database of extracts of texts regarding exposure-related disease (NIOSH-Tic*)

    The cumulative opinions of Occ-Env-Med-L international forum listserv, including both its present-day members and the collected discussions over 10 years of archived discussion;

    The case database[†] of the Association of Occupational and Environmental Clinics.

Establishing Work Restrictions

Authoring justifiable and protective, health-motivated communications to management without disclosing medical diagnoses can be challenging. The case examples of these communications that follow can be adapted to other clinical settings.

Case 1

A middle-aged worker in a manufacturing facility with hazardous machinery has type 1 diabetes with poor control of blood sugar. Potential work restrictions and accommodations for this worker that need to be communicated to management might include:

---

*Available at: <http://outside.cdc.gov/niotic/>.
[†] Available at: <http://www.aoec.org/epid.htm>.

- No unscheduled overtime
- No frequent workshift changes
- No skipped meal breaks
- Access to unscheduled snacks during work hours
- No work alone and co-worker monitoring or contact every 15 minutes
- No work assignment with unprotected high hazards, including electrical, chemical, height, or mechanical dangers
- No operation of vehicles or hazardous powered equipment.

If neuropathy, retinopathy, cataracts, peripheral vascular disease, or coronary artery disease has developed, then other restrictions and accommodations may be necessary, including:

- No climbing ladders
- Practical vision testing for visually demanding assignments
- No strenuous physical activity
- Custom-fit, steel-toed shoes for all non-office work.

Case 2

A young worker entering a new work situation in a chemical packaging plant has mild intermittent asthma. Even if this employee's physical exam is normal, work restrictions and accommodations may need to include:

- No exposure to respiratory irritants, such as chlorine, ozone, and smoke
- No work with diisocyanates or where these compounds have recently been used
- No tasks requiring respirators—medical evaluations may be needed to evaluate the need for this restriction
- No work in IDLH (Immediate Danger to Life or Health) environments that require respirators.

Case 3

A worker who developed a lumbar strain outside of work may be permitted to work in a modified assignment, with restrictions and accommodations for 5 days, possibly including:

- No lifting, carrying, pushing, or pulling of 25 lb (force, not weight)
- No sustained crouching, stooping, or kneeling
- Frequent position changes, including changes from sitting to standing

- Optional posture (employee's choice of sitting or standing) for half of any work hour.

Developing work restrictions and accommodations includes consideration of risk assessment, pathophysiology, and familiarity with job demands as well as the culture of the employer and employees.

CASE MANAGEMENT AND SUPERVISED REHABILITATION

Occupational health clinicians often coordinate and monitor care provided by others, especially for patients receiving workers' compensation, in order to reduce miscommunication, delay, and even fraud. A case manager, sometimes an insurance company employee, shortens delays, improves communication among specialists, and informs caregivers of opportunities for workers to return to modified work. Care monitoring is often achieved by telephone contacts, but sometimes nurses accompany patients on visits to specialists to ensure that treatment and rehabilitation plans are received and acted upon. The patient needs to recognize that the nurse's role is observational and passive and that the employer has complex motives.

SENTINEL HEALTH EVENTS: RECOGNIZING THE PUBLIC HEALTH IMPACT OF INDIVIDUAL CASES

Sentinel health events are individual or multiple cases of occupational disease or injury that have significant public health importance. Clinicians need to report these in order to trigger investigations and intervention measures that are designed to protect a larger population of workers. For example, when a worker is diagnosed with a toxic neuropathy, the clinician needs to report the problem so that the employer can control or eliminate the responsible agent, assess co-workers, and establish a comprehensive plan to deal with the problem.

HEALTH PROMOTION

The primary goal of health promotion is to help people stay healthy and optimize their health potential. Emphasis is placed on developing positive health behaviors, recognizing personal responsibility for health, and engaging families and communities in health promotion and disease prevention

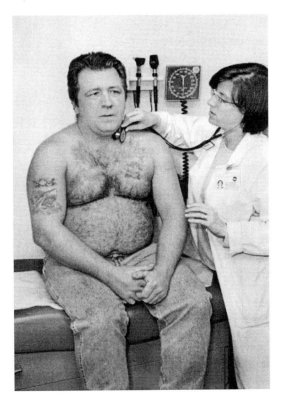

FIGURE 12-1 ● Occupational health services provide opportunities for physicians to identify a wide range of health risks, including nonoccupational risks such as obesity. (Photograph by Earl Dotter.)

activities (Fig. 12-1). The framework of *Healthy People 2010* provides 28 focus-area objectives, each with targeted objectives. The goal for the occupational safety and health focus area (no. 20) is to "promote the health and safety of people at work through prevention and early intervention."[11] This focus area has 11 objectives, each with baseline and target measures (Table 12-1). Preventing occupational disease and injury may require changes in work practices, engineering controls, worker monitoring, workplace surveillance, worker education, and supportive management.

Occupational and environmental health practice is a population-based specialty within public health practice. Thus, the goals of health promotion and health protection are inextricably linked to prevention of illness and injury. The Core Functions Project, a working group within the U.S. Public Health Service, has developed a Health Services Pyramid (Fig. 12-2) that depicts five levels of population-focused public health programs; em-

phasis placed at the lower and broader levels of the pyramid tiers serves to prevent morbidity and related risk factors, thereby reducing the need for more and more costly services at the upper levels.[12]

As described below, occupational and environmental health care providers practice at all three levels of prevention, working to ensure the employee's best interests and health regardless of the source of the provider's compensation for these services. *Primary prevention services* are those intended to prevent illness or injury. Because occupational health is a preventive health specialty, primary preventive services distinguish occupational health from other types of health care that address only curative services. Primary prevention incorporates both health promotion and protection and is accomplished by enhancing the well-being of individuals or groups of employees and the company in general, eliminating hazardous exposures, and protecting workers against remaining exposures and their effects. Primary preventive services include programs designed to enhance coping skills and good nutrition, knowledge about potential health hazards both in and outside the workplace, and immunizations and use of devices to prevent needlesticks. Primary preventive strategies include making walk-through assessments of workplaces to identify hazards, to modify work environments in order to reduce hazards, or to supply personal protective equipment to workers when hazardous exposures cannot otherwise be controlled. Although industrial hygienists, ergonomists, and safety specialists may have leading roles in primary prevention, occupational health care providers often work closely with them to identify potential health hazards that require correction.

Secondary prevention services are those intended to detect illness or injury at a relatively early stage, often before symptoms or clinical signs are noticed. When disease is detected at this early stage, it may be possible to take measures to slow, arrest, or reverse the disease process. For employees with potential work-related exposures, early detection uses preplacement examinations, health surveillance, and periodic screening activities to identify illness at the earliest possible stage and to eliminate or modify a hazard-producing agent or condition.[13] Because the interventions are likely to be both clinical and workplace–based, secondary prevention explicitly shows the need for occupational health clinicians to work with employers in a role that extends beyond their clinical role. For example, a worker at a battery manufacturing plant

TABLE 12-1

Healthy People 2010 Objectives in Occupational Safety and Health

Objective 20-1: Reduce deaths from work-related injuries.

	Deaths per 100,000 workers > 16 years of age	
	1998 Baseline	2010 Target
All industry	4.5	3.2
Mining	23.6	16.5
Construction	14.6	10.2
Transportation	11.8	8.3
Agriculture	24.1	16.9

Target setting method: 29 percent improvement

Objective 20-2: Reduce work-related injuries resulting in medical treatment, lost time from work, or restricted work activity.

	Injuries per 100 full-time workers > 16 years of age	
	1997 Baseline	2010 Target
All industry	6.6	4.6
Construction	9.3	6.5
Health services	7.9	5.5
Agriculture, forestry, and fishing	7.9	5.5
Transportation	7.9	5.5
Mining	5.7	4
Manufacturing	8.9	6.2
Adolescent workers	4.8	3.4

Target setting method: 30 percent improvement

Objective 20-3: Reduce the rate of injury and illness cases involving days away from work due to overexertion or repetitive motion.

Injuries per 100 full-time workers > 16 years of age	
1997 Baseline	2010 Target
675	338

Target setting method: 50 percent improvement

Objective 20-4: Reduce pneumoconiosis deaths.

Deaths among those > 15 years of age	
1997 Baseline	2010 Target
2,928	1,900

Target setting method: 10 percent fewer than the number of pneumoconiosis deaths projected for 2010 based on a 15-year trend (1982–1997)

Objective 20-5: Reduce deaths from work-related homicides.

Deaths per 100,000 workers > 16 years of age	
1997 Baseline	2010 Target
0.5	0.4

Target setting method: 20 percent improvement

(continued)

TABLE 12-1 (Continued)

Healthy People 2010 **Objectives in Occupational Safety and Health**

Objective 20-6: Reduce work-related assault.

Assaults per 100 workers > 16 years of age	
1987–1992 Baseline	**2010 Target**
0.85	0.6

Target setting method: 29 percent improvement

Objective 20-7: Reduce number of persons who have elevated blood lead concentrations from work exposures.

Blood concentrations of > 25 μg/dL per million persons > 16 years of age	
1998 Baseline	**2010 Target**
93	0

Target setting method: Total elimination

Objective 20-8: Reduce new cases occupational skin diseases or disorders among full-time workers

Skin disorders per 100,000 full-time workers > 16 years of age	
1997 Baseline	**2010 Target**
67	47

Target setting method: 30 percent improvement

Objective 20-9: Increase the proportion of worksites employing 50 or more persons that provide programs to prevent or reduce employee stress.

Stress reduction programs per worksites with > 50 employees	
1992 Baseline	**2010 Target**
37%	50%

Target setting method: 35 percent improvement

Objective 20-10: Reduce occupational needlestick injuries among health care workers.

Annual needlestick exposures	
1996 Baseline	**2010 Target**
600,000	420,000

Target setting method: 30 percent improvement

Objective 20-11: Reduce new cases of work-related, noise-induced hearing loss.

No data—Developmental

---

is screened for lead exposure, and results indicate that the worker has significantly elevated blood lead levels. The clinical response is to assess target organ function and determine whether chelation therapy is indicated. However, this case is a sentinel health event, indicating excessive lead exposure in the workplace. In addition to providing clinical care, the health care provider should contact the employer to report the exposure, alerting the employer to the need for making workplace changes to reduce or eliminate the exposure. Secondary prevention usually addresses ailments that are not yet symptomatic. These ailments typically are detected through screening examinations, some of which are required by OSHA for workers exposed to specific hazards. OSHA may also use the "general duty" clause of the Occupational Safety and Health Act to require medical surveillance for other occupational exposures (see Chapter 6). In addition, screening for generally nonoccupational medical problems,

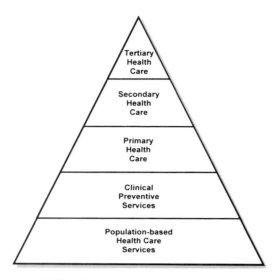

FIGURE 12-2 • Health services pyramid.

such as high blood pressure, is another example of secondary prevention, as is referral for counseling and treatment of an employee with an emotional or mental health problem whose work performance has deteriorated.

Tertiary prevention services are provided after injury or illness has occurred and are intended to provide for rehabilitation and optimal recovery. Tertiary preventive services include clinical care for occupational injuries and illnesses. Those who provide this care need to plan for the employee's ultimate return to work. Rehabilitation strategies, such as return-to-work programs after a heart attack or traumatic injury or transitional duty programs after treatment of a cumulative trauma disorder, are examples of tertiary prevention. This may require initial return to a modified or alternative job with reduced demands and with a graduated return to the original (or similar) job. It may also be necessary to modify the original job to correct ergonomic or other problems that would otherwise lead to reinjury or exacerbation of an illness. Clinicians should coordinate this process with employer representatives to ensure that needed workplace changes are made. Tertiary preventive measures also include continued rehabilitation of employees with substance abuse problems through hospitalization or outpatient treatment, counseling of employees with chronic obstructive pulmonary disease regarding smoking cessation, and special monitoring for employees with noise-induced hearing loss.

ETHICS

Literature from the United States and elsewhere frequently reflects on the ethical problems encountered by occupational and environmental health professionals in their work. Because the environments in which these health and safety professionals function can be characterized by competing goals and interests and differential power structures, thorny ethical issues are common (see Chapter 5).

Ethical conflict is nothing new in occupational and environmental health practice. Traditional concerns about maintaining confidentiality of employee health records, hazardous workplace exposures, issues of informed consent, risks and benefits, and dual-duty conflicts have been added to newer concerns of genetic screening, worker literacy and understanding, work organization issues, and untimely return to work.[1,14,15]

REFERENCES

1. Rogers B. Occupational health nursing: Concepts and practice. St. Louis: W.B. Saunders, 2003.
2. Dietchman S. Occupational health services. In: Levy B, Wegman D, eds. Occupational health: Recognizing and preventing work-related diseases and injury. 4th ed. Philadelphia: Lippincott Williams & Wilkins, 2000: 297–308.
3. American Board of Occupational Health Nurses. Certification in occupational health nursing. Hinsdale, IL: ABDHN, 2004.
4. Smith TJ, Schneider T. Occupational hygiene. In: Levy B, Wegman D, eds. Occupational health: Recognizing and preventing work-related disease and injury. Philadelphia: Lippincott Williams & Wilkins, 2000: 161–71.
5. NIOSH. Elements of ergonomic program. Cincinnati, OH: NIOSH, 1997. (NIOSH pub. no. 97–117.)
6. Sluchak TJ. Ergonomics: Origins, focus, and implementation considerations. AAOHN J 1992;40:105–12.
7. Twitchell KT. Bloodborne pathogens: What you need to know. AAOHN J 2003;51:38–46.
8. NIOSH. NIOSH Alert: Preventing needlestick injuries in health care settings. Cincinnati, OH: NIOSH, 2000. (NIOSH pub. no. 2000–118.)
9. CDC. Guidelines for the use of anti-retroviral agents in HIV-infected adults and adolescents. MMWR 1998;47 (RR-5):43–82.
10. CDC. Updated U.S. Public Health Service guidelines for the management of occupational exposures to HBV, HCV, and HIV and recommendations for postexposure prophylaxis. MMWR 2001;50(RR-11):1–52.
11. U.S. Department of Health and Human Services. Healthy people 2010. Washington, DC: USDHS, 2001.
12. U.S. Public Health Service. The core functions project. Washington, DC: Office of Disease Prevention and Health Promotion, 1993.
13. Rogers B, Livsey K. Occupational health nursing practice in health surveillance, screening, and prevention activities. AAOHN J 2000;48:92–9.

14. Rawbone RG. Future impact of genetic screening in occupational and environmental medicine. Occup Environ Med 1999;56:721–4.
15. Koh D, Jeyaratnam J. Biomarkers, screening, and ethics. Occup Med 1998;48:27–30.

BIBLIOGRAPHY

Boles M, Pelletier B, Lynch W. The relationship between health risks and work productivity. JOEM 2004;46:737–45.
   Provides evidence about higher health risks (smoking, diet control) and work productivity. Occupational health professionals need to consider these influences in planning an overall comprehensive health program that will benefit the workforce and employer.
Brodkin CA, Frumkin H, Kirkland KH, et al. Choosing a professional code for ethical conduct in occupational and environmental medicine. [Editorial] The AOEC Board of Directors. Association of Occupational and Environmental Clinics. J Occup Environ Med 1998;40:840–2.
   A useful resource concerning ethics in this field.
Glass LS, ed. Occupational medicine practice guidelines. 2nd ed. Beverly Farms, MA: OEM Press, 2004.
   American College of Occupational and Environmental Medicine consensus and evidence-based guidelines provide essential information, step-by-step guidance, and practical aids for the diagnosis, evaluation, and management of injured workers.
Greenberg GN. Internet resources for occupational and environmental health professionals. Toxicology 2002;178:263–9.
   Refers to a valuable set of materials.
Rogers B, Randolph S, Mastroianni K. Occupational health nursing guidelines for primary clinical conditions. Beverly, MA: OEM Press, 2003.
   An excellent resource guide that that provides more than 135 guidelines for common clinical conditions typically seen in the occupational health setting and programmatic guides. Occupational health resource aids are also provided.

Hazardous Exposures

CHAPTER 13

Chemical Hazards

Michael Gochfeld

Chemical hazards range from very simple molecules, such as carbon tetrachloride, to large complex molecules, such as those found in the toxins of many marine organisms. There are several terms for toxic chemicals: The word *toxin* refers to a poisonous substance of biological origin, including animal venoms and many plant chemicals. *Toxicant* is a technical term for hazardous substance but is awkward for common usage. The word *toxic* is sometimes used as either an adjective or a noun for a chemical with hazardous properties. This chapter uses the terms *hazardous chemical, toxic chemical*, and *toxic substance* interchangeably. The term *xenobiotic* is used to describe any foreign substance that gains entry to the body. Toxic chemicals vary in potency or toxicity, from potent toxins causing profound damage at low doses to very ordinary compounds that only cause damage at extremely high doses. Chemicals that are highly toxic to one species may be only slightly toxic to another that has mechanisms for detoxifying or eliminating it or is resistant because of a genetic or biochemical factor. Chemicals may cause harm that is apparent shortly after exposure or harm that may not be apparent until years after exposure.

This chapter covers basic principles of toxicology, including how chemicals enter and move through the body and how they exert pathophysiologic effects on target organs. It includes several classifications of chemicals but is not a catalogue of toxic effects or a compendium of individual toxic compounds. There is an abundant literature on toxic chemicals and their effects, including the Toxicologic Profiles published by the Agency for Toxic Substances and Disease Registry (ATSDR), which are extensive monographs on more than 200 individual chemicals commonly encountered at hazardous waste sites and elsewhere. The Integrated Risk Information System (IRIS) of the Environmental Protection Agency (EPA) is also a valuable source of information. The National Institute for Occupational Safety and Health (NIOSH) maintains a series of valuable reference databases on its Web site. The following Web sites are useful and free resources:

<www.atsdr.cdc.gov/toxpro2.html>
<www.epa.gov/iriswebp/iris/index.html>
<www.cdc.gov/niosh/database.html>

Of the more than 80,000 chemicals, many of which find some use in industry and commerce, few have had adequate toxicity testing. For 2,863 organic chemicals produced or imported into the United States at 1 million lb or more per year, there is no basic human or animal toxicologic data for 43 percent; and only 7 percent have a complete Screening Information Data Set (SIDS) covering acute and chronic toxicity, developmental and reproductive effects, mutagenesis and cancer, ecotoxicity, and environmental fate and transport.[1] Therefore, health professionals, workers, employers, and the public are severely hampered in dealing with chemicals. Even the requirement of the Occupational Safety and Health Administration (OSHA) Hazard Communication Standard for employers to provide material safety data sheets (MSDSs) is made ineffective if basic information on the chemicals is unavailable.

This chapter includes five cases, with commentaries, that highlight aspects of some major categories of toxic substances. (See Boxes 13-1 through

13-5.) Box 13-1 presents cases of carbon monoxide poisoning among workers on an onion farm. Box 13-2 presents two cases of birth defects in children of mothers exposed to chemicals at work. Box 13-3 presents a case of a car painter with nonspecific central nervous system symptoms due to organic solvents. Box 13-4 presents a case of recurrent stomach pains in a bridge repair worker exposed to lead. Box 13-5 presents cases of acute poisoning among greenhouse workers exposed to pesticides.

All chemicals have properties or characteristics that affect their fate and transport in the environment, the circumstances under which they come in contact with a living organism, the routes of absorption into that organism, and their distribution, metabolism, storage, and excretion after entering the organism. (See Chapter 9 for a description of how chemical exposures are measured in the workplace and ambient environment.)

Aerosol Size Definitions

The *inhalable fraction* of an aerosol consists mainly of particles smaller than 100 μm. The *thoracic fraction* of an aerosol consists of inhaled particles that pass the larynx, mainly smaller than 10 μm. The *respirable fraction* of an aerosol consists mainly of particles smaller than 4 μm. EPA defines particles greater than 10 μm as supercoarse, from 2.5 to 10 μm as coarse, from 1.0 to 2.5 μm as fine, and smaller than 1.0 μm as ultrafine. Particles (particulate matter; PM) smaller than 10 μm are designated as the PM_{10} fraction and particles smaller than 2.5 μm as the $PM_{2.5}$ fraction. (See Figure 9-8.)

TOXICOLOGY

Toxicology is the study of the harmful effects of chemicals, including drugs, on living organisms. Toxicologists explore these effects using techniques ranging from whole-animal dosing studies to molecular biology.

Toxic chemicals enter and move through the environment (air, water, soil, and food) at various concentrations until they:

- contact a receptor individual;
- enter the body by inhalation, ingestion, or skin absorption;
- are absorbed into the bloodstream (uptake), reaching a certain concentration;
- undergo metabolism; and

- are delivered to target organs, where they affect some molecular, biochemical, cellular, or physiologic target to produce an adverse effect, or end point.

Many toxic substances occur naturally, including many metals and their compounds, whereas others are anthropogenic, or synthetic, in origin, created deliberately or inadvertently, such as through human agricultural or industrial activities. Among the most dangerous toxics are biocides, used deliberately for their toxic effects on certain forms of life. Some biocides are natural in origin, such as the pyrethrins extracted from members of the daisy family.

Around 1500 BC, natural venoms were used for therapeutic purposes. In medieval times, a variety of poisons were similarly used, many of botanical origin, such as aconitum. The birth of toxicology is often ascribed to Paracelsus (1493–1541), who recognized that a substance that was physiologically inactive at a very low dose might be toxic at a high dose, and even therapeutic at an intermediate dose.[2] Modern science emerged in the mid-1600s, but it was not until the latter half of the 1800s that the chemical industry arose, especially for the development of dyes and paints. In the early 20th century, modern toxicology emerged, largely due to warfare, pest control, drug development, and food safety.

Toxicology has become a very broad discipline, embracing virtually all aspects of biology and many aspects of chemistry. It has played an important role in the development of pharmaceuticals and pesticides, chemicals used deliberately and with relatively high concentrations of active ingredients. Industrial toxicology focuses on the hazardous properties of raw materials, intermediates, products, and waste products. Occupational exposures to these chemicals are not deliberate but may involve high concentrations. Data generated by toxicologists play important roles in risk assessment and regulation, even for residential and community exposures that are inadvertent and often occur at very low concentrations. Areas within toxicology focus on organs (such as neurotoxicology), functions (such as behavioral toxicology), and organizational levels (such as genetic toxicology). *Molecular toxicology* is aimed at understanding the most basic level at which xenobiotics interact with organisms and also provides biomarkers of exposure and effect.

BOX 13-1

Asphyxiants: Carbon Monoxide Poisoning Among Workers at an Onion Farm

James Melius

In December, a 50-year-old woman was brought to the emergency department of a small rural hospital after collapsing at work at an onion farm. She reported no previous episodes of syncope or chest pain and had no significant past medical history other than treatment for mild hypertension. She was doing her ordinary work at the farm's packing shed, preparing onions for shipment, when she suddenly became dizzy and passed out. Her electrocardiogram (ECG) showed mild ischemic changes, and she was admitted to the intensive care unit for observation.

The next afternoon, two other workers from the same farm were brought to the emergency department complaining of headaches, dizziness, and nausea. Blood samples were drawn for determination of carboxyhemoglobin concentration, and both workers had slightly increased levels (about 10 percent). Interpretation was complicated by the fact that more than 30 minutes had elapsed before the two patients reached the hospital from the farm, and it was unclear whether they had been treated with oxygen during that time. The emergency physician contacted the farm owner, who reported that he had called the gas company to check the propane heaters used in the barn. They had tested the barn with a "gas meter" and found no problem with carbon monoxide (CO) or other gases.

The two workers went back to work the next morning and again became ill. They returned to the emergency department. This time, their carboxyhemoglobin levels were between 14 percent and 16 percent. A nurse from a local occupational health program was notified and visited the farm that afternoon. In discussing the situation with the farmer and other workers, she found a number of potential problems. Temperatures in the barn were kept very cold, and there was little ventilation. Several small propane heaters provided some heat. More importantly, a propane-powered forklift was used intermittently in the barn. Because of weather conditions, the doors to the barn had been kept closed for the last several days.

The nurse requested that an industrial hygienist visit the facility to conduct further air sampling. He arrived the next day. Long-term personal samples taken that day showed acceptable CO levels—up to 24 ppm, compared with the Occupational Safety and Health Administration (OSHA) standard of 50 ppm. However, short-term samples showed levels up to 100

ppm at some locations, especially around the forklift. Doors in the facility were kept open during the day that sampling took place. Based on these findings, the farmer obtained a battery-powered forklift and took steps to improve ventilation in the facility.

CO, a by-product of combustion, is the most common chemical asphyxiant. Most exposures can be related to a combustion source such as a heating device or a gasoline engine. CO has a very strong affinity for hemoglobin, forming carboxyhemoglobin, which interferes with oxygen transport and delivery to tissues. In acute exposure, the first symptom is usually headache, progressing to nausea, weakness, dizziness, and confusion. CO exposure should be considered in patients who collapse at work or report sudden headaches, lightheadedness, dizziness, or nausea. More severe poisoning can lead to unconsciousness and death.

The standard laboratory test for CO exposure is determination of the carboxyhemoglobin concentration in the blood; this reveals the proportion of hemoglobin that is bound to CO. Normal levels in nonsmokers range up to 4 percent, and smokers can have levels as high as 8 percent. Serious medical problems usually do not develop unless levels exceed 20 percent. However, patients with ischemic heart disease are especially susceptible to the effects of CO. After CO exposures that raise their carboxyhemoglobin levels only slightly exercise, can lead to ischemic ECG changes. Interpretation of carboxyhemoglobin levels is challenging, because they return to normal within hours (even faster in patients who have been given oxygen). Therefore, if a patient collapses at work, is given oxygen, and is then brought to the emergency department, the carboxyhemoglobin level measured in the emergency department may be well below the peak level the patient reached during the exposure.

Hyperbaric oxygen therapy is used for severe CO poisoning, but even with such treatment permanent neurologic damage may occur.

Intermittent or episodic exposures to increased concentrations of CO can increase the risk of cardiovascular disease among groups such as tunnel workers and highway toll collectors. However, such exposures can be difficult to detect. In the case presented here, the original testing by the "gas meter" might

(continued)

BOX 13-1

Asphyxiants: Carbon Monoxide Poisoning Among Workers at an Onion Farm (Continued)

have occurred when the ventilation was especially good (such as with a breeze blowing through the barn), or the instruments might have been insensitive to slight CO elevations. Similarly, a worker's exposure from the forklift could vary with time and location in the facility. In this case, sampling with better instrumentation revealed the source of CO.

Asphyxiants usually are grouped into two major categories. Simple or inert asphyxiants, such as propane or hydrogen, act by displacing oxygen in the atmosphere. The most common scenario for this type of asphyxiation is work in a confined space, such as a manhole or a storage tank. OSHA requires special precautions for work in confined spaces, such as warning signs, air testing before entry, and the use of supplied-air respirators.

Chemical or toxic asphyxiants include a number of chemicals that interfere with the transport, delivery, or use of oxygen in the body. In addition to CO, common examples include hydrogen sulfide and hydrogen cyanide. Although these materials are sometimes used in a workplace, more commonly they are produced as a result of some other process, such as combustion or chemical mixing, and the asphyxiation occurs accidentally as a result of that process.

Hydrogen cyanide exposure may occur in several industries, including electroplating and production of certain specialty chemicals. Hydrogen cyanide is most commonly produced when acids come into contact with cyanide compounds. The burning of acrylonitrile plastics can also produce significant levels of hydrogen cyanide. This chemical acts by inhibiting the enzyme cytochrome oxidase, which is necessary for tissue respiration. Exposure to levels of about 100 ppm for 30 to 60 minutes can be fatal. Initial symptoms include headache and palpitations, progressing to dyspnea and then convulsions. Treatment with sodium nitrite, sodium thiosulfate, and amyl nitrite can be effective but must be started almost immediately. Blood cyanide levels can be used to monitor the effectiveness of treatment.

Acute hydrogen sulfide poisoning may occur in a number of workplace settings, including leather tanning, sewage treatment, and oil drilling. Hydrogen sulfide is a common cause of work-related fatalities in oil fields in the southwestern United States, where it occurs naturally as a contaminant of natural gas.

Hydrogen sulfide acts by interfering with oxidative enzymes, resulting in tissue hypoxia. Although at lower concentrations hydrogen sulfide has a characteristic "rotten egg" odor, at levels higher than 100 to 150 ppm olfactory sensation is diminished, which can provide a false sense of security. Initial symptoms of acute exposure include eye and respiratory irritation progressing to dyspnea and convulsions (from anoxia). As with hydrogen cyanide, rapid treatment with nitrites is effective. Delayed pulmonary edema has also been reported in some people after acute exposures.

The outbreak of CO poisoning described in this case, along with the consideration of other asphyxiants, highlights several important principles. First, not every toxic exposure is exotic. Such familiar items as a forklift can cause fatal exposures. Second, occupational medicine can be directly applicable to the general environment. For example, many cases of CO poisoning occur in the home and are caused by faulty heaters. Third, workers, when exposed to an asphyxiant or intoxicant, become less alert and less able to react briskly to hazards. This is a form of synergy, which increases the risk of injuries, further exposures, and other mishaps on and off the job. Fourth, in an environment with very high gas concentrations, every breath boosts the blood level of the gas, and toxicity can develop remarkably rapidly. Such acute toxicity is common in enclosed spaces, affecting not only the primary victims but co-workers who rush to provide assistance. Fifth, when a worker is found dead or unconscious after an unknown exposure, a blood sample should always be taken. Carboxyhemoglobin levels and evidence of other toxicities can be determined.

Perhaps the most important principle illustrated by the asphyxiants is the primacy of prevention. Asphyxiation can almost always be anticipated; the hazards of confined spaces, forklifts, and other sources are well recognized. Once anticipated, exposures can be prevented by some combination of usual measures: minimizing the formation of the asphyxiant, proper ventilation, personal protective equipment, proper work practices, and worker training.

BOX 13-2

Teratogens: Birth Defects in Children of Mothers Exposed to Chemicals at Work

James Melius

Case A

A 19-year-old woman, who worked in the reinforced plastics industry and whose husband was a 26-year-old carpenter in the same factory, gave birth to her first child, a 3,900-g, 54-cm boy, 18 days before her predicted delivery date. The child was found to have congenital hydrocephalus, anomaly of the right ear, and bilateral malformations of the thoracic vertebral column and ribs. Antibody tests for rubella, *Toxoplasma*, and *Listeria* in mother and child, and for mumps and herpes simplex in the mother, were negative.

In the third month of pregnancy the mother had had bronchitis, and she was given 3 days of sick leave and treated with penicillin. Otherwise her pregnancy was normal, and she had taken no drugs except for iron and vitamin preparations. The mother worked regularly during pregnancy; she ground, polished, and mended reinforced plastic products and was exposed to styrene, polyester resin, organic peroxides, acetone, and polishes. In her second trimester, she was heavily exposed to styrene for about 3 days when she cleaned a mold without a facemask.

Case B

A 24-year-old woman, who worked in the reinforced plastics industry and whose husband was a 22-year-old welder-plater in the metal industry, gave birth to her first child, a 2,200-g, 47-cm girl, 6 weeks before her predicted delivery date. The baby died during delivery; anencephaly was diagnosed. Serologic tests of the mother for *Toxoplasma* and *Listeria*, and placental culture for *Listeria*, were all negative.

The pregnancy had been normal except for contractions during the second month. At that time, 10 mg of isoxsuprine was prescribed three times daily for 7 days. Slight edema occurred in the seventh month of pregnancy, and 50 mg of chlorthiazide per day was prescribed for 7 days. The mother worked during most of her pregnancy. In the third month of pregnancy, she did manual laminating for about 3 weeks with no facemask and was then exposed to styrene, polyester resin, organic peroxides, and acetone. After this she did needlework in the same workshop for about 1 month and then did lamination again at varying intervals.[1]

These two cases were identified during an investigation of congenital malformations in Finland. They were reported after the investigators found that workers in the reinforced plastics industry were overrepresented among parents of affected infants.

Teratogenesis caused by industrial chemicals may well have occurred in these cases. Styrene (vinyl benzene) is metabolized to styrene oxide, a known bacterial mutagen. Styrene is also a structural analogue of vinyl chloride, which is associated with lymphocyte chromosomal aberrations and hepatic angiosarcomas among exposed workers (see Chapter 24). These molecules are sufficiently fat-soluble to cross membranes and could have passed from the maternal to the fetal circulation. In both cases, the women had multiple chemical exposures, and the possibility of combined effects cannot be excluded.

In these cases, as is typical when a chemical exposure is clinically associated with teratogenic or carcinogenic effects, causation is difficult to establish. For any particular substance, it may be impossible ever to assemble a large enough group of exposed subjects to conduct an epidemiologic study that would yield statistically significant results (see Chapter 8). Health professionals therefore must use available toxicologic knowledge to evaluate case reports such as this one, identify potential hazards, and advise their patients regarding appropriate precautionary measures.

Reference

1. EPA. US EPA/Chemical Hazard Data Availability Study. Washington, DC: Environmental Protection Agency, Office of Pollution Prevention and Toxics, 1998. Available at: <www.epa.gov/chemrtk/hazchem.pdf>.

BOX 13-3

Organic Solvents: A Car Painter with Nonspecific Central Nervous System Symptoms

James Melius

During a routine medical examination, a 24-year-old man reported problems with concentration. He frequently lost his train of thought, forgot what he was saying in midsentence, and had been told by friends that he seemed to be forgetful. He also felt excessively tired after waking in the morning and at the end of his workday. He had occasional listlessness and frequent headaches. At work he often felt drunk or dizzy, and several times he misunderstood simple instructions from his supervisor. These problems had all developed insidiously during the previous 2 years. The patient thought that other employees in his area of the plant had complained of similar symptoms. He had noted some relief during a recent week-long fishing vacation. He denied appetite or bowel changes, sweating, weight loss, fever, chills, palpitations, syncope, seizures, trembling hands, peripheral tingling, and changes in strength or sensation. He was a social drinker and denied drug use and cigarette smoking.

The patient had worked for approximately 3 years as a car painter in a railroad car repair garage. On his physician's urging, he compiled a list of substances to which he had been exposed:

Paint Solvents	Paint Binders	Other Substances
Toluene	Acrylic resin	Organic dyes
Xylene	Urethane resin	Inorganic dyes
Ethanol	Bindex 284	Zinc chromates
Isopropanol	Solution Z-92	Titanium dioxide
Butanol		Catalysts
Ethyl acetate		
Ethyl glycol		
Acetone		
Methylethyl-ketone		

His plant had been inspected by OSHA 1 year previously, and only minor safety violations had been noted.

Physical examination, including a careful neurologic examination, was completely normal. The erythrocyte sedimentation rate was 3 mm/hour. Routine hematologic and biochemical tests, thyroid function studies, and heterophile antibody assay were all negative, except for slight elevations of serum γ-glutamyl transpeptidase (SGGT) and alkaline phosphatase.

This case illustrates some of the many problems that confront a health care provider in applying occupational toxicology. The patient reported vague, nonspecific symptoms, which a busy clinician might easily dismiss. However, many toxins have just such generalized effects. Furthermore, the patient had multiple chemical exposures, and no one toxin could readily be identified as the culprit. This patient was unusual in that he was able to provide a list of his exposures, but even this list had its limitations. Note the presence of two (fictional) trade names on the list; their identities are unknown and may be elusive even to an inquiring physician. The absence of OSHA citations 1 year earlier may mean that all exposures were then at permissible levels, but one cannot be certain of this fact. The inspection might have been directed only at safety hazards, the plant may have been temporarily cleaned up for the inspector's benefit, conditions could have deteriorated in the subsequent year, and new production processes could have been initiated or new materials introduced. In any event, all the symptoms reported by this patient have been associated with "safe" levels of solvent exposure, so even a well-maintained plant might offer cause for concern.

Organic solvents are commonly used industrial chemicals. Exposures occur in a variety of workplace settings, including oil refining and petrochemical facilities, plastics manufacturing, painting, and building maintenance. Often, several different solvents

(continued)

BOX 13-3

Organic Solvents: A Car Painter with Nonspecific Central Nervous System Symptoms *(Continued)*

are used in a given product, and multiple products containing solvents may be used in a facility. Some products, such as paints, glues, and pesticides, are mixtures containing substantial portions of solvents. The formulation of products containing solvents has changed over time because of economic factors and concern about the toxicity of specific solvents. These factors may make identification of the specific exposure of an individual worker difficult to ascertain.

As illustrated in this case, many organic solvents target the nervous system, causing both acute effects (narcosis) and chronic neurobehavioral effects in some persons. In addition, several specific solvents, including carbon disulfide, *n*-hexane, and methyl *n*-butyl ketone, cause a peripheral neuropathy characterized by loss of distal sensation, progressing to include motor weakness and even paralysis. The disease may progress for several months after exposure has ceased, and permanent damage may occur (see also Chapter 26).

Several organic solvents cause other toxic effects. Benzene was commonly used as an industrial and commercial solvent in the past. High exposures suppress bone marrow production, sometimes leading to anemia or pancytopenia. Benzene is also a potent carcinogen, leading to leukemia and other hematopoietic malignancies (Chapter 30). Because of this toxicity, benzene is used much less commonly today, although exposures continue to occur in the petrochemical industry and in some other industries. Some other

hydrocarbons, including ethylene oxide, the chloromethyl ethers, and epichloro-hydrin, are also known carcinogens. Many other solvents are suspected of being carcinogenic, including several halogenated compounds.

Several organic solvents are hepatotoxic. Carbon tetrachloride, chloroform, and tetrachloroethane can cause hepatic necrosis. Long-term exposure to carbon tetrachloride has been associated with the development of cirrhosis. Dimethyl formamide and 2-nitropropane have caused outbreaks of chemically induced liver disease in exposed workers (Chapter 30).

Several organic solvents, including the glycol ethers and ethylene oxide, have been shown to affect the reproductive system. Skin irritation also commonly results from solvent exposures. These chemicals dry the skin by removing natural skin oils. Many organic solvents are also acute respiratory irritants.

The diagnosis of health problems related to solvent exposure depends strongly on a thorough exposure history. Biological monitoring may be helpful for ongoing exposures, but it is not useful for evaluating past exposures, because most solvents are metabolized and cleared from the body relatively quickly.

Control of solvent exposure is based on a careful evaluation of how the exposure occurs. Work procedures and practices are often important determinants of solvent exposure for many persons who work with organic solvents (such as painters). Personal protective equipment, a switch to a less toxic alternative, and/or changes in work practices may be needed to limit exposures. In some settings, traditional engineering methods such as ventilation may also be useful.

BOX 13-4

Metals: Recurrent Stomach Pains in a Bridge Repair Worker

James Melius

A 29-year-old laborer who worked intermittently for a construction firm that did bridge repair work complained to his family physician of intermittent stomach pains of several weeks' duration. The pain was not associated with meals. Onset had been gradual, and he had no associated systemic or gastrointestinal symptoms. He had not experienced any unusual stress at home or at work. He reported drinking one or two cans of beer per day. His physician treated him with antacids.

Approximately 9 months later, the patient saw his physician again with the same complaints. His earlier pains had resolved approximately 1 month after treatment, and he had been feeling fine until a few weeks earlier, when his stomach pains started to recur. This time, the pains were more severe and were associated with loss of appetite and generalized fatigue. There was no consistent association with meal times or with other activities. He had no other significant symptoms and reported no recent changes in his personal life or habits. His physical examination was normal. His doctor sent him for an upper gastrointestinal series that was scheduled approximately 1 week later. He was again treated with antacids and dietary restrictions.

The doctor saw the patient again approximately 1 week after the x-ray studies. The results had been normal, and the patient's symptoms had improved slightly over the past week. He was seen again 4 weeks later, with continued improvement. However, he still reported intermittent epigastric pains. At this time, his physician became concerned about possible exposures to lead from his occupation. Although the patient knew that lead had been an ingredient in gasoline, he was unaware that the paint on bridges could contain lead. He reported no other hobbies that might expose him to lead. The physician ordered a complete blood count and a blood lead level (BLL). The blood count showed slight anemia, and the BLL was 20 μg/dL. The physician continued antacid and dietary treatment.

Approximately 2 months later, the patient returned complaining of more severe epigastric pains, this time associated with abdominal cramping, headaches, and fatigue. He had been getting better but then started work at a new site, where he had used an oxyacetylene torch to remove paint from sections of an old bridge before welding. In reviewing the history of his episodes of pain, the patient

reported that all three had occurred a few weeks after he started a similar type of job. After consultation with an occupational physician, the family physician obtained another BLL, which was 53 μg/dL. The patient stopped doing paint removal work, and his symptoms gradually improved. Within 2 weeks, his BLL was reduced to 43 μg/dL. The contractor arranged a ventilation system for use when paint was being removed from bridges, and quarterly monitoring of the patient's BLL showed a gradual decline.

Although the use of lead pigment was discontinued in most paints by the 1970s, older lead-containing paints still cover many interior and exterior surfaces in older buildings and continue to be used on steel structures such as bridges. Not only does this exposure account for many cases of childhood lead poisoning, but also painters and other workers conducting renovation work on buildings with lead paint can be significantly exposed to lead. Burning or torching of the surface to remove the paint produces a lead fume that is readily absorbed through the respiratory tract.

Most occupational lead exposures occur by inhalation, although ingestion may also contribute, especially through contamination of food or cigarettes at work. Lead is initially absorbed into the blood and then gradually stored in the bones. BLL determinations are a good indicator of recent exposure but may not reflect past exposures. Newer x-ray fluorescence techniques provide a better assessment of lead storage in bones, but they are not widely available.

Most metals, including lead, exert their biological effects through enzyme ligand binding, and for many metals excretion can be hastened by chelation therapy with agents such as dimercaptosuccinic acid (DMSA; succimer), dimercaprol (British antilewisite; BAL), or ethylenediaminetetraacetic acid (EDTA). Beyond these generalizations, however, metal toxicology is as varied as the metals themselves.

Lead affects a number of organ systems, including the hematopoietic, renal, and nervous systems. Typical early signs of exposure in adults include abdominal colic, headache, and fatigue. At higher levels of exposure, lead may cause a peripheral motor neuropathy with wrist or foot drop. Higher levels of exposure may also lead to

(continued)

BOX 13-4

Metals: Recurrent Stomach Pains in a Bridge Repair Worker (Continued)

an anemia related to the inhibition of several enzymes involved in hemoglobin production. Chronic exposure to lead can cause renal tubular damage and, eventually, renal failure. Lead exposure is also associated with adverse reproductive effects in both men and women.

The current OSHA lead standard is 50 μg/m^3 over an 8-hour day. Regular exposure at this level yields an average BLL of about 40 μg/dL. The standard requires routine BLL monitoring and removal of a worker from exposure if the BLL becomes elevated. This standard applies equally to general industry, where routine lead exposure occurs in such operations as battery manufacturing, and to the construction industry, where many lead poisoning cases are being reported, especially in workers who remove lead paint from highway bridges and similar structures.

Mercury is another important metal used in the manufacture of monitoring instruments and in certain industrial processes. It is important to distinguish the form of mercury (metallic, inorganic, or organic) when evaluating toxic effects. Metallic and inorganic mercury affect the nervous system and the kidneys. At high doses, exposed persons undergo personality changes such as irritability, shyness, and paranoia (a syndrome called erethism); tremor; and peripheral neuropathy. Lower doses cause more subtle forms of these problems, such as visual-motor changes on neurobehavioral testing and slowed nerve conduction velocity. The kidney toxicity can manifest as both tubular and glomerular dysfunction; patients show proteinuria and in severe cases impaired creatinine clearance. Gingivitis is another classic sign of severe mercury poisoning. Exposure to metallic mercury is usually monitored through determinations of urine mercury levels, although blood levels may also be useful.

Organic mercury compounds (usually methyl mercury) are sometimes encountered in workplace settings, but they are better known from outbreaks related to environmental contamination (usually human exposure to contaminated fish). These exposures have been associated with severe neurologic disease (both central and peripheral) and birth defects in children of pregnant women exposed to high levels of methyl mercury.

Arsenic is used in some industrial and chemical processes. Exposure also occurs in the smelting of some metal ores. Exposure to arsenic can cause a symmetrical distal polyneuropathy. High exposures cause liver damage and skin lesions. Arsenic is also carcinogenic, causing lung, liver, bladder, kidney, and skin cancer. Exposure to arsenic is usually monitored through urinary arsenic levels.

Cadmium exposure occurs in many different industrial processes. Its main effect is on the renal system, leading to renal tubular dysfunction as cadmium accumulates in the kidney. Cadmium also causes lung cancer. Cadmium exposure can be monitored with either urine or blood concentrations.

Beryllium is a metal used in electronics and some other industrial applications. Exposure leads to a fibrotic lung disease similar to—and often mistaken for—sarcoidosis. Lymphocyte transformation testing of blood or bronchoalveolar lavage can assist with the early diagnosis of this illness.

Other important toxic metals include nickel, which is carcinogenic and is a very common cause of contact dermatitis; chromium, which similarly causes contact dermatitis and is believed to be carcinogenic, but only in the hexavalent form; and manganese, which causes a neurologic condition similar to Parkinson disease.

Prompt medical diagnosis is extremely important in the control of metal poisonings. Many current exposures occur in small businesses or involve exposures secondary to other work (such as lead exposure from removing lead paint). Biological monitoring and a careful exposure history are critical for proper diagnosis and follow-up of people working in these industries. In larger industries, routine industrial hygiene control techniques are applied, including better ventilation and use of personal protective equipment.

BOX 13-5

Pesticides: Acute Poisoning in Greenhouse Workers

James Melius

A 38-year-old woman was seen in the emergency department of a rural hospital on Saturday evening, complaining of a severe rash. The rash had initially appeared on her forearms several weeks earlier, but during the last 2 weeks it had become more severe, spreading to her face and neck. She indicated that the itching from the rash had become so severe that she had hardly slept for the last three nights. She came to the hospital on a Saturday night because that was the only time she had off from work. She had no previous history of any skin problems. On questioning, the patient suspected that the rash might have resulted from chemical exposures at work. She worked at a greenhouse, where she had contact with pesticides, fungicides, fertilizers, and cleaning materials. Physical examination showed a severe maculopapular rash on her hands, forearms, face, and neck. The emergency room physician treated her with topical steroids and an antihistamine for the itching and referred her to a local community clinic for follow-up.

Two weeks later, the patient was seen at the community clinic. The rash was still quite severe. She had used up the medication provided at the hospital but was unable to fill her prescriptions because they were expensive. The physician asked her about the chemicals used at work, but she could not identify any of them by name. She did not apply pesticides or fungicides herself but was exposed to them when the greenhouses were sprayed before she arrived at work and when she handled the flowers. The physician provided her with medication for her dermatitis, advised her to return in 2 weeks, and asked her to try to get the names of the pesticides and fungicides that were used at work.

The physician from the community clinic treated the patient for the dermatitis, which slowly cleared up. After two more workers from the greenhouse came to the clinic reporting episodes of acute illness (headaches and nausea), the physician reported the problem to the state pesticide enforcement agency, which then inspected the facility. Although it found problems with labeling of the pesticides used at the facility and with disposal practices, no serious violations of current regulations were found. The owner did change some application practices, and the patient was later able to return to work in another area of the facility without problems.

Pesticides and fungicides include a wide range of chemicals used to control various undesirable species. Although most pesticide use occurs in agricultural settings, people may also be occupationally exposed from the use of these chemicals for structural pest control. Pesticides, as a class of chemicals, affect almost every organ system, but individual pesticides usually have a more limited and more specific toxicity.

Pesticides can be absorbed by all three routes: inhalation, ingestion, and skin absorption. Skin absorption is an important route for many pesticides, especially among workers who have extensive contact with sprayed plants or crops. Organophosphate pesticides are among the types most widely used in agricultural and structural applications. These compounds act by inhibiting the enzyme acetylcholinesterase at the nerve-to-nerve synapse or at the nerve-to-muscle motor end plate, leading to increased levels of the neurotransmitter acetylcholine at many different sites in the body.

The worker in this case probably was acutely exposed to one of the organophosphates. Any of these pesticides can be absorbed via the respiratory, percutaneous, and gastrointestinal routes. The exposure in this example probably included both inhalation (from the pesticide fogging) and dermal exposure from contact with pesticide-contaminated plants and surfaces. Once absorbed, organophosphates are metabolized by hepatic microsomal enzymes. For one of the most studied of these pesticides, parathion, the first major conversion it undergoes is replacement of its sulfur by oxygen to form paraoxon, the actual anticholinesterase. Subsequent oxidation and hydrolysis result in detoxification.

Paraoxon binds with acetylcholinesterase molecules at cholinergic nerve endings, both centrally and peripherally. The organophosphates and the carbamates both act through this mechanism, but carbamate complexes dissociate spontaneously, whereas organophosphate complex formation is virtually irreversible. As a result, organophosphate poisoning causes a predictable constellation of muscarinic, nicotinic, and central nervous system symptoms. Severe cases can progress to coma and death.

(continued)

BOX 13-5

Pesticides: Acute Poisoning in Greenhouse Workers (Continued)

Typical symptoms include miosis, salivation, sweating, and muscle fasciculation; at higher exposures, diarrhea, incontinence, wheezing, bradycardia, and even convulsions may occur. Cholinesterase inhibition can be measured with cholinesterase levels, but these tests are difficult to interpret for several reasons: people vary widely in their normal levels, laboratories vary widely in their measurements, and levels may quickly return to normal after exposure ceases. Cholinesterase levels are most useful for ongoing monitoring (if baseline levels are known) and in monitoring recovery from acute toxicity. Acute poisoning can be treated with atropine with or without pralidoxime.

A delayed neurotoxicity syndrome, with weakness, paresthesias, and paralysis of the distal lower extremities, has been found in persons exposed to organophosphate pesticides, and other chronic neurotoxicity syndromes also have been reported. These syndromes usually occur in people with chronic exposure or after a very severe acute exposure.

Another frequently used category of pesticides is the carbamates. Carbamates also inhibit the enzyme acetylcholinesterase, but this inhibition is more readily reversed than that caused by organophosphate pesticides. Hence, effects tend to be less severe. Because of the rapid reversal, serum and red blood cell cholinesterase levels tend to be less useful in the diagnosis of exposure to this type of pesticide.

Organochlorine pesticides, such as dichlorodiphenyltrichloroethane (DDT), were more widely used in the past, but their use has been limited owing to their persistence in the environment. However, some (such as lindane) are still commonly used. Organochlorine pesticides are metabolized very slowly and accumulate in fat and other tissues. Their major toxic effects involve the nervous system, leading to anorexia, malaise, tremor, hyperreflexia, and convulsions. In addition, evidence (mostly from animals) suggests that organochlorines and other persistent organic pollutants may have hormonal effects. If this is true, these agents could contribute to impaired reproductive function, developmental abnormalities in children, and increases in hormone-responsive cancers such as those of the breast and prostate. The endocrine disrupter hypothesis is the subject of intense research.

Many other individual pesticides have significant toxicity. Paraquat (an herbicide) can cause a severe pulmonary fibrosis. Dibromochloropropane (DBCP), used in the past to control nematodes, caused sterility among male workers exposed to high levels of this chemical (see Chapter 29). Many pesticides are carcinogenic. A series of studies found a high incidence of non-Hodgkin lymphoma among midwestern U.S. farmers who used large amounts of herbicides. Dermatitis is also common among people working with pesticides, although some of this incidence is a result of exposure to other materials mixed with the pesticides.

Finally, although many fungicides and herbicides have low toxicity, others present a range of toxic effects. For example, skin problems may result not only from insecticides and the solvents used to dilute them for application but also from fungicides and herbicides. In the case described, the patient had probably developed skin sensitization to fungicides used in the cultivation of the flowers.

The diagnosis of pesticide-related illnesses can be very difficult. A high index of suspicion and a very careful medical and exposure history are essential. Laboratory testing is helpful for some pesticides, as noted previously. Prevention strategies for control of pesticide-related health risks are discussed in Chapter 32.

EXPOSURE

Hazardous materials, including both naturally occurring and anthropogenic (or synthetic) chemicals, can be released to the environment where they become contaminants in air, water, soil, dust, and food. Humans are exposed to (come into proximity or actual contact with) such chemicals, which gain access to the body by inhalation, ingestion, dermal absorption, or, rarely, by injection. In Table 13-1, which is an exposure matrix, each cell represents a potential exposure pathway. Those that are highlighted in bold are the main concerns in occupational health. Table 13-2 similarly illustrates pathways that are important in residential or community exposures; in this case, soil ingestion by toddlers is often the highest intake to a sensitive recipient. Chemicals can also be inadvertently brought home by workers (see drawing on page 306).

Figure 13-1 illustrates an exposure pathway from source to exposure to toxicokinetics in the body, resulting in a dose to the target organ. It is this dose to the target organ that determines the health effect, but many factors intervene, including those governing (a) fate and transport in the environment; (b) absorption efficiency in the respiratory and gastrointestinal systems and the skin; and (c) metabolism, distribution, storage, and excretion. Activity modifies absorption; for example, exercise that increases respiratory rate increases inhalation of contaminants.

Chemicals may exert their toxic effect at the site of contact (skin, eyes, mucous membranes, or lungs) or may be absorbed into the bloodstream and distributed to target organs where they cause damage. Some chemicals, such as carbon monoxide, cause damage by affecting blood flow or delivery of oxygen to cells. Some enter cells and interfere with crucial life processes, such as hormone synthesis. Some interfere with cell cycling, disrupting the genetic activities of the cell and preventing the cell from undergoing normal division. Some kill all cells or only specific ones. Some, which are carcinogens, directly damage the DNA in the cell or interfere with normal regulatory processes of cell division, resulting in cancer.

Assessment of Exposure to Chemicals

Exposure assessment is the discipline that develops and applies measurement techniques and models to quantify human exposure to hazards in the home, community, and workplace (see Chapter 9).

The task of measuring the amount or concentration of a substance in an environmental medium, such as by air sampling, is relatively easy, requiring appropriate collection and analytic instrumentation. For example, the degree of exposure of an individual exposed to an airborne chemical can be determined by breathing-zone measurements.

TABLE 13-1

Generic Exposure Matrix[a]

	Air	Water	Soil/Dust	Food
Inhalation	**Very important for occupational health**	Volatiles when cooking or showering	**Both workplace and residential**	Not a common pathway
Ingestion	Airborne deposition on foods or crops	A major residential pathway	**Gardeners, and workers who eat at work or without washing**	A major residential pathway
Dermal	A few gases penetrate skin	**Important for a few chemicals or mixtures**	Some direct contact with workplace chemicals	Not a pathway
Injection	Not a pathway	Not a pathway	Some sharp solid objects can penetrate	Not a pathway

[a] Exposures prevalent in the workplace are in boldface.
Source: Exposure Matrix modified from M. Gochfeld (©). A matrix of routes and media of exposure for risk assessment scenarios. Piscataway, NJ: Environmental and Occupational Health Sciences Institute, 1991.

TABLE 13-2

Exposure Matrix for Residential or Community Exposure[a]

	Air	Water	Soil/Dust	Food
Inhalation	**Important for community air pollution or indoor contaminants**	Volatiles when cooking or showering	Final dust particulates	Not applicable
Ingestion	Airborne deposition on foods or crops	**A major residential pathway, particularly with private wells**	**Toddlers and gardeners**	**A major residential pathway for garden crops, wildlife, and fish**
Dermal	A few gases penetrate skin; now a bioterror concern	Important for a few chemicals or mixtures; also for some household chemicals through direct contact	Some direct household chemicals or pesticides	Not a pathway
Injection	Not a pathway	Not a pathway	Some sharp solid objects can penetrate	Not a pathway

[a] Major pathways shown in bold.

Source: Exposure Matrix modified from M. Gochfeld (©). A matrix of routes and media of exposure for risk assessment scenarios. Piscataway, NJ: Environmental and Occupational Health Sciences Institute, 1991.

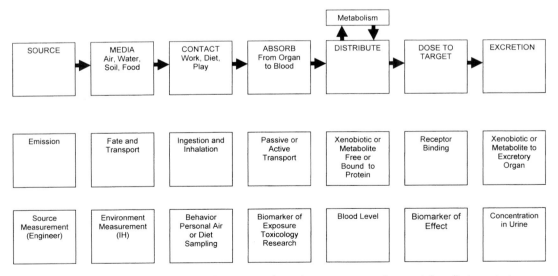

FIGURE 13-1 ● An exposure pathway from source through one or more environmental media to contact, absorption, and distribution in the body, eventually reaching a target organ as well as excretory organs. Top rectangles identify the components of the pathway. Middle rectangles indicate the movement of the contaminant. Bottom rectangles indicate what can be measured. (Source: Environmental and Occupational Health Sciences Institute.)

However, direct measurement of absorption is challenging and usually requires extensive research. Therefore, methods have been developed to infer absorption by measuring biomarkers. In the case of lead, the best biomarker is the blood lead level. It is highly specific; only lead can influence the blood lead level. Similarly, exhaled ethanol, a reflection of recent ethanol intake and current blood alcohol level, forms the basis of the breath-testing of intoxicated motorists. Many organic compounds are only transiently in the bloodstream before being metabolized or excreted. Therefore, to estimate exposure, it may be necessary to measure a specific metabolite in the urine. Because benzene is rapidly metabolized, measurement of the blood benzene level is not useful; however, a common metabolite, phenol, can be measured in urine and can be a useful biomarker. One problem, however, is that there are other sources of urinary phenol, including phenol in some cough preparations. Therefore, urinary phenol is a sensitive, but not specific, biomarker of benzene exposure. Serum or urinary cotinine, a breakdown product of nicotine, is a good biomarker of exposure to cigarette smoke.

ROUTES OF ABSORPTION

Chemicals can enter the body through the skin (*dermal absorption*), the gastrointestinal tract (*ingestion*), the respiratory tract (*inhalation*), and, in some cases, by injection or penetration. Special sites of absorption include the mucous membranes of the eyes, nose, and throat; the placenta; and the blood–brain barrier. In contrast, many chemicals to which humans are exposed do not enter the body.

Crossing Membranes

To move through the body, chemicals must cross various membranes. For example, in the lung a chemical must pass from inhaled air in the alveolar sac through the membrane that separates the alveolus from the adjacent capillary. Once in the bloodstream, the chemical may pass to a metabolic organ, such as the liver; an excretory organ, such as the kidney; or a target organ. In each case, it must again pass through a capillary membrane into interstitial space and then through a cell membrane. Membranes are not inert "plastic bags" but rather have active physical and chemical structures of lipid and protein, with different features in different organs. Some substances pass mainly through membrane pores (as seen under scanning electron microscopes); others are transported by transporter molecules; and some actually remain in the membrane, bound to receptors on the cell surface. Pore transfer often involves passive diffusion along a concentration gradient. Active transport involves processes that use energy to move a substance through a membrane, often against a concentration gradient with the aid of transporter molecules. In addition, membranes can be target organs for chemicals that cause lipid peroxidation and alter membrane fluidity.

Inhalation

Inhalation is the primary route of entry in industrial workplaces and in areas with high levels of ambient air pollution. It can also be a serious and occasionally fatal route of entry in homes, where, for example carbon monoxide may be a hazard. A typical adult may take about 12 breaths a minute, each with a tidal volume of 500 ml (of which 150 ml is the "dead space" of the upper airway). This amounts to 4,200 ml (12 × 350 ml), or 4.2 liters per minute (6,000 liters per day) of air exchange in the lung—6 cubic meters of air for a resting adult. With activity, both breathing rate and volume increase, and 20 cubic meters of air is used to estimate how much airborne contaminant a moderately active person could breathe in a day. To put this in perspective, at the standard of 0.1 asbestos fibers per milliliter of air, a person at rest would breathe in about 600,000 fibers per day.

As air passes through the nose, large particles (dusts) are trapped by nasal hairs or may impact on the mucous membranes of the pharynx. Smaller particles enter the tracheobronchial tree where they may land on the ciliated epithelium that lines the walls of larger airways. A thin layer of mucous covers the cilia; particles trapped in this mucous are moved upward by the rhythmic wave-like action of the cilia until they reach the throat, where they are either expectorated or swallowed. *In vitro* experiments show that a puff of tobacco smoke paralyzes this mucociliary escalator, interfering with an important defense against particulates. The trachea divides or bifurcates into two branches (main stem bronchi) and these divide again and again (about 27 generations) until the alveolar duct ends in the alveolus. The smallest particles eventually reach the alveoli, where they are likely to be engulfed by pulmonary macrophages, which secrete enzymes that destroy many kinds of particles. Particle size, shape, speed, and density all influence the extent to which particles are able to penetrate distally into the alveoli. For example, asbestos fibers up to 200 μm in length, but with thin diameter, become entrained in laminar air flow. By contrast, pollen grains, which are spherical and in the range of 20 μm in size, are scrubbed out in the nasopharynx and do not enter the lungs. Particle toxicity may also be related to shape or to intrinsic toxicity. Some particulates stimulate the macrophages to secrete cytokines that invoke a local inflammatory response, followed by formation of a microscopic fibrotic area. Recurrent exposure to such substances may lead to more fiber deposition, until eventually the elasticity of the lung is compromised by interstitial fibrosis, leading to restrictive lung disease. Inhalational exposures to nonparticulate chemicals in vapor or gas form typically exert effects more proximally (in the upper airways) if water-soluble and more distally (in the alveoli) if not. Water-soluble chemicals cause proximal irritation that triggers local reflex responses, which generally limit distal deposition, such as crying, coughing, sneezing, and reflex bronchoconstriction. Many substances are filtered out at the nose or trapped by the mucociliary defenses of the tracheobronchial tree, and cause mainly local irritation, such as coughing. Substances that evade these defenses can reach the alveoli, where, depending on their properties, they may pass readily through the alveolar-capillary membrane and enter the systemic circulation. Phosgene does not cause upper airway irritation and passes to the alveoli, where it causes an irritant response and potentially fatal pulmonary edema, which usually takes several hours to develop.

Dermal Absorption

The skin is a very effective barrier for many chemicals, but some organic chemicals, such as methylmercury, readily pass through intact skin and enter the bloodstream. The mucous membranes are less effective barriers, and substances can be absorbed in the nasal passages or pharynx. Both the skin and mucous membranes, including those of the eyes, can also be target organs. There are remarkably few data on skin absorption of chemicals. Some nonpolar compounds pass through the skin, whereas polar compounds do not.

A tragic example of dermal absorption occurred in a chemist, who died after 3 to 5 drops of dimethylmercury were spilled on her latex gloves. Prior to her death, no studies had been conducted to determine the barrier protection offered by different gloves, and she had no way of knowing that latex gloves offered no protection from the compound. Dimethylmercury quickly passes through latex gloves and is readily absorbed through the skin. Because mercury has a specific gravity of 13, 1 cc of mercury weighs about 13 g of which over 11 g is mercury, and three drops, therefore contains about 1.6 g (1,600,000 μg) of mercury. Thus, three absorbed drops were sufficient to be fatal.

Ingestion

Many chemicals enter the body in the food we eat or the water or other liquids we drink. Many nonpolar compounds readily pass through the wall of the gastrointestinal tract into the bloodstream and are carried first to the liver (in the *first pass*) in which they may undergo metabolic activation or deactivation. From the liver, ingested nutrients and xenobiotics enter the venous circulation and are subsequently distributed throughout the body. Risk assessment assumes a default value of 2 liters per day to represent drinking water intake to a homebound adult.

Transplacental Absorption

The placenta is a complex organ with several cell layers and provides oxygen and nutrients to the fetus, removes fetal waste products, and maintains the pregnancy through hormonal secretion. The placenta maintains active transport for necessary nutrients, such as vitamins, amino acids, calcium, and iron. Xenobiotics pass through the placenta mainly by passive diffusion unless they are similar in structure to a transported substance. Although it is customary to speak of a placental barrier, there are many infectious agents (especially viruses) and chemicals that readily cross the placenta to reach the fetal circulation. Nonpolar compounds, such as methylmercury and polychlorinated biphenyls (PCBs) readily pass the placenta. Xenobiotics that are bound to proteins or are conjugated are less likely to enter the placenta.

Passage Through the Blood–Brain Barrier

The blood-brain barrier, with its low permeability, restricts entrance of many compounds into the brain. It exists because capillary cells in the central nervous system (CNS) form a tight endothelial layer with few pores. There are also tightly wound glial cells that impede passage of chemicals into the brain from the circulation. In addition, the protein concentration in the CNS is lower than in other organ systems, restricting the amount of protein available to bind and transport xenobiotics. The blood–brain barrier is poorly developed at birth, and thus fetuses and young infants are particularly vulnerable to toxicants that can reach the brain. Although methylmercury crosses the blood–brain barrier, one would not predict that inorganic mercury would do so. However, inorganic mercury is bound by cysteine in cell membranes and can pass through the barrier in this bound form.

TIME COURSE OF EXPOSURE AND TOXICITY

The *time course* of exposure to a chemical can range from a one-time, acute, short-term exposure, lasting minutes to hours, to continuous, chronic exposure lasting for years (Fig. 13-2). *Acute toxic effects*

occur in the first 24 hours after a single dose. *Subchronic effects* usually occur after repeated dosing for 10 percent of the life span. *Chronic exposure* is defined as exceeding 10 percent of an animal's life span. Despite the use of these terms, there is a continuum in the duration and frequency of exposure. Most occupational exposures are somewhat intermittent, occurring only during working hours or during particular activities within those working hours. The tradition of averaging exposures over an 8-hour period (as a time-weighted average; TWA) ignores peaks that may contribute to acute damage.

An analogy is a person who has a bottle of 30 pills to take once a day for a month. Taking all the pills on the last day yields the same monthly total, but could have very different toxic consequences. Taking 10 pills three times a month is not likely to achieve the desired pharmacologic outcome, but 3 pills taken every 3 days might achieve it. Such mixing of frequency and duration is difficult to

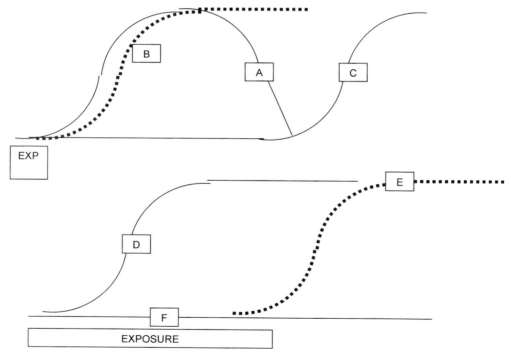

FIGURE 13-2 ● Time course of exposure and response, showing acute versus chronic exposures as well as acute and chronic responses with both short and long latency demonstrated. Solid line is duration and intensity of exposure; dashed line is the response or health effect. Curves A, B, C show responses to a single acute, high-level exposure. (**A**) An acute self-limited effect; (**B**) an acute and persistent effect; (**C**) a long-delayed effect beginning after a long latency after the acute exposure. Curves D, E, F show response to a chronic, lower level exposure. (**D**) A chronic condition arising shortly after onset of exposure, and probably idiosyncratic; (**E**) a chronic condition beginning after a long period of cumulative exposure; (**F**) no appreciable response even after long-term, low-level exposure. (Source: Environmental and Occupational Health Sciences Institute.)

model, and there are relatively few studies that address this important topic. Thus, in permissible and recommended exposure limits, there are often two measures: an 8-hour TWA and a 15-minute short-term exposure limit (STEL).

The terms *acute* and *chronic* can also refer to the outcome (Fig. 13-2). There is usually a time lag between a dose and its effect, which is referred to as latency. *Latency* is the period between the start of exposure and when disease is apparent. Latency may change, depending on the techniques used to diagnose the disease. For example, new early diagnostic tests for cancer may result in a shorter apparent latency. Some latencies are only seconds in duration, such as the effects of hydrogen sulfide. On the other hand, the latency start of asbestos exposure and onset of mesothelioma may be 40 years or more. There is a general principle that the latency period shrinks as the cumulative dose of a carcinogen increases. Long-term chronic exposure may reach a point where the cumulative dose has become sufficient to trigger an adverse health effect. An acute dose may cause damage, which eventually leads to an adverse health effect after a long latency. In general, the longer the latency, the harder it is to connect an effect to an exposure.

Progressive, Permanent, and Reversible Effects

A pathophysiologic effect caused by a toxic chemical exposure may be progressive, permanent, or reversible. Progressive changes worsen as exposure continues. In some cases, damage, such as cancer, may progress even after the exposure has ceased. In other cases the damage persists, without progressing, after cessation of exposure. Once the exposure (insult) is removed, many pathophysiologic changes have some degree of reversibility, often complete. Reversibility is a function of cumulative dose; that is, a change, such as neurologic or renal damage, may be reversible until it reaches a point where definite structural damage occurs. For example, methylmercury poisoning produces a variety of symptoms and signs, beginning with tingling sensations on the lips and progressing to visual, auditory, and gait impairments, and culminating in blindness, coma, convulsions, and death. The early changes are reversible; but once blindness occurs, complete recovery is not possible.

Different organ systems have different possibilities of total repair. Death of a cell is not reversible,

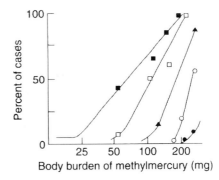

FIGURE 13-3 ● A series of dose–response curves for different end points of methylmercury toxicity reflecting a major poisoning episode from contaminated grain in Iraq For each end point, a separate dose–response curve can be drawn, and these are nested from the least serious on the left (paresthesias occurring at the lowest dose) to death on the right, compared to the estimated body burden of methylmercury. Solid squares, paresthesias; open squares, ataxia; solid triangles, dysarthria; open circles, deafness; solid circles, death. (Source: Modified from Takizawa Y. Epidemiology of mercury poisoning. In: J Nriagu J, ed. The biogeochemistry of mercury in the environment. Amsterdam: Elsevier, 1979.)

but almost all organs are capable of replacing damaged cells by regeneration, which is not always perfect. For example, after viral or toxic hepatitis, the liver regenerates, but the healing often results in cirrhosis, because new liver cells have interposed fibrous tissue that compresses cells and interferes with function. Similarly, after lung inflammation, the healing process involves formation of fibrous tissue that eventually impairs respiratory function.

When DNA is damaged, there are repair enzymes capable of restoring the genetic material, although not always in the same order as the original. DNA repair mechanism(s) become less efficient in the elderly, and this is believed to be one of the factors associated with the increased cancer rate with age. Figure 13-3 shows a variety of dose–response curves.

TOXICOKINETICS

Figure 13-4 summarizes the movement of substances from environmental media into and out of various body compartments. Toxicologists distinguish toxicokinetics (what the body does to a chemical) from toxicodynamics (what the chemical does to the body). Toxicokinetics refers to a series of phenomena that govern the uptake, metabolism, distribution, and elimination of a toxic substance and

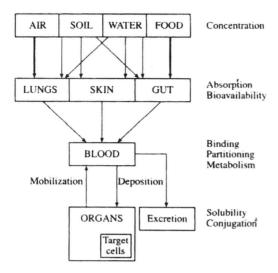

FIGURE 13-4 ● A multicompartment model of toxicant distribution showing the relationship among uptake, metabolism, distribution, storage, and excretion. (Modified from Gochfeld M. Principles of toxicology. In JM Last, RB Wallace, eds. Maxcy-Rosenau-Last's public health and preventive medicine. Norwalk, CT: Appleton & Lange, 1992. Source: Environmental and Occupational Health Sciences Institute.)

its metabolites and the dose delivered to target organs. As researchers provide data on partitioning coefficients and metabolic rates, it becomes possible to develop models that predict how much of a chemical will circulate through each organ, using data on the perfusion rate (amount of blood delivered per minute). These are called physiologically based pharmacokinetic (PBPK) models, patterned after models that predict the fate of pharmaceutical agents in the body.

Absorption

Absorption occurs mainly through the lungs, gastrointestinal tract, and skin. When the skin or mucous membranes (mucosa) lining the respiratory or gastrointestinal tract come in contact with a contaminated medium, there is an opportunity for transfer of contaminants across the skin or mucosa into the bloodstream. For every chemical, there is a characteristic absorption pattern across the skin (usually very low) and mucosa (sometimes very high), depending on the chemical and physical attributes of the chemical, including its polarity, solubility, and size. Small, nonpolar compounds tend

to be lipophilic and readily pass through membranes. The skin and mucosa prevent the ingress of most large, polar molecules. In addition, there are differences among organs. Elemental mercury is volatile at room temperature, and mercury vapor is readily absorbed through the lung. However, the same amount of elemental mercury, if swallowed, would pass through the intestinal tract with negligible absorption. On the other hand, if methylmercury were ingested, there could be almost complete absorption.

The superficial linings of the skin, lungs, and gastrointestinal tract form barriers that retard the exchange of water and solutes between the environment and the extracellular and intracellular compartments. Material crosses membranes in various ways, by free diffusion (mainly of polar molecules), through small pores, and by transporter molecules (mainly for polar compounds).

There can be individual variability and variability related to age or other factors. For example, children can absorb about 50 percent of the lead they ingest, whereas adults absorb usually less than 10 percent. Women who have depleted iron stores absorb a much higher proportion of ingested cadmium than men or women with normal iron stores. Transporter molecules are specific carriers of certain toxics, and their presence and efficiency varies among people, in part due to genetic factors. Transporters serve a normal physiologic function; for example, metallothionein proteins regulate movement of zinc, an essential element, through the body. Cadmium, a xenobiotic, strongly binds to metallothionein, which carries it to other organs, including the kidney where it is excreted.

Bioavailability

Whereas absorption for any chemical is a property of the organ, *bioavailability* refers to the matrix properties, especially of soil and food, which may bind a toxic and interfere with absorption. Even a chemical that is readily absorbed in pure form may not be absorbed from a particular environmental medium. For example, organic matter in water or soil may bind toxic chemicals, impeding their absorption. The relatively sandy soil of Times Beach, Missouri, readily yielded dioxin when fed to animals by gavage, while the the oil-contaminated soil of Newark, New Jersey, bound the dioxin tenaciously, so that little could be extracted and absorbed in the gastrointestinal tract. Thus, for any chemical, the amount absorbed depends on the characteristics of both the contact organ and the chemical in its environmental medium or matrix.[3]

Transport

Once a xenobiotic has entered the bloodstream, it is transported by the blood to many organs. Chemicals absorbed from the gastrointestinal tract are carried first to the liver through the portal circulation—sometimes referred to as the *first pass*. In contrast, many volatile chemicals absorbed through the lung are delivered immediately to all organs, including the brain and kidneys. Substances can be carried in free form or bound to transporter molecules, especially proteins. Once a substance reaches an organ, its transfer from the capillaries of the organ out into the extracellular fluid or into cells is partially governed by how strongly it is bound in the bloodstream.

Metabolism

Metabolism consists of the processes organisms use to handle foreign substances that have been absorbed. It is divided into two phases: *Phase I* includes a series of transformations involving mainly oxidation or reduction that make the absorbed compound more water soluble, and *Phase II* involves adding a larger molecule to the original substance by conjugation. A xenobiotic that is carried to any organ, but especially the liver, may undergo metabolic alteration. Sometimes, the metabolic change reduces the toxicity (*detoxification*); in other cases, it increases it (*bioactivation*). Metabolism may also make a compound more (or occasionally less) water soluble, thereby enhancing the ability of the kidney to eliminate the chemical. Because metabolism is not usually 100 percent effective, there can be a complex situation with both the absorbed chemical and one or more metabolites circulating at the same time. The ratio of metabolite to parent compound in the blood is called the metabolic ratio, whereas is sometimes used to measure the efficiency of metabolism in humans. Genetic differences among people in certain enzyme efficiencies can be reflected in the metabolic ratio. Slow metabolizers have a low metabolite:parent compound ratio, whereas rapid metabolizers have a high ratio.

INTERMEDIARY METABOLISM (BIOTRANSFORMATION)

Many xenobiotics are subject to metabolism in various organs, especially the liver. Metabolites may have greater or lesser toxicity than the parent compound. Whereas the liver detoxifies some xenobiotics, it metabolically activates many others, usually through an enzymically mediated, oxidative reaction. In general, metabolites are more polar, hence more water soluble, than the parent compound. Oxidized metabolites, often referred to as reactive intermediates, can "attack" cell membranes as well as intracellular membranes and macromolecules.

Phase I reactions cause hydrolysis or hydroxylation, form epoxides, and lead to other outcomes. The cytochrome P450–dependent enzyme system plays a major role in Phase I reactions. Phase II links a metabolite to a glucuronide (glutathione) or adds acetyl or methyl radicals. Phase II reactions usually increase the hydrophilic nature of the substance, facilitating its excretion in urine.

Metabolic enzymes are found in most organs, beginning with the nasal passages, but the greatest variety and quantity are in the liver. Within cells, these enzymes are found mainly in the microsomal component of the endoplasmic reticulum but also in the cytosol and other organelles. Certain xenobiotic compounds are metabolized by intestinal flora. Many of the metabolic responses begin with an oxidation step (Fig. 13-5).

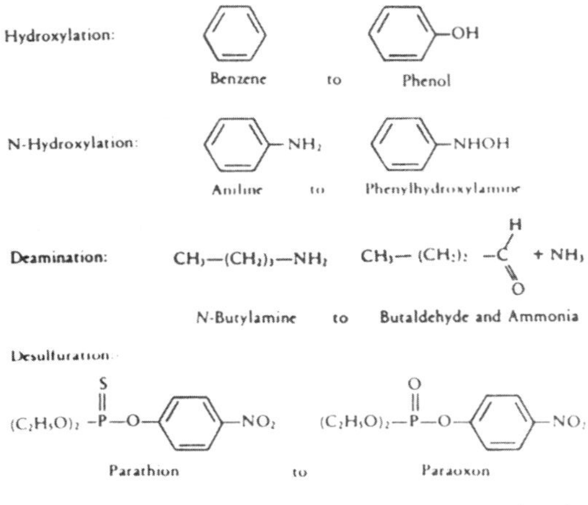

FIGURE 13-5 ● Examples of oxidation reactions in metabolism of several common industrial chemicals.

Cytochrome P450

Among Phase I metabolic enzymes are a large group of enzymes known as *cytochrome P450s* (or P450s, for short). These occur in many families in all organisms, and an entire subdiscipline has arisen to study the classification of P450s and their variation among species and organs, the different substrates on which they act, their specificity (or lack thereof), and the metabolites they produce. Once known as *liver microsomal oxidases* or *mixed function oxidases*, the various metabolic functions are now being assigned to particular P450s, only a few of which are discussed in detail below.

P450s are found in most tissues, although the greatest amount and variety occur in the liver. They have a general feature of adding oxygen to their substrate. Sometimes the addition of oxygen forms a highly reactive epoxide and sometimes a less reactive hydroxide. Oxygen can be involved in breaking double-bonds, cleaving esters, and in dehalogenation reactions. As new forms of these enzymes are discovered, they are assigned to major families and subfamilies. Much of the research on P450 has come from the pharmaceutical industry investigating how drugs are metabolized. For example, the P450 that metabolizes caffeine is referred to as P450 1A2 (often abbreviated as CYP1A2). This enzyme also metabolizes some toxic chemicals with very variable efficiency among individuals. Its intrinsic activity can be evaluated by the caffeine breath test. Subjects are given a dose of caffeine labeled with carbon-13, and the amount of C-13 carbon dioxide ($^{13}CO_2$) in exhaled breath is measured over a 2-hour period. A high percentage recovery of labeled $^{13}CO_2$ indicates high CYP1A2 activity and decreases susceptibility to polychlorinated aromatic compounds, such as dioxins and furans.

Enzyme Polymorphisms and Susceptibility

Studies of enzyme polymorphisms[*] have helped explain why people can vary widely in their metabolic activity and toxic responses after similar exposures: the sequence of nucleotides in the DNA of a gene code for a specific sequence of amino acids in a protein that determines its action as an enzyme. A mutation at some point in the gene may result

in the substitution of one amino acid for another, which, in turn, may reduce or eliminate the activity of the resulting protein. Heritable deficiencies of P450 activity can arise from single nucleotide polymorphisms (SNPs). Although in any population, most people share identical gene sequences for enzymes, a small percentage of individuals may have an abnormal sequence causing them to produce an abnormal enzyme. However, rarer mutant forms of an enzyme may place a few individuals at high risk. Polymorphism in the genes that code for various P450 proteins has been shown to result in different metabolic phenotypes. Great interest has focused on CYP2D6 because it was identified as the enzyme metabolizing the drug debrisoquine; however, it also metabolizes a variety of other xenobiotics.

People whose CYP2D6 phenotype makes them poor metabolizers of debrisoquine are at risk of various adverse drug reactions, whereas extensive metabolizers are at increased risk of lung cancer, probably because of carcinogenic metabolites they produce. Thus CYP2D6-deficient people are protected from certain environmentally caused cancers, such as lung, bladder, and liver cancer, because of their failure to activate certain procarcinogens. About 5 to 10 percent of Caucasians, but less than 1 percent of Japanese, have a mutant CYP2D6 that is inefficient at metabolizing debrisoquine to its hydroxide form. The metabolic ratio, which is defined as:

$$\text{Metabolic ratio} = \frac{\text{Debrisoquine-OH}}{\text{Debrisoquine}}$$

can therefore serve as a measure of metabolic efficiency. Those who are poor metabolizers of debrisoquine (low metabolic ratio) are also poor metabolizers of other substances acted on by CYP2D6. This phenomenon was first discovered because about 5 percent of patients receiving debrisoquine developed prolonged hypotension, due to failure to metabolize the drug.

Tissue Specificity

There is important variability in where a P450 is expressed, as significant metabolic activation or detoxification may occur in target tissues. Thus, CYP1A2 is expressed in the liver, but not other organs, whereas CYP1A1 is low in the liver of most mammals, but high in other tissues. Both are induced by polyaromatic hydrocarbons (PAHs) and indoles. Because the two CYPs catalyze

---

[*] *A polymorphism is an allele type that, by convention, occurs in more than 1 percent of a population.*

different reactions, a single substrate may follow different metabolic pathways in different tissues. This is a rapidly evolving area of research, with important applications to pharmacology and toxicology. Another example is the 10-fold variation in the liver content of CYP3A4, which influences the metabolism of many steroids and xenobiotics. This may add credence to the use of a 10-fold uncertainty factor in risk assessment to try to protect the most susceptible individuals.

Flavin-Containing Monoxygenases

The flavin-containing monoxygenases (FMOs) represent another family of oxidizing enzymes that are NADPH-dependent. They act on nitrogen-, phosphorus-, or sulfur-containing substrates, such as amines, organophosphates, or thiols. FMOs have different isoforms that are distributed differently among species and organs. FMO1 occurs at high levels in rat and rabbit liver, with low levels in mouse and human liver; FMO3 occurs at a high concentration in human and mouse liver but at low concentrations in rat and rabbit liver. Liver cells of female mice have higher amounts of FM01 and FMO3 than do male mice.

Examples of Metabolic Activation

An example of the importance of metabolic activation is the case of 1-methyl-4-phenyl-1,2,5,6-tetrahydropyridine (MPTP), an accidental by-product in the production of a designer narcotic. The narcotic was sold "on the street" and was used by many young people, several hundred at a dangerous level. MPTP is oxidized by monomine oxidase to MPP+, which is transported by the dopamine transporter and concentrates in dopaminergic neurons, where it inhibits cellular respiration and causes cell death. Hundreds of those affected develop irreversible parkinsonism. MPTP then became an important model drug for research producing parkinsonism in animals.

Many chlorinated and aromatic hydrocarbons, such as vinyl chloride and trichlorethylene, undergo metabolic activation by formation of a reactive epoxide intermediate. The P450 system also metabolizes the analagesic, acetaminophen, to a quinone that causes centrilobular necrosis of the liver. Acetaminophen is acted on by prostaglandin H synthase in the kidney, producing a nephrotoxic free radical. In the bladder, the prostaglandin H synthase

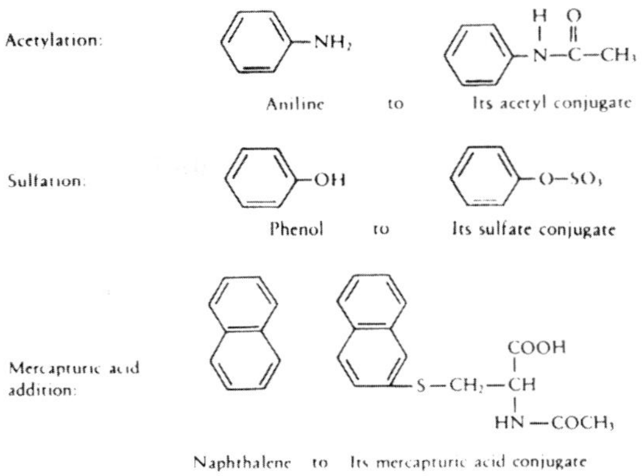

FIGURE 13-6 ● Examples of Phase II (conjugation reactions).

system metabolizes a variety of aromatic amines into genotoxic metabolites that can induce bladder cancer. In rats these same organic amines undergo N-hydroxylation in the liver and cause mainly liver cancer.

Phase II Reactions

Phase II reactions include several important conjugation reactions. Metabolites from Phase I reactions can undergo conjugation with other molecules, which facilitates their transport and excretion in urine. There are several types of conjugation reactions, among which conjugation to reduced glutathione (GSH) is particularly common (Fig. 13-6). This effects a wide range of electrophilic substrates and is accelerated by glutathione-S-transferase (GST) enzymes. Glucuronidation involves connecting the metabolite to a glucuronide moiety, by various enzymes called glucuronosyltransferases that are found in various mammal tissues. The low-molecular-weight glucuronide complexes are excreted in the urine, although some forms are excreted in the bile.

Polymorphisms at the GST loci result in variable efficiencies of the conjugation reaction. Divalent cations, such as many metals, readily bind with sulfhydryl groups, including GSH. Exposure to mercury increases the activity of several enzymes involved in the synthesis of GSH and the reduction of oxidized glutathione (GSSG). Conversely, acetaminophen depletes GSH levels in liver. Both the depletion and the subsequent hepatotoxicity are inhibited by diallyl sulfone, a metabolite of garlic, which inhibits CYP2E1, the enzyme that activates acetaminophen.

However, conjugation can be harmful if it occurs in excess and depletes the body of essential constituents. Sulfation is the major means of preparing phenol for excretion. It is also used for alcohols, amines, and other categories of chemicals. Sulfation and acetylation exemplify the sequential processing of substances by Phase I and Phase II reactions. Phenol and aniline can be metabolites of other toxins and can then be conjugated and excreted. The addition of mercapturic acid (*N*-acetylcysteine) is a multistep process that proceeds through the addition of glutathione and subsequent cleavage to cysteine derivatives. This reaction is extremely important in handling reactive electrophilic compounds that result from exogenous exposure or endogenous metabolic processes. PAHs and polyhalogenated hydrocarbons are predominantly excreted in this manner.

N-Acetyltransferase

Aromatic amines or hydrazines with a nitrogen atom can be metabolized by attaching acetate to the nitrogen (N-acetylation). This is accomplished by *N*-acetyltransferases (NATs) and serves as a major degradation pathway. There are at least three forms of NAT, and a deficiency in either activity or structure of NAT2 results in slow acetylation of certain drugs, such as isoniazid. This deficiency occurs in about 70 percent of the Middle East population, 50 percent of Europeans, and 20 percent of Asians.

Sequestration or Storage

A chemical or its metabolite circulating in the bloodstream can be delivered to many organs simultaneously—excretory organs, target organs, or storage organs. Chemicals may be stored for days, months, or decades in storage organs, usually while manifesting little evidence of harm. For example, lead is stored in bone, where it is fairly innocuous; lead exerts its primary toxic effects in the nervous system and other organ systems. Organochlorines, such as polychlorinated biphenyl compounds (PCBs), are stored in fat. They generally do not harm fatty tissue; but, if a person mobilizes fat rapidly, there may be a massive release of PCBs and a potentially harmful dose to sensitive target organs. Cadmium is stored mainly in the kidney, its primary target organ; even when exposure is terminated, the cadmium is eliminated from the kidney very slowly.

Elimination or Excretion

Once a xenobotic or its metabolites is circulating in the bloodstream, it can be delivered to an excretory organ. Excretion is mainly through the urine and feces, but volatile compounds can be excreted in exhaled breath or in sweat. Many biomarker tests rely on measuring the concentration of a chemical in urine or exhaled breath. Some chemicals, especially those that are lipophilic, are readily transferred to breast milk, potentially posing more of a hazard for an infant than its mother. Some compounds, particularly metals, concentrate in skin or hair and are lost through the natural sloughing of epidermal cells or hair growth. Substances that are water-soluble—or become water-soluble—through conjugation are excreted via the kidney; however, they may be toxic to the kidney or bladder because they are concentrated in these organs during urine production. Lipophilic substances or complexes may be secreted into bile and then excreted in the feces; some compounds excreted in the bile—in what is referred to as an enterohepatic cycle—may be reabsorbed in the intestine, thereby retarding elimination and enhancing toxicity.

The bloodstream delivers toxic substances to the renal glomerulus where most are filtered with water and many other substances, forming the glomerular ultrafiltrate. Only cellular elements and large proteins, such as albumin and substances bound to them escape the filter and remain in the blood. Some of these may be secreted into the renal tubule. As the filtrate leaves the glomerulus and begins to pass down the tubule, the concentration of the toxic substance is similar to its concentration in the bloodstream. However, by the time the filtrate has traversed the tubular system and enters the collecting duct, about 99 percent of the water has been reabsorbed, so that the toxic substance is about 100 times more concentrated in the urine than in the blood. In this form, it is delivered to the bladder, where it may reside for hours before being eliminated. The liver also plays a prominent role in excretion by producing bile, which may incorporate nonpolar compounds that are not easily excreted by the kidney. Bile carries toxic compounds with it into the intestinal tract.

The rate of elimination of a toxic substance from the body is an important variable. As long as it equals or exceeds the rate of intake, the substance will not build up in the body. Excretion is widely used in biomonitoring. Blood and urine concentrations are measured for many compounds. Hair and fingernails have been used to monitor metals, because they are composed of keratin, which is rich in sulfydryl groups that readily bind certain metals, such as mercury. Comparing concentrations in two or more fluids or tissues provides information on the nature of the chemical. Thus, organic mercurial compounds, such as methylmercury, are readily deposited in hair or are excreted in the feces, whereas inorganic forms of mercury are eliminated mainly in the urine. People who have high blood and urine mercury levels, but low hair mercury levels, probably have been exposed to inorganic, rather than organic, mercury. On the other hand, patients who have consumed much fish may have high blood and hair mercury, but low urine mercury.

Biological Half-Life

The amount of a toxic substance that is circulating in the bloodstream at any time or the amount delivered to target organs represents a balance between (a) uptake and (b) elimination or storage. If exposure were terminated, the amount of the toxic substance in the body would gradually decrease. Some substances with short biological half-lives are rapidly excreted, whereas others with long biological half-lives tend to remain in the body for long periods. Many chemicals have a biphasic or even triphasic elimination pattern, with very rapid elimination for the first few days after exposure, followed by very gradual elimination as the substance is re-released from organs and delivered to the kidney. There can be substantial interindividual variation in the biological half-life of a given chemical; for example, cadmium may have a biological half-life ranging from a few years to many decades.

Delivery to Target Organ

While a chemical is being delivered to storage or excretory organs, some is delivered to target organs, where the toxic substance enters cells. The rate of delivery determines the dose to target, or the internal dose. This depends on the blood perfusion rate of the organ and the movement of the substance across the cell membrane—either by passive diffusion or a variety of active-transport mechanisms. The diffusion rate, following Fick's principle, is proportional to the concentration gradient, the membrane surface area, and a compound-specific coefficient (which depends on the membrane condition and the octanol:water partitioning coefficient, with lipophilic compounds passing membranes more quickly than hydrophilic ones). The diffu-

sion coefficient is approximately related to the cube root of the molecular weight of the compound, with smaller molecules therefore passing through membranes much more easily than large ones.

END POINTS

Health professionals are concerned with identifying and preventing morbidity and mortality end points—ranging from skin lesions to death, and involving molecular, biochemical, anatomic, physiologic, behavioral, or other effects. For example, Fig. 13-3 shows a series of dose–response curves for different end points of methylmercury toxicity, reflecting a major poisoning episode in Iraq due to contaminated grain. For each end point, a separate dose–response curve can be drawn; these are nested from the least serious on the left, occurring at the lowest dose, to death on the right.

Traditionally, toxicologists have used the LD_{50} as the primary end point. This is the lethal dose for 50 percent of the animals tested. The LD_{50} has also been used to assess the efficacy of antibiotics and pesticides. The potency of chemicals can be ranked on the basis of the LD_{50}. Other end points can be quantified the same way, yielding an ED_{50} (the dose that produces a particular effect in 50 percent of the animals) or an ED_{10} (the dose that produces the effect in 10 percent). The ED_{10} is sometimes referred to as a benchmark dose. However, most often we are interested in doses that affect only 1 to 10 percent of the population—the most sensitive people. Many recent studies use a broad range of biochemical, physiological, behavioral, and other end points. The ED_{50} and the ED_{10} can be calculated from data generated in animal studies using computer programs.

DOSE–RESPONSE CURVES

The *dose–response curve* describes how any particular response increases as the dose increases. Figure 13-7 represents a series of dose–response curves, with dose plotted on the x axis and the response on the y axis. The y axis may be the number of cells killed, the amount of a biomarker released, the number of animals affected, the percent of people with a particular symptom, or the number who die. The most common dose–response curve has a sigmoid shape with three zones: *subthreshold*, *rapid increase*, and *maximal effect* or *plateau*. If the toxic effect is *idiosyncratic*, relying on the underlying susceptibility of individuals to a great extent, the sigmoid curve may not be a good representation.

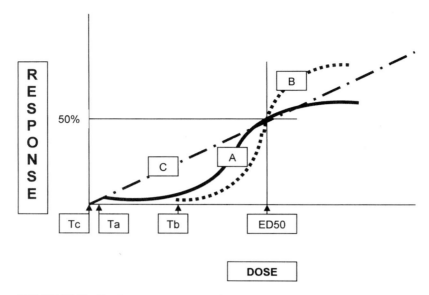

FIGURE 13-7   ●   Dose–response curves for three hypothetical chemicals. Curves A and B are typical sigmoid curves differing in potency and efficacy. C is a linear, no-threshold curve presumed to be characteristic of the causation of cancer by ionizing radiation. B has a higher threshold than A. Thresholds are indicated by "t". ED_{50s} represent the dose corresponding to a 50 percent response. (Source: Environmental and Occupational Health Sciences Institute.)

The central portion of the dose–response curve can rise with varying degrees of steepness, reflecting differences in susceptibility of the target population. A chemical that induces the same effect in all people, with little differential susceptibility, will have a much steeper rise than one for which individual responsiveness differs greatly. Dose is usually measured as amount of chemical, such as in milligrams, per kilogram of body weight. This works reasonably well for systemic exposures and effects but does not adequately describe some toxic phenomena, such as skin sensitization.

Threshold

A *threshold* is the lowest dose at which the response can be detected, usually in the most susceptible individual. For any given chemical, the threshold may vary, depending on conditions of exposure and individual susceptibility. The threshold can be used as a basis for guidelines or standard-setting. Thresholds must be defined in terms of a particular form of a chemical time course of exposure, target population, and response.

Most toxicologic experiments use at least three doses (including a zero control), but relatively few studies use as many as five doses. Thus, knowledge of the actual threshold may be crude, as it seldom corresponds exactly to the dose used. Thus, experiments yield a *lowest observed adverse effect level* (LOAEL), which is the lowest dose, above the control value, at which the effect is detected. In some studies, this may correspond to the lowest dose tested. A *no observed adverse effect level* (NOAEL) is the lowest level above the zero control dose at which no effect can be detected. LOAELs and NOAELs are used in risk assessment and standard-setting.

Although for most chemicals and most responses it is possible to detect a threshold, this is not always possible. Radiation carcinogenesis is generally assumed to follow a nonthreshold pattern. For childhood blood lead levels, there is no detectable NOAEL for neurobehavioral effects; one study, in fact, surprisingly found that the response slope was steeper in the 5 to 10 μg/dL range than above 10 μg/dL. Because there is no known beneficial role for lead in the body, it is not surprising that any amount of the chemical may be harmful. Because the threshold is the dose below which no effect is detected, it is possible—and indeed likely—that for lead any apparent threshold was due to the insensitivity of testing rather than to lack of adverse effect.

Chemical carcinogens vary in their mechanism of action. A major controversy in toxicology is whether the linear nonthreshold model is an appropriate description of the dose–response relationship for chemical carcinogens. At present, this model is used for genotoxic carcinogens. In developing its risk assessments for cancer, EPA uses a linearized multistage model to account for cancer arising not only from induction (chemical alteration of the genetic material) but also from factors governing promotion and proliferation.

Hormesis

Chemicals have multiple end points with multiple dose–response curves (see Fig. 13-3). A special issue in dose–response is *hormesis*, best exemplified by pharmaceutical agents or nutrients, such as vitamin A and copper, which not only have a therapeutic, but also a toxicologic, threshold. Ideally, these two thresholds are far apart. However, where they are close—and thus there is a small margin of safety—toxicity can occur. Many drugs, for example, have been removed from the market, or never make it to market, because of a low margin of safety.

The concept of hormesis emerges from studies of radiation, where low doses of radiation have sometimes been associated with increased longevity. However, the dose–response curve for radiation-induced mutation is independent of any beneficial dose–response curve that might exist. Critics of low-dose extrapolation argue that it ignores hormesis. Hormesis is thus highly controversial, including in a political context. One must be cautious in interpreting arguments based on hormesis.

CHEMICAL INTERACTIONS

When an individual is exposed simultaneously to two or more chemicals or to a mixture of chemicals, a variety of interactions may occur, both outside and inside the body. These interactions are generally grouped into three categories: (a) independence and additivity, (b) synergism, and (c) antagonism.

If chemical A and chemical B each produce their effects independent of the other chemical, then the there is no interaction. There is no interaction when chemicals affect different organs or produce different end points. *Independence* can occur when two chemicals follow different metabolic pathways, bind to different receptors, and do not compete. *Additivity* occurs when the two chemicals contribute to the same end point but show no interaction.

Synergism—a multiplicative effect—is of great practical importance, although there are remarkably few documented examples. In *synergism*, one chemical enhances the effect of another (or vice versa), such that their combined effect on some end point is greater than would be expected from their independent dose–response curves. Chemical A may enhance the effect of chemical B, enhance its activation, or interfere with its degradation and elimination. The best documented example of synergism is based on a study of lung cancer in relation to smoking and occupational exposure to asbestos.[4] Smoking increased lung cancer risk about 10 times; asbestos, about 5 times, and both about 50 times.

Antagonism occurs if chemical A reduces the effect of chemical B. For example, they may compete for the same activating metabolic pathway or for the same receptor. Chemical A may inhibit the uptake of chemical B or its delivery to the target organ. If both A and B are activated by the same pathway, A may saturate the enzyme, preventing B from being activated.

Susceptibility

Individuals vary in their physiologic responses to chemicals, their immunologic responsiveness to various allergens (hypersensitivity), and in their subjective responses to stresses, odors, noise, and discomfort. At the extreme, individuals can be labeled as *hypersusceptible* to chemicals—not to be confused with *hypersensitivity* to allergens.

There are several ways of graphically representing susceptibility, such as with a dose–response curve in which the y axis is the percent of individuals manifesting a particular end point. Typically susceptibility is either (a) bimodal, with some individuals susceptible and others not, or (b) log-normal in distribution. *Hypersusceptibility* refers to people at the extreme end of the susceptibility spectrum. In 1938, the geneticist J.B.S. Haldane suggested that someday, genetic screening might allow identification of hypersusceptible workers—but he emphasized that in the meantime, industrial hygiene controls were needed.[5] In 1967, H.E. Stockinger actively lobbied for genetic screening of workers for glucose-6-phosphate dehydrogenase (G6PD) deficiency, sickle cell anemia, and alpha-1-antitrypsin deficiency.[6] Over the ensuing decade, some companies experimented with mandatory or voluntary genetic screening tests; however, like pre-employment back x-rays, most were abandoned because of lack of predictive value, high potential for discrimination, and lack of cost-effectiveness. Genetic screening for susceptibility has resurfaced with completion of the human genome process, and serious ethical and legal issues have been raised. Some states have legislated that genetic information cannot be used to deny health insurance or treatment but have not excluded its use in life insurance.

Hypersensitivity

Exposure to allergenic compounds will eventually sensitize some workers so that they respond immunologically, developing either dermal or respiratory symptoms. Some allergens, such as chromium, are potent sensitizers, quickly affecting a small proportion of people who contact them. On the other hand, workers who care for research animals in vivariums gradually build up allergic responsiveness that requires them to switch to other species until they become responsive to those as well. Workers who become allergic to particular chemicals at work usually will require relocation; desensitization is seldom an option. However, if an allergen is encountered only infrequently and predictably, then special personal protective equipment can be put on before exposure.

Adaptation, Tolerance, and Hardening

At the opposite end of the spectrum are workers who show very little response to a chemical at a dose that would produce symptoms in most co-workers. These people are said to be tolerant or resistant. In other cases, repeat exposure to a chemical results in physiologic adaptation (the opposite of sensitization) at the metabolic or target tissue level. People who build up tolerance to a chemical may no longer experience its acute effects. Thus, smokers, who are chronically exposed to CO from cigarettes, are less likely to experience headaches at CO levels that cause headaches in non-smokers. Work hardening is the deliberate process of allowing workers to adapt to conditions or exposures. It is used effectively when workers are transferred to high altitudes or extreme environmental temperatures, when a week or more is required to regain full physiologic and physical functioning. Tolerance to chemical exposures can also be developed, but is not considered an appropriate alternative to industrial hygiene controls.

Extrapolation from Animals to Humans

For some common industrial chemicals, there is a database of dose–response information based on studies of acute and chronic exposures among workers. To estimate environmental effects, we customarily use data from the relatively high workplace exposures and extrapolate down to levels found in communities. Most industrial chemicals, however, do not have a good database on adverse effects in humans, hence we must rely on animal studies. (Animal studies are also helpful because they allow use of high doses of a chemical.) Due to different metabolism and susceptibility, interspecies differences in response may be very great. For example, even among experimental rodents, response to a xenobiotic varies by the species, strain, age, and sex of the test animals as well as the exposure circumstances. Similar genetic factors influence human responses.

A general principle of toxicology relies on the extrapolation from the results of animal studies to effects on humans. The biochemical, physiological, and organ structure of humans is very similar to that of other mammals—and to vertebrates in general. Although there are unique differences between humans and other mammals mainly at the cognitive level, other organ functions are remarkably similar. Although amino-acid sequences in major functional proteins have changed over long periods of time, the basic hormonal and enzyme functions have changed little and data on avian and mammalian toxicity have been particularly useful in understanding human toxicology.

CLASSIFICATION (TAXONOMY) OF CHEMICAL AGENTS

Chemicals can be classified according to their structures, their sources, their economic roles, their mechanisms of action, and their target organs. Sometimes, the only information we have on a chemical is the class to which it belongs, such as pesticide or solvent. The lists below are intended to be illustrative, not exhaustive.

Classification by Structure

Structure–activity relationships (SARs) are often useful in inferring the toxicity of an unfamiliar chemical from the known activity of familiar or better-studied chemicals. Because only a handful

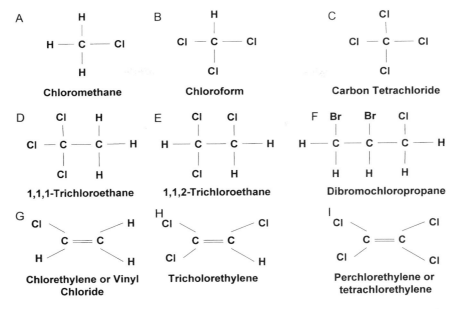

FIGURE 13-8 ● Examples of simple chlorinated hydrocarbons. Single carbon compounds are (a) chloromethane, (b) trichloromethane or chloroform, and (c) tetrachloromethane or carbon tetrachloride. Two carbon compounds with a single bond (alkanes) are (d) 1,1,1-trichloroethane, (e) 1,1,2-trichloroethane, and the three-carbon alkane (f) is 1,1-dibromo, 2-chloropropane, or DBCP. Two-carbon compounds with double bonds (alkenes) are (g) chloroethylene or vinyl chloride, (h) trichloroethylene (TCE), and (i) tetrachloroethylene or perchlorethylene.

of the thousands of chemicals in commercial use have been adequately tested, reliance on SARs may provide the only information. Yet one must be cautious because similar chemicals do not always have similar properties.

Thus, chlorinated hydrocarbons with simple chain structure (alkanes) tend to share the common property of central nervous system depression (Fig. 13-8). Their potency varies with structure (the number of carbons); the presence of double bonds; and the addition of chlorine, fluorine, or bromine, but the general effects are similar. Figure 13-8 shows several common chlorinated compounds that are, or have been, in widespread commercial use. Similarly, many heavy metals are toxic to the proximal kidney tubule, and many hallucinogenic compounds share a common active group. SARs are predictive of carcinogenicity, as identified by long-term animal bioassays.

Chemicals classified by structure are:

ORGANIC CHEMICALS

Aromatics, such as phenols and benzene derivatives

Aliphatics, such as ethanes and ethenes

Polyaromatic hydrocarbons (PAHs)

Chlorinated polyaromatics, such as dioxins, furans, and polychlorinated biphenyls (PCBs)

Chlorinated hydrocarbons, such as chlorinated alkanes and alkenes

Amines

Ethers

Ketones

Aldehydes

Alcohols

INORGANIC CHEMICALS

Acids

Bases

Anions and cations

Heavy metals, such as lead and mercury

Metalloids, such as arsenic and selenium

Salts.

Classification by Source

Toxin refers only to chemicals produced naturally by organisms. Many plants and animals secrete chemicals designed to keep them from being eaten. Butterflies, such as Monarch butterflies, may incorporate plant alkaloids in their own tissues, rendering themselves inedible. Beetles may squirt cyanide compounds to deter predators. Plants that have been partially eaten by herbivores may load increased levels of distasteful tannin compounds in newly regenerated leaves. Similarly, many fungi may secrete chemicals that inhibit bacterial growth. Snakes have developed a variety of neurotoxic and hematotoxic venoms for immobilizing prey. There is great diversity of toxins produced in the terrestrial or marine environment by organisms ranging from fungi and dinoflagellates to fish. A wide variety of these naturally occurring bioactive substances, or toxins, have been adapted into some of our most familiar pharmaceuticals, such as antibiotics.

Chemicals classified by source are:

NATURAL OR BIOLOGICAL COMPOUNDS (TOXINS)
Plant
Bacterial
Invertebrate
Vertebrate

SYNTHETIC COMPOUNDS
Industrial reagent, by-product, or product
Pharmaceutical
Pesticide.

Classification by Use

Very often, the first thing one wants to learn about a chemical exposure is the type of compound. Thus, a person trying to commit suicide may be brought to an emergency department with "an overdose of sleeping pills"; a worker may have been overcome while "using a solvent"; or a homeowner may report "some pesticide spray" making him or her ill. Examples of common-use classes of materials that may have toxic effects include:

Solvents
Fuels
Paints, dyes, and coatings
Glues
Pesticides
Pharmaceutical agents
Detergents and cleansers
Acids and bases.

Pharmaceuticals and abused substances are grouped together because of the tendency for very high concentrations of bioactive agents to be deliberately introduced into the body. In fact, many abused substances originally developed as pharmaceuticals, such as amphetamines, barbiturates, and narcotics, have profound toxic effects—quite apart from their addictive properties. By whatever route and whether legal or illicit, these chemicals are used because of their high level of bioactivity. Even when the dosage used is in the therapeutic range, there may be undesired side effects that are manifestations of toxicity. These may occur in most users, such as the soporific effects of diphenhydramine, or rarely, such as anaphylaxis from penicillin. The most widespread toxic exposures involve the chronic inhalation of tobacco smoke by the smoker and bystanders and chronic overconsumption of ethanol. Because many pharmaceuticals affect the same enzymes that metabolize industrial chemicals, it is important to evaluate the drugs a person may be taking in order to assess whether there may be dangerous interactions with chemicals at work, in hobbies, or at home.

Classification by Mechanism of Action

Much exciting research in modern toxicology focuses on the mechanism by which a bioactive substance interacts with and alters its targets to produce its adverse effects. Chemicals can be classified by mechanism of action. Asphyxiants interfere with oxygen uptake or use. For example, methane and other gases that are toxicologically inert, can function as simple asphyxiants by displacing oxygen from inhaled air, thereby decreasing the oxygen saturation of the blood and reducing its availability to cells. Chemical asphyxiants, interfere with oxygen transport (CO) or cellular respiration (cyanide). Carbon monoxide, for example, has a strong affinity for hemoglobin, and the resulting carboxyhemoglobin is unable to transport oxygen from the lungs to the cells. Chemicals classified by mechanism of action are:

Enzyme inducers
Metabolic poisons and asphyxiants
Macromolecular binders to, for example, DNA or protein
Cell membrane disrupters
Competitive binders of active sites or receptors
Formers of free radicals/active oxygen
Chemicals causing redox reactions
Chemicals interfering with signal transduction
Chemicals interfering with hormone activity
Sensitizers
Irritants.

Classification by Target Organ

Toxics can act on any organ system in the body.[7] This classification includes:

Neurotoxins
Hematotoxins
Nephrotoxins
Hepatotoxins
Cardiotoxins
Pulmonary toxins
Metabolic toxins
Endocrine disruptors
Dermatotoxins
Reproductive agents
Genotoxins, including mutagens
Carcinogens, including initiators and promoters
Teratogens.

PROPERTIES OF CHEMICALS

Chemical Species

A chemical variant of a metal is called a *species*. Trivalent chromium (Cr-III) and hexavalent chromium (Cr-VI), which differ in oxidation state, also differ in toxicity, carcinogenicity, and ability to pass through cell membranes. They represent different chromium species, yet they are interconvertible, depending on whether they are in an oxidizing or reducing environment. Cr-III is an essential nutrient, whereas Cr-VI is a potent lung carcinogen. The difficulty in reliably analyzing the concentrations of Cr-III and Cr-VI in soil presents a problem. Depending on how the soil sample is collected, transported, and analyzed, Cr-III can be oxidized and appear spuriously as Cr-VI when analyzed; or Cr-VI might be inadvertently reduced to Cr-III and analyzed as such.

The same chemical, such as mercury, may exist in several different chemical species. Slight modifications may have profound effects. Elemental mercury, often referred to as quicksilver, is a dense silvery liquid, with a specific gravity of 13. It is one of the few elements that is liquid at ambient temperature and also volatile, giving off an odorless, colorless, but highly toxic vapor that is readily inhaled and absorbed into pulmonary capillaries. Mercury compounds used in industry are often inorganic salts, whereas many of the biocidal mercurial compounds, such as phenylmercuric acetate, are organic chemicals. The methylmercury species produced from elemental or inorganic mercury in aquatic sediments by anaerobic bacteria biomagnifies in the food chain, causing organic mercury poisoning in people who consume large amounts of fish.

In general, organic forms of metals have a different spectrum of toxicity than the inorganic forms of the same metals. Thus, organic mercury and organotin compounds are more highly toxic than the corresponding inorganic compounds. Both have been used extensively as biocides, especially in antifouling paints used for ships to discourage the growth of barnacles. As the mercury and tin have leached out of the paints into the sea, contamination of marine organisms has become a problem. There are exceptions to the rule; for example, organic arsenic compounds, especially arsenobetaine, are substantially less toxic than inorganic arsenic.

Isomers and Congeners

Two chemical compounds that have the same chemical formula, but differ in structure, are called *isomers*. Figure 13-9 reveals isomers of the common lighter fuel, butane, which as a four-carbon chain can appear as either normal (linear) butane or branched isobutane. *Congeners* have the same basic structure but different numbers of atoms. For instance, dichlorophenol and trichlorophenol are congeners, whereas 2,4-dichlorophenol and 2,5-dichlorophenol are isomers. There are 209 different congeners of polychlorinated biphenyls (PCBs), differing in the number and position of chlorine atoms on the two attached benzene rings. Several of these compounds have four chlorines and are thus isomers of tetrachlorobiphenyl. The behavior in the body and the toxicity of isomers and

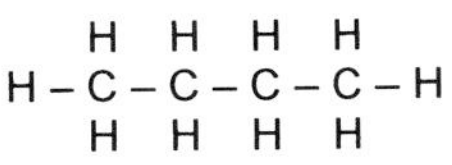

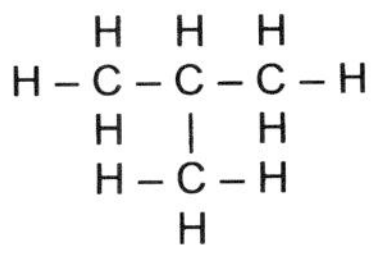

FIGURE 13-9 ● Isomers of butane showing normal (*n*-butane) and isobutane.

congeners may vary greatly. Thus, different chlorinated dibenzodioxins vary by orders of magnitude in their toxicity.[3] The most toxic of these is 2,3,7,8-tetrachlorodibenzodioxin (TCDD), which, among other sources, was a contaminant in the production of the herbicide, 2,4,5-trichlorophenoxyacetic acid (2,4,5-T). Each of the dioxin congeners can be assigned a toxicity potency (toxic equivalency factor, or TEF) relative to TCDD, which is given a value of 1.

MECHANISMS OF TOXICITY

Mechanism refers to the manner in which a chemical causes damage, usually at the subcellular or molecular level. Understanding mechanisms is useful in risk assessment, such as in choosing between different extrapolation models for nongenotoxic, as opposed to genotoxic, carcinogens. Toxic substances can interact with different parts of macromolecules, such as nucleic acids and proteins. They may bind to receptors, causing overactivation or inhibition of normal activation. The explosion of knowledge in cell and molecular biology, including the mapping of the human genome, gene expression and transcription, cell-cycle regulation, enzyme polymorphisms, cytokines, transcription factors, and cascades of signaling molecules, have greatly increased the opportunity to understand toxicologic mechanisms.

Metabolic and Cellular Poisons

Chemicals, such as cyanide, that interfere with cellular respiration are among the oldest known poisons. A chemical may cause enzyme inhibition by binding to a site on an enzyme, altering its three-dimensional structure, and distorting its active site(s) so that it is no longer functional. Some chemicals alter the structure or function of intracellular membranes, such as membranes of the endoplasmic reticulum or the mitochondria. For many toxic substances, swelling of the mitochondria, with loss of detailed structure, is an early histologic sign of damage. Others, such as the hemolysins of certain snake venoms, cause lysis of cells. Some chemicals, especially metals, may bind to the sulfhydryl groups of the cell membrane protein, disrupting its structure and increasing membrane fluidity.

Enzyme Induction

The body does not maintain a complete inventory of all the enzymes that it may need. Some con-

stitutive enzymes are always present, but most enzymes must be induced by introduction of their substrate; it may take up to 24 hours before there is sufficient enzyme to metabolize a xenobiotic completely. Thus, the amount of enzyme in a cell may increase by several orders of magnitude. Some enzyme systems are highly specific and act only on a single substrate; others are nonspecific, catalyzing reactions on a wide range of substrates. Conversely, different substrates vary in their potency at inducing enzymes. Enzyme induction plays an important role in metabolizing xenobiotics. However, sometimes the most important consequence of enzyme induction is the greatly accelerated metabolism of endogenous bioactive compounds.

Enzyme inhibition is a common mode of action for toxic substances. Both cyanide and hydrogen sulfide interfere with the function of cytochrome oxidase, thereby inhibiting oxidative phosphorylation that is necessary for cellular respiration. Heavy metals, which have a strong affinity for sulfur in proteins, are able to break the disulfide bridges that confer the tertiary structure necessary for normal function. Yet, because of differences in their atomic radius, different metals tend to inhibit different enzymes. Thus, several enzymes in the pathway for making hemoglobin, such as delta-aminolevulinic acid dehydratase, are inhibited strongly by lead, but weakly by mercury. Therefore, induction can be accomplished, albeit with different efficiencies, by a range of substrates. CYP1A2 is induced by a variety of polyaromatic hydrocarbons (PAHs). Before its identity was known, it was referred to as aryl hydrocarbon hydroxylase—its induction triggered by the substance binding to the aromatic hydrocarbon (Ah) receptor. Conversely, a single chemical can be acted upon by more than one of the P450s.

Receptors

Many toxic effects involve the binding of a xenobiotic or metabolite to a receptor, usually on a cell membrane. Receptors vary in their degree of specificity. Advances in receptor biology are proceeding rapidly. Many hormone effects are mediated by attachment of the hormone to a specific receptor. Some endocrine-active substances act by binding to the endogenous receptor without initiating the appropriate response. The effects of TCDD (a dioxin) are partially mediated by binding to the Ah receptor. Related substances that bind to the Ah receptor have effects similar to TCDD but with vastly different dose–response curves due, in part, to their binding affinity. In animal studies, dioxin binds to estrogen receptors in the breast tissue, interfering with normal estrogenic stimuli, and possibly (and ironically) reducing the likelihood of estrogen-stimulated breast cancer.

Under normal circumstances, a signal molecule binds to a receptor and initiates a response. The signal molecule is then removed from the receptor, usually by an enzyme, and another molecule attaches, which allows a sustained response. Abnormal molecules may bind to the receptor and not release, thereby blocking any further impulses and responses. Acetylcholinesterase secreted at a presynaptic terminal binds to special receptors on the postsynaptic terminal, initiating a nerve impulse, and then is immediately removed by acetylcholinesterase. Some chemicals block the enzyme and others bind irreversibly to the receptor, in both cases preventing further nerve transmission.

Oxidative Stress and Free Radicals

Oxygen is sometimes referred to as highly toxic, because of its ability to alter molecules and change their function. Many bioactivation reactions involve oxidation. Normally, there is a balance between oxidative and antioxidant reactions. Oxidative reactions play important roles in inflammation, aging, carcinogenesis, and other aspects of toxicity. Research is discovering an increasing number of toxicants for which oxidative stress is an important mechanism. For example, chromium increases the formation of superoxide anion and nitric oxide in cells and enhances DNA single-strand breaks.

Toxicologists speak of reactive oxygen species, some of which are free radicals. Oxygen can receive an electron and form superoxide anion radical, which can, in turn, react with hydrogen to form hydrogen peroxide, which reacts with free electrons and hydrogen ion to form water and a highly reactive hydroxide radical. An asterisk is used to designate these radicals.

$$O\text{-}O + e^- \_ > O\text{-}O^* \text{(superoxide radical)}$$

$$O\text{-}O^. + e^- + H^+ \_ > H\text{-}O\text{-}O\text{-}H \text{ (hydrogen peroxide)}$$

$$H\text{-}O\text{-}O\text{-}H + e^- + H^+ \_ > H_2O + {}^*OH \text{ (hydroxy radical)}$$

In the course of these reactions, the highly reactive free radicals, especially the hydroxy radical, are available to attack macromolecules, initiating a variety of toxic effects. The superoxide anion radical is formed in many oxidation reactions, where oxygen acts as an electron receptor. In response to the

potential harm these reactive oxygen species may cause, the body has evolved antioxidant defenses, including water-soluble vitamin C and lipid-soluble vitamins E and A. Superoxide dismutase, a metalloprotein, and glutathione-dependent peroxidases, in association with glutathione reductase, serve to scavenge free radicals. Excess nitric oxide production increases intracellular free radicals, enhancing neuronal degradation.

A new area of interest is oxidative damage to proteins through the binding of oxygen to various sites on the protein, forming protein carbonyls. Oxidizers, such as reactive oxygen species and nitric oxide, can bind to proteins, altering their configuration and activity. The amount of oxidation correlates with aging and, in some cases, disease severity. It is not clear if it can be a useful marker of toxic damage.

Lipid Peroxidation

One of the consequences of the formation of free radicals is reaction with lipids, including those in cell and organelle membranes, to form lipid peroxides, which, in turn, lead to cell damage and dysfunction. Some cytotoxicity of chlorinated hydrocarbons, such as carbon tetrachloride, is mediated by peroxidation of membrane lipids, which can be caused by a variety of reactive oxygen species. An active area of research involves identifying naturally occurring and synthetic compounds that cause or interfere with lipid peroxidation.

EFFECTS ON SIGNAL TRANSDUCTION

Cell cycles are regulated by molecules that serve as signals to activate certain genes or receptors that influence the expression of other genes. Signal transduction pathways typically alter gene expression or modify gene products, either enhancing or inhibiting their function. Many endogenous signal chemicals, such as hormones and xenobiotics, can alter gene expression by activating transcription factors, which, in turn, promote the transcription of certain genes.

Macromolecular Binding and Adduct Formation

Many chemicals bind to the macromolecules, hemoglobin, proteins, and nucleic acids, resulting in adduct formation. DNA-repair enzymes may remove adducts, but some adducts persist long enough to interfere with DNA activity during cell division. Adducts have been linked to cancer induction, and DNA adducts have been investigated as possible markers of genotoxic or carcinogen exposure. (Interpretation of the frequency of adducts, however, is difficult, partly due to the propensity for repair. Some adducts are repaired within hours, whereas others persist.) For example, smokers have higher levels of benzo[*a*]pyrene adducts to DNA than nonsmokers. DNA-protein cross-linking is promoted by a variety of genotoxic chemicals, including hexavalent chromium. Detecting adducts has not yet been useful in screening other populations. New techniques may greatly improve the sensitivity and utility of testing for adducts.

Genotoxicity

Damage to germ cells may be heritable; damage to somatic cells is not. Various chemicals and ionizing radiation damage nucleic acid directly or interfere with chromosomal replication and cell division. People are constantly bombarded with a natural background of ionizing radiation from cosmic, terrestrial, and endogenous sources. Normally the damage such radiation causes is repaired quickly, and only some of the unrepaired damage goes on to become cancer.

Mutagens are substances that cause point mutations (replacement of one base nucleotide with another), chromosomal damage (breakage or translocations), or interference with meiosis, mitosis, or cell division. A variety of tests can measure chromosomal aberrations, aneuploidy, sister chromatid exchange, translocation, micronucleus formation, glycophorin A, and T-cell receptor genes. New genetic techniques allow sequencing of genes and detection of changes at specific codons. (A *codon* is a sequence of three nucleotides.)

Genetic analysis can reveal changes such as GC or AT base-pair substitutions, deletions, or duplications at a single gene locus in individuals. The relative frequency of the different mutations is influenced by dose and the conditions of exposure. Whereas GC substitutions are more common in nonsmokers, there is an increased frequency of AT substitutions in smokers. After radiotherapy, there is a substantial increase in rearrangements and deletions that can persist for several years.

Genotoxic chemicals may cause mutation in proteins called *proto-oncogenes*, producing a mutant oncogene that encodes for a modification of the natural protein product. Some changes, such as that in the *ras* proto-oncogene, increase cell susceptibility to cancer. The p21 protein (so-called because

it has a weight of 21 kilodaltons) binds with a receptor on the inner cell membrane and mediates responses to growth factors. Mutation at codon 13 "locks" the protein into the active form such that it no longer responds to other cell signals. With signal transduction impaired, this permanent activation is associated with malignant transformation and proliferation.

Another important phenomenon is the role of tumor suppressor genes, such as *p53*. Mutant forms of *p53* allow unbridled cell proliferation. "Knockout mice," which lack *p53*, develop cancer at an early age. Some patients with hepatocellular carcinoma have a specific mutation at the 249th codon of *p53*. The same mutation also occurs in people exposed to aflatoxin B_1, suggesting that the toxin may cause liver cancer by this highly specific mutation.

Carcinogenesis

Carcinogenesis typically involves three steps: initiation, promotion, and proliferation. Many carcinogens exert direct action on DNA and are referred to as genotoxic, but others seem to cause or allow cancer without a direct genotoxic mode of action. The genotoxic damage stage is called *initiation*. When initiated cells are exposed to certain promoter compounds, they may begin to undergo cell division. Proliferation occurs when there is unbridled and uncontrolled cell division accompanied by a proliferation of capillaries that supply the growing tumor with blood (see Chapter 24).

Some scientists believe that there must be a threshold for cancer as there is for other toxicologic reactions. Others argue, on theoretical grounds that because no threshold (below which no cancer risk exists) has been demonstrated, there is no threshold for cancer. Most scientists are probably undecided about the no-threshold concept for carcinogens or believe that there may be thresholds for some, but not all, carcinogens. In the light of the ongoing controversy, some governmental regulatory agencies have concluded that until it is more certain, it is prudent to act as if there were no threshold for carcinogens. Thus, the application of a no-threshold approach to carcinogens can be viewed as a policy decision rather than a scientific decision.

Apoptosis

Apoptosis, or *programmed cell death*, is a necessary part of the life history of a cell. Activation leads to proteins that prepare the cell to die. This is followed by phagocytosis of cell fragments. The important feature of this natural form of cell death, compared with cytotoxicity, is that the former proceeds without invasion of inflammatory cells. Apoptosis is an essential phenomenon during development, allowing the remodeling of tissues. Apoptosis also selectively eliminates cells with damaged DNA and also counters the clonal expansion of neoplastic cells. Inhibition of apoptosis, such as by estrogens, allows mutations to accumulate and tumor proliferation to occur. Hormone-dependent tumors expand when the hormone inhibits apoptosis, whereas an anti-estrogenic drug, like tamoxifen, allows apoptosis to occur. Conversely, the tumor-promotor phenobarbital inhibits apoptosis. Some chemicals appear to inhibit apoptosis, thus enhancing the proliferative phase of carcinogenesis. New approaches to cancer chemotherapy focus on exploiting apoptosis to destroy tumor cells.

Immunotoxins

Immunotoxins act by activating or suppressing the immune system. Some alter the expression of immunoglobulins, and others affect lymphocytes. T lymphocytes mature in the thymus and are the main factor in cell-mediated immunity. B lymphocytes are responsible for producing antibodies (humoral immunity). T cells are classified by their surface antigens, and techniques exist for quantifying types and subtypes of different T populations in order to identify which functions are depressed. Some agents interfere with the production, function, or life span of T and B lymphocytes.

Substances known to interfere with the immune system include (a) polyhalogenated aromatic compounds, such as dioxins; (b) metals, including mercury; (c) pesticides; and (d) air pollutants, such as oxides of nitrogen and sulfur. Tobacco smoke has constituents that are immunotoxic. Mercury causes autoimmune damage and glomerulonephritis in rats due to depletion of the $RT6^+$ subpopulation of T-lymphocytes.

Sensitizers or allergens induce an increased immune response. The main target organs are the skin and the respiratory system. Nickel and poison ivy (*Rhus*) contact dermatitis are common examples of such skin sensitization. Occupational asthma reflects sensitization of the lung and airways to aerosols.

Reproductive Effects

The processes of gametogenesis, fertilization, implantation, embryogenesis and organogenesis and postnatal development are complex and subject to many environmental insults. Major errors incompatible with life generally result in spontaneous abortion (miscarriage), which can be viewed as a quality-control procedure. All stages are vulnerable to chemical hazards, including the failure to form gametes, such as azoospermia, and formation of abnormal gametes. Chemical workers at a chemical plant in California suffered testicular toxicity from the nematocide dibromochloropropane (DBCP; see Fig. 13-9). Those men with azoospermia (no sperm in the semen) did not recover spermatogenesis, whereas those diagnosed with oligospermia (reduced sperm count) gradually recovered over several years. Many other chemicals, such as lead, have also been implicated in toxicity to the male reproductive system (including interfering with spermatogenesis, semen quality, erection, and libido). The list of chemicals affecting females includes cancer chemotherapeutic agents, other pharmaceuticals, metals, insecticides, and various industrial chemicals (see Chapter 29).

Endocrine Disruptors

In the past decade, there has been an intense research and policy focus on endocrine disruption by chemicals that exert endocrine activity leading to unfavorable alterations in reproduction and/or behavior.[7] Endocrine-active substances can mimic hormones, leading to overactivity, or can bind with high affinity to endocrine receptors, thereby inhibiting normal endocrine functions. Chemicals can lead to overexpression or underexpression of genes governing hormone or receptor synthesis, and chemicals can exert effects on the target tissues influencing their response. The potency of these compounds is influenced by environmental persistence and bioamplification, bioavailability, as well as binding affinities. Endocrine disruption was well recognized by the 1970s, when the ability of DDT to alter estrogen metabolism through enzyme induction was described. Although major concerns were raised regarding the effect of chemicals on human reproductive function, clearer effects on a wide range of animals have been demonstrated, including development, maturation, reproduction, and cancer.[8]

Many endocrine disruptors occur naturally in vegetables (*phytoestrogens*), including a group of isoflavonoid and lignin polycyclic compounds. At the same time that concern is voiced regarding interference with reproduction and development, their beneficial features are being exploited. One isoflavenoid, coumesterol, antagonizes estrogen during embryonic development, leading to reproductive abnormalities in behavior and hormone function. Others, such as genistein, protect against (a) certain hormone-dependent breast cancers by competing with estrogens or (b) other cancers by inhibiting proliferation, differentiation, or the vascular supply.

The bioengineered yeast estrogen screen (YES) is being used to screen for the endocrine disruptor action of xenobiotics.

Teratogenesis

Development from conception to birth involves a remarkable sequence of carefully timed interactions among cells through chemical signals, which results in the differentiation of a few primordial embryonic cells into different tissues and organs. Cells multiply, migrate, connect, and often die, to be replaced by other cells—a necessary part of complex developmental biology. Chemicals may interfere with morphogenesis in varying ways. They may inhibit necessary signals or alter the timing of signals so that cells migrate and differentiate before the appropriate time. The effect of a particular chemical depends on the stage of embryogenesis and fetogenesis, as well as dose. Different chemicals cross the placental barrier with different efficiencies.

Chemicals may have no effect, produce subclinical alterations, or cause major birth defects or fetal death. For example, some effects on the developing nervous system from lead or methylmercury may disrupt the migration, maturation, and connections of nerve cells, leading to a viable baby with cognitive impairment, which may only be apparent when the child has learning difficulties in school or when he or she is subjected to psychometric testing. Recognition of this phenomenon has given rise to a field of *behavioral teratology*, which focuses on studying the impact of fetal exposure or to lead or alcohol on development and behavior.

Approximately 3 percent of live births have detectable congenital abnormalities. In general, chemical exposure prior to implantation is likely to be lethal. Exposure during organogenesis begets birth defects or embryolethality. Later in fetal life, there can be intrauterine growth retardation, fetal death, or functional changes that interfere with birth or postnatal development.

TOXICOLOGIC CONSIDERATIONS IN CLINICAL EVALUATION

Occupational and environmental exposures to toxic chemicals occur frequently, and adverse health effects are not rare. Clinicians are frequently confronted by patients who have symptoms that they ascribe to, or suspect are caused by, some chemical or event. It is easy to be skeptical, especially when histories are complex and exposures uncertain. However, a high index of suspicion is a hallmark for success in diagnosing true illness or reassuring patients. Many chemical exposures have specific end points (such as marrow depression due to benzene) and nonspecific end points (such as light-headedness due to benzene). Some effects are acute, whereas others develop only after long periods of exposure.

First, one must establish whether the reported symptoms are typical of, or even likely to be associated with, the putative exposure. If not, one is likely to look for a different causal explanation, which may often be a different chemical or biological agent. *General causation* is the process of determining if a chemical can cause a given adverse health effect.

Second, one must establish exposure. A careful history can often confirm exposure. If exposure is recent or ongoing, clinical testing may reveal a biomarker of exposure. In addition, environmental measurements can be made to document the presence of the chemical. However, often many months—and many physician visits—have passed before the patient reaches a clinician who understands occupational and environmental disease. By this time, the trail may be cold, and only the history is available to provide information. The clinician must then determine if the specific individual's illness was due to this chemical (*special causation*).

For toxicity due to metals, one can often use chelation to help determine specific causation, given the propensity of metals to bind to sulfhydryl (–SH) groups. A variety of drugs with high concentrations of sulfur can be used to circulate through the body and bind any metal encountered. This can be used in a provocative mode to try to extract stored metal from prior exposures. A baseline urine measurement is obtained; then, the chelator is administered (usually intramuscularly or intravenously, although some oral medications, such as DMSA, are now available). Urine is then measured, usually at 12-, 24-, and 72-hour intervals. There should be a rapid increase in excretion of the metal, followed by a gradual return to baseline. Although chelation can be useful to treat heavy metal poisoning, it is often misused by clinicians who perform a chelation challenge, but compare the resulting urine concentration with the range of values derived from non-provoked urine samples. This results in many false-positive results and unnecessary anxiety and inappropriate treatment.

Biomarkers

A biomarker can be measured, usually in blood or urine, to provide information about exposure or pathophysiology (Table 13-3). *Molecular epidemiology* is the study of biomarkers in human populations. There are numerous applications of biomarkers in estimating internal dose. They can be defined as end points in a dose–response assessment. Some biomarkers reflect exposure, some reflect damage, and some can identify susceptibility. DNA adducts are biomarkers of exposure to carcinogens or mutagens; the carcinogenic polyaromatic hydrocarbon, benzo[*a*]pyrene, forms a specific adduct with DNA. Although adduct formation is believed to be part of carcinogenesis, and smokers who have high exposure to benzo[*a*]pyrene have an increased rate of adduct formation, this marker has not had sufficient predictive value to support widespread use. Familiar biomarkers include blood lead level (a biomarker of exposure) and zinc protoporphyrin (a biomarker of effect from lead exposure). (The Board on Environmental Studies and Toxicology of the National Research Council has a Committee on Biologic Markers that has published monographs on markers in pulmonary toxicology, reproductive toxicology, urinary toxicology, and immunotoxicology.)

CAUSALITY: ENVIRONMENAL CHEMICAL EXPOSURE AND HEALTH EFFECTS

An important role for the clinician, the epidemiologist, and the industrial hygienist is to identify a causal relationship between a chemical exposure and an adverse health effect. Laboratory experiments using sound experimental design can con-

TABLE 13-3
Examples of Biomarkers

Biomarkers of exposure
    Specific chemical agents[1]
    Metabolites
Biomarkers of effect
    Male reproductive disorders
        Sperm motility
        Semen quality
        Müllerian-inhibiting factor
        Chromosomal aberrations
        DNA adducts in sperm
    Female reproductive disorders
        Chorionic gonadotropin assay
        Urinary progesterone metabolites
    Pulmonary disorders
        Pulmonary function testing
        Airway reactivity (challenge tests)
        Pulmonary cytology
    Immunology disorders
        Immunoglobulin levels
        Lymphocyte ratios (T and B cells)
        T-helper cells
        T-suppressor cells
        Natural killer cells
        Lymphocyte functional assays
        T cell–dependent antibody response
        Plaque-forming assays
        Lymphocyte proliferation tests
        Interleukin-2 activity
        Specific receptor expression assays
        Macrophage/leukocyte respiratory burst response
    Lead poisoning
        Zinc or erythrocyte protoporphyrin
        Delta amino levulinic acid in urine
        Delta amino levulinic acid dehydratase activity

tribute to causality assessment, but health professionals need to make causal inferences with incomplete data. This is especially challenging for conditions with long latency periods or where hazardous susbstances are part of a mixture. In addition, the health effect may not be specific because many illnesses manifest as a complex of many symptoms or signs, each of which has multiple causes.

TABLE 13-4

Bradford Hill's (1965) Postulates for Establishing a Causal Relationship Between an Exposure and a Disease[9]

Criterion	Explanation	Application
Strength	First on his list is "strength of association." "Enormous" excess of a disease in a particular industry. Scrotal cancer mortality in chimney sweeps was 200 times greater than other workers. Lung cancer death rate in smokers is 10 times greater than nonsmokers.	Useful. Hill cautioned that even a small relative excess might indicate causation when there is a large exposed population.
Consistency	"Has it been repeatedly observed by different persons, in different places, circumstances and times?"	Important, but Hill cautioned that inconsistency did not refute causation.
Specificity	Association of a particular disease with a particular type of work.	"We must not, however, over-emphasize the importance?" Hill linked specificity to strength of association. If one outcome showed a much stronger association than others, it could be considered specific.
Temporality	Which comes first, exposure or outcome? Does work cause a disease or do people with a predilection for that kind of work have a susceptibility to the disease?	The only essential standard: that the putative cause precedes the outcome.
Biological gradient	Dose–response is helpful if the "association is one which can reveal a biological gradient."	Dose–response is helpful for most toxic reactions, but idiosyncratic sensitivities will not follow the typical dose–response curve.
Plausibility	"It will be helpful if the causation we suspect is biologically plausible. But this is a feature I am convinced we cannot demand."	Is it biologically realistic? Do we have a known mechanism? But must take into account that there will always be a first case.
Coherence	"...the cause-and-effect interpretation of our data should not seriously conflict with generally known facts. ..." Also includes histologic verification of preclinical conditions in similarly exposed workers.	Very similar to plausibility.
Experiment	Does a preventive action reduce the frequency of the association? "...the strongest support for the causation hypothesis may be revealed."	An effective intervention is good evidence.
Analogy	"With the effects of thalidomide and rubella before us we would surely be ready to accept slighter but similar evidence with another drug or another viral disease in pregnancy."	Based on what we know, we may accept by analogy, even before definitive evidence accumulates.

Simply defining what the health effect is can be time-consuming and frustrating, and establishing specific causation may be impossible.

Establishing a scientific basis for causality often relies on the *Bradford Hill postulates*, which were presented by Sir Austin Bradford Hill, a British statistician, in the mid-1960s (Table 13-4).[9] These nine items have been widely cited—and often miscited. To establish general causation does not depend on meeting all nine; only temporality—the cause must precede the effect—is essential.

However, even when scientists and clinicians believe they understand the probable cause of a work-related condition, courts may require different interpretations for toxic tort cases. In addition, different judicial jurisdictions have different standards of evidence and different criteria for establishing causation and liability. "Reasonable probability" that A caused B is the standard in some jurisdictions, while "more probable than not" is the standard in others. "But for" may require a determination that without exposure to A, health effect B would not have occurred. In many states, workers' compensation requirements are less stringent than those in tort law. In New Jersey, for example, an exposure that causes, aggravates, or accelerates a condition is eligible for workers' compensation. In the future, it seems likely that experts will be asked to estimate attributable risk, so that costs can be assigned to different parties in proportion to their contribution to causation of an illness. Finally, in some cases, causation is assumed unless proven otherwise. For example, the U.S. Congress required the Veteran's Administration to give veterans the benefit of the doubt in cases involving herbicide exposure; certain diseases, such as soft tissue sarcoma, in exposed veterans are presumed to be related to herbicide exposure and qualify for compensation.

TOXICITY TESTING

A wide variety of systems and paradigms are used to test chemicals in order to predict their effects on human health or the environment. Under the Toxic Substances Control Act, new chemicals must undergo extensive safety testing (see Chapter 37). It is important to select the appropriate animal model or *in vitro* test system and to have well-chosen controls, which could include *positive controls* (controls known to manifest a particular end point readily). Animal researchers need to choose the appropriate species, genetic strain, gender, and age as well as exposure route. The dosage schedule may be single or multiple; and acute, subchronic, or chronic. Duration of a study should be longer than the longest expected latency period. Dosages must be chosen to span the suspected threshold, if one is thought to exist. The route of administration should be relevant to natural conditions of exposure.

Toxicity testing must be subject to good quality assurance and quality-control procedures.

Quality assurance includes use of trained (and, in some cases, certified) personnel, buying and maintaining appropriate equipment and standards, maintaining laboratory hygiene and avoiding cross-contamination, documenting procedures, maintaining records, and participating in interlaboratory testing programs. *Quality control* refers to laboratory procedures of calibration using blanks and known standards, as well as running replicate samples and analyzing spiked samples.

Good laboratory practices describe animal care, dosing, and data management. Many commercial laboratories have been found to have faulty laboratory procedures, especially for documentation of exposure, side effects, and outcomes.

The National Toxicology Program (NTP), operated by the National Institute for Environmental Health Sciences, sponsors long-term rodent studies to detect the carcinogenic and other toxic properties of chemicals. Chemicals are selected on the basis of data needs of governmental agencies and in response to public input. The standard protocol is two species (rat and mouse), both sexes, and a minimum of 50 individuals for each category, with oral dosing over a 2-year "life span." These 2-year bioassays can provide information on metabolism; genetic, reproductive, and developmental toxicity; and toxic effects on various organ systems. NTP bioassays screen new chemicals for carcinogenic activity and classify them with respect to human carcinogenicity. However, their main application has been to provide tumor incidence data in risk assessment.

ANIMAL WELFARE AND ANIMAL RIGHTS

Animal studies have played an important role in human toxicology and in the development of drugs that are safe for humans and for animals as well. Advances in toxicology have included the exploration of alternative testing procedures, including reducing the number of animals, using animals other than mammals, and developing *in vitro* techniques. Toxicologists have become increasingly attentive to animal welfare, due to the recognition that reducing stress for animals makes them more reliable subjects, as well as pressure from animal welfare activists. Proponents of animal rights argue that animals have intrinsic rights that, in the extreme, should protect them from any and all use in experimental research. The Animal Welfare Act, administered by the Animal and Plant Health Inspection

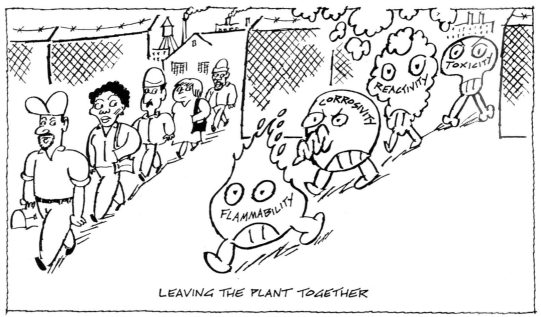

LEAVING THE PLANT TOGETHER

Workers can inadvertently bring toxic chemicals home with them. (Drawing by Nick Thorkelson.)

Service of the U.S. Department of Agriculture, applies to all mammals, except mice and rats. Toxicologists generally agree that experimental animals should not be exposed to unnecessary stress, discomfort, or pain. Researchers using animals must consider animal-care guidelines. Most universities and other animal-testing organizations have animal-use committees that review all research protocols to minimize unnecessary stress and pain, inspect conditions under which animals are kept, and assure availability of veterinary care.

The concern over animal welfare reaches its peak when primates are used. Primates are expensive to acquire and maintain; and most primate studies can afford only a few animals who often live under unnatural and extremely stressful conditions. The capturing of huge numbers of primates for medical research and industrial applications has had a drastic impact on the survival of several species in the wild.

The assumption that primates are the best models for humans makes sense, when cognitive performance is studied, but does not take into account great differences in diet, as most primates are herbivorous. Thus, extrapolation from primates to humans is not always more appropriate than extrapolation from other animal models. Statistical interpretation of primate research is thwarted by small

sample sizes, and, in some cases, by re-use of the same animals in sequential experiments. Over the past two decades, many primate laboratories have been closed, and, with few exceptions, primate research can be expected to play a diminishing role in future toxicology.

SUBSTITUTION

Substitution of hazardous substances or processes with safe ones is the first choice in prevention (Chapter 7). Caution is needed in the substitution process because the substitute may have unanticipated toxic effects. Thus, tributyltin was substituted for organic mercury in marine antifouling paints to protect the marine ecosystem from mercury (Box 13-6). However, because the organotin compound proved equally damaging, new alternatives are being developed. Many uses of asbestos have been replaced by man-made mineral (synthetic vitreous) fibers, although the full health consequences of this substitution remain to be determined; preliminary studies show that some of the synthetic fibers may also be carcinogenic.

The global move to phase out all uses of chlorine is controversial. Many chlorinated solvents are probable human carcinogens. Exposure to chlorination products in drinking water has been linked, in

BOX 13-6

Mercury Contamination in the Brazilian Amazon: An Ecosystem Approach to Health

Donna Mergler

During the past 10 years, an interdisciplinary team of Canadian and Brazilian researchers from the natural, health, and social sciences have used an ecosystem approach, with a strong participatory research component, to examine the pathways of mercury contamination, human exposure and health effects, and mitigation measures and their efficiency, in collaboration with communities living along the Tapajós River, a major tributary of the Amazon in Brazil. Previous reports of high levels of mercury in fish and in humans attributed the source to gold mining.

The study revealed that large-scale deforestation, mainly from "slash-and-burn" agricultural practices, was the major culprit, through soil erosion and lixiviation (washing the soluble matter), releasing mercury into the river. The deforested areas are increasing in size due to large in-migration and the need to clear the forest to grow food to feed the growing population. Climatic conditions and aquatic vegetation are optimal for mercury methylation, accelerating the incorporation of mercury into the trophic chain and contaminating the fish, a dietary mainstay of this population. Measurements of hundreds of fish samples showed that mercury concentrations varied greatly, depending on feeding habits, growth rate, age, and location. Mercury in humans, measured in hair samples, cut in centimeters, provided a chronological portrait of exposure. Exposure increased with fish consumption, was higher among those who ate more piscivorous (fish-eating) fish, and varied seasonally. Evaluation of nervous system functions showed significant declines in motor and visual functions in relation to increasing exposure.

The integrated results were returned to the communities and village workshops examined short-, medium-, and long-term solutions with respect to diet, fishing, and farming practices. Because fish is a highly nutritious food and the major source of animal protein, a positive slogan, inviting people to "Eat more fish that don't eat other fish" was adopted. In addition, a chart with drawings of 42 fish species in red (high mercury), yellow (medium levels), and green (low mercury) was posted in every house.

Reassessment of fish consumption, exposure, and neuro-outcomes 5 years later showed that the villagers ate the same amount of fish but had reversed the proportion of herbivorous to piscivorous fish. Exposure had decreased by 40 percent! There was improvement in motor functions, but visual functions continued to decline in correlation with previous exposure levels.

To further foster maximizing nutritional input from fish and minimizing toxic risk, an extensive dietary study was undertaken with 26 village women, coordinated by the village midwife; for 13 months, they kept daily food-frequency diaries. Comparison of monthly hair mercury levels with food intake, after controlling for fish consumption, showed that those who ate more fruit had lower mercury. This positive influence of fruit consumption was confirmed in an epidemiological study of more than 400 persons.

Ongoing health studies are examining the progression of visual decline and the possible role of selenium. The environmental team is working with fishers to identify "hot spots" for methylation and with farmers to modify agro-forestry practices to reduce soil erosion. Analysis of communication networks within the villages is helping to identify how to implement programs for improving the environment and health. The success of this project is attributed to the synergy of scientific inputs, coupled with community participation and an ecosystem approach to human health.

some studies, to low birthweight and small head circumference and possibly to intestinal cancer. Chlorine will probably not be totally eliminated, but many nonessential uses are already being reduced.

The removal of organic lead from gasoline was a major success in applied toxicology. Figure 13-10 tracks the dramatic decline in blood lead levels coincident with the reduction of leaded gasoline use in the United States. However, its proposed

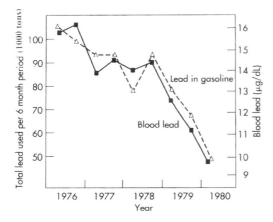

FIGURE 13-10 ● This graph tracks the dramatic decline in blood lead levels coincident with the reduction of leaded gasoline production in the United States (1976–1980). The decline reached 2.9 ug/dL by 1990 and has continued so that the mean blood lead level is below 2 ug/dL. (Source: U.S. Environmental Protection Agency, based on publication by Annest JL et al. Chronological trend in blood lead levels between 1976 and 1980. N Engl J Med 1983;308:1373–77.)

replacement, methylcyclopentadienyl manganese tricarbonyl (MMT), may greatly increase exposure to manganese, a potent neurotoxin that causes parkinsonism. Since 1977, MMT has been used in Canada, where urban pigeons have higher levels of manganese than rural ones, consistent with traffic-related contamination. Canada attempted to phase out the use of MMT but was sued successfully by the chemistry industry. Thus far in the United States, despite a court-ordered lifting of the EPA ban on MMT in gasoline, petrochemical companies have taken a precautionary approach and decided to withhold MMT as an antiknock agent for now.

REFERENCES

1. EPA. US EPA/Chemical Hazard Data Availability Study. Washington, DC: Environmental Protection Agency, Office of Pollution Prevention and Toxics, 1998. Available at: <www.epa.gov/chemrtk/hazchem.pdf>.
2. Gallo MA. History of toxicology. In: Klaassen C, ed. Cassarett and Doull's toxicology. 6th ed. New York: McGraw Hill, 2001.
3. Umbreit TH, Hesse EJ, Gallo MA. Bioavailability and cytochrome P-450 induction from 2,3,7,8-tetrachlorodibenzo-*p*-dioxin contaminated soils from Times Beach, Missouri, and Newark, New Jersey. Drug Chem Toxicol 1988;11:405–18.
4. Hammond EC, Selikoff IJ, Seidman H. Asbestos exposure, cigarette smoking and death rates. Ann N Y Acad Sci 1979;330:473–90.
5. Haldane JBS. Heredity and politics. New York: Norton, 1938.
6. Stokinger HE, Mountain JT. Progress in detecting the worker hypersusceptible to industrial chemicals. J Occup Med 1967;9:537–42.
7. Colburn T, Dumanoski D, Myers TJ. Our stolen future. New York: Dutton, 1996.
8. Miyamoto J, Burger J. Implications of endocrine active substances for humans and wildlife. SCOPE/IUPAC Conference. Pure Appl Chem 2003;75:1617–2615.
9. Hill AB. The environment and disease: Association or causation? Proc Royal Soc Med 1965;58:295–300.

BIBLIOGRAPHY

Agency for Toxic Substances and Disease Registry. Toxicological Profiles. Atlanta: Centers for Disease Control and Prevention. Available at: <http://www.atsdr.cdc.gov/toxpro2.html>.
Exhaustive monographs and reviews of more than 200 chemicals most commonly found at "Superfund Sites."
Brooks S, Gochfeld M, Herzstein J, et al. Environmental medicine. St Louis: Mosby, 1995.
Introductions to clinical and exposure aspects of toxicology.
Environmental Protection Agency. Integrated Risk Information System Web site. Available at: <http://www.epa.gov/iriswebp/iris/index.html>.
Reference doses and documentation of literature reviewed by the EPA.
Greenberg MR, Hamilton P, McClusky GJ. Occupational, industrial, and environmental toxicology. St. Louis: Mosby, 2003.
Valuable chapters on industrial chemicals.
Klaassen CD. Casarett and Doull's toxicology: The basic science of poisons. 6th ed. New York: McGraw-Hill Medical Publishing, 2001.
A textbook for toxicology students with detailed coverage of toxicokinetics and toxicodynamics and mechanisms of toxicity as well as organ systems and groups of chemicals.
Mendelsohn ML, Mohr LC, Peeters JP. Biomarkers: Medical and workplace applications. Washington, DC: Joseph Henry Press, 1998.
Many papers describing different applications and the strengths and limitations of biomarkers.
NIOSH. NIOSH Pocket Guide to Chemical Hazards. Rockville MD: National Institute for Occupational Safety and Health. Available at: <http://www.cdc.gov/niosh/npg/npg.html>.
Concise information on different toxicity levels recommended by NIOSH (more protective than OSHA standards), including levels Immediately Dangerous to Life and Health (IDLH).
National Institute for Occupational Safety and Health. Available at: <http://www.cdc.gov/niosh/database.html>.
A collection of databases on toxicity, workplace hazards, industrial hygiene methods, and protective equipment.
Plog BA, Niland J, Quinlan PJ. Fundamentals of industrial hygiene. 4th ed. Itasca, IL: National Safety Council, 1996.
More than the fundamentals of industrial hygiene including the anticipation, recognition, control, and evaluation of exposure to workplace hazards.
Sheehan HE, Wedeen RP. Toxic circles: Environmental hazards from the workplace into the community. New Brunswick, NJ: Rutgers Press, 1993.
Eight detailed case studies that provide a feel for occupational toxicology problems.
Sipes IG, McQueen CA, Gandolfi AJ. Comprehensive toxicology. New York: Pergamon, 1997.
This very expensive 13-volume set (available on CD-ROM) was the most exhaustive reference on toxicology, with

hundreds of excellent review chapters. Still valuable for researching specific organ systems and chemical groups in depth.

Sullivan JB, Krieger GR. Clinical environmental health and toxic exposures. 2nd ed. Philadelphia: Lippincott, 2001. *Readable chapters on toxicology with an emphasis on environmental exposures.*

APPENDIX

DEFINITIONS

Aerosol: Either fine liquid droplets or solid particles dispersed in the air. Depending on their size, they may be respirable and may reach the alveoli. The effective aerodynamic diameter is not always the same as the actual droplet or particle size.

Bioavailability: The ability of a substance that enters the body to be liberated from its environmental matrix, especially soil or food, thereby gaining access to enter the bloodstream.

Biotransformation: Intermediary metabolism consisting of metabolic processes that change the structure of a chemical. It may increase (activate) or decrease (detoxify) the harmful properties of a chemical.

Carcinogenicity: The ability of a chemical to cause cancer. Carcinogens can be genotoxic chemicals that damage the nucleic acid leading to unbridled cell replication (induction) or chemicals that enable induced cells to undergo rapid cell divisions (promotion).

Concentration: The level of a chemical present in an environmental medium or in a body organ or fluid, often expressed on a mass basis, such as micrograms per gram or parts per million, or a volume basis, such as micrograms per liter of water or micrograms per cubic meter of air.

Dose: The amount of a chemical that reaches a target organ or the amount administered (external dose); the amount crossing a specific absorption barrier (absorbed dose).

Effect Dose 50% (ED_{50}): The dose of a chemical that produces a specific effect in 50 percent of the animals studied.

Exposure: (a) Proximity and/or contact with a source of a disease agent in such a manner that effective transmission of the agent or harmful effects of the agent may occur; (b) the amount of a factor to which a group or individual was exposed; or (c) the process by which an agent comes into contact with a person or animal in such a way that the person or animal may develop the relevant outcome, such as disease.

Fumes: Very fine solid particles, usually generated when a heated vapor condenses. Many metals form fine fumes. These fine particles readily reach the alveoli.

Lethal dose 50% (LD_{50}): The dose of a chemical that causes death in 50 percent of the animals studied.

Lipophilic: A chemical (nonpolar) that is much more soluble in organic solvents than in water can readily move through membranes and can concentrate in lipid-rich tissues. (See definitions of polar and nonpolar compounds below.)

Mechanism: The way in which toxic substances act at the molecular and cellular levels to cause morbidity and mortality. Toxic substances include metabolic poisons and cytotoxic poisons that disrupt cell membranes, interfere with chemical reactions, or bind to nucleic acids.

Mutagenicity: The ability of a substance to damage genetic material either by disrupting chromosomal structure or changing the sequence of nucleotides on the nucleic acid molecule.

Pathway: The combination of media and route of exposure, such as ingestion of contaminated soil. (See Tables 13-1 and 13-2.)

Polar and nonpolar compounds: Polar compounds (such as many inorganic salts) tend to be soluble in water. Nonpolar compounds (many organic compounds) tend to be soluble in organic solvents, such as toluene and lipids, but have very low water-solubility. The standard for describing this is the *octanol-to-water partitioning coefficient* (solubility in octanol, divided by solubility in water). Nonpolar compounds pass through the skin and cell membranes more readily than polar compounds. Polar compounds are more readily excreted in urine.

Susceptibility: The vulnerability of an individual or population to be harmed by an agent. It is influenced by many factors including age, sex, genetic polymorphisms, nutrition, prior exposure, and overall health status.

Teratogenicity: The ability to interfere with normal fetal development, resulting in birth defects.

Threshold: The lowest dose of a chemical that has a detectable effect. For any given chemical, each cellular, biochemical, physiologic, or clinical response may have a threshold. Some effects occur without a known threshold. Because susceptibility varies among animal species and among humans, the threshold is approximated.

Thresholds are often used to categorize or rank chemical toxicity.

Toxicity: The intrinsic ability of a substance to harm living cells or processes, organisms, or ecosystems.

Toxicodynamics: What the chemical does to the organ, including the biochemical and physiological mechanisms of action on affected target molecules and tissues. This includes binding to and activating (agonistic) or blocking (antagonistic) receptors.

Toxicokinetics: What the body does to a xenobiotic in terms of metabolism, conjugation, transport, storage, and excretion.

Xenobiotic: Any substance foreign to the body, including all synthetic chemicals as well as many pharmaceuticals and essential nutrients.

CHAPTER 14

Physical Hazards

This chapter describes physical exposures that occur over time that can cause human illness. These hazards transfer energy in a variety of forms, such as sound waves, vibration, heat transfer (into or away from individuals), electromagnetic energy, and increased or decreased atmospheric pressure. Safety hazards, which result in the acute transmission of uncontrolled energy to a vulnerable individual, are classified separately because they result in instantaneous effects, or injuries, rather than illnesses—although the distinction is one of convenience and definitions may overlap (see Chapters 10 and 22). Biomechanical hazards, such as the repetitive lifting, stooping, and reaching that result in musculoskeletal disorders, are also addressed separately (see Chapters 11 and 23), although again, some people classify them together with physical hazards.

The underlying science that explores measurement and intervention to reduce physical exposures is based in physics, the study of the relationship between energy and matter.

The sections included in this chapter address the physics of noise (acoustics), vibration, thermal stress (both hot and cold), and both ionizing and non-ionizing electromagnetic radiation. These exposures are widespread in industry, in nature, and in various community and medical settings. Additional physical hazards addressed are low-pressure and high-pressure environments.

—The Editors

Noise

John J. Earshen

M uch impairment to hearing is produced by excessive exposure to noise as well as to oto-toxic chemicals. Enhanced synergistic effects by both also occur. Although immediate damage can be caused by high amplitude noise, the predominant process encompasses cumulative chronic occupational and non-occupational exposures. Exposure to high levels of noise can also have other adverse physiological effects (see also Chapter 27).

PROPERTIES OF SOUND AND PERTINENT METRICS

Perceived sound is a dynamic pressure fluctuation superposed on the relatively static atmospheric pressure. It is generated by vibrating surfaces immersed in air (or a liquid) that produce pressure fluctuations. (No sound can be produced if the surface is in a vacuum.) Another process by which sound is generated is the turbulent flow of a medium, commonly air, such as whistles, organ pipes, or the exhaust of a jet engine producing broadband noise. Distinct tonal or pitch properties of organ pipes are produced by built-in, frequency-selective resonances, acting on broadband sound generated by turbulence. Yet another process by which sound is generated is the sudden change in pressure, such as by puncturing a balloon or triggering an explosion.

Variables and metrics pertaining to the physics of sound reflect these properties. There is a related, but distinct, set of properties that describe human factors. Care must be exercised to distinguish between the two to avoid misinterpretations especially when similar terminology is employed, as shown by the following examples.

Sound observed at a point in space exhibits a variable pressure. In the physics of sound, the amplitude of pressure is stated in pascals, newtons/m^2, or pounds/in^2. In terms of the human factors of hearing, the amplitude of pressure is stated in (nondimensional) decibels—and rarely in physical units. Although decibel notations are functionally applied to many aspects of science and engineering, a set applied to hearing contains mutations related to properties of human perception of loudness.

Loudness tends to vary logarithmically with pressure rather than linearly, so doubling the amplitude of pressure of a perceived sound does not double its loudness. Decibel (dB) functions are logarithmic and are applied to measurements of sound pressure. The functional relation that applies to hearing is

$$\text{decibels} = 10 \log_{10} [p/p_o]^2 = 20 \log_{10} [p/p_o]$$

where p is sound pressure and p_o is the nominal threshold of normal hearing at 1,000 Hz. (Both p and p_o are in the same units; in the SI system, both are in pascals [newtons/m^2].) The reference pressure used is 20 micropascals. Note that 0 dB corresponds to 20 (not zero) micropascals. In addition, some individuals can have thresholds lower than 20 micropascals, corresponding to -10 or more decibels. (A value of -10 dB equals 6.32 micropascals; 0 dB corresponds to 20 micropascals.)

Except for extremely high levels, such as gunfire, explosions, and rocket motors, there are no universally identified sound levels that cause immediate hearing damage. Nevertheless, damaging durations at levels above approximately 115 dB can be very short.

Susceptibility varies among individuals and is influenced by frequency content, temporal waveform, and cumulative exposure. Regulatory limits and professionally recommended guidelines generally limit unprotected exposures to levels below 110 or 115 dB. Limits for short-duration transients (impulses) of less than 1 second duration are stated at 140 dB. Regulatory requirements typically limit extended unprotected exposures, starting at 85 dBA. But extended exposures to levels below 85 dBA can still be hazardous.[1,2] Potential exposures should be carefully evaluated for residual risk as well as regulatory compliance.

A basic type of sound is a pure tone having a constant amplitude sinusoidal waveform. It can be generated by a steadily vibrating surface. As the surface is displaced into the neighboring air mass, an increase in pressure occurs; when it reverses, a decrease in pressure occurs. The number of times per second that a cyclic excursion occurs (from maximum to minimum, and back to maximum) is the frequency, given in cycles per second (cps), or hertz (Hz). All possible sound waveforms can be represented by an appropriately adjusted summation of pure tones. Based on this principle, hearing perception of any sound waveform can be derived from the response to pure sinusoidal tones over a specified frequency range. The nominal range of normal hearing spans the frequency range of 20 to 20,000 Hz.

The perception of loudness for pure tones having constant pressure amplitudes varies with frequency. In addition, proportionality between pressure amplitude and loudness changes with frequency. This property of hearing affects how sounds composed of many frequencies are perceived if the composite amplitude is varied without changing the relative amplitudes at each component frequency. At low levels, the ear has poor sensitivity at low frequencies and better sensitivity at medium and high frequencies. As the composite amplitude is raised, sensitivity becomes more uniform, and thus loudness perception becomes largely independent of frequency.

To illustrate the effect on perception, consider listening to a recording of a symphony orchestra, with contributions from all instruments played at a high volume. As the volume is reduced substantially, the quality of the sound deteriorates and become "tinny" due to reduction of bass content. This is a result of reduced sensitivity of hearing at low frequencies.

Potential damaging effects of noise are not uniform at all frequencies, with contributions at low frequencies being less harmful. Criteria for exposure and measurements of hazardous noise stipulate sound levels measured in decibels as *A-weighted* (dBA). This means that the level is formulated or measured to incorporate a frequency-selective filter having the defined shape of A-weighting. The origins of such a filter stem from the Fletcher–Munson curves. The susceptibility to hearing damage is not explicitly related to the perceived loudness. The loudness-derived, A-weighting response has served as a sorting aid, discovered empirically to relate to damage potential. It can be derived through controlled audiometric measurements on subjects having "normal" hearing (Fig. 14A-1). Each of the solid line plots is obtained during a separate audiometric test. The curves shown, however, represent processed averages obtained from large numbers of screened subjects.

The procedure for obtaining each plot is to instruct a subject that a sequence of two sounds will be perceived. The first will be a reference, followed by a second exploratory stimulus. The first will always be at a fixed frequency (1 kHz), the second will be at a changed frequency set by the operator. The subject has a "loudness control." After exposure to each sequence, the subject is instructed to adjust the control to make the two stimuli equally loud. Both stimuli initially have equal acoustic pressure. The reference stimulus at 1 kHz has an amplitude of 20 micropascals (0 dB). Although the second stimulus initially also has equal amplitude, the departure from 0 dB shows the adjustment necessary by the subject to approach equal loudness at frequencies other than 1 kHz.

In subsequent tests, the reference level is increased by 10 dB and the procedure is repeated. For the highest reference levels, such as 100 dB, the equal loudness plots show the least variability as frequency drops below 1 kHz. In contrast, examine the plot for threshold perception referenced to 0 dB and compare it to the high level plot referenced to 100 dB. Note the approximate 60 dB change in threshold sensitivities at 1 kHz, as compared to 35 Hz for the first plot. This represents a ratio of intensities of 1 million! In contrast, at a reference level of 100 dB, little change over frequency reduction is observed. At frequencies above 1 kHz, the shapes of the equal loudness

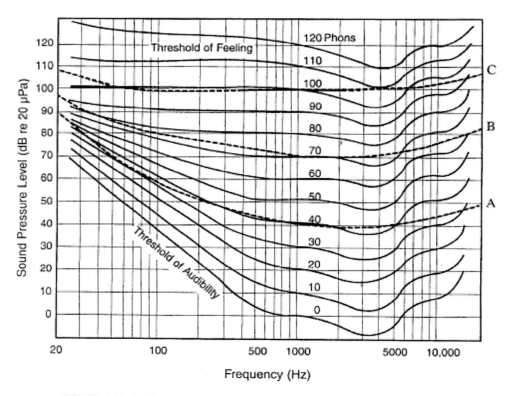

FIGURE 14A-1 ● Fletcher–Munson curves with weighting filter response overlay.

curves are not significantly changed at individual frequencies.

Historically, plots were derived to specify frequency selective filters for instruments intended to obtain single number "loudness ratings" for sounds having different overall levels. Figure 14A-1 shows three dashed curves superimposed on the Fletcher–Munson plots. The lowest, designated A, was established for characterizing sounds of low amplitude. It approximates the 40 dB reference equal loudness curve (convention is to designate the reference levels in *phons*). The next higher is designated *B* and is an approximation of the 70 phon equal loudness curve. The highest is designated *C* and relates to the 100 phon equal loudness curve.

The A-weighted filter response is related to very low sound levels. For example, this is similar to background noise levels in a quiet suburban area. The B filter has characteristics similar to loud speech levels. Finally, the C is similar to what are considered hazardous industrial workplace levels. Figure 14A-2 shows the frequency response of filters used in sound level meters (SLMs).[3]

The use of A-weighting for measuring and stipulating exposure levels is not related to the loudness

metric from which it was derived. The application derives from empirical correlation with measurements made to quantify hazardous exposures.

METRICS PERTAINING TO NOISE EXPOSURES

Noise exposure can be measured and quantified in units of pressure in relation to units of time (in seconds or hours). In prevailing practice, these data are not reported in physical units when relating the exposure to noise-induced permanent threshold shift (NIPTS). Instead, nondimensional metrics (such as decibels) are used. It is to this practice that "change in notation" refers. Examples of the metrics relate to:

1. Waveforms of the sound (continuous steady-state, slowly varying, interrupted, and short-duration transients identified as impact or impulsive noise).
2. Averaged level over defined periods (averaging performed by a variety of processes).
3. Noise dose (percentage) and time-weighted average (TWA).
4. Statistical properties.

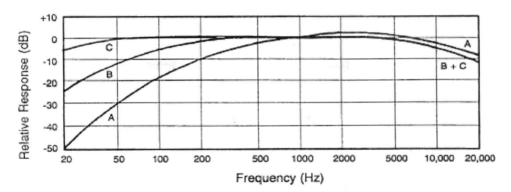

FIGURE 14A-2 ● SLM weighting curves (ANSI S1.4-1983).

There is no single criterion for evaluating or specifying acceptable exposures, so a practitioner must be aware of and understand the pertinent regulatory or protective criterion applied in a particular instance and the meanings and derivations of applicable metrics.

A widely applied criterion states the permissible exposure in dBA as a criterion level for a work shift (commonly 8 hours). Because actual exposure levels vary, the limits on permissible exposure are changed by trading levels for exposure duration. When the level is increased, the permissible exposure duration is decreased, and vice versa. For example, given an exchange rate of 3 dB, an increase of 3 dB above the criterion level requires a cut in half of permissible exposure to 4 hours; a decrease of 3 dB allows a doubling of exposure time to 16 hours. Complying with the exchange rate results in equal exposures. In different regulatory environments or under some recommended guidelines, the following have been used: criterion levels of 90 and 85 dB and exchange rates of 3, 4, and 5 dB. The relationship between permissible exposure levels and durations is detailed in high-resolution incremental tables.

The rationale for using incremental tables relates to the fundamental limitations of the traditional monitoring instrument used, the SLM. This instrument, in its basic configuration, is only capable of indicating steady or minimally varying sound levels. Accordingly, the traditional approach has been to attempt to break lengthy exposure periods into short increments of time during which measurements have small excursions—not always possible when sound levels vary rapidly. With modern instruments (integrating/averaging SLMs and dosimeters), noise level variability is not an obstacle. Continuous real-time processing to apply the

selected criterion eliminates the need for segmentation.

A common metric employed in protective guidelines and regulatory practice is *noise dose* expressed in percentages, with 100 percent constituting a limit of acceptable exposure without the use of hearing protection. For worker exposures to other agents, the concept of a dose is directly related to a physical measure. For example, a 100 percent dose of exposure during a work period to a toxic or carcinogenic agent may be stated as the number of nanograms that are inhaled or absorbed. In contrast, a noise dose is a function of noise level in dB and exposure time. Note that dB are nondimensional, and, accordingly, no direct physical interpretation of a noise dose is indicated.

A sound level in dB is based on a specific sound intensity expressed in units of sound power per unit area. Power has the dimensions of energy transfer per unit time. Accordingly, when exposure to a noise level in dB for 8 hours is stipulated as a limit, it is equivalent to stipulating the exposure to the corresponding intensity of a sound for 8 hours. Such an exposure corresponds dimensionally to an accumulated sound energy, the limit of which must not be exceeded. In defining a particular 100 percent noise dose, a criterion sound level and a criterion exposure time are given. The two identify a quantity of sound energy that constitutes 100 percent noise dose. Accordingly, the accumulation of a smaller amount of energy constitutes a lower dose and a larger amount constitutes a higher dose.

If an actual exposure duration at a fixed level listed in an exchange rate table departs from the permissible duration, the associated noise dose is proportional to the ratio of actual duration to permissible duration. For example, under OSHA, 100 percent noise dose is accumulated in 8 hours at a level of 90 dBA.[4] For exposure at that level during a 16-hour shift, the accumulated dose is 200 percent.

The general expression for determining noise dose using an exposure table for a sum of exposures at different levels and different durations is

$$D = 100 \ (C_1/T_1 + C_2/T_2 + \ldots C_n/T_n)$$

where C_n indicates exposure duration at a specific noise level (listed in an exposure table), and T_n indicates the permissible duration for that level. To illustrate properties of different exchange rates, consider Table 14A-1, which lists permissible noise exposures for a 5-dB exchange rate (current OSHA standard) and a 3 dB exchange rate (1989 NIOSH proposed standard).[1]

The following are other metrics pertaining to exposures[5]:

Average level (dB): Noise levels cannot be arithmetically averaged. Consider an example in which a compressor is on for 5 minutes, then off for 5 minutes. At a nearby work location, during operation of the compressor, the sound level is 100 dBA, and when it is off, the sound level is 60 dBA. The average level is not 80 dBA (the arithmetic average), but 97 dBA, the logarithmic average. (There is additional bias if the averaging pertains to levels obtained with exchange rates other than 3 dB.)

Time-weighted average (TWA), or equivalent continuous level (ECL): A fixed sound level at which exposure for 8 hours will produce the same noise dose as exposure to a variable sound level for a work shift of arbitrary length. The TWA level and the average level are not equivalent, except when the exposure duration is exactly 8 hours. In addition, TWA represents the same information about a particular exposure as the noise dose. The two are completely interchangeable, recognizing, however, that there is a change in notation.

Action level: In regulatory practice, this stipulates a level above which certain actions are required, such as mandating that those exposed wear hearing protectors. It is important to determine whether a sound level or a TWA is specified for the action.

OCCUPATIONAL NOISE REGULATIONS IN THE UNITED STATES

Noise regulations pertaining to individuals in the United States vary depending on the agency or branch of government having jurisdiction.

Occupational Safety and Health Administration (OSHA) Standard for Manufacturing

For manufacturing, OSHA mandates[4]:

1. For a TWA exceeding the action level of 90 dBA, no unprotected exposure is permitted (equivalent to limiting unprotected exposure to 100 percent noise dose). To prevent such exposures, engineering or administrative controls must be implemented. Engineering controls require reducing the noise level; administrative controls reduce accumulated exposure by rotating workers during the work shift to locations having adequately lower noise levels. There is an absolute limit of 115 dBA for unprotected exposure to steady or slowly varying sound levels. There is a separate absolute limit of 140 dB for impulsive noise. (Frequency weighting, such as A or C, of the sound pressure level is not stated.) Such noise has a duration of less than 1 second and is not repeated more often than once per second. This definition is ambiguous, and the conservative action is to avoid unprotected exposure at any level above 115 dBA. Instruments that correctly incorporate all contributions up to 140 dB

TABLE 14A-1

Permissible Noise Exposures

Hours per Day	Sound Level dBA	
	5-dB Exchange	3-dB Exchange[a]
8	90	90
6	92	—
4	95	93
3	97	—
2	100	96
1.5	102	—
1.0	105	99
0.5	110	102
0.25	115	105

[a] To avoid confusion in the comparisons, the non–time doubling increments are omitted because they have fractional dB levels.

in computing noise dose or TWA will provide information necessary for appropriate action.[6] If controls are not technically or economically feasible, hearing protective devices (HPDs) must be employed. The effective protection must reduce the exposure below action level.

2. Workers potentially exposed to TWA above 85 dBA must be placed in a hearing conservation program (HCP), which requires establishing baseline audiograms for the included workers and annual reexaminations. The objective is to obtain information to determine if workers are experiencing unacceptable threshold shifts, despite protective measures having been taken. Workers exposed to TWAs above 85 dBA, but below 90 dBA, are not required to use HPDs, but must be provided with them.[4,7]

Other United States Regulations

Occupational noise regulations vary with the agency or branch of government having jurisdiction and type of occupation. An informative summary of key requirements among the various regulations is provided in Table 14A-2. In 2004, the Federal Railroad Administrative published a proposed rule that would include mandatory HCPs.

Engineering Controls

When there is a potential for overexposure to noise at specific locations in a workplace, the preferred solution is to reduce noise levels at those locations by implementing engineering controls, using procedures such as the following[5]:

1. Reduce noise emitted by individual sources, such as by modifying machines or changing their operating cycles or by enclosing sources with acoustical shielding. (In most cases, enclosure will require adding a means of cooling. Openings necessary to circulate cooling air by convection or blowers require addition of acoustical silencers.)
2. Specify limits on noise emission for new acquisitions or replacement of sources. (A clause specifying such limits is routinely added to purchase orders by large manufacturers with an established HCP.)
3. Acoustically shield affected workers if sources cannot be modified or enclosed. Such shielding can range from providing an insulated control room to providing full or partial booth enclosure for an exposed worker.
4. Install acoustical absorbers on walls or ceilings may be useful if exposed workers are distant from noise sources, and thus in a reverberant field. However, in most situations, such installations yield little or no improvement. A simple way to determine if these absorbers may be useful is to scan the workplace with an averaging sound level meter to determine if there is noticeable change in sound level as contributing sources are approached. Small or no variations in level are indicative of a reverberant environment. Most often, however, workers are close to machines that they operate and hence are not in a reverberant environment.
5. Place partial barriers between noise sources and workers, although less effective than complete enclosure, may be sufficient to reduce noise dose to an acceptable level. For example, at a work station where a TWA of 90 dBA or noise dose of 100 percent is accumulated, a reduction by 3 dBA results in a dose reduction of 50 percent for an exchange rate of 3 dBA, or 34 percent for an exchange rate of 5 dBA.
6. Obtain assistance from qualified acoustical engineers, technicians, and appropriate manufacturers. Although there are many approaches and devices that can potentially be used to reduce source noise, selection on the basis of intuition should be avoided. Unfortunately, failure to produce desired results is often discovered only after nonrecoverable expenditures are made.

Use of Hearing Protective Devices

Resorting to use of HPDs is a suboptimal approach to reducing exposures. Their principal deficiency is the highly variable degree of unpredictable protection that they provide. Field studies in workplaces have discovered substantial differences between actual noise attenuation and attenuation claimed by manufacturers.[5] Factors contributing to reduced performance include (a) worker discomfort, especially in hot and dirty work environments; (b) workers' reluctance to wear them for a full work shift; and (c) the tendency to remove HPDs to readjust or clean them, leading to incorrect positioning. To achieve maximum protection, HPDs must be correctly fitted and installed—not simple tasks—and workers must be motivated to use them correctly.

TABLE 14A-2

Occupational Noise Regulations in the United States

Agency and Worker Type	Exchange Rate	Action Level*	Permissible Exposure Level*	Hours Allowed at A-weighted Sound Level in Columns B and C	Threshold of Measurement*	Maximum Continuous Sound*	Maximum Impulse Noise*	Mandatory Hearing Conservation above 85 Time Weighted Avg.
	A	B	C	D	E	F	G	H
OSHA manufacturing	5	85	90	8	80[1]	115	140	Yes
OSHA construction	5	90	90	8	90	115	140	Yes[2]
Other civilian employees	5		90	8	80	115	140	No
MSHA, all mining	5	85	90	8	90	115	140	Yes[3]
FRA, trainmen	5		87	12		115		No
USCG, commercial vessels	5		82	24	80		140	No
FHWA, motor vehicles	5		90					No
DOD	3,4[4]	85	85	8			140	Yes

*A-weighted sound level in dB.

[1] A-weighted sound level of 80 dB for hearing conservation; 90 dB for engineering and administrative controls. An executive order by President Reagan permits industry to use hearing protection without doing engineering or administrative controls if the TWA is less than 100 dB.

[2] Although this regulation does not provide any details for a hearing conservation program, some requirements have been recently proposed.

[3] Above 105 TWA, dual protection is required. Engineering controls are required.

[4] Navy uses 4 dB doubling rate.

OSHA is the Occupational Safety and Health Administration, a part of the Department of Labor (DOL) of the U. S. Government.

MSHA is the Mine Safety and Health Administration, also part of DOL.

FRA is the Federal Railroad Administration, part of the Department of Transportation (DOT).

USCG is the U. S. Coast Guard, also a part of DOT.

FHWA is the Federal Highway Administration, also a part of DOT.

DOD is the Department of Defense, with separate Army, Navy, and Air Force regulations.

From Bruce RD, Wood EW. The USA needs a new national policy for occupational noise. Noise Control Eng J 2003;51:162–5.

Commercially available HPDs are certified to have noise reduction ratings (NRRs), obtained by skilled technicians under carefully controlled laboratory conditions. But, in actual workplace situations, the degree of noise reduction provided is often less. For example, an HPD rated at NRR 30 was found in multiple field tests to actually provide approximately 13 dBA of attenuation, and another type rated at NRR 18 was found to actually provide only 4 dBA of attenuation.

Another factor contributing to these findings derives from the basic definition of NRR, which is a composite approximate attenuation, based on an assumed spectral content of workplace noise. Even under ideal conditions, if, for example, the noise encountered is predominantly at low frequencies in comparison to NRR test levels, the HPD may not be as protective as claimed by the manufacturer. Comparing reexaminations to baseline audiograms can provide information on the effectiveness of the HCPs and their HPD use.

Instruments for Surveys

Sound (dynamic pressure) is the physical agent that presents a threat to hearing. Measurements of sound, in time and space, provide a basis for predicting and quantifying adverse impacts of noise and developing means of control. Because data from such measurements have little utility in their crude form, two transformations of these data are required to apply them usefully. One is in the form of the derived metrics, which can then be directly interpreted for impact. The other is a spatial representation so that conclusions can be drawn on the relation between accumulated exposure and movements of affected workers.

The basic instrument for surveys is the sound level meter (SLM), which converts pressure measurements into decibel levels. Such an instrument, as a minimum, has a built-in, A-weighted filter (and sometimes also a selectable C-weighted filter). When sound levels do not vary rapidly, a surveyor using a basic SLM can observe and transcribe readings by time and location, which can later be reduced to noise dose or TWA.[3] The surveyor cannot respond quickly enough to record rapid variations and must resort to more advanced SLMs having real-time exposure-processing capability. The basic SLM cannot respond quickly enough to measure exposure of short duration, but more advanced SLMs have supplementary capability. To accumu-

late data for use in engineering controls or special HPDs, other versions of SLMs are available that have built-in octave or fractional-octave band filters to sort surveyed sound into multiple frequency bands.

A typical workplace will have a variety of work stations. Some workers will be constrained, such as at production lines, where spot measurements with SLMs can be sufficient, provided that there is no rapid fluctuation of noise level. If there is rapid fluctuation, one may need to use integrating/averaging SLMs, which have built-in data-processing functions that can obtain averages in time and space. (Most of these instruments perform averaging on the basis of a 3-dB exchange rate; others have selectable exchange rates.) Workers who are highly mobile might need to have surveyors document their shift-long exposures by tracking them closely during an entire shift—not an attractive option. An alternative is placing personal dosimeters on workers.[6]

Dosimeters are available with extensive memory capacity for acquiring a wide range of exposure data. The most basic dosimeter computes accumulated noise dose, or TWA, for a worker over an entire workshift. A more advanced dosimeter records exposure level by time for an entire workshift, with time resolution as low as 1 second—accumulating a very large file. Associated software, however, is very flexible and one can compress information into increments of various durations. These data can help detect and identify important sources of noise exposure.

Exposure Determination

Determining and classifying exposures of many workers can be time-consuming and can require many dosimeters. If groups of workers have similar shift-long exposures, the number of measurements may be reduced. To plan surveys of worker exposure to noise, one must first determine prevailing noise levels and work stations where noise levels may exceed the OSHA action level (85 dBA).

OSHA requirements and practices make no explicit allowance for interpreting and taking protective actions based on statistical sampling and inferences. Strict interpretation of existing rules mandates certainty in assigning worker exposure levels. Although individual monitoring of all workers will provide useful information, the variance of results obtained still presents a problem in interpretation. A conservative approach is to increase estimated individual exposures levels by a safety factor and apply results in formulating HCP plans.

Another question affecting determination of potential exposure level for a specific worker is raised when exposure conditions are temporary, such as in seasonal work and work on a short project. There is no explicit directive addressing such conditions. Accordingly, strict interpretation requires compliance based on a worst-case scenario.

To apply any plan for simplifying and reducing the scope of a survey, one must understand the conditions and factors influencing the magnitudes and variability of individual noise exposures. One way to simplify assigning expected exposures is to segregate workers in cohorts, in which individual workers are considered to experience similar shift exposures. When this is possible, exploratory surveys are made of a few workers likely to have the highest exposures. From these surveys, exposures of those most highly exposed are designated to represent conservatively each worker in the cohort.

Use of task-based analyses is another approach to explore commonality of noise exposure among workers. Noise exposures are collected for each task performed. Provided that tasks can be well defined and proper noise exposures for performance of each task are determined, combination exposures can be computed for individual workers. Use of computer processing can greatly expedite exposure documentation for large numbers of workers.

Before applying the procedure, critical factors that can invalidate results must be considered and evaluated for cost-effectiveness. For example, there can be significant exposure differences among workers performing a given defined task, depending on individual style of performance. Furthermore, the nature and duration of tasks must be accurately defined. For highly structured and regimented production lines, this is feasible. In many other work environments, tasks are highly variable in performance and duration.

ENVIRONMENTAL EXPOSURES

The potential for hazardous exposures to noise extends beyond the workplace (Fig. 14A-3). Clinicians who see patients exposed to excessive noise at work can identify similar hazards in the community at large. Because noise-induced hearing loss is cumulative, exposures acquired outside the workplace can result in hearing impairment not predictable by workplace monitoring alone. Clinicians should obtain quantitative information about the scope of nonoccupational exposures to noise. Such information can facilitate additional preventive measures in the workplace, including educational programs. Some employers permit and encourage use of company-provided HPDs for protection outside the workplace.

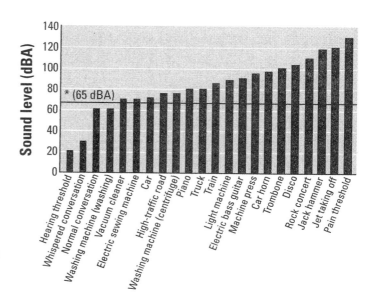

FIGURE 14A-3 ● Sound levels (in dBA) for various typical environmental noise exposures. (Source: Frenzilli G, Lenzi P, Scarcelli V, et al. Effects of loud noise exposure on DNA integrity in rat adrenal gland. Environ Health Perspect 2004;112:1671–2.)

Live rock concerts are known to expose not only performers, but also members of the audience, to levels above 115 dBA. A permanent threshold shift even after a single performance is possible. Although the audience members may be considered to be participating voluntarily in a hazardous activity, workers at a concert often face unprotected exposures to loud noise that would not be permitted even by the least stringent of guidelines. Members of the audience who experience modest exposures to noise in their jobs may be exposed beyond acceptable limits. Although people are qualitatively aware about the adverse effects of such loud noise, clinicians should provide cautionary advice to avoid unprotected exposure to high levels of sound. Examples would include rock concerts, indoor exposures to music reproduced at high levels, use of firearms, automobile boom boxes, motorized lawn mowers, chainsaws, and stock car races. Useful indications that ambient sound is excessive include the following. If conversation at a separation distance of 3 feet is difficult or impossible even when shouting, the level is excessive. After excessive exposure such as at a rock concert, stock car race, or gun range, a temporary threshold shift will occur. Another effect that individuals can detect after exposure to excessive noise is tinnitus. These effects should be explained to individuals and they should be instructed to detect them.

Noise produced by magnetic resonance imaging (MRI) equipment can produce noise levels above 115 dBA in the bore of toroidal magnets. Patients are usually provided simple HPDs, the effectiveness of which is not certain. Care should be exercised to limit actual exposures because individual patients may already have hearing impairment and increased susceptibility due to use of cisplatin and other ototoxic drugs.

REFERENCES

1. NIOSH. Criteria for a recommended standard-occupational exposure to noise. Cincinnati: NIOSH, 1998.
2. American Conference of Governmental Industrial Hygienists. TLVs and BEIs threshold limit values and biological exposure indices. Cincinnati: ACGIH, 2004.
3. American National Standards Institute. Specification for sound level meters (ANSI S1.4-1983) (R2001). New York: ANSI, 1997.
4. OSHA. Occupational noise exposure, 1910.95. OSHA regulations (Standards - 29 CFR). Sub part number G title: Occupational health and environmental control. Washington, DC: OSHA, 1983.
5. Berger EH, Royster LH, Royster JD, et al., eds. The noise manual. Fairfax, VA: American Industrial Hygiene Association, 2003.
6. ANSI: Specification for personal noise dosimeters (S1.25-1991) (R2002). New York: ANSI, 1991.
7. Royster JD, Royster LH. A guide to developing and maintaining an effective hearing conservation program. Raleigh, NC: North Carolina Department of Labor, 1998. (NC-OSHA Industry Guide #15.) Available at: <www.nonoise.org>.

BIBLIOGRAPHY

ANSI: Determination of Occupational Noise Exposure and Estimation of Noise-Induced Hearing Impairment (S3.44-1996) (R2001). New York: ANSI, 1997.
This is a basic reference presenting statistical data relating noise exposure to noise induced hearing premanent threshold shift (NIPTS). Of significant interest are separate data for an otologically normal population ("highly screened"). The latter offer insight into presbycusis effects up to age 60.

Bies DA, Hensen CH. Engineering noise control, theory and practice. London and New York: Spon Press, 2003.
This text presents a comprehensive discussion of theoretical principles and concepts of acoustics and noise control aimed at practicing engineers and students. Of significant interest to others, it contains lucid discussions of the hearing mechanism, psychoacoustic effects, and noise criteria and metrics.

The Hearing Review, 1999, Vol. 6, No. 9.
A special issue containing a broad spectrum of articles pertaining to hearing conservation of interest to occupational health practitioners. The articles address measurement and control of noise exposures, regulatory standards and practices, hearing protectors, and conduct and evaluation of hearing conservation programs.

Rossing TD. The science of sound. New York: Addison-Wesley, 1990.
There is a gap between physical acoustics and the acoustics of hearing that requires bridging. This text is designed for an undergraduate-level course focused on musical acoustics. It provides broadly based descriptions and definitions of metrics regarding the perception of sound. It is an effective bridge between the two disciplines. Of particular utility are instructive descriptions of experiments to illustrate perception effects. It also presents a foundation for the study of sound quality that has become prominent.

Office of Noise Abatement and Control. Information on levels of environmental noise requisite to protect the public health and welfare with an adequate margin of safety (550/9-74-004). Washington, DC: U.S. Environmental Protection Agency, 1974:7–8.
Even after many years, this document is still referenced in many publications pertaining to community noise.

Vibration

Martin G. Cherniack

Vibration is traditionally divided into *whole-body vibration*, having particular pertinence to vehicle seat design, and *segmental vibration*, affecting the hand and arm. For segmental vibration, health effects are usually related to energy transfer to the upper extremity from either powered tools or from stationery sources producing oscillatory vibration, such as mounted drills and pedestal grinders. There are parallel physical principles that apply to both sound and vibration, and in the case of whole-body vibration, the psychological and physiological effects of sound and vibration are often intertwined.

Vibration is a complex physical exposure, which lends itself to electro-physical measurement. There are also well-accepted methodologies for exposure measurement and for the evaluation of human health effects. Chronic vibration from hand tools is associated with Raynaud's phenomenon, a signature disorder of blood vessels, and peripheral nerve mechanoreceptor dysfunction in the fingertips. There is both overlap with and distinction from other work-related musculoskeletal, neuromuscular, and neurovascular disorders that affect the upper extremity.

Adverse health effects from segmental vibration involving measurable neurological and arterial dysfunction have led to the development of quantitative approaches to surveillance and industrial control. In 1986, the International Standards Organization (ISO) published methods for measuring segmental vibration and controlling its exposure (ISO 5349 [1986]).[1] In the same year, the American National Standards Institute (ANSI) adopted this approach.[2] The ISO standards were recently revised with sim-

ilar, but even stricter, recommendations.[3,4] Consensus standards emphasize specific quantitative medical tests and the transformation of tool-based measurements into exposure limits and metrics for disease prevention. These accepted international approaches to measurement reflect the technical feasibility of translating the vibration from hand tools into physical principles: the frequency distribution of oscillations; the direction, velocity, and acceleration of those oscillations; and the impulsiveness, or force range, expressed in each impact cycle. Each of these physical characteristics has a bearing on symptoms and tissue injuries, especially in the palms and digits, but also more proximally in the shoulder and neck.

The approach to measurement for whole-body vibration (WBV) is similar in principle, although exposure magnitudes and targeted frequencies are considerably lower. The association with health effects is, however, quite different. There is a general delineation between acute physical and psychological effects that involve loss of proficiency or fatigue and chronic health effects, the most important being low-back disorders. Because low-back disorders are common and have many causes, their association with WBV is more challenging to assess.

Segmental vibration does not exist as an independent phenomenon. Workers with hand-tool exposure are subject to the same combination of biomechanical and intrinsic risks that accompany other forms of hand-intensive work. As a consequence, the successful reduction of segmental vibration as a physical exposure may not reduce other disorders, which may complicate recognition and attribution.

SEGMENTAL (HAND–ARM) VIBRATION

A Brief History

The deleterious effects on the peripheral nerves and small vessels of the upper extremity from hand-transmitted vibration produced by power tools have been documented for almost a century. The clinical recognition and environmental control of hand–arm vibration is based on the reduction of the most prominent sign and symptom complex: cold-related finger blanching (Raynaud's phenomenon). In 1918, the pioneering occupational medicine physician Alice Hamilton first described this disorder in the United States among Indiana quarry workers using air-powered tools.[5] Subsequent studies have confirmed a strong effect between duration and intensity of vibration exposure and the onset of acquired neurological and vascular symptoms.[6]

There are a variety of tool types and qualities of exposure that are associated with vibration-related upper extremity disorders. The most recognized sources are air-powered rotary tools, such as grinders, sanders, and cutting wheels. However, gasoline-powered oscillating tools, such as chainsaws and brushcutters, have a classic association with disease in the forestry industry. In addition, electrical power tools, although narrower in bandwidth than air tools, often generate forces in ranges that are deleterious to human tissue. Power tools, such as chipping hammers and pavement breakers, have greater impact (cycles that are defined by transient peak levels of force followed by rapid diminution). In the past three decades, characterization of the exposure–response relationship, disease identification, and antivibration tool design have helped to reduce exposure and cumulative incidence of traumatic vasospasm and vibration white finger (VWF). By the mid-1980s, investigators had recognized that the typical vascular disorder could occur independent of injuries to fingertip mechanoreceptors, experienced as paresthesias and reduced hand function. Thus, the term *hand–arm vibration syndrome* (HAVS) came into general use, with the accompanying Stockholm Workshop Scale designed to independently assess vascular and neurological effects.[6,7] The Stockholm Workshop Scale provided a consensus rating system for the two hallmark disorders: (a) vasospasm and disturbances of digital circulation and (b) diffuse digital neuropathy. There has been less agreement about associations with other disorders, including

(a) carpal tunnel syndrome (CTS), which is often confounded by biomechanical factors[8]; (b) a pattern of upper extremity muscle weakness[9]; and (c) bone and joint disorders, such as traumatic osteoarthritis and problems with the elbows, shoulders, and neck, which are potential sites of energy absorption.[10]

HAVS poses more than an incidental problem. In 1990, the National Institute for Occupational Safety and Health (NIOSH) warned that up to 2 million American workers were exposed to vibration at magnitudes and frequencies sufficient to provoke injury with a symptom prevalence approaching 40 percent.[6] The general decline in metalworking in industrial countries, coupled with antivibration tools having damping and balancing features, has significantly reduced symptom rates in specific industries, most notably in forestry. In the longest established longitudinal study of vibratory disease, Finnish forest workers were regularly resurveyed from 1972 to 1990.[11] Vibration exposures were reduced after the introduction of antivibration chainsaws. During this same interval, VWF prevalence declined from 40 percent to 5 percent of the population, and prevalence of hand and finger numbness from 78 percent to 28 percent, with remaining symptoms more suggestive of CTS. Although the physiologic response to vibratory stimuli is only partly understood and the use of high-frequency oscillatory devices continues to occur in small-scale occupations, such as bone prosthetic preparation and dental hygiene, HAVS in traditional work settings is largely preventable.

Exposure and Its Measurement

Vibration is a physical factor, expressible in precise units: frequency in Hz, acceleration in m/s^2 (g), and cycles in milliseconds. This offers highly accessible measurement with available instrumentation, principally accelerometry and frequency spectrum analysis. The ISO has taken a consensus regulatory approach to tool design by assuming a relationship between the relative hazards presented by vibration at different frequencies. This is achieved by (a) frequency weighting the acceleration-time history, $a_w(t)$, and (b) temporal summation, by means of energy averaging over the duration of an 8-hour work shift. Customarily, frequency-specific acceleration is reported at one-third octave bands and downweighted above 16 Hz, so that frequencies above 250 Hz have minimal effect on exposure calculations. (NIOSH had recommended that this downweighting be abandoned.) The implications are significant. For example, a small burring machine that produced a frequency-weighted acceleration of 5.6 m/s^2 was found to have an unweighted acceleration of 146.8 m/s^2.[12] Appreciating that these differences are substantial is not a critique of international standardization but helps to explain why future scientific controversy is likely. ISO Standards 5349.1 and 5349.2 are central to consensus measurement of exposure. ISO standard 5349.1 defines vibration parameters, such as acceleration; a hand-oriented coordinate system; a hand–arm measurement filter; and a dose–response relationship.

Although ISO has presumed an exposure–response relationship, translating exposure from laboratory measurement into the work environment is not straightforward. Vibratory characteristics are highly tool-specific. Chainsaws and drills, for example, are primarily oscillatory and continuous-energy tools; impact wrenches and rivet guns have large physical displacements and are highly impulsive; tools such as nut runners have major nonvibratory biomechanical features. Thus, simple generic measurements may not capture the extent of a potential tool-specific hazard.

Frequency, direction of vibration, and the position of the arm and hand all have an effect on impedance to and absorption of vibration energy. Push and pull as well as grip force affect transmission and are, in turn, altered by the characteristics of vibration: impulsiveness and frequencies.[13] Perhaps the most problematic area involves high-impulse acceleration. The ISO and ANSI weighted curves treat all vibration as harmonic, ignoring impact forces and instantaneous peak accelerations that may exceed 10^5 m/s^2 (10,000 g). The dramatic reduction in vascular symptoms occurring with the introduction of antivibration chainsaws in the 1970s was better explained by the flattening of high transient accelerations than by a reduction in root mean squared (rms).[14] Also vascular symptoms, which were consistently underestimated by ISO 5349 for pedestal grinding and stone cutting, were better accounted for when high-peak impulsivity was factored into the exposure model. This is consistent with, but does not fully explain, the high prevalence of VWF in platers and riveters, who use high-impulse tools for only a few minutes a day.[15] A similar problem arises in the setting of tools that oscillate at very high frequencies, such as small precision drills and saws. Most measurement protocols exclude frequencies that exceed 1,500 Hz. There are sound reasons for this: (a) energy transfer is directly related to velocity, so that its first derivative, acceleration, is seemingly discounted at high frequencies; and (b) there is no physiological evidence that the Pacinian corpuscle, the principal fingertip mechanoreceptor, responds above 1,500 Hz. Nevertheless, neurologic and vascular symptoms have been highly concentrated in select working populations using these types of tools.

Perhaps because of these complexities, the European Community has advanced practical regulations that set a low action level for vibration of $a_w(t)$ at 2.5 m/s^2 and daily exposure limit of 5.0 m/s^2. The European Committee for Standardization (CEN) approach emphasizes tool design and exposure control and is based on expert opinion and more loosely on epidemiology to reflect feasibility and a presumed modest risk of disease in less than 10 percent of those exposed. This simplifies the dimensions of human exposure and sets a threshold where disease is expected to be uncommon.

Pathology

Sensorineural symptoms in the hands are generally the most common clinical presentation in industrial workers exposed to vibratory tools. Sensory nerve conduction velocity (SNCV) in the digits of vibration-exposed symptomatic workers is slowed, especially in proximal segments.[16,17] These deficits in the function of distal myelinated nerve fibers are distinct from the characteristic slowing in the wrist-palm segment that occurs in CTS. Injuries to small nerve fibers in the fingertips are distinct from demyelinating nerve compression disorders, such as CTS, that affect larger nerve fibers. When changes in tactile function associated with occupational use of vibratory tools are examined in each of the three mechanoreceptor populations at a fingertip—Meissner corpuscles, Merkel disks, and Pacinian corpuscles—the chronic changes in thresholds, determined by vibrometry, occur differentially among the three populations (Table 14B-1).[18] It appears that at least transient deficits in mechanoreceptor function occur at higher oscillatory frequencies (125 Hz or more) than are emphasized in international standards. Mechanoreceptor dysfunction impairs both sensation and muscular responses, such as grip.

The hallmark symptom associated with segmental vibration, digital vasospasm, predominates in

TABLE 14B-1

Mechanoreceptors and Their Function

Type	Property	Mechanoreceptor	Location	Innervation	Sensation	Peak Response (Hz)
A-Beta	Slow Adapting SA I	Merkel's neurite	Basal layer epidermis	Single nerve	Fixed touch Edge and gap Braille receptor	4.8
A-Beta	Fast Adapting FA I	Meissner's corpuscle	Dermal papillary ridge	Multiple nerves	2-point Slippage 5 mm gap	26–32
A-Beta	Fast Adapting FA II	Pacinian corpuscle	Deep dermal and subcutaneous	Single nerve (lamellar)	Movement and pressure	125

the hand most exposed. However, companion vasoconstriction in the hand not exposed to vibration suggests central sympathetic mechanisms affecting peripheral blood vessels.[19] The characteristic clinical finding is a local blanching of the skin of the fingers that is well demarcated from surrounding skin and occurs in paroxysmal attacks, usually induced by exposure to cold. Dramatic reductions in digital artery diameter provoked by cold, measured either by ultrasound or plethysmography, present similarly, whether or not Raynaud's phenomenon is work-induced, idiopathic, or secondary to a systemic collagen vascular disease.[20] Sensitive and specific tests include plethysmographic measurement of cold-induced arterial effects through the use of (a) strain gauges that measure finger systolic blood pressure (FSBP) and (b) locally applied cold provocation.[21] Although intimal injury has been identified in finger biopsy on a few advanced cases,[22] this is exceptional; arteriography and baseline noninvasive studies are usually normal. Thus, pathology is best understood in physiologic terms.[23]

There are two limitations to this type of measurement: (a) specialized devices are uncommon, and more conventional ice-water baths are unreliable; and (b) plethysmography measures full finger perfusion, which may be intact in nutritive capillaries while cutaneous blood flow is reduced. Thus, laser Doppler, a method that primarily measures cutaneous flow, produces significantly more abnormal tests than plethysmography,[24] and, in subjects with VWF, blood pressure appears to normalize in the setting of cold stress, whereas skin temperature (cutaneous perfusion) and symptoms remain unchanged.[25] Accordingly, (a) conventional non-invasive vascular measurements, such as Doppler, pulse volume, and photoplethysmography, are without value in the absence of controlled cold provocation; and (b) crude immersion challenge and measurement of skin temperature is not an adequate procedure.

Clinical Presentation and Diagnoses

The hallmark sign of clinical disease related to hand–arm vibration is a well-delineated patchwise blanching of the fingers, occurring at sites of greatest exposure, after exposure of the hands or the whole body to a cold environment. VWF signs and symptoms are a subset of those designated by the acronym HAVS. VWF includes:

1. White fingers;
2. Peripheral neuropathy, with or without increased cold sensitivity;
3. Distal compressive and demyelinating neuropathies of digital nerves, the median nerve at the carpal tunnel, and, less plausibly, the ulnar nerve; and

4. Musculoskeletal disturbances, such as weakness, lancinating forearm pain, and bone and joint degeneration.

Finger blanching and small fiber neuropathy are fairly specific, but nerve compression disorders and musculoskeletal pain and joint degeneration are nonspecific. Diagnosis of a case of HAVS is based on clinical assessment: a history of exposure and complaints, physical examination, and, often, laboratory studies. To some extent, the diagnosis of HAVS is exclusionary, as peripheral nerve dysfunction and Raynaud's phenomenon can reflect serious underlying disorders that are unrelated to exposure to vibration.

Even classic VWF can be problematic as pathology may arise in either the arterial or cutaneous circulation. In addition, temperature sensitivity and hand weakness may be representative of injury to small nerve fibers or to compression-related conduction block. In cases where CTS has been ruled out, a finding of diffusely distributed reduction of skin sensitivity and/or paresthesia and an increased sensitivity to cold are more likely due to mechanoreceptor injury. This type of injury, in contrast to typical CTS, is aggravated acutely by exposure to vibratory tools, is less intermittent, and is induced by arm position. The association between segmental vibration and upper extremity osteoarthritis is more ambiguous; bone and joint changes are very difficult to differentiate from the effects of other ergonomic hazards or aging.

In patients with early symptoms of classical VWF, there is the possibility of other, even multiple, pathologies. These patients often present with symptoms that are more diverse than is anticipated by conventional diagnostic criteria. Their complaints may be due to vibration damage or other pathology but also to variants of normal vascular physiology. In an industrial population already self-selected by hand-intensive work, it is relatively uncommon to uncover underlying systemic diseases, such as thyroid disease, diabetes, early presentations of collagen vascular disease, or vascular symptoms attributable to circulating cold agglutinins or cryoglobulins.

Reduction of exposure magnitude through tool design or transfer of individuals showing symptoms, or even a subclinical stage of the disorder, has produced a shift in the tenor of differential diagnosis. As vibratory exposures are contained and job tasks diversified, pure HAVS cases may be replaced by more obscure presentations. Because there are recoverable components, diminished exposure can produce a pattern where the incidence of new symptoms is balanced by symptom recovery. This changes the pattern from a purely exposure–response disease and toward a cumulative trauma disorder.

In a setting where exposures to hand–arm vibration are high or where there is a need for legal–administrative criteria, the accent is necessarily on HAVS-specific medical history questions and on tests that are also specific to vibration-related disease, such as small-fiber nerve tests and cold-challenge tests. However, exposure control, longer employment duration before symptom onset, and the conflicting presence of biomechanically induced or naturally occurring injury change the context of diagnostic testing. A lower prevalence of hallmark HAVS sequelae and a higher prevalence of mixed disorders require a broader and nonexclusionary approach to differential diagnosis. These issues are demonstrated in the two cases presented below.

Case 1: Typical Case of HAVS

A man who had worked 27 years as a shipyard welder, having worked 2 to 3 hours a day on a pneumatic grinder and needle gun, had a 10-year history of cold intolerance and a 5-year history of blanching of his fingers when the temperature was less than 10°C. He had nocturnal paresthesias in all of his fingers and paresthesias at work, resolving 4 to 8 hours after a work shift. He also noted diminished grip strength and clumsiness while attempting fine coordinated movements. On physical examination he had a positive Tinel sign, cold hands, and diffuse musculotendon pain. Anti-nuclear antibodies (ANA) and rheumatoid factor were negative. Nerve conduction velocity revealed a sensory latency of 4.4 m/s² in both the right and left distal median nerve. Grip strength was 30 kg for the right hand and 25 kg for the left hand. Two-point discrimination was 5 to 6 mm, monofilaments were 0.2 g.

Case 2: Atypical Case of Possible HAVS

A man who had worked 15 years as a carpenter, with intensive use of electric sanders, drills, and saws, had a 5-year history of cold intolerance with no clear blanching of his fingers. He tended to avoid cold exposure whenever possible. He had nocturnal paresthesias and moderate paresthesias at work with pinching of his thumb and second and third fingers. All the time at work, however, he had mild paresthesias in all of his fingers. He also noted hand cramps with painless claw-like rigidity and diffuse joint pain. On physical examination, he had a positive Tinel sign at the wrist and elbow, a positive Adson sign, and decreased range of motion at the wrists. He had arthralgias in his carpometacarpal joints and lateral epicondylar pain. Nerve conduction velocity tests revealed a sensory latency of 4.7 m/s^2 in the distal right median nerve and 4.2 m/s^2 in the distal left median nerve, and 4.1 m/s^2 in the distal right ulnar nerve and 4.2 m/s^2 in the distal left ulnar nerve. His grip strength was 25 kg in his right hand and 42 kg in his left hand. Two-point discrimination was 5.6 mm, monofilaments were 2.0 g.

In Case 1, there is a classic pattern of long exposure to air-powered tools, typical cold-induced finger blanching, a pattern of hand paresthesias, and dysfunction that is not clearly attributable to nerve compression. In Case 2, exposures are more diverse, and there is a strongly suggestive pattern of CTS. The raised sensory latency, diminished strength in the dominant hand, and nighttime paresthesias and positional relief are all typical for median nerve compression at the wrist. Also present are the type of chronically acquired musculoskeletal injuries, such as epicondylitis and proximal nerve compression, that occur more commonly in manual work and may have a waxing-and-waning course. In Case 2, HAVS cannot be assumed, which raises an issue of specialized diagnosis.

Although clinicians experienced in the treatment of neuromuscular disorders may regret the insufficiencies of diagnostic tests, HAVS is unique among occupationally related upper extremity disorders because of the availability of signature tests, such as (a) cold-challenge plethysmography or other cold-provocation tests for the diagnosis of Raynaud's, and (b) quantitative sensory tests (QSTs) for detecting small-fiber neuropathies. Nerve conduction studies, used in the diagnosis of work-related entrapment neuropathies, are notably less specific and less physiologic in their application to this type of injury. However, specialized tests are not generally available, and it is an error to proceed to specialized functional tests in the absence of judgment based on clinical anamnesis and a detailed physical exam.

An approach to evaluation is summarized in Box 14B-1. The extensiveness of the test battery will depend on several considerations, including the clinical presentation, medicolegal criteria, and the likelihood that a patient will be available for sequential follow-up. Thus, the list can be regarded as either complete or contingent.

In the classical case of white fingers and neurological disturbances due to damage of small nerve fibers, there are few therapeutic options. Therapeutic interventions are available but should be provided only under experienced clinical supervision.

The goal of rehabilitation should always be to transfer the affected worker to an alternative job, where hands are not exposed to hand-transmitted

---

BOX 14B-1

Standard Diagnostic Measures for HAVS Evaluation

- Case history;
- Physical examination of the upper extremity focused on vascular, neurologic, and musculoskeletal signs;
- Provocative clinical tests: Tinel (wrist and elbow), Adson, Roos, and Wright;
- Standardized and exclusionary criteria for clinical diagnosis of proximal disorders of the shoulder and neck;
- Tests of individual muscle strength and pinch and grip strength;
- Electromyographic studies, cold-challenge tests (finger systolic blood pressure), and quantitative sensory tests (VTT and temperature thresholds), as indicated;
- Radiographic imaging of cervical spine and shoulders, as indicated;
- Blood tests (complete blood count, sedimentation rate, blood viscosity, glucose, uric acid, rheumatoid factor, cryoglobulins, serum protein electrophoresis, immunoglobulins), as clinically indicated;
- Autoimmune serology (such as antinuclear antibodies, anti-DNA antibodies, animucleolar antibodies, anticentromere antibodies, ENA antibodies, and anticardiolipin antibodies), as clinically indicated.

vibration. In such a situation, disability assistance services would also come into play.

WHOLE-BODY VIBRATION

WBV is transmitted to the anatomic supporting surfaces, especially the legs when standing and the buttocks and back when sitting. A major emphasis for risk evaluation and remediation has been on vehicular seating in forklifts, construction vehicles, and off-road vehicles. Although transient alterations in psychomotor, physiological, and psychological function have been attributed to WBV, the greatest concerns and controversies involve chronic low back pain. Common sources of WBV are listed in Table 14B-2.

Exposure and Its Measurement

The principles involved in measuring WBV are analogous to those employed for segmental vibration. The control of human exposure is dependent on frequency, magnitude (expressed as rms acceleration), and duration of contact. An ISO standard sets reproducible conditions for measurement and prevention.[26] There is a separate ISO draft standard that addresses sound and vibration coming from rail systems.[27] As is the case for segmental vibration, measurements proceed in three orthogonal directions; however, the planes are adapted to the trunk, rather than the hand and arm. Measurements include one longitudinal direction (buttocks to head, or az) and two transverse directions (chest to back, or ax; and right to left side, or ay). The

TABLE 14B-2

Sources of Whole-Body Vibration

Activity	Source
Warehousing and material handling	Forklifts
Construction	Cranes, power shovels, bulldozers, off-road trucks, and tractors
Farming	Tractors
Transportation	Metros, buses, trains, helicopters, and tractor-trailers
Buildings	Metro and rail vibration and ventilation systems

standard provides numerical limits for exposure to vibrations transmitted from solid surfaces to the human body in the frequency range of 1 to 80 Hz. This is a critical distinction, differentiating WBV from HAVS, for which ISO recommends frequency measurement through 1,200 Hz.[1]

Health Effects of WBV

The lower frequencies characteristic of WBV involve potential resonant frequencies affecting the musculosketal system. Parts of the human body have their own resonant frequencies and do not vibrate as a single mass. The resulting response to exposure is complex, as amplification or diminution of the vibratory input will be affected differentially by different parts of the body due to intrinsic resonant frequencies. The most effective exciting frequency for vertical vibration delivered to the feet or buttocks occurs at 4 and 8 Hz.[28,29] Vibratory frequencies between 2.5 and 5.0 Hz generate strong resonance in the vertebrae of the neck and lumbar region with amplification up to 240 percent. Between 4 and 6 Hz, resonance in the trunk may be doubled. Vibrations between 20 and 30 Hz set up the strongest resonance between the head and the shoulders, with amplification up to 350 percent. In a human body, this may create chronic stresses and sometimes even permanent damage to the affected organs or body parts.[30] Thus, principal health effects are expected and measured at frequencies that are below those of hand–arm exposure.

The ISO standard on WBV exposure is directed to three different areas of health effects: reduced comfort, fatigue-decreased proficiency, and exposure limits. Reduced comfort boundary is applicable where passenger comfort is of concern, such as on trains, subways, and buses. Fatigue-decreased proficiency boundary is applied to the situations where maintaining operator efficiency of a vehicle is of concern, where, for example, work demands include reading gauges and screens, performing fine manipulation, and maintaining cognitive function. Exposure limit applies to situations where worker health and safety may be compromised by chronic injuries to the back, neck, and internal organs.

Fatigue-decreased proficiency and exposure-related health effects are the outcomes of primary interest in occupational settings. The exposure limit is calculated by multiplying accelerations by 2. For an 8-hour work shift, rms acceleration of 0.315 m/s^2 is the upper boundary if fatigue-decreased

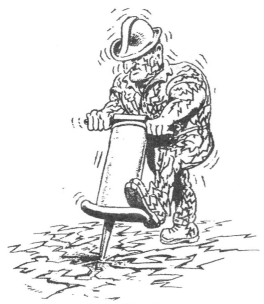

(Drawing by Nick Thorkelson.)

proficiency is the criterion and 0.63 m/s^2 if health effects determine an exposure limit. These limits are often exceeded under field conditions when earth-moving equipment is used.

Databases on WBV exposure from industrial vehicles are available online.[31] Profiles based on new equipment are misleading. Vehicle age and maintenance, the terrain, seat and cab design, and the presence of other vibrating equipment on the vehicle also determine the WBV magnitude of exposure in field settings. Exposure from WBV is not the only factor affecting equipment operators. Awkward sitting postures often required by drivers can adversely affect back health. Drivers must also resort to side and outside views and drive backwards, forcing twisted postures. Depending on shift and overtime schedules, drivers may work continuously for over 12 hours. Awkward postures, repetition, long duration, and/or forceful exertion are considered risk factors for the development of musculoskeletal disorders (see Chapters 11 and 23). In addition, poor ergonomic designs of cabs and seats as well as inaccessible control gear, such as pedals and steering wheels, will adversely affect workers. Cab and seat design modification most commonly address acceleration to the spine occurring in az axis. However, chest–back and side–side exposures are expected to produce more adverse effects at similar levels of exposures.

There appears to be an association between WBV and low-back pain but no established dose–response relationship.[32] The damaging effects from WBV on other organ systems are less clear. One study demonstrated reduced gastric motility after exposure on a vibrating platform, but the magnitude of exposure (2 m/s^2) and the frequencies (10 to 40 Hz) were relatively high[33]; however, reduction occurred at lower levels of exposure after eating. The clinical significance is unclear. More serious concerns have been raised about fetal injury, based on exposures to pregnant animals.[34]

Vibration in Buildings

One of the most important concerns with WBV includes low-level exposure in buildings. Other human health effects are presumed to be subtle and largely psychological or psychophysical. The extent of the exposed population and the importance of cognitive acuity makes this an area for targeted investigation. Vibration in buildings can be constant, intermittent, or impulsive and can occur as typical vertical WBV from the floor, or more commonly as a composition of gross structural vibration and reaction. Resonance occurs at very low frequency in tall buildings (1 Hz), but wood-framed walls may resonate at 10 to 25 Hz and masonry at 50 Hz. Current ISO and ANSI standards set exposure limits well below the point where WBV is expected to produce fatigue or generate loss of proficiency; but in residential buildings, vibration often proves irritating just above the level of perception.

Prevention and Remediation

The control of WBV rests more on selection of the appropriate measurement standard and prophylactic design rather than on health surveillance or medical evaluation. For example, in transportation the use of absorbent or "air-ride" seats reflects a focused effort to reduce vertical vibration. However, more sophisticated designs that provide front–back attenuation, cab isolation, and vehicle suspension represent a more effective integrated approach. In the industrial environment, antishock mounting of machinery, remote manipulation, and vibration-isolated pulpits provide additional measures of protection. Independent of etiology, in construction and earth-moving, low-back pain can be alleviated by seat and cab design. Even if the origins and pathology of low-back pain remain unidentified, a work environment protected against WBV can reduce symptoms and preserve function.

REFERENCES

1. ISO: Mechanical vibration—Guidelines for the measurement and the assessment of human exposure to hand-transmitted vibration. Geneva: International Organization for Standardization (ISO). (Ref. No. ISO 5349-1986.)
2. ANSI: Guide for the measurement and evaluation of human exposure to vibration transmitted to the hand. New York: American National Standards Institute, 1986. (ANSI S3.34.)
3. ISO 5349-1. Mechanical vibration—Measurement and evalaution of human exposure to hand-transmitted vibration; Part 1: General Requirements. Geneva: International Organization for Standardization, 2001.
4. ISO: Mechanical vibration—Measurement and evaluation of human exposure to hand-transmitted vibration—Part 2: Practical guidance for measurement in the workplace. Geneva: International Organization for Standardization, 2001. (5349-2).
5. Hamilton A. A study of spastic anemia in the hands of stone cutters. Washington, DC: US Bureau of Labor Statistics, 1918. (236:Ind Accidents and Hyg Series 1918, No. 191:53–66.)
6. NIOSH. Criteria for a recommended standard "occupational exposure to hand-arm vibration 1989. (DHHS [NIOSH] Publication No. 89-106).
7. Gemne G, Pyykko I, Taylor W, et al. The Stockholm Workshop scale for the classification of cold-induced Raynaud's phenomenon in the hand-arm vibration syndrome. Scand J Work Environ Health 1987;13:275–8.
8. Koskimies K, Farkkila M, Pyykko I, et al. Carpal tunnel syndrome in vibration disease. Br J Ind Med 1990;47:411–6.
9. Koskimies K. Hand grip force among forest workers. J Low Freq Noise Vib 1993;12:1–7.
10. Gemne G, ed. Stockholm Workshop 1986. Symptomatology and diagnostic methods in the hand-arm vibration syndrome. Scand J Work Environ Health 1987;13S:265–388.
11. Koskimies K, Pyykko I, Starck J, et al. Vibration syndrome among Finnish forest workers between 1972 and 1990. Int Arch Occup Environ Health 1992;64:251–6.
12. Letz R, Cherniack M, Gerr F, et al. A cross-sectional epidemiologic survey of shipyard workers exposed to hand-arm vibration. Br J Ind Med 1993;49:53–62.
13. Griffin M. Measurement, evaluation, and assessment of occupational exposures to hand-transmitted vibration. Occup Environ Med 1997:S4:73–89.
14. Starck J. High impulse acceleration levels in hand-held vibratory tools. Scand J Work Environ Health 1984;10:171–8.
15. Dandanell R, Engstrom K. Vibration from riveting tools in the frequency range 6 Hz to 10 MHz and Raynaud's phenomenon. Scand J Work Environ Health 1986;12:38–42.
16. Sakakibara H, Hirata M, Hashiguchi T, et al. Affected segments of the median nerve detected by fractionated nerve conduction measurement in vibration-induced neuropathy. Indus Health 1998;36:155–9.
17. Cherniack M, Brammer AJ, Lundstrom R, et al. Segmental nerve conduction velocity in vibration exposed shipyard workers. Int Arch Occup Environ Health 2004; 77:159–76.
18. Brammer AJ, Piercy JE, Nohara S, et al. Vibrotactile thresholds in operators of vibrating hand-held tools. In: Okada A, Taylor W, Dupuis H, eds. Hand-arm vibration. Japan: Kyoei Press, 1990;221–3.
19. Hyvarinen J, Pyykko I, Sundberg S. Vibration frequencies and amplitudes in the aetiology of traumatic vasospastic diseases. Lancet 1973;i:791–4.
20. Maricq HR, Diat F, Weinrich MC, et al. Digital pressure responses to cooling in patients with suspected early vs definite scleroderma (systemic sclerosis) vs primary Raynaud's phenomenon. J Rheumatol (Canada) 1994;21:1472–6.
21. Olsen N. In: Gemne G, Brammer AJ, Hagberg M, et al., eds. Hand-Arm Vibration Syndrome. Diagnostics and Quantitative Relationships to Exposure. Finger systolic blood pressure during cooling in VWF; value of different diagnostic categories for a routine test method. pp 65–69. Stockholm Workshop '94. Stockholm, Arbete och Hälsa 1995:05
22. Takeuchi T, Imanishi H. Histopathologic observations in finger biopsy from thirty patients with Raynaud's phenomenon of occupational origin. J Kumamoto Med Soc 1984;58:56–70.
23. Gemne G. Pathophysiology and pathogenesis of disorders in workers using hand-held vibrating tools. In: Pelmear P, Taylor W, Wasserman D, eds. Hand-arm vibration. New York: Van Nostrand Reinhold, 1992;41–76.
24. Allen JA, Doherty CC, McGrann S. Objective testing for vasospasm in the hand-arm vibration syndrome. Br J Indus Med 1992;49:688–93.
25. Cherniack M, Brammer AJ, Meyer J, et al. Skin temperature recovery from cold provocation in workers exposed to vibration: A longitudinal study. Occup Environ Med 2003;60:962–8.
26. ISO 2631: Evaluation of human exposure to whole body vibration. International Organization for Standardization. Geneva, 1985. (Ref. No. ISO 2631/1-1985.)
27. ISO 14837: Mechanical Criteria Ground-borne Noise and Vibration Coming from Rail Systems. Geneva: ISO, 2004. (ISO/PWI 14837/1-3.)
28. Boshuizen HC, Bongers PM, Hulshof CT. Back disorders and occupational exposure to whole body vibration. Int J Ind Ergon 1990;6:55–9.
29. Wilder DG. The biomechanics of vibration and low back pain. Am J Ind Med 1993;23:577–88.
30. ANSI S3.18.1979–99 ACGIH standard for whole-body vibration (1996–99). New York: American National Standards Institute.
31. WBV/HOME.html. Centralized European database for whole-body vibration. 2004. Available at: <umetech. niwl.se/vibration/WBV/Home.htm>.
32. Lings S, Leboeuf-Yde S. Whole-body vibration and low back pain: A systematic critical review of the epidemiological literature 1992–1999. Int Arch Occup Environ Health 1999;73:290–7.
33. Miyazaki Y. Adverse effects of whole-body vibration on gastric motility. Kurume Med J 2000;47:79–86.
34. Peters A, Abrams R, Gearhardt K, et al. Acceleration of the fetal head induced by vibration of the maternal abdominal wall in sleep. Am J Ob Gyn 1996;174:552–6.

BIBLIOGRAPHY

ISO 5349-1. Mechanical vibration—measurement and evalaution of human exposure to hand-transmitted vibration—General requirements. Geneva: International Organization for Standardization, 2001.

ISO: Mechanical vibration—Measurement and evaluation of human exposure to hand-transmitted vibration—Part 2: Practical guidance for measurement in the workplace. Geneva: International Organization for Standardization, 2001. (5349-2.)
These two recent publications on hand–arm vibration from the International Standards Organization (ISO) are essential documents, reflecting international consensus among investigators on the nature of morbidity and exposure–response prediction and on the appropriate methods of measurement. There are extensive references.
Koskimies K, Pyykko I, Starck J, et al. Vibration syndrome among Finnish forest workers between 1972 and 1990. Int Arch Occup Environ Health 1992;64:251–6.
This is a useful summary of the Suomussalmi forest worker prospective study, which is a landmark epidemiological investigation.
ISO: Evaluation of human exposure to whole body vibration. Geneva: International Organization for Standardization, 1985. (Ref. No. ISO 2631/1.)
This is a standard publication on the measurement of whole-body vibration.
Wilkstrom B, Kjellberg A, Landstrom U. Health effects of long-term occupational exposure to whole-body vibration: A review. Int J Ind Ergon 14:273–92.
This article is a thorough review of the literature on chronic health effects from whole-body vibration.

APPENDIX

DEFINITIONS

Acceleration: Time rate of change in velocity (expressed as m/s^2 or as gravity, g); the second derivative of displacement with respect to time. Force from vibratory tools is usually expressed in terms of accleration.

Frequency: Number of oscillations per unit of time; 1 hertz (Hz) = 1 cycle/s. Oscillatory vibration is defined as ≥ 125 Hz.

Mechanoreceptor: A sensory nerve organelle that records dimensions of touch, including gap, texture, and movement. The three best-known mechanoreceptors are the SAI (Merkel disk), FAI (Meissner corpuscle), and FAII (Pacinian corpuscle).

Raynaud's phenomenon: A sometimes painful condition, affecting the fingers or toes, that is due to compromised circulation and is provoked by the cold. It causes the digits to turn white because of lack of blood supply. It is commonly divided into an idiopathic, or primary, condition and secondary Raynaud's phenomenon. The responses associated with vibratory exposure—occupational Raynaud's phenomenon or vibration white finger (VWF) disorder—belong to the category of secondary Raynaud's phenomenon.

Root mean square (rms): The square root of the arithmetic mean of the squares of a series of numbers. rms is a traditional way of reporting multifrequency magnitudes, such as tool acceleration.

Weighted curves: The progressive filtering, or downweighting, of accelerations as they exceed 16 Hz, commonly expressed as a_w. Vibration is usually reported as a weighted (filtered) or unweighted acceleration.

Extremes of Temperature

Ann M. Krake

This section of the chapter deals with extremes of temperature and their adverse health effects. Box 14C-1 deals with physical hazards related to hyperbaric and hypobaric environments and their adverse health effects.

HOT ENVIRONMENTS

Environmental Heat Stress and Strain

An 86-year-old woman is found unresponsive in her bedroom. She has no known medical history, but her grandson reports that she kept her bedroom windows closed for the week during a heat wave and had no fan or air conditioning. A rectal temperature taken at the hospital is 42.2°C (108°F). Heat stroke is listed as the primary cause of her death.

A 43-year-old man hikes down a trail in the Grand Canyon National Park during the hottest part of the day. He is carrying water but has brought nothing to eat. He is found later that evening by park rangers wandering around the campground "in a state of shock." His pulse is approximately 100 beats per minute and his oral temperature is 39.2°C (102.6°F). He is treated for hyponatremia (decreased serum sodium) with intravenous fluids, kept under observation overnight, and medically evacuated the following morning. He later reports the following: When told by hikers coming up the trail there was no water or shade along the 7-mile route, he decided to continue even more quickly to his destination, the campground at Phantom Ranch; he noticed that

although he was drinking and urinating frequently, his urine became clearer the farther he hiked; and when asked why he did not try to cool off by getting into the creek running alongside the campground, he told the rangers he did not think to do that and hardly noticed it was there.

From 1979 through 1999, there were 8,015 deaths attributed to exposure to excessive heat in the United States. Almost half (48 percent) were "due to weather conditions," 5 percent were "of man-made origins" (such as heat generated in vehicles, kitchens, boiler and furnace rooms, and factories), and the rest were of "unspecified origin."[1]

During a typical year in the United States, heat waves, which have been defined as consecutive days of air temperatures 90°F (32.2°C) or greater,[1] kill more people than all other natural disasters combined.[2] During the 1990s, two heat waves struck the city of Chicago, killing more than 1,000 people. Hundreds of people also died throughout Europe during the summer of 2003, with the early onset of hot weather, unusually high temperatures, and prolonged heat-stress conditions. Advanced age and the inability to care for oneself are found to be major contributing factors for heat-related deaths. In Rome, the greatest mortality increases were seen in people aged 65 years or older and living in the most economically disadvantaged areas of the city. Other factors that may have had an impact on health include poor-quality housing, lack of air conditioning, lack of access to social services and health care, and behaviors such as drinking alcohol and taking medication.[3]

BOX 14C-1

Physical Hazards Related to Hyperbaric and Hypobaric Environments and Their Adverse Health Effects

John Halpin

The physiology of the human body is well suited and well adapted to functioning at an atmospheric pressure equal to 760 mm Hg. This pressure has been designated as a standard reference point of 1 Atmosphere Absolute (1 ATA). Above or below this pressure (under hyperbaric or hypobaric conditions), the body is subject to various physical hazards due to the change in pressure or as a direct result of high or low pressure.

Hyperbaric environments are most commonly encountered in a diving setting but include any situation in which compressed air is required, including caisson operations, underwater tunneling, and tending patients in a hyperbaric chamber. The most common health problem occurring in hyperbaric environments is known as *barotrauma*, which involves an imbalance in pressure of air cavities and sinuses within the body as they are subjected to an acute change in pressure. A classic example is middle ear barotrauma, in which a pressure imbalance develops between the middle ear and the external ear canal causing tympanic membrane trauma and acute ear pain. A related but much more serious form of barotrauma is known as *pulmonary overinflation syndrome*, in which the lungs become overinflated due to expansion of the air within them during ascent. This overinflation can reach a breaking point at which alveolar capillaries rupture, leading to pneumothorax, mediastinal emphysema, and arterial gas embolism. Arterial gas embolism, resulting from the introduction of compressed air into the arterial bloodstream, has various neurologic manifestations, including confusion, weakness resembling a stroke, or loss of consciousness.

While functioning in hyperbaric conditions, the lungs absorb increased amounts of nitrogen into the bloodstream in the form of a dissolved gas. When ambient pressure is reduced rapidly upon ascent, nitrogen can reform into gas bubbles in the blood and lead to impaired circulation. The resulting array of clinical symptoms is commonly known as *decompression sickness* (DCS). Pain alone, typically in the joints and muscles, is a mild form of DCS that often occurs about 4 to 6 hours after ascent from depth, and is known as type I DCS. Involvement of the neurologic and cardiopulmonary systems represents a more serious form, type II DCS. It can manifest as paralysis, severe cough, and severe shortness of breath, and may be fatal. It requires immediate oxygen therapy and recompression in a hyperbaric chamber.

Two other disorders related to hyperbaric environments occur as a direct result of the increased partial pressure of gas at depth: nitrogen narcosis and oxygen toxicity. At increased partial pressures, nitrogen can exert a narcotic effect—similar to the effects of alcohol intoxication, which increases as depth increases. Even at 1 ATA, but especially under increased partial pressure at depth, oxygen can become neurotoxic, manifest by paresthesias, tinnitus, visual changes, confusion, nausea, vertigo, and sometimes seizures. Preventive measures in hyperbaric environments include managing time spent at depth and carefully controlling the rate of descent and ascent. More specific recommendations can be found by referring to dive tables and instructions at the Divers Alert Network (<www.diversalertnetwork.org>) and the National Association of Underwater Instructors (NAUI) (<www.naui.org>).

Hypobaric environments are commonly encountered by those in high-altitude mountain settings as well as pilots and passengers in unpressurized aircraft. At altitudes greater than 2,500 m (about 8,000 ft) the partial pressure of oxygen becomes significantly reduced, and altitude-related illness can begin to occur, especially in those who have not acclimatized because of ascending too rapidly. The most common form of altitude illness, known as *acute mountain sickness* (AMS), is characterized by headache, nausea, vomiting, fatigue, and loss of appetite. It is thought to occur due to an imbalance between hypoxic-induced cerebral vasodilation and hypocarbia-induced cerebral vasoconstriction. It is best treated with administration of oxygen while lowering the victim to an altitude where symptoms resolve, and can be prevented by use of acetazolamide and dexamethasone.

(continued)

BOX 14C-1

Physical Hazards Related to Hyperbaric and Hypobaric Environments and Their Adverse Health Effects (Continued)

A more serious manifestation of altitude illness affects the lungs: *high-altitude pulmonary edema* (HAPE). It is believed to occur as a result of hypoxic-induced vasoconstriction and pulmonary capillary leakage. Onset is usually insidious and occurs within 24 to 60 hours of arrival at high altitude, with initial symptoms including shortness of breath, cough, weakness, tachycardia, and headache, which may progress to cough productive of bloody sputum, low-grade fever, and pulmonary congestion. If untreated, coma may ensue as a result of the most serious manifestation of

altitude illness: *high-altitude cerebral edema* (HACE). Prior to onset of coma, the development of cerebral edema may be suspected by symptoms of severe headache, confusion, ataxia, or hallucinations. As with acute mountain sickness, descent with administration of oxygen is the best form of treatment for both HAPE and HACE, although symptoms may also respond to the use of dexamethasone. Preventive measures for hypobaric environments include proper acclimatization, along with an understanding and recognition of symptoms that indicate that descent is warranted. More specific recommendations can be obtained by contacting the International Society for Mountain Medicine at <www.ismmed.org>.

During heat waves, the following measures are recommended:

- Make frequent (daily) checks on homebound neighbors, friends, and relatives, especially if they are elderly or disabled.
- Never leave children or pets alone in a car, even with the windows "cracked" and even on seemingly cool or cloudy days.
- Encourage those without air-conditioned homes to seek out cool places, such as shopping malls and theaters, during the hottest parts of the day.
- Encourage the drinking of nonalcoholic and noncaffeinated beverages.
- Reduce or eliminate strenuous activities during a heat wave.

Occupational Heat Stress and Strain

There are an estimated 5 to 10 million workers in industries where heat stress is a potential safety and health hazard (Fig. 14C-1).[4] In all industries from 1992 to 2002, exposure to environmental heat killed 291 workers, and contact with hot objects or substances killed an additional 141 workers.[5] On average, approximately 400 people die each year in the United States from exposure to excessive heat in work, home, and community settings.[6]

Heat-related occupational illness, injuries, and strain occur in any situation where total heat load (environmental heat plus heat generated by the body's metabolism) exceeds the capacity of the

body to maintain normal bodily functions. Situations that have increased potential for causing heat strain include high ambient air temperatures, radiant heat sources (such as the Sun, ovens, and foundry furnaces), direct physical contact with hot objects, high humidity, and strenuous physical activity. A hot, humid environment, which impedes evaporative cooling, combined with heavy work activity, poses the highest risk for workers because the metabolic load placed on the body generates even more heat; however, work in cooler, less strenuous environments can also pose a risk, depending on an individual's heat-tolerance capabilities.

Total heat stress is defined by the National Institute for Occupational Safety and Health (NIOSH) as the sum of the heat generated by the body (metabolic), plus the heat gained from the environment, minus the heat lost from the body to the environment (primarily through evaporation). Heat strain is defined as the body's response to the heat stress it experiences. Many bodily responses to heat stress are desirable and beneficial because they help regulate internal temperature and, in situations of appropriate repeated exposure, help the body adapt (acclimate) to the work environment. However, at some individually determined stage of heat stress, the body's compensatory measures cannot maintain internal body temperature at the level required for normal functioning. As a result, the risk of heat-induced illnesses, disorders, and accidents substantially increases.[4]

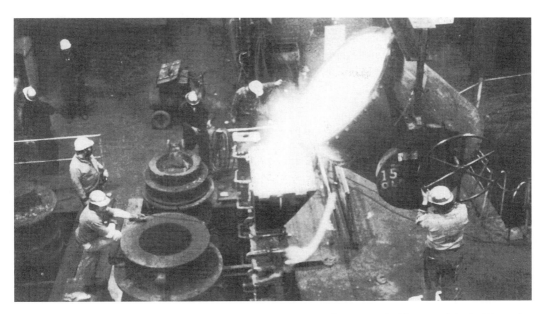

FIGURE 14C-1 ● Foundry workers with exposure to excessive heat at work. (Photograph by Earl Dotter.)

An essential requirement for continued normal body function is that deep core body temperature be maintained within the acceptable range of approximately 98.6°F (37°C) ± 1.8°F (1°C). Achieving this equilibrium requires a constant exchange of heat between the body and the environment. The amount of heat to be exchanged is a function of the total heat produced by the body (metabolic heat) and the heat gained from the work environment. The rate of heat exchanged with both hot and cold environments is a function of air temperature, humidity, skin temperature, air velocity, evaporation of sweat, radiant temperature, and type, amount, and characteristics of clothing.[4] The basic heat balance equation, which can also be used to evaluate situations of extreme cold, is

$$S = (M - W) \pm C \pm R - E$$

where S is change in body heat (either lost or gained by the body), (M – W) is heat produced by metabolism minus heat produced by external work, C is convective and conductive heat exchange, R is radiative heat exchange, and E is body heat lost by evaporation.

Each of the terms in the equation represents a rate of energy transfer—positive values for any of the variables signify that the body is gaining heat in that manner, whereas negative values indicate a loss of heat. When the body is not thermally challenged, as in homeostasis, there will be no net gain or loss of heat, and S will equal zero. An S greater than zero indicates a heat imbalance that may lead to heat strain and subsequent heat-related illnesses. The quantity $(M - W)$ describes total body heat produced by combining the metabolic heat gained from the work effort minus the heat lost due to the external work effort. The metabolic heat value, M, is a combination of the energy expended in doing the work and the energy transformed into heat,[4] which must be removed rapidly from the muscles. When muscle workload is high, so is the body's heat production. A high workload can cause heat gain even when environmental temperatures feel cool to those conducting less strenuous activities. Therefore, it is extremely important to consider the metabolic rate when evaluating the heat stress of those performing physically demanding work.[7] W represents the amount of energy that is successfully converted from chemical energy to mechanical work, which is usually only about 10 percent of M. Therefore, because W is small relative to the other routes of heat exchange, this value is usually ignored.[7]

The major modes of heat exchange between workers and their environment are convection, radiation, and evaporation. Convection refers to the rate of heat exchange between the individual's skin and the air immediately around the skin, assuming the air is moving. Its value is a function of the difference between the skin and air temperatures and the rate of air movement over the skin. Skin temperature is normally assumed to be 95°F (35°C). Therefore, for a worker wearing a single layer of clothing (long-sleeved work shirt and trousers), an ambient air temperature of greater than 95°F will cause the body to gain heat from the air, whereas an ambient air temperature of less than 95°F will cause the body to lose heat into the air, all by convection. Conduction, which is the transfer of heat to the skin from direct contact (touch) with hot equipment or floors or from hot liquids, plays a minor role in heat stress other than for brief periods of time when the body may come into contact with such objects. Radiative heat exchange also refers to heat that is transferred between the skin and solid surfaces or objects, cold or hot, but without direct skin contact. Working in direct sunlight is one example of radiative heat exposure. Evaporation of water from the surface of the skin (sweating) is the body's primary method of regulating internal body temperature. Evaporative cooling also occurs from the lungs, but with the exception of hard work in very dry environments, its contribution to overall heat reduction is minor.[4] The evaporative capacity of the body is a function of ambient air velocity and the water vapor pressure difference between the ambient air and the wetted skin at skin temperature, which is assumed to be 95°F. To solve the equation, measurement of metabolic heat produced, air temperature, air water-vapor pressure, wind velocity, and mean radiant temperature are required.[4]

Health Effects of Exposure to Hot Environments

The level of heat stress at which excessive heat strain will result is highly individual and depends on the heat-tolerance capabilities of each individual. Age, weight, degree of physical fitness, degree of acclimatization, metabolism, use of alcohol or drugs, and a variety of medical conditions, such as hypertension and diabetes, all affect a person's sensitivity to heat. At greatest risk are unacclimatized workers, people performing physically strenuous work, those with previous heat illness, older people, people with cardiovascular or circulatory disorders (diabetes, atherosclerotic vascular disease), those taking medications that impair the body's cooling mechanisms, people who abuse alcohol or are recovering from recent use, people in poor physical condition, and those recovering from illness. A core body temperature increase of only 1.8°F above normal encroaches on the brain's ability to function.[8]

Heat disorders and health effects of individuals exposed to hot working environments include (in increasing order of severity) irritability, lack of judgment and loss of critical thinking skills, skin disorders (such as heat rashes and hives), heat syncope (fainting), heat cramps, heat exhaustion, and heat stroke. Heat syncope (fainting) results from blood flow being directed to the skin for cooling, resulting in decreased supply to the brain, and most often strikes workers who stand in place for extended periods in hot environments. Heat cramps, caused by sodium depletion due to sweating, typically occur in the muscles employed in strenuous work. Heat cramps and syncope often accompany heat exhaustion, or weakness, fatigue, confusion, nausea, and other symptoms that generally prevent a return to work for at least 24 hours. The dehydration, sodium loss, and elevated core body temperature (CBT) above 100.4°F of heat exhaustion are usually due to individuals performing strenuous work in hot conditions with inadequate water and electrolyte intake. Heat exhaustion may lead to heat stroke if the patient is not quickly cooled and rehydrated.

Whereas heat exhaustion victims continue to sweat as their bodies struggle to stay cool, heat stroke victims cease to sweat as their bodies fail to maintain an appropriate core temperature. Heat stroke occurs when hard work, hot environment, and dehydration overload the body's capacity to cool itself. This thermal regulatory failure is a life-threatening emergency requiring immediate medical attention. Signs and symptoms include irritability, confusion, nausea, convulsions or unconsciousness, hot dry skin, and a CBT above 106°F. Death can result from damage to the brain, heart, liver, or kidneys.[7]

Prolonged increase in CBT and chronic exposures to high levels of heat stress are associated with disorders such as temporary infertility (male and female), elevated heart rate, sleep disturbance, fatigue, and irritability. During the first trimester of pregnancy, a sustained CBT greater than 102.2°F may endanger the fetus. In addition, one or more occurrences of heat-induced illness predisposes a person to subsequent injuries and can result in temporary or permanent loss of their ability to tolerate heat stress.[4,9]

Acclimatization

Acclimatization is a low-cost, highly effective way to improve the safety and comfort of employees in heat-stress situations.[7] Acclimatization allows the employee to withstand heat stress with a reduction in heat strain by a series of physiological adaptations. Acclimatized individuals are able to perspire more abundantly and more uniformly over their body surface and they also start to sweat earlier than nonacclimatized individuals, resulting in lower heat storage (lower CBT) and lower cardiovascular strain (lower heart rate). In addition, acclimatized individuals lose less salt through sweating and are therefore able to withstand greater water loss.[10]

Working at even a moderate rate in a heat-stress situation brings about physiological changes that substantially improve comfort and safety for those who are in general good health. Exposure to heat only, however, will not bring about acclimatization—an elevated metabolic rate, such as happens during work activities, is required. The ability of a worker to tolerate heat stress requires integrity of cardiac, pulmonary, and renal function, the sweating mechanism, the body's fluid and electrolyte balances, and the central nervous system's heat-regulatory mechanism. Impairment or diminution of any of these functions may interfere with the worker's capacity to acclimatize to the heat or to perform strenuous work in the heat once acclimatized.[4] Acclimatization at a certain temperature is effective only at that temperature—a person exposed to higher levels of heat stress will not be fully acclimatized at that level, only to the lower

one.[7] Empirical data suggest that fewer than 5 percent of workers cannot adequately acclimatize to heat stress.[4]

There are three phases of heat acclimatization. Initially, consecutive exposures to heat in the first few days, with the requisite rise in metabolic rate for 2 hours (such as doing work or exercising), cause the body to reach 33 percent of optimum acclimatization by the fourth day of exposure. The intermediate phase is marked by cardiovascular stability, and surface and internal body temperatures are lower, reaching 44 percent of optimum by day 8. During the third phase, a decrease in sweat and urine osmolality and other compensations to conserve body fluids and restore electrolyte balances are seen, and 65 percent of optimum is reached by day 10, 93 percent by day 18, and 99 percent by day 21.[7] Figure 14C-2 describes a typical acclimatization schedule for employees working a 10-hour shift.

Although heat acclimatization for most individuals begins early in a period of working in the heat, it is also quickly lost if the exposure is discontinued. The loss of acclimatization begins when the activity under those heat-stress conditions is discontinued, with a noticeable loss occurring after only 4 days. This loss is usually rapidly made up so that by Tuesday, workers who were off on the weekend are as well acclimatized as they were on

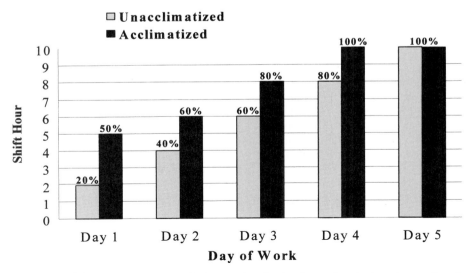

FIGURE 14C-2 ● Work schedule for heat acclimatized and unacclimatized employees. (Based on a 10-hour shift.) (Adapted from: NIOSH. Criteria for a recommended standard: Occupational exposure to hot environments, rev. Cincinnati, OH: U.S. Public Health Service, Centers for Disease Control and Prevention, National Institute for Occupational Safety and Health, 1986, p. 69. [DHHS publication no. [NIOSH] 86–113.])

the preceding Friday. However, if there is no exposure for 1 to 2 weeks, full acclimatization can require up to 3 weeks of continued physical activity under heat-stress conditions similar to those anticipated for the work.[7] Chronic illness, the use or misuse of pharmacologic agents, a sleep deficit, a suboptimal nutritional state, or a disturbed water and electrolyte balance may reduce the worker's capacity to acclimatize. In addition, an acute episode of mild illness, especially if it entails fever, vomiting, respiratory impairment, or diarrhea, may cause abrupt transient loss of acclimatization.[4]

Evaluating and Assessing Heat Stress

Assessing heat stress in workers involves measuring environmental temperatures at the work location and assessing metabolic work rates for each task. The wet-bulb globe temperature (WBGT) index, most commonly used to assess the environmental contribution to heat stress, accounts for the combined effects of air movement, temperature, humidity, and radiative heat.[4] The WBGT index gives an idea as to how the worker feels or perceives the work environment and is a function of dry-bulb (ambient air) temperature, natural wet-bulb temperature (simulates the effect of evaporative cooling), and a black-globe temperature, which estimates radiant (infrared) heat load. Individual and task metabolic rates can be estimated using the NIOSH table, "Estimated metabolic heat production rates by task analysis," in the NIOSH document, *Occupational Exposure to Hot Environments*, or by using the work rate categories of the American Conference of Governmental Industrial Hygienists (ACGIH).[11]

Many heat-stress guidelines have been developed to protect people against heat-related illnesses. The objective of any heat stress index is to prevent a person's CBT from rising excessively. The World Health Organization concluded that "it is inadvisable for CBT to exceed 38°C (100.4°F) or for oral temperature to exceed 37.5°C (99.5°F) in prolonged daily exposure to heavy work and/or heat."[8] According to NIOSH, a core body temperature of 39°C (102.2°F) should be considered reason to terminate exposure even when core body temperature is being monitored. This does not mean that a worker with a CBT exceeding those levels will necessarily experience adverse health effects; however, the number of unsafe acts committed by workers increases as

does the risk of the occurrence of illness from heat stress.

Currently, the Occupational Safety and Health Administration (OSHA) does not have a specific heat stress standard; however, acceptable exposure to heat stress is enforced by the U.S. Secretary of Labor under the General Duty Clause [Section 5(a)(1)]. The OSHA technical manual (Section III, Chapter 4: Heat Stress) provides investigation guidelines that approximate those found in the 1992–1993 ACGIH publication, *Threshold Limit Values (TLVs) for Chemical Substances and Physical Agents and Biological Exposure Indices*. NIOSH recommends that total heat exposure be controlled so that unprotected healthy workers who are medically and physically fit for their required level of activity and are wearing, at most, long-sleeved work shirts and trousers or equivalent, are not exposed to metabolic and environmental heat combinations exceeding the applicable NIOSH criteria, as follows: Almost all healthy employees, working in hot environments and exposed to combinations of environmental and metabolic heat less than the NIOSH recommended action limits (RALs) for nonacclimatized workers or the NIOSH recommended exposure limits (RELs) for acclimatized workers, should be able to tolerate total heat stress without substantially increasing their risk of incurring acute adverse health effects. And, no employee shall be exposed to metabolic and environmental heat combinations exceeding the applicable ceiling limits (C) of the RELs and RALs without being provided with and properly using appropriate and adequate heat-protective clothing and equipment.[4]

ACGIH guidelines require the use of a decision-making process that provides step-by-step situation-dependent instructions that factor in clothing insulation values and physiological evaluation of heat strain (Fig. 14C-3). ACGIH WBGT screening criteria (Table 14C-1) factor in the ability of the body to cool itself (considering clothing insulation value, humidity, and wind), and, like the NIOSH criteria, can be used to develop work/rest regimens for acclimatized and unacclimatized employees. The ACGIH WBGT-based heat exposure assessment was developed for a traditional work uniform of long-sleeved shirt and pants and represents conditions under which it is believed that nearly all adequately hydrated, unmedicated, healthy workers may be repeatedly exposed without adverse health effects. Clothing insulation values and the

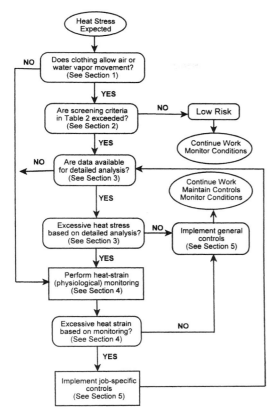

FIGURE 14C-3 ● Evaluation scheme for heat stress. (From American Conference of Governmental Industrial Hygienists [ACGIH]. 2004 TLVs and BEIs: Based on the documentation of the threshold limit values for chemical substances and physical agents & biological indices. Cincinnati, OH: ACGIH, 2004, p. 168. Reprinted with permission.)

appropriate WBGT adjustments, as well as descriptors of the other decision-making process components can be found in ACGIH's *Threshold Limit Values for Chemical Substances and Physical Agents and Biological Exposure Indices*. The ACGIH TLV for heat stress attempts to provide a framework for the control of heat-related disorders only. Although accidents and injuries can increase with increasing levels of heat stress, the TLVs are not directed toward controlling these.

NIOSH and ACGIH criteria can only be used when WBGT data for the immediate work area are available and must not be used when encapsulating suits or garments that are impermeable or highly resistant to water vapor or air movement are worn. Further assumptions regarding work demands include an 8-hour work day, 5-day work week, two 15-minute breaks, and a 30-minute lunch break,

with rest area temperatures the same as, or less than, those in work areas, and "at least some air movement." NIOSH and ACGIH guidelines do not establish a fine line between safe and dangerous levels but require professional judgment and a heat-stress management program to ensure protection in each situation.

Evaluating and Assessing Heat Strain

Physiological monitoring for heat strain becomes necessary when impermeable clothing is worn, when heat stress screening criteria are exceeded, or when data from a detailed analysis, such as the ISO required sweat rate (SRreq), shows excess heat stress.[11]

One indicator of physiological strain, sustained peak heart rate, is considered by ACGIH to be the best sign of acute, high-level exposure to heat stress. Sustained peak heart rate, defined by ACGIH as 180 beats per minute (bpm) minus an individual's age, is a leading indicator that thermal regulatory control may not be adequate and that an increase in core temperature has, or will soon, occur. Sustained peak heart rate represents an equivalent cardiovascular demand of about 75 percent of maximum aerobic capacity. During an 8-hour work shift, even if sustained peak demands do not occur, there may still be excessive demand placed on the cardiovascular system. These "chronic" demands can be measured by calculating the average heart rate over the shift. Decreases in physical job performance have been observed when the average heart rate exceeds 115 bpm over the entire shift. This level is equivalent to working at roughly 35 percent of maximum aerobic capacity, a level sustainable for 8 hours.

According to ACGIH, an individual's heat-stress exposure should be discontinued when any of the following excessive heat-strain indicators occur: Sustained (over several minutes) heart rate is in excess of 180 bpm minus the individual's age in years, for those with normal cardiac performance; core body temperature is greater than 38.0°C (100.4°F) for unselected, unacclimatized personnel and greater than 38.5°C (101.3°F) for medically fit, heat-acclimatized personnel; recovery heart rate at 1 minute after a peak work effort exceeds 110 bpm; or there are symptoms of sudden and severe fatigue, nausea, dizziness, or lightheadedness. An individual may be at greater risk of heat strain if: (a) profuse sweating is sustained over

TABLE 14C-1

Screening Criteria for Heat-Stress Exposure (WBGT Values in °C)

Work Demands	Acclimatized				Unacclimatized			
	Light	Moderate	Heavy	Very Heavy	Light	Moderate	Heavy	Very Heavy
100% Work	29.5	27.5	26		27.5	25	22.5	
75% Work, 25% rest	30.5	28.5	27.5		29	26.5	24.5	
50% Work, 50% rest	31.5	29.5	28.5	27.5	30	28	26.5	25
25% Work, 75% rest	32.5	31	30	29.5	31	29	28	26.5

Wet-bulb globe temperature (WGBT) values are expressed in °C and represent thresholds near the upper limit of the metabolic rate category.
If work and rest environments are different, hourly time-weighted averages (TWAs) should be calculated and used. TWAs for work rates
  should also be used when the work demands vary within the hour.
Values in this table are applied by reference to the "Work-Rest Regimen" section of the *Documentation* and assume 8-hour workdays in a
  5-day work week with conventional breaks, as discussed in the *Documentation* (see reference 7). When workdays are extended, consult
  the "Application of the TLV" section of the *Documentation*.
Because of the physiological strain associated with very heavy work among less fit workers regardless of WBGT, criteria values are not
  provided for continuous work and for up to 25 percent rest in an hour. The screening criteria are not recommended, and a detailed analysis
  and/or physiological monitoring should be used.
From American Conference of Governmental Industrial Hygienists (ACGIH). 2004 TLVs and BEIs: Based on the documentation of the
  threshold limit values for chemical substances and physical agents & biological indices. Cincinnati, OH: ACGIH, 2004, p. 171. Reprinted
  with permission.

several hours; (b) weight loss over a shift is greater than 1.5 percent of body weight; or (c) 24-hour urinary sodium excretion is less than 55 millimoles.

There is a variety of equipment available for monitoring heat strain in an individual. One of the simplest devices is a standard body-weight scale. Employees should weigh themselves fully clothed, without equipment belts, just prior to starting a shift and again, wearing the same clothing, just before the shift has ended. Weight loss over the shift (hydration status) can then be calculated by subtracting postshift weight from preshift weight and dividing that total by preshift weight. Multiplying by 100 gives percent body weight lost or gained. Weight loss should not exceed 1.5 percent of total body weight in a work day. If it does, fluid and food intake should be increased until a return to baseline is achieved. (The thirst mechanism is usually not strong enough to drive an individual to drink enough to replace the water lost in sweat; therefore, the palatability of fluid replacement is important to ensure adequate rehydration. Adding sweeteners to drinks has been shown to increase consumption, facilitate sodium and water absorption, and provide energy for muscular activity for vigorous activities. Ideally, about 5 oz of fluid at 50–60°F should be consumed every 15–20 minutes.)

Another simple and inexpensive method for monitoring heat strain is to use a heart rate monitor. Currently, two types are available. One consists of a wireless strap worn around the chest that sends a signal to a read-out display, usually worn on the wrist. The second type is also worn on the wrist and requires the user to place two fingers on the sensors. Heart rate is displayed after a few seconds. Measurements should be taken at appropriate intervals covering at least a full 2-hour period during the hottest parts of the day and again at the end of the day to ensure a return to baseline.[4]

There are also currently two methods of monitoring internal (core) body temperature. Both involve swallowing disposable sensors that send a signal to a data logger with direct read-out capabilities worn by the worker. One sensor incorporates a crystal that vibrates in direct proportion to the worker's CBT, whereas the other is a thermistor-based system. Both offer radio-frequency capabilities and can monitor CBT and heart rate in multiple workers in direct line of sight.

Prevention of heat stress and strain is still the best method of keeping workers safe. This can be accomplished a number of ways. Administratively, employers can evaluate ways to reduce the physical demands of the work and limit work for hot jobs to morning and evening hours. Employees should be allowed to acclimatize to a hot work environment, which may require additional staffing for the same job until all workers are acclimated. Employers should institute preplacement and periodic (medical surveillance) exams that include individual aerobic capacity testing and also assess mental and medical qualifications. Those with low heat tolerance and/or poor physical fitness should be excluded from hot jobs. Continuing education programs can provide employees with information regarding the hazards of heat stress, awareness of signs and symptoms in themselves and other employees, and the dangers of using drugs and alcohol while working in hot and physically demanding environments.

One of the most important administrative steps an employer or supervisor can take to prevent heat stress and strain is to allow employees to take breaks when they feel they need to, thereby self-limiting their exposure. Employees can also help themselves by ensuring they are well hydrated, nourished, and not sleep-deprived. Those working in hot, dry environments will also benefit from soaking their clothing with water before and during their shift to aid in evaporative cooling. Equipment such as ice vests and capillary cooling systems worn under air-and vapor-impermeable protective suits will help keep workers cooler during certain short-term, high-intensity tasks.

COLD ENVIRONMENTS

Workers' compensation claims for cold injury from the Bureau of Labor Statistics and the Industrial Commission of Ohio were found to be reflective of an expected association between environmental factors and reported cold injuries. The study results showed that both nationally and in Ohio, the highest injury rates occurred in the oil and gas industry; trucking and warehousing; protective services; interurban and local transportation; electric, gas, and sanitation; auto repair, service stations, and dealers; food and kindred products; and heavy construction.[12] Further analysis of the Ohio data showed that most of those injured were men under 35 years old, and that approximately 92 percent of the claims were for frostbite that resulted from "routine outdoor work."[13] There was a significant correlation of injuries with periods of extreme cold, and as wind speed increased, rate of injury increased. On a single day when wind speeds exceeded 32 kilometers per

hour (kph) (20 miles per hour [mph]), the rate of cold injury was 80 times higher than on days when average wind speeds ranged from 8 to 14.5 kph (5 to 9 mph).[12]

Cold stress–related occupational illnesses, injuries, and reduced productivity result from a net body heat loss (decrease in core body temperature [CBT]) or heat loss from parts of the body such as limbs, feet and hands, or the head. Hypothermia (abnormally low body temperature) causes approximately 700 deaths a year in the United States, half of which occur in people aged 65 and older.[14] Workers in agriculture, transportation, oil and gas extraction, construction, warehousing, food products, utilities industries, and specifically those who work outdoors, as open-water divers, and in cold storage, are at increased risk of cold-stress injuries. Heat loss occurs by radiation (up to 65 percent), conduction (up to 15 percent, but greater in cold water where body heat is lost up to 25 times faster), convection (as the wind increases), respiration, and evaporation, with the last two depending on the ambient temperature and relative humidity.[15] Conditions of low temperatures, high winds, and wet clothes or body pose the highest risk of developing cold stress injuries and illnesses for workers. However, hypothermia can result even when air temperatures are above freezing and when water temperature is below normal body temperature, 98.6°F (37°C).

The CBT of a worker must remain within 1 to 4 percent of normal body temperature (no lower than 36°C [96.8°F]). This is the temperature at which the body's metabolic rate increases in an attempt to compensate for heat loss and is just slightly above the point at which maximum shivering begins. For single, occupational exposures, a drop in CBT to no lower than 35°C (95°F) is permissible under the ACGIH guidelines.[16] However, core body temperature is maintained at the expense of other parts of the body as peripheral blood flow decreases to reduce heat lost from the skin's surface, so extra care must be taken to protect the extremities from discomfort and damage.

Health Effects of Exposure to Cold Environments

Exposure to a cold environment causes intense stimulation of the sympathetic nervous system, which results in reduced heat loss through the skin (vasoconstriction), and pain and numbness of the fingers and toes may be felt. Cold injuries to peripheral body parts include both freezing and nonfreezing of the tissue. The most common nonfreezing injuries are chilblain (pernio) and immersion (trench) foot. With chilblain, neuronal and endothelial damage result, usually on the backs of the hands and the tops of the feet, from repetitive exposure to dry cold. Trench foot, which can progress to gangrene, is caused from repetitive exposure to a cold, wet environment above the freezing point, conditions that are common in the commercial fishing industry. Symptoms include tingling or itching, burning, swelling, and blisters in more extreme cases.[17] Frostbite occurs when the skin tissue itself falls below 0°C (32°F) and can happen when workers touch cold metal or chemicals or wear constrictive clothing or shoes. Frostbite is classified in degrees and can be superficial, causing some redness and numbness (first degree), or deep, affecting bone and muscle tissue (fourth degree).[14] Freezing in deeper layers of tissue causes the affected area to look waxy and pale and feel hard to the touch.

If exposure to the cold continues and CBT falls to around 36°C (96.8°F), metabolic rate, respiration, and pulse increase, and blood pressure is elevated in an attempt to maintain homeostatsis. At a CBT of 35°C (95°F), maximum shivering occurs, and physical work and mental processes are impaired. Workers should be removed from the environment when shivering, the most inefficient way of producing heat, becomes evident.[16] Severe hypothermia results if CBT falls below 33°C (91.4°F). Consciousness becomes clouded and progressively lost, respiration and pulse decrease, and blood pressure falls and becomes difficult to measure. The skin becomes cold and may turn bluish in color. When CBT reaches 28°C (82.4°F), loss of consciousness with little or no breathing may occur, and ventricular fibrillation is possible. Worker fatalities from exposure to cold have almost always resulted from failure to escape from low-air- or low-water-temperature environments.[16]

Workers at greatest risk of cold stress are the elderly, those with cardiovascular or circulatory disorders (diabetes, atherosclerotic vascular disease, hypothyroidism), and those taking medications that interfere with body temperature regulation or reduce tolerance to working in the cold. The danger of hypothermia is also increased in people who use alcohol and other central nervous system depressants. Workers routinely exposed to temperatures below −25°C (−11.2°F) at wind speeds less than 2 m/s (5 mph) or air temperatures below −18°C (0°F) at wind speeds less than 2 m/s (5 mph) should be medically qualified for work in such environments.[16]

Workers suffering from cold stress should be moved to a warm, dry area, and any wet or tight clothing should be removed. It is important to protect the affected body parts from further trauma, including not rubbing to rewarm the part, because rubbing causes damage to the affected tissue. Affected areas should be soaked in a warm water bath for approximately 25–40 minutes and then dried and wrapped. The skin may blister and appear puffy, and medical attention should always be sought as soon as possible even though normal movement, skin color, and feeling may have returned. In cases of hypothermia, give the worker warm, sweet, nonalcoholic, noncaffeinated drinks and high-calorie food if they are alert. If the worker can move, have them do so to warm up muscles. If they cannot move, place warm water bottles or packs in the armpits, groin, neck, and head areas. Keep the victim awake and provide medical attention as soon as possible.

Assessing the Work Environment

Whenever environmental temperatures are expected to go below 16°C (60.8°F), the air temperature should be monitored, and workers performing barehanded tasks for more than 20 minutes should be provided with ways to warm their hands. These may include radiant heaters or warm air jets. When they fall below −1°C (30.2°F), air temperatures should be monitored at least every 4 hours, and metal tool handles and control bars should be wrapped in insulating material. Wind speed should also be monitored when it exceeds 2 m/s (5 mph) or whenever air temperatures drop below −1°C.[16] Workers should be provided with anticontact gloves, such as those made of silk, to prevent contact frostbite from surfaces that are less than −7°C (19.4°F). Workers in an environment that is continually at or below −7°C (19.4°F) should be provided a work-warming regimen. Table 14C-2 is an example of a work/warm-up schedule for a 4-hour work shift. Heated shelters stocked with warm, noncaffeinated drinks and food should be readily available. Workers should remove their outer layer of clothing while in the shelter. (The work rate should not be so high that heavy sweating results; however, dry clothing should be available if necessary to prevent a return to the work environment in wet clothing.)

Threshold Limit Values (TLVs) Work/Warm-up Schedule for a 4-Hour Shift

Air Temperature, Sunny Sky		No Noticeable Wind		5 mph Wind		10 mph Wind		15 mph Wind		20 mph Wind	
°C (Approx.)	°F (Approx.)	Max. Work Period	No. of Breaks	Max. Work Period	No. of Breaks	Max. Work Period	No. of Breaks	Max. Work Period	No. of Breaks	Max. Work Period	No. of Breaks
−26 to −28	−15 to −19	(Norm. breaks) 1		(Norm. breaks) 1		75 min	2	55 min	3	40 min	4
−29 to −31	−20 to −24	(Norm. breaks) 1		75 min	2	55 min	3	40 min	4	30 min	5
−32 to −34	−25 to −29	75 min	2	55 min	3	40 min	4	30 min	5	Nonemergency work should cease	
−35 to −37	−30 to −34	55 min	3	40 min	4	30 min	5	Nonemergency work should cease			
−38 to −39	−35 to −39	40 min	4	30 min	5	Nonemergency work should cease					
−40 to −42	−40 to −44	30 min	5	Nonemergency work should cease							
−43 and below	−45 and below	Nonemergency work should cease									

Schedule applies to moderate to heavy work activity with warm-up breaks of 10 minutes in a warm location. For light to moderate work (limited physical movement), apply the schedule one step lower. For example, at −35° C (−30°F) with no noticeable wind (step 4), a worker at a job with little physical movement should have a maximum work period of 40 minutes with 4 breaks in a 4-hour period (step 5).

The following is suggested as a guide for estimating wind velocity if accurate information is not available: 5 mph, light flag moves; 10 mph, light flag fully extended; 15 mph, raises newspaper sheet; 20 mph, blowing and drifting snow.

If only the wind chill cooling rate is available, a rough rule of thumb for applying it rather than the temperature and wind velocity factors given above would be (1) special warm-up breaks should be initiated at a wind chill cooling rate of about 1,750 W/m². (2) all nonemergency work should have ceased at or before a wind chill of 2,250 W/m². In general, the warm-up schedule provided above slightly undercompensates for the wind at the warmer temperatures, assuming acclimatization and clothing appropriate for winter work. On the other hand, the chart slightly overcompensates for the actual temperatures in the colder ranges, as windy conditions rarely prevail at extremely low temperatures.

TLVs apply only for workers in dry clothing.

From American Conference of Governmental Industrial Hygienists (ACGIH). 2004 TLVs and BEIs: Based on the documentation of the threshold limit values for chemical substances and physical agents & biological indices. Cincinnati, OH: ACGIH, 2004, p. 164. Reprinted with permission. Adapted from Occupational Health and Safety Division, Saskatchewan Department of Labour.

When temperatures in the work environment are at or below $-12°C$ ($10.4°F$), workers should pair up or be under constant protective observation. Workers new to the environment should be allowed to acclimate. They should not be required to work full-time in the cold during the first few days while they adjust to the conditions and protective clothing.[16]

Workers should also be educated about the symptoms of cold-related illnesses and should be encouraged to seek shelter and medical attention if they or fellow workers experience pain, numbness or tingling, severe shivering, or drowsiness. In general, workers who are provided with insulated protective clothing, in work areas where drafts and wet conditions are minimized, and who have adequate breaks with access to a warm shelter and food, are far less likely to suffer ill effects from exposure to cold.

REFERENCES

1. Centers for Disease Control and Prevention. Heat-related deaths - Chicago, Illinois, 1996–2001, and United States, 1979–1999. MMWR 2003;52:610–3.
2. Klinenberg E. Heat wave: A social autopsy of disaster in Chicago. Chicago: The University of Chicago Press, 2002.
3. Centers for Disease Control and Prevention. Impact of heat waves on mortality - Rome, Italy, June-August 2003. MMWR 2004;53:369–71.
4. NIOSH. Criteria for a recommended standard: occupational exposure to hot environments, rev. Cincinnati, OH: U.S. Public Health Service, Centers for Disease Control and Prevention, National Institute for Occupational Safety and Health, 1986. (DHHS (NIOSH) publication no. 86–113.)
5. BLS. Bureau of Labor Statistics. Tabular data, 1992–2002: Census of fatal occupational injuries (1992–2002). Fatalities by detailed event or exposure, all industries, exposure to environmental heat and contact with hot objects or substances. Available at: <http://data.bls.gov/>.
6. Centers for Disease Control and Prevention. Heat-related deaths - Four states, July–August 2001, and United States, 1979–1999. MMWR 2002;51:567–70.
7. ACGIH. Heat stress and strain: Documentation of the TLVs and BEIs with other worldwide occupational exposure values CD-ROM–2003 (2001 Supplement). Cincinnati, OH: American Conference of Governmental Industrial Hygienists, 2003.
8. WHO. Health factors involved in working under conditions of heat stress. Geneva, Switzerland: World Health Organization, 1969. (Technical Report Series No. 412.)
9. OSHA. Technical manual, section III: Chapter 4, heat stress, 1999. Available at: <http://www.osha-slc.gov/dts/osta/otm/otm_iii/otm_iii4.html>.
10. Malchaire J, Kampmann B, Havenith G, et al. Criteria for estimating acceptable exposure times in hot working environments: A review. Int Arch Occup Environ Health 2000;73:215–20.
11. ACGIH. 2004 TLVs and BEIs: Threshold limit values for chemical substances and physical agents & biological exposure indices. Cincinnati, OH: ACGIH, 2004.
12. Sinks T. Mathias CG, Halperin W, et al. Surveillance of work-related cold injuries using workers' compensation claims. J Occup Med 1987;29:504–9.
13. Sinks T. A joint NIOSH/Division of Safety and Hygiene study identified workers at greatest risk of frostbite and hypothermia. Ohio Monitor 1987;Jan:12–15.
14. Braunwald E, Fauci AS, Kasper DL, et al., eds. Harrison's principles of internal medicine (15th ed.) New York: McGraw-Hill, 2001.
15. OSHA. The cold stress equation. 2004. Available at <http://www.osha.gov/Publications/OSHA3156.pdf>.
16. ACGIH. Cold stress: Documentation of the TLVs and BEIs with other worldwide occupational exposure values CD-ROM-2003 (2001 Supplement). Cincinnati, OH: ACGIH, 2003.
17. OSHA. Protecting workers in cold environments. Available at <http:www.osha.gov/pls/osaweb/owadisp.show_docment?p_table=FACT_SHEETS&p=186&p_text_vversion=FALSE>.

BIBLIOGRAPHY

ACGIH. Heat stress and strain: Documentation of the TLVs and BEIs with other worldwide occupational exposure values CD-ROM2003 (2001 Supplement). Cincinnati, OH: American Conference of Governmental Industrial Hygienists, 2003.

NIOSH. Criteria for a recommended standard: Occupational exposure to hot environments, revised. Cincinnati, OH: U.S. Public Health Service, Centers for Disease Control and Prevention, National Institute for Occupational Safety and Health, 1986. (DHHS (NIOSH) publication no. 86-113.)

These two publications are the best technical guides for keeping workers safe from the effects of heat stress and strain. The NIOSH document also covers international and foreign standards and recommendations.

ACGIH. Cold stress: Documentation of the TLVs and BEIs with other worldwide occupational exposure values CD-ROM-2003 (2001 Supplement). Cincinnati, OH: ACGIH, 2003.

This is a useful summary of the issues relevant to protecting workers from the effects of cold on the body.

Braunwald E, Fauci AS, Kasper DL, et al., eds. Harrison's principles of internal medicine. 15th ed. New York: McGraw-Hill, 2001.

This reference provides a good overview of hypothermia and, more importantly, the exact steps to take when you are faced with a victim of cold stress.

The findings and conclusions in this chapter are those of the author and do not necessarily represent the views of the Centers for Disease Control and Prevention.

Ionizing and Non-ionizing Radiation

John J. Cardarelli II

T he word "radiation" brings about certain feelings and responses in different people based on their past experiences and knowledge of the subject. Although humans evolved in an environment with background radiation for millions of years, mankind only became aware of this invisible energy in 1895, when Wilhelm Conrad Roentgen announced his discovery of x-rays. The following year, Antoine Henri Becquerel discovered that uranium emits another form of invisible energy, which was later given the name *radioactivity* by Marie Curie, who was also a pioneer in the field of radiation. Since 1895, these discoveries have led to thousands of beneficial uses of radiation in the medical, industrial, and agricultural industries, which have employed millions of workers. But perhaps the most common association with radiation today is the terror and images brought about through the nuclear weapons industry and the lingering adverse health effects of the workforce that fueled that industry. In addition, highly publicized negative events all too often are the basis from which populations judge the acceptance of radiation in society. The atomic bombings of Hiroshimi and Nagasaki (1945), nuclear power plant accidents at Three Mile Island (Pennsylvania, 1979) and Chernobyl (Soviet Union, 1986), the criticality at a nuclear fuels fabrication facility in Tokaimura, Japan (1999), the dispersion of a radioactive source from a teletherapy machine in Goiania, Brazil (1987), and the recently perceived terrorist threats with radioactive "dirty bombs" contribute to the fear associated with radiation.

The impact to the psychological, social, and economic sectors of society from these radiation events leaves little doubt that radiation could be an effective terrorist weapon. However, since September 11, 2001, the United States has placed a priority on preventing biological, chemical, and radiological attacks and, in doing so, created a new category of workers that not only defend against such attacks but are also exposed to radiation in the course of their work (Fig. 14D-1). These workers are categorized as "security-based" workers that use radiation technology to prevent terrorist attacks. They use computed tomography (CT) technology to scan checked baggage at U.S. airports for explosive materials, operate gamma-emitting equipment to detect illegal contraband, and use special backscatter and transmission technologies to view through clothing and body cavities.[1]

These workers join the ever-increasing workforce that uses radiation or radioactive materials in their jobs (Table 14D-1). In 1989, the National Council on Radiation Protection and Measurements (NCRP) published summary statistics on the average radiation exposures to various occupations in the United States.[2] Occupations that received the largest annual doses included underground uranium miners, commercial nuclear power plant workers, fuel fabricators, physicians, flight crews, industrial radiographers, and well loggers. Although these data are more than 15 years old, the general trends of an ever-increasing number of workers combined with a reduction of the average individual exposure likely continues today. Two exceptions to this statement exist for occupations in the commercial nuclear power plant industry and medical

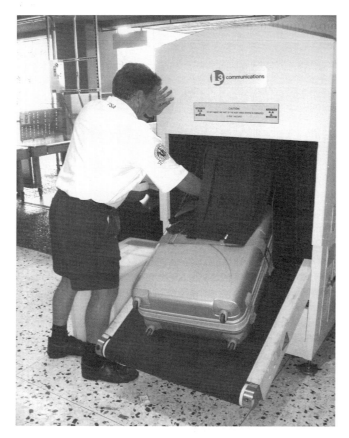

FIGURE 14D-1 ● Transportation Security Administration worker exposing his hands to x-rays while reaching into an explosive-detection system to extract a piece of luggage. (Photograph by John Cardarelli II.)

industry. The commercial nuclear power plant industry has had limited growth because no new plants have been built since the 1970s. Workers in health care may be exposed to higher radiation exposures due to a tremendous growth and use of new imaging technology, especially digital imaging.

The risk that all these occupations assume remains controversial among the radiation-control community because most of the recorded doses are well below regulatory limits, where the risks are not well characterized. The controversies were further enhanced when the United States enacted legislation to compensate workers in the nuclear weapons industry whose average doses were among the lowest when compared to other industries with radiation exposure.[3] According to a report recently published by the National Academies, the smallest doses are presumed to pose a potential risk of cancer,[3a] so it remains a priority of those in occupational and environmental health to anticipate, recognize, evaluate, and control exposures to prevent radiation injuries and illnesses.

IONIZING RADIATION

Ionizing Radiation Basics

The multiple units and scientific terminology used to define radiation do little to bring understanding to those outside the field. These problems have been around for decades and will continue to exist until scientific organizations, industry, and international governments work more actively toward harmonization. Scientific organizations are leading the way by publishing internationally recognized standards via the International Commission for Radiation Protection (ICRP) and the International Atomic Energy Agency (IAEA). Industry falls behind by continuing to produce instrumentation that provides results in the conventional units, and government regulations struggle to keep up with the changing recommendations due to lengthy legislative processes. As this field approaches more consistent use of units and terminology (Table 14D-2), those outside the field will begin to better understand the basics of radiation.

TABLE 14D-1

Types of Workers Who May be Exposed Occupationally to Ionizing Radiation

Accelerator personnel

Department of Defense (DOD) workers

Department of Energy (DOE) workers

Contractor employees

Reactor facility employees

Weapons fabrication personnel

Office workers

Uranium fuel cycle workers

Miners

Millers

Fuel fabricators

Fuel processors

Uranium enrichment workers

Educational institution workers

Radiographic (nondestructive testing) workers

Manufacturing workers

Distribution workers

Well-logging workers

Health care workers

Other hospital workers

Veterinary workers

Nuclear power plants workers

Commercial workers

Naval (fleet and shipyard) workers

Transportation workers

Screening personnel

Trucking and other shipping workers

Inspectors and other regulatory workers

Researchers

Adapted from National Council on Radiation Protection and Measurements. NCRP Report No. 101: Exposure of the U.S. Population from Occupational Radiation, NCRP, Washington, DC, 1989.

Some of the most important concepts to understand in the field of radiation are ionizing and non-ionizing radiation, exposure and dose, half-life and activity, and risk. *Ionizing radiation* is caused when an electron is ejected from its atomic structure. *Non-ionizing* radiation does not eject electrons, but causes the molecules to vibrate. *Exposure* represents the amount of radiation that is absorbed in air. *Dose* refers to the amount of energy absorbed in a specified material other than air, usually tissue. The difference is due to the different densities of air and the specified material. *Half-life* is the amount of time it takes for half of the radioactive material to decay. *Activity* represents the decay rate or how quickly that radioactivity material decays. *Risk* is defined as the increment of some adverse health affect associated with a known amount of cumulative radiation dose.

TABLE 14D-2

Radiation Units

Parameter	Conventional Units	SI Units
Exposure	Roentgen (R) = 87.6 ergs per gram (air) = 2.58×10^{-4} Coulomb/kg (air)	Coulomb/kg
Dose	rad = 100 erg per gram (tissue) = 0.01 Gy	Gray (Gy) = 100 rad
Dose equivalent	rem = 1 rad × w_r[a] = 0.01 Sv	Sievert (Sv) = 100 rem
Activity	Curie (Ci) = 3.7×10^{10} decays per second	Becquerel (Bq) = 1 decay per second

[a] w_r = radiation weighting factor: a dimensionless number that depends on the way in which the energy of the radiation is distributed along its path through the tissue. In general, it is 20 for alpha particles, 1 for beta particles and gamma and x-rays, and 5 to 20 for neutron exposures.

Types of Ionizing Radiation

The various types of radiation and how they interact with matter can be described by our understanding of the atom. *Alpha radiation* (α) is a helium nucleus (contains only two protons and two neutrons) and is typically associated with heavy elements like radon, radium, uranium, and plutonium. It is a large, positive-charged particle and easily interacts with other atoms to quickly deposit its energy. Depending on its energy (measured in units called million electron-volts; MeV), an alpha particle can travel up to 10 cm in air, but most only penetrate 1 to 3 cm (less than 5 MeV) before being absorbed. Alpha particles with at least 7.5 MeV can penetrate the nominal protective layer of the skin (0.07 mm), but only 13.7 percent of all known alpha emissions (N = 1,999) occur above this energy and most of these are human-made. Therefore, alpha radiation does not pose an external hazard to humans because they are easily shielded (by air, skin, or paper) but can be hazardous if the emitting radionuclide is inhaled, ingested, or injected in the body where there is little protection to living tissue.

Beta radiation (*β*) is an electron emitted by an atom. Relative to the mass of a single proton, the beta particle mass is 1/1,836 the size and can penetrate further into materials or tissue.[4] Due to their smaller size and charge as compared to an alpha particle, beta particles can travel about 12 feet per MeV in air and need only 0.07 MeV to penetrate the skin. Most beta particles do not normally penetrate beyond the top layer of skin, but exposure to higher energy beta particles (>0.07 MeV) can cause skin burns. Beta radiation is easily shielded with plastic, glass, or metals, but layers of plastic materials are preferred in the occupational environment to reduce the production of x-rays. These characteristics make beta radiation both an external and internal hazard to humans.

Photon radiation (gamma or x-ray) is a form of electromagnetic radiation like light, except with energies high enough to cause ionization. There are several differences between these two forms of radiation with the foremost being their point of origin. *Gamma rays* originate from within the nucleus, and *x-rays* originate from surrounding orbital electrons. Gamma ray emissions are very specific and are often used to identify radionuclides with special instruments. X-ray emissions are generally not specific because they are produced artificially by the rapid slowing down of an electron beam (*bremsstrahlung radiation*). Because the rate of slowing is not specific, the various x-ray energies exist within a continuum of energies that peak at the maximum energy of the incident electron beam or beta particle. Characteristic x-rays are one exception where x-rays with specific energies are emitted due to the specific energy levels between electron shells. An electron shifting from a higher energy shell to a lower energy shell will emit an x-ray of a fixed energy equal to the energy difference between shells. Finally, gamma rays commonly encountered in the occupational environment (medical and industrial) are generally higher in energy than x-rays.

Neutron radiation is essentially zero for background radiation levels at ground level and is only an occupational concern at commercial nuclear power plants, research facilities, and high-altitude activities (airline industry and space exploration). Neutrons have no charge, therefore they are not influenced by other charged particles and can easily penetrate materials. Water or concrete are effective shielding materials because they contain many similar sized atoms close to that of a neutron (hydrogenous materials). As the neutrons penetrate these materials, they interact with the atomic nuclei of the material like billiard balls. Neutron radiation is also capable of creating radioactive materials through a process called *activation*. When a neutron is absorbed by an atomic nucleus, the atom becomes "excited" and often releases the excess energy in the form of other types of radiation, especially protons. Because atoms are identified by the number of protons in the nucleus, any change in this number will change the element and its chemical properties. The most common activation product encountered in various industries is cobalt-60. It is important to understand that alpha, beta, gamma, and x-radiation do not cause the body to become radioactive, but most materials in their natural state (including body tissue) contain measurable amounts of radioactivity.

External and Internal Exposures

External exposures occur when the body is irradiated by a radioactive source outside the body. Dose measurements from external exposures are relatively simple to measure using pocket ion-chambers (PICs); film; or thermolumenscent (TLD), optically stimulated luminescence (OSL), or electronic personal dosimeters (EPD). All these technologies can be arranged to differentiate between the types of radiation exposure (beta, gamma, or neutron) and their respective energies. Choosing the most appropriate dosimeter should be done by a qualified individual who can assess the advantages and limitations for the given application (Table 14D-3). Additional considerations include the type of radiation encountered, the monitoring frequency (immediate, hourly, weekly, monthly, quarterly), the required sensitivity, processing time, and cost.

Internal exposures occur when a radioactive material enters the body via inhalation, ingestion, injection, or absorption through the skin. Doses from internal exposures are more difficult to assess than external exposures because individual characteristics, such as diet, health status, and age, vary greatly within a population. In an attempt to standardize the dosimetry methodology, ICRP has developed sophisticated human reference models to estimate internal doses.[5,6] These models often govern the airborne radiation concentration limits, called derived air concentrations (DACs), for occupational environments. Internal dose estimates are determined

TABLE 14D-3

Advantages and Limitations of Dosimeter Types

Dosimeter Type	Advantages	Limitations
Pocket ion chambers	Immediate read-out Reusable Cost efficient Some can differentiate between gamma and neutrons	False positives (impact sensitive) Requires minor maintenance
Film	Provide a permanent record of dose (re-readable). Can differentiate between beta, gamma, and neutron exposures Provides integrated dose Can estimate energy level of radiation Simple design	Sensitive to light Higher limit of detection Measurement must be processed Variation from batch emulsions Chemical processing variables
Thermoluminescent (TLD)	Can differentiate between beta, gamma, and neutron exposures Provides integrated dose Can estimate energy level of radiation Lower limit of detection Simple design	Measurement must be processed Not a permanent record Some TLD materials subject to fading (result in under reporting of dose) Potential for false-positives
Optically stimulated luminescence (OSL)	Similar to TLDs Identify static vs. dynamic exposure conditions Provides a permanent record (reanalysis; dose verification) Quicker read-out (within seconds) Reduce potential false-positive	Measurement must be processed Sensitive to light
Electronic	Immediate read-out Can differentiate between beta, gamma, and neutron exposures Provides integrated dose Can estimate energy level of radiation Lower limit of detection Datalogging capabilities Some provide visual and audible warnings Telemetry	Cost (expensive) Requires calibration and maintenance Availability may be suspect Sophisticated design

by either direct measurements, biological sample analyses, or a combination of the two. Direct measurements of, for example, thyroid, whole body, or bone, employ very sensitive instruments that measure photon radiation (gamma rays or characteristic x-rays) emitted from within the body. Specific gamma energies identify the radionuclides while the measurement estimates the amount internally deposited. These data are then used with the knowledge of the initial time of exposure and the ICRP standardized models to estimate the dose. Biological samples, such as urine, feces, exhaled breath, sweat, and hair, are used when the type of exposure, chemical properties (soluble versus insoluble), and radionuclide is known. The amount of radioactive material measured in these samples can estimate internal dose via the ICRP models. In the occupational environmental, both methods are used to refine internal dose estimates as more information on the individual's biological clearance process is obtained.

Background Radiation and the Environment

Background radiation levels vary all around the world from less than 0.005 milli-roentgen per hour (mR/hr) to more than 2.5 mR/hr. This results in an annual dose of about 0.4 mSv (40 mrem) to 220 mSv (22,000 mrem). This large dose range is due to various deposits of naturally occurring radioactive materials (NORM), altitude, and longitude positions on Earth. The Biological Effects of Ionizing Radiation Committee (BEIR V) reports an average annual background dose of about 3.6 mSv (360 mrem) to people living in the United States. Radon exposure is responsible for about 55 percent of background dose (about 2.0 mSv) and is highest where NORM material (uranium and thorium) is found. Cosmic radiation accounts for about 8 percent (0.27 mSv) of background levels and increases at higher altitudes and at longitude positions closer to the poles. Terrestial radiation (rocks and soil) also account for about 8 percent (0.28 mSv). Internal exposures (radioactive substances inside the body, particularly potassium-40) account for about 11 percent (0.39 mSv). Human-made radiation sources (medical procedures and consumer products) account for about 18 percent (0.63 mSv). Other sources (occupational, nuclear fuel cycle, fallout, and artificial sources) account for the remaining 0.3 percent (0.03 mSv).

Health Effects

Health effects from radiation exposures vary with the type, amount, and duration of exposure. When radiation exposes a cell, it may (a) pass through without doing any damage, (b) interact and damage the cell, with later repair by the cell, (c) interact and damage the cell in such a way that it continues to reproduce itself in a damaged state, or (d) kill the cell. The death of a single cell may not be harmful, but if many cells are killed within an organ then that organ may not function properly. The likelihood of damage is also related to the mitotic cycle of the cell.

In 1906, the Law of Bergonie and Tribondeau concluded that the most radiosensitive cells have a high division rate, long dividing future, and are not of a specialized type. In general, tissues that are young and rapidly growing are most likely radiosensitive. Therefore, mature lymphocytes are more radiosensitive than (in order) intestinal crypt cells, mature spermatocytes, erythrocytes, and nerve cells.

Acute effects, sometimes referred to as *nonstochastic effects*, are those in which the severity of the effect varies with the dose and occur shortly (minutes to days) after exposure. If the dose is kept below a given threshold, usually about 0.25 Gy (25 rad), no effect will be observed. Above this value, especially above 1 Gy (100 rad), a group of clinical syndromes known as *acute radiation sickness* develop. These include the hemopoietic syndrome, gastrointestinal syndrome, and central nervous system syndrome. Another called cutaneous radiation syndrome may occur simultaneously with the others and often complicates the recovery process of the exposed individual due to an increase potential for infection. The hemopoietic syndrome occurs with penetrating gamma or x-ray doses ranging between 2 to 10 Gy (200 to 1000 rads) and is characterized by deficiencies of WBC, lymphocytes, and platelets. It consists of four phases: prodromal phase (nausea, vomiting, and anorexia lasting up to 48 hours); latent phase (asymptomatic but will begin to show changes in blood elements lasting up to 3 weeks); bone marrow depression; and recovery (Figure 14D-2). The gastrointestinal syndrome occurs with penetrating gamma or x-ray doses greater than 10 Gy (1,000 rads) and an immediate, prompt, and profuse onset of nausea, vomiting, and diarrhea, followed by a short latent period. Severe dehydration is caused by the massive denuding of the gastrointestinal tract. Most patients do not survive. The central nervous syndrome occurs with penetrating gamma or x-ray dose above 100 Gy (10,000 rads) accompanied by vomiting and diarrhea within minutes of exposures, confusion, disorientation, hypotension, and hyperpyrexia resulting in death within a short time. Cutaneous-syndrome severity is determined by the dose of beta radiation, the energy of the radiation, and the type of exposure (skin contamination, contact with contaminated clothing, or distant exposure). Effects depend on whether exposure is uniform or nonuniform and the location of contamination on the body. Most radiosensitive are moist areas (axilla, groin, and skin

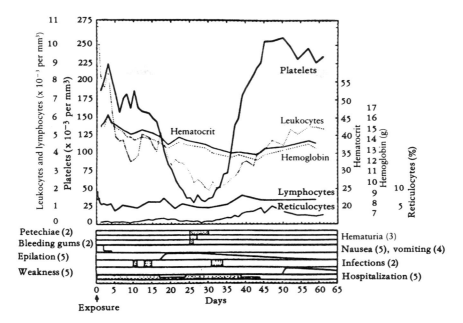

FIGURE 14D-2 ● Hematologic values, symptoms, and clinical signs in five men exposed to whole-body irradiation in a criticality accident. The blood counts are average values for the five men; the figures in parentheses denote the numbers showing the symptoms and signs indicated. (From Andrews GA, Sitterson EW, Kretchmar AL, et al. Criticality accidents at the Y-12 plant. In: Diagnosis and treatment of acute radiation injury. Geneva: World Health Organization, 1961:27–48.)

folds), followed by the inner aspect of the neck, the antecubital and popliteal spaces, and the flexor surfaces of the extremities, chest, abdomen, face, and back. Least sensitive are the nape of the neck, scalp, palms, and soles. The larger the area irradiated, less dose is needed for adverse reactions. Likewise, the smaller the area irradiated, more dose is needed for a similar reaction. A temporal scheme proposed by Rubin and Casarett classifies the effects as *acute effects* (within first 6 months), *subacute effects* (second 6 months), *chronic clinical period* (2 to 5 years), and *late clinical period* (after 5 years). Depending on dose, the skin will experience several stages of response. These include erythema (3–10 Gy; 14–21 days); epilation (>3 Gy; 14–18 days), dry desquamation (8–12 Gy; 25–30 days), moist desquamation (15–20 Gy; 20–28 days), blister formation (15–25 Gy; 15–25 days), ulceration (>20 Gy, 14–21 days), and necrosis (>25 Gy; >21 days). The commercial nuclear power industry presents a unique skin hazard of highly localized, radioactive material (usually cobalt-60 or cesium-137) called "hot particles," "fleas," or "specks." These particles range from 1 to 100 μm in diameter, deliver very high doses to a local area, and are difficult to remove. In the event of a

terrorist attack involving nuclear (involving fission) or radioactive (nonfissile) material, these particles may become a principal radiological concern but are not likely to result in whole-body doses leading to death.

Pregnancy Issues

Thousands of pregnant workers are exposed to ionizing radiation each year. The great anxiety and consideration of unnecessary termination of pregnancies are due to a lack of knowledge. These fears and concerns can be alleviated by understanding that the radiation risks throughout pregnancy are related to the stage of pregnancy and dose. Preconception irradiation of either parent's gonads has not been shown to result in increased risk of cancer or malformations in children. Radiation risks are most significant during organogenesis and in the early fetal period and become lower with each successful trimester. Malformations have a threshold ranging between 0.1 to 0.2 Gy (10 to 20 rad) and are typically associated with central nervous system problems. Fetal doses of 0.1 Gy are not reached even with 3 pelvic CT scans or 20 conventional diagnostic x-ray examinations. Radiation has been shown to increase the risk of leukemia in adults and children. The embryo/fetus is assumed to be at about the same risk for carcinogenic effects as children. For an individual exposed *in utero* to 0.01 Gy, the absolute risk of cancer at ages 0 to 15 years is about 1 excess cancer death per 1,700. This suggests that the probability of bearing a healthy child is very high, even if the pregnant worker receives a radiation dose that exceeds the occupational dose limit for nonpregnant workers. These risks must be taken into context with the abnormal affects in a pregnant population that are not exposed to radiation (that is, spontaneous abortion, more than 15 percent; incidence of genetic abnormalities, 4 to 10 percent; intrauterine growth retardation, 4 percent; and incidence of major malformation, 2 to 4 percent).

The dose ranges mentioned above are extremely rare in the workplace, especially if the woman declares pregnancy to her employer. The dose to a declared pregnant worker is limited to 0.005 Gy (0.5 rad) per gestation period in the United States (a factor of 10 lower than the nonpregnant occupational dose limit). ICRP states that pregnant workers may work in a radiation environment as long as there is reasonable assurance that the fetal dose can be kept below 0.001 Gy (0.1 rad), above background, during the pregnancy. This is about the same dose that all persons receive annually from penetrating natural background radiation (excluding radon) and a factor of 50 lower than the nonpregnant occupational dose limit.

Termination of pregnancy is rarely contemplated from the perspective of an occupational exposure but may become a dominant concern after a nuclear or radiological terrorist attack. Despite the political or religious arguments, the scientific literature provides some guidance on this issue. High fetal doses (0.1–1.0 Gy; 10–100 rad) during late pregnancy are *not* likely to result in malformations or birth defects because all the organs have been formed, and there is less than 1 percent chance that the exposed fetus will develop childhood cancer or leukemia with a dose of about 0.1 Gy (10 rad). For this reason, termination of pregnancy at fetal doses less than 0.1 Gy (10 rad) is not justified based on radiation risk. As the fetal dose increases to above 0.5 Gy (50 rad), there can be significant fetal damage based on the stage of the pregnancy. At fetal doses between 0.1 (10 rad) and 0.5 Gy (50 rad), decisions should be based on individual circumstances.[7]

Chronic effects, sometimes referred to as *stochastic effects*, are those in which the probability of the effect increases with increasing dose without threshold. Any dose has a probability of causing the effect, but the severity of the effect remains unchanged. Cancer and heredity effects are examples of chronic effects. The international scientific community has adopted a linear no-threshold dose–response model to set occupational dose limits based primarily on the atomic-bomb survivors and medically exposed individuals. There is little controversy about the linear response between adverse health affects associated with high cumulative doses ($>$1 Gy; 100 rad). However, controversy continues as to whether the linear no-threshold model is appropriate for lower cumulative doses and dose-rate exposures as found in the workplace.[8] Recently, the National Academies published a report that concluded that the current scientific evidence is consistent with the hypothesis that there is a linear dose-response relationship between exposure to ionizing radiation and the development of solid cancers in humans. It also concluded that it is unlikely that there is a threshold below which cancers are not induced, but at low doses the number of radiation-induced cancers will be small.[3a] Over the past several decades, several response models have been studied and proposed in the scientific literature. These include the linear quadratic model, threshold model, supralinear model, and hormesis models (Fig. 14D-3).

Radiation Protection

Radiation protection standards have evolved since the discovery of x-rays in 1895 and continue to undergo changes, additions, and revisions today. International and national organizations recommend scientifically based protection standards, and governments promulgate legislation setting occupational dose limits (Table 14D-4). The latest scientific recommendations differ from regulatory standards because the regulatory process cannot keep pace with the recommended changes by scientific organizations due to a complex promulgation process. The BEIR VII report by the National Academies recently concluded that the magnitude of estimated risks for total cancer mortality or leukemia has not changed greatly from estimates provided in past reports, such as BEIR V (1990) and recent UNSCEAR and ICRP reports. BEIR V reported that the cancer risk estimates had increased

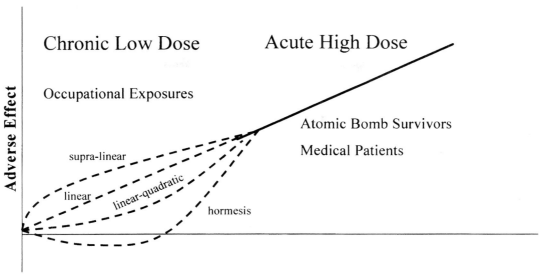

FIGURE 14D-3 ● Health effects associated with radiation dose.

TABLE 14D-4

Occupational Dose Limits or Recommendations

Dose Limits	DOE	NRC	OSHA	NCRP (1993)	ICRP[a] (1991)
Occupational	50 mSv per year (external plus internal doses)	50 mSv per year (external plus internal doses)	12.5 mSv per quarter for the whole body (head and trunk; active blood-forming organs or gonads)	50 mSv per year	20 mSv per year averaged over 5 years (100 mSv in 5 years), with a further provision that the effective dose should not exceed **50 mSv in any single year**
Lens of eye	150 mSv per year	150 mSv per year	12.5 mSv per quarter	150 mSv per year	150 mSv per year
Hands and forearms; feet and ankles	500 mSv per year	500 mSv per year	187.5 mSv per quarter	500 mSv per year	500 mSv per year
Skin	500 mSv per year	500 mSv per year	75 mSv per quarter	500 mSv per year	500 mSv per year
Cumulative	None	None	50 (N − 18) mSv N = age (years)	10 mSv × age **(years)**	100 mSv in 5 years

DOE, Department of Energy; NRC, Nuclear Regulatory Commission; OSHA, Occupational Safety and Health Administration; NCRP, National Commission on Radiological Protection; ICRP, International Commission on Radiological Protection.
[a] The 2005 ICRP recommendations continue to endorse these limits.

by a factor of about 3 for solid cancers (relative risk projection) and about 4 for leukemia from its previous BEIR III (1980) report, on which many regulatory standards are based. The regulatory dose limits are based on BEIR III or earlier scientific reports and were set to be commensurate with the basic philosophy that radiation workers ought to have at least the same level of protection as those in safe industries (about 1 death per 10,000 workers per year).[9]

Radon

Occupational exposure limits for radon and radon progeny (also known as *radon daughters*) were derived to protect the health of underground miners over a working lifetime of 30 years.[10–12] When radon gas and radon progeny are inhaled, the radiation dose is primarily caused by the short-lived radon progeny rather than by the radon gas. Because it was not feasible to routinely measure the individual radon progeny, the concept of the working level (WL) was introduced and defined as 1.3×10^5 million electron volts (MeV) of alpha radiation emitted from the short-lived radon progeny in 1 L of air. An exposure of 1 WL for a working period of 1 month (170 hours) results in a cumulative exposure of 1 working level month (WLM). A WLM is the common unit of measure for human exposure to radon progeny and is the basis for the occupational exposure limits. More information about occupational radon exposures is available from the International Atomic Energy Organization (http://www.iaea.org) and the National Institute for Occupational Safety and Health (http://www.cdc.gov/niosh/).

Protection Programs

The objective of a radiation protection program is to reflect the application of the management responsibility for radiation protection and safety through the adoption of policies, procedures, and organizational structures that are commensurate with the nature and extent of the risks. Three principles of radiation protection and safety include justifying, limiting, and optimizing exposures. Radiation exposures may be justified if the activity produces sufficient benefit to offset the harm it might cause the exposed worker, taking into account social, economic, and other relevant factors. Dose limitation is necessary to limit the risk of stochastic effects from exposures considered to be unacceptable. Protection and safety should be optimized to ensure that

the magnitude of worker doses, the number of workers exposed, and the likelihood of incurring exposure all be kept as low as reasonably achievable after accounting for social and economic factors. A "safety culture" is one key element that contributes to a successful radiation protection program. It depends on management commitment to encourage a questioning and learning attitude toward protection and safety and to discourage complacency. Studies have shown that a neutral or negative attitude toward radiological protection by management is one of six causes of unnecessary or excessive radiation exposure in the workplace. The other five are (a) inaccurate or incomplete radiation surveys, (b) inadequately prepared radiological work permits, (c) failure of the radiological technician to react to changing or unusual conditions, (d) failure of workers to follow procedures, and (e) lack of supervisor involvement. Whatever the situation, the basic structure of the radiation protection program should include the following:

1. Assignment of responsibilities to various levels of management.
2. Designation of controlled or supervised areas.
3. Local rules for workers to follow and the supervision of work.
4. Arrangement for monitoring workers and the workplace with appropriate dosimeters and instrumentation.
5. A system to record and report all relevant information to the appropriate decision makers.
6. Education and training programs on the nature of the hazards, protection, and safety.
7. Methods to periodically review and audit performance of the program.
8. Emergency response plans.
9. A health surveillance program.
10. A quality assurance and control program.

Emergency Response

Recent events have focused attention on preparedness to deal with large-scale radiological or nuclear threats and small-scale industrial accidents. In 2002, the United States established the Department of Homeland Security, consolidating many federal emergency response plans into a single national response plan and providing funding to states and local governments. Emergency response workers, such as police and firefighters, may be highly exposed to radiation at levels requiring additional precautions and medical intervention. Many of the medical, public health, and public safety decisions may be made by a variety of individuals ranging from personal physicians to political leaders. All the decisions require consideration of several factors, including law enforcement issues, mass casualties and damage to infrastructure, psychosocial impacts, and environmental concerns, the details of which are beyond the scope of this chapter.[13] However, a key concept for those in occupational and environmental health regarding emergency response is to always treat life-threatening injuries first before measures to address radioactive contamination or exposure. Even if the patient has been heavily irradiated or contaminated, he or she must be evaluated for other forms of injury, such as mechanical trauma, burns, and smoke inhalation. One should be especially cautious of wounds containing metallic objects, as these could be very high source of radiation. The best way those in occupational and environmental health can protect themselves during a radiological or nuclear response is to seek additional training in the field of ionizing radiation. Most of the basic training materials can be found at the following Web sites:

GOVERNMENT WEB SITES

- Centers for Disease Control and Prevention
  <http://www.cdc.gov/nceh/radiation/default.htm>
- EPA Radiation Protection Programs
  <http://www.epa.gov/radiation/>
- FDA Center for Devices and Radiological Health
  <http://www.fda.gov/cdrh/>
- Federal Emergency Management Agency
  <http://www.fema.gov/>
- International Atomic Energy Agency
  <http://www.iaea.org/>
- Occupational Safety and Health Agency
  <http://www.osha.gov/SLTC/radiation/index.html>

WEB SITES OF SCIENTIFIC ORGANIZATIONS

- American Association of Physicists in Medicine (AAPM)
  <http://www.aapm.org/>
- American Association of Radon Scientists and Technologists (AARST)
  <http://www.aarst.org/>
- Conference on Radiation Control Program Directors (CRCPD)
  <http://www.crcpd.org/>
- Health Physics Society (HPS)
  <http://www.hps.org/>

- International Commission on Radiological Protection (ICRP)
  <http://www.icrp.org/>
- International Radiation Protection Association (IRPA)
  <http://www.irpa.net/>

NON-IONIZING RADIATION

Non-ionizing radiation exposes every person, every day, throughout the world. It is both naturally occurring and human-made. It can be both beneficial and detrimental to those exposed. Like ionizing radiation, one cannot see it (outside visible light; 400 to 760 nm), taste it, or smell it. But unlike ionizing radiation, one may be able to feel it via heat or shock sensations. It is the energy absorbed by any material without causing ionization (ejection of electrons surrounding the atoms within the material). It is the energy of television and radio signals, radar, transmissions for cordless and cellular phones and pagers, microwaves, visible light, infrared and ultraviolet light, lasers, and other examples.

Non-ionizing radiation is one of the most common and fastest growing environmental and occupational influences, about which anxiety and speculation are spreading. Levels of exposure will continue to increase as technology advances combined with societal demands for the conveniences it brings. The universal aspect of this subject is too voluminous to capture in this text, so a brief introduction will be given on the basics, how to interpret measurement data, the associated health effects, and how to protect those exposed in an occupational environment. It will focus primarily on extremely low frequency (ELF) and radio-frequency (RF) radiation, because ELF and RF comprise most of the electromagnetic spectrum and expose the most people. Ultraviolet radiation, infrared radiation, and lasers are briefly addressed by summarizing industrial applications and their associated adverse health effects.

Non-Ionizing Radiation Basics

The electromagnetic spectrum includes ionizing and non-ionizing radiation (Fig. 14D-4). All non-ionizing radiation presents itself in electric and magnetic fields called electromagnetic fields (EMFs). EMFs can be described by the frequency

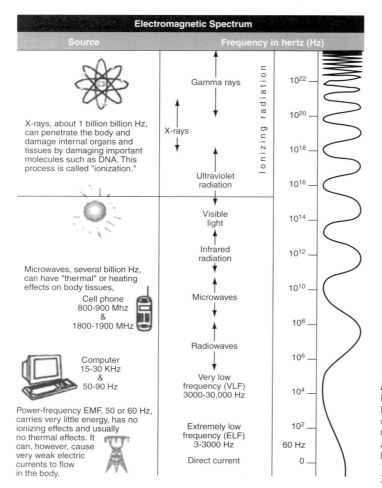

Electromagnetic Spectrum

Source | **Frequency in hertz (Hz)**

X-rays, about 1 billion billion Hz, can penetrate the body and damage internal organs and tissues by damaging important molecules such as DNA. This process is called "ionization."

Gamma rays — 10^{22}
X-rays
— 10^{20}
— 10^{18}
Ultraviolet radiation — 10^{16}

Ionizing radiation

Microwaves, several billion Hz, can have "thermal" or heating effects on body tissues,
Cell phone 800-900 Mhz & 1800-1900 MHz

Visible light — 10^{14}
Infrared radiation — 10^{12}
Microwaves — 10^{10}
— 10^{8}
Radiowaves — 10^{6}

Computer 15-30 KHz & 50-90 Hz

Very low frequency (VLF) 3000-30,000 Hz — 10^{4}

Power-frequency EMF, 50 or 60 Hz, carries very little energy, has no ionizing effects and usually no thermal effects. It can, however, cause very weak electric currents to flow in the body.

Extremely low frequency (ELF) 3-3000 Hz — 10^{2}
— 60 Hz
Direct current — 0

FIGURE 14D-4 ●
Electromagnetic spectrum. (From EMF in the Workplace. Department of Energy, National Institute for Occupational Safety and Health, and National Institute of Environmental Health Sciences, 1996. Note: ELF is defined as 3 to 300 Hz by NCRP Report 119.)

or the corresponding wavelength through the fundamental equation:

$$\lambda = c/f$$

where λ is wavelength in meters (m), c is velocity (usually the velocity of light, 3×10^8 meters per second; m/s), and f is frequency in cycles per seconds, commonly referred to as hertz (Hz), named after the German physicist Heinrich Rudolf Hertz.

Industrial applications span the entire EMF spectrum. For convenience, most of the non-ionizing radiation spectrum is partitioned into specified radio-frequency bands. Hazards potentially associated with exposure to EMFs in the various bands may result in (a) currents being produced within the body via contact with energized sources or induced within the body without contact with sources or nearby metallic objects, (b) increased internal body temperature, or (c) increased body surface temperature (Table 14D-5). How efficient

these fields interact with the body depends on several factors. For example, materials with a high water content (muscles) absorb EMF energy at a higher rate than dry materials. The absorption rate is higher when the incident electric field is parallel versus perpendicular to the body and higher when the incident magnetic field is perpendicular to larger cross-sectional areas versus smaller areas. Sharp corners, edges, and points concentrate electric fields. Depth of penetration decreases as conductivity increases and as frequency increases (shorter wavelengths).

Electric fields exist when electric charges exert forces on one another. *Electric field strength* describes the strength of forces on charges and has units of V/m. A good example of electric fields, their strengths, and shape is demonstrated in thunderstorms where the local build-up of electric charges in the atmosphere eventually reach a level that produce lightning. Lightning can illustrate the shape of the electric field but also provides the pathway

TABLE 14D-5

Frequency Bands and Their Associated Biological Impacts

Band	Frequency Range (Hz)	Wavelength Range (m)	Biological Impact
SELF (Sub-extremely-low frequency)	0 to 30	0 to 10^7	0–10^5 Hz 0–$3,000$ m
ELF (Extremely-low frequency)	30 to 300	10^7 to 10^6	Electrostimulation (primary dosimetric parameter is
VF (Voice frequency)	300 to 3,000	10^6 to 10^5	internal current density)
VLF (Very-low frequency)	3,000 to 3×10^4	10^5 to 10^4	
LF (Low frequency)	3×10^4 to 3×10^5	10^4 to 10^3	10^5 to 6×10^9 Hz
MF (Medium frequency)	3×10^5 to 3×10^6	10^3 to 10^2	3,000 to 0.05 m Specific absorption rates
HF (High frequency)	3×10^6 to 3×10^7	10^2 to 10	(heating effects)
VHF (Very high frequency)	3×10^7 to 3×10^8	10 to 1	
UHF (Ultrahigh frequency)	3×10^8 to 3×10^9	1 to 0.1	
SHF (Super-high frequency)	3×10^9 to 3×10^{10}	0.1 to 10^{-2}	Above 6×10^9 Hz
EHF (Extremely-high frequency)	3×10^{10} to 3×10^{11}	10^{-2} to 10^{-3}	Below 0.05 m Surface heating (Radiant)
SEHF (Supra-extremely-high frequency)	3×10^{11} to 3×10^{12}	10^{-3} to 10^{-4}	
Infrared radiation	IR-C	0.3 μm to 1 mm	Corneal burns, thermal skin
	IR-B	0.14 μm to 0.3 μm	burns
	IR-A	760 nm to 1,400 nm	Retinal burns, cataracts of lens, thermal skin burns
Visible light		400 to 760 nm	Retinal burns, thermal skin burns
Ultraviolet radiation	UV-A	400 to 320 nm	Cataract of lens, thermal skin burns
	UV-B	320 to 280 nm	Corneal injuries, cataracts of
	UV-C	280 to 200 nm	lens, photokeratitis, photoconjunctivitis, erythema

mm = millimeter (10^{-3} m); μm = micrometer (10^{-6} m); nm = nanometer (10^{-9} m).

for the electric charges to move through the atmosphere. Thus, an electric field can exist even when there is no movement, but once electric charges begin to move, magnetic fields also exert forces on charges moving through them.

Magnetic field strength has units of A/m and is associated with the strength of these additional forces on moving charges. The relationship between these fields is described by the term *power density*, defined as the power incident on a surface per unit surface area. It is given the abbreviation *S* and can be calculated from electric or magnetic field measurements by the following equation:

$$S = E^2/377, \text{ or } 377H^2$$

where *S* is power density in watts per square meter (W/m² or VA/m²), *E* is electric field strength measurement (V/m) or *H* is magnetic field strength measurement (A/m), and the constant 377 is the impedance of free space (ohms, Ω or V/A). However, near RF sources where the highest exposures occur, the impedance cannot be assumed to be 377 ohms. Thus, for near-field exposures below 300 MHz, both *E*- and *H*-field strengths must be measured. Near-field exposures exist within one-half of a wavelength from RF sources or metallic objects illuminated with an RF field.

Exposure Limits

The transfer of energy from electric and magnetic fields in any material is described in terms of the specific absorption rate (SAR). "Specific" refers to the normalization to mass of the material exposed, "absorption" refers to the absorption of the energy, and "rate" means the time rate of change of the energy absorption. The SAR has been found to be the most reliable indicator or predictor of the potential for biological effects in test animals and a measure of what is happening inside the human body. It is expressed in units of watts per kilogram (W/kg) or milliwatts per gram (mW/g). Because the SAR is difficult to evaluate or measure outside the laboratory, the measurable quantities of magnetic or electric field strengths and power density as well as induced and contact currents are used to define the RF environment and have been correlated with SAR to determine the maximum permissible exposure (MPE) levels (Table 14D-6). In the far-field (greater than one wavelength from RF source), measuring electric field strengths or power density provides reliable exposure assessments. In the near-field or

in contact with RF sources and/or other metallic objects (where many occupational exposures occur), induced and contact current measurements provide the most reliable exposure evaluations. Measuring field strengths or power density is unreliable near or in contact with RF sources or other metallic objects. The MPE values provided are those from the Institute of Electrical and Electronics Engineers Standard, which incorporate the latest scientific findings and recommendations for occupational exposures.[14] Guidelines for limiting RF exposure have also been developed by several other scientific organizations and government agencies, but the differences are minor and efforts are underway to harmonize the various exposure limits.[15-20] In the case of exposure of the whole body, a human adult (height = 175 cm) absorbs RF energy most efficiently when the wavelength is 40 percent of the long axis of the body and parallel to the incident *E*-field vector. This occurs at a frequency of about 70 megahertz (MHz). The RF exposure limits reflect this dependency on frequency and were derived from a SAR of 4 W/kg for those frequencies associated with heating affects (100 kilohertz to 300 gigahertz). In terms of human metabolic heat production, 4 W/kg represents a moderate activity level, such as housecleaning. A safety factor of 10 was applied resulting in a RF exposure limit of 0.4 W/kg, virtually an indistinguishable heating effect from normal temperature variation, exercise, or exposure to the Sun. RF exposures below this level are intended to prevent adverse health effects. However, exposures in excess of the limits are not necessarily harmful, yet without intended benefit, such as lifesaving or medical benefits, these situations are not recommended.

Interpreting RF Measurement Data

Occupational limits—sometimes referred to as *controlled environment*—apply to persons exposed as a consequence of their employment, provided they are fully aware of the potential for exposure and can exercise control over their exposure. There are three fundamental concepts that one should understand when interpreting measurement data: (a) the difference between exposure and emission limits, (b) spatial averaging, and (c) time averaging.

Emission limits are the maximum power output authorized by government authorities for companies or individuals. However, these transmitting signals are often not emitted at the maximum power

TABLE 14D-6

Maximum Permissible Exposure for the Occupational Environments

Frequency Range (MHz)	E-Field[a] Strength (V/m)	H-Field[a] Strength (A/m)	Power Density (S) (mW/cm)^2	Averaging Time (min)
0.003–0.1	614	163		6
0.1–3.0	614	16.3/f		6
3–30	1,842/f	16.3/f		6
30–100	61.4	16.3/f		6
100–300	61.4	0.163	1.0	6
300–3,000			f/300	6
3,000–15,000			10	6
15,000–300,000			10	616,000/f$^{1.2}$

[a] Institute of Electrical and Electronics Engineers (IEEE) report C95.1 1999 Edition.

output. This is especially true for cell-phone base stations or towers, as the amount of power used is proportional to the number of calls handled. For this reason, the emission limit (maximum power output) may not be directly related to exposure potentials. Unlike the emission limits, the exposure guidelines apply to exposure limits, and they are relevant only to locations that are accessible by workers.

Spatial Averaging

The *exposure limits* are based on the concept that the exposures are applied to a whole-body averaged SAR. This means that spot measurements exceeding the stated exposure limits do not imply noncompliance or harmful exposure scenarios if the spatial average of RF fields over the body does not exceed the limits. A *spatial average measurement* may consist of three or more measurements averaged together that span a length of an adult.

Time Averaging

Another feature of the exposure guidelines is that exposures may be averaged over certain periods of time with the average not to exceed the limit for continuous exposure. The averaging time for occupational (controlled environment) exposures is 6 minutes. To properly apply field measurements to the exposure limits, one must consider the length of time the individual is exposed. For example, with the occupational exposure, during any given

6-minute period, a worker could be exposed to twice the applicable limit for 3 minutes as long as they were not exposed at all for the preceding or following 3 minutes. Similarly, a worker could be exposed at three times the limit for 2 minutes as long as no exposure occurs during the preceding or subsequent 4 minutes.

Protective Measures

Engineering Controls

Protection of workers from unnecessary or excessive exposure to RF radiation is accomplished through engineering and administrative controls. Engineering controls are preferred because they eliminate or reduce the potential exposures at the source, but they require a sophisticated level of knowledge to install. Improperly installed controls may actually enhance worker exposures. Interlocks, shielding, bonding, grounding, and filtering are some of the more common controls employed. OSHA requires a lock-out/tag-out program for working with sources of hazardous energies, which may include installing many of the RF controls mentioned above.

The effectiveness of shielding materials varies with the material, geometry, frequency, and where the field reduction is measured. Some are more effective for reducing electric fields, whereas others are more suitable for reducing magnetic fields. One of the most recognizable types of shielding is that used on microwave ovens. The perforated screen is designed to allow penetration of visible light (wavelength about 0.7×10^{-6} to 0.4×10^{-6} m, 430,000,000 to 750,000,000 MHz), but prevents leakage of microwave radiation (wavelength about 12 cm, 2,450 MHz). Perforated or continuous shielding materials reduce exposures by reflection, absorption (attenuation), and internal reflection. The proper selection of material is complex and should be done by qualified individuals.

Techniques that may supplement the use of engineering controls include prudent placement of RF sources, resonant frequency shift, and personal protective equipment. Consideration should be given to building construction materials and layout when installing RF equipment to reduce or prevent unnecessary enhancement of reflected energy at the worker's location. If the operating frequencies are around 10 to 40 MHz, the whole-body SAR may be reduced by separating the body from the ground plane by a small distance with electrically insulating materials. This is known as a *resonant frequency shift*. It reduces worker's absorption characteristics by reducing the flow of current from the body to a grounded surface. This may be especially useful for dielectric heater (plastic sealer) operators by having them stand on a nonconductive platform made of wood or rubber. For plant worksites, metal-reinforced concrete floors act as ground planes. Footwear that reduces the grounding effect achieves the same effect as resonant frequency shift. The level of RF exposure reduction is dependent on the RF frequency and the types of shoes and socks worn by the worker. Wool socks and rubber-soled shoes show the greatest reduction for frequencies below 100 MHz. RF protective suits may be helpful when work must be done in "hot" areas, such as continual radar, onboard naval vessels, and in some communication and broadcast environments. The suit material is typically wool, polyester, or nylon impregnated with a highly conductive threaded metal. Some are more effective than others depending on frequency, orientation of the worker in the environment relative to the incident electric fields, and construction of openings for feet, hands, and head. Washing these suits may reduce their protective capabilities. Some experts also recommend against use of RF-protective suits because the suits may present a potential hazard to individuals near the wearer and increase the hazard to the wearer by allowing closer proximity to open circuits that may act as secondary sources.

Administrative Controls

Administrative controls include increasing the distance between the source and workers, controlling the duration of exposure, restricting access, placing warning signs, providing training commensurate with the level of potential hazard, and real-time monitoring via dosimetry. Increasing the distance between the source and the worker is perhaps the most frequently used control measure and easiest to bypass. Horizontal and vertical distance should be considered when determining the appropriate distance, which is often the distance that results in a radiation level equal to the limit. This is referred to as the *hazard distance*. There are no simple means to calculate the reduction of field strength with distance because the calculation depends on so many factors; however, some researchers have suggested that field strengths are reduced by $1/r^5$ for induction heaters[21] and $1/r^3$ for video display terminals.[22] Controlling the duration of exposure is achieved by applying the time-averaging technique discussed earlier. Installing warning signs, restricting access, and providing training heighten the awareness of those potentially exposed to RF radiation, which may prevent harmful exposures. Finally, real-time monitoring devices, called *dosimeters*, are especially useful in identifying harmful exposures. Actions taken after identifying harmful exposures can reduce exposures. They provide an audible and visual alarm when exposures exceed a predetermined alarming level, giving the wearer immediate notification of a potentially hazardous environment. This equipment also allows the wearer to quickly identify if changes occur during their work activities.

Health Effects

Exposures to electric and magnetic fields (below 300 MHz) emanating from the generation, transmission, and use of electricity have been studied extensively over the past two decades. The current findings and recommendations by various scientific organizations and regulatory agencies continue to acknowledge controversy regarding the potential health effects of chronic low-level EMF exposures to children and adults; yet there remains no clear, convincing evidence of an actual health risk.[23,24] One of the most comprehensive reviews of the scientific literature was published by the International Agency for Research on Cancer (IARC),[25] which found that there is:

1. Limited evidence in humans for the carcinogenicity of ELF magnetic fields in relation to childhood leukemia.
2. Inadequate evidence in humans for the carcinogenicity of ELF magnetic fields in relation to all other cancers.
3. Inadequate evidence in humans for the carcinogenicity of static electric or magnetic fields and ELF electric fields.
4. Inadequate evidence in experimental animals for the carcinogenicity of ELF magnetic fields.
5. No data relevant to the carcinogenicity of static electric or magnetic fields and ELF electric fields in experimental animals were available.

As a result of these findings, IARC concluded that ELF magnetic fields are possibly carcinogenic to humans, and that static electric and magnetic fields and ELF electric fields are not classifiable as to their carcinogenicity to humans.

More than 100 million Americans use wireless communication devices, and this number continues to grow at a rate of about 50,000 new users daily.[26] If the use of wireless communication devices is ever associated with even the slightest increase in risk of adverse health effects, it could become a significant public health problem. Exposures to EMF above 300 MHz have shown a variety of biological responses including varied cell proliferation; reproduction, development, and growth effects; calcium efflux; increases in ornithine decarboxylase (ODC) activity; thermoregulation; cell membrane effects; neural effects; nueroendocrine effects; cardiovascular effects; hematopoiesis and hematologic effects; immune response; biochemical effects; cutaneous effects; cataracts and other ocular effects; increased blood–brain barrier permeability; and changes in behavior.[27] Any measurable change in biological systems may or may not be associated with adverse health effects.

A report of the potential health risks of RF fields from wireless telecommunication devices states: "Scientific studies performed to date suggest the exposure to low intensity non-thermal RF fields do not impair the health of humans or animals. However, the existing scientific evidence is incomplete, and inadequate to rule out the possibility that these non-thermal biological effects could lead to adverse health effects."[28] Although the quality of these studies has improved over time, they continue to suffer from poor exposure assessment information, the lack of a clear biological metric to measure, and confounding factors, such as multiple sources.

The scientific community continues to debate the level of protection necessary to prevent long-term health effects from RF exposures. Many European countries and the World Health Organization promote a precautionary approach by discouraging the widespread use of mobile phones by children for nonessential calls because they may be more vulnerable due to their developing nervous system and longer lifetime of exposures.[29] The Russian National Committee on Non-Ionizing Radiation Protection endorses the WHO precautionary approach and extends the recommendations for children to pregnant women, those suffering from a list of diseases or disorders, and recommends that the duration of cellular phone calls be limited to a maximum of 3 minutes followed by a 15-minute break between calls. The United States does not necessarily endorse the precautionary approach because, without clear, convincing epidemiologic evidence that a health hazard exists from RF exposures, this approach could adversely affect economic development.

Infrared and Ultraviolet Radiation

Infrared radiation (IR) lies at frequencies higher than those of radar waves and microwaves. Nearly 50 percent of the Sun's radiant energy is emitted as IR. It is strongly absorbed by water and the atmosphere, invisible to the eye, and can be detected as warmth by the skin. All objects with temperatures above absolute zero emit IR. In industry, significant levels of IR are produced directly by lamp sources and indirectly by sources of heat, such as heating and drying devices. The primary biological effect is thermal due to absorption in tissue water. For this reason, IR cannot penetrate the skin, leaving a sensation of heat that often serves as an adequate warning sign to take protective action or risk skin burns. The lens of the eye is particularly vulnerable to IR because the lens has no heat sensors and a poor heat-dissipating mechanism. Cataracts may be produced by chronic IR exposure at levels far below those that cause skin burns. Occupations typically at risk of IR exposure include glass blowers, furnace workers, foundry workers, blacksmiths, solderers, oven operators, workers near baking and drying heat lamps, and movie projectionists. Like RF radiation, IR exposure limits are frequency-based, except they represent conditions under which it is believed that nearly all healthy workers may be repeatedly exposed without acute adverse effects. The limits for IR most recognized in the scientific community are published by ACGIH.[30] Control of IR hazards requires (a) shielding of the IR source and eye protection with appropriate IR filters, (b) maximizing the distance between workers and the IR source, and (c) reducing the time spent in areas with high levels of IR exposure.

Ultraviolet radiation (UVR) is produced by the Sun and artificially by incandescent, fluorescent, and discharge types of light sources. It is characterized by three distinct energy bands known as UV-A (400 to 320 nm), UV-B (320 to 280 nm), and UV-C (280 to 200 nm). The first two bands are principal UV components in sunlight, with nearly all of the UV-A reaching the surface of Earth, whereas most of UV-B is absorbed by the stratospheric ozone layer. UV-C is completely absorbed by the ozone layer and oxygen but is artificially produced on Earth. Industrial sources of UVR include arc welding, plasma torches, electric arc furnaces, germicidal and black-light lamps, and certain type of lasers. Because UVR wavelengths are so small, it presents a surface heating hazard.

The most common health effect from overexposure to UVR is the common sunburn (erythema). Chronic, low-level UVR exposure from the Sun is also associated with various skin effects including cancer (basal cell carcinoma, squamous cell carcinoma, and malignant melanoma), premature aging of the skin, solar elastosis (wrinkling), and solar ketatoses (premalignant lesions). Basal cell carcinoma and malignant melanoma are more strongly associated with a history of multiple sunburns, whereas squamous cell carcinoma is associated with total and occupational skin exposure. UVR exposures have also been associated with suppressing the immune system and developing cortical cataracts (UV-B exposure). Photosensitizing agents like coal tar, plants containing furmocoumarins and psoralens, such as figs, lemon and lime rinds, celery, and parsnips, and pharmaceuticals, such as chlorpromazine, chlorpropamide, and tolbutamide, can increase susceptibility to UVR. All these effects vary with individual susceptibilities and location with greater solar UVR exposures. Acute, high-level UVR exposures, especially from UV-B, result in eye injuries that are often realized several hours after the exposure. Photokeratitis (inflammation of the cornea) and photoconjunctivitis (inflammation

of the thin transparent mucous membrane lining the inner surface of the eyelids) are usually reversible within several days. Intense UVR exposure also has an indirect impact on health through its ability to cause photochemical reactions. Small amounts of oxygen and nitrogen can be converted into ozone and oxides of nitrogen, which are respiratory irritants. Halogenated hydrocarbon solvent vapors can decompose into toxic gases such as perchloroethylene into hydrogen chloride and trichloroethylene into phosgene.

Controlling UVR from chronic low-level exposures requires the use of protective clothing and eyewear, sunscreen lotions, and reduced time of exposure. Controlling UVR from acute, high-level photochemical exposures may require proper local exhaust ventilation and isolation of UVR sources from the solvent process. Only qualified personnel

TABLE 14D-7

Laser Classification

Class of Laser[a]	Hazard Potential
1	Pose no potential for injury. No safety measures required to either the eye or skin.
2; 2a	Visible beam posing no significant potential for injury. Blinking response limits exposure.
3; 3a; 3b	Modest potential for injury. Normal aversion response is not sufficient to limit eye exposure to a safe level. Skin hazards normally do not exist. May require safety precautions and personal protective equipment. Class 3b lasers require more safety precautions than Class 3a.
4	Serious potential for injury of the eye and skin. Requires safety precautions and personal protective equipment. Diffuse reflection viewing hazard. Potential fire hazard. Most laser systems for cutting, heat treating, and welding are Class 4.

[a] When Class 3 and 4 lasers are fully enclosed to prevent potentially hazardous laser radiation exposures, the system may be classified as a Class 1 system.

should determine the effectiveness of any particular form of personal protection.

Laser Radiation

Laser is an acronym for light amplification by the stimulated emission of radiation. Uses in industry include heat treatment, glazing, alloying, cladding, cleaning, brazing, soldering, conduction welding, penetration welding, cutting, hole drilling, marking, trimming, and photolithography.[31] Health and safety decisions are based on the class of laser and the wavelength of the laser source. The hazard classification system places lasers into four categories depending on their potential to cause harm from direct beam exposures (Table 14D-7). These exposures may result in at least four types of injury to the eyes and skin, each requiring a special consideration for selecting the appropriate personal protective equipment (Table 14D-8).

Nonbeam hazards, however, constitute the greatest source of noncompliance with United States federal safety codes. Some sources of nonbeam hazards include (a) improper electrical design, (b) lack of knowledge for production of laser-generated air contaminants (LGAC), (c) unwanted plasma radiation, (d) excessive noise levels, (e) inadequate venti-lation controls, (f) fire hazards, (g) explosion issues from high-pressure tubes, and (h) exposure to toxic chemicals and laser dyes. Most of these hazards are associated with Class 3b and Class 4 lasers. In practice, it is always desirable to totally enclose the laser and beam path to prevent direct beam and nonbeam exposures.

Unlike most other workplace hazards, there is generally no need to perform workplace measurements because of the highly confined beam dimensions, the minimum likelihood of changing beam paths, and the difficulty and expense of laser radiometers. However, measurements must be performed by manufacturers to ensure proper laser classification. Laser safety standards are published by government agencies and independent and industrial standards organizations. In the United States, the American National Standards Institute publishes general safety requirements for users ([ANSI] Z136.1 *Standard for the Safe Use of Lasers*). It is not law but forms the basis for state and OSHA requirements. Other laser safety standards and state-specific regulations exist, but these primarily apply to Class 3b and Class 4 installations and maintenance activities.

The ISO and the International Electrotechnical Commission (IEC) have published standards

TABLE 14D-8

Laser Injuries

Type of Hazard	Laser Wavelength (nm)	Target Tissue	Comment
UV photochemical injury	180 to 400 180 to 400 295 to 380	Skin Cornea Lens	Eye protection is required whenever a bluish-white light is seen at the laser focal point.
Blue-light photochemical injury	400 to 550	Retina	Retinal burn has been referred to as "eclipse blindness."
Thermal injury	400 to 1,400 1,400 nm to 1 mm	Retina Skin Cornea Conjuctiva	Nd:YAG lasers pose the greatest risk because the beam image can be intensified of the order 100,000. Most common injury from laser radiation exposure. Biggest concern with CO_2 lasers.
Near-IR thermal injury	800 to 3,000	Lens	Results from molten metal or large, heated surface during treatment. This hazard is only of concern for repeated, chronic exposures.

similar to those in the United States. Two requirements in the ISO documents that affect manufacturers are (a) all systems must be Class 1 during operation; and (b) the manufacturer must specify which materials the equipment is designed to process. Achieving a Class 1 laser rating can be done by installing appropriate engineering controls.

Controlling all aspects of potential laser exposures is complex and requires a qualified individual to assess the direct and nonbeam hazards. Control measures include process isolation, local exhaust and building ventilation, training and education, restricted access, proper housekeeping, preventive maintenance, and use of appropriate personal protective equipment.

REFERENCES

1. Shenk D. Watching you: The world of high-tech surveillance. National Geographic 2003;November:3–29.
2. NCRP. Exposure of the U.S. populations from occupational radiation. Report number 101. Bethesda, MD: National Council on Radiation Protection and Measurement, 1989.
3. Energy employees occupational illness compensation program act, in 20 CFR parts 1 and 30, 2001, pp. 28948–29003.
4. Turner JE. Atoms, radiation, and radiation protection. Pergamon Press, New York, 1986.
5. ICRP. International Commission on Radiological Protection publication 68: Dose coefficients for intakes of radionuclides by workers, Elsevier, New York, 1995.
6. ICRP. International Commission on Radiological Protection publication 66: Human respiratory tract model for radiological protection. Elsevier Health Publishing, New York, 1995.
7. ICRP. International Commission on Radiological Protection publication 84: Pregnancy and medical radiation. Elsevier Health Publishing, New York, 2001.
8. Parsons PA. Radiation hormesis: Challenging LNT theory via ecological and evolutionary consideration. Health Physics 2002;82:513–6.
9. Meinhold CB, Lauriston S. Taylor Lecture: The evolution of radiation protection—from erythema to genetic risks to risks of cancer to . . . ? Health Physics 2004;87:240–8.
10. NIOSH. A recommended standard for occupational exposure to radon progeny in underground mines. Washington, DC: NIOSH, 1987. (DHHS [NIOSH] Publication No. 88-11.)
11. IAEA. IAEA safety standards series: Occupational radiation protection. Safety guide no. RS-G-1.1. Vienna: International Atomic Energy Agency, 1999.
12. CFR. Code Federal Regulation, 29 CFR 1910.96. Washington, DC: U.S. Government Printing Office, Office of the Federal Register.
13. NCRP. Management of terrorist events involving radioactive material, report 138. Bethesda, MD: National Council on Radiation Protection and Measurement, 2001.
14. IEEE. IEEE Standard for safety levels with respect to human exposure to radio frequency electronmagnetic fields, 3 kHz to 300 GHz. New York: Institute for Electrical and Electronics Engineers, Inc., 1999.
15. NCRP. Biological effects and exposure criteria for radiofrequency electromagnetic fields, report 86. Bethesda, MD: National Council on Radiation Protection and Measurements, 1986, pp. 1–382.
16. ICNIRP. Guidelines for limiting exposure to time-varying electric, magnetic and electromagnetic fields (up to 300 GHz). Health Physics 1998;74:494–522.
17. NRPB. Board statement on restrictions on human exposure to static and time-varying electromagnetic fields and radiation, documents of the NRPB, vol. 4, no. 5. Chilton, Didcot, Oxon, UK: National Radiological Protection Board, 1993.
18. Hitchcock RT, Patterson RM. Radio-frequency and ELF electromagnetic energies. A handbook for health professionals. New York: Van Nostrand Reinhold, 1995, pp. 211–58.
19. OET. Evaluating compliance with FCC-specified guidelines for human exposure to radiofrequency electromagnetic fields, bulletin 65. U.S. Federal Communications Commission, Office of Engineering and Technology, 1997.
20. WHO. Framework for developing EMF standards. International EMF project. Geneva: WHO, 2003.
21. Conover DL, Murray WE, Lary JM, et al. Magnetic field measurements near RF induction heaters. Bioelectromagnetics 1986;7:83–90.
22. Walsh ML, Harvey SM, Facey RA, Mallette RR. Hazard assessment of video display units. Am Ind Hyg Assoc J 1991;52:324–31.
23. IEEE. Possible health hazards from exposure to power-frequency electric and magnetic fields—a COMAR technical information statement. IEEE Engineering in Medicine and Biology Magazine 2000;19:131–7.
24. AIHA. Position statement on extremely low frequency (ELF) fields, 2002. Available at: <http://www.aiha.org/GovernmentAffairs-PR/html/PosStatelf.htm>.
25. International Agency for Research on Cancer. IARC monographs on the evaluation of carcinogenic risks to humans. Non-ionizing radiation, part 1: Static and extremely low-frequency (ELF) electric and magnetic fields. Vol. 80. Lyon, France: IARC, 2002.
26. National Toxicology Program. Fact sheet: Studies on radiofrequency radiation emitted by cellular phones, 2003. Dept. of Health and Human Services, Washington, DC.
27. Michaelson SM, Lin JC. Biological effects and health implications of radiofrequency radiation. New York: Plenum Press, 1987.
28. The Royal Society of Canada. A review of the potential health risk of radiofrequency fields from wireless telecommunication devices. An expert panel report prepared at the request of the Royal Society of Canada for Health Canada, 1999. The Royal Society of Canada, Ottawa, Ontario.
29. Maisch D. Children and mobile phones . . . is there a health risk? J Australasian Coll Nutr Environ Med 2003;22:3–8.
30. American Conference of Governmental Industrial Hygienists. Threshold limit values for chemical substances and physical agents and biological exposure indices. Cincinnati, OH: ACGIH, 2004.
31. Ready JF, ed. LIA handbook of laser materials processing. Orlando, FL: Laser Institute of America; Manolia Publishing, Inc, 2001.

BIBLIOGRAPHY

Ionizing Radiation

Cember H. Introduction to health physics. 3rd ed. New York: McGraw-Hill, 1996.
This edition provides a basic understanding of the biophysical bases of ionizing radiation, safety standards, and the key factors in radiation protection. It includes coverage of non-ionizing radiation, laser and microwaves, computer use in dose calculation, and dose limit recommendations. The book emphasizes a problem-solving approach.

National Council on Radiation Protection and Measurement (NCRP). Exposure of the U.S. populations from occupational radiation. Report number 101. Bethesda, MD: NCRP, 1989.
This report provides an overview of occupations exposed to ionizing radiation, purposes for conducting radiation monitoring, and statistical data on average doses received by various work groups.

Non-Ionizing Radiation

National Council on Radiation Protection and Measurements (NCRP). Biological effects and exposure criteria for radio frequency electromagnetic fields, Report 86. Bethesda, MD: NCRP, 1986.
This report provides a basic understanding of the biological effects associated with exposures to radio-frequency radiation, epidemiologic findings, field applications, exposure criteria, and the rationale behind these criteria.

World Health Organization: International Agency for Research on Cancer (IARC). IARC monographs on the evaluation of carcinogenic risks to humans. Volume 80, Non-ionizing radiation, Part 1: Static and extremely low-frequency (ELF) electric and magnetic fields. Lyon, France: IARC, 2002.
This monograph provides a comprehensive review of non-ionizing radiation frequencies below 60 Hz including a description of the fundamental principles, sources, exposures, and animal and human health effects.

CHAPTER 15

Biological Hazards

Mark B. Russi

Infectious hazards in the workplace include a wide range of pathogens. Frequently exposed are health care and animal care workers as well as workers in some other occupations in which the usual microbial environment is altered (Figs. 15-1 and 15-2). High-risk workplaces include those where ill people are treated, those where there is contact with animals, those where contact with anthropod disease vectors or environmental fungi is likely, or those in which exposure to an altered range of diseases in the general environment occurs—such as going to work in a developing country or working (and living in close proximity to others) in the military.

In industrialized countries, the most important type of work setting in which there is increased contact with a broad range of human diseases is health care, where workers may be exposed to pathogens spread via direct contact, the airborne or droplet route, fecal–oral contact, or bloodborne transmission. Primary illnesses spread via the airborne or droplet route include tuberculosis, severe acute respiratory syndrome (SARS), pertussis, parvovirus B19, influenza, varicella, measles, and rubella. Principal bloodborne pathogens are human immunodeficiency virus (HIV), hepatitis B virus (HBV), and hepatitis C virus (HCV). Fecal–oral spread of *Salmonella* and *Shigella* species, enteroviruses, and hepatitis A virus (HAV) may occur in hospitals and other work settings. In addition, health care workers might be exposed to patients infected with bioterrorist agents, such as those that cause smallpox, anthrax, plague, tularemia, and viral hemorrhagic fevers.

Beyond health care, other infectious agents pose risks to a wide spectrum of workers. Zoonotic agent exposures may occur by direct contact with animals or their respiratory secretions or droppings. Veterinarians, farmers, cat and dog breeders, animal handlers, and several other types of workers are at heightened risk. Although arthropod-borne diseases and fungal infections occur in the general population, outdoor work settings may place specific occupational groups, such as forestry workers, farmers, construction workers, and landscapers, at increased risk of contact with mosquitoes or ticks or exposure to agents, such as *Coccidioides immitis* or *Histoplasma capsulatum*, in soil and dust. Finally, workers in developing countries may be exposed to endemic infectious diseases, such as malaria and other parasitic diseases.

BIOLOGICAL HAZARDS IN HEALTH CARE INSTITUTIONS AND LABORATORIES

Bloodborne Pathogens

More than 500,000 needlestick injuries occur annually in the United States, of which at least 5,000 involve HIV-contaminated blood. Unfortunately, there is frequent underreporting of exposures to blood and bodily fluids. For example, in operating rooms, where sharps injuries may occur in 15 percent of procedures, and where blood contact may occur in 50 percent, reporting rates are very low.[1,2] A study comparing incident reports of blood exposures with the actual frequency of such exposures observed at the operating table demonstrated that only 2 to 11 percent were reported.[3] Because early prophylactic therapy is indicated for certain

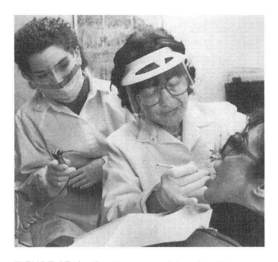

FIGURE 15-1 ● Dentists and dental technicians are at increased risk of exposure to HIV, hepatitis B and C viruses, and other pathogens. They require protection against pathogens in aerosols, blood, and saliva. The worker closest to the patient has eye, but no respiratory, protection (no mask), whereas the other worker has a mask but lacks eye protection. Both workers should have masks and eye protection. (Photograph by Marvin Lewiton.)

exposures, underreporting places health care workers at unnecessary risk of infectious disease.

Guidelines and regulations have been designed to reduce bloodborne exposures among health care workers. Universal Precautions, developed by the Centers for Disease Control and Prevention (CDC) in 1987, were incorporated into the Occupational Safety and Health Administration (OSHA) Bloodborne Pathogen Standard in 1991, along with a requirement for annual training, exposure reduction plans, engineering controls, and provision of hepatitis B vaccine to potentially exposed health care workers. In 1995, Standard Precautions were introduced, combining Universal Precautions with body substance isolation into a set of procedures for patient care and handling of blood and potentially infectious body fluids.

Needlestick injuries can be reduced through educational programs and by replacement of unsafe instruments with safer devices (Fig. 15-3). Significant reductions have been demonstrated with introduction of safety features on phlebotomy devices, adoption of needleless intravenous delivery

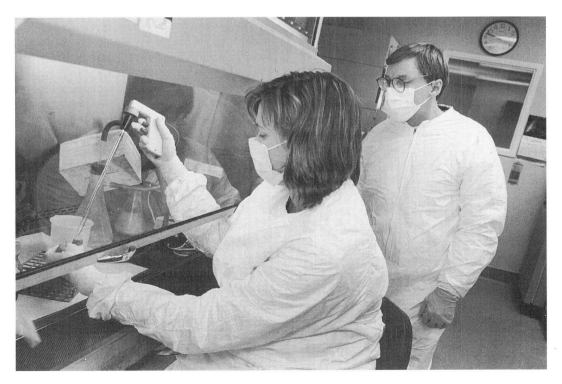

FIGURE 15-2 ● Workers in an HIV/AIDS laboratory are at risk of acquiring HIV infection. This photograph shows HIV/AIDS laboratory workers using personnel protective equipment and exhaust ventilation under a hood. (Photograph by Earl Dotter.)

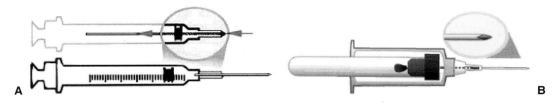

FIGURE 15-3 ● Shown above are two devices that help prevent accidental needlesticks (sharp sticks). (**A**) Syringe with retractable needle: After the needle is used, an extra push on the plunger retracts the needle into the syringe, thus removing the hazard of needle exposure. (**B**) Blunt-tipped blood-drawing needle: After blood is drawn, a push on the collection tube moves the blunt-tip needle forward through the needle and past the sharp needle point. The blunt point tip of this needle can be activated before it is removed from the vein or artery.

systems, use of blunt needles for certain procedures, and educational programs on needle safety. The Needlestick Safety and Prevention Act of 2000 recognized the potential for safer devices to reduce bloodborne pathogen exposures among health care workers and required OSHA to amend the Bloodborne Pathogens Standard to require that employers document consideration and implementation of appropriate commercially available and effective safer medical devices designed to minimize or eliminate occupational exposure.[4]

Although a broad range of infections can be transmitted percutaneously or mucocutaneously, the bloodborne pathogens of greatest significance for health care workers are HIV, HBV, and HCV.

HIV

As of late 2004, CDC had learned of 57 health care workers in the United States having become HIV-positive after occupational exposure, among whom were 24 nurses, 19 laboratory workers, 6 physicians, 2 surgical technicians, 2 housekeeping/maintenance workers, 1 dialysis technician, 1 respiratory therapist, 1 health aide, and 1 morgue technician. Forty-eight of them had percutaneous exposure; 5, mucocutaneous exposure; 2, both cutaneous and mucocutaneous exposure; and for 2, the exposure route was not known.

It is thought that there is an 0.3 percent risk of HIV infection after a needlestick exposure involving an HIV-positive patient. Characteristics associated with a higher risk of seroconversion include deep injury, visible contamination of the device with blood, needle placement directly into an artery or vein, or exposure to an individual with an elevated HIV titer. Risk of seroconversion after mucous membrane exposure to HIV has been estimated at 0.09 percent.[5] The risk of seroconversion

after isolated skin exposure has not been quantified but is likely to be extremely low.

The U.S. Public Health Service recommends prophylactic treatment of individuals exposed to HIV-contaminated blood or body fluids with antiretroviral medications. Several lines of evidence support use of prophylaxis. Health care workers who became HIV-positive after bloodborne exposure to HIV were significantly less likely to have used antiretroviral prophylactic medication (zidovudine).[6] Administration of zidovudine to HIV-positive pregnant women significantly lowered maternal–fetal transmission of HIV from 22.6 percent to 7.6 percent, suggesting that zidovudine may act prophylactically in the fetal circulation.[7] According to animal studies, drug efficacy is decreased if treatment is not begun until 48 or 72 hours after exposure or if the treatment course is only 3 or 10 days rather than 28 days.

A major challenge to effective use of antiretroviral therapy is drug resistance. A recent study showed that 39 percent of 41 source persons whose HIV was sequenced had primary genetic mutations associated with resistance to reverse transcriptase inhibitors.[8] Several seroconversions have occurred despite prophylaxis with one or more antiretroviral medications, potentially due to viral resistance, late initiation of therapy, inadequate length of therapy, or an overwhelming inoculum of virus. In prescribing combination antiretroviral therapy to exposed health care workers, probable patterns of viral resistance should be considered, based on source patient medication history. Drug toxicities also should be monitored closely in health care workers receiving prophylaxis. A broad range of side effects has been reported.[9] In addition, many workers experience concerns about their possibly placing sexual partners or other family members at risk, implications for future pregnancies, and career options. Clinicians treating exposed workers should counsel them—and sometimes partners and family members—on the use of barrier protection to prevent pregnancy and HIV transmission.

Health care workers exposed to HIV-infected blood or body fluids should receive prophylaxis as soon as possible after exposure. Health care workers traveling to work in HIV-endemic areas in other countries, where prophylactic medications may not be readily available, should be provided these medications before they leave, in case an exposure takes place.[10]

Hepatitis B

Due to the implementation in medical centers of Standard Precautions and widespread hepatitis B vaccination, the estimated incidence of hepatitis B infections among health care workers is approximately one-fifth that of the general population. Percutaneous exposure to HBV-infected blood is associated with a seroconversion risk of 1 to 6 percent if a source patient is e-antigen negative and to 22 to 31 percent if the source patient is e-antigen positive.[11] Viral titers may be as high as 1 billion virions per milliliter of blood or serous fluid but are generally several orders of magnitude lower in saliva, semen, and vaginal secretions. HBV is resistant to drying, ambient temperatures, simple detergents, and alcohol and may survive on environmental surfaces for up to 1 week.[12] A sharp object contaminated with HBV may pose a threat to health care workers for several days after last contact with a source patient.

Less than half of individuals who become infected with HBV manifest acute symptoms. Acute illness generally consists of several weeks of malaise, jaundice, and anorexia, but fulminant hepatitis develops in approximately 1 percent of patients. Chronic infection develops in approximately 5 percent of patients and is generally accompanied by the persistent presence of hepatitis B surface antigen (HB_sAg) in the blood for more than 6 months. In people whose infections do not become chronic, hepatitis B surface antibody (anti-HB_s) develops as HB_sAg levels fall. IgM antibodies to hepatitis B core antigen (HB_cAg) indicate current infection, whereas IgG core antibodies are a marker of past infection. The e-antigen (HB_eAg), which is separated from HB_cAg during intracellular processing, is a marker of core antigen production and viral replication. Cirrhosis develops in an estimated 20 to 35 percent of people with chronic

hepatitis B, about 20 percent of whom will develop hepatocellular carcinoma.

Administration of hepatitis B vaccine generates immunity in more than 90 percent of those who receive three vaccine doses. Once established, immunity persists even if anti-HB_s titers fall or become undetectable. The duration of immunity is not known, but there is no recommendation for periodic booster doses. Individuals who do not produce anti-HB_s after vaccination should have the series of three vaccine doses repeated. Those who do not mount an anti-HB_s response to the vaccine after repetition of the series should be counseled regarding their susceptibility to HBV and should receive hepatitis B immune globulin (HBIG)—and possibly additional vaccine if exposed percutaneously or mucocutaneously to HBV-contaminated blood or body fluids. HBIG, which should be administered as soon as possible after an exposure, is approximately 75 percent effective in preventing HBV infection in those without vaccine-induced protection.

The single most effective step to prevent HBV infection among health care workers is vaccination. Despite an OSHA requirement that employers provide vaccine free of charge to health care workers, a surprising number of workers remain at risk. A 1992 survey conducted at 150 hospitals revealed that slightly more than half of eligible employees had completed the vaccine series. A more recent survey of more than 100 hospitals demonstrated that approximately two-thirds of employees had completed the vaccine series.[13]

Hepatitis C

Prevalence of HCV infection among health care workers is about the same as in the general population—approximately 1.5 percent. After percutaneous exposure to infected blood, risk of seroconversion among exposed health care workers averages 1.8 percent.[14] Infection after mucocutaneous exposure appears to be much less common. The incubation period for hepatitis C varies from 2 to 24 weeks, and averages 6 to 7 weeks. Antibodies to HCV may be detected within 6 weeks of infection and may persist, regardless of whether or not HCV is actively replicating. The vast majority of those who become infected with HCV have no acute symptoms. Chronic hepatitis develops in approximately 85 percent of those infected.

No hepatitis C vaccine is available, and administration of immune globulin is ineffective.

Several studies have demonstrated the efficacy of interferon-alpha-2b in treating chronic hepatitis C; and treatment during acute infection or early in the course of chronic HCV infection may be associated with higher cure rates.[15] Patients with symptomatic acute hepatitis C are more likely to spontaneously clear HCV than are patients with asymptomatic infection.[16] For symptomatic acutely infected individuals, delaying therapy with interferon or interferon/ribavirin until approximately 12 weeks from the onset of symptomatic disease would lessen the likelihood of unnecessary therapy in individuals destined to clear virus spontaneously. Given the lower apparent likelihood of spontaneous clearance among individuals with asymptomatic acute infection, initiation of therapy may be prudent after infection is documented by polymerase chain reaction (PCR) assay and seroconversion. Given the high cure rates associated with acute therapy and the toxicities of interferon and ribavirin, there is no role for prophylactic therapy in individuals exposed percutaneously or mucocutaneously to HCV-infected blood or body fluids. Exposed individuals should be monitored at 6 weeks, 3 months, and 6 months for seroconversion. PCR testing can be used to detect early infection or to confirm the presence of HCV.

Other Infections

Tuberculosis

After a resurgence of tuberculosis (TB) in the United States during the 1980s and early 1990s, disease incidence has fallen in recent years, although TB remains the single most important infectious cause of death worldwide. It is important to distinguish between infection with *Mycobacterium tuberculosis*, the organism that causes TB, and active disease. Approximately 95 percent of individuals who become infected will wall off the organism through a healthy immune response and will never develop active disease. These individuals are considered to have latent infections and cannot infect others. Risk for developing active disease is highest within the first 2 years of infection. It is increased when the infected individual has compromised immune response, which may occur with HIV infection, malnutrition, diabetes mellitus, and other diseases, as well as cancer chemotherapy. In 2002 in the United States, 5.2 cases of active TB were reported per 100,000 population—a total of 15,075 cases, representing a 44 percent rate decrease compared to 1992, when cases most re-

cently peaked. The proportion of total U.S. cases among the foreign-born now exceeds 50 percent with a foreign-born case rate of 23.1 per 100,000—eightfold higher than that among persons born in the United States. In the 1997–2002 period, the top five countries of origin for TB cases in the United States were Mexico, the Philippines, Vietnam, India, and China. The proportion of patients with multidrug-resistant TB decreased from 2.5 percent in 1998 to 1.2 percent in 2002. Despite a currently decreasing population incidence, health care workers without appropriate engineering and administrative controls and personal protective equipment remain at risk.

In response to increasing TB rates in the late 1980s and early 1990s as well as occupational transmission in several medical centers, CDC issued guidelines in 1990 and 1994 recommending that health care facilities at high risk for TB transmission develop and implement programs to prevent occupational exposure to TB.[17] The guidelines addressed early identification of potentially infectious patients, engineering controls to minimize spread of TB within a medical center, use of personal protective equipment, and medical surveillance among health care workers. For the potentially infectious patient placed in negative pressure isolation, work practice controls included respiratory isolation signage, use of N95 respirators by all individuals entering the isolation room, and restriction of diagnostic and therapeutic procedures to negative pressure isolation settings. The National Institute for Occupational Safety and Health (NIOSH) has published a set of guidelines to assist health care facilities implement respiratory protection programs for TB; appendices of the document include names and addresses of respirator manufacturers, respirator fit testing procedures, and checklists useful for program evaluation.[18]

TB skin testing is based on a healthy immune response to the presence of *Mycobacterium tuberculosis* and may be positive in persons with latent infection as well as those with active disease. The most reliable type of skin testing utilizes intradermal injection of Purified Protein Derivative (PPD). A decreasing incidence of PPD conversion among health care workers during the past decade is testament to the success of administrative and engineering controls and personal protective equipment in health care facilities. A study, based on the experience of three hospitals in high TB-prevalence areas after implementation of the 1994 CDC Guidelines for Preventing the Transmission of Mycobacterium

Tuberculosis in Health-Care Facilities, found neither an elevation of PPD conversion rates among health care workers nor an association between TB care and PPD conversion.[19] Others have reported a similar experience. Administrative controls (early isolation of suspected tuberculosis patients) and engineering controls (adequate ventilation rates) have been strongly associated with the reduced rates of PPD conversion among health care workers.[20,21] Despite recent successes in TB control, it is important to recall past outbreaks in health care facilities, which caused substantial morbidity among health care workers. A review of 11 separate outbreaks during the 1928–1991 period showed skin test conversion rates ranging from 15 to 100 percent and active TB in 11 to 61 percent of skin test converters. This same review revealed that health care workers who were already PPD-positive at the time of exposure did not experience elevated risks of active TB due to the exposure in this outbreak.[22]

PPD skin testing is currently the method of choice for medical surveillance among health care workers. Guidelines recommend that health care workers with negative tuberculin tests be tested at time of hire. Because positive skin tests can wane with time, but may be "boosted" by repeated skin testing, those in whom testing has not been performed within the preceding year should receive a two-step test to ensure adequate test sensitivity. In addition to prior infection, vaccination with BCG, a live, attenuated form of *Mycobacterium bovis* used in many developing countries to reduce TB infection among children, sometimes produces a positive skin test initially or on two-step testing, particularly if BCG vaccination has been recent. It is important to establish accurate baseline skin testing results to avoid mistakenly identifying a "boosted" response as a new infection, as a new infection requires an intensive public health search for a source patient and carries with it different recommendations for chemoprophylaxis for the worker. Recommended frequency of ongoing testing is based on a risk assessment that considers community TB prevalence and frequency of inpatient TB admissions. Individuals with documented positive tuberculin tests should not be retested but should undergo monitoring for symptoms suggestive of active TB. Once a negative chest x-ray is documented after PPD conversion, serial screening chest x-rays should not be done. PPD skin reactions may be suppressed by some illnesses or medications and may be difficult to interpret in areas where non-

TB mycobacterial infections are common. Newer serologic tests, which have been developed to help address the shortcomings of PPD test interpretation, are being evaluated for clinical utility.

OSHA withdrew its proposed TB standard but has continued to require employers to meet the general duty of providing a workplace free of recognized hazards, which includes identifying potential respiratory hazards and providing respiratory protection. Based on the hazard, the employer is required to select an appropriate form of respiratory protection and to implement a formal program that includes fit testing and training.

Severe Acute Respiratory Syndrome

From November 2002 through July 2003, a total of 8,098 people worldwide were reported as having SARS, a newly recognized respiratory disease caused by a coronavirus. The disease, which appears to be transmitted primarily by droplets and direct contact, spread to more than 1,700 health care workers. In some hospital settings, primarily because of delayed recognition of the disease, attack rates among health care workers were nearly 60 percent. Worldwide, SARS caused 774 deaths in the 2002–2003 period, with a case fatality rate of 9.6 percent.

After an incubation period of about 2 to 10 days, clinical illness was characterized by fever, shaking, chills, headache, malaise, and sometimes diarrhea. Lower respiratory tract involvement followed, which was the usual cause of death in those who did not recover. Mortality rates varied widely, with one hospital outbreak having a case fatality rate of 3 percent among patients less than 60 years old, and 54 percent among patients 60 and older, many of whom had underlying illnesses.[23]

Transmission of SARS varied considerably. Although most patients with SARS did not transmit the disease to others, some were "superspreaders" who accounted for widespread transmission in certain settings, such as in hotels, apartment buildings, and hospitals, and on airplanes. One particular superspreading event, which occurred when a physician who had treated SARS patients in Guangdong Province of China stayed in a Hong Kong hotel, and was then admitted to a hospital, eventually infected approximately 100 workers at the hospital and gave rise to SARS epidemics in several other countries.

The key step in preventing transmission of SARS to health care workers is early recognition of disease and proper isolation of possibly infected

patients. SARS has often been spread from patients who had been hospitalized for many days before their infections with the coronavirus that causes SARS was recognized. In one such incident, an index patient possibly exposed 10,000 other patients and visitors and 930 hospital staff members, leading to a nationwide SARS outbreak in Taiwan. Since the SARS epidemic of 2003, there have been some cases associated primarily with laboratory exposures to the coronavirus, and secondary spread has been limited.

CDC guidelines recommend various measures to screen for SARS patients with respiratory symptoms or atypical pneumonia, depending on the local epidemiology of the disease. To minimize transmission in physicians' offices, clinics, and hospitals of respiratory pathogens, including the coronavirus that causes SARS, it has been recommended that symptomatic patients wash their hands and wear surgical masks. Even when health care workers have used personal protective equipment, certain patient care activities, such as intubation, have been associated with SARS transmission,[24] possibly due to improper wearing of equipment, inadvertent direct contact, or inadequate face seals with respirators that had not been fit tested.

Research is attempting to identify the origin of the virus that causes SARS, to improve diagnostic testing and treatment options, and to develop a vaccine against this disease. A virus very similar to the human SARS coronavirus has been found in several animals, including the Himalayan palm civet; antibodies to this virus have been detected in 40 percent of wild animal traders and 20 percent of tested animal slaughterers at a live animal market in China.[25] Antibodies to human SARS coronavirus and/or animal SARS-CoV-like virus have been detected in 1.8 percent of healthy adults in Hong Kong whose serum was banked in 2001—before the SARS epidemic in China.[26] Many believe the human SARS coronavirus mutated from viruses that have circulated among certain animals for some time. PCR testing may allow for early diagnosis of SARS, although maximal titers in respiratory secretions generally occur at day 10 of infection, with maximal stool titers generally at day 14 or later. False negatives and false positives may occur. Comparison of serum antibody levels at time of clinical presentation and 28 days after disease onset is the most accurate way to confirm a diagnosis. Research is being performed to develop a vaccine, but its development will probably take many years.

BIOLOGICAL HAZARDS IN SCHOOLS, HEALTH CARE INSTITUTIONS, AND OTHER WORKPLACES

Measles

The introduction of measles vaccine in 1963 was associated with a 99 percent decrease in measles incidence in the United States. However, from 1989 to 1991, more than 55,000 cases were reported in the United States, mostly in children under the age of 5 and disproporionately in unvaccinated Hispanic and African-American children. From 1989 to 1991, a total of 123 people died of measles-related illness, half of whom were under age 5 and 90 percent of whom had not been vaccinated. Since then, the incidence rate of measles has fallen, and, in 2000, expert consultants convened by CDC concluded that measles is no longer endemic in the United States, all U.S. cases appearing to have been imported, generally from Europe or Asia, with limited domestic spread due to high vaccine coverage. Health care institutions should nevertheless continue to maintain measles vaccination programs for their staff members, as several measles epidemics in the past have been linked to health care settings. Because measles may be spread by large droplets and via airborne transmission, airborne precautions must be used when caring for a measles patient. Hospitals, schools, and day care centers should be vigilant for imported measles cases, especially in children from Europe or Asia.

Rubella

Since the licensure of rubella vaccine in 1969, rubella cases in the United States have decreased from more than 57,000 (in 1969) to fewer than 300 (in 1999)—more than 80 percent of which occurred in adults, most of whom were born in Mexico, Central American countries, or elsewhere. The principal hazard of rubella virus is its potential to affect fetal development. In an outbreak reported in 1980, 47 health care workers at a Boston hospital developed rubella, and a pregnant health care worker elected to terminate her pregnancy. In another outbreak, 56 hospital employees developed rubella, and three women terminated their pregnancies. More recently, rubella outbreaks have tended to occur in workplaces (other than hospitals) that employ a large proportion of foreign-born workers.[27] Rubella virus is spread via droplets. It is most contagious at the time rash is erupting, although virus may be shed from 1 week before to 5–7 days after onset of the rash. Infants with congenital rubella may excrete virus for months to years. Droplet Precautions must be used when caring for patients with rubella. Health care workers should be vaccinated if they do not have evidence of rubella immunity.

Varicella (Chickenpox)

Varicella may be spread by contact with infected lesions or via the airborne route. Incubation is generally 2 weeks but may range from 10 to 21 days after exposure. Populations at risk for more severe disease include immunocompromised patients, pregnant women, and premature infants. Adults generally have more severe disease than children. From 1990 to 1994, fewer than 5 percent of varicella cases occurred among adults older than 20, but these patients accounted for 55 percent of varicella-related deaths. Outbreaks may occur in hospitals when staff members without immunity care for patients with unrecognized disease. Varicella vaccine is recommended for nonimmune health care workers, teachers of young children, day care workers, military personnel, those who work in institutional settings and prisons, and international travelers. It must not be given to pregnant women. Because the vaccine provides only partial protection in some individuals, many medical centers require that only health care workers with immunity from natural disease care for infected patients. As the epidemiology of varicella changes due to widespread vaccination of children, this practice will need to be revisited. Exposed hospital staff members without varicella immunity should be prevented from having patient contact between days 10 and 21 after contact with an infected patient.

Parvovirus B19

Parvovirus has been transmitted to health care workers infrequently. Risk of parvovirus infection among school and day care teachers generally exceeds that of health care workers. Parvovirus is spread via large droplets, direct contact, or fomites. Patients with erythema infectiosum (fifth disease) rash are infectious before the appearance of the rash. Infected adults generally suffer a self-limited viral arthropathy. Those with parvovirus-associated aplastic crisis are infectious for up to 1 week after onset of illness. Infected immunocompromised persons may be infectious for months or years. Patients hospitalized during a phase of disease when transmission may occur should be treated using droplet precautions. When women become infected during the first half of pregnancy, there is a small risk of fetal death due to hydrops or spontaneous abortion.

Pertussis

Pertussis is easily spread by droplets or direct contact, with an attack rate of 80 percent in unvaccinated individuals. Immunity from whole-cell pertussis vaccine has been shown to wane over 5 to 10 years. Immunity from acellular vaccine also appears to wane. Although clinical illness among adults is generally milder than that among children, many adults are at risk for disease, and no vaccine is licensed for use in those over age 7. Several outbreaks have involved health care workers.[28] Schoolteachers and day care workers are also at risk. A 2-week course of erythromycin is indicated for prophylaxis of those with close exposures to infected individuals. Resistance to erythromycin appears to be very rare, and CDC currently does not recommend routine resistance testing. Alternative prophylactic regimens include trimethoprim–sulfamethoxazole, clarithromycin, or azithromycin.

Influenza

In the United States each year, more than 110,000 people are hospitalized due to influenza or its complications, and an average of approximately 36,000 die each year from the disease. Hospitals represent workplaces at higher than usual risk of influenza transmission, which generally occurs via large droplets. Patients hospitalized with influenza should be treated using droplet precautions. In adults, virus may be shed from 1 day prior to illness to 7 days after onset. Children may excrete virus for longer periods. The most effective means of influenza prevention is annual vaccination, which is specifically recommended for health care workers. Vaccine consists of killed virus from three strains (H3N2, H1N1, and B strain) designed closely to match annually circulating strains. Generally, vaccine prevents disease in 70 to 90 percent of healthy immunized adults when the match of circulating and vaccine strains is close. Amantadine, rimantidine, and oseltamivir may be administered in outbreak settings to prevent influenza in nonimmunized adults. Amantadine, rimantidine, oseltamavir, and zanamavir may be used to reduce the duration of influenza by approximately 1 day, on average, if given during the first 24 to 48 hours of symptoms.

In 1997, the first instance of transmission of avian influenza virus (H5N1) to a person was documented. Since then, several transmissions have taken place, including transmissions in Vietnam and Thailand during the 2003–2004 influenza season. Mortality of avian influenza is high, but so far human-to-human disease transmission has been limited. An avian influenza strain capable of widespread transmission from human to human would represent a public health emergency of global proportion.

Hepatitis A

Although outbreaks of hepatitis A have occurred in health care facilities, the prevalence of hepatitis A antibodies among health care workers is similar to that of the general population. CDC currently does not recommend hepatitis A vaccine for health care workers. Transmission has occurred in hospitals during care of patients with diarrhea who were later discovered to be acutely infected with hepatitis A virus (HAV), as well as through contamination of food due to improper handwashing after patient-care activities (Box 15-1). Outbreaks may occur in day care centers, particularly in the setting of community transmission. However, staff members at day care centers do not have a substantially

---

BOX 15-1

Food Safety

Sherry L. Baron

Since the publication of Upton Sinclair's *The Jungle* 100 years ago, food safety has remained a major public health priority. Federal, state, and local public health agencies face challenges ranging from the routine maintenance of sanitation standards in community food service establishments to the complex challenges of protecting the food supply against inadvertent and deliberate contamination. CDC estimates that foodborne diseases cause approximately 76 million cases of illness, 325,000 hospitalizations, and 5,000 deaths in the United States each year.[1] Most individuals with a foodborne illness experience symptoms of mild gastroenteritis and often go undiagnosed; a small proportion may develop severe diarrhea, renal failure, neurological symptoms, or hepatitis. As with other environmentally related illnesses, young children and the elderly are often the most severely affected.

Toxic chemical contamination of food falls into three main categories:

- Residues of pesticides deliberately applied to crops or to stored or processed foods;
- Colorings, flavorings, or other chemicals deliberately added to foods during processing; and
- Chemicals that inadvertently enter the food supply, such as mercury, polychlorinated

biphenyls (PCBs), and persistent pesticide residues, such as DDT.

Pathogenic contamination of foods includes:

- Viruses, such as hepatitis A virus and Norwalk virus;
- Bacteria, such as *Salmonella* and *Campylobacter* species, and *E. coli* 0157:H7;
- Protozoa, such as *Toxoplasma gondii* and *Cryptosporidium* and *Cyclospora* species; and
- Aquatic microorganisms that elaborate toxins, such as *Pfiesteria* species and dinoflagellates responsible for producing red tides.

The global system of production and distribution of food products often makes the identification and control of foodborne disease outbreaks extremely complex. For example, in 1997 the CDC identified multiple clusters of cases of gastroenteritis caused by a protozoan, *Cyclospora*. Of the approximately 1,500 recognized cases, almost half occurred after about 50 catered luncheons held in various cities throughout the country. Most of the cases were eventually tied to raspberries from a single Guatemalan exporter obtained from five farms. Although the investigation never definitively identified the source of contamination, investigators believed it resulted from the use of contaminated irrigation water. A temporary ban on importation of Guatemalan raspberries was

(continued)

BOX 15-1

Food Safety (Continued)

implemented and a laboratory method for rapid identification of *Cyclospora* contamination was developed.[2]

Prevention of Foodborne Illnesses

The prevention of foodborne illness is accomplished most effectively through the routine use of safe food-handling techniques in private homes, retail establishments, and agricultural and food-processing facilities. Most foodborne illness can be prevented when individuals (a) wash fruits and vegetables with water to remove pathogens and pesticide residues; (b) avoid raw milk products, eggs, fish, and meat (especially by young and older people and those who are immunocompromised); (c) thoroughly cook meat, poultry, and eggs to assure that pathogens are killed; (d) when preparing poultry, wash with hot water and soap hands, cutting boards, and cooking utensils that come in contact with raw poultry; and (e) refrigerate prepared foods. The use of chemical agents is not more effective than soap and water in eliminating contamination.

Once an infection occurs, primary care practitioners play a key role in the early identification and eventual control of foodborne illnesses.[3] Every outbreak begins with an index patient who may not be severely ill. Clinicians who treat patients may be the only ones with the opportunity to make an early diagnosis that prevents further illness. Clinicians should contact state or local health department epidemiologists or others who are the best qualified to determine whether and how to initiate an outbreak investigation. Often, clinicians who collect the appropriate information can contribute the clue that ultimately leads to identification of the source of an outbreak

Clinicians must have a high degree of suspicion and ask appropriate questions. Important characteristics of the illness include (a) incubation period; (b) major clinical symptoms and duration of symptoms; and (c) the identification of others who may have similar symptoms. Clinicians seeing patients should specifically ask about the consumption of high-risk foods, such as raw or poorly cooked food items, unpasteurized milk or juices, home-canned goods, fresh produce, or soft cheeses made from unpasteurized milk. Other important potential risk factors include living on or visiting a farm; contact with pets; attending day care; working in certain occupations, such as animal handling; foreign travel; travel to coastal areas; camping excursions to mountains or other areas where untreated water is consumed; and attendance at group picnics or similar outings.

If foodborne illness is suspected, clinicians should submit appropriate specimens for laboratory testing. In most laboratories, routine stool cultures are limited to screening for *Salmonella* and *Shigella* species as well as *Campylobacter jejuni/coli*. Cultures for other organisms require additional media or incubation conditions; if such organisms are suspected, advance notification or communication with laboratory and infectious disease personnel is necessary.

U.S. government responsibility for the prevention of foodborne illnesses is shared by several agencies. The Department of Agriculture sets and enforces standards for the control of pathogens in meat, poultry, and egg products. The Food and Drug Administration (FDA) is responsible for establishing and enforcing most other food-related regulations, including those for the control of food additives. An extensive network of state and local public health agencies assist in enforcing food safety standards. The Environmental Protection Agency (EPA) prevents food contamination by controlling the level of permissible contamination of water sources that could result in contamination of fish, livestock, and crops. Finally, CDC, in conjunction with state and local health departments, is responsible for monitoring and investigating outbreaks of suspected foodborne illness.

(continued)

BOX 15-1

Food Safety (Continued)

References

1. Mead PS, Slutsker L, Dietz V, et al. Food-related illness and death in the United States. Emerg Infect Dis [serial online]. 1999;5:607–25. Available at: <www.cdc.gov/ncidod/eid/vol5no5/mead.htm>.
2. Herwaldt BL. Cyclospora cayetanensis: A review focusing on the outbreaks of cyclosporiasis in the 1990s. Clin Infect Dis 2000;31:1040–57.
3. Diagnosis and management of foodborne illnesses: A primer for physicians and other health care professionals. Produced collaboratively by the American Medical Association, American Nurses Association–American Nurses Foundation, CDC, Center for Food Safety and Applied Nutrition, FDA, Food Safety and Inspection Service, and U.S. Department of Agriculture. MMWR 2004;53(RR04):1–33.

Bibliography

<www. foodsafety.gov>
The official U.S. government food safety information Web site with comprehensive information regarding all aspects of food safety.

increased prevalence of HAV infection compared to control populations.[29]

Agents of Bioterrorism

After the attack on the World Trade Center in September 2001 and the distribution of anthrax spores in the U.S. mail system during October 2001, substantially increased attention has focused on preparedness for terrorism. Bioterrorism agents are viewed as credible threats, due to their capacity for widespread dissemination and their potential to make ill or kill many people. CDC classifies such disease agents into three categories: Category A diseases/agents are those that can be easily disseminated or transmitted from person to person, result in high mortality rates and have potential for major public health impact, might cause public panic and social disruption, and require special action for public health preparedness. Category B disease/agents are considered moderately easy to disseminate, result in moderate morbidity rates and low mortality rates, and require specific enhancements of diagnostic capacity and enhanced disease surveillance. Category C diseases/agents include those that could be engineered for mass dissemination in the future due to their availability, ease of production and dissemination, and potential for high morbidity and mortality rates.

Category A agents include *Bacillus anthracis* (anthrax), *Clostridium botulinum* toxin, *Yersinia pestis* (plague), variola major (smallpox), *Francisella tularensis* (tularemia), and the viruses that cause Ebola, Marburg, Lassa, and Machupo hemorrhagic fevers. Category B agents include *Brucella* species (brucellosis), Epsilon toxin of *Clostridium perfringens*, food safety threats (*Salmonella* species, *Escherichia coli* 0157:H7, and *Shigella* species), *Burkholderia mallei* (glanders), *Burkholderia pseudomallei* (melioidosis), *Chlamydia psittaci* (psittacosis), *Coxiella burnetii* (Q fever), ricin toxin, staphylococcal enterotoxin B, *Rickettsia prowazekii* (typhus fever), viral encephalitis (alphaviruses such as those that cause Venezuelan equine encephalitits, eastern equine encephalitis, western equine encephalitis), and water safety threats (*Vibrio cholerae* and *Cryptosporidium parvum*). Category C agents include Nipah virus and hantavirus and other agents that cause emerging infections.

Potential bioterrorism agents vary widely in their propensity for person-to-person transmission. For many agents, such as those that cause anthrax, tularemia, and Q fever as well as biological toxins, only Standard Precautions are required to prevent transmission from infected patients to health care workers. However, infected patients who have not been adequately decontaminated may harbor anthrax or other spores on their skin or clothing that could cause disease in health care providers. For some agents, for which the primary means of transmission is close contact, such as smallpox virus and the viruses that cause hemorrhagic fever, isolated examples of airborne spread dictate use of respiratory protection when providing patient care.[30,31] Anyone rendering care to a patient with smallpox should receive smallpox vaccine. Droplet Precautions should be employed by those caring for pneumonic plague and certain types of viral encephalitis. Contact precautions are indicated for the care of patients with brucellosis.

During the anthrax outbreak of 2001, a total of 23 people developed inhalational or cutaneous disease, of whom 6 died. Clinical presentations included fever, flu-like symptoms, cough, dyspnea, pleuritic chest pain, nausea or vomiting, headache, and chest discomfort. Presence of shortness of breath, nausea, and vomiting and lack of rhinorrhea (runny nose) helped to distinguish the initial clinical presentation of anthrax from influenza or influenza-like illness. For postal workers, the most important factor for survival was clinical suspicion of anthrax based on work history, which led examining physicians to obtain blood cultures during the initial visit. For approximately 10,000 people potentially exposed to anthrax who did not have symptoms, prophylactic regimens were offered,[32] most commonly 60-day courses of ciprofloxacin or doxycycline—although overall adherence was poor. The most common side effects of prophylaxis were nausea, vomiting, diarrhea, and abdominal pain.

Military personnel considered to be at risk of a bioterrorist attack with smallpox virus have been vaccinated. Health care workers who might be required to care for smallpox patients have also been offered the vaccines, but only a small percentage have chosen to be vaccinated, due to widespread concerns about the side effects of smallpox vaccine, which frequently include fever and less commonly include erythema multiforme, generalized vaccinia, myocarditis, and life-threatening conditions, such as eczema vaccinatum, progressive vaccinia, and post-vaccinia encephalitis. With only marginal acceptance by health care workers of pre-event vaccination, emphasis has switched to rapid vaccination strategies should actual smallpox cases occur.[33–35]

BIOLOGICAL HAZARDS ASSOCIATED WITH ANIMAL CONTACT

Many bacterial, fungal, parasitic, viral, and rickettsial diseases (zoonoses) are transmissible from animals to humans (Table 15-1). Workers who have frequent contact with wild animals, farm animals, or domestic pets are at highest risk of infection.

A wide range of workers, including park rangers, hunters, ranchers, forestry workers, trappers, fur traders, geologists, other scientific field workers, butchers, rendering workers, expedition leaders, and zoo workers have contact with wild animals, such as rats, mice, bats, rabbits, raccoons, skunks, deer, and bison. For some diseases, relatively close animal contact is required for transmission, while for others, illness may occur by ingesting small amounts of water or food contaminated by animal waste (such as giardiasis due to contaminated water) or by breathing animal waste–contaminated dusts (such as histoplasmosis). Diseases for which workers with wild animal contact may be at increased risk include brucellosis (bison, deer, and other wild animals), raccoon roundworm infestation (raccoons), giardiasis (many animals), hantavirus infection (wild mice), histoplasmosis (bat guano), lymphocytic choriomeningitis (house mice and other rodents), tuberculosis (deer, elk, and bison), plague (wild rodents), rabies (raccoons, skunks, and bats), and tularemia (rodents, rabbits, and hares).

Contact with macaque monkeys, which may occur in an animal laboratory setting or a monkey cell culture facility or among veterinarians, may lead to transmission of herpes B simiae virus to humans, causing an often-fatal encephalomyelitis. Transmission usually occurs by bites, scratches, or other exposures to the tissues or secretions of macaques. Immediate and thorough wound cleansing is indicated after a macaque bite. Prophylactic treatment with acyclovir or valacyclovir is indicated for percutaneous or mucocutaneous exposures to potentially infected animals.

Farm workers and those who process farm products, such as meat packers, butchers, and slaughterhouse workers, may be exposed to cattle, sheep, pigs, goats, domestic fowl, horses, and other animals. Because many farm workers live, eat, and sleep in the farm environment, their level of contact with livestock and/or livestock waste may be particularly high. Diseases that may be transmitted in the farm environment include brucellosis, *Campylobacter* gastroenteritis, cryptosporidiosis, *Escherichia coli* 0157:H7 infection, Q fever (due to *Coxiella burnetti* from cattle, sheep, and goats), rabies, ringworm infestation, salmonellosis (especially chicken and horses), and yersiniosis (due to *Yersinia enterocolitica* from pigs). Bovine spongiform encephalopathy (BSE, or *mad cow disease*) is a neurological degenerative disease of cattle, likely caused by a prion. Consumption of BSE-infected meat has been strongly associated with variant Creuzfeldt–Jakob disease in humans, but

TABLE 15-1

Zoonoses, Causative Agents, and Transmitting Animals and Situations

Zoonoses	Transmitting Animals and Situations
Bacterial Diseases	
Brucellosis (*Brucella* species)	Farm animals and dogs
Campylobacteriosis (*Campylobacter* species)	Cats, dogs, farm animals, and improper food preparation
Cat scratch disease or cat scratch fever (*Bartonella henselae*)	Cat scratches and bites
Escherichia coli O157:H7	Cattle and improper food preparation
Fish tuberculosis (*Mycobacterium* species)	Fish and aquarium water
Leptospirosis (*Leptospira* species)	Livestock, dogs, rodents, wildlife, and contaminated water
Lyme disease (*Borrelia burgdorferi* infection)	Dogs and ticks
Plague (*Yersinia pestis*)	Wild rodents, cats, and fleas
Psittacosis (*Chlamydia psittaci*)	Pet birds, including parrots and parakeets
Q fever (*Coxiella burnetti*)	Cattle, sheep, goats, dogs, and cats
Salmonellosis (*Salmonella* species)	Reptiles, birds, dogs, cats, horses, farm animals, and improper food preparation
Tuberculosis (*Mycobacterium tuberculosis*)	Deer, elk, bison, and cattle
Tularemia (*Francisella tularensis*)	Sheep and wildlife, especially rodents and rabbits
Yersiniosis (*Yersinia enterocolitica*)	Dogs, cats, farm animals, and improper preparation of chitterlings
Fungal Diseases	
Cryptococcosis (*Cryptococcus* species)	Wild birds, especially pigeon droppings
Histoplasmosis (*Histoplasma* species)	Bat guano (stool)
Ringworm (*Microsporum* species and *Trichophyton* species)	Mammals, including dogs, cats, horses, and farm animals
Parasitic Diseases	
Cryptosporidiosis (*Cryptosporidium* species)	Cats, dogs, and farm animals
Giardiasis (*Giardia lamblia*)	Various animals and water
Hookworm infestation (*Ancylostoma caninum, Ancylostoma braziliense*, and *Uncinaria stenocephals*)	Dogs and their environment
Leishmaniasis (*Leishmania* species)	Dogs and sand flies
Raccoon roundworm infestation (*Baylisascaris procyonis*)	Raccoons
Roundworm infestation (*Toxocara canis, Toxocaris cati*, and *Toxocaris leonina*)	Cats, dogs, and their environment
Tapeworm infestation (*Dipylidium caninum*)	Flea infections in cats and dogs
Toxoplasmosis (*Toxoplasma gondii*)	Cats and their environment
Viral Diseases	
Hantavirus pulmonary syndrome (hantavirus)	Wild mice
Herpes B infection (herpesvirus 1)	Macaque monkeys
Lymphocytic choriomeningitis	Rodents such as rats, guinea pigs, and house mice
Monkeypox	Suspected to be associated with prairie dogs, Gambian rats, and rabbits
Rabies	Mammals, including dogs, cats, horses, and wildlife
West Nile virus	Mosquitoes
Rickettsial Diseases	
Rocky Mountain spotted fever (*Rickettsia rickettsii*)	Dogs and ticks
Other (Possibly Due to a Prion)	
Bovine spongiform encephalopathy (BSE), or mad cow disease	Associated with cattle

farm workers are not at increased risk for this disease.

Enhanced contact with pet animals may occur among breeders, delivery personnel, veterinarians, pet-shop workers, and others. Illnesses associated with dogs include brucellosis (rarely), *Campylobacter* gastroenteritis, cryptosporidiosis, dipylidium (tapeworm) infestation, giardiasis, hookworm infestation, leptospirosis, Lyme disease, Q fever, rabies, ringworm infestation, Rocky Mountain spotted fever, roundworm infestation, salmonellosis, and *Toxocara* (roundworm) infestation. Many of the same illnesses are associated with cats; cat scratch disease (caused by *Bartonella henselae*), and plague (rarely) can also be transmitted from cats. Bird-associated illnesses may occur among veterinarians, pet-shop workers, poultry workers, and bird breeders, including psittacosis (from parrots and parakeets), Q fever (from ducks and geese), cryptococcosis (from wild bird/pigeon droppings), and salmonellosis (from chickens, baby chicks, and ducklings). Human cases of monkeypox have been reported in association with pet prairie dogs. Smallpox vaccine, which may be 85 percent protective for monkeypox, is recommended for workers investigating monkeypox outbreaks or involved in the care of infected people or animals.

BIOLOGICAL HAZARDS ASSOCIATED WITH ARTHROPOD VECTORS

Contact with arthropod vectors, especially mosquitoes and ticks, may occur frequently among many of the occupational groups at high risk for zoonoses. Park rangers, landscapers, nursery workers, farmers, ranchers, trappers, construction workers, and soldiers are at increased risk.

A number of types of encephalitis are transmitted in the United States by mosquito vectors. Eastern equine encephalititis, transmitted primarily from birds to humans by a mosquito bite, is very rare but has a case fatality rate of 35 percent. Coastal areas and freshwater swamps represent areas of high transmission. Western equine encephalitis, also rare, has a lower case fatality rate. La Crosse encephalitis, less rare, is typically transmitted from chipmunks or squirrels to humans via the treehole mosquito (*Aedes triseriatus*). Workers in woodland areas are at increased risk. St. Louis encephalitis is transmitted from birds to humans by primarily *Culex* mosquitoes. In temperate areas, St. Louis encephalitis occurs primarily during the late summer and early fall but may occur year-round in Southern states. West Nile virus, a flavivirus common in Africa, West Asia, and the Middle East and closely related to St. Louis encephalitis virus, has been introduced into the United States. It is transmitted primarily from birds to humans by mosquitoes, with outbreaks in temperate regions mainly in late summer and early fall. Year-round transmission takes place in milder climates. During 2003, a total of 9,862 West Nile cases were reported to CDC, with 2,866 of these people suffering encephalitis, meningitis, or meningoencephalitis.

Tick bites represent another occupational hazard for outdoor workers. The most important illnesses associated with tick vectors are Lyme disease, Rocky Mountain spotted fever, babesiosis, and ehrlichiosis. Lyme disease is caused by *Borrelia burgdorferi* and transmitted to humans by blacklegged ticks (*Ixodes scapularis* in the north central and northeastern United States and *Ixodes pacificus* on the Pacific Coast). Infection is most likely to be transmitted if the tick has fed for 2 or more days. Workers in woodland areas of the north central and northeastern Unites States, and in a limited region of the northwestern Pacific Coast, are at highest risk. Lyme disease can be effectively treated with oral antibiotics if recognized early. Rocky Mountain spotted fever is caused by *Rickettsia rickettsii* and spread either by the American dog tick, which predominates in central and eastern areas of the United States as well as along the coast of California, or the Rocky Mountain wood tick, which predominates in the Rocky Mountains. Most infections are transmitted from April through September. The greatest concentrations of cases have occurred in the South Atlantic states.

Babesiosis is caused primarily by the parasites *Babesia divergens* and *Babesia microti*. Disease is spread from mice to humans primarily by the *Ixodes scapularis* tick and is characterized by fever, chills, myalgia, hepatosplenomegaly, and hemolytic anemia. It is treated with clindamycin plus quinine or atovaquone plus azithromycin. Ehrlichiosis is caused primarily by three distinct bacterial species of the genus *Ehrlichia*. In the United States, ehrlichiosis due to *Ehrlichia chaffeensis* occurs primarily in the southeastern and south central states and is transmitted by the lone star tick, *Amblyomma americanum*. *Ehrlichia ewingii* has caused a few cases of human ehrlichiosis in Missouri, Oklahoma, and Tennessee. Human granulocytic ehrlichiosis is caused by a third *Ehrlichia* species and is transmitted by black-legged ticks (*Ixodes scapularis* or *Ixodes pacificus*).

Preventive measures, which should be used by outdoor workers to prevent transmission of mosquito- or tick-borne illnesses, include wearing lightly colored, long-sleeve shirts tucked into pants and lightly colored, long pants tucked into socks; using DEET-containing insect repellants; using mosquito netting when sleeping outdoors; avoiding outdoor work at dawn and dusk; and checking skin and hair for ticks daily. Permethrin-containing repellants may be used on clothing, shoes, bed nets, and camping gear.

TRAVELERS' HEALTH

Travelers are at risk of encountering disease in other countries. The most common cause of illness in travelers is contamination of food or water. Travelers' diarrhea can be due to bacteria, including *E. coli*, *Salmonella* species, and *Vibrio cholera*; viruses; or parasites. Many illnesses are transmitted to travelers via arthropod vectors, including malaria, yellow fever, dengue, filariasis, leishmaniasis, trypanosomiasis, and onchocerciasis. Schistosomiasis can be transmitted through the skin during swimming in fresh water. Travelers should wash their hands frequently, drink only bottled or boiled water or canned drinks, eat only thoroughly cooked food or self-peeled fruits and vegetables, comply with malaria prophylaxis recommendations, and protect themselves from mosquito bites (as described above). They should not eat food purchased from street vendors, drink beverages with ice, eat unpasteurized dairy products, handle animals, or swim in fresh water. Prior to departure, workers traveling to developing countries should consult with a travel medicine specialist. Prevention and treatment information can also be found at <www.cdc.gov/travel>.

REFERENCES

1. Centers for Disease Control and Prevention. Evaluation of blunt suture needles in preventing percutaneous injuries among health-care workers during gynecologic surgical procedures—New York City, March 1993-June 1994. MMWR 1997;46:25–9.
2. Quebbeman EJ, Telford GL, Hubbard S, et al. Risk of blood contamination and injury to operating room personnel. Ann Surg 1991;214:614–20.
3. Lynch P, White MC. Perioperative blood contact and exposures: A comparison of incident reports and focused studies. AJIC 1993;21:357–63.
4. Federal Register. 2001;66(18 Jan.):5317–25.
5. Bell DM. Occupational risk of human immunodeficiency virus infection in healthcare workers: an overview. Am J Med 1997;102(Suppl 5B):9–14.
6. Cardo DM, Culver DH, Ciesielski CA, et al. A case-control study of HIV seroconversion in health care workers after percutaneous exposure. N Engl J Med 1997;337:1485–90.
7. Sperling RS, Shapiro DE, Coombs RW, et al. Maternal viral load, zidovudine treatment, and the risk of transmission of human immunodeficiency virus type 1 from mother to infant. N Engl J Med 1996;335:1621–9.
8. Beltrami EM, Cheingsong R, Respess R, et al. Antiretroviral drug resistance in HIV-infected source patients for occupational exposures to healthcare workers [Abstract P-S2-70]. In: Program and Abstracts of the 4th Decennial International Conference on Nosocomial and Healthcare-Associated Infections. Atlanta, GA: CDC, 2000, p. 128.
9. Centers for Disease Control and Prevention. Serious adverse events attributed to nevirapine regimens for postexposure prophylaxis after HIV exposures—worldwide, 1997–2000. MMWR 2001;49:1153–6.
10. Russi M, Hajdun M, Barry M. A program to provide antiretroviral prophylaxis to health care personnel working overseas. JAMA 2000;283:1292–3.
11. Centers for Disease Control and Prevention. Updated U.S. Public Health Service Guidelines for the management of occupational exposures to HBV, HCV, and HIV and recommendations for postexposure prophylaxis. MMWR 2001;50(RR11):1–42.
12. Beltrami EM, Williams IT, Shapiro CN, et al. Risk and management of blood-borne infections in health care workers. Clin Microbiol Rev 2000;13:385–407.
13. Mahoney FJ, Steward K, Hu H, et al. Progress toward elimination of hepatitis B virus transmission among health care workers in the United States. Arch Intern Med 1997;157:2601–5.
14. Centers for Disease Control and Prevention. Recommendations for follow-up of health-care workers after occupational exposure to hepatitis C virus. MMWR 1998;47:603–6.
15. Jaeckel E, Cornberg M, Wedemeyer H, et al. Treatment of acute hepatitis C with interferon alfa-2b. N Engl J Med 2001;345:1452–7.
16. Gerlach JT, Diepolder HM, Zachoval R, et al. Acute hepatitis C: High rate of both spontaneous and treatment-induced viral clearance. Gastroenterology 2003;125:80–8.
17. Centers for Disease Control and Prevention (CDC). Guidelines for preventing the transmission of Mycobacterium tuberculosis in health care facilities, 1994. MMWR 1994:43: No. RR-13.
18. DHHS (CDC): TB respiratory protection program in health care facilities: Administrator's guide. Atlanta: DHHS, 1999. (DHHS publication no. 99–143.)
19. Tokars JI, McKinley GF, Otten J, et al. Use and efficacy of tuberculosis infection control practices at hospital with previous outbreaks of multidrug-resistant tuberculosis. Infect Control Hosp Epidemiol 2001;22:449–55.
20. Blumberg HM, Watkins DL, Berschling JD, et al. Preventing the nosocomial transmission of tuberculosis. Ann Intern Med 1995;122:658–63.
21. Menzies D, Fanning A, Yuan L, et al. Hospital ventilation and risk for tuberculous infection in Canadian health care workers. Canadian Collaborative Group in Nosocomial Transmission of TB. Ann Intern Med 2000;133:779–89.

22. Stead WW. Management of health care workers after inadvertent exposure to tuberculosis: A guide for the use of preventive therapy. Ann Intern Med 1995;122: 906–12.

23. Varia M, Wilson S, Sarwal S, et al. Investigation of a nosocomial outbreak of severe acute respiratory syndrome (SARS) in Toronto, Canada. Canadian Medical Association Journal (CMAJ) 2003;169:285–92.

24. Centers for Disease Control and Prevention. Cluster of severe acute respiratory syndrome cases among protected health-care workers—Toronto, Canada, April 2003. MMWR 2003;52:433–6.

25. Guan Y, Zheng BJ, He YQ, et al. Isolation and characterization of viruses related to the SARS coronavirus from animals in southern China. Science 2003;302:276–8. Published online 4 September 2003; 10.1126/science.1087139.

26. Zheng BJ, Guan Y, Wong KH, et al. SARS-related virus predating SARS outbreak, Hong Kong. Emerg Infect Dise 2004;10:176–8.

27. Centers for Disease Control and Prevention. Control and prevention of rubella: Evaluation and management of suspected outbreaks, rubella in pregnant women, and surveillance for congenital rubella syndrome. MMWR 2001;50:1–23.

28. Weber DJ, Rutala WA. Management of healthcare workers exposed to pertussis. Infect Control Hosp Epidemiol 1994;15:411–15.

29. Centers for Disease Control and Prevention. Prevention of hepatitis A through active or passive immunization: Recommendations of the Advisory Committee on Immunization Practices (ACIP). MMWR 1999;48(RR12): 1–37.

30. Carey DE, Kemp GE, White HA, et al. Lassa fever epidemiological aspects of the 1970 Epidemic, Jos, Nigeria. Trans R Soc Trop Med Hyg 1972;66:402–8.

31. Gelfand HM, Posch J. The recent outbreak of smallpox in Meschede, West Germany. Am J Epidemiol 1971;93:234–7.

32. Shepard CW, Soriano-Gabarro M, Zell ER, et al. Antimicrobial postexposure prophylaxis for anthrax: Adverse events and adherence. Emerging Infectious Diseases abbreviated as Emerg Infect Dis 2002;8:1124–1132.

33. Kaplan EH, Craft DL, Wein LM. Emergency response to a smallpox attack: The case for mass vaccination. Proc Nati Acad Sci USA 2002. Accessed at www.pnas.org/cgi/doi/10.1073/pnas.162282799.

34. Mack T. A different view of smallpox and vaccination. N Engl J Med 2003;348:460–3.

35. Bozzette SA, Boer R, Bhatnagar V, et al. A model for a smallpox-vaccination policy. N Engl J Med 2003;348:416–25.

CHAPTER 16

Occupational Stress

Joseph J. Hurrell Jr. and Carlos Aristeguieta

Nowhere are the rising costs of work-related chronic ill-health more evident than in the area of occupational stress. For example, claims for stress-related illnesses in California increased by approximately 560 percent over a 6-year period, inflating costs for individuals, organizations, and society at large.[1] Disability due to job stress alone—without evidence of any physical injury or illness—is now a compensable condition in about one-half of U.S. states.

Despite increased recognition by the legal, medical, and insurance communities, for many people—even scientists—stress remains an intuitively understandable yet nebulous construct, implying numerous events and processes. Although there are many definitions of job stress, it can be most simply viewed as the harmful physical and emotional responses that occur when the requirements of the job do not match the capabilities, resources, or needs of the worker.

Stress-related responses are ubiquitous in human society. This chapter focuses specifically on work-related stress. Other important sources of stress that impact individuals and communities include unemployment, poverty, environmental exposure, racial and ethnic discrimination, violence, and other factors that are beyond the scope of this chapter.

A BRIEF HISTORY OF JOB-STRESS RESEARCH

Occupational stress, as a field of inquiry examining job conditions and their health and performance consequences, is a relatively new research domain that crystallized in the early 1970s. Its conceptual roots can be traced to the animal research of Hans Selye and to Walter Cannon's work on the physiologic concomitants of emotion. In the early 1930s, Selye discovered that a wide variety of noxious stimuli—which he later referred to as *stressors*—such as exposure to temperature extremes, physical injury, and injection of toxic substances, evoked identical patterns of physiologic changes in laboratory animals. In each case, the cortex of the adrenal gland became enlarged, the thymus and other lymphatic structures became involuted, and deep-bleeding ulcers developed in the stomach and intestines. These effects were *nonspecific*; that is, they occurred regardless of the particular stressor and were superimposed on any specific effects associated with the individual agents. Some years later, Selye described this somatic response as the general adaptation syndrome (GAS) and defined stress as the nonspecific response of the body to any demand. His mention of *nervous stimuli* among the stressor agents capable of eliciting the GAS had an energizing effect on investigators working in the field of psychosomatic medicine. Cannon had laid the groundwork earlier for an understanding of how emotions affect physiologic functions and disease states in his description of the *fight-or-flight response.* This response, elicited by potentially dangerous situations, involved elevated heart rate and blood pressure, redistribution of blood flow to the brain and major muscle groups and away from distal body parts, and a decrease in vegetative functions. Perhaps equally important, Cannon advanced the concept of *physiologic homeostasis,* and developed an "engineering" concept of stress and strain—with stress as the "input" and strain as the response. In particular, Cannon proposed the notion of critical stress levels that were capable of producing strain in homeostatic mechanisms. Although he used the term somewhat casually, Cannon, like Selye, conceived of *stress* as involving physical as well as emotional stimuli.

In the 1960s and 1970s, Richard Lazarus and his colleagues added immensely to the study of stress by describing in specific terms how an organism's perceptions or appraisals of objective events determine their health valence. Cognitive appraisal was described by Lazarus as an intrapsychic process that translates objective events into stressful experiences. The importance of this formulation lies in its recognition that subjective factors can play a much larger role in the experience of stress than objective events. Indeed, any given objective event can at once be perceived positively by one person and negatively by another; that is, "One person's meat is another person's poison."

The study of occupational stress was given impetus in the early 1970s by the establishment of the National Institute for Occupational Safety and Health (NIOSH), whose goal is to conduct research to reduce work-related illnesses and injuries. The importance of behavioral and motivational factors was clearly acknowledged in certain research provisions of the Occupational Safety and Health Act (OSHAct). For example, Sections 20(a)(1) and 20(a)(4) explicitly directed NIOSH to include psychological, behavioral, and motivational factors in research on problems of worker safety and health and in developing remedial approaches for such problems. Job-related hazards were interpreted broadly to include conditions of a psychological nature—undue task demands, work conditions, or work regimens that, apart from or combined with exposure to physical and chemical hazards, may degrade workers' physical or mental health. Since its inception, NIOSH has not only sponsored, but also conducted, many research studies, which have helped shape the course of job-stress research in the United States. For example, in 1988, NIOSH proposed a national strategy for prevention of work-related psychological disorders. Key elements in this prevention strategy include abatement of known job (environmental) risk factors, research to improve understanding of these risk factors, surveillance to detect and track risk factors, education and training to facilitate recognition of risk factors and their control, and improved mental health services.[2]

In 1996, NIOSH identified "organization of work" as one of the 21 priority research topics for the next decade and developed a comprehensive research agenda for investigating and reducing occupational safety and health risks associated with the rapidly changing nature of work.[3] This document describes how macrolevel forces impact occupational stress levels. For example, national and international economic, legal, political, technological, and demographic forces influence production methods, human resource policies, management structures, and supervisory practices. These factors, in turn, directly impact the work context, influencing the nature of jobs and the tasks that compose them. For example, fueled by global competition, organizational downsizing and restructuring has influenced not only the way work is performed but also—as many laid-off workers can attest—whether work was available to perform.

A MODEL OF JOB STRESS AND HEALTH

Working conditions play a primary role in causing job stress. However, the role of individual factors cannot be ignored. Exposure to stressful working conditions (job stressors) can have a direct influence on worker safety and health.[4] But individual and situational factors can intervene to strengthen or weaken this influence (Fig. 16-1). Individual and situational factors can modulate the effects of job stressors on the risk of illness and injury in different ways: they can decrease or completely deflect them, leave them unchanged, or potentiate them.

Based on this view of job stress, a paradigm of stress was developed by researchers at NIOSH to guide efforts at examining the relationship between working conditions and health consequences (Fig. 16-2). In this paradigm, job stress is viewed as a situation in which job stressors—alone or in combination with other stressors—interact with individual worker characteristics and result in an acute disruption of psychological or physiologic homeostasis. This disruption (often called *job strain*) can be psychological (disruption in affect or cognition); physiological; or behavioral. Job strain, if prolonged, is thought to lead to a variety of disorders, including cardiovascular disease, psychological disorders, and musculoskeletal disorders. In addition, job stressors are probably linked to risk of

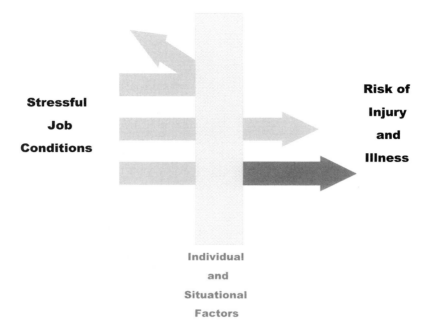

FIGURE 16-1 ● This NIOSH model of job stress illustrates the different roles that individual and situational factors can have in reducing the impact of job stress (top arrow), having no effect on job stress (middle arrow), or exacerbating job stress (bottom arrow). (Source: National Institute for Occupational Safety and Health. *Stress at work.* Washington, DC: NIOSH, 1999. [DHHS [NIOSH] publication no. 99-101.])

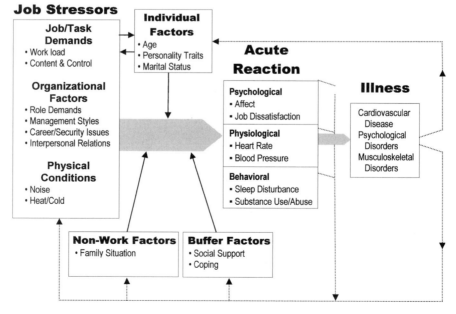

FIGURE 16-2 ● Detailed model of job stress and health.

workplace injury and violence. Job stressors also have strain consequences for organizations (often called *organizational strain*) in the form of increased absenteeism, decreased performance, increased rate of accidents, and increased likelihood of employees looking for alternative employment (turnover).

Job stressors generally fall into three very broad categories: job/task demands, organizational factors, and physical conditions. Examples of common stressors in each category are briefly described in the following sections.

Job and Task Demands

Workload is a feature of occupations that is easily recognized as stressful and has received substantial empirical attention (Figs. 16-3 and 16-4). The strains associated with being overworked have been found to be uniformly negative—psychologically, physiologically, and behaviorally. Working excessive hours or performing more than one job, for example, has been associated with a variety of health consequences, including poor perceived health, increased injury rates, and increased cardiovascular disease morbidity and mortality[5] (Box 16-1). Issues of workload and work pace become increasingly important in an environment where hours of work

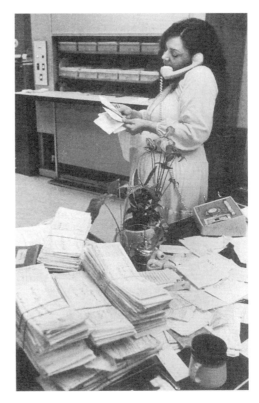

FIGURE 16-4 ● Secretaries often experience high levels of workload and report high levels of stress. (Photograph by Earl Dotter.)

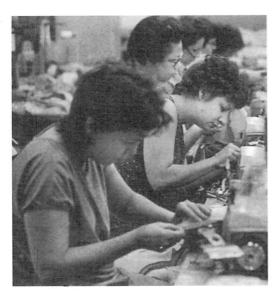

FIGURE 16-3 ● Garment workers, who often work on a piecework basis, can experience much stress at work. (Photograph by Earl Dotter.)

are increasing. In the United States, working couples have seen their average work year increase by nearly 700 hours in the past two decades, and 30 percent of workers are exhausted by the end of the workday.[3]

Shift work, a work-related stressor, is another job demand associated with health and safety consequences (Box 16-2). Working rotating shifts or permanent night work results in disruption of social activities and physiological circadian rhythms, impairing alertness and the sleep cycle.[6] For example, employees report that working nights or overtime affects their mental and physical health. The decreased alertness that occurs in these workers makes them more prone to errors and increases their risk for injuries. Most workers state that they work shifts because it is required by the job or because there was no other job available. Another source of stress comes from the friction between the shift schedule and the family and social life of the worker. Furthermore, rotating shift-work is associated with

BOX 16-1

Time, Work, and Stress on the Job and in Society

Sherry L. Baron

One of the most pronounced changes affecting working people and their families is how they experience and perceive time as a result of changes in demographics, society, technology, and work organization. Although the length of average workweek for full-time workers has not changed considerably over the past several decades, a substantial percentage of Americans—more than 26 percent of men and more than 11 percent of women—worked 50 or more hours per week in 2000. The sense of control of time at work, in the family, and in society has adverse effects on the health and well-being of workers, their partners, and their children—an important focus for research. Time demands can increase work stress, which is associated with both adverse mental and physical health outcomes (Chapters 16 and 26).

Although average working hours have not increased, several factors have transformed the way the overall family experiences time. The most dramatic change has been the rapid increase in women's participation in the workforce. In 1970, in only 35 percent of married couples, both spouses worked; today, 60 percent of married couples are dual wage-earners. In the same period, there has been an increase in single-parent families, from about 10 percent of all families in 1970 to about 20 percent today. The result is that spouses have less time with each other and parents have less time with their children.

The schedule challenges of the dual-earning and single-parent families are made worse by the increasing proportion of workers employed in jobs requiring work hours outside of the standard 9-to-5 workday and the Monday-to-Friday workweek. In one of three dual-earner families and one in five single-parent families with children under 14, a parent works either a rotating or a nonstandard work shift. Whether single mothers or dual-earner couples *choose* nonstandard work in order to trade off childcare responsibilities between themselves or with extended family members, or are forced into those jobs because they do not have other options, there may be adverse impacts on family activities—especially those that require parental interactions at school or other activities geared to standard schedules.

The experience and perception of time at work has changed as well. As the productivity rate in workplaces continues to increase, the introduction of new technology and the intensification of job tasks mean that employees experience greater job demands. For very different reasons and in quite different ways, both salaried and hourly wage-earners may experience a sense that there is never enough time and always too much stress. Downsizing and outsourcing often require professionals and managers to work longer hours and take work home. Increased demand for after-hour and weekend services, in addition to the increased productivity demanded in manufacturing, means that low-wage workers often have to work nonstandard workweeks and work shifts, including rotating shifts, night work, or split shifts. Whereas the status of salaried professionals allows them more flexibility to leave work early in the event of a family responsibility, hourly workers usually are not allowed such flexibility.

Bibliography

Jacobs JA, Gerson K. The time divide: Work, family and gender inequality. Cambridge, MA: Harvard University Press, 2004.

Presser HB. Working in a 24/7 economy: Challenges for American families. New York: Russell Sage Press, 2003.

increased rates of cardiovascular and gastrointestinal disease. These effects are sufficiently well established to provide the basis of labor law in the European Union, which regulates the scheduling of shifts and rest days.

Narrow, fragmented, invariant, and short-cycle tasks that provide little stimulation, allow little use of skills or expression of creativity are job characteristics that are considered stressors in the NIOSH model.[2] Robert Karasek's demand–control–social support model is perhaps the best known of all models relating such job characteristics to well-being.[7] This model proposes first that high job demands, lack of job control, and lack of social support predict strain outcomes. In addition, this model suggests that demands, control, and social support interact

BOX 16-2

Shift Work

David H. Wegman

Shift work is an imprecise concept, although it usually refers to a work-hour system in which a relay of employees extends the period of production beyond the conventional daytime third of the 24-hour cycle. There are four major types of work hours: day work, permanently displaced work hours, rotating shift work, and roster work.

Day work involves work periods between approximately 7 a.m. and 7 p.m. *Permanently displaced* work hours require the person to work either a morning shift (approximately 6 a.m. to 2 p.m.), an afternoon shift (approximately 2 to 10 p.m.), or a night shift (approximately 10 p.m. to 6 a.m.). *Rotating shiftwork* involves alternation between two or three shifts. Two–shift-work usually involves morning and afternoon shifts, whereas three–shift-work also includes the night shift. Three–shift-work is often subdivided according to the number of teams used to cover the 24 hours of the work cycle—usually three to six teams, depending on the speed of rotation (number of consecutive shifts of the same type). *Roster work* is similar to rotating shift work but may be less regular, more flexible, and less geared to specific teams. It is used in service-oriented occupations, such as transport, health care, and law enforcement. In most industrialized countries, approximately one-third of the population has some form of "non-day work" (shift work). Approximately 5 to 10 percent have shift work that includes night work.

Effects on Health and Well-being

Sleep

The dominant health problem reported by shift workers is disturbed sleep and wakefulness. At least three-fourths of shift workers are affected. The sleep loss is primarily taken out of stage 2 sleep and REM sleep. Furthermore, the time taken to fall asleep (sleep latency) is usually shorter. The level of sleep disturbances in shift workers is comparable to that seen in insomniacs.

Alertness, Performance, and Safety

Night-oriented shift workers complain as much of fatigue and sleepiness as they do about disturbed sleep. This is particularly severe on the night shift, hardly appears at all on the afternoon shift, and is intermediate on the morning shift. The maximum is reached toward the early morning (5 to 7 a.m.). Frequent incidents of falling asleep occur during the night shift, and this has also been documented through ambulatory EEG recordings in process operators, truck drivers, train drivers, pilots, and the like. Remarkably, even though one-fourth exhibit sleep incidents, most workers seem unaware of them. This suggests an inability to judge one's true level of sleepiness.

Performance on Night Shift is Impaired

A classic study showed that errors in meter readings over a period of 20 years in a gas works had a pronounced peak on the night shift. Other studies demonstrated that telephone operators connected calls considerably more slowly at night and that train engineers failed to operate their alerting safety device more often at night. Performance may be reduced to levels comparable with those seen in connection with considerable alcohol consumption. There is evidence that the Challenger space shuttle disaster and the nuclear power plant incidents at Chernobyl, Three Mile Island, the David Beese reactor in Ohio, and the Rancho Seco reactor in California were due to fatigue-related errors during night work. Concern about resident physician performance after prolonged shifts has led to changes in residency on-call rules. Recent studies have documented an increase of motor vehicle crashes after prolonged shifts.

Other Effects on Health and Well-Being

Gastrointestinal complaints are more common among night-shift-workers than among day workers. There is a higher incidence of coronary artery disease in male shift-workers than in men who work days. As with gastrointestinal disease, a high prevalence of smoking among shift workers might contribute to the increased risk of coronary artery disease, but smoking alone cannot explain the observed

(continued)

BOX 16-2

Shift Work (Continued)

elevated risk. A few studies of pregnant shift workers suggest an increased risk of miscarriage and lower birthweight of infants of mothers who worked irregular hours but did not suggest a risk of birth defects. Health problems in shift workers usually increase with age as exposure to shift work increases. Being a "morning-type" person, as opposed to an "evening-type" person, is associated with poorer adjustment to shift work. Gender is not related to shift-work tolerance, although the extra burden of housework may put women at a disadvantage. Good physical condition of the worker may facilitate shift work.

One of the major effects of shift work is the interference of work hours with various social activities. Thus, direct time conflict reduces the amount of time available to spend with family and friends or in recreation or voluntary activities.

Factors Affecting Adjustment

Shift-System Characteristics

Aside from the night shift per se, an important shift-system characteristic is the number of night shifts in a row. Most studies indicate that the circadian system and sleep do not adjust (improve) much across a series of night shifts even in permanent night workers. Thus, a series of more than four night shifts might be expected to be particularly taxing. On the other hand, if it is of major importance that performance capacity remain high during the night, it seems that a solution with permanent night shifts is preferable, in combination with other teams that work a two-shift system (with only morning and afternoon shifts).

With respect to the duration of shifts, there appears to be increased prevalence of extended (to 10 to 12 hours) work shifts, popular because they permit long sequences of free time and reduced commuting. On the other hand, having a second job may exacerbate the effects of long shifts or lack of recovery days.

Although there is still a question about the best direction of rotation for shifts, phase delays are easier to adjust to than phase advances. For the rotating shift-worker, this implies that schedules that delay (rotating clockwise: morning–afternoon–night) are preferable to schedules that rotate counterclockwise. There

have been, however, very few practical tests of this theory, particularly in relation to sleepiness.

Preventive Measures

The following preventive measures with respect to the organization of shift work deserve attention:

PRIMARY IMPORTANCE

- Avoid night work (and morning work if possible).
- Avoid quick changes.
- Maintain time between shifts, of at least 11 hours.
- Avoid double shifts or other greatly extended work shifts.
- Avoid very early morning shifts (starting before 6 a.m.).
- Intersperse rest days during the shift cycle.

CLEAR IMPROVEMENTS

- Schedule naps during the night shift.
- Provide long sequences of days off and few weekends with work.
- Avoid having a morning shift immediately after a night or evening shift.

PROBABLE IMPROVEMENTS

- Avoid long (more than three shifts) sequences of night or morning shifts (rotate rapidly).
- Introduce permanent night work as an alternative under certain conditions.
- Plan night shifts at the end of the shift cycle.
- Give shift workers older than 45 years of age the right to transfer to day work.
- Rotate shifts clockwise.

The most important individual preventive measure is good sleep hygiene, including sleeping in a dark, cool, sound-insulated bedroom; using ear plugs; and informing family and friends about one's sleep schedule. Another important preventive measure is strategic sleeping. For night shift-work, the sleep period should be between 2 and 9 p.m. If not socially feasible, the next-best alternative is to have a moderate morning sleep and then to add a 2-hour nap in the evening. Common sense suggests that the worker should avoid intake of major meals during the night shift.

Bibliography

Costa G. Shift work and occupational medicine: An overview. Occup Med 2003;53:83–8.
van der Hulst M. Long workhours and health. Scand J Work Environ Health 2003;29:171–88.

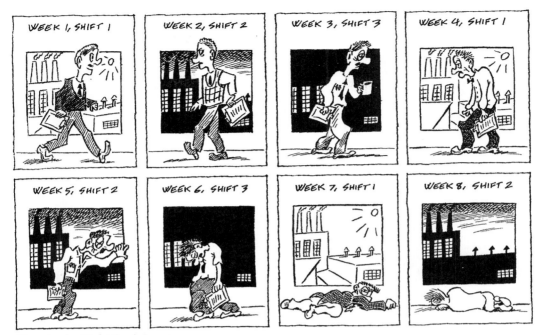

(Drawing by Nick Thorkelson.)

to predict strain, such that high control and high social support buffer the effects of job demands on strain outcomes.

Karasek postulated that the amount of work does not seem to be as critical to worker health as the interaction of workload with the amount of control or discretion the worker has over the work and related work processes (referred to as *decision latitude*). The ever-growing number of studies using the model suggests support for the first hypothesis—the main effects of demand, control, and social support—and limited support for the hypothesized interaction among these factors. The combination of low decision latitude and high psychological demands is a risk factor for cardiovascular mortality in most studies.[8] Indeed, it is widely accepted that worker control or discretion over working conditions is integral to worker health. The theoretical basis and specific mechanisms of the effects of control on health, however, are not clear.

Organizational Factors

Many studies have examined the psychological and physical effects of various role-related demands in organizations. *Role conflict* exists whenever individuals face incompatible demands from two or more sources. *Role ambiguity* reflects the uncertainty employees experience about what is expected of them in their jobs; the opposite of role ambiguity would be role clarity. *Inter-role conflict* exists when employees face incompatible demands from two or more roles. The most common form of inter-role conflict is work-family conflict, where the demands of work conflict, with the roles of parent and spouse. Each of these role-related stressors have been linked, in the job-stress literature, to strain and, in some cases, illness outcomes. Given the revolutionary changes in the way that work has been structured and performed in recent years, these stressors are also believed to be highly prevalent and problematic.[3]

Various management styles, including total or partial intolerance of worker participation in decision-making, lack of effective consultation, and excessive restrictions on worker behavior, are also stressful. Of these style characteristics, exclusion from decision-making has received the most research attention and has been shown to be related to a variety of strain outcomes, including lowered self-esteem, low job satisfaction, and overall poor physical and mental health. By contrast, studies have demonstrated that greater participation in decision-making has led to greater job satisfaction,

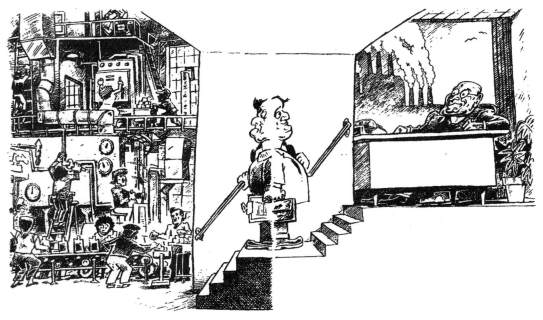

A supervisor's job may be highly stressful due to its high degree of role conflict. (Drawing by
Nick Thorkelson.)

lower turnover, better supervisor–subordinate relationships, and greater productivity. Increasing worker participation seems to result in reductions in work-related psychological strain.

Stressors include career-related concerns, such as job insecurity, fear of job obsolescence, under- and overpromotion, and more generally concerns about career development. The importance of job insecurity as a stressor in the workplace is highlighted by observations that the temporary or contingent labor force is rapidly increasing and that job tenure has declined for many workers.[3]

Recently, the development of the effort–reward imbalance model of job stress has focused attention on the role of organizational rewards as a job stressor.[9] In general, this model proposes that strain results when rewards are not consistent with efforts in the work environment. Efforts are described as the strivings of individuals to meet the demands and obligations of the job. Rewards are conceptualized as encompassing financial rewards, esteem rewards, and career rewards, including job security. The theory is based on the notion that workers attempt to maintain a state of equilibrium and cannot maintain an imbalance between effort and rewards over an extended period of time, and eventually this condition will result in ill health. Although initial studies

using cardiovascular risk as the outcome generally support the theory, a long-term evaluation is still needed.

Organizational culture and climate factors can be associated with worker stress, although the mechanism by which this happens is not known.

Interpersonal Relations

Poor interpersonal relations in the workplace are stressors that result in a variety of strain consequences. Violence and aggression as well as poor-quality leadership represent two forms of interpersonal relations that are stressors. Although incidents of physical violence are relatively rare, they have a dramatic effect on individual and organizational well-being. Aggression in the workplace, much more prevalent than violence, is associated with impaired physical and psychological health. Poor-quality leadership has been associated with increased levels of employee strain. Employees who perceive their supervisors as abusive experience low levels of job and life satisfaction, lower levels of commitment, increased work–family conflict, more psychosomatic symptoms, and psychological distress.

Physical Conditions

Adverse environmental conditions exacerbate overall job demands placed on employees, thus lowering worker tolerance to other stressors and decreasing worker motivation. Environmental conditions, including excessive noise, temperature extremes, poor ventilation, inadequate lighting, and ergonomic design deficiencies have been linked to employee physical and psychological health complaints as well as attitude and behavior problems. For example, outbreaks of mass psychogenic illness (often called *collective stress response*), when they rarely occur, are generally in workplaces that employees regard as physically uncomfortable. Psychological job stressors appear to produce increments in muscle tension that may exacerbate muscle loads and symptoms resulting from physical task demands.[10]

MODERATING FACTORS

Several personal and situational characteristics can modify the way individual workers exposed to a work environment perceive or react to it. These characteristics, known as "moderators," are depicted in Fig. 16-2, in the blocks labeled individual factors, nonwork factors, and buffer factors.[1]

Individual Factors

The most widely discussed personal characteristic related to stress at work has been the coronary artery disease-prone type A behavior pattern. Type A behavior is characterized by intense striving for achievement, competitiveness, time urgency, excessive drive, and overcommitment to vocation or profession. Although investigators in the past have reported the type A pattern to be independently associated with coronary artery disease, more recent studies have suggested that the variables of hostility, cynicism, anger, irritability, and suspicion may be the primary pathogenic component of type A found to be significant in earlier studies. Similarly, though earlier studies suggested an interaction between certain job stressors and type A characteristics that may lead to heart disease, overall the evidence that people with type A are more adversely affected by various job stressors is limited.

The hardy personality style and an internal locus of control are also thought to mediate the stressor–illness relationship. Hardy persons are believed to possess various beliefs and tendencies that are useful in coping with stressors, such as optimistic appraisals of events and decisive actions in coping. Hardy persons report less illness in the presence of stressors. Persons with an internal locus of control—a general belief that events in life are controlled by their actions—also have shown a consistent tendency to report better health than those who believe that life events are beyond their control.

Stage of career development, though little studied, may also moderate the stressor–illness relationship. For example, work experience (job tenure) seems to moderate worker responses to negative events at work. For workers in midcareer, job stressors lose potency in affecting physical health, but stressful events outside the job domain become increasingly deleterious to health.

Non-work Factors

Workers do not leave their family and personal problems behind when they go to work, nor do they forget job problems on returning home. Difficult transportation options, childcare needs, and available community resources may also moderate home and work stress. Nearly all models of job stress acknowledge extraoccupational factors and their potential interaction with work in affecting health outcomes. Few studies, however, have attempted to examine the respective health effects of job and extraorganizational stressors. Although some investigators have incorporated generic stressful life-events scales into job-stress surveys, these scales provide only crude indications of social, familial, and financial stressors. In future studies, more attention needs to be paid to nonwork factors. Interpersonal, marital, financial, and child-rearing stressors can exacerbate existing job stressors to promote acute stress reactions. Alternatively, the absence of extraorganizational problems may make stressful job situations more tolerable (that is, less stressful) and may impede the development of stress reactions. Environmental factors are recognized modifiers within the job-stress model. For example, a worker living in a noisy, high-crime neighborhood will be exposed to added stress and be unable to recover from stress endured at work. Or a worker facing a long commute by automobile, with traffic and construction delays, will be subjected to significant stress. In contrast, the environment a worker lives in can offer good opportunities to reduce stress, such as by biking, running, and walking, or to enhance social interaction among neighbors.

Buffer Factors

Social Support

Stress researchers have sought to identify factors that reduce or eliminate the effects of job stressors. These factors are termed *buffer factors*. One of the most extensively studied buffer factors has been the degree of social support an individual worker receives from work and nonwork sources. However, evidence for a buffering effect of social support has been mixed. Whereas some studies have found that social support buffers the relationship between a variety of job stressors and psychological symptoms, others have found no such buffering effect. These disparate results appear, at least in part, to be the result of differences among researchers in conceptualizing and measuring support.

Coping

Another potential buffering factor is coping. The literature on coping is voluminous, but until relatively recently little of this knowledge has been incorporated into studies of occupational stress and health. *Coping* is not a stable trait or disposition but rather seems to be a transactional process that is modified continuously by experience within and between stressful episodes. Further, a specific coping strategy that alleviates stress in one situation may not alleviate stress, or may actually increase perceived stress, in other situations. Clearly, the coping responses that people use are a function of the social and psychological resources at their disposal. Social supports and psychological resources, like mastery and self-esteem, are what people draw upon in developing coping strategies. Research has shown that these resources vary by socioeconomic status with people who are better educated and more affluent possessing more resources and a wider range of coping alternatives. It also appears that no single coping response is uniformly protective across work and nonwork situations. However, having a large and varied coping repertoire can be helpful in reducing stressor–strain relationships. Although various coping responses have been found to be effective in the areas of marriage, child rearing, and household finances, coping is sometimes strikingly ineffective when applied to occupational problems. This may be due to the impersonal nature of work and the lack of worker control over this class of stressors. Future research on coping would benefit from a clear delineation of the various types of coping strategies and their relative effectiveness across work and nonwork situations.

Lifestyle Factors

Lifestyle factors, such as physical fitness and exercise, smoking cessation, sound nutrition habits, and stress management, have the potential to buffer the health effects of job stressors, but clear evidence for such a buffering effect is lacking. However, such evidence could result from a new NIOSH initiative (Steps to a Healthier U.S. Workplace), which is creating an opportunity for occupational safety and health professionals and health promotion professionals to develop and implement collaboratively workplace programs that prevent occupational illness and injury, promote health, and optimize the health of U.S. workers.

PATHOPHYSIOLOGICAL CORRELATES OF JOB STRESS

Despite the amount of data linking stressful job conditions to poor health, surprisingly little is known about the actual pathophysiologic mechanisms that underlie the relationships between stress and disease. Both direct and indirect pathways have been described. The direct pathways that are thought to play a role are disregulations of the neurohormonal system (pituitary–adrenocortical axis), the autonomic nervous system, and the immune system. A combination of these pathways, influenced by genetic factors, probably links exposure to job stressors and adverse health effects. An indirect pathway links job and nonjob stressors first to high-risk behaviors, which then lead to adverse health effects. For example, strain effects from rotating shift-work directly influences the circadian rhythm, with resultant changes in the autonomic nervous system and the immune system.

To further complicate the relationships, job stressors can be seen as influencing the early development of disease, such as the precursors of coronary heart disease (CHD), or as a trigger for an ultimate event, such as an acute myocardial infarction. For example, acute stress elevates catecholamine levels, leading to increased heart rate and blood pressure, decreased plasma volume, coronary constriction, and increased lipid levels, platelet activity, coagulation, and inflammation. Chronically, stress causes autonomic imbalance, leading to decreased cardiovascular reactivity, neurohormonal changes, a pro-coagulant state, and increased lipid levels.

Immune system responses may mediate some of these relationships. Many animal studies have demonstrated that experimentally induced stress increases susceptibility to a variety of infectious agents and the incidence and rate of growth of certain tumors. Some human studies have shown that psychosocial factors, including stressful life events, are related to diseases under immune system regulation. And stress has been linked to changes in levels of circulating antibodies, lymphocyte cytotoxicity, and lymphocyte proliferation.

PREVENTION AND INTERVENTION

The gap between etiologic and intervention-related knowledge is great in the realm of occupational stress. Despite the ever-burgeoning literature on the nature, causes, and physical and psychological consequences of occupational stress, surprisingly little is known about intervention for occupational stress. Views differ regarding the importance of worker characteristics versus working conditions as "the" major cause of organizational stress; these views have, in part, led to the development and use of primary, secondary, and tertiary prevention (intervention) approaches for occupational stress. The aim of *primary prevention intervention* is to reduce risk factors or job stressors. The aim of *secondary prevention intervention* is to alter the ways that individuals respond to risks or job stressors. And the aim of *tertiary prevention intervention* is to heal those who have been traumatized. Research on primary and tertiary prevention intervention has been recently reviewed by this author,[12] and secondary prevention intervention has been the subject of reviews by Murphy[13] and van Der Klink and colleagues.[14] The following provides a brief overview of research findings for all three types of intervention.

Primary Prevention Interventions

Primary prevention interventions can be characterized as either psychosocial or sociotechnical. *Psychosocial interventions* focus *primarily* on human processes and psychosocial aspects of the work setting and aim to reduce stress by changing workers' perceptions of the work environment; they may also include modifications of objective working conditions. In contrast, *sociotechnical interventions* focus *primarily* on changes to objective working conditions and are considered to have implications

for work-related stress. Some interventions involve elements of both approaches.

Psychosocial Interventions

Most primary prevention interventions appear to be psychosocial. Many are based on the principles of participatory action research (PAR)—a methodology in which researchers and workers collaborate in a process of data-guided problem-solving to improve the organization's ability to provide workers with desired outcomes and to contributing to general operational knowledge. PAR involves workers and experts from outside the workplace, in an empowering process of defining problems (identifying stressors), developing intervention strategies, introducing changes that benefit employees, and measuring outcomes. Some PAR interventions have specifically focused on efforts to redesign work or work processes. In general, there is very limited evidence for the efficacy of PAR and other participatory-type interventions; studies evaluating its efficacy tend to be methodologically weak, difficult to interpret, and causally ambiguous. When found, the effects of the interventions have often been on job satisfaction and perceptions of the working environment; few effects on health-related outcomes have been reported. It is unclear whether the general lack of health benefits are due to ineffective interventions, the insufficient duration of the studies, or the nature of the health-outcome variables studied. Moreover, which effects are attributable to the act of participating in the intervention and which are attributable to changes in working conditions or processes resulting from the intervention are unclear.

There is, however, some evidence for the efficacy of psychosocial interventions focused on supervisors and managers rather than workers. Although few in number, these interventions resulted in positive organizationally relevant outcomes and found modest positive effects on individual well-being. An intriguing aspect is that the effects on well-being may extend beyond the supervisors and managers themselves, possibly representing a potentially effective and seemingly cost-efficient approach to primary prevention. No firm conclusions, however, can be drawn, and more research is needed.

Sociotechnical Interventions

In contrast, sociotechnical interventions are generally not a result of employee–employer or employee–employer–researcher collaboration.

Sociotechnical interventions have generally involved changing only a very limited variety of objective working conditions, such as the modification of workload, work schedules, and work processes. However, as a whole, sociotechnical intervention studies provide more consistent and robust evidence for the efficacy of the intervention than psychosocial intervention studies. In addition to incorporating self-report measures of affect, such as job satisfaction, anxiety, and depression, most of these studies have incorporated objective outcome measures, such as blood pressure, job performance, and sickness absence, in the study design. In general, these studies have also tended to use more rigorous experimental and quasiexperimental designs.

Secondary Prevention Interventions

Secondary prevention interventions, often termed *stress management,* involve techniques and procedures designed to help workers modify their appraisal of stressful situations and/or to deal with the symptoms of stress. Typically, such interventions are prescriptive, person-oriented, relaxation-based techniques such as biofeedback, progressive muscle relaxation meditation, and cognitive-behavioral skills training. They differ from other health-promotion programs in the variety of training techniques and wide range of health-outcome measures used to assess program effectiveness. In contrast to primary prevention interventions, they do not seek to alter the sources of stress at work (job stressors) through organizational change strategies or job redesign.

Cognitive-behavioral skills training, frequently used in stress management, involves techniques designed to modify the appraisal processes that determine perceived stressfulness of situations and to develop behavioral skills for managing stressors. It helps people to restructure their thinking patterns through cognitive restructuring. In general, it can reduce psychological strain, especially anxiety, and improve organizationally relevant outcomes, such as job satisfaction. However, it has not shown consistent improvement of physiological strains.

In contrast, muscle relaxation techniques can benefit some physiological strains, such as blood pressure, but not others. Such techniques involve focusing one's attention on muscle activity, learning to identify even small amounts of tension in a muscle group, and practicing releasing of tension from muscles.

Meditation methods used in worksite stress-management studies, often secular versions of Transcendental Meditation, involve sitting upright in a comfortable position, in a quiet place, with eyes closed, and mentally repeating a mantra while maintaining a passive attitude. The few studies that have examined the efficacy of such worksite-based meditation provide surprisingly consistent evidence that they reduce psychological, physiological, and behavioral strain. More research is needed on the efficacy of meditation methods.

Combinations of two or more stress-management approaches into a single intervention are frequently used, the most common combination and most effective of which seems to be muscle relaxation coupled with cognitive-behavioral skills training—apparently more effective than either technique used alone.

Tertiary Prevention Interventions

Tertiary organizational stress prevention is therapeutic—treatment of the physical, psychological, or behavioral consequences of exposures to job stressors. No comprehensive discussion of this subject is found in the stress literature—perhaps because so many individual physical, psychological, and behavioral illnesses are thought to be related to job stress. The following is an overview of tertiary stress interventions that are often based in organizations.

Medical Care

Many large companies have occupational medicine departments that offer services that include urgent medical care, employee examinations, disability reviews, health promotion activities, and referrals for medical treatment (see Chapter 12). In general, these departments are not structured to provide extensive or long-term care for stress-related illness or injury and must rely on making referrals to appropriate health care providers. Mental health problems related to job stress can present special challenges to occupational medicine departments that may not be well equipped either to deal with them or to make referrals.

Counseling and psychotherapy are commonly used methods to treat individuals suffering from work-related mental health problems. Common techniques of psychotherapy and counseling include behavioral and cognitive therapy, supportive counseling, and insight-oriented psychotherapy.

Counseling and psychotherapy can have marked benefits on symptom reduction, but it may not have beneficial impact on work performance (as measured by reduced absenteeism).

Many companies offer limited counseling at the workplace through employee assistance programs (EAPs) that often provide a variety of mental health–related services. Employees can refer themselves to EAPs or be referred by management. The goals of an EAP are to restore employees to full productivity by (1) identifying those with drug abuse and those with emotional or behavioral problems that result in deficient work performance; (2) motivating these employees to seek help; (3) providing short-term professional counseling assistance and referral; (4) directing employees toward the best assistance available; and (5) providing continuing support and guidance throughout the problem-solving period. Very few studies have addressed the cost-effectiveness of EAPs. There is little agreement on evaluation methodology. And, some have questioned whether there should be any economic evaluation of EAPs. However, reduced health claims, financial savings, lower absenteeism rates, and increased return on investment have been reported.

For many employees, a stigma continues to be associated with psychological treatment of any kind. This fear, along with concerns regarding confidentiality, may limit the use of workplace-based mental health resources. Employees may also feel that the company has a vested interest in their productivity that is of greater importance than their health. This concern may be exacerbated by the fact that EAPs are gatekeepers with financial biases not to refer employees for more sophisticated and long-term care and to refer to mental-health-care providers with limited training who may charge the employer less money. Indeed, who provides the care seems to be an important issue. For example, psychologists, psychiatrists, and social workers seem to achieve equally positive results, whereas results by other counseling professionals—who generally charge less money— do not appear to be as positive. There are paradoxes embedded in the very nature of EAPs, which lead to conflicting demands and to occupational stress for professionals on the staff of EAPs, such as conflicts of employer versus employee assistance and pressures to provide short-term individual solutions to what may be long-term structural problems.[15]

Implications for Practice and Policy

A tremendous gulf exists between our knowledge regarding job stress and the most efficacious and economical means of preventing it and treating its consequences in the workplace. There is only limited evidence that certain primary prevention interventions have worked, although it is unclear why they worked. Those that focus on a few stressors and those that do not introduce too many changes too quickly appear to be the most successful. Before primary prevention interventions are designed and implemented, the most prevalent and problematic stressors must be identified and prioritized according to their potency and amenability to meaningful change.[16] Practitioners and researchers should target appropriate objective and subjective outcomes by which to assess the efficacy of interventions and valid and reliable measures of these outcomes. Objective measures that are organizationally relevant need to be included, without which other organizations will be reluctant to engage in these interventions.

Regardless of whether they are primary, secondary, or tertiary in nature, job-stress interventions seem to be implemented in relative isolation from one another within an organization. For example, management, human resources, medical departments, and/or EAPs may be given the responsibility for an intervention, and there may be little involvement or cooperation of other organizational structures. Primary, secondary, and tertiary interventions for job stress should be integrated within the organization as a whole.

REFERENCES

1. Quick JC, Quick JD, Nelson DL, et al. Preventive stress management in organizations. Washington, DC: American Psychological Association, 1997.
2. Sauter SL, Murphy LR, Hurrell JJ Jr. Prevention of work-related psychological disorders: A national strategy proposed by the National Institute for Occupational Safety and Health (NIOSH). Am Psychol 1990;45:1146–58.
3. NIOSH. The changing organization of work and safety and the health of working people: Knowledge gaps and research directions. Washington DC: NIOSH, 2002. (DHHS [NIOSH] publication no. 2002-116.)
4. NIOSH. Stress at work. Washington DC: NIOSH, 1999. (DHHS [NIOSH] publication no. 99–101.)
5. NIOSH. Overtime and extended work shifts: Recent findings on illness, injuries and health behaviors. Washington DC: NIOSH, 2004. (DHHS [NIOSH] publication no. 2004–143.)
6. NIOSH. Plain language about shiftwork. Washington, DC: NIOSH, 1997. (DHHS [NIOSH] publication no. 97-145.)

7. Karasek RA, Theorell T. Healthy work: Stress, productivity, and the reconstruction of working life. New York: Basic Books, 1990.

8. Schnall PL, Belkic K, Landsbergis P, et al. eds. The workplace and cardiovascular disease. Philadelphia: Hanley & Belfus, Inc., 2000.

9. Siegrist J. Adverse health effects of high/low reward conditions. J Occup Health Psychol 1996;8:27–41.

10. Hurrell JJ Jr. Psychosocial factors and musculoskeletal disorders. In: Perrewe PL, Ganster DC, eds. Exploring theoretical mechanisms and perspectives. New York: JAI, 2001:233–57.

11. Hurrell JJ Jr, McClaney A, Murphy LR. The middle years: Career stage differences. Prevention in Human Service 1990;58:327–32.

12. Hurrell JJ Jr. Occupational stress intervention. In: Kelloway E, Barling J, Frone M, eds. Handbook of stress. Thousand Oaks, CA: Sage Publications, 2004:623–45.

13. Murphy LR. Stress management in work settings: A critical review of the health effects. Am J Health Promotion 1996;11:112–35.

14. Van der Klinck JJL, Blonk RWB, Schene AH, et al. The benefits of interventions for work-related stress. Am J of Public Health 2001;9:270–76.

15. Bento RF. On the other hand... the paradoxical nature of employee assistance programs. Employee Assistance Quarterly 1997;496–513.

16. Hurrell JJ Jr, Murphy LR. Occupational stress intervention. Am J Ind Med 1996;29:338–41.

BIBLIOGRAPHY

Sauter SL, Hurrell JJ Jr, Murphy LR. In: Stellman JM, ed. Encyclopedia of occupational health and safety. 4th ed. Geneva: International Labor Office, 1998:34.3–34.14.
A comprehensive review of job stressors and health effects and interventions.

Hurrell JJ Jr, Murphy LR. Occupational stress intervention. Am J Ind Med 1996;29:338–41.
A good, brief overview of available interventions.

APPENDIX

WEB SITES

<http://www.cdc.gov/niosh/topics/stress/>
This site, sponsored by NIOSH, provides information about job stress and health, and links to other sources of information on job stress.

The findings and conclusions in this chapter are those of the authors and do not necessarily represent the views of the National Institute for Occupational Safety and Health.

CHAPTER 17

Ambient Air Pollution

Isabelle Romieu, Mauricio Hernández-Ávila, and Fernando Holguin

In the mid-20th century, dramatic episodes of ambient (outdoor) air pollution in developed countries showed that air pollution could cause excess deaths. For example, during the London Fog of 1952, which was due mainly to smoke from coal-burning household stoves, an estimated 12,000 excess deaths occurred. Infants and young children as well as older people were at especially increased risk, and the proportion of deaths attributed to respiratory causes was increased.[1] Ambient air pollution has now been examined as a risk factor for respiratory morbidity and mortality in numerous epidemiologic studies,[2–5] and, even though ambient air pollution levels have now declined in developed countries, the epidemiologic evidence continues to indicate adverse effects on health at levels frequently reached now in many urban areas that were previously considered to be safe.[6,7] Recently, the World Health Organization (WHO) has estimated the burden of disease related to urban air pollution to 6.4 millions DALYs (disability-adjusted life years; accounting for years life lost to premature mortality as well as years of life lived with disability due to disease).[8]

NATURE AND SOURCES OF AMBIENT AIR POLLUTION

Ambient air pollutants are derived mainly from fuel combustion (Fig. 17-1). They include (a) primary pollutants (sulfur dioxide, nitrogen oxides, and particles), (b) secondary acidic aerosols and other particles, and (c) oxidant pollutants (primarily ozone) that are produced by photochemical reactions involving hydrocarbons and nitrogen oxides. In most areas where photochemical reactions are prevalent, the emissions of nitrogen oxides and hydrocarbons reflect urban sprawl, with heavy motor vehicle traffic that is often associated with high levels of particulates—especially in the large cities of developing countries.[3,7,9] In cities and some rural areas of developing countries, residential space-heating and cooking with solid fuels (biomass and coal) can also contribute significantly to ambient air pollution. Industrial processes also emit contaminants, such as volatile organic compounds, that may adversely affect health.

To comprehend health effects, it is important to have a basic understanding of the sources and properties of major ambient air pollutants, including sulfur dioxide, particulates, nitrogen oxides, ozone, volatile organic compounds, carbon monoxide, persistent organic pollutants, and lead.

Sulfur Dioxide

Sulfur dioxide (SO_2) is a water-soluble gas formed from the oxidation of sulfur, which contaminates coal and petroleum fuels. Consequently, sulfur dioxide is emitted by coal- and oil-fired power plants and by industrial processes involving fossil fuel combustion. Sulfur dioxide and particulate pollution are typically emitted together by combustion sources and exist as components of a complex mixture.[3] However, depending on the source, the proportion of particulates to sulfur dioxide varies greatly. For example, in areas where low sulfur fuel is used, the ambient sulfur dioxide level will be low. In contrast, in areas where high-sulfur fuel is used or where much coal is burned, such as China, the ambient level of sulfur dioxide will be high.

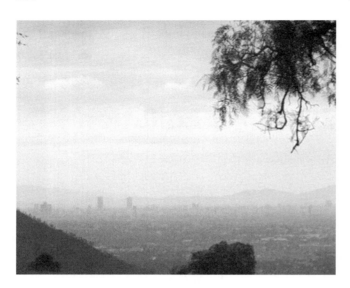

FIGURE 17-1 ● Air pollution in Mexico City. (Photograph by Dr. Matiana Ramirez.)

Particulates

Particulate air pollution refers to the mixture of solid and liquid particles suspended in the air, forming an aerosol. The particles in air vary in shape, size, composition, and origin. Typically, particles are classified according to their size (Fig. 17-2).[10] Particle size affects deposition in the respiratory tract and consequently the potential to cause adverse health effects. Particles less than 10 μm in diameter (PM$_{10}$) compose the *inhalable fraction* of airborne particles. Particles (particulate matter; PM) between 2.5 and 10 μm compose the *coarse fraction* and include mainly soil material, such as suspended road dust and windblown dust, and parti-

cles generated by handling, crushing, and grinding operations. Particles less than 2.5 μm (PM$_{2.5}$), the *respirable* or *fine fraction*, comprise all particles capable of entering the alveoli. They are produced from fuel and biomass combustion and the atmospheric reaction of gases. A subset of PM$_{2.5}$, *ultrafine particles* smaller than 0.1 μm, are formed by combustion exhaust.[10]

Nitrogen Oxides

Like sulfur dioxide, nitrogen dioxide (NO$_2$) and other nitrogen oxides (NO$_x$) are produced by high-temperature combustion processes and contribute

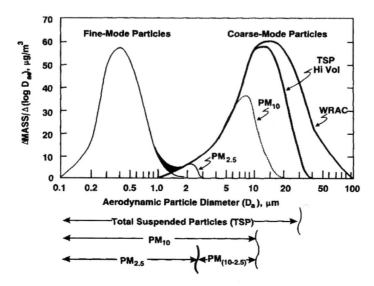

FIGURE 17-2 ● Example of a mass distribution of ambient PM as a function of aerodynamic particle diameter. (Source: USEPA. Air quality criteria for particulate matter. National Center for Environmental Assessment, 1996.)

to the formation of acid aerosols. Outdoors, nitrogen oxides are nearly always present together with other combustion pollutants. Initially, almost all emissions of nitrogen oxides are in the form of nitric oxide (NO), which is then oxidized in air to form nitrogen dioxide, a more toxic compound and a major precursor of photochemical smog.[10]

Ozone

Ozone (O_3) is a colorless gas that occurs naturally in the stratosphere, where it has the important function of filtering out ultraviolet (UV) radiation. At ground level in cities and many rural areas, it is the prime oxidant ingredient of smog, along with other oxidant species and fine particles. Ozone is a secondary pollutant formed as the product of the atmospheric photochemical reaction of primary emissions, such as nitrogen oxides and volatile organic compounds, in the presence of sunlight and accelerated at high temperature.[2] This photochemical pollution is especially prevalent in the many large cities with heavy vehicle traffic, especially those located in sunny regions and/or at high altitude, such as Mexico City.[7]

Volatile Organic Compounds

Volatile organic compounds (VOCs) are present in the atmosphere mainly as gases. They include a variety of hydrocarbons, such as alkenes, aldehydes, and aromatic hydrocarbons, such as benzene and toluene. Some VOCs are chlorinated compounds. The sources of VOCs include evaporation and combustion of fossil fuels, use of solvents, and industrial processes. Benzene, a VOC that has received much attention because of its carcinogenicity, is present in gasoline. Population exposure in urban areas to benzene depends on its concentration in the gasoline used in the area.[10]

Carbon Monoxide

Carbon monoxide (CO) is produced by the incomplete combustion of fossil fuels, mainly derived from mobile sources. Most of the carbon in automotive fuel is oxidized to carbon dioxide; only a small fraction is incompletely oxidized to carbon monoxide.[11]

Persistent Organic Pollutants

Persistent organic pollutants (POPs) are a subclass of air toxicants that persist for long periods in the environment. A recent international treaty aims to eliminate 12 of these compounds from the environment, including 8 pesticides (aldrin, chlordane, dieldrin, endrin, heptachlor, mirex, toxaphene, and DDT); an industrial chemical (hexachlorobenzene); and a group of industrial chemicals (polychlorinated biphenyls [PCBs]); and 2 by-products of combustion (dioxin and furans).[10] Because they are volatile, POPs travel great distances in the atmosphere, settling out in colder regions, where they become incorporated into the food chain. Exposure is primarily via ingestion.

Lead

Population exposure to lead, as a gasoline additive, is decreasing as leaded gasoline is being phased out in many countries. Leaded gasoline, however, is still used in many developing countries. The primary air pollutant is lead oxide, a product of gasoline combustion.

In the United States, removal of lead from gasoline lowered the average blood lead level between 1976 and 1980 from 13 to 3 μg/dL.[12] In Mexico City, control measures implemented from 1988 to 1998 to phase out lead from gasoline lowered the annual ambient lead level from 1.2 to 0.2 μg/m^3.[13] Simultaneously, an estimated 7.6 μg/dL average decline in blood lead level was observed in children living in Mexico City.[6]

AMBIENT AIR QUALITY STANDARDS AND GUIDELINES

In the past 30 years, much progress has been made in many countries to control ambient air pollution and thereby reduce adverse impacts on human health and the environment. In the United States, the Clean Air Act of 1970 mandated that the federal government develop and promulgate National Ambient Air Quality Standards (NAAQS), specifying uniform nationwide limits for certain major air pollutants (*criteria air pollutants*): carbon monoxide, lead, nitrogen dioxide, ozone, particulate matter, and sulfur dioxide. The Act has been amended several times, most recently in 1990.[14]

Under the Act, the EPA must identify pollutants that "may reasonably be anticipated to endanger public health or welfare" and issue air quality criteria for them—primary and secondary NAAQS for these pollutants. *Primary standards* set limits to protect public health, including the health of

TABLE 17-1

National Ambient Air Quality Standards, United States[a]

Pollutants	NAAQS Concentrations (ppm)	NAAQS Concentrations (μg/m^3)	Standard Type
Particulate matter <10 μm (PM$_{10}$)			
24-hr average		150	Primary and secondary
Annual arithmetic mean		50	Primary and secondary
Particulate matter <2.5 μm (PM$_{2.5}$)			
24-hr average		65	Primary and secondary
Annual arithmetic mean		15	Primary and secondary
Ozone (O$_3$)			
24-hr average	0.12	235	Primary and secondary
Annual arithmetic mean	0.08	157	Primary and secondary
Sulfur oxides			
24-hr average	0.14	365	Primary
Annual arithmetic mean	0.03	80	Primary
3-hr average	0.50	1,300	Secondary
Nitrogen dioxide (NO$_2$)			
Annual arithmetic mean	0.053	100	Primary and secondary
Carbon monoxide (CO)			
1-hr average	35	40	Primary
8-hr average	9	10	Primary
Lead (Pb)			
Quarterly average		1.5	Primary and secondary

[a] For detailed information on scientific bases and policy considerations underlying decisions establishing the National Ambient Air Quality Standards (NAAQS) listed here, see the AQCs, staff papers, and NAAQS Promulgation notices cited in text. Such information can also be obtained from several Web sites, such as <www.epa.glv/airs/criteria.html>, <www.epa.gov/oar/oaqps/publicat.html>, and <www.epa.gov/ncea/biblio.htm>.

sensitive populations, such as asthmatics, children, and older people. *Secondary standards* protect against other effects, such as decreased visibility and damage to animals, crops, vegetation, and buildings. Standards are set for both long-term (annual average) and short-term (24 hours or less) averaging times (Table 17-1). The act requires that NAAQS be reviewed periodically and revised, if appropriate. In 1997, the NAAQS for ozone was revised to 0.08 ppm measured over 8 hours and the NAAQS for PM$_{2.5}$ was added, which the EPA is currently revising.

The World Health Organization has developed air quality guidelines for international use, which can be obtained at <www.who.ch/pll/dsa>. These guidelines, consisting of concentration limits of air pollutants for certain averaging times that were recommended by international experts, are intended for consideration by national and international authorities in promulgating air quality standards.[14]

EXPOSURE ASSESSMENT

Individuals within a population differ considerably in their exposure to air pollutants. However, nearly all routine monitoring and regulation of air pollution is based on measurements that are conducted at fixed locations. Assessment of individual and population exposure to air pollution should consider variations of sources of exposure among individuals.[10] Personal exposure assessments encompass (a) identification of key sources of selected

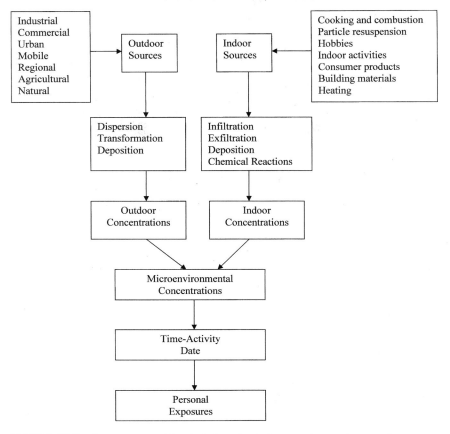

FIGURE 17-3 ● Sources and factors influencing indoor, outdoor, and personal exposures to air pollutants. (Source: Ozkaynak H. Exposure assessment. In: Holgate ST, Samet JM, Koren HS, Maynard RL, eds. Air pollution and health. London: Academic Press, 1999:149–162.)

pollutants, (b) their emission rates, (c) their concentration in outdoor and indoor air, and (d) the duration of contact with the pollutants (Fig. 17-3).[15] Knowledge of where people are and what they do during the course of a typical day is essential for determining personal exposure.

People living in North America spend, on average, approximately 87 percent of their time indoors. People living in urban areas of developing countries also spend most of their time indoors. When indoors, individuals are exposed to outdoor air pollutants that penetrate inside as well as to pollutants that are generated inside (see Chapter 18). If particles as small as 1 μm are considered, the correlation between indoor and outdoor air concentrations is very high. Penetration of outdoor air pollutants to indoor air is a function of the exchange rate, which is determined by type of construction and use of air conditioning. Carbon dioxide, sulfur dioxide, and nitrogen dioxide penetrate from out-

door to indoor air with great efficiency.[10] Ozone exposure is directly related to the amount of time spent outdoors.[10] An estimated 70 percent of fine particles (PM$_{2.5}$) from outdoors penetrates indoors in the absence of air conditioning.

Three factors govern the risk of toxic injury from pollutants and their metabolites: (a) their chemical and physical properties, (b) the dose that reaches critical tissues, and (c) the responsiveness of these sites to the pollutants and their metabolites. The physical form and properties, such as the solubility of airborne contaminants, influences distribution in the atmosphere and body tissues—and therefore the dose delivered to the target site. Dose is very difficult, if not impossible, to determine in epidemiological studies; therefore, surrogate measures are used, ranging from atmospheric concentration of pollutants to concentrations of biomarkers. For some pollutants, mathematical models of the relationship between exposure and dose can be used to develop

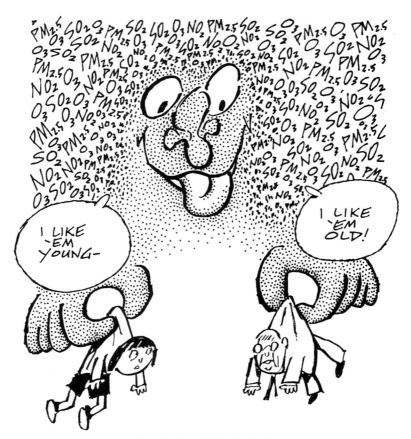

(Drawing by Nick Thorkelson.)

surrogate measures. The interaction of pollutants with biological receptors can trigger the mechanism of toxic response, which may act by direct stimulation or cascade of molecular and cellular events that ultimately damages tissues.[3,16] Different pathways of pollutant sources from exposure through inhalation to toxic effects are shown in Fig. 17-4.

GLOBAL CONCENTRATION PATTERNS OF AMBIENT AIR POLLUTION

During the past 25 years in developed countries, the generally measured indicators of urban air quality have tended to improve. In contrast, in many developing countries, rapid growth of urban population, development of industry, intensification of traffic, limited availability to clean fuel, and lack of effective control programs have led to high levels of ambient air pollution.[7,17] The Air Management Information System (AMIS) of WHO[17] provides comparative data from cities in more than 60 countries for major air pollutant levels (see <www. cepis.ops-oms.org/enwww/aire/amis.html>). Figure 17-5 presents data by country on the global distribution of PM_{10} concentrations and cumulative percentage of urban population exposed to these levels.[18]

ADVERSE HEALTH EFFECTS OF AMBIENT AIR POLLUTANTS

Adverse health effects ascribed to exposure to ambient air pollution include excess cardiorespiratory mortality, exacerbation of asthma, increased respiratory symptoms and illnesses, decreased lung function, and reduced host defense (Table 17-2).[2] The evidence linking these effects to air pollution comes from animal toxicology, human clinical-exposure, field-exposure, and epidemiological studies. Some of the outcomes listed in Table 17-2, such as increased deaths and hospitalizations,

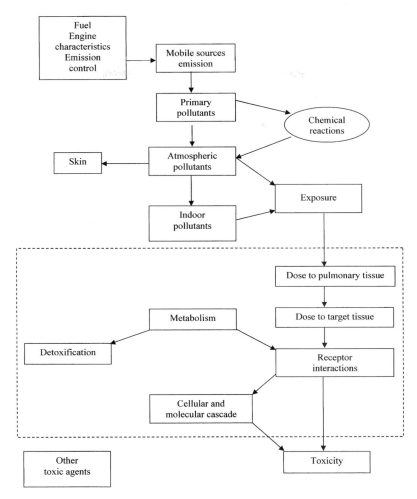

FIGURE 17-4 ● Pathway from motor vehicle pollutant sources to toxic effects in humans by exposure through inhalation. (Source: Watson AY, Bates RR, Kennedy D, eds. Air pollution, the automobile, and public health. Sponsored by the Health Effects Institute. Washington, DC: National Academy Press, 1988:21.)

are clearly adverse, whereas others are elevated levels of biomarkers, such as inflammatory mediators in bronchoalveolar lavage (BAL) fluid, which have uncertain clinical significance.[2]

Levels of ambient air pollutants usually correlate with one another, either because (a) emission sources are common to different pollutants—vehicles emit particles, nitrogen oxides, and carbon monoxide; or (b) pollutants interact in the atmosphere—as is the case of ozone and the secondary aerosols that are part of $PM_{2.5}$. Although the health effects of specific pollutants have been studied separately, and are regulated and controlled separately, mixtures of specific pollutants commonly occur and may be responsible for observed effects.[2] Such mixtures may lead to difficulties in interpreting epidemiological data. Correct interpretation of data on chronic human exposures often depends on (a) comparing results from different locations and/or (b) considering results of acute human exposures and/or animal experiments as indications of the adverse health effects of the primary pollutant.[10]

In the next section, we will consider only the adverse health effects of criteria air pollutants regulated by the NAAQS, except for lead, which is discussed in Chapters 13, 26, and 30 (see Table 17-3).

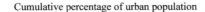

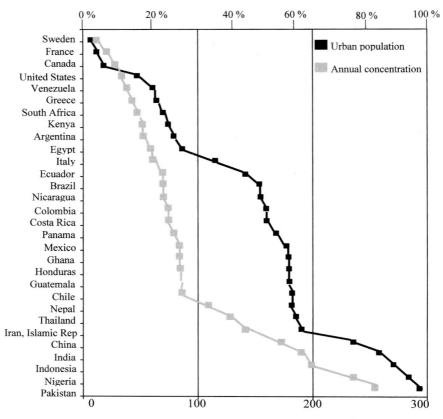

FIGURE 17-5 ● Cumulative percentage of PM_{10} (particulate matter less than 10 μm in aerodynamic diameter) and average annual concentration in urban populations, by country. Population-weighted concentrations are averages that take into account both air pollution levels and the number of people exposed in each country. For example, the average annual concentration of PM_{10} in cities in Pakistan is approximately 260 $\mu g/m^3$, and almost all of the world's urban population experiences less air pollution than do urban residents in Pakistan. Similarly, the average annual concentration of PM_{10} in cities in India is approximately 190 $\mu g/m^3$, and approximately 90 percent of the world's urban population experiences less air pollution than do urban dwellers in India. (Source: Holdren JP, Smith KR. Energy, the environment and health. In: Goldenberg J, ed. World energy assessment: Energy and the challenge of sustainability. New York: United Nations, 2000:61–110.)

Particulate Matter and Sulfur Dioxide

The health effects of particulate matter and sulfur dioxide are presented together because they are both products of fossil fuel combustion and are usually present together in complex mixtures.

Epidemiological studies suggest (a) an increase in mortality and morbidity associated with levels of airborne particles below the current standards and (b) approximately twice the previously reported effect of fine particles (smaller than 2.5 μm), which

appear to contain more of reactive substances linked to health effects.[19,20]

Experimental Studies

Sulfur dioxide may cause bronchitis-like pathology in animals exposed to levels far above ambient air concentrations. In asthmatics, exposure to 0.25 to 0.5 ppm elicits acute bronchoconstriction associated with increase airway resistance and decreased air-flow rates. Sulfur dioxide can also reduce various aspects of pulmonary defense.[21]

TABLE 17-2

Health Effects and Biological Markers of Response Associated with Air Pollution

Excess cardiorespiratory mortality
  Excess deaths from heart or lung disease
Increased health care use
  Increased hospitalization, physician visits, and
  emergency department visits
Asthma exacerbations
  Increased physician visits and medication use
  Decreased peak-flow measurements
Increased respiratory illness
  Increased upper and lower respiratory infections
  Increased physician visits and episodic symptoms
Increased respiratory symptoms
  Wheezing
  Cough/phlegm
  Chest tightness
Decreased lung function
  Acute reduction
  Chronic reduction
Increased airways reactivity
  Altered response to challenge with methacholine,
  carbachol, histamine, and cold air
Increased lung inflammation
  Influx of inflammatory cells, mediators, proteins
Decreased heart-rate variability
Increased systemic inflammatory markers
  Fibrinogen
  C-reactive protein
Increased plasma viscosity
Altered host defense
  Altered mucociliary clearance, macrophage function,
  and immune response
Eye, nose, and throat irritation

Fine particulates, especially ultrafine particles (<100 nm), are toxic to the lungs. This toxicity seems to result from their small size (rather than their content), particle surface area, number, particle surface chemistry, oxidative stress. and interstitialization of particles.[22] In addition, transition metals contained in particles may cause oxidative stress, augmented by the release of reactive oxygen species by the inflammatory cell influx that results from the primary interaction between the lung and particles. Short-term exposure to high levels of concentrated ambient particles (200 μg/m^3 PM$_{2.5}$) can induce a transient, mild pulmonary inflammatory reaction[22] and changes in both blood indices and heart rate variability.[23] Figure 17-6 summarizes the pathways by which deposition of particles in the airways can induce effects, both in the airways and systematically, that may lead to adverse health effects.[24]

In addition, combustion products may modulate the immune system, impairing inflammatory and host-defense functions of the lung and acting in synergy with allergens to enhance allergen-specific IgE production, initiate a TH$_2$ cytokine environment, and promote primary allergic sensitization.[25]

Population-Based Studies of Mortality

Acute exposure to airborne particulates increases mortality. Occurrence of deaths is related to daily changes in air pollution levels.[3,19] A study summarizing data from 20 cities in the United States reported an increase in total mortality of 0.51 percent per 10 μg/m^3 increase of PM$_{10}$ and in cardiovascular mortality of 0.68 percent.[26] Similar results were observed in European cities.[27] The relationship appears to be linear down to the lowest levels, without any threshold. People who otherwise might have survived for a substantial amount of time are among those affected. Daily mortality appears to be more strongly associated with concentrations of PM$_{2.5}$ than with concentrations of larger particles[20]—of great implication for urban areas of developing countries, where vehicular traffic with poorly maintained engines and extensive use of diesel fuel is a major source of particulate pollution. Increased infant mortality in these countries has been partially linked to exposure to airborne particulates.[7,9]

A recent summary estimate of these data suggests an increase of 1 percent of nonaccidental death in children less than 5 years of age per 10 μg/m^3 increase in PM$_{10}$.[28] Chronic exposure to fine particulates also increases mortality.[29] One study in the United States suggests that fine particulates and sulfur dioxide–related pollution are associated with mortality from all causes combined, cardiopulmonary diseases, and lung cancer. Each 10 μg/m^3 elevation in fine-particulate air pollution in this study was associated with a 4 percent increase in all-cause mortality, a 6 percent increase in cardiopulmonary mortality, and an 8 percent increase in lung cancer mortality.[30] Similar results were observed in

TABLE 17-3

Health Effects of Air Pollutants and Populations at Greatest Risk

Agent	Susceptible Population	Clinical Consequences	Comments
Particles (PM_{10}, $PM_{2.5}$)	Children	Increased acute cardiovascular and respiratory mortality	Effects seen alone or in combination with SO_2
	Chronic lung/ heart disease	Increased cardiovascular mortality with chronic exposure	Probable effects:
			Acute respiratory infections in children
	Asthmatics	Increased hospital admissions for respiratory and cardiac conditions	Decreased rate in lung function growth
		Increased respiratory symptoms	Low birthweight
		Decreased lung function	Post neonatal mortality
		Increased asthma exacerbations	
		Increased prevalence of chronic bronchitis	
		Increased risk of lung cancer	
		Increased blood fibrinogen	
		Increased inflammatory markers	
		Reduced heart rate variability	
Sulfur dioxide	Healthy adults and COPD patients	Increased respiratory symptoms	Highly soluble gas with little penetration to distal airways
		Increased respiratory mortality and increased hospital visits for respiratory disease	
	Asthmatics	Acute bronchoconstriction in asthmatics	Observations related to short-term exposures
Acid aerosols	Healthy adults	Increased respiratory illness	Currently not a criteria pollutant; no NAAQS established
	Children	Decreased lung function (Increased hospitalizations)	
	Asthmatics and others		Effects seen in combination with O_3 and particles
Ozone	Athletes, outdoor workers	Increased hospital admissions for acute respiratory illnesses	Effects found at or below current NAAQS; effects increased with exercise
	Asthmatics (and others with respiratory illnesses)	Aggravation of asthma Increased bronchial responsiveness	Effects seen in combination with acid aerosols and particles
		Decreased lung function	Probable effects: increase in mortality
	Children	Lung inflammation	Possible effects
			Aggravation of acute respiratory infections
		Increased respiratory symptoms	
		Decreased exercise capacity (Increased hospitalizations)	Chronic bronchiolitis with repetitive exposure

(continued)

TABLE 17-3 (Continued)

Health Effects of Air Pollutants and Populations at Greatest Risk

Agent	Susceptible Population	Clinical Consequences	Comments
Nitrogen dioxide	Asthmatic children	Increased respiratory morbidity	Effects occur at levels found indoors with unvented sources of combustion
	Young children	Increased airway reactivity Decreased lung function Increased respiratory symptoms Increased respiratory illness	
Carbon monoxide	Healthy adults	Increased cardiac ischemia	Effects increase with anemia or chronic lung disease
	Patients with ischemic heart disease	Decreased exercise capacity Decreased exercise capacity	Possible effect: low birthweight preterm birth

COPD, chronic distructive pulmonary disease; NAAQS, National Ambient Air Quality Standards.

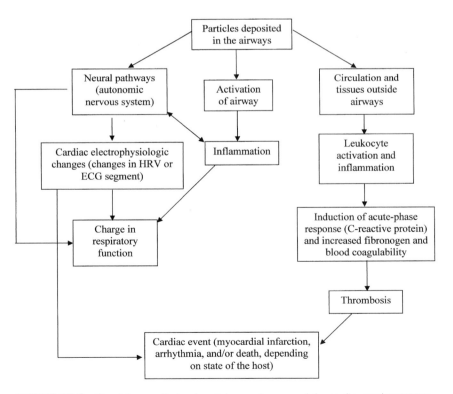

FIGURE 17-6 ● Adverse effects of particles on airways and the cardiovascular system: Possible pathways. (Adapted from Health Effects Institute. Understanding the health effects of components of the particulate matter mix: Progress and next steps. Boston, MA: Health Effects Institute, 2002. Available at: <http://www.healtheffects.org>.)

a study in The Netherlands, where cardiopulmonary mortality was associated with living near a major road.[31]

Population-Based Studies of Morbidity

Acute exposure to high concentrations of sulfur dioxide can cause bronchoconstriction, chemical bronchitis, and tracheitis. Asthmatics appear to be more sensitive. There is a linear exposure–response relationship.[3]

Acute exposure to particulates has been associated with morbidity in children and older people. Among children, particulates have been associated with emergency department visits and hospital admissions, increased respiratory illnesses (including upper respiratory infection and pneumonia), respiratory symptoms, and decrease in lung function.[3,32] Among older people, PM_{10} ambient levels have been associated with increased admissions for respiratory illnesses, including chronic obstructive pulmonary disease and pneumonia, and cardiovascular disorders, including ischemic heart disease.[26] Most studies show an increase of 1 to 2 percent in illness occurrence with each 10 $\mu g/m^3$ increase in PM_{10}. Ambient levels of particulates have also been associated with increases in systemic inflammatory markers, such as fibrinogen, C-reactive protein, and plasma viscosity, and decreases in neural control of heart function, such as decreases in heart rate and heart-rate variability.[24] Asthmatics appear to be more susceptible to the impact of PM_{10}, with increases in respiratory symptoms and decrease in lung function.[2,19] In addition, diesel particulates increase allergic response and might lead to the development of allergy and asthma.[5,6]

Long-term exposure to sulfur dioxide has been related to chronic bronchitis, especially in cigarette smokers.[3]

Long-term exposure to particulate air pollution has been associated with chronic cough, bronchitis, and chest illness—a 10 $\mu g/m^3$ increase in PM_{10} seems to be associated with a 5 to 25 percent increase in bronchitis or chronic cough and a 1 to 3 percent decrease in lung function.[4] Exposure to particulates may lead to a reduction in maximum attained lung function, which occurs early in adult life and, ultimately, to an increased risk of chronic respiratory illness.[32,33]

Adverse effects of particulates and sulfur dioxide on fetal growth, preterm birth, birthweight, and other pregnancy outcomes have been reported,[6,33] but further studies are needed.

Ozone

Ozone is a powerful oxidant that can react with a wide range of cellular components and biological material. Its biological effects are likely caused by intermediates, such as free radicals, lipid hydroperoxides, aldehydes, and hydrogen peroxide. The primary target organ for ozone is the lung, where exposure produces cellular and structural changes that reduce lung function.

Experimental Studies

Ozone causes oxidation or peroxidation of biomolecules via free radical reaction. Ozone reacts rapidly with substrates in the lung-lining fluid, preferentially with antioxidants; however, low content of lung-lining fluid antioxidant defense or high ozone exposure leads to the oxidation product responsible for adverse health effects. Lipoperoxidation of polyunsaturated fatty acids (PUFAs) of lung cells can release arachidonic acid subsequently converted into prostaglandin E2 (PGE_2) and prostaglandin F2-alpha, which will act on neuroreceptors in airways and induce an inflammatory response.[34]

Ozone damages the respiratory tract, increasing permeability and inflammation; causing morphological, biochemical, and functional changes; and decreasing host defenses. Ozone exposure causes a major lesion in the centriacinar area, thus affecting the efficiency of gas exchange. It causes fibrotic changes in animals,[35] which would be expected to cause airflow obstruction.

In humans, ozone induces an increase in the constituents of the bronchoalveolar lavage fluid. Levels of ozone frequently measured in urban areas in the United States reduce lung function. Decrement in lung function and physical performance, aggravation of respiratory tract symptoms, increased airway reactivity, and acute inflammation have been observed at exposure levels as low as 0.08 ppm. Acute reversible reductions in lung function have been observed in exercising children exposed to 0.12 ppm.[3,34] After repeated exposure to ozone, decrement in lung function observed after single exposures attenuated, suggesting adaptation, but airway inflammation persisted despite attenuation of some markers of inflammation.

These studies, taken together, show wide but reproducible variability among individuals' sensitivity to ozone and suggest that adults and children who engage in prolonged exercise or labor outdoors may be at risk of adverse health effects of ozone concentrations near the ambient standard.[36]

Population-Based Studies of Mortality

Ozone is related to daily mortality counts during the high-ozone season. A study showed that increases of 50 μg/m^3 (25 ppb) in ozone were associated with a 2.9 percent increase in daily deaths. A pooling of 15 recent time-series studies yielded an increase of 3.6 percent per 100 ppb.[37]

Population-Based Studies of Morbidity

Exposure of healthy individuals, including children, to relatively low concentrations of ozone can cause lung inflammation, acutely decreased lung function, and respiratory impairment, which lead to increases in emergency department visits and hospital admissions due to respiratory diseases, respiratory symptoms (such as cough, throat dryness, eye and chest discomfort, thoracic pain, and headache), and temporary lung function decrements. The combined relative risk estimate for respiratory-disease hospital admission from major time-series studies for all ages has been estimated to 1.18 per 100 ppb increase in daily 1-hour maximum ozone concentrations.[36] Asthmatics appear to be more sensitive to ozone exposure; increases in respiratory-related emergency department visits and symptoms and a decrease in lung function have been reported.[3,6] In clinical studies, ozone potentiates the effect of allergen exposure in sensitive asthmatics, perhaps as a consequence of increased penetrability of the respiratory epithelium from ozone exposure.[34]

Because of the acute health effects associated with short-term ozone exposure and the available studies on long-term animal exposure to ozone, there is concern that long-term exposure may have a cumulative human health impact. Long-term ozone-exposure studies suggest both a decrease in baseline pulmonary function and induction of new cases of asthma.[36] One study has linked ozone exposure to the incidence of asthma in children participating in heavy-exercise activities in communities with high-ozone concentration.[33]

Nitrogen Dioxide

Nitrogen dioxide is highly reactive and causes bronchitis and pneumonia and increases susceptibility to respiratory infections. Much exposure to nitrogen dioxide takes place indoors, where sources include cooking stoves and space heaters. Brief exposure to concentrations as high as 0.5 ppm may be experienced while cooking with gas stoves or driving in traffic.[37] In ambient air, nitrogen dioxide does not generally occur alone but as part of a complex mixture of primary and secondary pollutants. Consequently, characterizing the effects of nitrogen dioxide in ambient air has proved difficult. The contribution of nitrogen dioxide to secondary particles and its role in the formation of ozone may be more relevant to public health than any of its direct effects.

Experimental Studies

Animal experiments show that exposure to NO_2 concentrations of an order of magnitude greater than those generally found in ambient urban air can impair both the cellular and humoral immunological mechanisms of the lung.[38]

Population-Based Studies of Mortality

There is a significant positive association between daily deaths and nitrogen dioxide. Increases of 50 μg/m^3 (26.5 ppb) in nitrogen dioxide have been associated with a 1.3 percent increase in daily deaths. Nitrogen dioxide has also been associated with daily mortality in children under 5 years of age and intrauterine mortality.[6]

Population-Based Studies of Morbidity

Studies of short-term effects among children and adults related to outdoor exposure have been inconsistent. One study indicated an increase in asthma admissions related to ambient levels of nitrogen dioxide.[39] In certain occupations, workers are intermittently exposed to high concentrations of oxides of nitrogen. The spectrum of pathological effects in the lung resulting from occupational exposure to nitrogen oxides range from mild inflammatory response in the mucosa of the tracheo-bronchial tree at low concentrations to bronchitis, bronchopneumonia, and acute pulmonary edema at high concentration.[3]

Long-term exposure to outdoor nitrogen dioxide has been associated with increased chronic respiratory symptoms and infections among children and possibly to a decrease in lung function. A meta-analysis of 11 epidemiological studies reported an increase in respiratory illness in children under age 12, associated with long-term exposure to high concentration of nitrogen dioxide from gas stoves as compared with low concentrations.[40] One study showed a significant deficit in lung growth related to

TABLE 17-4

Predicted Carboxyhemoglobin Levels for People Engaged in Different Types of Work in Different Concentrations of Carbon Monoxide

CO Concentration			Predicted COHb Level for Those Engaged in:		
(ppm)	(mg/m³)	**Exposure Time**	Sedentary Work	Light Work	Heavy Work
100	115	15 min	1.2	2.0	2.8
50	57	30 min	1.1	1.9	2.6
25	29	1 h	1.1	1.7	2.2
10	11.5	8 h	1.5	1.7	1.7

CO: Carbon monoxide; COHb: carboxyhemoglobin. (Source: Romieu I. Reference 3.)

nitrogen dioxide and fine particulate exposure[33] and more frequent chronic cough and phlegm among children with asthma in communities with higher nitrogen dioxide exposure. Among adults, chronic nitrogen dioxide exposure has been associated with increased respiratory symptoms and reduced lung function.

Carbon Monoxide

High exposure to carbon monoxide now occurs primarily in certain occupations, such as firefighter, in suicide, and in unintended poisoning, such as defective or improperly used combustion devices. High exposure can cause acute poisoning, resulting in coma and death. Although most fatal carbon monoxide poisoning occurs in confined spaces, such as inside garages, automobiles, in weather-sealed houses, and ice skating rinks, episodes of fatal carbon monoxide poisoning have recently been documented in the outdoor setting among swimmers and others using recreational houseboats near generators and other gasoline-powered motor exhaust, prompting hazard warnings and boat redesign. Although outdoor exposures to carbon monoxide in urban settings are generally several orders of magnitude lower than those associated with intoxication or poisoning, some exposures during urban activities may adversely affect the heart and the brain, the most oxygen-sensitive organs.[3] People who suffer from cardiovascular disease, particularly those with angina or peripheral vascular disease, are much more susceptible to the health effects of carbon monoxide.

In the lungs, carbon monoxide is rapidly absorbed into the blood, where it binds to hemoglobin (Hb) and forms carboxyhemoglobin (COHb), which impairs the oxygen-carrying capacity of the blood. The dissociation of oxyhemoglobin is also reduced due to the presence of COHb in the blood, thereby further impairing the oxygen supply to tissues. (The affinity of Hb for carbon monoxide is about 240 times that of oxygen.) The main factors influencing the uptake of carbon monoxide are the intensity of physical activity, body size, the condition of the lung, and barometric pressure. Table 17-4 shows expected COHb levels after exposure to carbon monoxide concentrations between 10 and 100 ppm (11.5 and 115 μg/m³) during different types of physical activity. In the absence of carbon monoxide exposure, COHb is approximately 0.5 percent; one-pack-per-day cigarette smokers may achieve COHb saturations of 4 to 7 percent (Table 17-4).[3]

Experimental Studies

Carbon monoxide leads to a decreased oxygen-uptake capacity with decreased work capacity under maximum exercise conditions. A blood COHb concentration of approximately 5 percent is required to decrease oxygen-uptake capacity. An impairment in the ability to judge correctly slight differences in successive short time intervals has been observed at COHb levels of 3.2 to 4.2 percent. Headaches and dizziness occur at COHb levels between 10 and 30 percent. At COHb levels higher than about 30 percent, severe headaches, cardiovascular symptoms, and malaise occur. Above COHb levels of about 40 percent, there is considerable risk of coma and death (Table 17-5).[3]

People with previous cardiovascular disease are very sensitive to carbon monoxide exposure.

TABLE 17-5

Human Health Effects Associated with Low-Level Carbon Monoxide Exposure

Carboxyhemoglobin Concentrations (%)	Lowest Observed Effect Level (LOEL)
2.3–4.3	Statistically significant decrease (3–7%) in the relation between work time and exhaustion in exercising young healthy men.
2.9–4.5	Statistically significant decrease in exercise capacity (shortened duration of exercise before onset of pain) in patients with angina pectoris and increase in duration of angina attacks.
5–5.5	Statistically significant decrease in maximal oxygen consumption and exercise time in young healthy men during strenuous exercise.
<5.0	No statistically significant vigilance decrements after exposure to CO.
5–7.6	Statistically significant impairment of vigilance tasks in healthy experimental subjects.
5–17	Statistically significant diminution of visual perception, manual dexterity, ability to learn, or performance in complex sensorimotor tasks (such as driving).
7–20	Statistically significant decrease in maximal oxygen consumption during strenuous exercise in young healthy men.

(Source: Romieu I. Reference 3.)

Exposure to carbon monoxide sufficient to raise the concentration of COHb to 2 percent may produce adverse effects during exercise in patients with coronary artery disease. The length of time to onset of angina was reduced by 4.2 percent for a COHb level of 2 percent and by 7.1 percent at a COHb level of 3.9 percent. Similar results have been observed in patients with intermittent claudication from peripherial vascular disease.[3]

Population-Based Studies

Daily increases in carbon monoxide levels have been associated with increases in premature mortality and hospitalizations from congestive heart failure.[3] However, epidemiologic studies relating carbon monoxide with daily counts of mortality or hospital admissions need to be interpreted with caution. In contrast with other pollutants, carbon monoxide measurements from fixed monitors used for air surveillance correlate poorly with personal carbon monoxide measurements; therefore, carbon monoxide may be a proxy for other pollutants, such as fine particles.[3]

Carbon monoxide exposure may also affect the fetus directly through oxygen deficit without elevation of COHb level in fetal blood. During exposure to high carbon monoxide levels, the mother's hemoglobin gives up oxygen less readily, with a consequent lowering of the oxygen pressure in the placenta and in fetal blood. In animals, carbon monoxide causes low birthweight and developmental effects.[2] In humans, research has mainly focused on the effect of cigarette smoking during pregnancy, including decreased birthweight and retarded postnatal development.[3] Ambient carbon monoxide exposure during pregnancy has been associated with adverse outcomes, including intrauterine death and low birthweight.[6]

Susceptibility (Vulnerability) Factors

Susceptibility is a concern in the regulation of ambient air pollution. Susceptibility may include (a) intrinsic factors, such as age, gender, race, preexisting health impairment, and genetic factors, and (b) extrinsic factors, such as the profile of exposures to pollutants, concomitant exposure to other toxic living conditions, nutritional status, and lifestyle factors.[41]

Intrinsic Factors

Certain subgroups are more susceptible to the impact of air pollution, including children, older people, people with certain diseases, and those with certain genetic factors.

Several factors are responsible for the high susceptibility of children to ambient air pollutants. Children spend more time outdoors than do most adults and are often engaged in vigorous play. They also have higher respiratory rates than adults and therefore may receive higher doses of pollutants in proportion to body weight. Intensive growth and development processes create windows of great vulnerability to environmental toxicants. Older people are more likely to suffer from cardiovascular disease and impairment of immune response, both of which increase their susceptibility to air pollutants, especially fine particulates. In general, people with asthma are more responsive to short-term exposure to inhaled agents, especially particulates and ozone. People with preexisting chronic obstructive pulmonary disease or cardiovascular disease appear to be more susceptible to exposure to particulates.

Genetic factors can play a major role in responsiveness to air pollutants, especially to ozone and particulates.[2,42] Certain genetic polymorphisms affect synthesis of enzymes involved in the response to oxidative stress, such as glutathione-*S*-transferase, which could increase the susceptibility to ozone and enhance the allergic response to diesel exposure. These genetic factors might explain part of the large variability among individuals in response to ozone exposure.

Extrinsic Factors

Air pollutants appear to have both short-term and long-term effects, but there are no clear data on how patterns of exposure might influence the development of health effects. Most exposures are to air pollutants in complex mixtures. Failure to consider the presence of multiple pollutants may confuse interpretation of observed effects. Within vehicular exhaust emission, it has been difficult to assess the effect of individual pollutants, particularly fine particles and nitrogen dioxide. Some studies have reported a synergistic effect of ambient particulates and ozone and others a synergistic effect of ozone and diesel exhaust in increasing susceptibility to allergens.

Dietary antioxidants modulate the response to photo-oxidant exposure in animals and humans. Water-soluble antioxidants, ascorbate, urate, and reduced glutathione, are abundantly present in lung fluid and provide protection against damaging oxidation reactions in the extracellular components of this compartment. Within the cell, alpha-tocopherol and glutathione peroxidase may act to prevent the propagation of lipid peroxidation reactions. Vita-

min E may prevent ozone-induced peroxidation, especially in vitamin E–deficient animals. Vitamin E, vitamin C, and beta-carotene may protect against the adverse health effect of ozone on lung function.[43,44] Other micronutrients, such as omega-3 fatty acids, may decrease the adverse cardiovascular response to particulate exposure. Deficiency of these micronutrients could increase susceptibility to particulates and photo-oxidants, especially where populations are chronically exposed to high ambient air levels of pollutants.

Low socioeconomic status increases the association between air pollution and adverse health effects. Several factors, such as poor living conditions, poor nutrition, concomitant exposure, and limited access to health care, likely interact to increase the vulnerability to air pollutants.[45]

REFERENCES

1. Logan WP. Mortality in the London fog incident. 1952. Lancet 1953;1:336–8.
2. Bascom R, Bromberg PA, Costa D. Health effects of outdoor air pollution. Part I and Part II. Am J Respir Crit Care Med 1996;153:3–50;447–98.
3. Romieu I. Epidemiological studies of health effects arising from motor vehicle air pollution. In: Schwela D, Zali O, eds. Urban traffic pollution. London: E and FN Spon, 1999:9–69.
4. Pope III CA, Dockery D. Epidemiology of particle effects. In: Holgate ST, Samet JM, Koren HS, Maynard RL, eds. Air pollution and health. London: Academic Press, 1999:671–705.
5. Brunekreef B, Holgate ST. Air pollution and health. Lancet 2002;360:1233–42.
6. Romieu I, Hernandez M. Air pollution and health in developing countries: A review of epidemiological evidence. In: McGranahan G, Murray F, eds. Air pollution and health in rapidly developing countries. London, UK: Earthscan, 2003:49–67.
7. Romieu I, Korc M. Contaminación del aire exterior. In: Romieu I, Lopez S, eds. Contaminación ambiental y salud de los niños en América Latina y el Caribe. Cuernavaca, Mor, Mexico: Instituto Nacional de Salud Publica, 2003:109–29.
8. Vander Hoorns S, Ezzati M, Rodgers A, et al. Estimating attributable burden of disease from exposure and hazard data. In: Ezzati M, Lopez AD, Rodgers A, Murray CJL, eds. Quantification of health risks. Global and regional burden of diseases attributable to selected major risk factors. Geneva, Switzerland: World Health Organization, 2004:2129–90.
9. Romieu I, Samet JM, Smith KR, Bruce N. Outdoor air pollution and acute respiratory infections among children in developing countries. J Occup Environ Med 2002;44:640–9.
10. Brauer M. Sources, emissions, concentrations, exposures, and doses. In: Bates DV, Caton RB, eds. A citizen's guide to air pollution. Second ed. Vancouver, Canada: David Suzuki Foundation, 2002:11–47.

11. Holman C. Sources of air pollution. In: Holgate ST, Samet JM, Koren HS, Maynard RL, eds. Air pollution and health. London: Academic Press, 1999:115–48.

12. Annest JL, Pirkle JL, Makuc D, et al. Chronological trend in blood lead levels between 1976 and 1980. N Engl J Med 1983;308:1373–7.

13. Cortez-Lugo M, Tellez-Rojo MM, Gomez-Dantes H, et al. Tendencia de los niveles de plomo en la atmosféra de la zona metropolitana de la Ciudad de Mexico, 1988-1998. Salud Publica Mex 2003;45:S196–202.

14. Grant LD, Shoaf CR, Davis M. United States and international approaches to establishing air standards and guidelines. In: Holgate ST, Samet JM, Koren HS, Maynard RL, eds. Air pollution and health. London: Academic Press, 1999:947–82.

15. Ozkaynak H. Exposure assessment. In: Holgate ST, Samet JM, Koren HS, Maynard RL, eds. Air pollution and health. London: Academic Press, 1999:149–62.

16. Health Effects Institute. Diesel Work Shop: Building research strategy to improve risk assessment. 1999. Available at: <http://www.healtheffects.org>.

17. Krzyzanowski M, Schwela D. Patterns of air pollution in developing countries. In: Holgate ST, Samet JM, Koren HS, Maynard RL, eds. Air pollution and health. London: Academic Press, 1999:105–13.

18. Holdren JP, Smith KR. Energy, the environment and health. In: Goldenberg J, ed. World energy assessment: Energy and the challenge of sustainability. New York: United Nations Development Programme, 2000:61–110.

19. Pope III CA. Epidemiology of fine particulate air pollution and human health: Biologic mechanisms and who's at risk? Environ Health Perspect 2000;108:713–23.

20. Klemm RJ, Mason RMJ, Heilig CM, et al. Is daily mortality associated specifically with fine particles? Data reconstruction and replication of analyses. J Air Waste Manag Assoc 2000;50:1215–22.

21. Schlesinger RB. Toxicology of sulfur oxides. In: Holgate ST, Samet JM, Koren HS, Maynard RL, eds. Air pollution and health. London: Academic Press, 1999:583–611.

22. MacNee W, Donaldson K. Particulate air pollution: Injurious and protective mecanhisms in the lungs. In: Holgate ST, Samet JM, Koren HS, Maynard RL, eds. Air pollution and health. New York: Academic Press, 1999:653–72.

23. Ghio AJ, Huang YC. Exposure to concentrated ambient particles (CAPs): A review. Inhal Toxicol 2004;16:53–9.

24. Health Effects Institute. Understanding the health effects of components of the particulate matter mix: Progress and next steps. Boston, MA: Health Effects Institute, 2002. Available at: <http://www.healtheffects.org>.

25. Thomas PT, Zelikoff JT. Air pollutants: Modulators of pulmonary host resistance against infection. In: Holgate ST, Samet JM, Koren HS, Maynard RL, eds. Air pollution and health. New York: Academic Press, 1999:357–79.

26. Samet JM, Zeger SL, Dominici F, et al. The national morbidity, mortality, and air pollution study. Part II: Morbidity and mortality from air pollution in the United States. Res Rep Health Eff Inst 2000;94:5–70; discussion 71–9.

27. Aga E, Samoli E, Touloumi G, et al. Short-term effects of ambient particles on mortality in the elderly: Results from 28 cities in the APHEA2 project. Eur Respir J Suppl 2003;40:S28–33.

28. Cohen AJ, Anderson HR, Ostro B. Urban air pollution. In: Ezzati M, Lopez AD, Rodgers A, Murray CJL, eds. Quantification of health risks: Global and regional burden of diseases attributable to selected major risk factors. Geneva, Switzerland: World Health Organization, 2004:1353–1433.

29. Dockery DW, Pope III CA, Xu X, et al. An association between air pollution and mortality in six U.S. cities. N Engl J Med 1993;329:1753–9.

30. Pope III CA, Burnett RT, Thun MJ, et al. Lung cancer, cardiopulmonary mortality, and long-term exposure to fine particulate air pollution. JAMA 2002;287:1132–41.

31. Hoek G, Brunekreef B, Goldbohm S, et al. Association between mortality and indicators of traffic-related air pollution in the Netherlands: A cohort study. Lancet 2002;360:1203–9.

32. Schwartz J. Air pollution and children's health. Pediatrics 2004;113:1037–43.

33. Kunzli N, McConnell R, Bates DV, et al. Breathless in Los Angeles: The exhausting search for clean air. Am J Public Health 2003;93:1494–9.

34. Mudway IS, Kelly FJ. Ozone and the lung: A sensitive issue. Mol Aspects Med 2000;21:1–48.

35. Paige RC, Plopper CG. Acute and chornic effects of ozone in animal models. In: Holgate ST, Samet JM, Koren HS, Maynard RL, eds. Air pollution and health. New York: Academic Press, 1999:531–57.

36. Thurston GD, Ito K. Epidemiological studies of ozone exposure effects. In: Holgate ST, Samet JM, Koren HS, Maynard RL, eds. Air pollution and health. New York: Academic Press, 1999:486–510.

37. Bernard SM, Samet JM, Grambsch A, Ebi KL, Romieu I. The potential impacts of climate variability and change on air pollution-related health effects in the United States. Environ Health Perspect 2001;109:199–209.

38. Morrow PE. Toxicological data on NOx: An overview. J Toxicol Environ Health 1984;13:205–27.

39. Ackermann-Liebrich U, Rapp R. Epidemiological effects of oxides of nitrogen, especially NO2. In: Schwela D, Zali O, eds. Urban traffic pollution. London: E & FN Spon, 1999:561–84.

40. Hasselblad V, Eddy DM, Kotchmar DJ. Synthesis of environmental evidence: Nitrogen dioxide epidemiology studies. J Air Waste Manage Assoc 1992;42:662–71.

41. American Thoracic Society. What constitutes an adverse health effect of air pollution? Am J Respir Crit Care Med 2000;161:665–73.

42. Kleeberger SR. Genetic aspects of susceptibility to air pollution. Eur Respir J Suppl 2003;21:S52–56.

43. Grievink L, Smit HA, Brunekreef B. Anti-oxidants and air pollution in relation to indicators of asthma and COPD: A review of the current evidence. Clin Exp Allergy 2000;30:1344–54.

44. Romieu I, Trenga C. Diet and obstructive lung disease. Epidemiol Rev 2001;23:268–87.

45. O'Neill M, Ramirez-Aguilar M, Meneses-Gonzalez F, et al. Ozone exposure among Mexican City outdoor workers. J Air Waste Manage Assoc 2003;53:339–46.

BIBLIOGRAPHY

Brunekreef B, Holgate ST. Air pollution and health. Lancet 2002;360:1233–42.
This review discusses the evidence for adverse health effects of particulates and ozone as well as potential mechanisms for these effects.

Holgate ST, Samet JM, Koren HS, Maynard RL. Eds. Air pollution and health. London: Academic Press, 1999.
This is a major reference book on this subject.

Kleeberger SR. Genetic aspects of susceptibility to air pollution. Eur Respir J 2003;21(Suppl):S52–S56.
This review discusses recent findings on the genetic aspects of susceptibility to air pollution.

Romieu I, Hernandez M. Air pollution and health in developing countries: A review of epidemiological evidence. In G. McGranahan, F. Murray, eds. Air pollution and health in rapidly developing countries. London: Earthscan, 2003: 49–67.
This chapter provides an overview of the effects of major outdoor air pollutants with emphasis on developing countries.

U. S. Environmental Protection Agency. Draft report on the environment. (EPA 600-R-03-050). Washington, DC: USEPA, 2003. Available at: <www.epa.gov/indicators/>.
This report provides a section on outdoor air quality and presents information on outdoor air pollution levels in the United States, major sources, human health effects, and ecological effects of outdoor air pollution.

CHAPTER 18

Indoor Air Quality

Mark R. Cullen and Kathleen Kreiss

T he focus of occupational health has been transformed in many ways by the increasing proportion of the workforce employed in offices and other kinds of public facilities, merging in many respects with the concerns of environmental health. Once considered safe by crude comparison with industrial settings such as construction, mining, and agriculture, experience has proved that these indoor environments are not free of significant health hazards. Moreover, the workers engaged in these sectors are neither experienced with environmental risks, nor as well prepared in general to think about hazards of work as their industrial counterparts were even long before the modern regulatory era. Because almost all previous attention has focused on the kinds of conditions and hazards that arise in more traditionally dangerous settings, the regulatory framework has not evolved forms of controls that ensure, at least in law, that work will be safe. This chapter is divided into two sections. The first deals with the spectrum of problems that occur indoors in nonindustrial buildings, focusing on common features of implicated facilities. The second deals with the spectrum of clinical complaints related to low-dose chemical exposures (relative to doses that occur in industry), which have received increasing attention. Although these problems of chemical sensitivity most often occur in association with indoor nonindustrial environments, they may also be seen in a range of other work settings as well as in the nonwork environment. Their distinguishing feature is the occurrence of symptoms or other clinical problems at levels that are far below those at which knowledge of toxicology would predict effects and typically far below accepted standards in industry for human exposures (see Chapter 13). These somewhat vexing problems have challenged many of the cherished paradigms of occupational health about what is safe and what is not and form a special challenge for the occupational medicine specialist, as well as the primary care provider whose patients may complain about chemicals at levels deemed "safe."

BUILDING-RELATED CONDITIONS

Nonspecific Building-Related Illness

Since the 1970s, office workers worldwide have frequently complained of mucous membrane irritation, fatigue, and headache when working in specific buildings, with improvement within minutes to an hour of leaving the building. This constellation of symptoms, with tight temporal association to building occupancy, is called *sick building syndrome*, or, more recently, *nonspecific building-related illness*. It is the most frequent of the building-associated health complaints in industrialized countries, which also include diseases caused by infection, allergic hypersensitivity, or specific toxins. Researchers have estimated that as many as 30 percent of office workers report symptoms attributed to poor air quality, and workers in buildings not known to have indoor air-quality problems have many complaints attributed to the indoor work environment.

Despite the effects on productivity and employee morale when many workers in a building have building-related symptoms, the causes of these symptoms are incompletely understood. Early investigations of this phenomenon sometimes concluded that symptoms were caused by mass psychogenic illness because no specific contaminants were measured in concentrations that could account for symptoms. However, the endemic nature of complaints in specific buildings and the consistency of complaints from workers in tight buildings across the world did not satisfy diagnostic criteria for mass psychogenic illness. Fortunately, such attribution to psychological cause is no longer common or acceptable, although work stress is associated with reporting of symptoms among occupants of specific buildings (see Chapters 16 and 26). Occupants of buildings with high levels of complaints are often angry and fearful, in no small part due to resistance of managers to investigation of the cause(s) of their problems, inconclusive results of investigations that are conducted, or ineffectual remediation for a syndrome for which causes remain elusive.

The recognition of building-related complaints by public health authorities in the United States followed an energy crisis in the 1970s, during which ventilation standards were lowered to supplying 5 cubic feet of outdoor air per person per minute. This observation led to the hypothesis that building-related symptoms were attributable to lower rates of ventilation in relation to indoor contaminant sources. Some evidence exists, both in cross-sectional and experimental studies, that ventilation rates are related to the prevalence of nonspecific building-related complaints, especially for ventilation supplying outdoor air at less than 30 cubic feet per person per minute. Indoor air-quality consultants commonly measure carbon dioxide levels in buildings with high complaint rates. However, human occupants, who are the source of increased concentrations of carbon dioxide in recirculated indoor air, are not the likely source of contaminants that would explain sick building syndrome. Carbon dioxide level is not predictive of nonspecific building-related complaints.

The American Society of Heating, Refrigerating and Air-conditioning Engineers (ASHRAE) publishes consensus standards for ventilation of various types of buildings that are frequently adopted into building codes. These standards are not health-based, nor are they performance standards for operating ventilation systems. Rather, they stipulate ventilation rates for design purposes. The latest ASHRAE Standard (62.1-2004) recommends 17 cubic feet per minute of outdoor air per occupant in office buildings, in the absence of cigarette smok-ing. Measuring effective ventilation is technically difficult, expensive, and rarely done apart from research settings. Indoor air consultants examine ventilation systems for possible entrainment of contaminants in the outdoor air source; design and operation of air flow; filter condition and maintenance schedules; cleanliness of the cooling coils and drip pans, which commonly support microbial growth because of moisture and dirt; condition of the duct lining, which commonly supports microbial growth if wet; and postdesign changes in occupancy, activities, and layout that may impact air quality.

Interesting work on causes of nonspecific building-related illness comes from cross-sectional epidemiologic studies of occupants of buildings selected without regard to known indoor air-quality complaints. These studies suggest that certain building features and occupant characteristics are related to symptom prevalence. The variation in prevalence of building-related complaints among buildings suggests remediable causes. Occupants of buildings with air-conditioning have been shown to have higher rates of building-related symptoms than occupants of naturally ventilated buildings or buildings with mechanical ventilation that does not alter air temperature or humidity. This observation suggests that the ventilation system itself may be the source of poor air quality in some buildings. A double-blind multiple crossover trial of ultraviolet germicidal irradiation in office ventilation systems reduced microbial contamination of cooling coils and drip pans as well as work-related respiratory and mucosal symptoms.[1] Building dampness, associated with bioaerosols, is also frequently accompanied by nonspecific building-related illness. Measurable indices of bioaerosols are being intensively investigated as correlates of building-related illness, with some evidence implicating endotoxin, β-1,3-glucan, and culturable microbes, particularly in dust samples. Other environmental correlates include carpeting, high occupancy, and video display terminal use. Personal factors associated with building-related symptoms in many cross-sectional studies include female gender, allergies, and job stress or dissatisfaction.

Health care providers faced with the challenge of responding to indoor air-quality complaints must proceed without the benefit of a complete scientific understanding of what may be a multifactorial syndrome. No single measurement establishes whether air quality is adequate or inadequate, and a determination of the acceptability of indoor air quality rests with the occupants, and not a laboratory. In the difficult situation of indoor air-quality complaints, a multidisciplinary approach allows attention to design and maintenance of air-conditioning systems, exclusion of obvious contaminant sources or water damage in the occupied space, and reassurance of occupants that nonspecific building-related illness, in the absence of respiratory symptoms, is a self-limited condition. Indoor air-quality investigations customarily assess the ventilation in relation to occupant load by measuring carbon dioxide, identify remediable deficiencies in ventilation system maintenance and cleanliness, assess water damage and moisture incursion, and examine smoking policies. Health care providers, on a multidisciplinary team alongside industrial hygienists and ventilation engineers, have an important role to play in ruling out the possibility of less common, but more medically serious, building-related diseases, such as asthma and hypersensitivity pneumonitis, that frequently occur with a background of nonspecific building-related complaints among other workers.

Building-Related Allergic Disease

A 48-year-old social services eligibility technician began working in an office building in October. She had a history of sinus symptoms and a 15 pack-year history of cigarette smoking, having been an ex-smoker for 10 years. In January, she began to have insidious onset of dry cough, which, in March, was diagnosed as asthma. Skin prick tests were negative to common aeroallergens. She was referred to an occupational medicine clinic in August, when she noted symptom deterioration during the workday (when she needed to use inhaled bronchodilators) and recovery in the evenings and on weekends (when she did not need to use them). Her asthma became much worse when she manipulated dusty records while her desk was being moved. Self-monitoring of peak flow showed reproducible, striking air-flow limitation shortly after entering the building, with partial recovery during lunch breaks outside the building and full recovery on weekends (Fig. 18-1). Methacholine challenge testing in September and November, before a 16-day vacation, found the provocative concentrations (PC_{20}) for a 20% decrement in forced expiratory volume in 1 second (FEV_1) to be 0.29 mg/mL and after the vacation to be 0.47 mg/mL (normal $PC_{20} > 15$ mg/mL). These results confirmed a diagnosis of asthma and suggested slight improvement in airway hyperreactivity with a short work absence. Although she had notified her employer, her relocation to another building was delayed until late February, after her third course of prednisone treatment. After this relocation, her work-related air-flow limitation (documented by peak-flow measurements), her symptoms, and her need for asthma medications all resolved. Her PC_{20} normalized to above 25 mg/mL 3 months after her relocation.

Nine months later, she was moved back to the original building into a set of offices that shared no ventilation system with the offices that she had previously occupied. Over the next 6 weeks, she

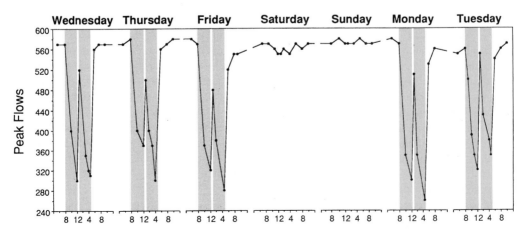

FIGURE 18-1 ● Peak-expiratory flow measurements, by hour and day, in a case of office building–related asthma. Stippled columns indicate time at work.

experienced increasing symptoms and air-flow limitation, once again requiring daily medication, and her PC$_{20}$ fell to 0.22 mg/mL. She was medically restricted from the implicated building, with resolution of her work-related decrements in peak flow, decrease of her medication requirements, and increase in her PC$_{20}$ to 5.19 mg/mL over the following 6 weeks. She has had no further difficulty with clinical asthma since then.

This building was built into an earthen bank, and workers reported musty odors and visible mold growth on the interior wall that abutted the bank. *Aspergillus* species of fungi were detected in the interior air but not in simultaneous measurements of outdoor air, suggesting amplification and dissemination of this fungus indoors. The presumed source of the woman's asthma was fungal bioaerosols associated with moisture coming in from the earthen bank.

Building-related asthma is infrequently recognized by physicians, although it can lead to chronic irreversible illness, unlike nonspecific building-related illness. Early recognition and removal from the building, as in this woman's case, can result in cure of asthma. Permanent asthma can result when recognition of occupational etiology is delayed and asthma becomes severe before the patient leaves the implicated exposure. Such sentinel cases of asthma imply risk for other workers. In this case, public health investigation after two sentinel cases showed that co-workers had nearly five times the prevalence of physician-diagnosed asthma with onset or exacerbation since building occupancy, compared with workers in another social service agency.[2]

Building-related asthma occurs in water-damaged buildings and in relation to microbially contaminated humidifiers or biocides used in them. Biological aerosols containing mold spores and possibly bacteria are the sensitizing agents. Characterization of bioaerosols is difficult because few laboratories have expertise in identifying saprophytic fungi, in contrast to fungi that cause human infection. In addition, no air measurement of viable fungi or spore count has been shown to predict hazard in the nonindustrial environment. An indoor source of microbial amplification and dissemination can be inferred from looking at the rank order of mold species concentrations indoors compared to outdoors, but no quantitative standards exist or are likely to be developed based on exposure–response studies. Experts counsel that visible mold

(Fig. 18-2) and moldy smells should be remediated without demonstrating specific mold air levels by culture or air sampling. Despite the difficulty in characterizing the exposure, the affected individual's symptom history and peak-flow measurements can be valuable in documenting the occupational nature of building-related asthma. Cases of building-related asthma may occur along with cases of hypersensitivity pneumonitis in water-damaged buildings.

A 46-year-old pediatrician had been followed by an allergist for 10 years for upper respiratory and chest complaints after moving into an office suite. At first, he complained of sinus drainage and a sore feeling in his nose and throat. Over the years, he had acquired achiness in his chest associated with fever, productive cough, chest tightness, wheezing, fatigue to exhaustion, and shortness of breath on exertion. His forced vital capacity (FVC) fell within 3 years of building occupancy, consistent with a restrictive pattern. He had been treated with nasal cromolyn, inhaled steroids, bronchodilators, theophylline, antibiotics, and intermittent oral corticosteroids, without receiving a diagnosis. A year before his referral to an occupational medicine specialist, he had noted exacerbation of his chest symptoms when he returned to his office suite after a week away from work. He then began to suspect an office-related cause to his symptoms, with increased cough, chest tightness, and achiness when he entered his suite, and resolution over hours after leaving and improvement on weekends. He noted a musty smell and fungal discoloration of wall board in the suite bathroom, which resulted from leaking pipes.

On referral, he was found to have basilar rales, bronchial hyperreactivity on histamine-challenge testing, and reduced exercise tolerance with excessive respiratory rate at rest and excessive minute ventilation for oxygen consumption. Chest x-ray was normal, but a high-resolution CT scan showed fine centrilobular nodules. Bronchoalveolar lavage showed a lymphocytic alveolitis compatible with hypersensitivity pneumonitis. A transbronchial lung biopsy showed a mild, patchy lymphocytic interstitial pneumonitis. His symptoms resolved with prednisone and removal from the office suite.

However, 2 months later, chest aching, exertional shortness of breath, profound fatigue, and chilly feelings recurred within 45 minutes of using a musty restaurant bathroom that had been water-damaged from recurrent roof leaks. He had a prolonged

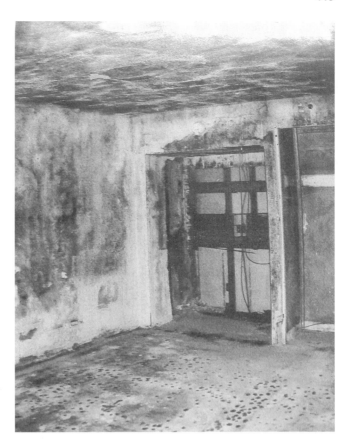

FIGURE 18-2 ● Extensive mold growth in a room of a former hotel in New Orleans. (Photograph courtesy of Michael R. Gray.)

recovery time, requiring systemic steroids for 7 months. A year after this acute exacerbation, he again had a recurrence of chest symptoms, within hours of handling medical records from his previous office suite that had become wet while stored in his basement (because of a hot water heater leak). He again required months of prednisone use and did not fully recover his health until 1 year later.

This case of building-related hypersensitivity pneumonitis illustrates the typical medical delay in suspecting and diagnosing a building-related etiology for symptoms. Few physicians are aware that office settings can be associated with diseases related to organic antigens. In contrast to building-related asthma, however, there are many published case reports and epidemic investigations of hypersensitivity pneumonitis and humidifier fever.[3] Typically, people with hypersensitivity lung diseases may not be able to reoccupy a building in which they were sensitized to biological aerosols from humidifiers, ventilation systems, or water-damaged materials on which fungal growth has occurred. Even

after remediation of the conditions that led to sensitization and disease, low levels of exposure can trigger recurrent symptoms. Because hypersensitivity pneumonitis can lead to irreversible lung fibrosis after recurrent acute episodes or prolonged exposure, early recognition and restriction of affected people from the implicated building are the best measures for preventing progression. Remediation is warranted to prevent cases in co-workers who are not yet sensitized. Occupational medicine physicians can encourage specialists to proceed with diagnostic tests before the affected individuals develop classic late-stage abnormalities, such as those evident on chest x-rays. The above case suggests that this pediatrician was sensitized to an antigen that was not unique to his water-damaged office setting. Cases of hypersensitivity pneumonitis are often accompanied by systemic symptoms of myalgia, fever, and profound fatigue. These symptoms are not usually present in asthma, although both diseases commonly share chest symptoms, such as cough, chest tightness, and wheezing. In contrast to asthma and hypersensitivity pneumonitis, sick building syndrome alone is not accompanied by chest symptoms. When indoor air-quality complaints exist, health care providers should evaluate occupants for building-related asthma and hypersensitivity pneumonitis. The occurrence of building-related chest disease dictates evaluation for sources of fungal and bacterial growth and means of dissemination from areas of water damage or from the ventilation system. The presence of chest disease also requires more aggressive medical restriction from the building to prevent irreversibility of the condition.

Many patients report that they have building-related nose and sinus symptoms. Allergic rhinosinusitis can occur, in a way analogous to the response of airways and lung tissue to building-related antigen exposure. Little research has been done on this common clinical complaint to determine its epidemiology, to distinguish it from non-immunologic mucous membrane complaints in sick building syndrome, or to link it to exposures in implicated buildings. Unfortunately, there are no practical ways of measuring antigens related to indoor microbial bioaerosols, although research is underway on antigen identification, measurement, and size differentiation. However, rhinitis may precede or exacerbate asthma. If the temporal association suggests that the nasal or sinus symptoms are building-related, the same attention to identifying and removing sources of water damage and attending to the maintenance of the heating, ventilation, and air-conditioning system is needed as for building-related chest diseases. In residential environments, allergic disease commonly occurs in relation to indoor allergens, which are more diverse than those in office settings. Antigens from dust mites, cockroaches, and animal danders are implicated in asthma beginning in childhood. Environmental intervention to lower these antigen exposures, such as by using antigen-impermeable mattress covers, vacuum cleaners equipped with high-efficiency particulate air (HEPA) filters, HEPA air purifiers, and professional pest control, can reduce childhood asthma morbidity when they are tailored to the sensitizers affecting an asthmatic child.[4]

Building-Related Infection

In 1976, a total of 182 cases of a mysterious pneumonia occurred among members of the American Legion attending a convention in Philadelphia. After months of laboratory investigation, a newly discovered bacterial organism, *Legionella pneu-*

mophila, was found to be the responsible agent. We now know that, in the absence of vigorous attempts to eradicate it, this common environmental organism frequently grows in the warm water of building cooling towers. When contaminated cooling tower mists are entrained in air intakes of large buildings, cases of infection with this organism (legionellosis) can occur. Outbreaks have also been recognized as a result of contaminated industrial water sprays, hospital shower heads, and hot tubs.

When legionellosis occurs, molecular biology techniques are now used to identify specific strains by DNA fingerprinting. Possible sources can be tested for the same strain in environmental reservoirs. This matching of aerosol source with clinical cases can help prioritize environmental controls through disinfection of hot water systems and avoidance of entrainment of contaminated aerosols.

In addition to pneumonia, *Legionella* organisms have been associated with another building-related disease called *Pontiac fever*, which is a self-limited disease characterized by fever, chills, headache, and myalgia. This disease was first described in 1968, in a building-related epidemic of 144 cases in a county health department in Michigan. The attack rate was nearly 100 percent, with an average incubation period of 36 hours.

In addition to infections that cannot be spread to other people, such as *Legionella* pneumonia, building ventilation characteristics are important to the spread of infections that can be passed on to other people, such as viral respiratory infection. Military studies have shown that types of housing with different ventilation characteristics, such as air-conditioned buildings (as compared with tents or naturally ventilated barracks), are associated with increased incidence of respiratory symptoms and signs of communicable disease in troops. Other airborne infectious diseases, such as tuberculosis, pneumococcal disease, varicella, and measles, may be affected by ventilation rates. A major concern in hospitals, prisons, and shelters is control of tuberculosis, for which ventilation and air disinfection techniques are critical (see also Chapter 15).

Building-Related Complaints Due to Specific Toxic Agents

Health professionals responding to building-related complaints must also consider specific toxic exposures as a possible explanation. This is particularly important when complaints differ from those of nonspecific building-related illness or occur in epidemic—rather than endemic—fashion. For example, complaints of headache and nausea dictate consideration of carbon monoxide poisoning, which can occur when internal combustion sources are not exhausted to the outdoors or when air intakes entrain fumes from loading docks, parking garages, or boiler stack emissions. Building-related itching without rash can occur with fibrous glass exposure, which can result when air-duct lining is entrained in the airstream entering the occupied space. Epidemic coughing, dry throat, and eye irritation can result from detergent residues after the misapplication of carpet cleaning products. In instances of building-related complaints associated with specific exposures, a careful evaluation of types of symptoms, their distribution among building occupants by location or job, and their temporal onset may point investigators to the cause and to remediation resources.

Environmental tobacco smoke may contribute to the irritant symptoms of sick building syndrome. In many buildings, environmental tobacco smoke is circulated throughout the building as air is recirculated, with modest dilution from outdoor air ventilation. In buildings with indoor air-quality complaints, restriction of smoking to areas with separate exhaust ventilation can result in improved air quality for the remainder of the building. In addition to mucous membrane irritation, environmental tobacco smoke contributes to exacerbation of asthma, accelerated decline in lung function, and increased occurrence of infections in infants and children.

INDOOR CARCINOGEN EXPOSURE

Environmental tobacco smoke has been the most common indoor carcinogen, but public tolerance of this exposure is decreasing across the United States, as reflected in state and municipality ordinances prohibiting smoking in workplaces, restaurants, and bars. Sometimes building-related carcinogen exposures do not lead to occupant symptoms but nonetheless pose a health risk. For example, radon gas emitted from building materials, water, and soil surrounding foundations poses increased risk of cancer. Radon exposures can be measured with simple devices. The Environmental Protection Agency (EPA) has guidelines for elevated exposures and effective remediation, such as sealing of foundations and subsurface ventilation. Similarly, asbestos in insulation and some building

materials in older buildings poses risks of cancer of the lung and other sites (as well as nonmalignant lung disease) if it is disturbed during occupant activities or renovation. Because of latency and dose–response considerations, occupational health specialists and other health professionals are often called to help communicate risks of asbestos exposure to building occupants or the public during removal of asbestos from older buildings. Most states license asbestos abatement professionals who are trained to protect remediation workers with respirators and other personal protective equipment, while maintaining negative pressure in asbestos removal areas to prevent asbestos fibers from entering occupied spaces. For all of these carcinogens, primary prevention is through identification and management.

MULTIPLE CHEMICAL SENSITIVITIES

Since the 1980s, a new clinical syndrome has been recognized in occupational and environmental health practice characterized by occurrence of multisystem symptoms after exposure to low levels of synthetic chemicals. Diagnoses and treatment are uncertain and controversial. Unlike any other building-related illness, this disorder recurs in affected people in a diverse array of environmental situations and cannot be readily reversed by attention to any single exposure situation. The following is a representative example of what is now most widely referred to as multiple chemical sensitivities (MCS):

A 46-year-old library worker enjoyed good health until the onset of eye, nose, and throat irritation and recurrent headache associated with a renovation of the library where she worked. She and many co-workers complained primarily of dust and paint fume exposures, which were initially poorly controlled. After several weeks of effort, the employer succeeded in establishing temporary ventilation for the work area and conducting most of the construction activities at night. Almost all of the patient's co-workers improved dramatically after these changes were instituted. She, however, felt no better and began experiencing similar symptoms in her car, at various stores, and whenever she was around anything she termed "scented," especially experiencing these symptoms in the office. She believed she was experiencing effects from the small residual levels of construction-related exposures, but temporary transfer to another part of the library brought no relief. New symptoms, including difficulty breathing, muscle and joint aches, and confusion occurred both at work and at home, triggered by an increasing list of offensive odors, irritants, and products. Efforts to clean her house of such materials, as well as a trial leave of absence from work (without the benefit of workers' compensation), resulted in only minimal improvement.

On clinical evaluation, the patient appeared well and had no abnormal physical findings. Laboratory tests, including workup for respiratory and central nervous system abnormalities, were unrevealing. Consultations in pulmonary medicine, rheumatology, and neurology were obtained but were unhelpful. Attempts at empirical therapy with various inhalers, nonsteroidal anti-inflammatory agents, and migraine therapies also failed to relieve her symptoms. Because of the disparity between complaints and findings, the patient was referred to a psychiatrist who confirmed some depressive features but could not explain the patient's symptoms. A trial of selective serotonin reuptake inhibitor (SSRI) antidepressants was initiated but was not tolerated by the patient, who discontinued the drugs after 3 days.

Finally, frustrated by unsympathetic physicians and her employer, the patient took advice she obtained from the Internet and sought evaluation from a non-traditional environmental medicine physician, who advised total avoidance of all chemical exposures, including quitting her job, and a variety of nontraditional remedies, based on results of blood and hair tests in an alternative laboratory, which reported organic chemicals and heavy metals as well as immunologic responses to a range of widely found chemicals, such as formaldehyde. She remains highly symptomatic.

Although this case occurred in the setting of building-related illness, MCS may develop in occupational and nonoccupational settings, and in people who have experienced one or more episodes of chemically induced illnesses, due to solvents, pesticides, or other chemicals. Once the problem begins, however, affected individuals experience symptoms they associate with many types of environmental contaminants in air, food, or water at doses well below those that clinically affect others. Although there may not be measurable impairment of specific organs, the complaints are associated with dysfunc-

tion and disability. Although MCS as severe as in the above case is not common, it is prevalent enough to have generated substantial controversy. However, research has not yet elucidated its cause and pathogenesis, nor ways to treat or prevent it.

Multiple Chemical Sensitivities: Definition and Diagnosis

There is no general consensus on a definition for MCS, but certain features are sufficiently characteristic to raise suspicion and differentiate it from other occupational and nonoccupational health problems. Its major features are as follows:

- Symptoms usually occur after an occupational or environmental inhalation or toxic exposure. This precipitating event may be a single episode, such as an exposure to a pesticide spray, or recurrent, as in the case presented previously. Often the initial event or reaction is mild and may merge without clear demarcation into the syndrome that follows.
- Symptoms resembling those associated with the preceding exposure begin to occur after exposures to surprisingly lower levels of various materials, including chemicals, perfumes, and other common work and household products, especially materials that have a pungent odor or are irritating.
- Symptoms appear referable to many organ systems. Central nervous system problems, such as fatigue, confusion, and headache, occur in almost every case.
- Complaints of chronic symptoms, such as fatigue, cognitive difficulties, and gastrointestinal and musculoskeletal disturbances, frequently complicate the temporal relationship between specific exposures and effects. These more persistent symptoms may even predominate over acute reactions to chemicals in some cases.
- Objective impairment of the organs that would explain the pattern or intensity of complaints is typically absent.
- No other diagnosis easily explains the range of responses or symptoms. Although the patient may, in fact, have other physical or emotional ailments, such as allergy or anxiety, symptoms related to MCS will often not resolve despite appropriate treatment of these concurrent illnesses. However, because illnesses such as asthma and panic attacks are both treatable and potentially life-threatening, it is important to make a positive diagnosis and to treat them when found.

Not every patient meets these criteria precisely. But because the diagnosis of MCS is, in the end, based on subjective information, each point should be carefully considered. Each serves to rule out other clinical disorders that MCS may resemble, such as generalized anxiety disorder, classic sensitization to environmental antigens (such as occupational asthma), late sequelae of organ system damage (such as reactive airways dysfunction syndrome after a toxic inhalation), or systemic disease (such as systemic lupus erythematosus). On the other hand, the diagnosis of MCS does not require the exclusion of all other possibilities, and exhaustive testing is not required in most cases.

In practice, diagnostic problems are seen in two clinical situations. Early in the course of the disorder, it is often difficult to distinguish MCS from occupational or environmental health problems that may have preceded it. For example, patients who have experienced symptomatic reactions to pesticide spraying indoors may find that their reactions persist even when they avoid direct contact with these chemicals. In this situation, a clinician might assume that significant exposures could still be occurring and may focus entirely on altering the environment further, which usually does not relieve the recurrent symptoms. This is especially troublesome in an office setting, where MCS may develop as a complication of nonspecific building-related illness. Although most co-workers improve after steps are taken to improve air quality, the patient who has acquired MCS continues to experience symptoms despite the lower exposures achieved. Later in the course of MCS, diagnostic dilemmas arise because of the chronic aspects that may obscure the patient's intolerance to common odors and chemicals. After many months, patients with MCS are often depressed, anxious, and frustrated about their health. Physical inactivity, often with weight gain, sleep disturbances, and significant social dysfunction are common. These phenomena demand considerable attention therapeutically.

Pathogenesis

The sequence of pathologic events that leads from apparently self-limited episodes of an environmental exposure to the development of MCS in certain people is not known. There are several current hypotheses.

A group of nontraditional environmental medicine physicians, initially called clinical ecologists, have hypothesized that MCS is a form of immune dysfunction caused by insidious accumulation of exogenous chemicals over a lifetime. They propose susceptibility factors that include nutritional deficiencies (such as vitamins and antioxidants), the presence of subclinical infections (such as candidiasis), or other host factors. In this approach, the precipitating exposure or exposures are important because of their contribution to lifelong chemical overload.

Another biologically oriented hypothesis is that MCS represents an atypical biological sequela of chemical injury, such as a new form of neurotoxicity due to solvents or pesticides, or injury to the respiratory tract after an acute inhalational episode. In this approach, MCS is seen as a final common pathway of different primary disease mechanisms.

A more recent concept has focused on the relationship between the mucosa of the upper respiratory tract and the limbic system, especially the close anatomic proximity of the two in the nose. Under this view, relatively small stimulants to the nasal epithelium could result in amplified limbic responses (as occurs in addicted people to the substances to which they are addicted), explaining the dramatic and sometimes stereotypic responses to low-dose exposures. This hypothesis also may explain the prominent role of stimuli with strong odors, such as perfumes, in triggering responses in many patients.

Many investigators and clinicians with experience have invoked primarily psychological mechanisms to explain MCS, linking it to other anxiety or affective disorders. Some believe that MCS is a variant of post-traumatic stress disorder or a conditioned response to a toxic experience. One hypothesis suggests MCS is a late-life response to early childhood traumas, such as sexual abuse. In these hypotheses, the precipitating illness plays a more symbolic than biological role in the pathogenesis of MCS. Host susceptibility is obviously very important in these approaches, particularly the predisposition to somaticize psychological distress.

Although there is much published literature, few clinical or experimental studies have been presented or published to support strongly any of these views as the single best explanation for MCS. Research has been hampered by variously defined study populations, inappropriately matched control groups, and lack of "blinding" of subjects and investigators. As a result, most available data are descriptive. Perhaps most difficult of all, debate over the etiology of MCS has been heavily dominated by dogma. Major financial decisions, such as patient benefit entitlements and physician reimbursement, may depend on how MCS is viewed. These theories may be well-known to patients as well, and they may also have very strong views.

Epidemiology

Detailed information about the epidemiology of MCS is not available. Estimates of prevalence in the U.S. population range as high as 6 percent; the rate found in military "controls" for veterans of Gulf War I was about 2.5 percent, while veterans of the conflict suffered MCS-like symptoms twice as frequently. Although many people find chemicals and other odors objectionable and report life modifications to avoid exposure to them, MCS in clinically overt form remains uncommon. Although much available data come from case series by various practitioners who treat patients with MCS, some general observations appear recurrently in the reports:

• MCS occurs most commonly in midlife, although patients of virtually all ages have been described.
• Workers in higher socioeconomic status jobs seem more often affected, whereas economically disadvantaged workers seem underrepresented; this may be an artifact of differential access to occupational and environmental health services or a diagnostic bias.
• Women are more frequently affected than men.
• Some host factor or susceptibility is important because mass outbreaks have been uncommon, and only a small fraction of victims of chemical overexposures acquire MCS or anything like it. Although few host factors have been adequately studied, common atopic allergic disorders do not appear to be an important risk factor for MCS.
• Several classes of chemicals have been commonly implicated in the initial presentation of MCS, specifically organic solvents, pesticides, and respiratory irritants, perhaps a function of the widespread exposure to these materials. The other commonplace setting in which many cases occur is in the "sick building" situation, with some patients evolving from nonspecific building-related illness into MCS, as in the patient described in the previous case. Although the two illnesses have much in common, their epidemiologic features serve to distinguish them: Nonspecific building-related illness usually affects a high proportion of

people sharing a common environment, whereas MCS occurs sporadically and is not location-specific.

Finally, there is great interest in whether MCS is a new disorder or a new presentation of an old one. Views on this are divided, much as is opinion on the pathogenesis of MCS. Those favoring a biological role for chemicals argue that MCS is a "20th-century disease" with rising incidence related to widespread chemical usage. Those who support psychological mechanisms see MCS as an old somatoform disorder with a new societal metaphor—the social perception of chemicals as agents of harm.

Natural History

MCS has not yet been studied enough to delineate its clinical course completely, although reports of large series of patients have provided some clues. The general pattern is early progression as the process evolves, followed by less predictable periods of small improvements and exacerbations. These modest changes are often perceived by the patient in relation to environmental factors or treatments, but no scientific basis for such relationships has been established.

Two important observations have been made. First, there is little evidence that MCS is a progressive disorder. Patients do not get worse from year to year in any demonstrable physical way or have resultant complications, such as organ system failure, unless there is intercurrent illness. Despite patients' perceptions, MCS is not lethal—a basis for a hopeful prognosis and reassurance. Unfortunately, complete remissions are unlikely, given current treatment (or lack thereof). Although significant improvement may occur, this is usually related to better patient function and sense of well-being. The underlying tendency to react to chemical exposures persists, although symptoms may become tolerable enough to allow a normal or near-normal lifestyle.

Clinical Management

There remains no established treatment for MCS. Many traditional and nontraditional strategies have been tried, although few have been subjected to the usual scientific standards to document success or failure, such as a blinded clinical trial. Approaches to treatment of the disorder have followed theories of pathogenesis. Those who believe that MCS is caused by biological consequences of large burdens of exogenous chemicals have focused attention on avoidance of further exposures through the use of "natural" products and the radical alteration of lifestyle. Diagnostic tests of unproved significance, including body fluid assays for trace organic chemicals and antibodies to common chemicals, have been developed as a basis to attempt to develop desensitization approaches. Dietary supplements, such as vitamins and antioxidants, have been recommended to improve host resistance to chemical effects, again without evidence of efficacy. A more radical treatment involves elimination of toxic chemicals from the body by chelation or accelerated turnover of fat, where lipid-soluble pesticides, solvents, and other organic chemicals may be concentrated. Unfortunately, serious side effects have occurred with some alternative therapies, including repeated chelation (renal damage), ozone therapy (anemia), and high levels of pyridoxine (peripheral nerve damage). In the absence of proven benefit, a major tenet should be to do no harm.

Those who take to a psychological view of MCS have tried approaches consistent with these theories. Supportive individual therapies and behavioral modification techniques have been described, although the efficacy of these therapies remains unproved, and some approaches, such as group therapy or breathing exercises, may be counterproductive. These patients tend to be intolerant to pharmacologic agents used to treat affective and anxiety disorders, making treatment plans much more difficult.

Despite limitations of current knowledge, certain treatment principles can be synthesized:

- To the extent possible, the search to "get to the bottom" of MCS in an individual patient should be minimized—it is counterproductive to starting support and treatment. Many patients have already had considerable medical evaluation by the time MCS is first recognized, and further evaluation, unless necessary to exclude treatable diseases, is often a distraction.
- Whatever the particular beliefs of the clinician, the existing knowledge and uncertainty about MCS should be explained to the patient, including that its cause is unknown.
- The patient must be reassured that consideration of psychological complications that commonly

arise does not mean that the illness is not real, serious, and worthy of treatment.
- The patient may also be reassured that MCS is neither progressive nor fatal, but that complete cures are not likely with current modalities.
- Uncertainty about pathogenesis aside, it is most often necessary to modify patients' work environments to remove them from triggers of symptoms. Although radical avoidance is counterproductive to the goal of enhancing function, regular and severe symptomatic reactions must be limited to allow the patient to begin the supportive care he or she needs in a trusting doctor–patient relationship. Often this requires a job change. Workers' compensation may be appropriate in the perspective of MCS as a complication of a work exposure, which often appears to be the case.

The goal of all therapy must be improvement of function because the underlying problem cannot be changed given current knowledge. Psychological problems, such as adjustment difficulties, anxiety, and depression, must be treated, as should coexistent clinical disorders, such as atopic allergies. Because patients with MCS do not tolerate chemicals in general, nonpharmacologic approaches may be necessary. Most patients need direction, counseling, and reassurance to adjust to life with an illness such as MCS. Whenever possible, patients should be encouraged to increase activities to their premorbid level. Passivity and dependence, common responses to the disorder, should not be reinforced by prescriptions of avoidance, however well intended.

Prevention and Control

Primary prevention strategies cannot be developed without knowledge of the pathogenesis of the disorder or the host risk factors that predispose some people to become affected. However, reduction of opportunities in the workplace for the overexposures that seem to lead to MCS in some people, including especially respiratory irritants, solvents, and pesticides and the products of war, may reduce the occurrence of MCS. Better ventilation in offices and other nonindustrial workplaces would also help.

Secondary prevention would appear to offer some greater control opportunities, although no specific interventions have been studied. Because psychological factors may play a role in victims of occupational overexposures, careful and early management of people seeking care after acute toxic exposures or symptoms related to buildings is advisable even when the prognosis from the exposure itself is good. Patients seen in clinics or emergency departments immediately after acute exposures should be assessed for their reactions to the events and should probably receive very close follow-up when undue concerns of long-term effects or persistent symptoms are noted. Obviously, efforts should be made for such patients to ensure that preventable recurrences do not occur because this may be an important risk factor for MCS by whatever mechanism is causal.

REFERENCES

1. Menzies D, Popa J, Hanley JA, et al. Effect of ultraviolet germicidal lights installed in office ventilation systems on workers' health and wellbeing: Double-blind multiple crossover trial. Lancet 2003;362:1785–91.
2. Hoffman RAE, Wood RC, Kreiss K. Building-related asthma in Denver office workers. Am J Public Health 1993;83:89–93.
3. Kreiss K, Hodgson MJ. Building-associated epidemics. In: Walsh PJ, Dudney CS, Copenhaver ED, eds. Indoor air quality. Boca Raton, FL: CRC Press, 1984:87–106.
4. Morgan WJ, Crain EF, Gruchalla RS, et al. Results of a home-based environmental intervention among urban children with asthma. N Engl J Med 2004;351:1068–80.

BIBLIOGRAPHY

Black DW, Doebbling BN, Voelker MD, et al. Multiple chemical sensitivity syndrome. Symptom prevalence and risk factors in a military population. Arch Intern Med 2000;160:1169–76.
Institute of Medicine. Damp Indoor Spaces and Health. Washington, DC; The National Academies Press, 2004.
This interdisciplinary review of the scientific evidence on associations between exposure to "dampness" in buildings and health effects concludes that many respiratory symptoms are associated with dampness, but that the mechanisms and environmental measurements predicting risk are unknown.
Gibson PR, Elms AN, Ruding LA. Perceived treatment efficacy for conventional and alternative therapies reported by persons with multiple chemical sensitivity. Environ Health Perspect 2003;111:1498–504.
Mendell MJ. Nonspecific symptoms in office workers: A review and summary of the epidemiologic literature. Indoor Air 1993;3:227–236.
Describes the conclusions about risk factors for sick building syndrome that can be drawn from the literature through the lenses of methodologic strength of design and consistency of findings among investigations.
Seiber WK, Stayner LT, Malkin R, et al. The National Institute for Occupational Safety and Health indoor environmental evaluation experience: Part three. Associations between environmental factors and self-reported health conditions. Appl Occup Environ Hygiene 1996;11:1387–92.
A report of systematic investigations of 2,435 respondents in 80 buildings with indoor air quality complaints, summarizing the environmental risk factors that were associated with symptom prevalence.
Sparks PJ, Daniell W, Black DW, et al. Multiple chemical sensitivity: A clinical perspective. I. Case definition, theories of pathogenesis, and research needs. J Occup Med 1994;36:718–30.
Sparks PJ, Daniell W, Black DW, et al. Multiple chemical sensitivity: A clinical perspective. II. Evaluation, diagnostic testing, treatment, and social considerations. J Occup Med 1994;36:731–7.
These two papers represent a refereed review of MCS.

The findings and conclusions in this chapter are those of the authors and do not necessarily represent the views of the National Institute for Occupational Safety and Health.

CHAPTER 19

Water Quality

Jeffery A. Foran

Lack of access to water—for drinking, hygiene and food security—inflicts enormous hardship on more than a billion members of the human family. Water is likely to become a growing source of tension and fierce competition between nations, if present trends continue.
—Kofi Annan, UN Secretary-General.

Water is essential for life and the earth has more than 1 billion cubic kilometers—2.6×10^{20} gallons or 240 million cubic miles—of it. But only a very small percentage is fresh water, and even less is available for human use. Effectively, only about 0.01 percent of all of the water in the world is usable, and this water is not evenly distributed among countries and regions.

The average person needs a minimum of 5 liters (1.3 gallons) of water per day to survive in a moderate climate at an average activity level. The minimum amount of water needed for drinking, cooking, bathing, and sanitation is between 50 and 100 liters (13 to 26 gallons) per day. Global, individual water use rates are markedly different. For example, the average person in Somalia uses only 8.9 liters (2.3 gallons) of water per day, whereas the average person in the United States uses between 250 to 300 liters (65 to 78 gallons) of water per day for drinking, cooking, bathing, and watering domestic property.

In 1995, the World Health Organization (WHO) reported that more than 1 billion people in low- and middle-income countries lacked access to safe water for drinking, personal hygiene, and domestic use, and nearly 2 billion people lacked access to adequate sanitation facilities. Annually, lack of access to clean drinking water has led to nearly 250 million cases of water-related disease and between 5 and 10 million deaths.

As of 2000, 3 percent of the world's population faced "water scarcity" situations (less than 1,000 cubic meters of water available per person per year) and 5 percent faced "water stress" (1,000 to 2,000 cubic meters of water available per person per year). By 2025, a projected 7 percent of the world's population will face water scarcity and 31 percent will face water stress. The total population in countries facing water stress or water scarcity is projected to grow from 480 million in 2000 to nearly 3 billion in 2025.[1]

The WHO projects that water scarcity will not affect all countries and regions in the same ways. For example, population increases and growing demands are projected to push all West Asian countries into water scarcity. By 2025, nearly 230 million Africans will face water scarcity and 460 million will live in water-stressed countries, with much of the burden falling on North Africa and sub-Saharan Africa.

After water availability, the single greatest hazard associated with drinking water worldwide is microbial contamination. Access to safe water (treated, or untreated but uncontaminated) is unevenly distributed throughout the world. An estimated 900 million people suffer from water-related diarrheal illness each year, resulting in 2 million deaths. Many of these people live in low- and middle-income countries. Those at greatest risk are children and older people. Many more suffer from other water-related diseases, such as cholera, elephantiasis, and hookworm infestation. The United

Nations reports that, overall, water-related diseases kill more than 5 million people each year. More than 2 billion people suffer from diseases linked to contaminated water, while 60 percent of infant mortality worldwide is linked to water-related infectious and parasitic diseases.

Advanced water treatment in many developed countries has reduced pathogen concentrations to levels that pose little threat to public health. However, pathogen contamination of water supplies has not been eliminated in developed countries, including those that employ sophisticated water-treatment technologies. In some of these countries, including the United States, pathogen contamination is a reemerging threat as a result of relatively new and newly discovered pathogens, such as *Cryptosporidium*, which are resistant to conventional treatment, and new sources of water contamination, such as bioterrorism.

Human health has also suffered as a result of chemical contamination of water supplies in developed as well as developing countries. Chemical contaminants in surface and ground water may occur naturally or from industry, agriculture, and other human activities (Fig. 19-1). The nature and sources of chemical contamination may be similar in some cases and may differ greatly in others between developed and developing countries.

Water quantity and quality profoundly affect quality of life. The global disparities in access to clean, fresh water are readily apparent, and the effects of these disparities on human health as well as on society and ecosystems are becoming better, although not yet fully understood. This chapter, which addresses water quality and its effects on health, provides overviews of pathogen and chemical contamination of surface and ground water, contaminant sources, effects of exposure to contaminants on human health, approaches to treatment of sanitary waste and drinking water (Boxes 19-1 and 19-2), and selected regulatory and nonregulatory approaches to address contamination of surface, ground, and drinking water.

CONTAMINANTS OF GROUND AND SURFACE WATER

There are myriad contaminants of ground and surface freshwater from both natural and human sources. Discharges of pathogenic and chemical contaminants from industry and wastewater treatment plants; runoff of pesticides, nutrients, and pathogens from agriculture regions; household use of cleaners and pesticides; leaking septic systems; and storm-water runoff contaminate ground and surface water. Human exposure to water contaminants occurs from two primary sources: direct exposure through ingestion of drinking water, dermal absorption, and inhalation; and accumulation of contaminants in aquatic organisms and human consumption of those organisms. The sources, exposure routes, and health effects of a representative set of contaminants in ground and surface water are discussed below.

Pathogens

Human history has been plagued by disease and suffering associated with pathogen-contaminated drinking water. John Snow identified contaminated drinking water as the source of a cholera epidemic that killed thousands of people in London in 1854. Ultimately, water treatment, primarily with chlorine, became widespread and reduced pathogen-associated diseases extensively. However, many developing countries continue to have inadequate water treatment capability and cholera, typhoid, and other diseases associated with pathogen-contaminated drinking water continue to be significant public health threats.

Pathogen contamination of drinking water is not just a problem in developing nations and regions. Pathogen-associated disease reemerged during the 1990s as an important public health threat in countries and regions with advanced water treatment. A 1993 outbreak of cryptosporidiosis in Milwaukee affected 400,000 people and killed approximately 100. The outbreak was likely due to runoff from agricultural areas polluted with cattle or other animal feces and water treatment that was not adequate

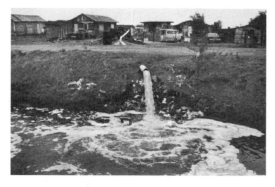

FIGURE 19-1 ● Water pollution from residential area for maquiladora plant workers in Matamoros, Mexico. (Photograph by Earl Dotter.)

BOX 19-1

Generalized Steps in the Treatment of Sanitary Waste Prior to Its Discharge to Surface Waters

Screening: Removal of items, such as wood, rocks, and dead animals, prior to wastewater entering the treatment plant. Most of these materials are sent to a landfill.

Pumping: Gravity moves sewage from homes and businesses to the treatment plant. If the plant is built above the ground level, wastewater has to be pumped up to the aeration tanks, where gravity moves wastewater through the treatment process.

Aeration: Aeration causes some dissolved gases that cause taste and odor problems, such as hydrogen sulfide, to be released from the water. Wastewater then enters a series of long, parallel concrete tanks. Each tank is divided into two sections. In the first section, air is pumped through the water. As organic matter decays, it uses up oxygen. Aeration replenishes oxygen. Bubbling oxygen through the water also keeps the organic material suspended while it forces grit (coffee grounds, sand, and other small, dense particles) to settle out. Grit is pumped out of the tanks and taken to landfills.

Sludge removal: Wastewater then enters the second section or sedimentation tanks. The sludge, the organic portion of the sewage, settles out of the wastewater and is pumped out of the tanks. Some of the water is removed in a step called thickening. The sludge is processed in large tanks called digesters.

Scum removal: As sludge is settling to the bottom of the sedimentation tanks, lighter materials, termed scum, float to the surface. This scum includes grease, oils, plastics, and soap. Slow-moving rakes skim the scum off the surface of the wastewater. Scum is thickened and pumped to the digesters along with the sludge. After solids are removed, the liquid sewage is filtered through a substance, usually sand, by the action of gravity. This method removes almost all bacteria, reduces turbidity and color as well as odors, reduces the amount of iron, and removes most other solid particles from the water. Water is sometimes filtered through carbon particles to remove organic particles.

Disinfection: Finally, the wastewater flows into a tank where chlorine is added to kill bacteria. The chlorine is mostly eliminated as the bacteria are destroyed, but sometimes it is neutralized by adding other chemicals. This protects fish and other aquatic organisms as the treated waste is discharged to surface waters. The treated water, called effluent, is then discharged to a local river, lake, or the ocean.

Residuals: Treating wastewater includes dealing with the solid-waste material. Solids are kept for 20 to 30 days in large, heated enclosed tanks, called digesters, where bacteria break down (digest) the material, reducing its volume and odors and removing organisms that can cause disease. The finished product is sent to landfills or is sometimes used as fertilizer.

Source: <ga.water.usgs.gov/edu/wwvisit. html>.

to kill *Cryptosporidium* oocysts. Parts of Milwaukee have taken steps to improve treatment capacity to prevent future *Cryptosporidium* outbreaks, including the use of advanced filtration, ozonation, and UV treatment. However, other emerging problems associated with pathogen contamination of water threaten public health in both developing and developed nations.

Bioterrorism

A potential source of pathogen contamination of drinking water supplies is bioterrorism.[2] Pathogens such as *Clostridium perfringens* and the bacteria that cause anthrax and plague and biotoxins such as botulinum, aflatoxin, and ricin have been weaponized, are potentially resistant to disinfection by chlorination, and are stable for relatively long periods in water.[3] Although water supply systems provide some dilution, sophisticated technologies such as microcapsules can be used to disperse human pathogens in drinking water systems. Effectiveness of an attack can be enhanced by introduction of the agent in the distribution system.

Although the probability of a terrorist threat to drinking water is extremely low, the consequences

---

BOX 19-2

General Steps Used in the Treatment of Drinking Water

Aeration: Water is mixed to liberate dissolved gases and to suspend particles in the water column.

Flocculation: Materials and particles present in drinking water (clay, organic material, metals, and microorganisms) are often quite small and will not settle out from the water column without assistance. To help the settling process, "coagulating" compounds are added to the water. Suspended particles stick to these compounds and create large and heavy clumps of material.

Sedimentation: Water is left undisturbed to allow the heavy clumps of particles and coagulants to settle out.

Filtration: Water is run through a series of filters that trap and remove particles still remaining in the water column. Typically, beds of sand or charcoal are used to accomplish this task.

Disinfection: Water, now largely free of particles and microorganisms, is treated to destroy any remaining disease-causing pathogens, commonly done with chlorination (the same process used to eliminate pathogens in swimming pools), ozone, or ultraviolet radiation. Water is now safe to drink and is sent to pumping stations for distribution.

---

could be very severe; therefore, preventing human exposure to pathogens is critically important and requires rapid detection in real-time in source water and water distribution systems. Rapid detection technologies such as DNA microchip arrays, immunologic techniques, microrobots, optical technologies, flow cytometry, and molecular probes are under development although none is available commercially, and none have been tested in large drinking water systems.

Contamination at Swimming Beaches

Although exposure to pathogens is typically through consumption of contaminated drinking water, ingestion of pathogen-contaminated water while swimming has become a public health concern. Swimming beaches in the United States are visited by more than one-third of all Americans. During 2001, there were at least 13,400 days of closings and advisories, 46 extended closings and advisories (6 to 12 weeks), and 73 permanent closings and advisories (more than 12 weeks) at beaches nationwide. This is not a new development. Since 1988, there have been more than 60,000 closings and advisories at beaches throughout the United States, although the number of closings has increased during recent years, due, in part, to more monitoring and sampling.

Beach closings and advisories are most often a result of elevated bacteria levels in water where people swim. During 2001, 87 percent of beach closings and advisories were based on water quality monitoring that detected elevated bacteria levels; the rest were precautionary, or due to pollution or reports of human disease.

Public health agencies typically take the lead in monitoring water quality at swimming beaches. Monitoring focuses almost exclusively on *Escherichia coli* or fecal coliforms, although monitoring of other parameters such as pH, nutrients, and temperature is also done. *E. coli* and fecal coliforms occur in the gastrointestinal tracts of higher animals and, as a result, are common in animal feces. Although the strain of *E. coli* commonly found in fecal-contaminated water and fecal coliforms do not cause human disease, they are used as indicators of other human pathogens, such as *Giardia* and *Cryptosporidium*.

There are many sources of contaminants that cause closings and advisories at beaches, including polluted storm-water runoff, spills and overflows of sewage from wastewater treatment plants and collection systems, discharges from boats, leaking septic systems, and feces from birds and other wildlife. However, little is known about sources of contaminants at more than half of U.S. beaches at which closings or advisories occur.

Contamination of water at swimming beaches causes, or has the potential to cause, a variety of human diseases, including ear, nose, and throat infections (such as swimmer's ear; otitis externa), respiratory infections, and diarrheal disease. Some of these disorders may be life-threatening to young children, older people, and individuals with compromised immune systems.

Uniform requirements for monitoring and standards for beach closings and advisories have not been implemented at U.S. swimming beaches, although the Beach Act of 2000 required that states adopt standards by 2004. Many states, however, have not yet come into compliance with the Beach Act of 2000, and as monitoring of water quality at swimming beaches increases, the nature and extent of the problem are likely to increase as well.

Chemical Contaminants

Lead

Lead occurs naturally in the earth's crust and is used in a variety of industrial applications. Previous use of lead in gasoline in the U.S. contaminated surface waters, although at very low levels that have not likely resulted in significant human exposure.

Because of its malleability and corrosion-resistance, elemental lead has been used in water supply pipes since Roman times. (The word "plumbing" comes from the Latin for "lead.") In older cities, public water supply pipes may still contain lead although more than 99 percent of all public drinking water systems have lead concentrations less than 0.005 ppm. However, lead concentrations in the water of homes and other buildings may be significantly higher and may pose a considerable threat to human health. Indeed, homes built before 1986 are more likely to have lead pipes, joints, and solder although new homes are also at risk: even pipes that are considered "lead-free" may contain up to 8 percent lead and can leave significant amounts of lead in the water for the first several months after their installation. The acidity of drinking water plays an important role in the availability of lead, with higher concentrations occurring in waters that are acidic. Acidic water (water with pH below 6.0) corrodes leaded pipes and solder and results in leaching of lead into the water distribution system; when water is acidic and remains in contact with the pipe for hours, the lead concentration in the first draw may be considerable.

The U.S. Environmental Protection Agency (EPA) Maximum Contaminant Level Goal (MCLG) for lead in drinking water is zero. However, EPA has not developed a Reference Dose (RfD) or Maximum Contaminant Level (MCL) for lead in water because health effects occur at very low levels and likely lack a threshold. EPA requires drinking water systems to install or improve corrosion control to minimize lead levels at the tap, install treatment to reduce lead in source water entering the distribution system, and replace lead service lines when more than 10 percent of targeted tap samples exceed lead concentrations of 15 μg/L. Drinking water systems are also required to conduct public education programs if levels remain above 15 μg/L after reduction actions are taken. Where lead contamination occurs as a result of plumbing, removal of the existing plumbing and installation of lead-free plumbing and fixtures should prevent further exposure. When this is not practical, running water for 15 to 30 seconds before drinking or cooking will reduce the lead concentration considerably, particularly when water has not been used for a prolonged period.

Arsenic

Arsenic, an element that occurs in soil and rock, is released to the environment naturally via leaching to water and from anthropogenic sources, including ore-smelting operations. The average concentration of arsenic in surface and ground water is about 1 ppb, although much higher concentrations can occur locally.

Arsenic in water can be lethal at concentrations of 50–60 ppm, and concentrations as low as 300 ppb can cause nausea, vomiting, and diarrhea. Chronic exposure to lower levels of arsenic can cause skin changes, including darkening and small corns or warts. The International Agency for Research on Cancer (IARC), EPA, and the National Toxicology Program (NTP) have classified arsenic as a known human carcinogen. Arsenic causes cancer of the liver, bladder, kidney, skin, and lung. The EPA has set an MCL for arsenic in drinking water of 10 μg/L (ppb).

Arsenic has been found in ground water throughout the United States (Fig. 19-2), in some cases at concentrations greater than the EPA drinking water standard. However, the public health toll associated with these concentrations pales in comparison to the environmental and public health disaster that occurred in Bangladesh and in West Bengal, India, where millions of people drink from ground water heavily contaminated with arsenic from geologic structures.

Bangladesh and West Bengal have some of the highest rates of waterborne infectious disease worldwide, including shigellosis, typhoid, cholera, and viral hepatitis. To address this problem, well water was heavily promoted and developed as a safe alternative to untreated surface water and people were instructed to rely on ground water as their primary drinking water source. As a result, the incidence of waterborne infectious disease declined dramatically. However, in the 1980s evidence of arsenic contamination was found in ground water,

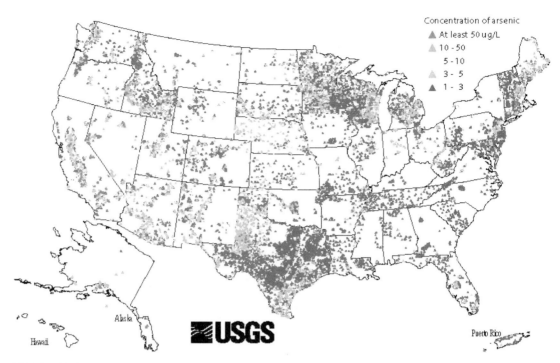

FIGURE 19-2 ● Arsenic concentrations in ground water in the United States. (Source: Ryker SJ. Mapping arsenic in groundwater. Geotimes 2001;46:34–6.)

and during the mid-1990s, the issue gained broad public attention. WHO estimates that more than 30 million people may be exposed to arsenic concentrations in drinking water greater than 50 ppb (Fig. 19-3).

WHO also estimates that drinking arsenic-contaminated water in Bangladesh has caused more than 100,000 cases of skin disorders. Ultimately, skin and internal cancers caused by arsenic exposure will become major health concerns with considerable associated social and economic hardship. Extensive water quality testing and on-site mitigation, with use of deep, arsenic-free wells, rainwater harvesting, installation of treatment plants, and extensive training and education have been implemented. However, the efficacy of these programs in reducing arsenic exposure and the risk of associated disease has not been assessed.[4]

Atrazine

Atrazine, a triazine pesticide, has been used for more than 35 years and is applied to more than 65 percent of U.S. corn acreage, as well as sorghum, sugar cane, macadamia nuts, and conifer trees.

In the United States, approximately 10 million pounds of this restricted-use pesticide are applied annually.

The use of atrazine results in runoff, leaching, and volatilization from agricultural soils, and transport to surface and ground water as well as the atmosphere. EPA estimates that atrazine is present in more than 1,500 community water supplies and more than 70,000 rural domestic wells nationwide. Atrazine has been detected in drinking water in more than 40 percent of municipal wells tested in Midwestern states and in more than 31 percent of drinking water wells tested in Maine. It has been found in more than 98 percent of samples collected from Midwestern streams, rivers, and lakes after it was used on crops. It was also the most commonly detected pesticide in southern Florida canals.

As would be expected of a broad-spectrum herbicide, atrazine is toxic to primary producers (plants and algae) in surface waters. Chronic, lower-level atrazine exposure causes changes in the community structure and function by changing species composition of aquatic plant and algal communities and the productivity of these systems. In turn, the

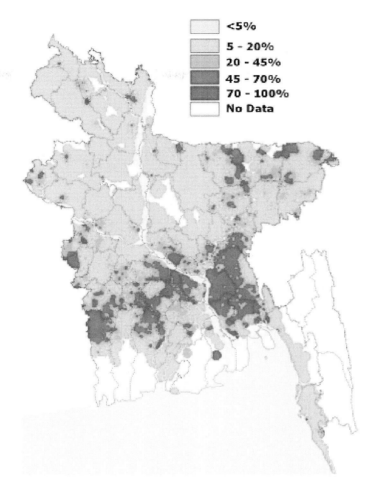

FIGURE 19-3 ● Probability of groundwater concentration exceeding 50 ppb (μg/L). (Source: McArthur JM, Ravenscroft P, Safiullah S, Thirlwall F. Arsenic in groundwater: Testing pollution mechanisms for sedimentary aquifers in Bangladesh. Water Resources Res 2001;37:109–17.)

feeding behavior and efficiency of organisms that consume plants and algae are affected resulting in changes in species assemblages and communities at higher levels in the food chain.

Atrazine has relatively low mammalian acute toxicity (LD_{50} in rats is greater than 1,000 mg/kg); however, because of its widespread use and its occurrence in surface and ground water, concern has arisen over adverse effects in humans and on aquatic or semiaquatic organisms associated with chronic, low-level exposures. Atrazine may cause cancer in humans and affect human reproduction and development via disruption of the endocrine system. Atrazine also causes developmental and reproductive toxicity in laboratory animals and in naturally occurring amphibians.

Because of its widespread use, its occurrence in ground and surface water systems, and concern with its potential to cause cancer, endocrine disruption, and reproductive and developmental effects in

human and nonhuman organisms, there have been calls to further restrict or ban the use of atrazine in the United States. These calls have been resisted by the pesticide's manufacturers and users, and a highly charged debate about atrazine's regulation has ensued (Box 19-3).

Mercury

Mercury is an important contaminant of many surface water systems and accumulates in fish and other aquatic organisms that feed high in the food chain. People consuming mercury-contaminated aquatic organisms (primarily fish)—the most important, nonoccupational source of human exposure to mercury—may be exposed to concentrations that pose threats to health.

Mercury is a naturally occurring element that is found in the earth's crust. It occurs in surface waters as a result of direct solubilization and from direct and indirect industrial discharges. Discharges

BOX 19-3

The Debate Over Regulation of Atrazine

Although a variety of adverse health effects have been associated with low-level, chronic exposure to atrazine, the most controversial are the potential to cause cancer and adverse effects on reproduction and development (in humans and amphibians) via disruption of the endocrine system. In 2003, EPA stated that atrazine is "not likely to be carcinogenic in humans," despite a different conclusion of its Science Advisory Board (SAB). Studies that EPA and the SAB evaluated showed significantly elevated rates of prostate cancer among men exposed to atrazine in a pesticide manufacturing plant; however, enhanced detection through aggressive screening impaired definitive determination of atrazine's potential carcinogenicity. Despite confounding effects of screening and limitations of sample size, the SAB stated that there was sufficient evidence to conclude that atrazine played a role in the increased cancer rate at the plant and that screening was only a partial explanation for the cancer increase.

Studies have also demonstrated an elevated risk of intrauterine growth retardation (IUGR) in the offspring of women who obtained water from atrazine-contaminated wells. However, although atrazine's reproductive and developmental toxicity as well as its endocrine disruption characteristics have been confirmed in studies of laboratory animals, a definite causal relationship between IUGR and human atrazine exposure has not been established because other pesticides in drinking water have also been correlated with IUGR.

Atrazine's endocrine-disrupting potential and its reproductive and developmental toxicity

are noteworthy in that they appear to also affect animals in the wild, with attendant concern for ecological effects. Atrazine has been associated with endocrine disruption and developmental abnormalities in amphibians. EPA conducted an assessment of the literature on these adverse effects and concluded that "there is sufficient evidence to formulate a hypothesis that atrazine exposure may impact gonadal development in amphibians but there are currently insufficient data to confirm or refute the hypothesis." Despite relatively extensive literature that describes these effects, debate among academic, government, and industry scientists continues around atrazine's potential to cause developmental abnormalities in amphibians.

In 2003, EPA approved a reregistration request for atrazine in the United States in light of scientific uncertainties and despite the conclusions of the SAB regarding human carcinogenicity and reproductive and developmental toxicity of atrazine in humans and amphibians. Although allowing continued use of atrazine, EPA has requested additional information and studies of the pesticide's effects in humans and amphibians. In contrast, the European Union and several European countries have banned the use of atrazine because of its widespread occurrence in drinking water and its potential health effects in humans and amphibians—a decision based on the Precautionary Principle for the management of potentially hazardous chemicals.[1]

Reference

1. Renner R. Controversy clouds atrazine studies. Environ Sci Technol 2004;38:107A–108A.

from chloralkali plants, leaking landfills, incineration of mercury-containing products, and combustion of coal are important sources of mercury contamination of surface water. Although some of these discharges are direct and result in local contamination, incineration of mercury-containing products, such as in medical waste, and combustion of coal used for electrical generation discharges mercury to the atmosphere, where it is transported long distances and deposited in lakes. Nearly 80 percent of anthropogenic emissions of mercury to the air come

from fossil fuel combustion, mining and smelting, and from incineration of waste.

Inorganic mercury that enters lakes is relatively insoluble; however, it is readily transformed by bacteria to its organic form (methyl mercury), which accumulates in the tissues of aquatic organisms, including fish. Because biomagnification (accumulation and concentration up the food chain) is the predominant mechanism of accumulation in aquatic ecosystems, mercury concentrations are highest in fish that feed at the top of the food chain, such as

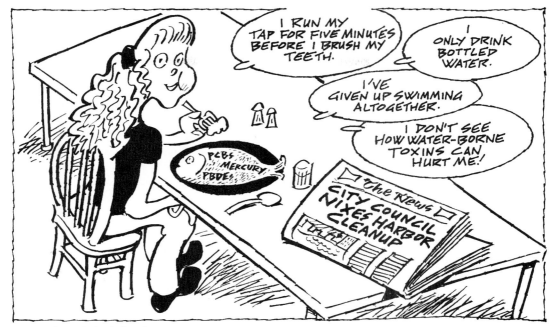

(Drawing by Nick Thorkelson.)

pike, shark, tuna, and swordfish. Mercury concentrations in these fish may be magnified as much as 100,000 times over concentrations found in surface water. Concentration of mercury in aquatic food chains is influenced by pH, with more accumulation occurring in water with lower pH. Acid precipitation, which results from the discharge of sulfates and nitrates from combustion of fossil fuels, may therefore play an important role in mercury accumulation in organisms in acidified lakes.

At high concentrations, mercury can damage the brain, kidneys, and other organs. Chronic exposure to lower concentrations of methyl mercury in adults impairs the immune and reproductive systems and may cause cardiovascular disease. Prenatal exposure to mercury and exposure of infants via breast milk may cause developmental disorders, such as delayed onset of walking, and abnormalities of language, attention, and memory.

Although a contaminant of many foods, most adult intake of mercury occurs from seafood. Concentrations of mercury in shark, swordfish, tile fish, mackerel, and albacore tuna occur at levels that have triggered warnings to women of childbearing age, pregnant women, nursing mothers, and young children to avoid consumption of these fish.[5] Similarly, 30 state natural resource and health agencies in the United States have advised these same individuals to reduce or avoid consumption of fish, including perch, northern and walleye pike, musky, and other species caught recreationally.[6]

Polychlorinated Biphenyls

Polychlorinated biphenyls (PCBs) are representative of a class of nonpolar, chlorinated organic compounds that include DDT, chlorinated dioxins, and toxaphene, among many others. PCBs and other compounds in this class are relatively insoluble in water; persistent in some environmental compartments, such as sediments; and accumulative to a high degree in animals and plants. Although they are present in water at extremely low concentrations, they occur at very high concentrations in aquatic organisms, such as fish, posing health risks to humans who consume contaminated fish and other organisms.

PCBs were manufactured and sold in the United States from 1929 to 1977, when Congress banned their manufacture. During this period, more than 1 billion pounds were produced. Despite a ban on the manufacture of PCBs, they continue to be encountered in various products and applications, including transformers and capacitors, heat transfer fluids, flame retardants, inks, adhesives, carbonless duplicating paper, paints, pesticide extenders, plasticizers, and wire insulators. They have also been found in more than 500 hazardous waste sites in the United States.

PCBs concentrate in the lipids of aquatic organisms, including fish. Bioconcentration and biomagnification of PCBs in upper levels of the food chain can lead to concentrations in the tissues of predatory fish that are more than 1 million times greater than concentrations in surrounding water. As a result, fish are the most significant exposure source of PCBs to the general public as well as other fish-eating animals.

PCBs are classified as probable human carcinogens by IARC, EPA, and NTP. The hepatotoxic effects of PCBs include induction of microsomal enzymes, liver enlargement, increased serum levels of liver-related enzymes and lipids, altered porphyrin and vitamin A metabolism, and histopathologic alterations that progress to noncancerous lesions and tumors. PCBs also cause adverse dermal effects (chloracne), ocular effects (hypersecretion of the Meibomian glands and abnormal pigmentation of the conjunctiva), and immunological effects (including increased susceptibility to respiratory tract infections, increased prevalence of ear infections in infants, decreased antibody levels, and changes in T lymphocytes). PCB exposure has also been associated with adverse effects on sperm morphology and production and menstrual disorders. Anthropometric effects, including reductions in head circumference and birthweight, and neurobehavioral abnormalities, including decreased neuromuscular maturity, abnormal reflexes, reduced psychomotor scores, impairment of short-term memory, decreases in visual recognition, and reduced activity levels, have been observed in children exposed to PCBs *in utero*. Some of these effects have persisted into later childhood.

As a result of high PCB concentrations in the tissues of many fish species, warnings have been issued to reduce consumption of the most contaminated fish species, including many salmon, trout, and walleye caught by recreational anglers in the Great Lakes and from other inland water bodies. Concern has also been raised recently around PCB contamination in farm-raised Atlantic salmon.[7]

Polybrominated Dipheynl Ethers

Polybrominated diphenyl ethers (PBDEs) are a relatively new class of compounds used as flame retardants in many commercial and household products. The use of PBDEs has increased dramatically over the last several years, with annual sales reaching more than 70,000 metric tons. Widespread use has resulted in migration from commercial products to the environment, including surface water and aquatic organisms (primarily fish), with human exposure occurring through consumption of contaminated fish. PBDEs are present in human blood, milk, and fatty tissues. Concentrations in people have increased 100-fold over the past 30 years, with a doubling time of about 5 years; and concentrations in North Americans are significantly higher than concentrations in Europeans.[8]

PBDEs are relatively insoluble in water but highly lipophilic; thus, they bioaccumulate in fish and other aquatic organisms as well as terrestrial species, including humans, that consume aquatic organisms. Concentrations of PBDEs in fish are highly variable depending on the type of fish and its location. PBDE concentrations in fish from Europe are about 10 times lower than in fish from North America, likely due to the proximity of fish feeding areas to PBDE sources. Regional distribution of PBDEs may also be associated with Europe's more aggressive approach of banning PBDE manufacture and use.

Some PBDE congeners are metabolically active and induce hepatic cytochrome P450 IIB1 and IA1. They also have weak or moderate binding affinity to the aryl hydrocarbon (Ah) receptor. PBDEs disrupt spontaneous behavior, impair learning and memory, and induce other neurotoxic effects in adult mice exposed neonatally. PBDEs are endocrine disruptors, altering thyroid hormone homeostasis and causing a dose-dependent depletion of thyroxine. PBDEs are agonists of estrogen receptors (both ERα and ERβ), an effect that may be enhanced by *in vivo* metabolism. PBDEs have not been demonstrated to be carcinogenic in rodent bioassays, although some concern for PBDE carcinogenesis continues to be raised. If humans are as sensitive as experimental animals to the adverse effects of PBDEs, current concentrations in humans may leave little or no margin of safety—arguing for close evaluation of the management of PBDEs and potentially aggressive regulation.

Disinfection By-products

Disinfection by-products (DBPs) are created by the interaction of organic matter in source waters with chlorine and other water disinfectants. Disinfection by-products include trihalomethanes, such as chloroform; haloacetic acids, such as trichloroacetic acid; bromate, which is formed when ozone is used for water disinfection; and chlorite, which is formed when chlorine dioxide is used for disinfection. The health effects of exposure to these substances include carcinogenicity (primarily bladder, colon, and rectal cancer) and reproductive and developmental effects including spontaneous abortions, stillbirths, neural tube defects, preterm births, intrauterine growth retardation, and low birthweight.

DBPs are formed by treatment of drinking water. Without treatment, the occurrence of pathogens that cause cholera, typhoid, cryptosporidiosis, and other diseases would increase with commensurate threats to public health. To address the DBP problem, EPA issued the Stage I Disinfectants and Disinfection Byproducts Rule in 1998, which requires drinking-water treatment plants to attain certain levels of disinfection and, at the same time, reduce DBPs to specified levels prior to distributing water. The rule also sets goals for the complete removal of some DBPs, although deadlines to achieve these goals have not been specified. Treatment plants that use surface waters with high concentrations of organic materials are also required to reduce the concentrations of these materials to specified levels prior to treatment in order to decrease or avoid the formation of DBPs.

EPA estimated that the nationwide cost of complying with the rule was about $700 million—the most affected households would see their annual water bill increase by about $12. It also suggested that the benefits of implementation of the rule, which included the prevention of cancer as well as reproductive and developmental disorders, would far outweigh the costs. EPA has proposed stage II of the rule, which would require DBP monitoring and assessments to determine compliance with the contaminant levels established in stage I.

REGULATING AND MANAGING WATER QUALITY

Water quality and the adverse health effects associated with water pollution can be managed by (a) preventing pollution before it occurs, (b) treating water after pollution has occurred, and (c) implementation of public health practices that reduce or eliminate human exposure when pollution prevention and treatment have not occurred or are ineffective.

Treatment-Based Approaches

The primary statutes to manage water quality in the United States are the Clean Water Act and the Safe Drinking Water Act. The Clean Water Act, adopted in 1972, emphasizes treatment of wastes before they are discharged to surface water. Treatment thresholds are guided by chemical-specific water quality criteria, which are risk-based contaminant concentrations that, if not exceeded, should prevent adverse effects of pollutants on human health and the environment. Treatment thresholds are also based on technology guidelines that require industrial sectors to install the best available, economically achievable levels of water treatment to remove pollutants prior to their discharge to surface waters. The Clean Water Act (CWA) has been successful in reducing toxic chemicals, such as PCBs, and pathogenic pollutants, such as bacteria and viruses, discharged from *point sources*—waste pipes of industrial facilities and wastewater treatment plants. As a result, surface waters are considerably cleaner than prior to the adoption of the CWA. However, the focus of the CWA on point sources has addressed only a portion of surface water quality problems in the United States.

Nonpoint source pollution, also called *polluted runoff*, enters lakes and streams from farms and animal feeding operations, leaking hazardous and sanitary landfills, septic systems, storm-water runoff that carries pollutants on city streets and sidewalks to surface waters, and the atmosphere. Nonpoint contaminants, such as PCBs (from contaminated sediments), mercury (atmospheric deposition), atrazine (from agricultural runoff), and many pathogens (from animal feeding operations, leaky septic systems, and runoff from urban areas) enter surface waters relatively uncontrolled by the Clean Water Act.

Prior to 1972, discharges of pollutants, such as PCBs from paper mills, occurred with little control and accumulated to very high concentrations in the sediments of lakes and rivers. They have persisted in sediments and are resuspended in surface waters during floods and other disturbances—a particularly challenging nonpoint pollutant source. In the Great Lakes region, dozens of hotspots have been identified, where sediments are highly contaminated with persistent, bioaccumulative toxicants, such as PCBs. In only a few cases are efforts underway to cap or remove contaminated sediments, often at very significant expense. However, without cleanup, these contaminants will continue to accumulate in fish and other organisms that will be consumed by humans and wildlife.

The Safe Drinking Water Act (SDWA), passed in 1974, is a treatment-based statute designed to control and reduce toxic and pathogenic compounds in drinking water, which in the United States is provided by more than 170,000 treatment plants. The act gives EPA the authority to set national, health-based standards for both naturally occurring drinking-water contaminants, such as bacteria and viruses, and contaminants of anthropogenic origin, such as lead and atrazine. Implementation of the standards occurs typically at the treatment plant, with enforcement provided either by states or by EPA. Although much of the SDWA focuses on treatment to reduce contaminant concentrations at the tap, revisions in 1996 gave EPA and the states greater authority to protect ground and surface water that serves as a source of drinking water. The SDWA also requires water suppliers to notify the public when there is a contamination problem in a drinking water system and treatment plants to provide annual reports to their users on the quality of their tap water.

On occasion, an approach to manage water quality or to protect human health leads to unintended consequences. In 2002, Washington, DC, discovered elevated lead concentrations in water serving more than 6,000 homes. Chlorination of the city's water to kill pathogens, as required by the Safe Drinking Water Act, created carcinogenic disinfection by-products. To reduce formation of disinfection by-products, also required by EPA under the SDWA, chlorine was replaced with chloramines, inadvertently mobilizing lead in its aging pipes and resulting in lead concentrations in the drinking water of some homes 20 times greater than EPA's recommended level. Ultimately, 23,000 lead-containing water service pipes will need to be replaced, although, to date, Washington, DC, has replaced only about 500 of these pipes. In the interim, the city is taking steps to notify individuals served by the pipes and providing recommendations to reduce lead exposure. It is also attempting to optimize corrosion control.

Exposure Reduction

The Clean Water Act has been relatively effective in regulating the discharge of contaminants from point sources, and the Safe Drinking Water Act has accomplished much of its goal of ensuring that contaminants do not occur in drinking water. However, these statutes have not addressed the vast quantities of in-place pollutants (in sediments) and other nonpoint sources of pollutants, such as leaking hazardous waste landfills or the atmosphere. As a result, PCBs, mercury, and other bioaccumulative contaminants have become concentrated in the tissues of fish and other aquatic organisms, posing threats to human health and the environment. Regulation of contaminants in fish sold commercially, such as PCBs and mercury, occurs under the Federal Food Drug and Cosmetic Act (FFDCA). The Food and Drug Administration (FDA) sets regulatory thresholds called tolerance levels for PCBs, mercury, and other compounds in fish. When the concentration of a contaminant in fish or other foods exceeds a tolerance level, the FDA can remove the food from commercial markets or it can issue a consumption warning, such as it did in 2001 for mercury in shark, swordfish, tilefish, and mackerel. However, many fish are caught and consumed by sport or recreational anglers, and the contaminants in these fish are not regulated by the FDA.

The EPA has developed methods to manage the health risks of toxicant exposure through consumption of contaminated fish caught by sport or recreational anglers. Its risk-based method is used to develop fish consumption advisories for compounds that are commonly found in fish, such as PCBs and mercury. Consumption advisories are typically issued by states and warn anglers and their families to restrict or eliminate consumption of particular species and size classes, based on tissue concentrations of individual contaminants and combinations of contaminants. The risk-based approach to consumption advisories developed by EPA conflicts, in many cases, with the tolerance levels set by FDA for commercially sold fish. (One important exception is mercury, for which FDA and EPA have developed a consensus approach for management in fish tissues.) For example, a PCB concentration of 1 mg/kg (ppm) will trigger stringent, do-not-eat consumption advice for a recreationally caught salmon, while the same salmon may be sold in commercial markets without restriction, as this concentration is below the FDA tolerance level for PCBs (2 mg/kg). This issue gained significant attention in 2004 when some types of commercially sold farmed salmon were found to have concentrations of PCBs, toxaphene, dieldrin, and other contaminants at levels that would trigger stringent

EPA-based consumption advice, but no action by FDA.[7] The difference in the two approaches is attributable to the reliance of EPA on a public health protective, risk-based approach to the development of fish consumption advisories, whereas FDA incorporates considerations not based on health, such as economic benefit and analytical detection capabilities in the development of tolerance levels. FDA has also fallen behind in updating its tolerance levels for most contaminants in fish; for example, the 20-year-old tolerance level for PCBs is one of the most recent levels established by FDA.

Source Control/Prevention

Water quality managers have recognized the limitations of end-of-pipe, treatment-based controls as a water quality management tool. This approach is not useful for many of the nonpoint sources that plague surface water. It also becomes cost-prohibitive as toxicant concentrations have been reduced to very low, but still harmful, levels. As a result, attention has turned to prevention-based approaches for the management of water quality. In 1992, a cooperative project of more than 80 public, private, and nonprofit groups brought together by the Water Environment Federation produced a consensus report, "A National Water Agenda for the 21st Century." Popularly known as Water Quality 2000, the project produced a vision statement and goal for the nation's waters of protecting and enhancing water quality that supports society and natural systems. To achieve this goal, it called for (a) consideration of all phases of the water cycle in the structuring of management approaches; (b) consideration of water as one part of a total environmental management plan to avoid transferring problems from one environmental medium to another; (c) consideration of the link between land use and water quality; (d) consideration of the relationship between water quality policy in the United States and global environmental issues; (e) promotion of source reduction and waste minimization; and (f) water conservation and reuse.

Promotion of source reduction and waste minimization are underway in industry, agriculture, and in many communities. Recycling and reuse of industrial waste has reduced point sources of pollutants and, concurrently, saved money by decreasing the need for purchase of unused resources. Similarly, measures in agriculture are being implemented to change crop rotation and tillage practices to reduce the need for large quantities of pesticides. Organic farming practices and produce from organic farms are increasing in popularity, with the concurrent benefit of reducing both leaching of pesticides to ground water and runoff to surface water.

THE FUTURE OF WATER QUALITY MANAGEMENT

Water quality management is being challenged by a convergence of water quality and water quantity issues, placing a focus on water conservation and reuse. Many technologies are available that can save enough water to reduce stress on threatened natural resources while still allowing adequate water for agricultural, industrial, and residential use.[1] By 2020, enough water can be saved from indoor residential use to meet the needs of more than 5 million people, and proper irrigation can save 450,000 acre feet of water per year, enough to satisfy the needs of another 3.6 million people. Water that is conserved is also water that does not have to be treated and discharged, eliminating the costs and adverse effects of treatment and discharge processes.

Although conservation will play an important role in addressing water quantity and some water quality issues worldwide, management of water quality will be challenged further by emerging stressors, such as global climate change. The United Nations Environment Programme Intergovernmental Panel on Climate Change predicts that continued increases of greenhouse gases will cause significant increases in global mean temperature. Presently, climate change may account for up to 20 percent of the global increase in water scarcity. Ultimately, global climate change will (a) disrupt traditional weather and runoff patterns and could increase the frequency and severity of drought and floods; (b) change snowfall and snowmelt patters leading to changes in the timing and amount of runoff; (c) threaten coastal aquifers and water supplies as a result of rising sea levels; and (d) threaten fish and other organisms, and harm critical habitat, such as wetlands, by increasing temperatures in lakes and streams, melting permafrost, and reducing water clarity.[1]

Global climate change, the threat of bioterrorism, unmanaged stressors such as nonpoint sources of contaminants, and a growing population relying more heavily than ever before on the 0.01 percent of water worldwide that is usable, pose formidable challenges for health professionals and water quality managers—and indeed all humankind.

REFERENCES

1. Gleick P. The world's water: The biennial report on freshwater resources, 2002–2003. Washington, DC: Island Press, 2002, 334.
2. Foran JA, Brosnan T. Early warning systems for hazardous biological agents in potable water. Environ Health Perspect 2000;108:993–5.
3. Burrows WD, Renner SE. Biological warfare agents as threats to potable water. Environ Health Perspect 1999;107:975–84.
4. Smith AH, Lingas EO, Rahman M. Contamination of drinking water by arsenic in Bangladesh: A public health emergency. Bull World Health Org 2000;78:1093–1103.
5. U.S. Environmental Protection Agency. What you need to know about mercury in fish and shellfish. Washington, DC: USEPA, 2004. Available at http://www.cfsan.fda.gov/~dms/admehg3.html.
6. U.S. Environmental Protection Agency. Fish advisories: Where you live. Washington, DC: USEPA, 2005. Available at http://epa.gov/waterscience/fish/states.htm.
7. Hites RA, Foran JA, Carpenter DO, et al. Global assessment of organic contaminants in farmed salmon. Science 2004;303:226–9.
8. Hites RA. Polybrominated diphenyl ethers in the environment and in people: A meta-analysis of concentrations. Environ Sci Technol 2004;38:945–56.

BIBLIOGRAPHY

Adler RW, Landman JC, Cameron DM. The Clean Water Act, 20 years later. Washington, DC: Island Press, 1993.
A review of the Clean Water Act: successes and failures.

ATSDR. Toxicological profile for lead. Washington, DC: U.S. Department of Health and Human Services, Public Health Service, 1999.
A comprehensive review of the toxicology and health effects of lead.

ATSDR. Toxicological profile for mercury. Washington, DC: U.S. Department of Health and Human Services, Public Health Service, 1999.
A comprehensive review of the toxicology and health effects of mercury.

ATSDR. Toxicological profile for PCBs. Washington, DC: U.S. Department of Health and Human Services, Public Health Service, 2000.
A comprehensive review of the toxicology and health effects of PCBs.

ATSDR. Toxicological profile for atrazine. Washington, DC: U.S. Department of Health and Human Services, Public Health Service, 2001.
A comprehensive review of the toxicology and health effects of atrazine.

Foran JA. Regulating toxic substances in surface water. Boca Raton, FL: Lewis Publishers/CRC Press, 1993.
An overview of approaches to the management of toxic substances in surface waters.

Natural Resources Defense Council (NRDC). Testing the waters: A guide to water quality at vacation beaches 12th ed. New York: NRDC, 2002.
A report on U.S. beach closings: extent, frequency, and causes.

Water Quality 2000. A national water agenda for the 21st century. Phase III report. Washington, DC: Water Environment Federation, 1992.
A forward-looking document intended to guide water management decisions in the 21st century.

World Bank Arsenic Mitigation Project. Available at: <http://web.worldbank.org/external/projects/main?pagePK=104231&piPK=73230&theSitePK=40941&menuPK=228424&Projectid=P050745>.
A summary of World Bank efforts to address arsenic contamination of drinking water in Bangladesh.

World Health Organization. Water, sanitation, and health. Available at: <http://www.who.int/water_sanitation_health/en/>.
A general overview of global water, sanitation, and health issues.

West Bengal and Bangladesh Arsenic Crisis Information Center. Available at: <http://bicn.com/acic/>.
Provides *information on arsenic contamination in drinking water.*

CHAPTER 20

Hazardous Waste

Denny Dobbin, Rodney D. Turpin, Ken Silver, and
Michelle T. Watters

Humans have been generating waste since earliest times. Prehistoric waste was largely food-related, including that related to hunting and gathering: piles of discarded shells and animal bones, broken pottery, and primitive tools. Only since the Industrial Revolution of the 19th century has waste become a significant societal problem: solid waste from industrial processes in addition to waste materials dumped into water, and gases, smoke, and vapors dispersed into the air. Unmanaged garbage supported proliferation of vectors, such as rodents and insects, that transmitted many pathogens. Waste increasingly became recognized for its effects on public health, the environment, and land use. In the 20th century, advances in chemical technology, especially synthesis of organic chemicals, brought an exponential increase in the volume of highly toxic material and resultant waste. And attempts to harness nuclear energy led to much radioactive and highly toxic—and long-persistent—waste that has been very difficult to manage.

As we make, use, and discard products, waste may be generated at each stage, "cradle-to-grave." We process raw materials, creating waste. We produce and package goods, creating waste. We consume or otherwise use products, creating waste. And we discard products at the end of their useful life, creating a waste that needs to be treated and disposed.

Hazardous waste adversely affects workers and community residents. Workers are at risk of harm at each of the cradle-to-grave stages. They are engaged in production, where hazardous waste is generated. They are engaged in treatment, storage, and disposal of waste. They are engaged in remediation of uncontrolled hazardous waste sites. And, they respond to emergencies, including spills of hazardous materials. Emergency responders are perhaps at the greatest risk because of the urgent and chaotic nature of situations they face. Community residents most often affected by hazardous waste are disproportionately those who are poor and of minority status. They usually have multiple environmental stressors and suffer a variety of adverse health effects, ranging from chronic disease to loss of the value of their property. Compared to those of workers, exposures of community residents tend to be at lower levels but of greater duration.

DEFINITION OF HAZARDOUS WASTE

Hazardous waste is officially defined as discarded solid or liquid material that may, directly or indirectly, cause adverse health effects, unless properly treated, stored, or disposed—in a manner that meets specific governmental regulatory definitions. For example, radioactive waste, composed of discarded materials and products that emit harmful radiation, can include spent nuclear fuel rods, high-level radioactive material left over from producing nuclear weapons, uranium-related (transuranic) waste, mill tailings from processing uranium ore, and low-level radioactive waste. The sense of waste as refuse, detritus, dregs, garbage, or trash can be traced to the 15th century. Unserviceable material remaining from any process of manufacture or extraction may include unused raw materials, useless by-products, or products so damaged as to be useless or unsaleable.

In legal terms, industrial waste is not defined as hazardous. It may include manufacturing waste, waste from mining and other mineral extraction, coal combustion, and gas and oil production. Municipal solid waste includes household garbage, food waste, and trash from public and commercial buildings in communities. Medical waste comes from clinics, hospitals, biomedical research laboratories, and elsewhere.

The Environmental Protection Agency (EPA) estimates that, by volume, 94 percent of waste is industrial waste; 5 percent, hazardous waste; and 1 percent, municipal solid waste. Radioactive and medical waste represent, by volume, less than 0.1 percent of total waste. Typical per-capita daily generation of waste in the United States includes about 4 lb per day of municipal waste, about 10 lb of hazardous waste, as much as 300 lb of industrial waste, and as little as 1 oz of medical waste.

Each year in the United States, as much as 700 million tons of legally defined waste is produced by as many as 200,000 generators. Chemical manufacturers generate approximately 80 percent of the total. Greater than 90 percent of hazardous waste is discharged as wastewater from industrial production streams. The remaining 10 percent includes inorganic solids as contaminated soil, metal, and other material; organic solvents in liquid form; and sludge and other residues from water- and air-pollution control systems.

All chemical wastes are toxic, but only those that are specifically designated as such by regulation are legally considered hazardous. In regulatory practice, hazardous waste has very precise legal meaning in statutes enacted to control threats to the environment and human health. Defining or listing a material as hazardous waste sets in motion a series of controls and actions to contain the material. However, just because a chemical is *defined* as not hazardous does not mean that it *is* not hazardous. Lobbying by special-interest trade associations has led to excluding some chemicals from hazard regulation. Economic hardship and market conditions are often cited as reasons for keeping chemicals off hazardous waste lists to avoid the cost of special handling required by legislation.

A waste may be classified as hazardous if it meets one of the following four characteristics:

• Ignitability: the relative likelihood that a chemical will burst into flame; that is, has a flashpoint at or less than 140°F.

• Corrosivity: the potential of strong acids (with a pH of 2 or less) and strong bases (with a pH of 12.5 or more) to eat through steel or burn living organisms.

• Reactivity: the potential for a chemical waste to explode or give off highly toxic gases.

• Toxicity: the capability of poisoning life forms.

ADVERSE HEALTH EFFECTS

When confronted with the problem of evaluating the adverse health effects of industrial chemicals discharged or dumped into the environment as waste, some extrapolation from occupational data may be helpful. However, standard assumptions and methods that apply to workplaces must be adapted in order to evaluate adverse health effects of exposures to the general public, who, for example, are generally exposed to much lower levels of chemicals than in the workplace and to complex mixtures of chemicals. Occupational exposure standards for chemicals, designed primarily to protect healthy, working men for 8-hour work shifts, are not sufficient to protect community residents who are exposed to chemicals—including children, pregnant women (and their fetuses), older people, and people homebound with chronic illnesses (Fig. 20-1).

As is the case in occupational epidemiology, nondifferential misclassification of exposure can obscure exposure–disease relationships. Patterns of exposure to chemicals in the environment can be especially difficult to characterize in time and space, due to variations in daily activities of people as well as episodic and seasonal fluctuations in highly complex physical processes, such as flow of groundwater and change in atmospheric conditions.

Compared to industry-wide studies that may enroll thousands of workers, epidemiologic studies of hazardous waste sites tend to be based on small, neighborhood-sized populations, which often makes it difficult to obtain statistically significant findings. Agencies and cleanup consultants often construct computer-based risk-assessment models, based on a small number of actual exposure measurements. Cleanup priorities are strongly influenced by predictions based on these models, typically in the form of a 1-in-10,000 (10^{-4}) to one-in-a-million (10^{-6}) risk of cancer. Seldom do epidemiologic studies or personal health data inform cleanup decisions.

Investigations of possible health effects from hazardous waste sites are performed in the most

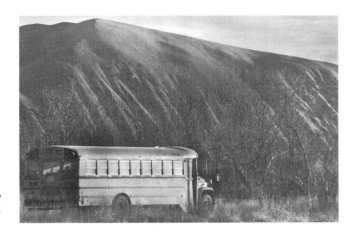

FIGURE 20-1 ● School bus travels by lead mine waste in rural area of Oklahoma. (Photograph by Earl Dotter.)

public of settings. Residents of a community often want scientists to confirm that their health effects are associated with exposure to hazardous waste.[1] Ideally, cluster investigations, which may be necessary initially, lead to mutual education among scientists and community residents on the desirability and feasibility of population-based epidemiologic studies. Early stages of this dialogue can be marked by conflict between residents with real-life tragedies, and scientists and regulators with their cool rationality. To respond to communities effectively, teams of public health professionals need to manifest a wide array of skills—in educating the public and health care providers, listening actively, and respectfully supporting the detective work of community residents ("popular epidemiology").[2,3] Health officials accustomed to doing "just science" often quickly discover they must share power with citizens' groups.[4]

The term *hazardous waste* is a social construct—its meaning changing with societal perceptions and concerns. Originally, it denoted industrial liquid chemicals leaking from corroded barrels at disposal sites, and migrating into the drinking water, backyards, basements, and sumps of nearby residences. Love Canal, a community built on a hazardous waste site in Upstate New York, was the site of a signal event in the 1970s, when residents noted a wide range of adverse health effects that seemed to be related to the site. Over time, however, it was recognized that any garbage dump that was active before about 1985 might, in fact, be a hazardous waste site. One-third of the hazardous waste sites on the current federal Superfund list were once "sanitary" landfills.

The term *hazardous waste* also applies to problems as disparate as one-time environmental re-

leases of chemicals, such as by spills, leaks, fires, and explosions, and long-term problems, such as the presence of radioactive and chemical wastes from the Cold War Era at facilities of the U.S. Department of Energy. The wide variety of contaminants, settings, and populations available for study has challenged scientists, required innovation, and generated a social movement that has facilitated cooperative projects among communities and public health scientists.

With the enactment of federal community right-to-know legislation in 1986, which required industrial facilities emitting toxic substances to file public reports, the term *hazardous waste* expanded to include air and water pathways of factory pollution. Increasingly, stringent disposal regulations spurred the expansion of a "treatment, storage, and disposal" industry for chemical wastes. This industry generally took the path of least resistance and expanded into minority communities—both urban and rural—and the environmental justice movement was born.[5]

To overcome the limited statistical power of neighborhood-sized populations, environmental epidemiologists seek ways to increase the size of study groups and/or the numbers of countable events. Registries of adverse birth outcomes have revealed associations between (a) proximity to hazardous waste sites and (b) low birthweight and certain congenital anomalies, including neural tube and cardiac defects.[6–10] A crude exposure surrogate of proximity to hazardous waste sites enables epidemiologists to include geographic areas large enough to capture many rare outcomes. Alternatively, many countable events can be identified by studying symptom clusters in neighborhood-sized populations.[11,12] Recall bias and confounding are major challenges in symptom prevalence surveys. However, as illustrated by one such study, some increased self-reports of complaints among exposed residents persist, even after controlling for recall bias and confounding.[13] Innovations in geographic methods have allowed for exploratory studies of possible associations between environmental exposures and various health outcomes. For example, use of the Geographic Information Systems (GISs) has furnished strong evidence of the disproportionate presence in minority communities of hazardous waste generators.[14]

Biological markers show promise as refined measures of individuals' exposures to synthetic organic chemicals. For example, in a longitudinal study of a Native American community, the impact of public health advisories recommending pregnant women reduce their fish intake was measured by a decline in breast-milk concentration of PCBs.[15] However, the use of biological markers as precursors of disease still presents major interpretative challenges. Application of a battery of immune markers may reveal statistically significant associations with an exposure, the clinical importance of which may be unknown.[16] Among genetic markers, chromosomal abnormalities are generally recognized as steps in—or very near to—causal pathways to cancer and to certain congenital anomalies; however, the clinical significance of sister chromatid exchanges and point mutations in specific genes is poorly understood. Standardized batteries of neurobehavioral and reproductive tests developed for use in hazardous waste site investigations rest on solid clinical foundations but, when used in field investigations, may face the full range of epidemiologic study design issues, such as recall bias and confounding.[17,18] Psychosocial influences on recall bias of living near a notorious hazardous waste site are probably real but have been poorly quantified.[19]

HAZARDOUS WASTE MANAGEMENT

Hazardous waste handling and management is regulated. Management methods include treatment, storage, and disposal and may also include reclamation and incineration, depending on technology, cost, regulation, and physical and chemical properties. Treatment methods include technologies that can alter the chemical and physical composition of the waste to make it less potentially harmful, such as diluting or neutralizing a strong acid or base to

make the waste less hazardous. Treatment could also include filtering, solidifying, or evaporating the waste. Waste treatment is very often done in surface impoundments, such as diked lagoons or ponds, where hazardous waste is temporarily contained. These sites, which are open-surface facilities that can hold liquid or partially solidified hazardous waste, can range in size from a basketball court to many acres. Barriers of clay or other impermeable material to prevent leakage must line these holding areas, and groundwater must be monitored for possible contamination. Hazardous waste may also be stored for variable periods before treatment or disposal. For example, a treatment operator may hold a volume of waste targeted for reclamation until markets are favorable for the reclaimed product.

Disposal is defined as hazardous waste burial. Methods of land disposal of hazardous waste, which is regulated, include injection in deep wells, land filling, or land farming. *Well injection* requires wells with depths greater than the drinking-water aquifers; this method is used for disposing of about 10 percent of hazardous waste. Abandoned oil and gas wells in Louisiana and Texas are often used for this purpose. *Land fills* are defined as holes below ground level where hazardous waste may be permanently stored. Land fills must be lined with impermeable material, such as clay. Leached-out liquids must be collected and treated. Groundwater must be periodically tested by monitoring wells surrounding the site.

Some hazardous wastes are banned, and generators are required to treat the waste to lessen its toxicity before it is sent to the land fill. *Land farming*, which relies on bacterial decomposition of hazardous waste, is used in some cases, where appropriate. Waste, such as that from petroleum refineries, is sprayed on land that is then tilled to mix waste, soil, and oxygen from the air with nutrients and bacteria. The resulting mixture enhances the breakdown of waste into safer substances.

Incineration, defined as thermal decomposition of material, is a method used for hazardous waste composed of organic compounds that can be broken down to simpler chemical components in kilns containing a flame at 1,600°F or higher. Although waste volume is greatly reduced, resultant emissions contaminate the air and ashes may contain high concentrations of toxic heavy metals, such as mercury. Because incineration is relatively expensive, less than 1 percent of hazardous waste in the United States is treated in this manner.

Incinerators come in a variety of forms that are appropriate to the waste being treated. For example, rotary kilns are used for solids; injection incinerators for liquids; and specially designed furnaces for explosives. Properly operating incineration—with accurately controlled temperature, turbulence, and oxygen concentrations—breaks down organic waste into carbon dioxide, water, and ash. If combustion is incomplete, carbon monoxide may form. Measurement of carbon monoxide in flue gas is used to determine the effectiveness of incinerator performance. Inorganic material in incinerated waste may change form, but emerge from treatment in reduced volume in the form of a hazardous waste product.

Finally, hazardous waste may be reclaimed in the form of a commercially useful product. Heavy metals, such as lead, can be reclaimed or recycled from discarded lead-acid batteries; silver can be reclaimed from certain types of photographic processes; and spent degreasing solvents can be cleaned and reclaimed. Pollution prevention and toxic use reduction rely on rehabilitation of hazardous waste that would otherwise be discarded. Some hazardous waste can be reclaimed in other than original form. One popular means is to use combustible hazardous waste as fuel in kilns to produce cement. Further attempts at waste minimization, cradle-to-grave stewardship, recycling, and reclamation can reduce hazardous waste volumes and increase efficiency of production.

The Resource Conservation and Recovery Act (RCRA) of 1976, administered by the EPA, is the primary federal legislation for managing solid waste, including hazardous waste. RCRA is structured around controlling hazardous waste from cradle to grave, including generation, treatment, storage, and disposal. RCRA covers waste from mines, municipalities, oil and gas production, manufacturing, and coal production facilities (see Chapters 3 and 37).

REMEDIATING ABANDONED AND ILLEGAL HAZARDOUS WASTE SITES

Public awareness of hazardous waste was heightened in the second half of the 20th century with reports of abandoned and uncontrolled hazardous waste sites and spilled, or illegally dumped, hazardous waste that posed a threat to public health or the environment. Too often, extensive sites were

abandoned with no one to hold responsible for cleaning them up. A series of legislative acts to address the problem became known as the *Superfund Law*. To support remediation of abandoned sites, a fund was established from taxes on waste generators, under the theory that the polluter should pay. Superfund began with enactment of the Comprehensive Environmental Response, Compensation and Liability Act (CERCLA) in 1980, and was later updated and improved by the Superfund Amendments and Reauthorization Act (SARA) in 1986. Administered by EPA, Superfund established (a) liability, in the event of releases or spills for generators, transporters, and managers of hazardous waste; and (b) a nearly $9 billion fund, which has been used for remediation of hazardous waste sites when those responsible for them cannot be identified or lack resources to conduct cleanup. Superfund excludes petroleum products and radioactive material waste (see Box 20-1 and Chapters 3 and 37).

Superfund cleanup is based on a 10-step approach:

1. *Site discovery*: Sites that require remediation are identified.
2. *Preliminary assessment*: Information on a discovered site is assessed to determine Superfund eligibility.
3. *Site inspection*: Preliminary data and samples are collected to determine the degree of threat that the site presents to public health and if emergency action is required.
4. *Hazard ranking system*: Site data is accumulated and used for ranking of the site to determine its inclusion on the National Priorities List.
5. *National Priorities List (NPL)*: Because Superfund resources are to be directed toward remediating the sites with the greatest public health hazards, EPA maintains a list ranked by the degree of threat to human health and the environment. Sites on the NPL list are eligible for cleanup funding.
6. *Remedial investigations/feasibility studies*: After listing of a site on the NPL, in-depth analyses of the site are conducted to (a) establish with greater detail and specificity the nature and extent of its health and safety risks and (b) develop recommendations for cleanup.
7. *Remedy selection:* After analysis of recommended alternatives, a preferred remedial

---

BOX 20-1

Key Components of Superfund

COMPREHENSIVE ENVIRONMENTAL RESPONSE, COMPENSATION, AND LIABILITY ACT (CERCLA)

- Enacted 1980. Trust fund of $1.6 billion is authorized over 5 years.
- Amended by the Superfund Amendments and Reauthorization Act (SARA), enacted 1986. Trust fund of $8.5 billion is authorized over 5 years.
- Extended to 1994. Additional $5.1 billion is authorized.

For more information: <www.epa.gov/superfund/action/law>.

NATIONAL OIL AND HAZARDOUS SUBSTANCES POLLUTION CONTINGENCY PLAN (NCP) (IMPLEMENTS SUPERFUND)

- Revised in 1982 to incorporate CERCLA requirements.
- Amended in 1986 by SARA.
- Revised 1990 in response to CERCLA Section 105.

HAZARD RANKING SYSTEM (HRS)

- Promulgated 1982 as Appendix A of the NCP.
- Revised 1990 in response to CERCLA Section 105(c) added by SARA.
- Effective date 1991.

For more information: <www.epa.gov/superfund/programs/npl_hrs/hrsint.htm>.

NATIONAL PRIORITIES LIST (NPL)

- Promulgated 1983 as Appendix B of the NCP.
- Last sites proposed under original HRS promulgated 1991.
- First sites proposed under revised HRS 1991.
- First sites added to the NPL under the revised HRS 1992.

For information on the NPL site listing process: <www.epa.gov/superfund/sites/npl/npl_hrs.htm>.

CONSTRUCTION COMPLETION LIST (CCL)

- Category activated 1991.
- List activated 1993.

For more information: <www.epa.gov/superfund/action/process/ccl.htm>.

---

action is proposed and made available for public comment in a "record of decision" document. After considering public comment, officials choose a specific remedy.

8. *Remedial design:* After the remedy is chosen, an engineering phase begins to plan and design the remediation.
9. *Remedial action:* The remedy is implemented in the construction phase.
10. *Project close-out:* After the remediation is complete, the project is ended and the site removed from the NPL.

From 1980 to 2004, EPA and its state and tribal partners investigated nearly 45,000 potentially contaminated Superfund sites. More than 33,000 sites (74 percent of the total investigated) have been removed from the original Superfund inventory. More than 7,000 emergency and short-term cleanup actions have been taken to stabilize sites and respond to immediate risks to human health and the environment.

Of the approximately 1,500 sites placed on the NPL for cleanup, almost 900 have been cleaned up

or referred to another federal agency for cleanup. Of the remaining 650 sites, most are in the construction, study, or design phase of cleanup. Since 1980, parties responsible for contamination and pollution have committed more than $21 billion for cleanup, and the federal government has paid out many billions more.

THE ROLE OF THE U.S. PUBLIC HEALTH SERVICE AND OTHER FEDERAL AGENCIES

Congress recognized the significance of the public health impact of unregulated hazardous waste and releases as it enacted legislation. Superfund has helped address public health issues by establishing appropriate federal programs to be responsive in areas where there was a need. For example, a basic research program was established at the National Institute of Environmental Health Sciences (NIEHS) to answer questions about preventing health effects related to hazardous waste. Congress recognized the need to protect workers who would be involved in hazardous waste operations and emergency response and directed the Occupational Safety and Health Administration (OSHA) to promulgate protective workplace standards and occupational safety and health training. As part of worker protection, Congress also provided for model training programs to be supported through grants administered by NIEHS.

Congress also recognized the need to address the health concerns of communities and, as a follow-up to CERCLA, established the Agency for Toxic Substances and Disease Registry (ATSDR) in 1980. ATSDR, part of the U.S. Public Health Service in the Department of Health and Human Services, has a multidisciplinary staff of about 400 employees, including epidemiologists, toxicologists, physicians, and public health educators. There are also 10 regional offices that support the corresponding EPA offices in their Superfund and emergency response activities. The mission of the ATSDR is "To serve the public using the best science, taking responsive public health actions, and providing trusted health information to prevent harmful exposures and disease related to toxic substances." To achieve this mission, ATSDR works with communities; health care providers; tribal, state, and local governments; industry; and EPA and other federal agencies. ATSDR is not a regulatory agency, but makes public health recommendations to EPA that may support enforcement actions.

In sum, CERCLA was designed to address past hazardous waste disposal activities, even if disposal was considered or the substance was not considered hazardous in the past. EPA was mandated to investigate the sites, develop cleanup plans, and negotiate payment by responsible parties. ATSDR was designed to work with EPA by assessing the adverse public health impacts of these sites.

In addition to conducting health assessments for every site on, or proposed for, the NPL, ATSDR provides health consultations and technical advice (a) on non-NPL sites, (b) on sites petitioned by concerned citizens and organizations, and (c) in response to accidental releases (see Box 20-2). It performs surveillance and epidemiologic studies to increase understanding of the relationship between exposure and adverse health outcomes. ATSDR maintains four subregistries: for people exposed to trichloroethylene (TCE), trichloroethane (TCA), benzene, and dioxin. It established the World Trade Center Health Registry to understand the long-term health effects of those who worked, lived, or were present near the World Trade Center on

September 11, 2001. It publishes toxicological profiles of hazardous chemicals found at NPL sites and provides health education to communities and health care providers on the adverse effects of hazardous substances.

With the Association of Occupational and Environmental Clinics (AOEC) and EPA, ATSDR developed the Pediatric Environmental Health Specialty Unit (PEHSU) program. Eleven PEHSUs across the United States address pediatric environmental health issues, including evaluation and treatment of children with environmental illnesses, training of pediatricians and other health care providers, and research on children's environmental health problems.

In 2003, the ATSDR was consolidated administratively with the National Center for Environmental Health (NCEH) at the Centers for Disease Control and Prevention (CDC). Several NCEH divisions maintain shared and complementary goals in environmental public health with ATSDR. Since federal law created ATSDR, a federal mandate is required to merge the two organizations; however, even without a formal merger, consolidation of administration and management provides for an enhanced joint approach to environmental policy, emergency response, and protection of the public's health from environmental hazards.

Federal Plans for Hazardous Waste–Related Emergency Response

Unplanned spills and releases of hazardous waste present special problems for public health protection, depending on the toxicity and physical characteristics of the chemicals involved. Congress anticipated these emergency situations as it enacted hazardous waste–related legislation and provided means to address these situations through governmental agencies.

For multimedium accidental chemical releases, oil spills, and terrorist activities, fire and police personnel are universally recognized as first responders. Specific events—train derailments, chemical plant explosions, aerospace accidents, natural disasters, and terrorist attacks—may require other professionals to participate with first responders on a case-by-case basis, yet these individuals are not generally recognized as first responders.

The National Oil and Hazardous Substance Pollution Contingency Plan (NCP) was first

BOX 20-2

Asbestos in Libby, Montana

In the early 1920s, a vermiculite mine was opened in Libby, a small community in northwest Montana. The mine was eventually purchased by W.R. Grace & Company. During its 70 years of operation, the mine produced millions of tons of vermiculite. The vermiculite ore was processed for many commercial and consumer applications including insulation, garden products, and building material. Dust from the processing facility settled in homes, children would play on waste piles created from processing the ore, and community members would use waste ore and contaminated vermiculite in their gardens, driveways, and homes. Until the mine's closing in 1990, Libby vermiculite ore was also shipped to more than 240 locations throughout the United States for processing and packaging.

Although most vermiculite products pose no health problems, the raw vermiculite ore mined at Libby contained as much as 26 percent naturally occurring asbestos. Asbestos refers to a group of silicate minerals consisting of thin, separable fibers. The fibers are resistant to heat, fire, and chemical or biological degradation. Inhalational exposure to asbestos is associated with several serious health problems, including, but not limited to, asbestosis, pleural plaques, lung cancer, and mesothelioma.

In 1999, the environmental and health problems in Libby received national attention after articles about it appeared in a Seattle newspaper. ATSDR was asked by the Department of Health and Human Services, after requests from EPA and the Montana Congressional delegation, to evaluate the health concerns related to asbestos exposure in Libby. ATSDR performed a mortality review for Libby using death certificate data for the 20-year period from 1979 to 1998. It found that deaths from asbestosis were 65 to 80 times higher than for the rest of the United States. Lung cancer was 20 to 30 times higher than expected, and mesothelioma mortality was also elevated.

Interviews, chest x-rays, and pulmonary function tests were performed on more than 7,300 people who had lived or worked in Libby for at least 6 months before 1991. Of those tested, 18 percent had pleural abnormalities

consistent with asbestos exposure. The risk of having a lung abnormality were increased in former mine or mill workers, smokers, and those who had played on the vermiculite piles. A computed tomography (CT) study of 353 Libby residents exposed to asbestos-contaminated vermiculite who had indeterminate chest x-rays demonstrated that 28 percent of the people tested had lung abnormalities. On the basis of medical testing results, ATSDR committed to develop the Tremolite Asbestos Registry for people exposed to asbestos in Libby.

The adverse health effects in Libby in workers and community members suggested that other W.R. Grace & Company sites processing or packaging asbestos-contaminated vermiculite from Libby were also at risk for adverse health effects. The ATSDR National Asbestos Exposure Review was established to work with other federal, state, and local environmental and public health agencies to identify past and present exposure pathways and to determine what actions are needed to protect public health. In partnership with state health agencies, ATSDR is conducting health consultations at 28 selected sites for initial review. Sites were selected if EPA required further action or if the site was an exfoliation (expansion of vermiculite by high heating) facility that processed more than 100,000 tons of Libby vermiculite ore. Collectively, the 28 sites represent 80 percent of the total tonnage shipped from Libby from 1964 to 1990.

In addition to the facilities and surrounding communities that received and processed the Libby vermiculite, there is public concern about the use of the vermiculite products, especially attic insulation products, sold under the brand name Zonolite. Many homes in the United States, especially those built before the early 1970s, may contain vermiculite building products contaminated with asbestos. Although the products do not normally present a health hazard, disturbing them may release fibers that may become airborne and subsequently inhaled. The EPA is evaluating the scope of the asbestos problems in homes. Additional information concerning Zonolite/vermiculite insulation can be found at <www.epa.gov/asbestos>.

promulgated in the 1968 Clean Water Act and has been refined over the years with the passage of various laws, including Superfund, the Clean Water Act, and the Oil Pollution Act. The original NCP reflected the lessons learned from the 37-million-gallon crude oil spill from the Torrey Canyon in 1967. (For comparison, in Alaska in 1989, the Exxon Valdez spilled 11 million gallons of crude oil.) The NCP was the first comprehensive system of accident reporting, spill containment, and cleanup requirements. It established the requirements for response headquarters and national and regional reaction teams, which were the precursors to National Response Team (NRT) and Regional Response Teams (RRTs) today. The NCP identifies the responsibilities of up to 16 participating federal agencies during a specific emergency. The NRT is responsible for the administration and implementation of the NCP and the planning and coordination of all national response activities.

By 1992, the federal government's emergency response activities ranged from natural disasters, such as floods and hurricanes, to accidental releases, such as chemical and oil spills. Several federal agencies developed response plans similar to the NCP, including the Federal Radiological Emergency Plan, the Mass Migration Response Plan, and the U.S. Government Interagency Domestic Terrorism Concept of Operations Plan. State and local governments also developed response teams capable of handling local emergencies. Therefore, the Federal Response Plan (FRP) was published in 1992 to establish the mechanism and structure by which the federal government would mobilize to address consequences of any major disaster or emergency that overwhelmed the capabilities of state and local governments. By signing the letter of agreement, the federal departments and agencies agreed to:

- Support the FRP concept of operations and carry out their assigned functional responsibilities;
- Cooperate with the Federal Coordinating Officer appointed by the President;
- Make maximal use of existing authorities to reduce disaster relief costs;
- Form partnerships with counterpart state agencies, voluntary organizations, and the private sector to take advantage of all existing resources; and
- Develop headquarters and regional planning, exercise, and training activities.

Twenty-seven federal departments and agencies have signed the FRP.

Until September 11, 2001, FRP response activities fit nicely into specific emergency support function activities for floods, hurricanes, oil spills, chemical spills, and urban search and rescue situations. If an emergency is a hazardous material event, then EPA is the lead agency and the NCP represents the primary rules of engagement.

Just as the NCP and FRP addressed emergency response events of their time, the September 11 attack and subsequent events demonstrated the need for a better, more comprehensive federal plan. The Department of Homeland Security has taken the first step in developing a new all-inclusive National Response Plan (NRP).

REFERENCES

1. Ozonoff D, Boden LI. Truth and consequences: Health agency responses to environmental health problems. Sci Technol Human Values 1987;12:70–7.
2. Brown P. Popular epidemiology and toxic waste contamination: Lay and professional ways of knowing. In: Illness and the environment: A reader in contested medicine. In: Kroll-Smith S, Brown P, Gunter VJ, eds. New York: NYU Press, 2000:364–83.
3. Clapp R. Popular epidemiology in three contaminated communities. Ann Am Acad Political Social Sci 2002;584:35.
4. Till JE. Building credibility in public studies. Am Sci 1995;83:468–73.
5. Brown P. Race, class and environmental health: A review and systematization of the literature. Environ Res 1995;69:15–30.
6. Baibergenova A, Kudyakov R, Zdeb M, et al. Low birth weight and residential proximity to PCB-contaminated waste sites. Environ Health Perspect 2003;111:1352–7.
7. Dolk M, Vrijhedi M, Armstrong B. Risk of congenital anomalies near hazardous-waste landfill sites in Europe: EUROHAZCON study. Lancet 1998;352:423–7.
8. Orr M, Bove F, Kaye W, et al. Elevated birth defects in racial or ethnic minority children of women living near hazardous waste sites. Int J Hyg Environ Health 2002;205:19–27.
9. Vrijhedi M, Dolk M, Armstrong B. Chromosomal anomalies and residence near hazardous waste landfill sites. Lancet 2002;359:320–2.
10. Croen LA, Shaw GM, Sanbonmatsu L, et al. Maternal residential proximity to hazardous waste sites and risk for selected congenital malformations. Epidemiology 1997; 8: 347–54.
11. Baker DB, Greenland S, Mendlein J, et al. A health study of two communities near the Stringfellow Waste Disposal site. Arch Environ Health 1988;43:325–34.
12. Dayal H, Gupta S, Trieff N. Symptom clusters in a community chronic exposure to chemicals in two Superfund sites. Arch Environ Health 1995;50:108–11.
13. Ozonoff D, Colten ME, Cupples A. Health problems reported by residents of a neighborhood contaminated by a hazardous waste facility. Am J Ind Med 1987;11:581–97.
14. Maantay J. Mapping environmental injustices: Pitfalls and potential of Geographic Information Systems in

assessing environmental health and equity. Environ Health Perspect Suppl 2002;110(Suppl 2):161–71.

15. Fitzgerald EF, Hwang SA, Bush B. Fish consumption and breast milk PCB concentrations among Mohawk women at Akwesasne. Am J Epidemiol 1998;148:164–72.

16. Vine MF, Stein L, Weigle K. Effects on the immune system associated with living near a pesticide dump. Environ Health Perspect 2000;108:1113–24.

17. Sizemore OJ, Amler RW. Characteristics of ATSDR's adult and pediatric environmental neurobehavioral test batteries. Neurotoxicology 1996;17:229–36.

18. Scialli AR, Swan SH, Amler RW. Assessment of reproductive disorders and birth defects in communities near hazardous chemical sites. II. Female reproductive disorders. Reprod Toxicol 1997;11:231–42.

19. Lipscomb JA, Goldman LR, Satin KP. A follow-up study of the community near the McColl waste disposal site. Environ Health Perspect 1991;94:15–24.

BIBLIOGRAPHY

Anderson SH, Beiswenger RE, Purdom PW. Environmental science, 4th Ed. New York: Macmillan, 1993.
This textbook presents environmental science as a living subject, and focuses on living systems and their interaction with the environment; human interactions especially regarding air and water; management of the environment and human use of resources; environmental toxins and their effect on ecosystems and human health; and protecting the environment and human communities that interact with it.

National Oil and Hazardous Substance Pollution Contingency Plan. Title 40 Code of Federal Regulations Pt. 300.2003. Available at: <http://access.gpo.gov/nara/cfr/waisidx_03/40cfr300_03.html>.

U.S. Federal Emergency Management Agency. Federal response plan. 1999. (9230.1-PL.)

Agency for Toxic Substances and Disease Registry. Public health assessment for Libby asbestos site, Libby, Lincoln County, *Montana.* Atlanta: ATSDR, 2003. Available at: <http://www.atsdr.cdc.gov/>.

Wagner T. In our backyard: A guide to understanding pollution and its effects. New York: Van Nostrand Reinhold, 1994.
This primer presents information concerning the types and sources and effects of pollution in an understandable and unbiased manner.

CHAPTER 21

Global Environmental Changes

Anthony J. McMichael, Simon Hales,
and Robyn M. Lucas

Global environmental changes are large-scale changes that are occurring systemically or ubiquitously to the world's natural environment as a result of human action. They are an increasingly important addition to the spectrum of environmental hazards to human health. Only in recent decades has the size and intensity of the human enterprise become sufficiently great to begin to change, and disrupt, the natural environment on this global scale. This reflects the combined impact of unprecedented population size, intensity of economic activity, and the prevailing types of technology. In other words, the aggregate environmental impact of humankind is so great that it is beginning to alter the earth system on a planetary scale.

We live in a world that is undergoing widespread and rapid globalization—the extension and intensification of various social, economic, cultural, technological, and political interconnections among human societies around the globe. Economic globalization, characterized by the increasingly integrated and "liberalized" (deregulated) worldwide systems of markets, capital flows, and trading, has adversely affected the natural global environment. However, globalization and global environmental change, which are strongly associated at present, need not always be closely connected. We could imagine a future in which there is yet greater globalization, though managed in an environmentally sustainable manner.

The best known of the global environmental hazards to health are those resulting from two major changes to the atmosphere:

1. *Depletion of stratospheric ozone by various anthropogenic gases, primarily halocarbons*: The resultant increased flux of solar ultraviolet radiation (UVR)—and the biological hazards that it poses to humans—are generally well understood. Although this depletion continues at present, if the necessary remedy is implemented, the stratospheric ozone layer should begin to recover over the next decade.

2. *Amplification of the natural greenhouse effect, by anthropogenic emissions of carbon dioxide and other greenhouse gases*: This process, which has increased the heat-trapping capacity of the lower atmosphere, appears to have contributed to recent world climate change. Climate scientists believe that this human-induced climate change will continue for many decades, even if we soon take effective international action to substantially curtail greenhouse gas emissions.

Although global climate change has attracted much recent attention from scientists and policymakers, other categories of global environmental change pose similarly serious risks to current and future human societies (Box 21-1). These categories include:

- Biodiversity losses, often with resultant disturbances of ecosystems;
- Land degradation;
- Disruption of other major elemental cycles, such as those of nitrogen, sulfur, phosphorus, and carbon;
- Depletion of freshwater supplies; and
- Global dissemination of persistent organic pollutants.

BOX 21-1

Global Environment Changes:
Context and Definition

This "global" category of human-induced environmental change is defined by both scale and its systemic character (alteration to basic life-supporting systems). Such changes to the structure and function of large natural biophysical and ecological systems diminish the capacity of the natural environment to supply "services," such as replenishing resources, and absorbing and recycling the waste products of humans and domesticated animals.

The earth system, comprising physical, chemical, biological, and human components, is self-regulating. Global environmental changes alter the forcings (drivers) and feedbacks that constitute the system's internal dynamics. In addition, earth system dynamics are characterized by critical thresholds and abrupt changes. Indeed, the earth system has operated in different states over the past 500,000 years, during which time abrupt transitions—within a decade or less—have sometimes occurred. Our understanding of these natural dynamics has advanced greatly in recent years, enabling more confident assessment of the consequences of human-induced change, including the possibility that human activities could inadvertently trigger abrupt changes with severe consequences.

Global environmental changes derive from multiple point sources of human economic activity. They are "global" in the sense of either (a) being integrated, thus becoming "systemic" changes to a global process, such as changes to

the world's climate system and to global elemental cycles; or (b) occurring by the worldwide aggregation of local changes, such as land degradation.

The main types of human-induced global environmental changes are:

1. Changes to atmospheric composition and, therefore, function:
   - Greenhouse gas accumulation, leading to climate change
   - Stratospheric ozone depletion
2. Changes to elemental cycles, such as of nitrogen, phosphorus, sulfur, and carbon.
3. Land degradation.
   - Land cover and soil fertility
   - Deforestation and reforestation
   - Habitat fragmentation
   - Desertification
4. Changes to the hydrological cycle, and depletion of supplies and quality of freshwater.
   - Water projects
5. Changes to coastal and marine ecosystems.
6. Biodiversity changes.
   - Loss of local population/extinction
   - Redistribution of species
   - Internal rearrangements (balance)
7. Worldwide dissemination of persistent organic pollutants and heavy metals.
8. Urbanization
   - Water supply and sanitation
   - Local air pollution
   - "Ecological footprint" (versus the available carrying capacity).

The public health significance of these global environmental changes is that the health of populations is increasingly being influenced by changes that originate beyond the boundaries of a given population's immediate living space (Fig. 21-1). In addition, major—perhaps irreversible—changes to the biosphere's life-support system, such as those due to climate change and biodiversity loss, increase the likelihood of adverse impacts on the health of future generations.

Periods of social and environmental upheaval have often been accompanied by infectious disease outbreaks, which, in turn, have often gener-

ated social and political changes. Since 1976, approximately 30 infectious diseases have emerged, demonstrating that such diseases can arise suddenly and spread rapidly, adversely affecting livelihoods, trade, travel, and tourism. In the past three decades, previously unknown infectious diseases have emerged at an unprecedented pace, prompting the suggestion that this is the fourth and largest of the great historical transitions in the relationship between microbes and humans.[1,2] Sometimes a single infectious disease arrives at a time of particular population vulnerability, with devastating consequences, as occurred with the bubonic plague in

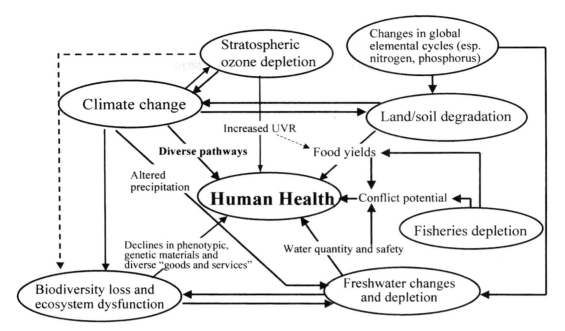

FIGURE 21-1 ● Interrelationships between major types of global environmental change, including climate change. Note that all of them impinge on human health and—though not shown here explicitly—there are various interactive effects between jointly acting environmental stresses. (Adapted from McMichael A, Campbell-Lendrum D, Corvalan C, et al. Climate change and human health: Risks and responses.Geneva: WHO, 2003.)

the 14th century, influenza at the end of World War I, and the HIV/AIDS epidemic, especially in sub-Saharan Africa. Sometimes infectious diseases arrive or intensify as a group, as occurred with urban epidemics of tuberculosis, smallpox, and cholera in England in the early 19th century.

Global environmental changes differ from many other familiar environmental concerns that are due to localized toxic or microbiological hazards. They indicate that we have begun to live beyond the biosphere's capacity to supply, absorb, and replenish. The challenges these changes pose are therefore a major part of the environmental health research agenda.

GLOBAL CLIMATE CHANGE

Compared to other planets, Earth has a distinctive atmosphere. Its high concentration of oxygen is a direct consequence of photosynthesis. Various trace gases in the atmosphere, especially carbon dioxide, produce a natural *greenhouse effect*, which warms Earth by around 30°C and keeps the planet comfortably above freezing point.

Most human societies today, especially in developed countries, have greatly escalated economic activity in ways that have increased the atmospheric concentration of various gases, several of which enhance the atmosphere's heat-trapping capacity. These *greenhouse gases* (GHGs)—primarily carbon dioxide, methane, nitrous oxide, and various human-made halocarbons—increase the atmospheric absorption of infrared radiation passing outward from Earth's surface. More radiative energy therefore accumulates in the lower atmosphere, and the surface of Earth warms.

In its *Third Assessment Report* (2001), the United Nations' Intergovernmental Panel on Climate Change (IPCC) stated: "There is new and stronger evidence that most of the warming observed over the last 50 years is attributable to human activities."[3,4] During the 20th century, the average surface temperature of the earth increased by approximately 0.6°C; approximately two-thirds of this warming has occurred since 1975. Concurrently, climate variability has increased in various regions of the world—just as climate modelers predicted.

The IPCC has estimated that the average surface temperature of Earth will increase by 2°C to 5°C during this century.[3] Two major types of uncertainty underlie this estimate: (a) how the climate system will respond to continuing change in atmospheric composition, and (b) what social, technological, demographic, and behavioral changes will occur in human societies in future decades.

Climate scientists believe that temperature increases will be greater at higher latitudes, on land (more than at sea), and at night. Global climate change will likely alter rainfall patterns, with rain increasing over the oceans but decreasing over much of the land surface—especially in (a) various low-to-medium latitude, midcontinental regions (such as central Spain, the midwestern United States, the African Sahel, and Amazonia); and (b) already-arid areas in northwest India, the Middle East, northern Africa, and parts of Central America. And rainfall events will likely intensify, with more frequent extreme events that will increase the likelihood of floods and droughts.

Surprise events may also occur. There is a small possibility that large sections of the Antarctic ice mass will melt, thus raising sea level by several meters. But this may not be likely because it appears that disintegration did not occur during the warm peak of the last interglacial period, about 120,000 years ago, when temperatures were apparently 1°C to 2°C higher than now. Another possibility is that the northern Atlantic Gulf Stream—that section of the huge, slow "conveyor belt" circulation that distributes Pacific-equatorial warm water around the world's oceans—might weaken, and eventually even shut down, if increased melt water from the great Greenland glacier disturbs its dynamics.[3] Some weakening of the Gulf Stream may have occurred over the past 25 years. Northwestern Europe, relative to same-latitude Newfoundland, currently enjoys around 5°C of bonus heating from this heat source. If weakening of the Gulf Stream occurred in the future, Europe would cool, even as the rest of the world warmed. With substantial weakening, glaciation could occur in northern Europe.

Potential Health Impacts of Climate Change

Global climate change is influencing the functioning of many ecosystems and the biological health of plants and creatures. Given standard forecasts of climate change, an estimated one-third of terrestrial plant and animal species will become extinct by 2050.[5] On the other hand, there will probably be beneficial health impacts for some populations. For example, milder winters would reduce the seasonal

wintertime peak in deaths that occurs in temperate countries, whereas in currently hot regions a further increase in temperatures might reduce the viability of disease-transmitting mosquitoes. Overall, however, scientists consider that most of the health impacts of climate change will be adverse (Fig. 21-2).[4]

Direct health impacts could occur from:

- Changes in exposure to weather extremes, such as heat waves and winter cold;
- Increases in other extreme weather events, such as floods, cyclones, and droughts; and
- Increased formation of certain air pollutants and aeroallergens, such as spores and molds.

Acting via less direct pathways, climate change would affect (a) transmission of many infectious diseases, especially waterborne, foodborne, and vectorborne diseases; and (b) regional food productivity, especially cereal grains. In the long term, these indirect effects of climate change are likely to be greater than direct impacts.

For vectorborne infectious diseases, the distribution and abundance of vectors, such as mosquitoes and ticks, and intermediate hosts are affected by (a) various physical factors, such as temperature, precipitation, humidity, surface water, and wind; and (b) biotic factors, such as vegetation, host species, predators, competitors, and human interventions. In addition, warming-related changes in the life-cycle dynamics of vectors and pathogens (protozoa, bacteria, and viruses) tend to increase the transmission of many vectorborne diseases, such as malaria (transmitted by mosquitoes), dengue fever (transmitted by mosquitoes), and leishmaniasis (transmitted by sandflies). However, the incidence of schistosomiasis (transmitted by water snails) may decrease because warmer water adversely affects snail survival.

Mathematical and statistical models have been used for making such projections. For example, from various computer-based modeling studies, it seems likely that the geographic range of potential transmission for many vectorborne diseases will be significantly extended due to global climate change in this century. Modeling studies, based on predicted future trends in trade and economic development, have also estimated the impact of climate change on yields of grain, which accounts for two-thirds of food energy worldwide. Models indicate that climate change over the next 50 years will slightly decrease grain yields—especially in food-insecure regions in South Asia, Africa, and Central America. Such a decrease would increase the

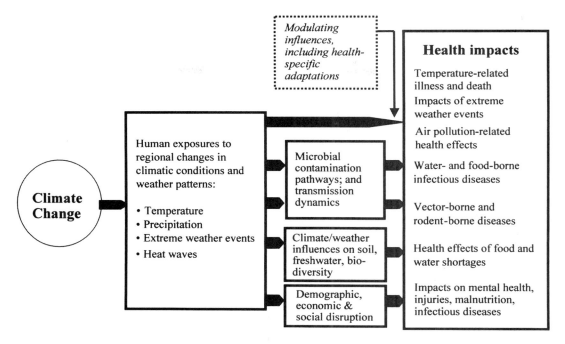

FIGURE 21-2 ● The main pathways whereby climate change causes direct and indirect effects on human health. The impact-modifying role of various modulating factors, and, specifically, adaptation measures is also shown. (Adapted from McMichael A, Campbell-Lendrum D, Corvalan C, et al. Climate change and human health: Risks and responses. Geneva: WHO, 2003.)

number of malnourished people globally by tens of millions above the otherwise projected number of up to 800 million.

Climate change over the past 25 years may well have had various incremental impacts on some health outcomes.[6] However, detection is a matter both of statistical power and reasonable—but difficult—judgment about attribution. The former depends on numbers of observations and the extent of divergence between observed and expected rates or magnitudes of health outcomes. The latter includes pattern recognition. If, for example, a particular infectious disease changes in occurrence in multiple geographic locations, each associated with local climate changes, then we can be much more confident that there is a climatic influence than if we were to see such a change in occurrence in just one setting.

STRATOSPHERIC OZONE DEPLETION

Ozone first appeared in Earth's atmosphere about 2 billion years ago. Oxygen produced by photosynthesis in water-based plants spilled over into the atmosphere and, in the upper atmosphere,

was chemically converted, by incoming solar ultraviolet radiation (UVR)* to ozone. This stratospheric ozone chemically filtered out the harmful short wavelengths of UVR, eventually allowing the progression from aqueous to land-based life.

Surface-level ambient UVR consists of: (a) most of the incident solar UVA, which penetrates the atmosphere almost fully; (b) less than 10 percent of incoming solar UVB, most of which is filtered out by stratospheric ozone; and (c) no shortwave UVC, which is completely absorbed in the atmosphere. The adverse health effects of ozone depletion will thus be largely confined to those associated with increases in UVB radiation, rather than with UVR per se.

Ninety percent of Earth's ozone is in the stratosphere; the remaining 10 percent is in the troposphere. Dobson units (DUs) are a measure of the total number of ozone molecules between the top of the atmosphere and Earth's surface, or the

---

*UVR is that part of the electromagnetic spectrum with wavelengths just shorter than the violet component of visible light. UVR comprises longer wavelength UVA, intermediate wavelength UVB, and shorter wavelength UVC. In general, the shorter the wavelength, the potentially more biologically damaging is the radiation (see Chapter 14D).

"thickness" of the ozone layer. Total column ozone is least at the Equator (less than 300 DUs) and increases at higher latitude, with greater overall column amounts at high latitude in the Northern than the Southern Hemisphere. There are seasonal and yearly fluctuations in total column ozone due to wind transport and stratospheric circulation of ozone.

Chlorofluorocarbons (CFCs) were developed in the 1920s as safe, nontoxic, nonflammable replacements for toxic, flammable refrigerants then in use, such as ammonia. They were further developed for use in the automotive industry and as propellants for aerosol cans. As propellants and as discarded refrigerants, CFCs eventually entered the atmosphere.

In 1974, scientists first theorized that free chlorine atoms released from atmospheric CFCs (by reaction with UVR at low atmospheric temperatures) might catalytically destroy stratospheric ozone (Box 21-2). Within 10 years, international action was taken in the United States and Europe to decrease the use of CFCs, especially in aerosols. The Vienna Convention for the Protection of the Ozone Layer was signed in 1985 by 20 nations, preceding by 2 months the first reports of measurable ozone loss (less than 220 DUs) in Antarctica— subsequently called the *ozone hole*. A rapid international response ensued, with the Montreal Protocol (1987) and its subsequent amendments providing global phase-out schedules for CFCs and their less-damaging substitutes, the halons and hydrochlorofluorocarbons (HCFCs).

CFCs have long atmospheric half-lives, so that, despite the relatively prompt international action to limit CFC production and consumption, atmospheric CFCs have continued to accumulate—with increasing destruction of stratospheric ozone. In the most recent United Nations Environmental Program (UNEP) assessment, ozone changes in the tropics appear to be minimal; ambient terrestrial levels of UVR are estimated to have increased by over 10 percent at mid-to-high latitudes since 1980 but now appear to be leveling off.[1] At high latitudes, in the Arctic and in Antarctica, ozone levels have been highly variable. In the spring of 2002, the ozone hole over Antarctica was the smallest since 1988, with earlier resolution, sparking some hope that this might signal recovery of the ozone layer. However, the spring ozone hole in 2003 was the second largest ever recorded—covering 11.1 million square miles, almost as large as the record ozone hole of 11.5 million square miles in 2000. Atmo-

---

BOX 21-2

Chemical Reactions in the Destruction of Ozone

Ozone "absorbs" UVR in the UVB band when UVB breaks an ozone molecule into an oxygen molecule and an oxygen atom. This atom then combines with another oxygen molecule to regenerate ozone. The result of these reactions is the conversion of solar UVB into heat energy.

Ozone formation:

$$O_2 + UVC \rightarrow O + O$$

$$O_2 + O \rightarrow O_3$$

Absorption of UVB: $O_3 + UVB \rightarrow O_2 + O + heat$

$$O_2 + O \rightarrow O_3$$

Although the reaction of ozone with UVR results in the regeneration of ozone molecules, as a catalyst, free chlorine radicals are regenerated postreaction to destroy further ozone molecules.

$$Cl + O_3 \rightarrow ClO + O_2$$

$$ClO + O \rightarrow Cl + O_2$$

---

spheric levels of most CFCs appear to have peaked and some have started to decrease.[7] If current trends continue, the Antarctic ozone hole is anticipated to disappear in about 50 years.

Health Effects

There are three important determinants of the individual UVR dose received:

- *The ambient UVR level and its relative wavelength constitution*: This is determined by season, latitude, and the level of stratospheric ozone. Ground-level measurements of UVR differ from satellite measurements of ambient UVR due to variations in cloud cover and lower atmospheric pollution.
- *Culture and behavior*: Although the usual outdoor exposure may only be 5 to 10 percent of daily erythemal UVR, for any ground level measurement of UVR at any location, there may be a 100-fold difference in individual exposure due to differences in sun-exposure habits.

Even in low-latitude countries, such as Sweden, most adults and adolescents report sunburn from outdoor tanning.

- *Skin pigmentation*: Human skin pigmentation is quite variable. Deeply pigmented skin has a natural sun protection factor (SPF) of approximately 13; the dose of erythemally weighted UVR required to produce barely discernible erythema in people with deeply pigmented skin is 33 times that in people with lightly pigmented skin.[8] For any level of UVR exposure, the biologically damaging effect will be much greater in fair skin than in more deeply pigmented skin.

UVB does not penetrate tissues as deeply as UVA, so that its main adverse effects on human health are on superficial tissues: the skin and the eye. UVB is absorbed by DNA, causing characteristic chemical changes (pyrimidine dimers) that, as mutations, may be critical in the initiation of carcinogenesis. UVB exposure also has beneficial health effects. The main source of vitamin D is from UVB-induced conversion of precursors in the skin. This essential vitamin is important for skeletal health, especially the prevention of rickets, osteomalacia, and osteoporosis. Vitamin D insufficiency has also been associated with hypertension and increased risks of breast and prostate cancer and non-Hodgkin lymphoma. UVR exposure causes local and systemic immunosuppression and this may be protective against the development of autoimmune diseases, especially multiple sclerosis.[9]

Adverse Effects of UVB on the Eyes, Skin, and Immune System

The eye is the only part of the human body not shielded from harmful UVB radiation by the protective layer of the skin. The vulnerability of the eye to environmental hazards is the price we pay for being able to see. Acute high-dose UVB exposure results in acute inflammation of the cornea and conjunctiva (photokeratitis and photoconjunctivitis, or snow blindness). Chronic UVB exposure is one risk factor for the development of pterygium (a fleshy wing-shaped growth on the surface of the eye) and for squamous cell carcinoma of the cornea and conjunctiva.

There is a causal relationship between "senile" cataract and UVR—especially UVB—exposure. Cataracts are extremely common, particularly in older people, and may cause visual impairment including complete blindness. They are associated with an increased risk of mortality. UVR exposure has been implicated in the causation of all three types of cataract: cortical and posterior subcapsular cataracts with chronic UVR exposure, and nuclear cataracts with high-level, early-life exposure.[10] (The evidence is strongest for cortical cataracts.)

Under normal circumstances, the anterior parts of the eye and the vitreous humor filter out most UVB radiation. However, a retinal "sunburn" (phototoxic retinopathy, solar retinopathy, or eclipse retinopathy) can occur if the sun is viewed directly, such as by sun-gazing or looking at the Sun during a solar eclipse. The acute vision loss usually resolves over weeks or months but occasionally progresses to permanent visual impairment.

Sunburn is the immediate result of acute overexposure of the skin to sunlight. UVB is three to four times as effective as UVA in causing erythema in humans. The longer term risk is that of cancer. Chronic or repeated UVR exposure is the strongest risk factor for the development of cutaneous malignant melanoma (CMM), squamous cell carcinoma (SCC), and basal cell carcinoma (BCC).[1] These cancers are particularly common in regions where pale-skinned populations are exposed to high levels of UVR, such as at lower latitudes. Although cumulative lifetime UVR exposure appears to be most important in the development of SCC, both BCC and CMM may be more closely associated with a pattern of intermittent high level exposure; in addition, there may be critical ages of exposure.[11] Although UVA may also be important in the development of CMM, the DNA damage associated with UVB absorption is particularly implicated in SCC and BCC. The modeling of skin cancer incidence in North American and European populations as a function of increased ground-level UVR exposure due to stratospheric ozone depletion during the early decades of this century indicates that a 5 to 10 percent excess incidence would occur during the second quarter of this century.[12]

Increased UVB exposure due to stratospheric ozone depletion may have both beneficial and detrimental effects on immune function. UV exposure may suppress autoimmune disorders, such as type 1 diabetes and multiple sclerosis,[9] but may impair vaccine efficacy and possibly increase susceptibility to a range of infections. UVB exposure appears to dampen the activity of T helper 1 lymphocytes, which are important in the body's reaction to simple chemicals, intracellular infections (such as those caused by viruses), and tumor growth, and in the development of autoimmune disorders. There appears to be either little effect on or enhancement of T helper 2 lymphocytes, which are important in the immune response to extracellular infections, such as those caused by most bacteria.[8]

Ecological Effects

Increased UVB will adversely affect terrestrial and aquatic ecosystems, which may indirectly affect human health.[1] Increased UVB exposure may be associated with decreased plant height and leaf area and may be responsible for changes in species composition and biodiversity of bacteria and fungi growing on plants. Chemical changes in plant tissue may affect the intensity and specificity of pathogen attack. UVB may impair photosynthesis. In aquatic ecosystems, increased solar UVB may reduce productivity, impair reproduction and development, and increase the mutation rate in phytoplankton, fish eggs and larvae, and in zooplankton, as well as primary and secondary consumers of these life forms. Stratospheric ozone depletion and resultant increased UVB radiation will also affect biogeochemical cycles, including oceanic carbon cycles, nitrogen availability to plants, and levels of tropospheric ozone by producing carbon monoxide from decomposition of plant matter and enhanced release of nitrogen oxides.[1]

BIODIVERSITY LOSS

Biodiversity underpins the resilience of the ecosystems on which human societies depend. Biodiversity loss is now occurring at an unprecedented rate that appears to be at least as great as in any of the five great extinctions that have occurred over the past 500 million years, since the advent of multicellular organisms. This loss is being driven by human-induced overexploitation of productive ecosystems, land use changes, climate change, pollution events (such as oil spills), transboundary migration of pollutants, introduced species, and biotechnology.[13] Loss of biodiversity threatens vital ecosystem services, including food, fuel and fiber, fresh water, nutrient cycling, waste processing, flood and storm protection, and climate stability. The potential consequences of ecosystem disruption on human health are discussed below.

Despite the fundamental importance of ecosystem services for human health, links between biodiversity loss and human health are difficult to demonstrate epidemiologically.[14] This difficulty is partly because biodiversity loss affects health through complex, indirect pathways.

Local social conditions can modulate the effects of ecosystem disruption. Human societies have adapted to natural fluctuations in ecosystem services and, especially in developed countries, have developed efficient methods of buffering communities, such as systems of trade, agriculture, and water storage. Especially in countries dominated by market economies, these adaptations are often designed to minimize short-term, local ecological changes, while maximizing profits. This means that large-scale unintended consequences of human economic activity tend to be displaced geographically (such as the costs of overconsumption by developed countries) or postponed into the future (such as the long-term consequences of climate change or desertification).

FOOD

The health of human populations depends crucially upon the services of food-producing ecosystems. This is most obvious in developing countries, especially in rural areas, where food is derived almost exclusively from local sources. Human dependence on ecosystems for nutrition is less apparent—but ultimately no less fundamental—in urban communities of developed countries. Historically, loss of productive ecosystem services has led to collapse of whole civilizations. For example, the Mayan empire collapsed about 1,000 years ago as a result of soil erosion, silting of rivers, and drought collectively leading to agro-ecosystem failure.[13,15]

Undernutrition remains a major health problem in developing countries, where poverty is a consistently strong underlying determinant.[16] The World Health Organization estimates that about one-fourth of the global burden of disease in the poorest countries is attributable to childhood and maternal undernutrition. Worldwide, undernutrition accounts for nearly 10 percent of disability-adjusted life-years (DALYs).[16] Among developed countries, diet-related risks (mainly overnutrition) in combination with physical inactivity, accounts for one-third of the burden of disease.

Aggregate food production is currently sufficient to meet the needs of all. However, of the current world population of just over 6 billion, an estimated 840 million are undernourished—while hundreds of millions are overfed. This unequal distribution of access to food has been driven primarily by political and economic factors, although ecological problems may play an increasingly important role in the future.

In poor countries, the number of people per hectare of arable land increased from three in 1961–1963 to five in 1997–1999.[17] Poverty and hunger have tended to force people onto marginal, drought-prone lands, with poor soil fertility. Agricultural production has tripled in the past four decades, mainly through growth in yield. However, food production has not kept pace with population increase in many countries, and improvements in yield appear to have slowed.[13,17]

Today, almost one-fourth of usable land has undergone reduced productivity. About 1 billion people are affected by land degradation through soil erosion, water logging, or salinity of irrigated land. Providing sufficient food for an expected human population of 8 to 9 billion people by 2050 will require, if it is to be achieved sustainably, profound changes in (a) production methods and technologies and (b) the distribution of resources (wealth, knowledge, and power).[18]

In many countries, agricultural production is increasingly dependent on irrigation. This situation is likely to lead to armed conflict where there are existing tensions over access to freshwater supplies. Many river systems with scarce water resources are shared uneasily among neighboring countries in unstable regions of the Nile, the Ganges, the Mekong, the Jordan, and the Tigris and Euphrates rivers. "Water wars" have therefore been postulated as increasingly likely in future, as population pressures and demands increase, including among countries in the Middle East, and between Ethiopia and Egypt, Lesotho and South Africa, and India and Bangladesh.[19]

FRESH WATER

Currently, 1.1 billion people lack access to safe water supplies and 2.4 billion people lack adequate sanitation. Lack of improved water and sanitation is strongly associated with poverty, although this relationship varies among regions.[16] Along with sanitation, water availability and quality are well recognized as important risk factors for infectious diarrhea and other major diseases, especially in children.[20] The associated effects on human health are severe. Poor countries, with inadequate provision of water and sanitation are most vulnerable to these effects.

Fresh water is a key resource for human health; it is used for growing food, drinking, washing, cooking, and for the recycling of wastes. Worldwide, almost 4 percent of the global burden of disease is currently attributable to unsafe water, sanitation, and hygiene.[20] In this century, water resources will be strongly affected by trends in population, land use, and the management of freshwater ecosystems. Increasing demand for food, in particular, will worsen water scarcity. By 2025, an estimated one-half of the world's population will live in river basins where water is scarce, and 70 percent of readily available water supplies will be used.[17] Water scarcity can lead to use of poorer quality sources of freshwater, which are more likely to be contaminated, tending to cause increases in water-related diseases.

FUEL

Most of the world's population has limited or no access to electricity supplies and about 2 billion people rely on biomass (wood, dung, and agricultural residues) for heating and cooking. Energy consumption per capita is about 25 times higher in rich countries than in poor countries.[17] Lack of clean, safe power contributes to a range of health impacts.

Outdoor air pollution, resulting from the combustion of fossil fuels for transport, power generation, and industry, aggravates heart and lung disease. Indoor air pollution causes much respiratory disease in adults and children. About one-half of the world's population still uses solid fuels for cooking, and 3 percent of the global burden of disease in DALY's has been attributed to indoor air pollution from this source. Urban air pollution has accounted for an additional 1 percent of global DALYs.[16]

Energy supplies are a fundamental factor in sustainable development and are also needed to provide and maintain modern health services. The need to spend considerable time collecting fuel can preclude proper education, with indirect adverse effects on health through illiteracy, lost work opportunities, and large family size. Finally, energy use is indirectly linked to adverse health effects through desertification, acidification, ambient air pollution, and climate change.

NUTRIENT MANAGEMENT AND WASTE MANAGEMENT, PROCESSING, AND DETOXIFICATION

Well-functioning ecosystems absorb and remove contaminants. For example, wetlands can remove excess nutrients from runoff, preventing damage to downstream ecosystems. Inadequate sanitation (management of solid waste) increases human exposure to infectious disease agents, such as by fecal contamination of water, or by disease transmission by rats, leading to a range of communicable diseases, especially diarrheal illness.[21]

When recycled appropriately, human waste can be a useful resource that promotes soil fertility.[22] However, where waste contains persistent chemicals, such as organochlorines or heavy metals, recycling onto land can lead to the accumulation of these pollutants and increased human exposure to them through food and water, possibly contributing to various chronic diseases.

Application of agricultural fertilizers and organic wastes, including sewage, can improve agricultural yields but may also lead to increased concentrations of nitrogen and phosphorus in surface waters and coastal sea areas. Resultant nitrates can cause methemoglobinemia and possibly certain cancers, such as stomach cancer. Another, more frequent, consequence is eutrophication in both marine and freshwater ecosystems, resulting in overgrowth of bacteria, phytoplankton, and algae—leading, in turn, to increases in waterborne diseases and poisoning from harmful algal blooms.[23] There are likely to be other ecological mechanisms by which increased nutrients can influence human disease risks, but further research is required to clarify these.

CLIMATE REGULATION

Climate regulation is an important property of Earth's natural systems. Each ecological service will be affected by climate change. For example, climate change may increase by 500 million by 2025 the number of people affected by water stress. Water-related disasters, due to droughts and floods, will likely have severe health impacts. The frequency of heavy rainfall events is likely to increase, leading to an increase in the magnitude and frequency of floods and a decrease in low-river flows.[3]

Healthy ecosystems provide a buffer against the damaging effects of climate extremes. For example, forests absorb rainfall and provide a buffer against increases in runoff, thereby reducing flooding and soil erosion. A combination of deforestation and increased heavy rainfall events could have much more severe ecological and health consequences than either would alone. Healthy coral reefs and mangroves stabilize coastlines, limiting the damaging effect of storm surges. A combination of overfishing, local pollution, sea temperature increase, and sea level rise could damage coral reefs and, in turn, increase the vulnerability of small island communities to extreme weather events. For example, the flooding of the Yangtze River Basin in China in 1998 was attributed to a complex web of factors, including heavy rain associated with an El Niño event, deforestation that increased water runoff, and more intensive cultivation of lakes and wetlands in the river basin, which reduced their "sponge" function.

Heavy rainfall due to climate change can adversely affect water quality by increasing chemical and biological pollutants flushed into rivers and overloading sewers and waste-storage facilities. Increases in temperature would worsen water quality by increasing the growth of microorganisms and decreasing dissolved oxygen. In some parts of the world, climate change also may increase requirements for irrigation water because of increased evaporation.

URBANIZATION

Since early in the 19th century, the proportion of the world's human population living in cities or large towns has increased from approximately 5 to 50 percent.[24] This radical transformation of human ecology continues apace, entailing changes in social organization, family relations, housing conditions, transport choices, dietary patterns, occupational environments, access to educational and health care services, and the transmission of infectious disease agents.[25]

Some health risks are obvious, such as hospitalizations for asthma during air pollution crises and road traffic injuries. Others are more subtle, such as sustained exposure to environmental lead (from car exhaust, leaded house paint, and emissions from smelters and other industrial facilities) that lowers the intelligence of young children. Physical aspects of the urban environment may affect seasonal patterns of morbidity and mortality. For example, housing quality, including dampness and inside temperature, may contribute to early-life exposure to fungal spores and to house-dust mites, both of which are a likely cause of asthma in children.

As modern cities expand, transport systems become increasingly prominent. Car ownership and travel has escalated over the past 50 years in much of the world. In addition to the problem of exhaust gas emissions—which cause local air pollution and contribute to acid rain and to greenhouse gas emissions—other major public health impacts of car-based systems include injuries, reduced physical activity (and resultant obesity), disruption of neighborhoods, and increased noise levels.

Urban air pollution has become a worldwide public health problem. The earlier industrial/domestic air pollution from coal-burning, characteristic of much of 19th-century Europe and North America, has been largely replaced by pollutants from motorized transport. These form photochemical smog in summer and a heavy haze of particulates and nitrogen oxides in winter.

Cities have increasingly large "ecological footprints." There are ecological benefits of urbanism, including economies of scale, shared use of resources, and opportunities for reuse and recycling. But, there are great "externalities." Urban populations depend on food grown elsewhere, on raw materials and energy sources (especially fossil fuels) extracted elsewhere, and on disposal of their voluminous wastes elsewhere. For example, the estimated consumption of wood, paper, fibers, and food by 29 cities of the Baltic Sea region requires a total area many hundred times greater than the combined area of the 29 cities.[26] For all these reasons, urban populations—often with little awareness—are a major and growing source of pressure on the biosphere.

ENVIRONMENTAL CONFLICT AND SECURITY

As human populations have expanded over the millennia, there has been increased exploitation of natural resources and increased territorial expansion, often leading to armed conflict between rival groups. Although the causes of such conflicts have been multifactorial, complex, and contentious, the competition for natural resources has been a key factor.[27] The World Commission on Environment and Development has stated that nations have often fought to assert or resist control over raw materials, energy supplies, and land.[28] The risk of conflict may significantly increase in the near future because of increased scarcity of natural resources, much of it due to declining environmental capacities. The Persian Gulf War of 1991 is a recent example of major conflict triggered by concern over an environmental resource—oil. Other recent, but lesser known, resource-associated conflicts include those in India, the Philippines, and the West African states of Mauritania and Senegal.[29]

Even if the "sustainability transition"[25] gains momentum, it is still likely that the per capita availability of water, arable land, and other critical environmental resources will decline. Spectacular technological improvements in the exploration and recovery of oil have not relieved concerns that the end of cheap oil is likely in this century. Therefore, oil wars are also possible.

More speculatively, climate change may interact with natural resource stresses (such as water scarcity) and expanding human populations to increase the possibility of armed conflict. Many parts of Africa already experience a less-than-favorable agricultural climate and, under various standard climate change models, this situation is forecast to deteriorate in the second half of this century,[30] increasing the likelihood of armed conflict.

Global warming may intensify the El Niño Southern Oscillation (ENSO).[31] Stronger, more frequent El Niños and La Niñas would be likely to increase adverse social, economic, and health consequences in different regions.[32] These, in turn, would tend to increase the risk of conflict in resource-scarce areas, such as by increasing regional food scarcity through intensified droughts.

Loss of biodiversity may not so obviously appear to potentiate conflict. The loss of genetic diversity will reduce the isolation of useful chemicals and the discovery of potentially useful biological compounds but is unlikely to lead to war. However, reduced ecosystem function, due to biodiversity loss, may interact with climate change to cause further deforestation and ecosystem collapse, such as by the loss of "keystone species" or changing the flowering and fruiting patterns of the tropical rainforest canopy. These changes could exacerbate local and regional tensions.

There are numerous other mechanisms by which damaged ecosystems providing essential "goods and services" may cause economic harm, and thus increase the risk of armed conflict. Several

BOX 21-3

Health Risks Arising from Contemporary Global Trade Patterns

1. Perpetuation and exacerbation of income differentials, both within and among countries, thereby creating and maintaining poverty-associated conditions for poor health.
2. Fragmentation and weakening of labor markets as internationally mobile capital acquires greater relative power. The resultant job insecurity, substandard wages, and "lowest common denominator" approach to occupational and environmental conditions and safety can jeopardize the health of workers and their families.
3. The consequences of global environmental changes, including changes in atmospheric composition, land degradation, depletion of biodiversity, spread of "invasive" species, and dispersal of persistent organic pollutants.

Other, more-specific examples of risks to health include:

- Spread of smoking-related diseases as the tobacco industry globalizes its markets.
- Diseases of dietary excess as food production and food processing become intensified and as urban consumer preferences are shaped increasingly by globally promoted images.
- Diverse public health consequences of the proliferation of private car ownership, as car manufacturers extend their marketing.
- Continued widespread rise of urban obesity as daily living patterns of eating and physical activity evolve.
- Expansion of the international drug trade, exploiting the inner-urban poor.
- Increasing prevalence of depression and mental disorders in aging and socially fragmented urban populations.
- Infectious diseases that now spread more easily because of increased travel worldwide.

Source: McMichael AJ, Beaglehole R. The changing global context of public health. Lancet 2000;356:495–9.

worst-case scenarios could even lead to global conflict, including (a) runaway global warming; (b) food scarcity, leading to nuclear war involving South Asia or China; and (c) disruption of the Gulf Stream, which would disrupt European agriculture and greatly increase European energy needs.[33,34]

GLOBAL TRADE AND DEVELOPMENT

Income is a strong predictor of health status, especially among low-income populations. In the past 50 years, coincident with economic growth, there have been widespread increases in life expectancy and decreases in fertility rates.[35] In recent years, economic gains have been greatest in Western Europe, North America, Oceania, and some Asian countries.[36] Yet during this period, income inequality has increased both within and among countries. The ratio of income earned in countries with the richest fifth of the population, compared to poorest fifth, widened from 30:1 in 1960, to 60:1 in 1990, to 74:1 in 1997.[37]

There is a strong coupling of the political and economic processes driving global economic inequality and ecologically unsustainable resource use. International trade and development policies have contributed substantially to the present global social and ecological predicaments (Box 21-3). For example, "liberalized" trading structures and practices have contributed to the emergence and spread of infectious diseases. Overall, globalization of the food market has unavoidably accentuated the movement of pathogens from one region to another—and has also amplified the redistribution of microbial resistance genes.

A primary stimulus for the great increase in migration internationally is the urge to enter the cash economy, with its demand for both skilled and unskilled workers in a globalizing marketplace. Rapid urbanization, often characterized by informal housing and periurban slums, tends to increase the occurrence of "old" infectious diseases like childhood pneumonia, diarrhea, tuberculosis, and dengue. Urbanization can also facilitate the spread of various emerging diseases. For example, poor-quality, high-rise housing creates new risks, as occurred with severe acute respiratory syndrome (SARS) in Hong Kong in 2003. Overcrowded, poor-quality housing may be associated with family breakdown, drug abuse, and antisocial behaviors—and, in turn, increases in infections transmitted by sex and intravenous drug use, including HIV.[38]

West Nile virus, a newly emergent infectious agent in North America, illustrates the epidemiological impact of long-distance trade and travel. It originated in Africa and has been detected sporadically in the Middle East and parts of Europe. It was unknown in North America until it arrived in New York in summer 1999, probably via an infected mosquito on an airplane. Birds were first infected, then humans. The apparently favorable conditions for viral propagation within New York City included:

- Early season rain and summer drought, providing ideal conditions for *Culex* mosquitoes;
- The warmest July on record for New York City;
- Suburban/urban ecosystems supporting large populations of selected avian host and mosquito vector species adapted to these conditions;
- Large populations of susceptible bird species, especially crows; and
- Suburban/urban ecosystems conducive to close interaction of mosquitoes, birds, and humans.

West Nile virus then spread rapidly across the United States and has now established itself as an endemic virus, harbored by animals, including birds and horses, and transmitted via mosquitoes. The virus could spread more rapidly in Central and South America than in North America because countries there have warmer climates, large bird populations, and year-round mosquito breeding.

RISK ASSESSMENT AND RISK MANAGEMENT

The risk to human health from global environmental change is a function, at the individual, community, regional, and global levels, of (a) the level of exposure to risk; (b) vulnerability (sensitivity, coping capacity, and adaptive capacity); and (c) adaptation responses.

The level of exposure to risk depends on the weather and climate characteristics of the geographic region, whereas sensitivity, coping capacity, and adaptive capacity depend on characteristics of the individual, the population, and the region. The developmental status and demographic structure moderate the current exposure response profile of the population.[37] *Coping capacity* is a measure of the current ability of an individual or population to manage risk exposure, and *adaptive capacity* is "the ability of a system to adjust to climate change (including climate variability and extremes) to moderate potential damages, to take advantage of opportunities, or to cope with the consequences."[4] In human societies, adaptive capacity varies with wealth, access to technology, education and information, skills levels, societal infrastructure, access to resources, management capabilities, and developmental status. There will almost certainly be increasing disparities between the ability of developed and developing countries to adapt to global environmental change.

Risk assessment aims to identify and quantify the risk of a particular exposure to human health and well-being. By assessing the exposure and knowing the likely health impact (a function of vulnerability) in a particular population, we can estimate the magnitude and frequency of the risk and who would be most affected. An assessment can be made of the current coping capacity, especially to deal with risks that gradually increase (such as shrinking water supplies) and of future adaptive capacity. Risk communication then becomes important for increasing the awareness and tolerance of risk at the local, regional, and national level. Using a common metric for "risk" may help determine risk-management priorities: For whom, how quickly, to what extent, and in which order risks should and could be reduced? Recent estimates by WHO of the environmental burden of disease[16] are an example of quantitative risk assessment, using DALYs to measure both current and projected health risks from environmental exposures. Risk assessment should include ongoing monitoring and evaluation of the effectiveness of any risk-decreasing interventions.[39]

Classically, *risk management* integrates the information derived from risk assessment with other information, including socioeconomic and political concerns, to formulate public health actions to decrease or eliminate the risk. However, global environmental changes represent a public health challenge that is already too far advanced, too wide-reaching, and too complex for actual elimination of risk to be possible. For global environmental changes, therefore, risk management seeks to minimize—rather than eliminate—risk.

It comprises two main strategies: (a) mitigation to decrease the level of future environmental health hazards and (b) adaptation to reduce the adverse effects of exposure to the hazard. For example, because of the momentum and time delays in the climate-change process, immediate cessation of excess greenhouse gas emissions (mitigation) cannot preclude some level of climate change; that is, past and current emissions have already committed us to future global climate change (entailing warming of around 0.7°C).

ADAPTATION VERSUS MITIGATION

Mitigation strategies to halt and reverse global environmental changes require participation by the global community. Although developed countries have largely driven global environmental change, mitigation cannot be fully effective unless all countries are prepared to make the necessary changes to decrease the production of greenhouse gases, explore different energy sources, and conserve water and other renewable resources. Adaptation can be somewhat country-specific, but it is also a strategy that may be dependent on wealth, because the poorest countries are generally least able to adapt to the consequences of global environmental changes. Adaptation can be responsive (to particular and immediate risks) or anticipatory (actions taken in advance of climate change effects). But while both adaptation and mitigation decrease risk, only mitigation decreases risk exposure; adaptation alters the exposure–response relationship.

Potential for Mitigation

Mitigation appears likely to have been an effective strategy in reversing the effects of CFC accumulation and stratospheric ozone depletion. However, it seems less likely that mitigation will effectively reverse the effects of greenhouse gas accumulation. Carbon cycle models indicate that to stabilize atmospheric carbon dioxide (CO_2) concentration at 450 ppm, anthropogenic CO_2 emissions would need to drop below 1990 levels within a few decades. (Before the 19th century, atmospheric CO_2 concentration was stable for many centuries at around 280 ppm.) Further delays in effective mitigation will mean atmospheric CO_2 stabilizing further into the future and at higher levels.[4] Reduction of CO_2 emissions to 1920s levels (about one-third of current emissions) would likely be required to prevent serious damage to ecological and other biophysical systems.[40] The Kyoto Protocol is a first attempt to slow greenhouse gas accumulation.

Much of the difficulty in establishing policies for climate change mitigation is due to the complex, multisphere nature of the problem. Climate change involves "complex interactions between climatic, environmental, economic, political, institutional, social and technological processes."[4] These interactions occur at individual, community, national, and international levels.

There is a wide variation in the mitigation capacity of nations. Mitigation strategies will need to include financial arrangements that allow greater access to more advanced technologies, training, and information for poorer countries.

Potential for Adaptation

Based on information from risk assessment, adaptive measures include the development of strategies, policies, and technology to allow populations to cope better with adverse health risks of environmental exposures that are not amenable to elimination. Global environmental changes with a single exposure route or a single health outcome present a relatively straightforward situation for adaptation. Thus, adaptations to stratospheric ozone depletion through behaviors to avoid excess UVR exposure, such as sunscreen, clothing, and avoiding sunburn, are easier to advocate and implement than adaptations to the widespread and somewhat ill-defined effects of climate change due to greenhouse gas accumulation. In addition, the potential for adaptation is greater for human systems than natural systems and for humans in more developed countries than in less developed countries.

Adaptation can be considered in terms of primary, secondary, and tertiary prevention of adverse health effects. Examples of primary prevention (avoiding the exposure, or removing the hazardous element of the exposure) include early warning systems for extreme events. Secondary prevention or reactive adaptation includes rapid response to disasters. Tertiary prevention includes better treatment of an established disease, such as malaria.[6]

Adaptation builds on current coping capacity, including baseline strategies for dealing with risk exposure. In addition to being reactive or anticipatory, adaptation can be autonomous (actions of individuals) or planned (for whole populations) through policy decisions.

CONCLUSION

Global environmental changes, both of systemic and worldwide mosaic kinds, are now occuring to the world's environment as a result of human actions. The aggregated environmental impact of humankind is now so great that it is beginning to change conditions of life on Earth. There is clear evidence of rising global temperatures, loss of stratospheric ozone, loss of biodiversity, and depletion of freshwater supplies. These changes pose new and escalating risks to human population health.

Climate change and ozone depletion are the best-known examples of global environmental change. Other categories of change, less appreciated but no less important, include urbanization, ecological disruption, land degradation, disruption of elemental cycles (such as nitrogen, sulfur, and phosphorus), depletion of freshwater supplies, and the global dissemination of persistent organic pollutants. There are important, complex, interactions between many of these categories of global environmental change. For example, biodiversity loss is driven by a combination of factors, including overexploitation of productive ecosystems, other land use changes, and climate change. In turn, biodiversity loss threatens vital ecosystem services, including the provision of food, fuel, and fiber, the quality and supply of freshwater, waste processing, flood protection, and climate stability.

Remedying stratospheric ozone depletion is a global cooperation "success" story, although recovery of the ozone layer will take several decades. Greenhouse gas emissions, disruption of elemental cycles, global dissemination of persistent organic pollutants, and the problems associated with biodiversity losses are more complex environmental change processes to study and are much more economically and politically challenging.

There is considerable overlap in the political and economic processes that drive both global economic inequality and ecologically unsustainable resource use. For example, international trade and economic development policies have contributed to various of today's global social and ecological predicaments. Relatedly, the risk of conflict is likely to increase because of regional resource scarcity, arising in part from damage to environmental "goods and services." Hence, it is in the self-interest of humans everywhere, including those in powerful nations, to reduce these large-scale environmental changes and their attendant risks to human social well-being, health, and survival.

REFERENCES

1. UNEP. Environmental effects of ozone depletion and its interaction with climate change: 2002 assessment. Photochem Photobiol Sci 2003;2:1–72.
2. McMichael AJ. Environmental and social influences on emerging infectious diseases: Past, present and future. Philos Trans R Soc London Ser B Biol Sci 2004;359:1049–58.
3. Intergovernmental Panel on Climate change. Climate change 2001 (IPCC third assessment report). Cambridge: Cambridge University Press, 2001.
4. Intergovernmental Panel on Climate Change. Climate change 2001: Impacts, adaptation and vulnerability. Contribution of working group II to the IPCC third assessment report. Cambridge: Cambridge University Press, 2001.
5. Thomas C, Cameron A, Green RE, et al. Extinction risk from climate change. Nature 2004;427:145–8.
6. McMichael A, Campbell-Lendrum D, Corvalan C, et al., eds. Climate change and human health: Risks and responses. Geneva: WHO, 2003.
7. Levinson D, and Waple AM, (eds). State of the climate in 2003. Bulletin of the American Meteorological Society 2004;85:S1–S72. Available at: <http://ams.allenpress.com/pdfserv/10.1175%2FBAMS-85-6-Levinson>.
8. Clydesdale GJ, Dandie GW, Muller HK. Ultraviolet light induced injury: Immunological and inflammatory effects. Immunol Cell Biol 2001;79:547–8.
9. Ponsonby AL, McMichael A, van der Mei I. Ultraviolet radiation and autoimmune disease: Insights from epidemiological research. Toxicology 2002;181–182:71–8.
10. Neale RE, Purdie JL, Hirst LW, et al. Sun exposure as a risk factor for nuclear cataract. Epidemiology 2003;14:707–12.
11. Armstrong BK, Kricker A. The epidemiology of UV induced skin cancer. J Photochem Photobiol B Biol 2001;63:8–18.
12. Slaper H, Velders GJ, Daniel JS, et al. Estimates of ozone depletion and skin cancer incidence to examine the Vienna Convention achievements. Nature 1996;384:256–8.
13. UNEP. Global environmental outlook. Nairobi: United Nations Environment Programme, 2002.
14. Corvalan C, Hales S, McMichael A, eds. Health synthesis report of the Millennium Ecosystem Assessment. Geneva: World Health Organization (in press).
15. Haug GH, Gunther D, Peterson LC, et al. Climate and the collapse of Maya civilization. Science 2003;299:1731–5.
16. WHO. The world health report 2002. Geneva: WHO, 2002.
17. WEHAB. A framework for action. Johannesburg: World Summit on Sustainable Development, 2002.

18. Mellor J. Poverty reduction and biodiversity conservation: The complex role for intensifying agriculture. Washington, DC: World Wide Fund for Nature, 2002.

19. Gleick P. The world's water. The biennial report on freshwater resources. Washington, DC: Island Press, 2002.

20. Pruss A, Kay D, Fewtrell L, et al. Estimating the burden of disease from water, sanitation, and hygiene at a global level. Environ Health Perspect 2002;110:537–42.

21. Cairncross S. Sanitation in the developing world: Current status and future solutions. Int J Environ Health Res 2003;13:S123–131.

22. Esrey S. Philosophical, ecological and technical challenges for expanding ecological sanitation into urban areas. Water Sci Technol 2002;45:225–8.

23. UNESCO. Manual on harmful marine macroalgae. Paris: UNESCO, 2003.

24. McMichael AJ. Human frontiers, environments and disease: Past patterns, uncertain futures. Cambridge: Cambridge University Press, 2001.

25. McMichael AJ. The urban environment and health in a world of increasing globalization: Issues for developing countries. Bull World Health Org 2000;78:1117–26.

26. Folke C, Larsson J, Sweitzer J. Renewable source appropriation. In R Costanza, O. Segura (eds.). Getting down to Earth. Washington, DC: Island Press, 1996.

27. Homer-Dixon T, Blitt J, eds. Ecoviolence. Links among environment, population and security. Lanham, Maryland: Roman & Littlefield Publishers, 1999.

28. WCED. Our common future, World Commission on Environment and Development. Oxford: Oxford University Press, 1987.

29. Homer-Dixon T. Environmental scarcities and violent conflict: Evidence from cases. Int Security 1994;19: 5–40.

30. Parry M, Rosenzweig C, Iglesias A, et al. Climate change and world food security: A new assessment. Global Environ Change Human Policy Dimensions 1999;9: S51–S67.

31. Timmerman A, Oberhuber J, Bacher A, et al. Increased El Niño frequency in a climate model forced by future greenhouse warming. Nature 1999;398:694–7.

32. Bouma MJ, Kovats RS, Goubet SA, et al. Global assessment of El Nino's disaster burden. Lancet 1997;350: 1435–8.

33. Broecker WS. Thermohaline circulation, the Achilles' heel of our climate system: Will man-made CO_2 upset the current balance? Science 1997;278:1582–8.

34. Butler C. Personal perspective: Epidemiology, australians and global environmental change. Australasian Epidemiologist 2001;8:13–16.

35. McMichael AJ, Beaglehole R. The changing global context of public health. Lancet 2000;356:495–9.

36. Labonte R. Nailing health planks into the foreign policy platform: The Canadian experience. Med J Aust 2004;180:159–62.

37. United Nations Development Programme. Human development report 1999: Globalization with a human face. New York: Oxford University Press, 1999. Available at: http:/hdr.undp.org/reports/global/1999/en/default.cfm.

38. Cohen A. Urban unfinished business. Int J Environ Health Res 2003;13(Suppl 1):S29–36.

39. Kovats S, Ebi KL, Menne B. Methods of assessing human health vulnerability and public health adaptation to climate change. Health and global environmental change. WHO, WMO, UNEP, Health Canada: 2003:1–111.

40. McMichael A, Powles J. Human numbers, environment, sustainability and health. Brit Med J 1999;319: 977–80.

BIBLIOGRAPHY

Environmental Health Criteria 160. Available at: <www.who.int/uv/publictions/EHC160/en/>.
This is a comprehensive review of the effects of ultraviolet radiation on human health and the environment. Although it is now 10 years old, it provides an excellent basis for understanding the range of health effects associated with excessive UVR exposure. A more recent review, focusing more strongly on effects on the immune system and beneficial effects of UVR exposure, is available at: <http://www.mja.com.au/public/issues/ 177_11_021202/luc10478_fm.html>.

IPCC. Climate change 2001: Synthesis report. A contribution of working groups I, II, and III to the Third Assessment Report of the Intergovernmental Panel on Climate Change. Cambridge: Cambridge University Press, 2001. Available at:<http://www.grida.no/climate/ipcc_tar/vol4/index.htm>.
IPCC assessments attempt to answer such general questions as: Has Earth's climate changed as a result of human activities? In what ways is climate projected to change in the future? How vulnerable are agriculture, water supply, ecosystems, coastal infrastructure, and human health to different levels of change in climate and sea level? What is the technical, economic, and market potential of options to adapt to climate change or reduce emissions of the gases that influence climate? Climate Change 2001: Synthesis Report provides a policy-relevant, but not policy-prescriptive, synthesis and integration of information contained within the Third Assessment Report and also draws upon all previously approved and accepted IPCC reports that address a broad range of key policy-relevant questions. For this reason, it will be especially useful for policymakers and researchers.

McMichael AJ. Human frontiers, environments and disease: Past patterns, uncertain futures. Cambridge: Cambridge University Press, 2001.
The expansion of human frontiers—geographic, climatic, cultural, and technological—has encountered frequent setbacks from disease, famine, and dwindling resources. However, recognition of how environmental change can limit health and survival has been slow. Over many millennia, disease and longevity profiles in populations have reflected changes in environmental conditions and, often, exceedances of carrying capacity. Today, population growth and the aggregated pressures of consumption and emissions are beginning to impair various global environmental systems. The research tasks in detecting, attributing, and projecting the resultant health effects are complex. Have recent health gains, in part, depended on depleting natural environmental capital?

McMichael AJ. Population, environment, disease, and survival: Past patterns, uncertain futures. Lancet 2002;359: 1145–8.
This paper summarizes the main arguments in the above book. It argues for a higher level understanding of the relationship between demographic, social, and environmental conditions and their effects on population health. Over decadal time, health is an "ecologically" determined property of a population. When the size of a population's "ecological footprint" exceeds the available environmental carrying capacity then population levels of health and survival will, later if not sooner, be reduced.

UNEP. Environmental effects of ozone depletion and its interaction with climate change: 2002 assessment. Nairobi: UNEP, 2003. Available at: <http://www.gcrio.org/ OnLnDoc/pdf/unep_ozone2002.pdf>.
The four earlier assessments on Environmental Effects of Ozone Depletion, between 1989 and 1998, dealt almost

exclusively with increasing ultraviolet radiation and its effects. The current assessment gives an update on these same problems, but with a special emphasis on the interactions with climate change. Depletion of the stratospheric ozone layer and climate change are both aspects of global atmospheric change, but the measures needed for phasing out ozone-depleting chemicals and for limiting the increasing greenhouse effect are distinctly different. For the time period that these two threats coexist, it is likely that their interactions will have consequences for human health and the environment.

McMichael A, Campbell-Lendrum DH, Corvalan C, et al (eds.). Climate change and human health: Risks and responses. Geneva: World Health Organization, 2003.
Climate change poses a major, and largely unfamiliar, challenge. This publication describes the process of global climate change, its current and future effects on human health, and how our societies can lessen those adverse impacts, via adaptation strategies and by reducing greenhouse gas emissions. A summary is available from <http://www.who.int/globalchange/publications/cchhsummary/en/>.

Adverse Health Effects

CHAPTER 22

Injuries

Dawn N. Castillo, Timothy J. Pizatella,
and Nancy A. Stout

ccupational injuries are caused by acute exposure in the workplace to physical agents, such as mechanical energy, electricity, chemicals, and ionizing radiation, or from the sudden lack of essential agents, such as oxygen or heat. Examples of events that can lead to worker injury include motor vehicle crashes, assaults, falls, being caught in parts of machinery, being struck by tools or objects, and electrocutions. Resultant injuries include fractures, lacerations, abrasions, burns, amputations, poisonings, and damage to internal organs.

Occupational and nonoccupational injuries represent a serious public health problem (Box 22-1). More than 5,500 workers died from occupational injuries in the United States in 2002.[1] Another 4.4 million workers sustained nonfatal injuries in 2002[2]; this estimate is conservative because it relies on employer reporting and excludes important groups of workers, such as the self-employed, workers on small farms, and government employees. An estimated 3.9 million workers were treated in an emergency department for a work-related injury or illness in 1999, with an estimated 70,100 of these workers being hospitalized. Although these data include illnesses, more than 90 percent are injuries.[3] The direct cost of serious occupational injuries and illnesses in the United States in 2001 was $45.8 billion[4]; this amount includes only wages and medical payments to workers whose injuries resulted in more than 5 days away from work.

CAUSES OF INJURY

Although the immediate cause of injury is exposure to energy or deprivation from essential agents, injury events arise from a complex interaction of factors associated with materials and equipment used in work processes, the work environment, and the worker. These factors include physical hazards in the workplace or setting, hazards and safety features of machinery and tools, the development and implementation of safe work practices, the organization of work, the design of workplaces, the safety culture of the employer, availability and use of personal protective equipment (PPE), demographic characteristics of workers, experience and knowledge of workers, and economic and social factors.

An 18-year-old laborer, working for a brick and masonry contracting business, was cleaning a portable mortar mixer at the end of the workday at a residential construction site. The laborer used a garden hose to spray water on the paddles and inside of the mixing drum while the engine was running and paddles were rotating. A painter working for another employer at the same site heard a scream and saw the laborer's arm being pulled into the mixer. The painter was unable to turn off the mixer and yelled for help. The laborer's co-worker ran to the machine and turned it off, but the laborer had already been pulled into the machine, with just his leg protuding. The laborer died from asphyxia due to compression of neck structures.[5]

This case illustrates how the occurrence of occupational injury events can be influenced by a variety

unsafe procedure had been used previously. Reportedly, the victim was using a procedure that was different from what was demonstrated during a hands-on training by the company owners, in which a safety guard would have been placed over the mixing drum. Training was informal and not documented. The company did not have a written safety program that specified safe work practices and the potential for injury if not followed. Given the young age of the laborer, he likely did not have other training and work experience that would have helped him recognize the hazards of cleaning the machine while the engine was running without the guard in place. It is not clear if the company owners or foreman had previously observed this unsafe practice or if the laborer had been provided feedback to correct this unsafe practice. The procedure the victim was using also differed from that specified in the manufacturer's operator's manual, which specified that the spark plug should be disconnected prior to cleaning inside the mixing drum.

When manufactured, the portable mortar-mixing machine comes with warning labels including a label for safe cleaning procedures, a label that the engine should be stopped when cleaning, and a label that the machine should not be operated without the cover. These labels were not visible on this machine which had been purchased approximately 5 years prior to the incident. Replacement labels that are available from the manufacturer may have helped foster safer working procedures. The absence of clear labeling on the machine and an obvious mechanism for shutting off the machine may have contributed to the painter not being able to quickly turn off the machine. The nature of the work environment (a residential construction site) and work (only one other employee who was working at another part of the site) precluded a quick response to the victim being pulled into the mixer. The portable mortar mixer did not include safety features that would prevent operation when the guard or cover were not in place. The employer was a small business in which two co-owners employed five laborers. A number of factors may have accounted for the absence of a comprehensive safety and training program, including the employer's perceptions that workers know how to conduct work safely and need little guidance or training and the cost to hire workers with safety and health expertise.

This case illustrates how injury events can arise from a complex array of factors, not all of which contribute equally to an injury event. In addition,

of factors and circumstances. Some of the contributory factors are clear, others are surmised. The victim was using a hazardous piece of equipment that he and co-workers had used without serious incident in the past. It is not unlikely that the same

the responsibilities for a safe work environment and safe work practices are not borne equally by all involved parties. Employers bear the greatest responsibilities, as they are responsible for providing a safe work environment, including the identification of potential safety hazards and the implementation of hazard controls and safe work practices and procedures. Workers are responsible for following established procedures and for reporting safety hazards to employers.

THE EPIDEMIOLOGY OF INJURIES

Occupational injuries are not random events. They cluster or are associated with specific types of workplaces and jobs, workplace exposures, and worker characteristics. Because occupational injuries are not random, they can be anticipated, and steps can be taken to prevent them.

Epidemiologic data allow those involved in injury prevention efforts to target groups and settings with high numbers or rates of occupational injuries and to anticipate and take steps to prevent injuries in specific workplaces or settings. Epidemiologic data on fatal and nonfatal occupational injuries differ and thus are addressed separately. Both categories of injuries require attention: fatal injuries, because they represent the most severe consequence of occupational injury and are devastating to families, communities, and workplaces; and nonfatal injuries, because of the sheer volume and aggregate costs to workers, families, employers, and society as a whole.

Fatal Injuries

The distribution and risks for fatal occupational injury differ by demographic characteristics of workers. Men account for more than 90 percent of occupational fatalities and have occupational fatality rates approximately 10 times higher than those for women.[1,6] Approximately 71 percent of occupational fatal injuries are among white, non-Hispanic workers, 15 percent among Hispanic workers, 9 percent among black, non-Hispanic workers, and 2 percent among Asian workers. Hispanic workers have the highest occupational injury fatality rates—27 percent higher than black workers and 43 percent higher than white workers.[1] Hispanic workers are a priority population for fatal occupational injury prevention (Box 22-2). Of all fatal occupational injuries, 66 percent occur to workers

between 25 and 54 years of age, with approximately 10 percent of the fatalities among workers younger than 25 years of age and 23 percent of the fatalities among workers 55 years of age and older. Rates of fatal occupational injury generally increase with age, with the highest rates among workers 65 years of age and older.[1,6] Decreased ability to survive injuries may account for some of the increased fatality rates among older workers.

Of all occupational injury deaths, 81 percent are among wage and salary workers; the remainder are among the self-employed, whose fatality rate is approximately three times greater than that of wage and salary employees.[1] The types of jobs held by self-employed workers explain some of this difference.[7] For example, high proportions of the self-employed work in agriculture and construction, two industries with the highest rates of fatal injury.[7,8]

Transportation-related events accounted for 43 percent of the 5,524 occupational injury deaths in the United States in 2002. These events involved motor vehicles and mobile equipment, such as tractors and forklifts; occurred on and off the highway; and included pedestrians and bystanders as well as operators and drivers.[1] Work-related road crashes provide unique challenges and opportunities for prevention (Box 22-3). Assaults and violent acts accounted for 15 percent of fatalities in 2002, with most of them involving homicides and some involving suicides. Violence-related injuries occur in a variety of work situations, and consequently prevention strategies vary (Box 22-4). Contact with objects or equipment accounted for 16 percent of the fatalities, including being struck by falling objects, being caught in running equipment or machinery, and being caught in or crushed by collapsing materials, such as in trench cave-ins or collapsing buildings. Falls, mostly to a lower level, accounted for 13 percent of fatalities. Exposure to harmful substances or environments, such as electric current, temperature extremes, hazardous substances, and oxygen deficiency, accounted for 10 percent of fatalities, with more than half of these being electrocutions. Fires and explosions accounted for 3 percent of the fatalities.[1] Demographic characteristics vary; for example, homicide is frequently the leading cause of death for women.[1,6,8]

The incidence of occupational injury deaths varies by industry division (Table 22-1), and among subgroups of industries within industry divisions. The occupational injury fatality rate averaged

BOX 22-2

Hispanics Are a Priority Population for Occupational Injury Prevention

Concomitant with increases in the U.S. population of Hispanics, the proportion of Hispanics in the workforce has increased and is expected to continue to increase. The number of Hispanics in the U.S. workforce increased 43 percent between 1990 and 2000 and is expected to increase another 36 percent by 2010 to nearly 21 million employed Hispanic workers.

Hispanics work more frequently in the most hazardous jobs, which helps explain their higher rates of fatal and nonfatal injuries. Fatality rates are highest for foreign-born Hispanic workers, while native Hispanic workers have occupational fatal injury rates comparable to those of the U.S. workforce. Most of the fatally injured foreign-born Hispanic workers are from Mexico, with fewer but substantial numbers from Central America and the Caribbean. It is not known to what extent language, literacy, culture, and vulnerable employment situations (such as work as a day laborer and illegal immigration status) contribute to the high injury death rate among foreign-born Hispanics. NIOSH and NIEHS have funded research projects to identify unique risks for Hispanic and immigrant workers and to develop and evaluate unique prevention approaches, such as using community-based organizations to communicate safety and health information to Spanish-speaking and immigrant workers.

Many groups are responding to the need for communication of occupational safety and health information to Spanish-speaking and foreign-born workers, addressing issues of language, literacy, and culture.

Bibliography

Bureau of Labor Statistics. BLS Releases 2000–2010 employment projections. Washington, DC: Department of Labor, Bureau of Labor Statistics, USDL 01-443, 2001.

National Research Council. Safety is seguridad: A workshop summary. Washington, DC: National Research Council, National Academies Press, 2003.

Occupational Safety and Health Administration. Fact sheet: OSHA Hispanic outreach efforts. Available at: <http://www.osha.gov/SLTC/spanish/hispanic_outreach.html>.

Richardson S, Ruser J, Suarez P. Hispanic workers in the United States: An analysis of employment distributions, fatal occupational injuries, and non-fatal occupational injuries and illnesses. In: Safety is seguridad: A workshop summary. Washington, DC: National Research Council, National Academies Press, 2003.

across all industries in the United States in 2002 was 4.0 per 100,000 workers.[1] Dozens of specific industries have injury rates far in excess of the average for all industries.[1,6,8,9]

The incidence and patterns of injury death also vary by occupation. Table 22-2 provides information on the incidence and patterns of fatal injury for occupations, selected to be illustrative of occupations with a range of fatality rates and injury patterns. In some occupations, one type of injury predominates, such as highway transportation incidents among truckers; in other occupations, such as groundskeepers/gardeners, a variety of events contribute to injury death. Data on additional occupations are available from several sources.[1,6,8,9]

Nonfatal Injuries

The two primary national sources of data on nonfatal work-related injuries are data from emergency departments[3] and the Bureau of Labor Statistics (BLS) annual survey of employers.[10] The BLS annual employer survey excludes the self-employed, farms with fewer than 11 employees, and government employees. Data on worker demographics and the circumstances of injuries are available only for lost workday cases in the BLS survey. Information on industry and occupation are not currently available in the emergency department data. Illnesses, such as dermatitis, are included in both the emergency department data and lost workday data from the BLS employer survey, but they represent less than 10 percent of cases in both systems.

Although not as dramatic as for fatal injuries, differences are seen across demographic categories for nonfatal injuries. Men account for approximately 70 percent of nonfatal work-related injuries, and based on data from emergency department visits, have rates approximately 1.6 times higher than those for women. Data on race and ethnicity are

---

BOX 22-3

Unique Challenges for Prevention of Roadway Occupational Deaths and Injuries

Roadway crashes are the leading cause of occupational fatalities in the United States. Between 1992 and 2000, nearly 12,000 workers died in roadway crashes, nearly four deaths daily. Truck drivers account for more roadway fatalities than any other occupational group and have the highest rates for roadway worker deaths. However, work-related roadway crashes are not limited to the transportation industry, and many workers in occupations that are not related to transportation are killed each year. Some workers are killed while using vehicles provided by their employers, and others are killed driving their own vehicles to perform their jobs.

Preventing work-related roadway crashes is especially challenging. Unlike most workplaces, the roadway is not a closed environment. Although employers cannot control roadway conditions, they can take a number of steps to help keep their workers safe when driving, such as:

- Implementing and enforcing mandatory seat belt use policies.
- Ensuring that no workers are assigned to drive on the job if they do not have valid driver's licenses, appropriate for the types of vehicles to be driven.
- Providing fleet vehicles that offer the highest possible levels of occupant protection in the event of a crash.
- Maintaining complete and accurate records of workers' driving performance. (In addition to driver's license checks for prospective employees, periodic rechecks after hiring are critical.)
- Incorporating fatigue management into safety programs.

- Ensuring that workers receive the training necessary to operate specialized motor vehicles or equipment.
- Offering periodic screening of vision and general physical health for all workers for whom driving is a primary job duty.
- Avoiding requiring workers to drive irregular hours or to extend their workday far beyond their normal working hours as a result of driving responsibilities.
- Establishing schedules that allow drivers to obey speed limits and follow applicable hours-of-service regulations.
- Setting safety policy in accordance with State graduated driver licensing laws[a] so that company operations do not place younger workers in violation of these laws.
- Assigning driving-related tasks to young drivers in an incremental fashion, beginning with limited driving responsibilities and ending with unrestricted assignments.

Employees can also take steps to increase their safety while driving in the performance of their work, including:

- Using safety belts.
- Avoiding placing or taking cell phone calls while operating a motor vehicle, especially in inclement weather, unfamiliar areas, or heavy traffic.
- Avoiding other activities, such as eating, drinking, or adjusting noncritical vehicle controls, while driving.

[a] *Graduated driver licensing (GDL) laws exist in many states to address high crash and injury rates among teenage drivers. A GDL is a phased licensing process that gradually eases restrictions off teenage drivers as they become more experienced at driving.*
Excerpted from Pratt SG. NIOSH hazard review: Work-related roadway crashes: Challenges and opportunities for prevention. Cincinnati: NIOSH, 2003. (DHHS [NIOSH] publication no. 2003-119.)

---

missing from more than 20 percent of records in nonfatal work-related injury databases.[3,10] Most nonfatal injuries (50 to 63 percent) occur among white, non-Hispanic workers; with fewer among black, non-Hispanic workers (9 to 12 percent), Hispanics (6 to 13 percent), Asians or Pacific Islanders (2 percent), and American Indians or Alaskan natives (less than 1 percent). An analysis of emergency department data that did not separate out Hispanic ethnicity found that black workers had an injury rate approximately 1.3 times that of white workers.[11] Most nonfatal injuries

BOX 22-4

Workplace Violence: A Complex Workplace Injury Phenomenon

Homicide is a leading cause of occupational injury death and accounts for many nonfatal injuries each year. Because of news coverage of sensational and more "newsworthy" events, many assume that disgruntled co-workers and former employees account for the bulk of these injury statistics. In reality, violence caused by co-workers or former employees is a relatively small part of the workplace violence problem.

Violence in the workplace has been categorized into four different types of events:

- *Type I: Criminal intent:* These situations are typically associated with crimes such as robbery, shoplifting, and loitering. A preexisting relationship does not exist between the employee and the perpetrator, and the perpetrator does not have a legitimate reason for being in the workplace.
- *Type II: Customer or client:* These situations involve customers or clients who have a legitimate reason for being in the workplace. The violence is associated with a business transaction or service. Perpetrators include customers, clients, patients, and inmates.
- *Type III: Worker-on-worker:* These situations involve violence between co-workers or violence perpetrated against an employee by a former employee.
- *Type IV: Personal relationship:* In these situations, the perpetrator has a pre existing relationship with the employee and the violence is associated with the relationship rather than the business. These situations include acts of domestic violence against the employee while they are at work.

Workplace violence occurs in a variety of workplaces and occupations, although there are some worker groups at increased risk for the more common type I and II events, including police, corrections officers, taxi drivers, health care providers, and employees in retail settings.

Although workplace violence is a complex phenomenon, there are a variety of strategies that employers and workers can take to reduce the risks for violence. Some are specific to work settings and tasks, and others are more general. Workplace violence prevention strategies include modifying the work setting and tasks to reduce the risks for robbery and/or assault (such as by posting signs in retail settings that minimal cash is kept on hand, providing physical barriers between employees and potential criminals or violent clients, and using surveillance cameras and/or security guards); establishing workplace policies for zero violence tolerance and procedures for reporting and following up on all threats or violent acts; and employee training on how to handle criminals or violent customers or clients.

Bibliography

Howard J. State and local regulatory approaches to preventing workplace violence. Occup Med State of the Art Rev 1996;11(2):293–301.

NIOSH. Current intelligence bulletin 57: Violence in the workplace: Risk factors and prevention strategies. Cincinnati: NIOSH, 1996. (DHHS [NIOSH] Publication No. 96-100.)

Peek-Asa C, Howard J, Vargas L, et al. Incidence of non-fatal workplace assault injuries determined from employer's reports in California. J Occup Environ Med 1997;39(1):44–50.

occur among workers 25 to 54 years of age—70 percent of injuries treated in emergency departments and 75 percent of injuries requiring at least 1 day away from work reported in an employer survey. Those younger than 25 years of age account for 23 percent of injuries treated in emergency departments and 14 percent of injuries reported by employers; those older than 54 years of age account for 7 percent of injuries treated in emergency departments and 11 percent of injuries re-

ported by employers.[3,10] Based on emergency department data, workers 18 to 19 years of age have the highest annual rates of injury (6 per 100 full-time workers). With the exception of workers 16 to 17 years of age, injury rates decrease with increasing age.[3]

Twelve percent of employer-reported cases occurred among employees who had worked for less than 3 months for the employer, 18 percent among employees with 3 to 11 months of service,

TABLE 22-1

Number and Rate of Fatal Occupational Injuries, by Industry Division, United States, 2002

Industry Division	Number of Fatalities	Fatality Rate[a]
Mining	121	23.5
Agriculture/forestry/fishing	789	22.7
Construction	1,121	12.2
Transportation/public utilities	910	11.3
Wholesale trade	205	4.0
Manufacturing	563	3.1
Retail trade	487	2.1
Services	680	1.7
Finance/insurance/real estate	87	1.0
Unknown	561	NA
Total/Overall	5,524	4.0

[a] Rate per 100,000 workers.

Source: Bureau of Labor Statistics. National census of fatal occupational injuries in 2002 [USDL 03-488]. Washington, DC: U.S. Department of Labor, Bureau of Labor Statistics, 2003.

33 percent with 1 to 5 years of service, and 25 percent with more than 5 years of service; length of service with the employer was not available for 12 percent of the reported injuries.[10]

The number and rate of nonfatal injuries by industry division varies greatly from the number and rate for injury deaths (Table 22-3). The occupational injury rate averaged across all industries in 2002 was 5.0 per 100 full-time workers. A number of specific industries have injury rates in excess of the average rate, including several in the manufacturing industry division. Workers in the manufacture of primary metal products, lumber and wood products, furniture and fixtures, and fabricated metal products have higher than average injury rates.[2] Because the BLS annual survey of employers excludes farms with fewer than 11 employees, the numbers and rates of nonfatal occupational injuries reported for agriculture/forestry/fishing should be considered as conservative estimates.

Table 22-4 provides information on the estimated incidence and patterns of nonfatal injury for selected occupations.[10] Many nonfatal injury events are common across a variety of occupations.

Clinical Presentation and Course of Injuries

Of all workers with occupational injuries, 34 percent are treated in emergency departments[12]; the remainder are treated at the workplace, physician's offices or clinics, or other medical treatment facilities. Table 22-5 provides information on diagnoses and anatomic sites of occupational injuries treated in emergency departments in the United States in 1999. Almost 2 percent of occupational injuries resulted in hospital admission.[3] Among an estimated annual average of 4 million work-related emergency department visits for occupational injuries in the United States in 1996, wound care was provided to 34 percent of patients, extremity x-rays were ordered or provided to 30 percent, and orthopedic care was provided to 21 percent of patients.[11]

Of the estimated 1.5 million injuries and illnesses with lost workdays in 2001, the median time away from work was 6 days. Among the more frequent injuries, median time away from work was highest for dislocations (30 days); amputations, excluding fingertips (24 days); and fractures (21 days).[10]

PREVENTION OF INJURIES

The Hierarchical Approach to Occupational Injury Control

Over the years, a number of models for occupational injury control have evolved. Many of these models categorize worker protection strategies based on a hierarchical approach,[13] such as the five-tier model (Table 22-6). William Haddon, Jr., proposed 10 basic strategies for injury prevention that have a number of similarities to the hierarchical approach, such as hazard elimination, hazard reduction, and use of barriers for protection.[14] Haddon also introduced the concept that injury causation was a chain of multifactorial events, each of which provided opportunities for intervention. Herbert Linn and Alfred Amendola suggested an approach that combines the public health model with safety engineering analysis for injury prevention.[15] The disciplines of epidemiology, safety engineering, biomechanics, ergonomics, psychology, safety management, and others form a multidisciplinary approach that is useful for identifying injury risk factors and developing control strategies.

TABLE 22-2

Fatality Rate and Frequent Events Leading to Occupational Injury Death for Select Occupations, United States, 2000

Occupation	Number of Deaths	Rate[a]	Frequent Events (Percent of Deaths)
Timber cutting and logging operations	95	143.9	74% struck by object
Extractive occupations	69	53.9	19% struck by object 13% caught in equipment or object 13% fire and explosions 12% highway transportation incident
Roofers	65	30.2	74% fall to lower level 11% contact with electric current
Farmers, except horticulture	251	28.4	39% nonhighway transportation 16% struck by object 11% caught in equipment or object
Construction laborers	288	28.3	29% fall to lower level 14% pedestrian 13% struck by object
Truck drivers	852	27.6	70% highway transportation incident
Firefighting, including supervisors	43	15.4	28% fires and explosions 26 % highway transportation incident
Groundskeepers and gardeners, except farm	130	14.9	25% struck by object 19% fall to lower level 12% nonhighway transportation 11% pedestrian
Laborers, except construction	178	13.2	16% pedestrian 15% struck by object 15% caught in equipment or object 12% fall to lower level
Electricians and apprentices	89	10.3	45% contact with electric current 17% fall to lower level
Supervisors and proprietors, salespeople	185	3.7	60% homicides 12% highway transportation incident
Machine operators, assemblers, and inspectors	237	3.2	23% caught in equipment or object 18% struck by object
Cleaning and building service workers	78	2.5	32% fall to lower level 15% homicides

[a] Rate per 100,000 workers.

Source: Bureau of Labor Statistics. Fatal workplace injuries in 2000: A collection of data and analysis (Report 961). Washington, DC: U.S. Department of Labor, Bureau of Labor Statistics, 2002.

The *hierarchical approach* focuses on (a) eliminating hazards through design; (b) using safeguards that eliminate or minimize worker exposure to hazards; (c) providing warning signs or devices to identify hazards; (d) training workers in safe work practices and procedures; and (e) using personal protective equipment (PPE) to prevent or minimize worker exposure to hazards or to reduce the severity of an injury if one occurs. Three main categories of control strategies correlate with the hierarchical

TABLE 22-3

Number and Rate of Nonfatal Occupational Injuries by Industry Division, United States, 2002

Industry Division	Number of Injuries	Injury Rate[a]
Construction	408,000	6.9
Manufacturing	1,029,000	6.4
Agriculture/forestry/fishing	90,000	6.0
Transportation/public utilities	362,000	5.8
Retail trade	878,000	5.1
Wholesale trade	312,000	5.0
Services	1,202,000	4.3
Mining	22,000	3.8
Finance/insurance/real estate	103,000	1.5
Total/Overall	4,406,000	5.0

[a] Rate per 100 full-time workers.
Source: Bureau of Labor Statistics. Workplace injuries and illnesses in 2002 [News Release USDL 03-913]. Washington, DC: U.S. Department of Labor, Bureau of Labor Statistics, 2003.

approach: engineering controls, administrative controls, and the use of PPE.

Engineering Controls

Engineering controls, also known as *passive controls*, involve eliminating hazards through design or the application of safeguards to prevent worker exposure to hazards. Effective hazard elimination and safeguarding are designed, or retrofitted, into equipment, work stations, and work systems to provide protection without direct worker involvement—thus the term *passive controls*. Experience has shown that to be most effective, engineering controls must be designed so that they do not adversely interfere with the work process or introduce additional hazards.

The optimal injury control strategy is to eliminate a hazard completely. Frequently, hazard elimination or the reduction of hazard severity can be accomplished through equipment design.

A 27-year-old male painter was fatally electrocuted when the aluminum ladder he was using contacted a 7,200-volt power line. The worker was standing on a 24-foot, fully extended, aluminum extension ladder while painting a gutter on an apartment building. The gutter was located 18 feet above the ground and approximately 9 feet horizontally from a 7,200-volt power line. The power line was parallel to the gutter and was 19 feet 6 inches above the ground. As the worker was moving the ladder to a new location on the gutter, the ladder came in contact with the power line and the worker was electrocuted.

Although a number of factors contributed to this worker's death, one of the National Institute for Occupational Safety and Health (NIOSH) recommendations was to use ladders made of nonconductive materials when working near energized power lines.[16] A ladder made of fiberglass greatly reduces the risk of electrocution in the event it contacts an energized electrical power source.

Because hazard elimination is not always possible, other control strategies in the hierarchy must be implemented to achieve worker protection. If a hazard cannot be eliminated completely, then the next control level should be to prevent worker exposure through protective safeguarding approaches. These types of safeguards prevent worker exposure to the hazard, as long as the control is in place and functions properly.

For example, many types of industrial equipment require power transmission units that include belts, pulleys, gears, shafts, and other mechanisms necessary for the equipment to function. Workers can be exposed to serious, or even fatal, injury hazards if they come into contact with these rotating or moving components. A fixed barrier guard that completely encloses the power transmission unit is an engineering control that protects workers from these types of hazards. As long as the barrier guard remains in place, the worker is protected from injury. Another engineering control is an optical sensor, also called a light curtain, used to protect the worker from injury when operating a mechanical power press (Fig. 22-1). The optical sensor is integrated into the press control mechanism so that if any part of the worker's body breaks the plane of light in front of the hazardous point of operation, the downward motion of the press ram cannot be initiated or, if motion has begun, the press ram is automatically disengaged.

Many engineering controls are interlocked to ensure that they cannot be removed without disabling the machine or equipment. An interlock is a device that is integrated into the control mechanism of a machine or work process to prevent the work cycle

TABLE 22-4

Incidence and Selected Events Resulting in Nonfatal Occupational Injuries and Illnesses Requiring Days away from Work for Selected Occupations, United States, 2001

Occupation	Estimated Number of Injuries	Most Frequent Events (Percent of Injuries, by Occupation)						
		Contact with Object	Fall to Lower Level	Falls to Same Level	Overexertion	Repetitive Motion	Exposure to Harmful Substances	Transportation
Truck drivers	129,068	18	10	10	29	1	2	13
Nursing aides, orderlies, and attendants	71,017	11	1	12	54	1	2	2
Laborers, except construction	68,896	33	4	8	30	3	4	4
Construction laborers	44,102	45	8	7	20	1	4	3
Janitors and cleaners	38,628	22	8	18	27	2	6	2
Carpenters	32,746	39	16	5	21	3	2	2
Assemblers	31,065	30	2	7	27	16	4	1
Cooks	27,819	27	2	23	14	1	23	—
Stock handlers and baggers	25,657	30	3	10	38	3	2	2
Registered nurses	24,719	11	3	15	43	1	5	4

Source: Bureau of Labor Statistics, Occupational injuries and illnesses; Counts, rates, and characteristics, 2001 [Bulletin 2560]. Washington, DC: U.S. Department of Labor, Bureau of Labor Statistics, 2003.

from being initiated until the interlock is closed, signaling the equipment that the work cycle can be initiated. Interlocks, which are usually electrical or mechanical controls, need to be designed so that they are not easily bypassed or disabled.

Although engineering controls should be viewed as primary tiers of prevention, it is not always possible to develop such controls for all potentially hazardous work situations. Administrative controls are the next tier for reducing or minimizing worker exposure to injury hazards.

Administrative Controls

Administrative controls are management-directed work practices or procedures that, when implemented consistently, will reduce the exposure to

hazards and the risk of injury. They are sometimes referred to as *active controls* because they require worker involvement to be effective. The use of warning signs and devices, along with worker training, is considered an administrative control because workers must be actively involved for this to be effective. Workers must adhere to warning signs that identify potential injury hazards and apply properly the training they have received. Another example of an administrative control is housekeeping procedures requiring that spills or debris be cleaned up quickly to reduce the potential for a slip, trip, or fall injury (Fig. 22-2). Implementation of a hazardous energy control policy for workers performing maintenance activities on a machine is also an example of administrative controls. Lockout/tagout procedures are important components of a hazardous

TABLE 22-5

Occupational Injuries Treated in Emergency Departments, by Diagnosis and Anatomic Site, United States, 1999

Diagnosis	Estimated Number	Percent of Total[a]	Part of Body Affected (Percent of Injuries, by Diagnosis)[a]					
			Trunk, Back, Groin	Leg, Knee, Ankle	Arm, Wrist Shoulder	Head, Face, Neck	Hand/ Finger	Other
Sprain or strain	1,033,400	26	45	22	20	7	4	2
Laceration	822,700	21	<1	6	10	15	67	2
Contusion, abrasion, or hematoma	736,800	19	14	17	16	21	20	12
Dislocation or fracture	229,700	6	9	14	21	2	36	18
Burn	142,600	4	<1	6	16	35	29	14
Other	974,400	25	13	7	10	26	27	17
Total	3,939,600	100	19	13	15	17	29	7

Source: NIOSH. Work-related injury statistics query system. Available at: <wwww2a.cdc.gov/risqs>.
[a] Percentages may not add to 100 because at rounding.

energy control policy (Fig. 22-3). However, to be effective, the procedures must be written and consistently implemented, and workers must be trained in their use.[17]

Personal Protective Equipment

PPE consists of devices worn by workers for protection by reducing (a) the risk that exposure to a hazard will injure the worker or (b) the severity of

an injury if one does occur. Although the hazard still exists, the potential for worker injury is mitigated by the use of PPE. The use of PPE in many work environments and situations is essential for worker protection. However, PPE is usually viewed as the

TABLE 22-6

Safety Hierarchy

Priority Rank	Safety Action
1	Eliminate hazard and/or risk
2	Apply safeguarding technology
3	Use warning signs
4	Train and instruct
5	Use personal protective equipment

Adapted from Barnett RL, Brickman DB. Safety hierarchy. J Safety Res 1986;17:49–55.

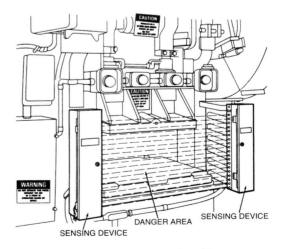

FIGURE 22-1 ● Photoelectric (optical) sensor installed on a mechanical power press to protect the point of operation. (Source: OSHA, Concepts and techniques of machine safeguarding. Washington, DC: OSHA, 1980.)

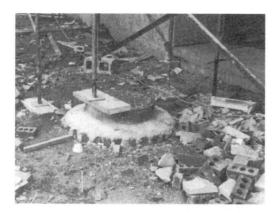

FIGURE 22-2 ● Example of poor housekeeping on a construction site. Loose bricks, lumber, and other debris create a potential tripping hazard for workers.

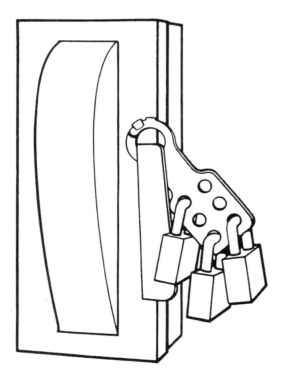

FIGURE 22-3 ● Lockout hasp on an electrical control panel, which provides a method for applying a lock (lockout) to the panel during maintenance or repair to ensure that the equipment is not energized until the work has been completed. The control panel should also be tagged (tagout) with a label indicating that work is being performed. Workers should be provided with individually keyed locks, and only the worker who applied the lock should remove it. (Source: OSHA, Concepts and techniques of machine safeguarding, Washington, DC: OSHA, 1980.)

lowest tier in the hierarchy of controls. If hazardous exposures cannot be eliminated through engineering controls or the application of administrative controls, then PPE provides another opportunity for worker protection. Examples of PPE designed to reduce worker injuries include protective hard hats, eyewear and face shields, steel-toed safety shoes, fall restraint devices, and personal flotation devices (Fig. 22-4). When worn properly and consistently, these devices can prevent, or at least reduce the severity of, traumatic injuries. Fall restraint devices, such as lanyards and body harnesses, do not prevent workers from falling but protect them from suffering more serious injuries or fatalities due to falls from elevations (Fig. 22-5).

Combined Application of Controls

A comprehensive approach to worker injury prevention efforts inevitably includes all tiers of the control hierarchy to achieve maximum worker protection. In most work environments, a combination of engineering controls, administrative controls, and PPE will be required to have a complete and effective injury prevention program. The following examples illustrate how the combined application of controls can be used to achieve an enhanced level of worker protection.

Tractors equipped with a rollover protective structure, an engineering control, significantly reduce the risk that the operator will be injured in a rollover event (Fig. 22-6). However, additional protection can be achieved if a seat belt, an administrative control, is worn to keep the operator within the protective envelope of the rollover protective structure. A similar example is the increased protection afforded by the combined use of seat belts, mandated in company safety policies and programs, in motor vehicles that are also equipped with air bags.

Training

Training refers to methods to assist individuals in acquiring knowledge (safety information on potential workplace hazards), changing attitudes (perceptions and beliefs regarding safety), and practicing safe work behaviors (organizational, management, or worker performance). Despite a paucity of data on the direct relationship between training and injury, evidence suggests a positive impact of training on establishing safe working conditions.[18]

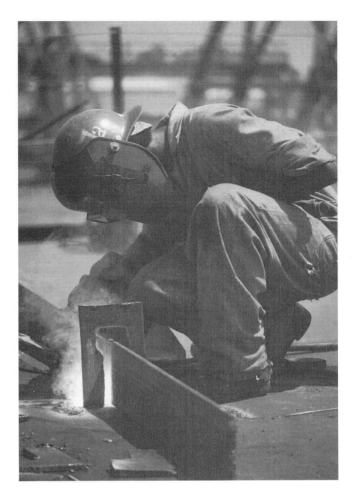

FIGURE 22-4 ● Example of worker using multiple forms of personal protective equipment: hard hat to minimize and protect the worker's head from falling objects; a shield and safety glasses to protect the worker's face and eyes from flying particles and damaging irradiation; and gloves to protect the worker's hands from burns, cuts, and flying particles. (Source: Photo Disc, Inc.)

Training is one of the key factors accounting for differences between companies with low and high injury rates. It is often critically important for developing and implementing effective hazard control measures.[18,19] Training increases hazard awareness and knowledge, facilitates adoption of safe work practices, and leads to other workplace safety improvements. Training is an administrative control, as workers must properly use training they have received on a consistent basis for it to be effective in preventing injuries.

The elements of effective training programs are (a) assessing training needs specific to the work task; (b) developing the training program to address these needs specifically; (c) setting clear training goals; and (d) evaluating the post-training knowledge and skills and providing feedback to the workers.[18] Other important characteristics of a successful program are management commitment to safety and training that is initiated as soon as a worker is hired and then is followed up with periodic retraining and reinforcement.[18,19]

Unique characteristics of the specific workforce must be considered when developing or implementing safety training programs. Language, literacy, cognition, and cultural issues may diminish the effectiveness of training when programs are not tailored to account for unique or diverse characteristics of the workforce. Workplace safety training appears to be most effective when it includes active learning experiences that stress worksite application and when it is developed and implemented in the context of a broader workplace-based prevention approach.[18]

Standards

Many *standards* aim at protecting workers from traumatic injury. These standards cover a multitude of hazards and address the work environment, work

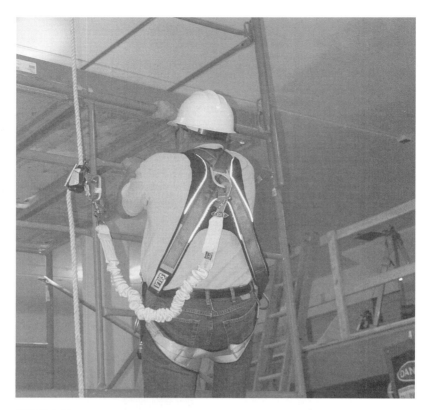

FIGURE 22-5 ● Worker wearing a full-body harness with attached lanyard (Photograph courtesy of the Construction Safety Council.)

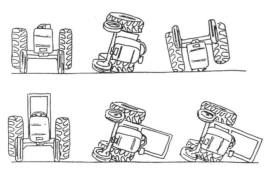

FIGURE 22-6 ● Tractor with a two-post rollover protective-structure (ROPS) frame installed. ROPSs are designed to reduce the risk of injury or death by preventing the tractor from rolling onto and crushing the operator. A properly fastened seat belt greatly improves the chances that the operator will stay within the protective envelope provided by the ROPS (the seat). (Source: NIOSH. Safe grain and silage handling. Washington, DC: NIOSH, 1995. [DHHS [NIOSH] publication no. 95-109.])

practices, equipment, PPE, and worker training. The two primary types of worker protection standards consist of (a) *mandatory standards*, such as those promulgated by the Occupational Safety and Health Administration (OSHA) or another regulatory agency, and (b) *voluntary standards*, such as those developed through independent organizations, such as the American National Standards Institute (ANSI), through a consensus process involving various stakeholders in an industry—typically including representatives from labor, management, and government. Numerous specifications, codes, and guidelines for machinery, equipment, tools, and other materials can also assist engineers and designers in developing safer products and systems, many of which have application in the workplace. Examples include the National Electric Code (NEC) published by the National Fire Protection Association (NFPA) and numerous consensus standards from the American Society of Mechanical Engineers (ASME) and the American Society for Testing and Materials (ASTM).

Injury Control: Roles and Responsibilities

Occupational injury prevention is not the sole responsibility of a single person or group. Employers, workers, regulators, and policymakers each share in the responsibility for prevention. A multidisciplinary approach involving interaction among diverse groups within an organization and active participation by both management and workers is crucial to an effective safety program.

Employers are responsible for establishing written safety policy, developing a comprehensive safety program, and effectively implementing that program at the workplace. A competent person or committee should be designated with responsibility for company safety policy. This person or committee should have sufficient knowledge concerning safety policy, standards, regulations, and hazard abatement and should actively participate with managers and workers in overseeing the safety program.

An effective safety program will strive to identify hazards through job safety analysis or other methods of systems safety analysis and eliminate or control identified hazards through the various approaches previously described. Workers, managers, and safety specialists should work together to analyze the job and potential hazards and to recommend changes or controls to abate them to avoid an injury event. In industries or jobs where the work environment is not constant, site hazard assessments should be performed prior to beginning work in any new environment. Occupations such as farming, logging, construction, and mining are characterized by frequently changing work sites and require a site hazard assessment prior to commencing work in any new or changed environment. This requirement is particularly important in construction, where work sites change not only from job to job, but also from day to day—even hour to hour, with constant potential for new hazards.

Employers are also responsible for ensuring proper maintenance of vehicles, equipment, and machinery and their safety features, such as machine guarding, interlocks, and barriers. Where job hazards cannot be eliminated or controlled, employers are responsible for providing appropriate PPE, such as fall-arrest systems, respirators, hearing protection, hard hats, or eye protection.

Employers must also ensure that workers receive appropriate training in minimizing their risk—including training on safety policy and practice, hazard recognition and control technologies, and the appropriate use of PPE. Enforcement of safety policy is also a crucial employer responsibility. The demonstrated commitment of management to safety is a major factor in successful workplace safety programs.[20-22] Employers who demonstrate concern and support for safety activities have top managers personally involved in safety activities and routinely involve workers in safety matters and decision making. These employers are more likely than others to have successful safety programs. As part of a comprehensive safety program, employers should require systematic reporting and tracking of occupational injuries and assessment of this information for corrective action to prevent similar occurrences.

Workers also play a vital role in workplace safety. Their participation is essential. Workers share in the responsibility for complying with safe work practices and policies, maintaining a safe work area, and using appropriate PPE when required by their employer to do so. Workers should also participate in company-sponsored training. They should report unsafe conditions for corrective action. As the experts in their jobs, workers should be involved in systems safety analysis and development of safe solutions. Workers input into recommended design or modification of safety controls, processes, or technology and into the development of safe work practices increases the acceptance of positive changes and, thus, the success of safety programs.

An effective workplace safety program that minimizes injuries results from a multidisciplinary effort that actively involves every level of the workforce, from the employer and upper-level managers to employee representatives and hourly workers. Each must assume some responsibility for safety and must work together interactively to achieve the common goal of preventing injuries.

Occupational injuries continue to exert too large a toll on the workforce. Although the rate of fatal injuries in the United States has decreased markedly over time, the rate of nonfatal injuries has not been reduced as much.[10] The prevention of workplace injuries requires concerted and consistent efforts from multiple parties using multiple strategies. In addition to the primary stakeholders in the workplace, additional groups can help reduce occupational injuries. These groups include manufacturers and distributors of industrial equipment and tools who design and promote safety features of equipment, insurers who provide monetary incentives for good safety records, and health care providers who provide their patients with information on preventing workplace injuries.

REFERENCES

1. Bureau of Labor Statistics. National census of fatal occupational injuries in 2002. News release USDL 03-488. Washington, DC: U.S. Department of Labor, Bureau of Labor Statistics, 2003.
2. Bureau of Labor Statistics. Workplace injuries and illnesses in 2002. News release USDL 03-913. Washington, DC: U.S. Department of Labor, Bureau of Labor Statistics, 2003.
3. National Institute for Occupational Safety and Health. Work-related injury statistics query system. Available at: <www2a.cdc.gov/risqs>.
4. Liberty Mutual. New study reveals financial burden of workplace injuries growing faster than inflation. Boston, MA: Liberty Mutual, 2003.
5. Division of Safety Research, NIOSH. Fatality assessment and control evaluation (FACE) report 2003–13. Morgantown, WV: NIOSH, 2004.
6. Marsh SM, Layne LA. Fatal injuries to civilian workers in the United States, 1980–1995: national and state profiles. Cincinnati, OH: U.S. Department of Health and Human Services (DHHS), Centers for Disease Control and Prevention (CDC), National Institute for Occupational Safety and Health, 2001. (DHHS (NIOSH) publication no. 2001-129S.)
7. Personick ME, Windau J. Self-employed individuals fatally injured at work. In: Fatal workplace injuries in 1993: A collection of data and analysis. Report 891. Washington, DC: U.S. Department of Labor, Bureau of Labor Statistics, 1995:55–62.
8. Bureau of Labor Statistics. Fatal workplace injuries in 2000: A collection of data and analysis. Report 961. Washington, DC: U.S. Department of Labor, Bureau of Labor Statistics, 2002.
9. Fosbroke DE, Kisner SM, Myers JR. Working life-time occupational risk of fatal injury. Am J Industr Med 1997;31:459–67.
10. Bureau of Labor Statistics. Occupational injuries and illnesses: Counts, rates, and characteristics, 2001. Bulletin 2560. Washington, DC: U.S. Department of Labor, Bureau of Labor Statistics, 2003.
11. McCaig L, Burt CW, Stussman BJ. A comparison of work-related injury visits and other injury visits to emergency departments in the United States, 1995–1996. J Occup Environ Med 1998;40:870–5.
12. Centers for Disease Control and Prevention. Surveillance for nonfatal occupational injuries treated in hospital emergency departments. MMWR 1998;47:302–6.
13. Hammer W. Occupational safety and management and engineering. 4th ed. Englewood Cliffs, NJ: Prentice-Hall, 1989.
14. Baker SP, O'Neill BO, Ginsburg MJ, Li G. The injury fact book. 2nd ed. New York: Oxford University Press, 1992.
15. Linn HI, Amendola AA. Occupational safety research: An overview. In: Stellman JM, ed. Encyclopaedia of occupational health and safety. Geneva: International Labor Office, 1998:60.2–60.5.
16. NIOSH. Preventing electrocutions of workers using portable metal ladders near overhead power lines. Cincinnati: NIOSH, 1989. (DHHS [NIOSH] publication no. 89-110.)
17. NIOSH. Request for preventing worker injuries and fatalities due to the release of hazardous energy. Cincinnati: NIOSH, 1999. (DHHS [NIOSH] publication no. 99-110.)
18. NIOSH. Assessing occupational safety and health training. Cincinnati: NIOSH, 1998. (DHHS [NIOSH] publication no. 98-145.)
19. Johnston JJ, Cattledge G.H, Collins JW. The efficacy of training for occupational injury control. Occup Med State of the Art Rev 1994;9:147–58.
20. Hofmann DA, Jacobs R, Landry F. High reliability process industries: individual, micro and macro organizational influences on safety performance. J Safety Res 1995;26:131–49.
21. Shannon HS, Mayr J, and Haines T. Overview of the relationship between organizational and workplace factors and injury rates. Safety Sci 1997;26:201–17.
22. Zohar D. A group level model of safety climate: Testing the effect of group climate on microaccidents in manufacturing jobs. J Appl Psychol 2000;85:587–96.

BIBLIOGRAPHY

American National Standards Institute Technical Report. Risk assessment and risk reduction—A guide to estimate, evaluate and reduce risks associated with machine tools. B11.TR3: 2000. McLean, VA: The Association For Manufacturing Technology, 2003.
A technical report that is part of the ANSI B11 series pertaining to the design, construction, care and use of machine tools. This report, published by the Association for Manufacturing Technology, provides a method for both machine suppliers and users to conduct a risk assessment (that is, analyze hazards) for industrial machinery and related components and includes guidance for selecting appropriate safeguarding to reduce the risk of worker injury.

Christoffel T, Gallagher SS. Injury prevention and public health: Practical knowledge, skills, and strategies. Gaithersburg, MD: Aspen Publishers, Inc., 1999.
A reference document that includes information on injury epidemiology and prevention strategies. The document includes chapters on conducting injury surveillance, developing an injury prevention program, and evaluating injury prevention efforts.

Hammer W. Occupational safety and management and engineering 4th ed. Englewood Cliffs, NJ: Prentice-Hall, 1989.
A good overall reference on occupational safety and health issues. Provides an overview of standards and codes for workplace safety; identifying and controlling hazards; analyzing safety hazards and conducting incident investigations; and developing and implementing workplace safety programs. Addresses both the engineering and management aspects of occupational injury and disease prevention.

NIOSH. Worker health chartbook, 2004. Cincinnati: NIOSH, 2004. (DHHS [NIOSH] publication no. 2004-146.)
A reference document that includes occupational injury data from multiple sources, including the Bureau of Labor Statistics' Census of Fatal Occupational Injuries and Annual Survey of Occupational Injuries and Illnesses. Data are presented in figures and tables and include charts on special topics, such as construction and agricultural injuries; young and older worker injuries; Hispanic worker injuries; fractures, burns and amputations.

Occupational Safety and Health Administration. Concepts and techniques of machine safeguarding. OSHA 3067. Washington, DC: U.S. Department of Labor, Occupational Safety and Health Administration, 1992 (revised).
An excellent reference for identifying potential hazards when working with industrial machinery. The publication also provides general principles of machine safeguarding to protect workers from injury.

Stout N, Borwegen W, Conway G, et al. Traumatic occupational injury research needs and priorities: A report by the NORA traumatic injury team. Cincinnati: NIOSH, 1998. (DHHS (NIOSH) publication no. 98-134.)
Provides a broad framework of research needed to begin filling gaps in knowledge and further progress toward the prevention of traumatic occupational injury in the United States. The recommendations target government agencies, academic institutions, public and private research organizations, labor groups, professional societies, and individual researchers, who could use the document as a basis for planning and prioritizing research efforts.

Wallerstein N, Rubenstein H. Teaching about job hazards: A guide for workers and their health providers. Washington, DC: American Public Health Association, 1993.
This comprehensive manual provides guidance for health and safety education to workers, including guidance specific to health care providers, as well as information for occupational safety and health training resources.

The findings and conclusions in this chapter are those of the authors and do not necessarily represent the views of the National Institute for Occupational Safety and Health.

CHAPTER 23

Musculoskeletal Disorders

Barbara Silverstein and Bradley Evanoff

Musculoskeletal disorders (MSDs) commonly involve the muscles, tendons, nerves, and supporting structures. The magnitude of the burden of musculoskeletal conditions is so large that the World Health Organization (WHO) and 750 associated organizations worldwide have proclaimed the 2000–2010 period as the Bone and Joint Decade to call attention to the discrepancy between the magnitude of the burden and the resources devoted to preventing and treating musculoskeletal disorders. *Work-related musculoskeletal disorders* (WMSDs) are soft-tissue disorders of nontraumatic origin that are caused or exacerbated by interaction with the work environment. Recognition of the work-relatedness of MSDs goes back at least to the early 1700s, when Ramazzini noted the harmful effects of unnatural postures and movements, such as the numbness in the upper extremity in scribes due to "incessant movement of the hand and always in the same direction," or sciatica in potters due to continual turning of the potter's wheel. Terms such as *washerwoman's sprain*, *telegrapher's cramp*, and *carpet layer's knee* speak to common lay knowledge of relationships between work and MSDs.

The most commonly reported body areas affected are the low back, the neck, and the upper extremity. There is increasing evidence of work-related hip and knee disorders. Tendonitis and tenosynovitis, the most common WMSDs, are an inflammation of the tendon or tendon sheath. Examples include rotator cuff tendonitis, epicondylitis, extensor and flexor tendonitis in the wrist, and peripatellar tendonitis in the knee. WMSDs can result in severe debilitating pain, burning, numbness, or tingling that, in turn, results in lost work time and less productivity while at work. Symptoms can initially be intermittent and may eventually lead to chronic pain, impairment, and disability. Attribution of musculoskeletal disorders to work activities can be difficult and controversial, as discussed in Box 23-1.

MAGNITUDE AND COST

In 2000, the Bureau of Labor Statistics (BLS) reported more than 577,800 WMSDs in private industry, which accounted for one-third of all injuries and illnesses requiring days away from work. The service and manufacturing sectors accounted for about half of the cases. Truck drivers, nursing aides and orderlies, and nonconstruction laborers accounted for one-fifth of all cases. Carpal tunnel syndrome cases had, on average, the most days away from work (median = 27).

Estimated workers' compensation costs for WMSDs in the United States vary between $13 and $20 billion annually in direct costs.[1] Liberty Mutual Research has estimated annual costs of "overexertion injuries" at work in the United States to be about $10 billion and costs of repetitive motion injuries to be $2.3 billion. Incidence and direct costs for workers' compensation cases of WMSDs by body area and specific conditions have been reported by Washington State (Table 23-1). Indirect costs range from two to five times direct costs. In addition to underreporting of cases in the BLS and workers' compensation data,[2,3] there is indication that lost time and diminished productivity

---

BOX 23-1

Plumber's Knee

James Stannard was forced to retire at age 50. He was a plumber for 32 years. He spent 65 percent of his work time kneeling and squatting. This was frequently combined with heavy lifting. This led to numerous knee surgeries.

- He first sought treatment for pain and swelling in 1980.
- Arthroscopic surgery to repair torn meniscus in the knees in 1985.
- Filed initial workers' compensation claim in 1983–1985.
- Filed another claim in 1998 because first surgery not fully successful.
- In 2003, the Vermont Supreme Court ruled that knee deterioration after 1995 was wholly attributable to the earlier injuries.

Source of case: Workplace Ergonomics News 2003;5:6.

Comment: There are at least three features of work-related musculoskeletal disorders that contribute to controversy over attribution: (a) gradual onset (days to years), (b) none are uniquely caused by work, and (c) ubiquity of risk factors. Figure 23-1 is adapted from the 2001 National Research Council Institute of Medicine report on MSDs and the workplace. The basic mechanism for these disorders appears to be overloading tissue tolerance with insufficient recovery time. A variety of individual (gender, age) and lifestyle (obesity, smoking, exercise), biomechanical, organizational and social factors may contribute to the tension between overload and recovery.

---

continue much longer than reported in official statistics.[4]

OVERALL APPROACH

Although WMSDs include a diverse group of disorders, the central concern for all these disorders is early recognition and appropriate treatment. Good management of MSDs requires early access to ap-propriate medical treatment, evaluation of patients' job exposures, and the provision of limited or modified work duties when necessary. Comprehensive programs that integrate ergonomic changes and medical treatment are effective in reducing the incidence and severity of WMSDs.

Early recognition and treatment of MSDs is essential because it allows earlier treatment of affected workers, at a time when treatment can

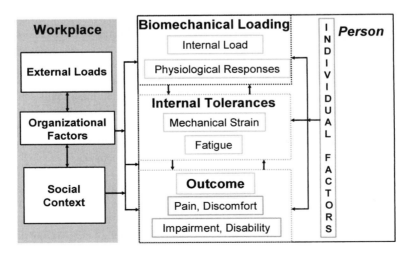

FIGURE 23-1 ● Conceptual model of contributors to musculoskeletal disorders. (Adapted from National Research Council–Institute of Medicine, 2001.)

TABLE 23-1

Washington State Fund Workers' Compensation Claims: WMSDs of the Neck, Back and Upper Extremity, 1993–2001

Type	Incidence per 10,000 FTEs	Median Lost Workdays	Median Cost
All	311.9	30	$610
Neck	36.0	34	$616
Back	166.0	18	$580
Sciatica	5.3	201	$18,687
Upper extremity	110.7	59	$538
Shoulder	37.7	59	$574
Rotator cuff syndrome	16.2	112	$3,108
Elbow/forearm	18.9	49	$420
Epicondylitis	11.3	73	$883
Hand/wrist	57.6	60	$555
Carpal tunnel syndrome	23.1	84	$5,235
Tendonitis	17.2	67	$842
Knee	1.2	45	$832
Tendonitis/bursitis	0.3	39	$568

WMSDs, work-related musculoskeletal disorders.
Note: Lost time and costs are for compensable (4+ lost days) claims. Cost adjusted to 2001 dollars.
Source: Silverstein B, Kalat J, Fan ZJ. Work-related musculoskeletal disorders of the neck, back, and upper extremity in Washington State, state fund and self insured workers' compensation claims 1993–2001. Tumwater, Washington: Washington State Department of Labor and Industries, 2003.

prevent progression to a more severe condition. Workers who are treated in the early stages of a disorder have a better prognosis and are less likely to have prolonged disability than workers treated only after prolonged duration of symptoms. Conservative management is most effective when begun in the early stages of these disorders.[5] With some disorders, such as carpal tunnel syndrome, patients can often be treated conservatively in the early stages of disease, whereas surgery is often necessary when patients present with advanced disease. Early detection is necessary to ensure that signs and symptoms of WMSDs are recognized and treated appropriately through medical management, administrative controls, and job evaluation/modification.

Both healthy and injured workers can potentially benefit from evaluation of their workplace for identification of physical stressors that can be reduced or eliminated. Simple modifications can often be made to a workplace that enables the work to be done with less effort on the part of the worker. Such modifications, where possible, can prevent injury

and can enable injured workers to safely return to their usual jobs more quickly. Clinical experience demonstrates that ergonomic evaluation and intervention is effective in the treatment of workers being treated for a WMSD, as earlier safe return to work is facilitated when clinicians have more information about a patient's job demands and exposures and when worksite modifications reduce physical exposures.[6]

Comprehensive ergonomic programs that incorporate primary prevention of MSDs through ergonomic changes in jobs, early detection of MSDs through surveillance, and early treatment of MSDs with an emphasis on early return to modified work have been endorsed by many corporations and by medical professionals. The American College of Occupational and Environmental Medicine (ACOEM) has recently released "Occupational Medicine Practice Guidelines," which describe its recommendations for best medical practice in the diagnosis and treatment of work-related disorders.[7] These recommendations include the application of ergonomic principles to job design in

---

BOX 23-2

Information about Work Requirements for Injured Workers is Important

Ideally, health care providers should have training or experience in ergonomics and the role of work modifications in the treatment of work-related musculoskeletal disorders. Effective diagnosis and treatment requires knowledge of specific job duties. The best way for a health care provider to get knowledge of job duties is through a worksite visit. Because this is impractical in some clinical settings, information about exposures and job duties can also be obtained through a written work description or a videotape of the job task. Employers should have a contact person with knowledge of job activities and the ability to coordinate appropriate job placement during a recovery period. Working knowledge of the industry and the specific workplace is also needed in order to make appropriate recommendations regarding temporary or permanent job modifications. Many employers will provide detailed information about job duties and physical exposures to the treating physician. It is difficult to provide optimal care for employees when this information is not available.

---

order to prevent MSDs and the use of work station or tool adjustment to avoid further aggravation of a disorder once it has begun. Return of workers to modified work that has reduced physical exposures is strongly recommended as part of treatment; the guidelines note that the best success with return to work is seen when workers go back to their original job with modifications to reduce physical exposures.

Although the main focus of prevention efforts should be on *primary prevention*—the reduction or elimination of workplace risk factors—it is also important to ensure that workers have access to appropriate and timely medical care if they do become injured. The goals of a medical management program should be to:

- Reduce or eliminate symptoms;
- Prevent progression of MSDs;
- Reduce the duration and severity of functional impairment; and
- Prevent or reduce the severity of disability.

Important elements of such a program include:

- Surveillance;
- Timely access to appropriate health care providers (Box 23-2);
- Job evaluation of injured workers;
- Availability of appropriate job modification; and
- Follow-up of treated workers and coordination with primary prevention efforts.

The vast majority of injured or symptomatic employees are able to return to productive work very quickly, as long as their work is modified to re-

duce physical exposures to the affected body parts. Such job modifications are frequently inexpensive and simple and can help employees safely return to work sooner and reduce risk of future injury. Examples of job modifications include:

- Training or retraining;
- Simple job changes to prevent awkward postures, such as a step stool or tilted work surface;
- Changes in tool design to reduce awkward postures and high hand forces;
- Preventive maintenance to reduce force in tool/equipment use;
- Changes in procedures, such as job rotation; and
- Use of conveyors, hoists, slides, and carts to reduce heavy lifting, pushing, pulling, and carrying.

Where there is no simple fix for a physical exposure that is causing or exacerbating a WMSD, temporary job transfer or restrictions are important to allow the patient's injury to heal. Examples of temporary restrictions include:

- Reduction in pace or quantity of work;
- Restriction of certain tasks; and
- Limitation of hours worked.

If an employee is to be transferred to a different job, the employer and the health care provider should assess the new job to be sure that the employee will not be exposed to relevant physical risk factors. When this cannot be accomplished, temporary removal from work will allow time for healing. In most cases, keeping an injured or symptomatic employee at work in an appropriate modified-duty position is preferable to lost work time.

Successful programs have decreased the length or severity of disability through improved early recognition and management of these disorders and integrating ergonomic interventions as part of medical treatment of injured workers.[8] For example, an integrated program designed for sheetmetal workers at an aircraft manufacturer combined preplacement evaluations of workers with ongoing surveillance for symptoms and signs of upper extremity MSDs. Job modification was implemented for those with signs of early disorders, through restriction of work hours and restriction of use of vibrating hand tools. This program reported decreased workers' compensation costs, decreased time loss, and decreased severity of injury after the implementation of this program for screening, surveillance, early medical evaluation, and job modification.[9]

There are also numerous industry case reports where the introduction of ergonomic or medical management interventions has reduced costs and injury rates. Most major corporations have ergonomics programs, in recognition that such programs are effective in reducing injuries. Successful approaches have most often used a combination of ergonomic principles for prevention, as well as improved recognition and management of those disorders that have occurred.

NECK AND UPPER EXTREMITY DISORDERS

Clinical, laboratory, and epidemiological studies have contributed to the current understanding of the pathophysiology of WMSDs of the upper extremity and neck. Five workplace physical factors are important in the etiology of these disorders:

- repetitive motions,
- forceful motions,
- mechanical stresses,
- static or awkward postures, and
- hand-arm vibration.

The effects of these physical load factors can be exacerbated by workplace psychosocial factors, such as the perception of intense workload, monotonous work, and low levels of social support at work.[10] The way in which work is organized largely determines the physical and psychosocial dimensions of the work. In assessing the role of workplace factors, it is important to consider the duration, frequency, and intensity of the individual and combined factors.

Physical Load Factors

Repetition and Force

Repetitive motions of the hands, wrists, shoulders, and neck commonly occur in the workplace. A data-entry operator may perform 20,000 keystrokes per hour; a worker in a meat-processing plant may perform 12,000 knife-cuts per day; and a worker on an assembly line may elevate the right shoulder above the level of the acromion 7,500 times per day. Such repetitive motions may eventually exceed the ability of the individual muscles and tendons to recover from the stress, especially if forceful contractions of muscles are involved in the repetitive motions.

Failure to recover usually implies some type of tissue damage or dysfunction , which may represent acute inflammation and may be totally reversible. Tissue damage may even lead, over time, to improved function—a *training effect*. Acute damage to muscle from overexertion often leads to muscle hypertrophy. In WMSDs, the sites of likely tissue damage are most commonly tendons, tendon sheaths, and tendon attachments to bones, bursae, and joints. It is probable that, over time, these tissue changes can in some cases lead to nerve compression, chronic fibrous reaction in the tendon, tendon rupture, calcium deposits, or fibrous nodule formations in a tendon.

Abrupt increases in the number of repetitive motions performed by a worker each day are well recognized clinically as a cause of tendonitis. New workers performing unaccustomed forceful or repetitive work are often at increased risk of developing MSDs.[11] Too many forceful contractions of muscles can cause corresponding tendons to stretch, compressing the microstructures of the tendons and leading to ischemia, microscopic tears in tendons, progressive lengthening, and sliding of tendon fibers through the ground substance matrix. All of these events can cause acute inflammation of tendons. Both laboratory and epidemiological studies have provided substantial evidence that high levels of exposure to the combination of repetitive and forceful movements is strongly associated with several MSDs of the upper extremity.[1,12] Repetitiveness has a number of components to be considered, including the velocity and acceleration of movement and the amount of recovery time within any repetitive cycle or task.

Posture, Stress, and Vibration

In addition to repetitive and forceful motions, three other exposure variables that influence the development of WMSDs are external mechanical stress, work performed in awkward or static postures, and segmental (localized) vibration.

Mechanical stress in tendons results from muscle contractions. It also arises from compression of a tendon, or other tissues, by contact between the body and an external object, such as by using the hand as a hammer. One of the major determinants of the level of the mechanical stress is the force of the muscle contractions. Posture is also very important because muscles are more susceptible to injury at longer muscle lengths, such as when the elbow extensor muscles are at long lengths. When combined with high forces, the amount of damage is even greater.[12] For example, a pinch that is very forceful is more stressful than one that is not very forceful. When it is combined with wrist flexion, the stress is increased and function more compromised. Another source of mechanical stress results from work surfaces or hand-held tools with hard, sharp edges or the ends of short handles that press on soft tissues. The tool exerts just as much force on the hand as the hand does on the tool. These stresses can lead, for example, to neuritis associated with the forceful contact between the edge of scissors handles or bowling ball holes with the sides of the fingers or thumb, and to cubital tunnel syndrome in microscopists who must position their elbows on a hard surface for long periods. Short-handled tools, such as needle-nosed pliers, can dig into the base of the palm and compress the superficial branches of the median nerve.

Work with the arm elevated more than 60 degrees from the trunk is more stressful for the rotator cuff tendons than work performed with the arm at the side. Work performed in static postures that require prolonged, low-level muscle contractions of the upper limb or trapezius muscle may also trigger chronic localized pain by an unknown mechanism—perhaps decreased blood flow to the muscle.

Segmental vibration is transmitted to the upper extremity from impact tools, power tools, and bench-mounted buffers and grinders. The mechanism by which localized vibration from power tools contributes to the development of work-related Raynaud phenomenon is not clear. Nevertheless, this syndrome has been associated with several types of power tools, including chainsaws, rock drillers, chipping hammers, and grinding tools.

Chronic or intermittent pain originating in muscles may be important in understanding several disorders, including tension neck syndrome (cos-toscapular syndrome) and overuse injuries in musicians. Two types of muscle activity may be important in work-related disorders: (a) low force with prolonged muscle contractions, such as moderate neck flexion while working on a video display terminal for several hours without rest breaks; and (b) infrequent or frequent high-force muscle contractions, such as intermittent use of heavy tools in overhead work. Sustained static contractions can lead to increases in intramuscular pressure, which in turn may impair blood flow to cells within the muscle.

It is hypothesized that if damage occurs daily from work activity, the muscle may not be able to repair the damage as fast as it occurs, leading to chronic muscle damage or dysfunction. The mechanism of this damage at the cellular level is not fully understood. Work activities that lead to sustained relatively low-level muscle activity or higher level muscular contractions may be a causal factor in some work-related musculoskeletal disorders.

Nonoccupational Factors

In addition to occupational risk factors or exposures, such as repetitive work, personal risk factors may influence the risk of developing WMSDs. For example, forceful repetitive activities, such as wrist extension, can occur in some recreational activities and contribute to the development of WMSDs; however, factors related to some specific disorders, such as rotator cuff tendonitis, have not been adequately studied. The nonoccupational factors for carpal tunnel syndrome (CTS) that have been most thoroughly studied include coexisting medical conditions, such as obesity, rheumatoid arthritis, diabetes mellitus, pregnancy, and acute trauma. Few, if any, personal factors are useful and strong predictors of susceptibility to WMSDs of the upper extremity.

Psychosocial Factors

In addition to the physical factors described, psychosocial factors may be important in both the initial development of these disorders and the subsequent long-term disability that sometimes occurs (see Chapter 16). Few studies have rigorously investigated both psychosocial and physical factors or their combined effects.[13] The effects of psychosocial factors may operate indirectly by altering muscle tension or other physiologic processes and decrease micropauses in muscle activity and, through the latter, may also influence the perception of pain.

Psychological factors may be particularly important in determining whether specific MSDs evolve into chronic pain syndromes due to responses of the central nervous system to high job stress. Overall, psychosocial factors appear to be somewhat more important in disorders of the neck and shoulder muscles than in tendon-related disorders of the forearm and the hand. Epidemiological studies of upper-extremity disorders suggest that the perception of an intense or stressful workload, monotonous work, and low levels of social support at work increase the risk of upper limb disorders. Different studies use a variety of measures to define intense or stressful workloads, such as lack of control over how work is done, perceived time pressure, deadlines, work pressure, or workload variability.[13] The causal role of psychosocial factors probably is not limited to particular job tasks, such as the use of computers in the office setting.

Studies that have addressed psychosocial factors have often used the demand–control–support model originally introduced by Robert Karasek and Tores Theorell.[14] In this model, high levels of psychological job demands may contribute to the development of WMSDs when they occur in an occupational setting in which the worker has little ability to decide what to do or how to do a particular job task and little opportunity to use or develop job skills. Further, these adverse effects are hypothesized to occur more frequently in a work environment in which there is little social support from co-workers or supervisors. Low job satisfaction has not been consistently identified as an important risk factor. Nonoccupational psychosocial factors could also be important.

It appears that when the exposure to several physical factors is high, then the risk of these disorders is substantially increased. When the level of exposure to physical factors is more moderate, then the overall level of risk may appear to depend more on the combination of personal attributes, physical factors, and psychosocial factors. As with many occupational exposures, the musculoskeletal risk is influenced also by nonoccupational factors.[1]

Diagnosis

This broad group of work-related disorders of the neck and upper extremity has a diverse set of symptoms and physical findings. The evaluation of a patient for a suspected work-related disorder should have three major components: (a) obtaining a his-

tory of present illness from the worker, (b) performing a physical examination of the upper extremity and the neck, and (c) assessing the work setting and tasks.[15]

The history of the present illness should fully characterize the symptoms by determining the location, radiation, duration, evolution, time patterns, and exacerbating factors. The worker's description of work activities is useful. The worker should describe the nature of specific work tasks by risk factors (forceful exertions, repetitive activities, and other adverse exposures). For example, a worker who for 8 hours a day uses a vibrating jack hammer to perform a task that is repeated every 30 seconds may be at high risk for CTS. Similarly, a repetitive job that requires the arms to be held overhead during most of the work shift may increase the risk of a rotator cuff shoulder tendonitis. Because specific job tasks can vary within even a high-risk occupation, a careful history of specific job tasks is important.

When a worker who has been performing the same job for a considerable period develops a disorder, the history should be directed not only at the chronic stable exposures but also at acute factors, such as changes in work tasks, tools, or materials. Other common acute risk factors are changes in work pace or length (longer or more frequent overtime, either by lengthening of the normal workday or by decreasing the number of days off); such changes may reduce the opportunity for recovery from fatigue and occult injury.

Determining whether the patient has a predisposing medical condition, such as previous injury to the symptomatic area, is also important. Nonoccupational exposure to risk factors can be a potential confounding influence and should be elicited during the worker interview. However, the cause of MSDs is frequently multifactorial, and the presence of a nonoccupational risk factor does not negate the importance of coexisting occupational exposures.

Surveillance and epidemiological studies have identified a number of industries and occupations associated with risks of CTS or other upper extremity disorders. Awareness of these findings can alert physicians to the industries and occupations in which adverse exposures are more common. Table 23-2 provides examples from Washington State workers' compensation data of the most frequent occupations in industries with more than 2.5 times the overall industry average rate for WMSDs. It is likely that there are also "high-risk" jobs in "low-risk" industries.

TABLE 23-2

Most Frequent Occupations in High-Risk Industries for Compensable WMSD Claims in Washington State

Industries	Occupations
Forest nurseries and forest product gathering	Nursery workers
	Laborers/farmworkers
	Production inspecting/packing workers
	Floral designers
Masonry, stonework, tile, plastering	Drywall installers
	Insulation installers
	Brickmasons
Roofing	Roofers
	Carpenters
	Laborers
Meat products	Butchers and meatcutters
	Laborers and freight stocking/handling
	Hand packers
Dairy products	Laborers and freight handlers/stockers
	Truck drivers
	Hand packers
Sawmills	Lumber handlers
Millwork	Laborers
	Woodworking machine operators
	Assemblers
	Cabinetmakers
Iron and steel foundries	Mold and core workers
	Furnace/oven workers
	Grind/polish machine operators
	Laborers
	Machine operators
Heating, ventilation, and air conditioning	Welders/cutters
	Assemblers/fabricators
	Laborers
	Grinding/polishing machine operators
Nursing and personal care facilities	Nursing aides and orderlies
	Health aides
	LPNs, RNs
	Maids/housekeeping
Local and suburban passenger transport	Emergency medical technicians
	Bus drivers
	Physician assistants/RNs
	Mechanics
	Taxi/drivers

(continued)

TABLE 23-2 (Continued)

Most Frequent Occupations in High-Risk Industries for Compensable WMSD Claims in Washington State

Industries	Occupations
Trucking and courier services	Truck drivers
	Freight handlers/stockers
	Refuse and recyclable collectors
	Graders/sorters
Air transportation scheduled and air courier services	Freight/stock handlers
	Flight attendants
	Couriers/messengers
	Transport/ticket/reservations
	Mechanics
Examples of high-risk occupations that cross over most industries	Housekeepers/janitors
	Data entry operators
	Stockers/receivers
	Assemblers/packagers

WMSD, work-related musculoskeletal disorder.
Source: Silverstein B, Kalat J, Fan ZJ. Work-related musculoskeletal disorders of the neck, back, and upper extremity in Washington State, state fund and self insured workers' compensation claims 1993–2001. Tumwater, Washington: Washington State Department of Labor and Industries, 2003.

The physical examination is an important part of evaluation of patients with WMSDs. An examination of the upper extremity typically involves inspection, assessment of the range of motion, palpation, and evaluation of peripheral nerve function.

One of the main objectives of the physical examination is to determine the precise structure or structures in the upper extremity that are the anatomic source of the symptoms. Numbness and paresthesias often result from peripheral nerve compression, but there are many other reasons why there might be numbness and tingling in the fingers. Increased pain on resisted movements often results from lesions in a tendon or at the insertion of a tendon. In some cases, it is not possible to determine the precise source of the pain in the upper extremity; in others it is possible to determine the specific disorder that is present. The severity of these disorders ranges from very mild, with no significant impairment of the ability to work, to very severe. Guidelines have been published to establish standardized methods for diagnosis, especially in epidemiological studies but also for clinicians.[15–18]

In addition to the disorders with specific findings on physical examination, workers in certain occu-pations, such as keyboard operators, musicians, and newspaper reporters, often have an increased rate of complaints of pain in the upper extremity or neck. These symptoms are similar to those of low-back pain because a specific anatomic source of the pain often cannot readily be identified on clinical evaluation. As with low-back pain, these pains are common, often intermittent in nature, and sometimes lead to substantial disability and impairment.

The diagnosis of a work-related musculoskeletal disorder is based on a three-step process:

1. Determination of whether the patient has a specific disorder, such as flexor tendonitis of the forearm. This is usually based on the history and physical examination.
2. Obtaining evidence from a detailed occupational history, or—better yet—from direct observation of the workplace or representative videotapes of substantial exposure to specific occupational risk factors, as well as from review of detailed job descriptions and job safety analyses. Although direct observation of the work is often required to determine more precisely the level of risk factor exposure in specific job tasks, descriptions

TABLE 23-3

Caution Zone Risk Factors, Washington State Ergonomics Rule/Guideline, 2000[a]

Awkward postures	Working with the hand(s) above the head, or the elbow(s) above the shoulders more than 2 hours total per day.
	Working with the neck or back bent more than 30 degrees (without support and without the ability to vary posture) more than 2 hours total per day.
	Squatting more than 2 hours total per day.
	Kneeling more than 2 hours total per day.
High hand forces	Pinching an unsupported object(s) weighing 2 or more pounds per hand, or pinching with a force of 4 or more pounds per hand, more than 2 hours per day (comparable to pinching half a ream of paper).
	Gripping an unsupported object(s) weighing 10 or more pounds per hand, or gripping with a force of 10 or more pounds per hand, more than 2 hours total per day (comparable to clamping light duty automotive jumper cables onto a battery).
Highly repetitive motions	Repeating the same motion with the neck, shoulders, elbows, wrists, or hands (excluding keying activities) with little or no variation every few seconds, more than 2 hours total per day.
	Performing intensive keying more than 4 hours total per day.
Repeated impacts	Using the hand (heel/base of palm) or knee as a hammer more than 10 times per hour, more than 2 hours total per day.
Frequent, awkward, or heavy lifting	Lifting object weighing more than 75 lb once per day or more than 55 lb more than 10 times per day.
	Lifting objects weighing more than 10 lb if done more than twice per minute, more than 2 hours total per day.
	Lifting objects weighing more than 25 lb above the shoulders, below the knees, or at arm's length more than 25 times per day.
Moderate to high hand–arm vibration	Using impact wrenches, carpet strippers, chainsaws, percussive tools (jackhammers, scalers, riveting or chipping hammers) or other tools that typically have high vibration levels, more than 30 minutes total per day.
	Using grinders, sanders, jigsaws, or other hand tools that typically have moderate vibration levels more than 2 hours total per day.

[a] Movements or postures that are a regular and foreseeable part of the job, occurring more than 1 day per week, and more frequently than 1 week per year.

by workers may identify many high-risk exposures with sufficient accuracy for a correct diagnosis. Analysis of health surveillance data, such as Occupational Safety and Health Administration (OSHA) logs or workers' compensation records from the specific workplace, may be particularly helpful in confirming that a particular job is associated with an increased risk of a work-related musculoskeletal disorder. Some employers, to facilitate return-to-work evaluations, now provide clinicians with a videotape of the job that the worker normally performs.

This may be useful in determining the approximate level of exposure. Table 23-3 provides an example of exposures of concern ("caution zone jobs") identified by Washington State as a standard/guideline for implementing ergonomics activities including employee awareness.[19] This is not an exhaustive list of exposures of concern but does provide a practical guide for frequently observed exposures in many workplaces.

3. Consideration of nonoccupational causes as possible primary causal factors or as extenuating factors based on the history and physical

examination. Review and analysis of surveillance and epidemiologic data of similar work may provide information on the relative contributions of occupational and nonoccupational factors in the causation of a specific WMSD in the patient's selected occupation and industry. With the exception of tests for abnormalities in nerve conduction, elaborate diagnostic or laboratory studies often are not necessary unless the patient has a history of trauma or symptoms suggestive of underlying systemic disease or fails to improve with conservative treatment.

The most difficult part of the diagnosis of WMSDs is determination of the relative contribution of occupational factors in the etiology of these disorders. As with other diagnostic evaluations of work-relatedness, the critical question is: Was the exposure of sufficient intensity, frequency, and duration to have caused or aggravated the injury or illness? Because intense periods of high exposure as short as days in duration can cause lateral epicondylitis or other WMSDs, attention should be directed to estimating the intensity and frequency of exposure. It is not uncommon for there to be exposure to multiple risk factors at the same time, such as repetitive and forceful exertions of the hands, shoulder abduction, and exposure to vibration from hand tools. There are no simple rules for assessing whether exposure has been of sufficient intensity, frequency, and duration to cause a specific disorder in a specific person.

Neck Disorders

Nonradiating neck pain is often called *tension neck syndrome*, suggesting muscular origin. Nonradicular radiating neck pain is often reported by patients with neck–shoulder pain. It is important to distinguish this pain from cervical osteoarthritis or cervical nerve root compression. Pain in the upper extremity on active or passive cervical rotation is often observed in nonradicular radiating pain.[16]

Neck disorders of nontraumatic origin are frequent and involve primarily muscles in the neck–shoulder region. Workers' compensation claims incidence is 36 per 10,000 full-time equivalent employees (FTEs) (see Table 23-1). Most of these involve nonspecific neck pain. Many studies of neck pain also include the neck/shoulder region primarily due to upper trapezius pain, and in some languages neck and shoulder are not differentiated. The annual

TABLE 23-4

Risk Factors for Nontraumatic Neck and Neck/Shoulder Disorders

Individual	Age
	Female gender (may be a function of gender segregation) Little physical exercise
Physical work factors	Prolonged seated work
	Neck flexion, rotation
	Prolonged shoulder shrugging
	Repetitive shoulder or hand work
	Inappropriate keyboard location
Psychosocial factors	Low decision latitude
	High demands
	High mental stress
High-risk job	Dental workers, microscopists, VDT workers, surgeons, Nurses/assistants, electronics assemblers

VDT, video display terminal.

incidence of neck pain lasting more than 1 week in office environments is about 34 percent, with radiating neck pain about 14 percent. Table 23-4 summarizes risk factors for neck and neck/shoulder disorders. Women office workers report neck pain about six times as frequently as men. Rating the ambient work environment as poor and inappropriate keyboard location increases risk slightly, whereas the interaction between high mental stress and limited physical exercise increases risk about sixfold. Sick leave due to neck pain has been predicted with prolonged neck flexion and rotation, low decision authority, and medium skill discretion.[20]

Among nurses, increased risk of neck/shoulder pain occurs with patient handling tasks involving pushing/pulling and reaching. When neck/shoulder complaints are combined with pressure tenderness, prevalence is about 7 percent and incidence about 2 percent, with those performing highly repetitive shoulder work (16 to 40 movements per minute) and/or forceful work at two to four times the risk when controlling for other factors.[20–22] Prolonged neck flexion and lack of recovery time from highly repetitive work in industrial populations also increase risk. Perceived job demands almost double the risk. Those experiencing a recent increase in exposure (prolonged VDT work or work above the shoulder) are more likely to seek health care than those who have been exposed long-term, suggesting a short induction time.

Shoulder Disorders

Rotator cuff tendonitis is one of the most frequent and costly upper extremity disorders associated with work activities. Average compensable claims cost around $21,000 in the late 1990s due to extensive lost work time and frequent surgical treatment. The rotator cuff is made up of four interrelated muscles arising from the scapula and attaching to the tuberosities that allow the humeral head to rotate: the supraspinatus that stabilizes and abducts the arm, and the infraspinatus, teres minor, and subscapularis muscles that stabilize and externally rotate the head of the humerus. The long head of the biceps muscle stabilizes and flexes the humeral head and the elbow. The supraspinatus is most active in the initial phase of abduction, whereas the deltoid is more active higher in the arc, but both are required for full power. Above 90 degrees, the rotator cuff force decreases, making the joint more susceptible to injury. The evolution of rotator cuff disease is episodic after more intensive shoulder activities, followed by remission with rest or treatment. It progresses to constant, particularly when combined with overhead and arm-length activities. Slow onset of localized pain that increases with activity suggests rotator cuff tendonitis, particularly with the pain located superiorly or laterally, whereas sudden onset suggests traumatic fracture, dislocation, or rotator cuff tear.

Table 23-5 summarizes risk factors for shoulder disorders. In the general population, rotator cuff disease is more common after age 40 (with onset around 55 years) and more frequently reported in men. Repetitive overhead activities and sports predispose to rotator cuff tendonitis. In working populations, repetitive work increases the risk of shoulder tendonitis threefold while combined with higher force; the risk is also increased somewhat more. Half of patients with shoulder tendonitis due to repetitive work recover within 10 months, but that recovery is slowed with increasing age. Newly employed workers are at increased risk of shoulder pain if they are lifting heavy weights, lifting with one hand, lifting above shoulder height, or pushing or pulling heavy loads. There is some indication that monotonous work and depression are indepen-

TABLE 23-5

Risk Factors for Nontraumatic Shoulder Disorders

Individual	Age
	Obesity
	Male gender
	Lack of physical exercise
Physical work factors	Repetitive shoulder work
	Repetitive hand work with tools
	High hand force
	Working above shoulder height
	Working in a bent posture
	Physically strenuous work
	Shoulder angle greater than 45 degrees static or repetitively
Psychosocial factors	Low decision latitude
	Monotonous work
	Mental stress
	High job demands
	Depression
Jobs with high-risk activities	Truck drivers, carpenters, welders, drywall installers, meatpacking assembly workers, masons, nursing assistants, freight handlers, garbage collectors

dent risk factors, but not as great as repetitive use of tools or low decision latitude. The 1-year incidence of rotator cuff in symptomatic computer users has been reported as 2.2 percent.

Bicipital tendonitis presents with pain in the anterior shoulder occasionally radiating down to the elbow. It is aggravated by activities requiring shoulder flexion, forearm supination, or elbow flexion. In the early stages, pain is worst at onset and completion of the activity, gradually becoming constant. On physical examination, pain is present in the bicipital groove with resisted arm flexion with a supinated forearm and full elbow extension, or on resisted supination. It is less frequently reported than rotator cuff tendonitis.

Elbow/Forearm Disorders

Epicondylitis is characterized by pain at the muscle–tendon junction or insertion points of the forearm flexor (medial) or extensor tendons (lateral). Pain is usually localized around the epi-condyle but may radiate distally to the forearm. Lateral epicondylitis (tennis elbow) is more frequently reported than medial epicondylitis (golfer's elbow)—five times more frequently in the Washington State workers' compensation data. Lateral epicondylitis is a result of inflammation at the muscular origin of primarily the extensor carpi radialis brevis, leading to microtears with subsequent fibrosis. Occasionally, the attachments of the other extensor tendons are involved. Medial epicondylitis involves primarily the flexor/pronator muscles at their origin on the anterior medial epicondyle; less often it affects other flexor tendons. Compression of the ulnar nerve in or around the medial epicondyle groove has been estimated to occur in 50 percent of cases.

Repetitive stress at the musculotendinous junction and its origin at the epicondyle cause an acute tendonitis and tendinosis in its more chronic form due to failure of the tendon to heal. Peak incidence is seen in patients 20 to 49 years of age with a 2:1 male:female ratio. Onset can accompany an acute injury but more commonly is associated with repetitive use of the extensor/supinator or flexor/pronator muscles. Work activities, such as using a screwdriver or hammer, have been reported to increase risk. In repetitive work environments, incidence of lateral epicondylitis is approximately 12 percent and it increases with age, number of other upper limb diagnoses, and "turn-and-screw" motions; gender has not been shown to be a significant predictor.[22,23] Prevalence of medial epicondylitis in a working population is 4 to 5 percent with annual incidence of 1.5 percent. Unlike with lateral epicondylitis, forceful work—but not exposure to repetitive work per se—has been shown to increase risk. Medial epicondylitis is often found in conjunction with other upper limb disorders in working populations. Approximately 80 percent of patients recover within 3 years. Table 23-6 summarizes risk factors for elbow/forearm disorders.

Diagnostic criteria include intermittent to continuous pain in the epicondylar area, pain on resisted wrist extension (lateral), or resisted pronation (medial). Although tenderness on palpation is often reported, there is low reliability and comparability of findings between examiners. It is not uncommon for symptoms to last up to 1 year, exacerbated by forceful gripping activities—irrespective of treatment. Poor prognoses are associated with intensive manual work and high baseline pain. A number of

TABLE 23-6	
Risk Factors for Nontraumatic Elbow/Forearm Disorders	
Individual	Age
	Number of other WMSDs
Physical work factors	Driving screws
	Tightening with force
Psychosocial factors	Low discretion
	High demands
	High mental stress
Jobs with high-risk activities	Carpenters, machinists, laborers, plumbers, assembly work with hand tools, hairdressers, drywall installers, hand packers, electricians, bus drivers, welders, grinders/polishers, butchers/meatcutters, kitchen/food preparation

WMSDs, work-related musculoskeletal disorders.

studies have reported elbow/forearm pain in occupational computer users.

Hand/Wrist Disorders

The most frequent hand/wrist diagnoses are tendonitis and carpal tunnel syndrome (CTS) (Fig. 23-2). The workers' compensation claims incidence for all nontraumatic hand/wrist disorders is 57.6 per 10,000 FTEs, with an average cost of almost $8,000. The claims incidence rate for tendonitis is 17.2 with an average cost of well over $9,000. Workers' compensation claims incidence is approximately 23 per 10,000 FTEs, with an average of 209 lost workdays and average cost of more than $16,000 (see Table 23-1).

Carpal Tunnel Syndrome

CTS comprises characteristic signs and symptoms, including pain, paresthesias, and sometimes weakness in the median nerve distribution of the hand, following entrapment of the median nerve in the carpal tunnel. Individual risk factors include a number of systemic conditions, such as diabetes mellitus, hypothyroidism, obesity, rheumatoid arthritis, older age, and female gender—but not smoking. In work-related CTS, the gender difference may

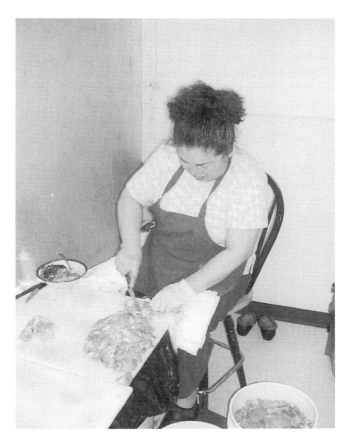

FIGURE 23-2 ● Woman in Nicaragua cutting meat. A high degree of hand force and frequent repetition combine to make this a high-risk job for development of carpal tunnel syndrome and tendonitis. In addition, this woman faces the potential hazards of cuts and neck strain. (Photograph by Barbara Silverstein.)

be a function of segregation of women in more repetitive work and men in more forceful work and a greater willingness among women to report symptoms. Work-related physical factors include highly repetitive or forceful hand work, particularly pinching, sustained awkward wrist postures and hand–arm vibration (Table 23-7). The more these factors occur simultaneously, the greater the risk. Although frequently reported in the mass media, CTS is not primarily associated with computer work. Among computer users, annual incidence of CTS is approximately 0.9 percent, compared to annual incidence of 14.7 percent for extensor tendonitis in the first dorsal compartment. Meatpackers, assembly-line workers, and other workers with high-force and high-repetition tasks appear to be at higher risk for CTS than computer users. There is a high incidence of CTS in workers doing repetitive work in the clothing (17.4 percent), food (15.3 percent), and assembly (10.9 percent) sectors. CTS has been associated with hand–arm vibration, but it is difficult to separate vibration from high hand

force. When workers are exposed to high force and high repetition simultaneously, the risk increases dramatically.

The basis for diagnosis of CTS increasingly includes electrodiagnostic criteria, but the presence of an abnormal electrodiagnostic test in the absence of symptoms does not appear to predict clinical CTS.[24] Electrodiagnostic testing has little utility in predicting outcomes of surgery but is possibly useful where clinical diagnosis is not clear.[25] The use of a hand map where the patient has marked the presence of pain/numbness/tingling in the palmar thumb, index finger, middle finger, and the radial half of the ring finger is recognized in almost all diagnostic criteria.

The case in Box 23-3 illustrates the intermittent and progressive nature of most work-related disorders of the upper extremity, especially of CTS—the best known of the common work-related disorders of the upper extremity.

Ulnar nerve entrapment at the wrist (Guyon canal) usually presents as a motor lesion. It is much

TABLE 23-7

Risk Factors for Nontraumatic Carpal Tunnel Syndrome, Tendonitis

Individual	Age
	Obesity
	Female gender, pregnancy
	Rheumatoid arthritis, diabetes, hypothyroidism, hypertension
Physical work factors	High force–high repetitive work
	Hand–arm vibration
	Repetitive pinching tightening/holding with force
	Repetitive hitting
Psychosocial factors	Low discretion
	Low job satisfaction
	High demands
	Poor social support
	High mental stress
Jobs with high-risk activities	Meat cutting, lumber turners, food processors, carpenters, assembly work with hand tools, foundry workers, hairdressers, kitchen workers, laborers, machine operators, sewing operators, hand packing, typist, stock handler/bagger, roofers

less frequently reported than median nerve entrapment in the carpal tunnel. Cubital tunnel syndrome (frequently called *student's elbow* or *Saturday night palsy*) results from compression of the ulnar nerve due to prolonged weight bearing on the elbow. Radial nerve entrapment is even less common than ulnar nerve entrapment and may be related to repetitive upper-arm activities requiring gripping and squeezing.

Hand/Wrist Tendonitis/Tenosynovitis

Tendonitis causes pain over the tendon close to where it is inserted in the muscle and worsens with repetitive motion. There can be mild swelling over the tendon. The highest risk of hand/wrist tendonitis is associated with a combination of high hand force and high hand repetition. There are a variety of different types of tendonitis associated with the many different tendons located in the hand and wrist. The most common type of tendonitis is DeQuervain's tenosynovitis, which presents with a history of repetitive pinching and pain along the

radial aspect of the wrist below the base of the thumb, particularly with the Finkelstein test (passive ulnar deviation with the thumb inside a closed fist). DeQuervain's tenosynovitis is common in computer users, who have an annual incidence of 15 percent. DeQuervain's, as is true for most other forms of tendonitis, becomes worse with activity and better with rest. The second most important location of tenosynovitis is the sixth dorsal compartment (extensor carpi ulnaris); it presents with wrist pain and dorsal swelling over the ulna, below the fifth finger. It occurs primarily in those with repetitive wrist motion, particularly with extension and ulnar deviation. *Trigger finger* (volar flexor tenosynovitis) presents with tenderness at the proximal end of the tendon sheath, in the distal palm, and with a catching of the tendon when the finger is flexed. There is frequently palpable tendon thickening and nodularity.

Treatment and Prognosis

The goals of treatment are elimination or reduction in symptoms and impairment and return of the employee to work under conditions that will protect his or her health. These goals can be most easily achieved by early and conservative treatment. Once pain becomes chronic, the choice of treatment changes more to increasing capacity to deal with pain. Treatment of WMSDs early in their course has several advantages: Such treatment is less difficult and less costly, surgical procedures can be avoided, periods of absence from work or stressful exposures are shorter, and the effectiveness of treatment is greater. Interaction among the health care provider, the patient, and the employer at a very early stage is critical to safe successful return to work. This early and safe return to work using ergonomics has shown impressive results for both back and upper limb workers' compensation claimants.[6,8]

The initial goals of treatment are to limit further tissue damage, dysfunction, and inflammation (if present) and to assist the repair of any tissue damage. Symptomatic relief is provided by the use of anti-inflammatory medications, rest (sometimes facilitated by splints), and application of heat or cold. Physical therapy techniques, such as stretching exercises, are used to assist in symptom relief, to ensure normal joint motion, and to recondition muscles after periods of rest or reduced use. If these more conservative measures fail to reduce symptoms and impairment for some conditions, such as CTS, steroid injections or surgical treatments can

BOX 23-3

Carpal Tunnel Syndrome Case

A 31-year-old, right-handed man had been employed in a variety of automobile manufacturing jobs for 13 years. Two years ago, he switched to a new plant and was assigned to a job that required him to manipulate a spot-welding machine beneath cars moving overhead. He completed four welds/minute on each car. The metal handles of the spot welder required substantial force for appropriate positioning, and were manually repositioned four times/car. The worker's wrists were in extreme extension for a substantial portion of the job cycle.

When the worker started on this job, the work shift was 9 hours 6 days per week. After 3 weeks on the job, he noted that he had pain in both wrists, numbness and tingling in the first four fingers of his left hand, at first only at night, a few nights each week, after he had fallen asleep. When he awoke at night with the numbness, it was alleviated by shaking his hands. Gradually, over the next several months, the numbness and pain worsened in both frequency and intensity. His left hand would feel numb by the end of the work shift, and any time he was driving his hands would become numb. Because he liked his job and did not want to be placed on restriction, which would mean he could not work overtime, he decided to visit his private physician rather than the company physician. He also was not sure that the company physician would be very sympathetic to his complaints.

The physician found on physical examination that the worker had decreased sensitivity to light touch in the left index and middle fingers and a positive wrist flexion-nerve compression test of the left hand. She suspected carpal tunnel syndrome (CTS) and believed that the disorder might be work-related because the patient was young, male, and had no other risk factors, such as diabetes, past history of wrist fracture, or recent trauma to the wrist. The physician discussed job changes with the patient. She also prescribed wrist splints to be used at night.

The splints relieved some of the nighttime numbness for a period. However, over the next 6 months, the symptoms became present most of the time, and he thought that his left hand was becoming weaker. Similar symptoms also developed in his right hand.

The patient felt he could no longer do his job and returned to his physician who ordered nerve conduction tests that showed slowing of median sensory nerve impulse conduction in the carpal tunnel, more so on the right than the left. She referred him to a hand surgeon.

One year after the problem was first noted, the worker had surgery, first on the left hand and then on the right. After surgery, the company placed him in a transitional work center for a 3-month period, where he worked at his own pace and had no symptoms. He then returned to the assembly line with the restriction that he not use welding guns or air-powered hand tools. When he worked on the line, he occasionally had symptoms, but they were substantially less intense and less frequent than before.

He later transferred to a warehouse, because he felt that he would have a better chance of avoiding long layoffs there. His job required use of a stapling gun to seal packages. Three weeks after beginning this job, his symptoms began to return with their former intensity. Through ordinary channels, he immediately sought and was given a transfer to a position driving a forklift truck. This change reduced, but did not eliminate, his symptoms. Currently, he has numbness, tingling, and pain in the fingers of both hands about twice a month. Playing volleyball usually triggers a severe attack. With the use of nighttime splints, he can sleep through most nights without awakening. Although he believes that his hands are weaker than before the symptoms developed, he still is able to perform his job. He has decided that he will continue working as long as the symptoms remain at no more than the current level.

---

be helpful. Surgery, even in CTS, may be ineffective if the worker is returned to the old job without an effort to reduce the occupational exposures that were present. Because few scientifically valid studies have evaluated the long-term effectiveness of the treatment of WMSDs of the limb and neck, an empiric approach is indicated. One year after carpal tunnel release surgery, distal sensory latencies remain abnormal in about 79 percent of patients.

Resting of the symptomatic part of the upper extremity is the most important part of the treatment program. In addition to engineering changes, restricted duty, job rotation, or temporary transfer may be effective. In order for job transfer or rotation to be effective, the new job duties must result in a net reduction in the level of exposure. It is often necessary to conduct an evaluation of the new duties to determine whether a reduction in exposure will occur. The magnitude of reduction required to facilitate recovery often is not known. In general, the more severe the disorder is, the greater the reduction in magnitude and duration of exposure that will be required. Because of the adverse consequences of complete removal from the work environment, this step should be taken only in severe cases or after less drastic measures have failed.

Splints and other immobilization devices may provide rest to the symptomatic region. However, they may increase the level of exposure if the worker must resist the device in order to carry out regular job tasks. Workers may also adapt to wearing a splint by altering their work activities in a way that leads to substantial stress on another region of the upper extremity, such as the elbow or shoulder. Immobilization or prolonged rest may have direct adverse effects if either leads to muscle atrophy. As a result, careful monitoring of the worker who is on restricted duty or job transfer or is wearing an immobilization device is indicated. In addition, because it is difficult to predict the clinical course of these conditions and because the empirical basis of many of the treatments is poorly understood, frequent follow-up is desirable. Failure of the treatment plan to produce improvement over several weeks should lead to thorough reevaluation of the plan and its underlying assumptions. Many of these conditions resolve within a few weeks with early treatment. The prognosis is generally good with early treatment and reduction in exposure. There is some indication from randomized clinical trials that a clinical population with moderate CTS does better with surgery than splinting at 1, 3, 6, and 12 months.[26]

Sometimes CTS and other conditions of the upper extremity follow a course similar to that of chronic severe low-back pain. With conservative treatment and appropriate adjustments in the work setting, most cases should improve enough so that the patient can successfully return to work, but a small minority of affected workers develop chronic symptoms and are very difficult to treat. In these cases, the physical capabilities of the worker, the work demands, and the psychosocial factors related both to the worker and the employer are important in determining whether the worker successfully returns to work.[6] The ways in which these factors interact are complex. The recognition that psychosocial factors—such as job satisfaction or negative self-fulfilling beliefs of the patient, the employer, or the health care provider—are important and should not lead to ignoring the role of occupational physical exposures or to "blaming the victim."[27] When the latter occurs, delayed recovery is often attributed to personal weakness, low job satisfaction, or desire for secondary gain. Critical to prevention of these persistent cases is early intervention—an important reason to eliminate barriers to early reporting of symptoms.

There has been a rapid development of comprehensive programs that ideally address the physical reconditioning of the worker, psychosocial factors, and workplace factors such as ongoing exposure.[28] A contract between the patient and the health care provider should be established early in the treatment process, with the explicit aim of returning the worker safely to work. The diagnosis and treatment of severe or chronic WMSDs is sometimes challenging. Identification of the level of exposure by patient history is difficult, and usually direct observation of work is the preferred approach. There is substantial uncertainty about how to best measure exposure in some occupational settings, especially in the office. There is a danger of both overdiagnosis and underdiagnosis—assuming either that every case of CTS is work-related or that no case of CTS is work-related. The danger exists of not recognizing when a case is becoming chronic and severe and when a multidisciplinary approach should be considered. Several observations are helpful when one is faced with challenges of diagnosing and treating these work-related conditions. A careful history and physical examination are important. An extensive objective assessment of the work environment may be required. In most cases, conservative treatment that (a) preserves normal physical conditioning, (b) relies on a reduction of the level of occupational exposure while the patient remains at work, and (c) incorporates careful monitoring of the patient is a reasonable initial approach and is effective. Prevention of these disorders requires the successful identification and remediation of adverse exposures.[29,30]

LOW-BACK PAIN

Low-back pain is among the most common health complaints among working-age populations worldwide, ranking second only to respiratory illnesses as a symptom-related reason for visits to a physician. Seventy to eighty percent of adults in the United States will experience a significant episode of low-back pain at least once in their lives; similar levels of lifetime prevalence are reported from other industrialized countries. There are more than 22 million cases of back pain annually in the United States that last 1 week or more, resulting in almost 150 million lost workdays.[31]

Low-back pain is a major cause of disability, limitation of activity, and economic loss in developed countries. Disability due to low-back pain is a complicated phenomenon influenced not only by the physical condition of an individual person but also by other personal factors and societal factors, including medical care, the work environment, and the workers' compensation system. Rapid rises in reported disability due to low-back pain in the 1970s and 1980s led some experts to describe an "epidemic" of low-back pain. More recent data have shown a 34 percent decrease in the number of low-back pain claims and an even sharper decline in workers' compensation payments for low-back pain in the United States between 1987 and 1995. BLS data have shown a decline over the past decade in the number of reported cases of back or spinal injury associated with lost workdays.

Nevertheless, low-back pain still accounts for a substantial burden of cost and disability. An estimated 1 percent of the working-age population in the United States is permanently disabled due to back pain, and, at any given time, up to 1 percent of workers are temporarily disabled due to back pain. Back disorders remain the most common chronic conditions causing activity limitation in people under age 45 in the United States. Back pain is the most common reason for filing a workers' compensation claim, reportedly accounting for 16 to 25 percent of all workers' compensation claims and 23 to 33 percent of all workers' compensation claim costs. Annual costs of low-back pain, in terms of workers' compensation claims, have been estimated at more than $9 billion. The total economic impact of low-back pain in the United States, including lost earnings and other uncompensated losses, has been estimated at $75 to $100 billion.[1] Estimates of the average workers' compensation

costs of low-back disorders and sciatica are shown in Table 23-1.

Although there is widespread agreement about the severity and widespread nature of low-back pain, there is much less agreement concerning its etiology or even its definition. One of the difficulties in interpreting the medical literature on low-back pain is the plethora of clinical definitions and different ways in which patients can be identified—such as by symptoms, medical treatment, or disability. Most people with symptoms of low-back pain do not come to medical attention. Most episodes of low-back pain that come to medical attention result in no change in work status. Most alterations of work status due to low-back pain do not lead to long-term disability. Very different pictures of low-back pain may thus emerge from differing case definitions. Interpretation of the literature is further complicated given the multifactorial origin of low-back pain. In a given patient, the onset, severity, reporting, and prognosis of low-back pain may be influenced by a variety of work and nonwork factors. The presence of personal risk factors in a patient does not rule out work-relatedness, just as work may not be the sole cause of an individual patient's symptoms.

Etiology

Comprehensive reviews of the scientific literature on work-relatedness of low-back pain, conducted by NIOSH and by the National Academy of Sciences, have concluded that there is strong evidence that low-back pain disorders are associated with work-related lifting and forceful movements, with whole-body vibration. heavy physical work, and work in awkward postures (bending and twisting; Table 23-8).[1,32] These reviews have also noted that psychosocial factors, such as job satisfaction, personality traits, perception of intensified workload, and job control, are associated with low-back pain.

Identified workplace factors include frequent bending and twisting, heavy physical labor, and prolonged sedentary work. Jobs requiring frequent lifting of objects weighing 25 lb or more seem to be associated with an increase in risk, as are sudden, unexpected maximal lifting efforts. The effect of lifting may be modified by individual fitness and strength capability and by the rate, position, distance, and height of the lifting task. The exposure to vibration that accompanies motor vehicle

TABLE 23-8

Jobs with High-Risk Activities for Sciatica, Washington State Fund Workers' Compensation Claims, 1993–2001

Nursing aides/orderlies	Nurses
Truck drivers	Construction laborers
Carpenters and apprentices	Garbage collectors
Maids and housekeeping cleaners	Glaziers
	Freight/stock handlers
Drywall installers	Brick masons
Carpet installers	

operation (4 to 6 Hz) is a risk factor for low-back pain. Truck drivers, manual material handlers, and nursing personnel are among the occupations with the highest rates of compensable back pain episodes.

The frequency and severity of low-back pain are also associated with a variety of personal and lifestyle factors, including age, gender, overall level of physical fitness, lumbar mobility, lumbar strength, tobacco use, nonwork physical activities, past history of low-back disorders, and congenital structural abnormalities, such as spondylolisthesis.[32–34]

Diagnosis and Evaluation

Low-back pain may arise from (a) any of the structures comprising the lumbosacral spine and its associated soft tissues or (b) abdominal, retroperitoneal, or pelvic structures. It may result from local or systemic processes. Even with clinical tests and imaging procedures, however, the causes of most episodes of low-back pain remain unclear, and perhaps as many as 85 percent of patients cannot be given a precise pathoanatomical diagnosis. Pain in these cases is typically assumed to be related to soft-tissue injury or to degenerative changes, and nonspecific terms, such as *sprain* or *strain*, are commonly used to describe the etiology of low-back pain. Given the idiopathic nature of most episodes of low-back pain, the primary goals of the evaluation are to identify:

- Any systemic or visceral cause of pain;
- Any neurologic compromise requiring urgent surgery;

- Any other findings that influence the choice of therapy or prognosis, including workplace exposures that may incite or exacerbate symptoms.

A limited diagnostic evaluation, combined with strong reassurance regarding prognosis and careful attention to the patient's concerns, best serves the needs of most patients. In cases of back pain that are work-related, it is also important to define work exposures that may need modification in order to improve functional recovery or prevent recurrence.

Current consensus guidelines and expert opinion on the appropriate diagnostic evaluations of low-back pain recommend that the evaluation focus on three questions:

1. Is the pain caused by a systemic disease?
2. Is there neurologic compromise that may require surgical evaluation?
3. Is there social or psychological distress that may amplify or prolong the pain?[35]

These guidelines, intended for general medical practice, give scant attention to issues of work-relatedness or fitness for work.

The most important immediate goal of the history is to determine if a patient has pain related to a serious local condition, such as a fracture, a systemic disorder (such as malignancy or infection), or a neurologic disorder requiring surgical evaluation (such as cauda equina syndrome). The history should focus on "red flags" that indicate the possible presence of a disorder more serious than nonspecific low-back pain, including:

- A history of trauma;
- Age over 50 or under 20;
- A history of malignancy or immune compromise;
- Pain that worsens when supine;
- Recent-onset bowel or bladder dysfunction or saddle anesthesia; and
- Severe or progressive neurologic deficit of the lower extremities.[36,37]

The vast majority of cases seen in a primary care setting or in an occupational medicine clinic will present with nonspecific low-back pain or with symptoms of sciatica. Past history of low-back disorders should be sought, as should information on the onset and time course of symptoms and any functional limitations due to symptoms. Location of symptoms should be determined, specifically radiation of pain or paresthesias to the distal lower extremity. Other important historical points include the temporal pattern, relation to work or other daily activities, other precipitating factors, and evidence of functional disability related to the syndrome. These factors are particularly important in planning the individual's return to work. Inquiry about alcohol or drug abuse and depressive symptoms may identify factors that amplify or prolong pain and are amenable to specific intervention.

Often neglected in the history is a description of the patient's work activities, including descriptions of awkward working postures, lifting requirements, other forceful movements, whole-body vibration, and need for bending and twisting of the back. Information on monotonous work, job control, and job satisfaction should also be sought. This information is essential for making determinations about work-relatedness, as well as for planning work restrictions and return to full work.

As with the history, the most important immediate goal of the physical examination is to seek physical signs that may indicate a serious medical condition. Examination of the lumbosacral spine includes musculoskeletal and neurologic components and should proceed according to an organized routine. Unfortunately, most of the items commonly assessed on physical examination have limited reproducibility between different examiners, as well as having limited prognostic significance.[36]

However, in addition to excluding serious disorders, a careful baseline physical examination is necessary to allow clinical progression to be assessed. Beginning with the patient disrobed and standing, the alignment, curvature, and symmetry of the spine, pelvis, and lower extremities are evaluated. The range of motion of the lumbosacral spine is assessed in flexion and extension. Visual estimation of range of motion is adequate for general clinical purposes, although goniometers can also be used for more precise measurement. Measurement of minimum distance from fingertips to floor is useful to assess the effect of treatment on combined lumbar and hip mobility. A lateral bending maneuver is performed to each side to assess symmetry and any resultant effect on symptoms. Toe raises, heel walking, and standing on one leg (Trendelenburg test) assist the evaluation of lower extremity muscle weakness. A thorough neurologic examination is also essential in patients with sciatica or lower extremity neurologic complaints.

Diagnostic tests play a very limited role in the initial management of acute low-back pain. In the absence of "red flags" on history, plain x-rays (radiographs) of the lumbosacral spine are unlikely to change diagnosis or therapy and are often overused. These x-rays are appropriate in cases of chronic or recurrent low-back pain but should be ordered acutely to rule out fracture or systemic disorder only if suggested by the history. For patients aged 20 to 50 with nonradicular back pain and no suggestive history of potentially serious underlying condition, it is most appropriate to wait 4 weeks before obtaining x-rays. If symptoms have not improved in 4 weeks, plain x-rays of the lumbar spine should be obtained, along with a complete blood count and erythrocyte sedimentation rate to help rule out an occult neoplasm or osteomyelitis.[38,39] If osteomyelitis or a neoplasm is suspected, but not detected on the plain x-rays, a bone scan or magnetic resonance imaging (MRI) of the spine should be performed.

Patients with radicular back pain may also derive little benefit from early diagnostic imaging, as many of these patients will have spontaneous resolution of their symptoms, and early surgical management is indicated only in cases of severe or progressive neurological deficits. Patients with persistent or progressive neurological deficits and an exam consistent with a nerve root impingement should be referred for MRI to evaluate the anatomic basis of the nerve root symptoms. Patients with more ambiguous nerve root involvement may benefit from electromyography in order to determine if nerve root impingement is present. Counseling and education of patients are important, as patients may request imaging that is inappropriate. The use of MRI is especially problematic because a substantial proportion of people without back pain have disk abnormalities that are revealed by MRI. Among asymptomatic adults, 22 to 40 percent have MRI evidence of disk herniation and 24 to 79 percent have evidence of a bulging disk. Therefore, anatomic abnormalities seen on MRI must be evaluated critically for their clinical importance in each patient.

Older adults with symptoms suggestive of spinal stenosis (pain or paresthesias in the legs relieved by spinal flexion, or pseudoclaudication) should be evaluated for the presence of this disorder. The diagnosis can usually be made on the basis of a computed tomography (CT) scan or an MRI; electromyography may be useful to determine the extent of neurologic impairment.

Treatment and Prognosis

Nonspecific Low-Back Pain

Evidence-based guidelines for the treatment of low-back pain have been provided by several expert panels and should be referred to for the management of most cases.[7,34] For acute cases, the health care provider should offer a confident and positive approach, which is justified by the generally good prognosis of acute low-back pain. Reassurance regarding prognosis should be provided, as many workers with low-back pain are apprehensive about the potentially disabling nature of their injury. Early return-to-work activities, with work modifications as necessary, and reestablishment of normal or near-normal activities of daily living are important aspects of care. Although unlikely to be of short-term benefit, measures to alter lifestyle factors associated with low-back pain, such as smoking, sedentary lifestyle, and obesity, should be implemented.

Nonsteroidal anti-inflammatory drugs (NSAIDs) are effective for relief of symptoms and provide adequate relief in most patients. Opioid analgesics may be considered in the small minority of patients who do not attain adequate symptom relief from NSAIDs; opioid drugs should be used with caution and for a clearly limited time. Muscle relaxants may also be of use in relief of symptoms, though clinical studies do not clearly identify which patients will benefit from these drugs. Sedation is a common side effect, although in patients who are having trouble sleeping due to back pain this can be used to therapeutic advantage by evening dosing. Physical therapy and spinal manipulation are also effective in providing temporary symptom relief in patients with acute or subacute low back pain. Many experts believe that use of manipulation or physical therapy should be delayed until 2 or 3 weeks after the onset of symptoms, because a substantial fraction of patients will improve spontaneously within this time. Back exercises do not seem to be useful in the acute phase, though there is evidence that exercise is helpful in chronic back pain and in the prevention of recurrence. Massage therapy has

not received extensive study but shows promise in clinical trials. A wide array of alternative therapies is advocated by practitioners but lack consistent evidence of effectiveness in clinical trials. These treatments include laser stimulation of trigger points, various injection therapies, acupuncture, reflexology, traction, and corsets.

In cases of chronic low-back pain, current clinical judgment favors use of an active exercise program. Treatment of chronic cases emphasizes strengthening and rangeofmotion exercises and aerobic conditioning in the context of formal assessment of baseline and progressive function (physical capacities evaluation). Maintaining patient adherence to an intensive exercise regimen may be difficult. Referral to a multidisciplinary pain center may be beneficial to some patients with low-back pain. Such centers usually employ multiple, simultaneous treatments, including supervised, graded exercise, cognitive or behavioral therapy, and patient education in concert with medical therapies. Antidepressants are useful in patients with depression (one-third of patients with chronic low-back pain), though there is conflicting evidence about their use in patients without clinical depression.

In workers who have been temporarily disabled from work due to low-back pain, decisions about return to work cannot be made in isolation from knowledge about their work and their workplace. The modification of physical job demands to facilitate early return to work is felt by many experienced clinicians to be a critical element in the prevention of longer term disability.[40] A combination of rehabilitation intervention along with the ergonomics intervention is the most successful in returning injured workers to work, with the ergonomics intervention contributing the most to the success. By facilitating return to usual work, ergonomics intervention appears to reduce progression to long-term disability. Intensive clinical and rehabilitation intervention alone have not significantly reduced the time of absence from regular work when applied separately from the ergonomics intervention.

Herniated Intervertebral Disc

In the absence of cauda equina syndrome or progressive neurologic deficit, conservative (nonsurgical) management should be pursued for at least 1 month in most cases. After 6 weeks of treatment, only about 10 percent of patients still have sufficient symptoms for consideration of surgical management. Early treatment parallels the treatment of nonspecific low-back pain with the caveat that the safety and effectiveness of spinal manipulation is not clear. Epidural corticosteroid injections offer temporary symptomatic relief in some patients, and their use may reduce rates of surgery in patients who otherwise would be candidates for surgical decompression.

In patients who still have significant pain or neurologic deficits after 4 weeks, discectomy should be considered in order to provide quicker symptom relief and return to function. Patients with herniated discs who undergo surgery do not return to work more quickly than those treated with nonsurgical therapy, though surgery appears to lead to improved functional and symptomatic outcomes at 1 year. Long-term outcomes are similar among patients treated with or without surgery. The result of surgical treatment of these patients is strongly related to the findings at surgery. The better defined the clinical syndrome is, the better the surgical outcome will be—with at least partial relief of sciatica in up to 90 percent of carefully selected patients. Approximately 70 percent of patients experience relief of back pain. Surgical outcomes also can be adversely affected by unrealistic patient expectations, depression, and substance abuse.

LOWER EXTREMITY DISORDERS

In comparison to low-back pain and upper extremity disorders, little attention has been paid to WMSDs of the lower extremities. Except for osteoarthritis, studies of work-related lower extremity disorders have mostly emphasized traumatic injuries. Although disorders such as Achilles' tendonitis, plantar fasciitis, and tarsal tunnel syndrome have been recognized as the result of chronic overuse in athletes, they have not been well characterized among working populations. Based on the few available studies, knee bursitis is associated with kneeling work. For example, floor laying has been recognized as an occupation with high rates of knee bursitis and other disorders of the lower extremities. There currently is no systematic evidence showing that occupational exposures cause other foot and ankle disorders. However, the absence of observed associations is due

to the paucity of studies in this area rather than the existence of studies that have not demonstrated associations.

The workers' compensation data from Washington State (see Table 23-1) indicate that nontraumatic knee disorders are infrequently accepted compared to other nontraumatic MSDs. The incidence rate for nontraumatic knee disorders was 1.2 per 10,000 FTEs and 0.3 per 10,000 FTEs for tendonitis/bursitis. The average costs were $11,468 for nontraumatic knee disorders and $8,502 for tendonitis/bursitis. The average cost of tendonitis was similar to epicondylitis and hand/wrist tendonitis. The industries with the highest claims rate for nontraumatic knee disorders were carpentry and floor work, plumbing, residential construction, and roofing. For knee tendonitis/bursitis, the high-risk industries were carpentry and floor work, plumbing, electrical work, masonry/stonework/tile setting, and roofing. The most frequently identified occupations of these claimants were carpenters, plumbers, electricians, carpet layers, and roofers.

The best-studied WMSD of the lower extremities is osteoarthritis of the hip and knee. Osteoarthritis is the most prevalent joint disease, the most common disabling medical condition among older adults, and a leading cause of disability among people during their working years.[41] The disease can affect one or several joints; common sites include the hips, knees, shoulders, and fingers. Among persons aged 55 or older, 5 to 15 percent have evidence of hip osteoarthritis, while knee osteoarthritis is even more common. Osteoarthritis has a wide range of severity, from an asymptomatic state evident only on x-rays to symptomatic states that severely limit an individual's working abilities and daily activities. Joint replacement may be performed in severe cases. Osteoarthritis is the leading indication for hip and knee replacement; an estimated 120,000 persons undergo total hip replacement annually in North America. In addition to the personal and social aspects of these diseases, the cost to society is enormous.

Most cases of osteoarthritis are idiopathic, and the biological or biomechanical processes underlying the disease are largely unknown. One hypothesis is that osteoarthritis occurs when repeated stresses at a joint exceed the ability of joint tissues to withstand those stresses, leading to "microtrauma" and cumulative damage. Heavy physical

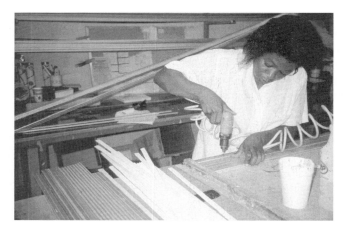

FIGURE 23-3 ● In jobs like this, reducing the load on the wrist, elbow, and shoulder can be accomplished by one or more of the following three methods: changing the tool, reorienting it (from vertical to horizontal, or vice versa), and changing the height of the work station—either elevating the worker or lowering the piece being worked on. (Courtesy of WISHA [Washington Industrial Safety and Health Act] Services Demonstration Project.)

loading from work or sports may thus play a causal role in osteoarthritis when they create imbalances between mechanical stresses and the ability of joint tissues to withstand those stresses.

There is evidence that heavy physical work is a risk factor for developing osteoarthritis of the hip.[42,43] Repeated heavy lifting and frequent stair climbing are associated with an increased risk of osteoarthritis requiring hip replacement. Osteoarthritis of the knee has been studied less often but has been found to be higher in occupations requiring frequent knee bending, squatting, heavy lifting, and frequent stair climbing.[44] However, some researchers have been critical of studies linking knee and hip osteoarthritis to work activities.

PREVENTION OF MUSCULOSKELETAL DISORDERS

Preventive strategies are largely experience-based and have not been comprehensively evaluated by scientific studies. The principles outlined here must be adapted to fit the specific characteristics of each working environment. They should be viewed as a guide rather than a blueprint. Reduction in exposures is the most important approach to prevention. This approach often requires changes in the work station, work process, or use of tools. Appropriate interventions must be specific to the biomechanical risk factors encountered in a particular workplace (Fig. 23-3).

In addition to these engineering controls, there is evidence to support the effectiveness of administrative controls (changing workplace culture), mod-

ification of individual risk factors through exercise programs, and the use of programs utilizing a combined approach. Multidisciplinary, participatory approaches that involve employers and employees appear to be successful and foster compliance and acceptance of changes.[45,46] Sometimes administrative changes, such as work restrictions, or job rotation are useful alternatives, either as preventive or as therapeutic interventions. Use of some types of personal protective equipment, such as palm pads and knee pads, are effective. However, one very popular device, lumbar corsets or back belts, do not seem to be effective in reducing the occurrence of low-back pain.

In order for work restrictions to be effective in the treatment of injured workers, the health care provider must be specific about the type of work activity that should be avoided or reduced. For example, it is better to limit repetitive hand activities to "fewer than 10 movements per minute for more than 2 hours per day" than to prescribe "no repetitive hand movements during the work shift." Developing specific recommendations for work restrictions is facilitated by viewing videotapes of the usual job of the worker or by obtaining detailed job descriptions from the employer. As a preventive intervention, job rotation of workers among jobs that require different types of motions of the upper extremity may simply expose an even greater number of workers to a considerable degree of risk.

To reduce exposure, the first step required for instituting changes in work stations or work processes is to analyze the specific characteristics of suspected high-risk jobs. Although an industrial engineer or occupational health professional with ergonomics training can conduct the job review, the involvement of those persons who are most knowledgeable about the job is important. Experience has shown that operators and supervisors with limited technical training can successfully identify many of the hazardous aspects of a specific job and that specific solutions may not be effective or accepted without the involvement of such persons in the job review and development of solutions.

The hand activity level (HAL) threshold limit value[47] is useful for assessing risk in monotask jobs looking at force and repetition. The strain index[48] for the distal upper extremity and the rapid upper limb assessment (RULA)[49] tools are useful in performing quick risk assessments. The NIOSH lifting equation[50] and the threshold limit value promulgated by the American Conference of Governmental Industrial Hygienists[51] provide guidance on acceptable lifting, depending on weight, location of the load, and frequency of handling.

After a job analysis has identified the potentially hazardous exposures associated with a particular job, specific solutions should be solicited from those who are knowledgeable about the job. With limited training in the control principles (discussed in the next section), engineers, production employees, and front-line supervisors often propose the most useful methods for eliminating hazardous risk factors. If several factors are present, it can be difficult to determine which is the most detrimental. Where possible, integrated solutions should be developed that reduce multiple risk factors at the same time.

Control of repetitiveness, forcefulness, awkward posture, vibration, mechanical contact stress, and cold are often possible, as illustrated in the following examples.

Control of Repetitiveness

1. Use mechanical assists and other types of automation. For example, in packing operations, use a device, rather than the hands, to transfer parts.
2. Rotate workers among jobs that require different types of motions. Rotation must be viewed as a temporary administrative control, one used only until a more permanent solution can be found.
3. Implement horizontal work enlargement by adding different elements or steps to a job, particularly steps that do not require the same motions as the current work cycle.
4. Increase work allowances or decrease production standards. Management rarely looks on this control strategy favorably.
5. Design a tool for use in either hand and also so that fingers are not used for triggering motions.

Control of Forcefulness

1. Decrease the weight held in the hand by providing adjustable fixtures to hold parts being worked on. Many conventional balancers are available to neutralize tool weight. Articulating arms are used in many plants to hold and manipulate heavy tools into awkward positions.
2. Control torque reaction force in power hand tools by using torque reaction bars, torque-absorbing overhead balancers, and mounted nut-holding devices. Control the time that a worker is exposed to torque reaction by using shut-off rather than stall power tools. Avoid jerky motions by hand-held tools.
3. Design jobs so that a power grip rather than a pinch can be used whenever possible. (Maximum voluntary contraction in a power grip is approximately three times greater than in a pinch.)
4. Increase the coefficient of friction on hand tools to reduce slipperiness, for example, by use of plastic sleeves that can be slipped over metal handles of tools.
5. Design jobs so that slides or hoists are used to move parts or people, to reduce the amount of lifting, handling, or carrying of parts by the worker (Fig. 23-4).

Control of Awkward Posture

The primary method for reducing awkward postures is to design adjustability of position into the job (Fig. 23-5). Wrist, elbow, and shoulder and back postures required on a job often are determined by the height of the work surface with respect to the location of the worker. A tall worker may use less wrist flexion or ulnar deviation than a shorter

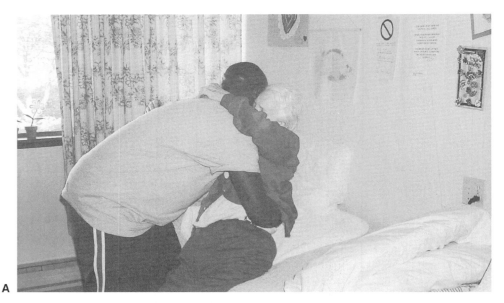

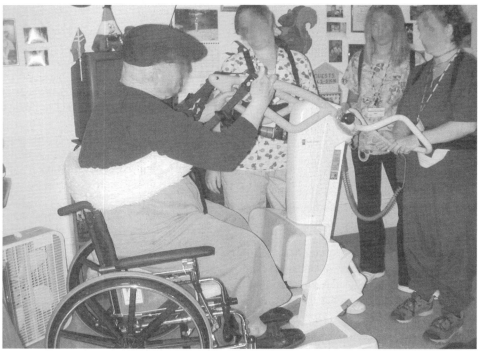

FIGURE 23-4 ● Risk of low-back injury can be reduced by using an electrical lifting device to reduce load and awkward postures. The photographs demonstrate lifting a patient without such a device (**A**) and with one (**B**). (Photographs by Barbara Silverstein.)

worker. Additionally, awkward postures can be reduced by the following procedures.

1. Alter the location or method of the work. For example, in automotive assembly operations,

changing the line location at which a particular part is installed may result in easier access.

2. Redesign tools or change the type of tool used. For example, when wrist flexion occurs with a piston-shaped tool that is used on a horizontal

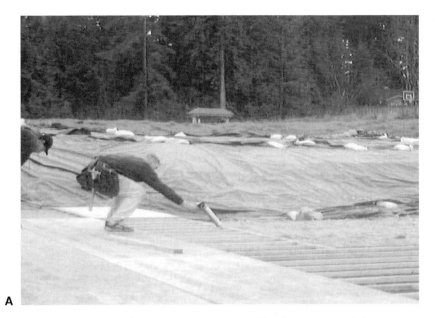

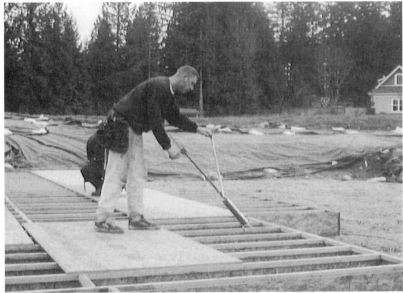

FIGURE 23-5 ● (**A**) Traditional method of applying glue to floor joists. (**B**) New method using commercially available extended gun ($50 retail). A handle was added to the gun to reduce hand/wrist fatigue (parts less than $10). Job times were the same for each of the two methods. (Photographs by Barbara Silverstein.)

surface, correction may involve use of an in-line type tool or lowering of the work station.

3. Alter the orientation of the work.

4. Avoid job tasks that require shoulder abduction or forward flexion greater than 45 degrees, elbow flexion greater than 110 degrees, wrist flexion more than 20 degrees, or extension greater than 30 degrees, or frequent neck rotation, flexion, or extension.

5. Provide support for the forearm when precise finger motions are required, to reduce static muscle loading in the arm and shoulder girdle.

Control of Vibration

1. Do not use impact wrenches or piercing hammers.
2. Use balancers, isolators, and damping materials.
3. Use handle coatings that attenuate vibrations and increase the coefficient of friction to reduce strength requirements.
4. Reduce exposure (intensity and duration of exposure) below the ACGIH standard[52] or Washington State ergonomics appendix B[19] using alternative tools.

Control of Mechanical Contact Stress

1. Round or flare the edges of sharp objects, such as guards and container edges.
2. Use different types of palm button guards, which allow room for the operator to use the button without contact with the guard.
3. Use palm pads, which may provide some protection until tools can be developed to eliminate hand hammering.
4. Use compliant cushioning material on handles or increase the length of the handles to cause the force to dissipate over a greater surface of the hand.
5. Use different-sized tools for different-sized hands.
6. Avoid narrow tool handles that concentrate large forces onto small areas of the hand.

Control of Cold and Use of Gloves

1. Properly maintain power tool air hoses to eliminate cold exhaust air leaks onto the workers' hands or arms.
2. Provide a variety of styles and sizes of gloves to ensure proper fit of gloves. Although gloves may protect the hands from cold exposures and cuts, they often decrease grip strength (requiring more forceful exertion), decrease tactile sensitivity, decrease manipulative ability, increase space requirements, and increase the risk of becoming caught in moving parts.
3. Cover only that part of the hand that is necessary for protection. Examples include use of safety tape for the fingertips with fingerless gloves and use of palm pads for the palm.

Other Prevention Strategies

A conditioning process that provides a period of time during which workers can gradually adapt their muscles and tendons to new demands can be a useful approach for workers in forceful or repetitive jobs. There is some evidence that exercise programs that combine aerobic conditioning with specific strengthening of the back and legs can reduce the frequency of recurrence of low-back pain.

Training of new workers in the most efficient and least stressful ways of performing their jobs may also be useful. Similarly, workers with symptoms may, with training, be able to adapt an equally efficient, but less stressful, work method. However, lifting-education programs have generally been ineffective at reducing the frequency of occurrence of low-back pain. Many other training activities have not been evaluated specifically. Several employers, perceiving long-term benefits from a "phasing-in period," have established transitional or training areas where employees may work at a reduced pace for a limited time. In a survey of 5,000 employers in Washington State, among those who took prevention steps, a larger percentage reported decreased number and severity of MSDs with engineering and administrative measures (such as task variety, reduced overtime) than with strictly personal controls (such as exercise programs, personal protective equipment).

Development of a replacement process to identify those persons who are at unusually high risk for development of a MSD is the least desirable prevention strategy because there are no scientifically valid screening procedures to identify which persons are at high risk. This shifts the cost of reducing the incidence of symptoms onto the workers (who are denied employment or placement) and increases the costs of the hiring and replacement processes. A recent study evaluating the practice of postoffer preplacement screening for CTS in new workers showed that this practice was not cost-beneficial to the employer.[25] Similarly, the use of preplacement screening with low-back x-rays should not be employed, as plain x-rays are not a useful predictor of future low-back disorders.

CONCLUSION

Work-related neck and low-back pain and disorders of the upper and lower extremities are together among the most common occupational health problems. Although scientific knowledge often limits our ability to determine precisely the role of occupational and nonoccupational factors in the diagnosis of these conditions, substantial progress can be made in reducing their severity by applying existing knowledge about the role of physical factors in these disorders, including forceful repetitive hand work and frequent lifting of heavy objects. Work should be designed to reduce exposure to the known physical risk factors. Encouraging employers to involve employees in decisions that affect the way they perform the job (decision latitude) and also reduce the psychological demands and increase social support will also improve employee health. Encouragement of prompt and appropriately conservative medical evaluation of workers with such disorders can contribute to secondary prevention. Early and safe return-to work made possible through ergonomic improvements and modified work regimes have had considerable success. Finally, for the minority of workers with disorders that do not respond to conservative treatment, including reduction in the level of exposure, treatment programs that address all psychosocial and physical aspects of the problem probably have the greatest chance of preventing permanent disability from these disorders.

REFERENCES

1. National Research Council and Institute of Medicine. Musculoskeletal disorders and the workplace: Low back and upper extremities. Washington, DC: National Academy Press, 2001.
2. Morse TF, Dillon C, Warren N, et al. The economic and social consequences of work-related musculoskeletal disorders: The Connecticut Upper-extremity Surveillance Project (CUSP). Int J Occup Environ Health 1998;4:209–16.
3. Silverstein BA, Stetson DS, Keyserling WM et al. Work-related musculoskeletal disorders: comparison of data sources for surveillance. Am J Ind Med 1997;31:600–608.
4. Evanoff B, Abedin S, Grayson D, et al. Is disability underreported following work injury? J Occup Rehabil 2002;12:139–50.
5. Rystrom CM, Eversmann WW Jr. Cumulative trauma intervention in industry: A model program for the upper extremity. In Kasdan ML, ed. Occupational hand and upper extremity injuries and disease. Philadelphia: Hanley and Belfus; 1991:489–505.
6. Arnetz BB, Sjogren B, Ryden B, et al. Early workplace intervention for employees with musculoskeletal-related absenteeism: a prospective controlled intervention study. J Occup Environ Med 2003;45:499–506.
7. Glass LS. Occupational medicine practice guidelines: Evaluation and management of common health problems and functional recovery in workers. 2nd ed. Beverly Farms, MA: OEM Press, 2004.
8. Loisel P, Lemaire J, Poitras S, et al. Cost-benefit and cost-effectiveness analysis of a disability prevention model for back pain management: a six year follow up study. Occup Environ Med 2002;59:807–15.
9. Melhorn JM, Wilkinson L, Gardner P, et al. An outcomes study of an occupational medicine intervention program for the reduction of musculoskeletal disorders and cumulative trauma disorders in the workplace. J Occup Environ Med 1999;41:833–46.
10. NIOSH. Musculoskeletal disorders and workplace factors: A critical review of epidemiologic evidence for work-related musculoskeletal disorders of the neck, upper extremity, and low back. Washington, DC: NIOSH, 1997.
11. Hakkanen M, Viikari-Juntura E, Martikainen R. Incidence of musculoskeletal disorders among newly employed manufacturing workers. Scand J Work Environ Health 2001;27:381–7.
12. Stauber WT. Factors involved in strain-induced injury in skeletal muscles and outcomes of prolonged exposures. J Electromyogr Kinesiol 2004;14:61–70.
13. Bongers PM, Kremer AM, Laak J. Are psychosocial factors, risk factors for symptoms and signs of the shoulder, elbow, or hand/wrist? A review of the epidemiological literature. Am J Ind Med 2002;41:315–42.
14. Karasek R, Theorell T. Healthy work: Stress, productivity, and the reconstruction of working life. New York: Basic Books, 1990.
15. Rempel D, Evanoff B, Amadio PC, et al. Consensus criteria for the classification of carpal tunnel syndrome in epidemiologic studies. Am J Public Health 1998;88:1447–51.
16. Sluiter JK, Rest KM, Frings-Dresen MHW. Criteria document for evaluating the work-relatedness of upper-extremity musculoskeletal disorders. Scand J Work Environ Health 2001;27:1–102.
17. Helliwell PS , Bennett RM, Littlejohn G, et al. Towards epidemiological criteria for soft-tissue disorders of the arm. Occup Med 2003;53:313–19.
18. Harrington JM, Birrell CL, Gompertz D. Surveillance case definitions for work related upper limb pain syndromes. Occup Environ Med 1998;55:264–71.
19. Washington State Department of Labor and Industries. WAC 296-62-051, Ergonomics, Washington State Department of Labor and Industries, Olympia, WA. 2000.
20. Ariens GA, Bongers PM, Hoogendoorn WE, et al. High physical and psychosocial load at work and sickness absence due to neck pain. Scand J Work Environ Health 2002;28:222–31.
21. Andersen JH, Kaergaard A, Frost P, et al. Physical, psychosocial, and individual risk factors for neck/shoulder pain with pressure tenderness in the muscles among workers performing monotonous, repetitive work. Spine 2002;27:660–7.
22. Andersen JH, Kaergaard A, Mikkelsen S, et al. Risk factors in the onset of neck/shoulder pain in a prospective study of workers in industrial and service companies. Occup Environ Med 2003;60:649–54.
23. Leclerc A, Landre MF, Chastang JF, et al. Upper-limb disorders in repetitive work. Scand J Work Environ Health 2001;27:268–78.
24. Descatha A, Leclerc A, Chastang JF, et al. Medial epicondylitis in occupational settings: Prevalence, incidence and associated risk factors. J Occup Environ Med 2003;45:993–1001.
25. Franzblau A, Werner RA, Yihan J. Preplacement nerve testing for carpal tunnel syndrome: Is it cost effective? J Occup Environ Med 2004;46:714–9.
26. Jordan R, Carter T, Cummins C. A systematic review of the utility of electrodiagnostic testing in carpal tunnel syndrome. Br J Gen Pract 2002;52:670–3.
27. Gerritsen AA, de Vet HC, Scholten RJ, et al. Splinting vs surgery in the treatment of carpal tunnel syndrome: a randomized controlled trial. JAMA 2002;288:1245–51.
28. Eakin JM, Clarke J, MacEachen E. Return to work in small workplaces: Sociological perspective on employers' and workers' experience with Ontario's strategy of self-reliance and early return. Toronto: Institute for Work

and Health/Institut de Recherche Sur Le Travail et La Sante, 2003. (Working paper #206.).

29. Parenmark G, Alffram P-A, Malmkvist A-K. The significance of work tasks for rehabilitation outcome after carpal tunnel surgery. J Occup Rehab 1992;2:89–94.

30. Silverstein BA, Fine LJ. Cumulative trauma disorders of the upper extremity: a preventive strategy is needed. J Occup Med 1999;33:642–4.

31. NIOSH. Elements of ergonomics programs. Washington, DC: NIOSH, 1997. (DHHS [NIOSH] publication no. 97–117.)

32. Guo HR, Tanaka S, Halperin WE, et al. Back pain prevalence in US industry and estimates of lost workdays. Am J Public Health 1999;89:1029–35.

33. Bernard BP. Musculoskeletal disorders and workplace factors: A critical review of epidemiologic evidence for work-related musculoskeletal disorders of the neck, upper extremity, and low back. Washington, DC: NIOSH, 1997. (publication no. 97–141.)

34. Dempsey PG, Burdorf A, Webster BS. The influence of personal variables on work-related low-back disorders and implications for future research. J Occup Environ Med 1997;39:748–59.

35. Bigos S, Bowyer O, Braen G. Acute low back pain problems in adults: Clinical practice guidelines no. 14. Rockville, MD: Agency for Health Care Policy and Research, 1994. (AHCPR publication no. 95-0642.)

36. Deyo RA, Weistein JN. Low back pain. N Engl J Med 2001;344:363–70.

37. Deyo RA, Rainville J, Kent DL. What can the history and physical examination tell us about low back pain? JAMA 1992;268:760–5.

38. Johanning E. Evaluation and management of occupational low back disorders. Am J Ind Med 2000;37:94–111.

39. Staiger TO, Paauw DS, Deyo RA, et al. Imaging studies for acute low back pain. Postgrad Med J 1999;105:161–72.

40. Loisel P, Abenhaim L, Durand P, et al. A population-based, randomized clinical trial on back pain management. Spine 1997;22:2911–18.

41. Parniapour M, Nordin M, Skovron ML, et al. Environmentally induced disorders of the musculoskeletal system. Med Clin North Am 1990;74:347–59.

42. Vingard E, Alfredsson L, Malchau H. Osteoarthrosis of the hip in women and its relation to physical load at work and in the home. Ann Rheum Dis 1997;56:293–8.

43. Lau EC, Cooper C, Lam D, et al. Factors associated with osteoarthritis of the hip and knee in Hong Kong Chinese: Obesity, joint injury, and occupational activities. Am J Epidemiol 2000;152:855–62.

44. Sandmark H, Hogstedt C, Vingard E. Primary osteoarthrosis of the knee in men and women as a result of lifelong physical load from work. Scand J Work Environ Health 2000;26:20–5.

45. Johanning E. Back disorder intervention strategies for mass transit operators with whole-body vibration: Comparison of two transit system approaches and practices. J Sound Vibration 1998;215(4):629–34.

46. Evanoff BA, Bohr PC, Wolf LD. Effects of a participatory ergonomics team among hospital orderlies. Am J Ind Med 1999;35:358–65.

47. ACGIH. Hand activity level. HAL-TLV & documentation. Cincinnati, OH: ACGIH, 1999.

48. Moore JS, Garg A. The strain index: A proposed method to analyze jobs for risk of distal upper extremity disorders. Am Ind Hyg Assoc J 1995;56:443–58.

49. McAtamney L. Corlett EN. RULA: A survey method for the investigation of work-related upper limb disorders. Appl Ergon 1993;24:91–9.

50. Waters TR, Putz-Anderson V, Garg A, et al. Revised NIOSH equation for the design and evaluation of manual lifting tasks. Ergonomics 1993;36:749–76.

51. ACGIH. Lifting TLV-NIE. American Conference of Governmental Hygienists Cincinnati, OH: ACGIH, 2003:115–19.

52. ACGIH. Hand arm (segmental) vibration. In ACGIH TLVs and BEIs. Cincinnati, OH: ACGIH Worldwide, 2005:122–5.

BIBLIOGRAPHY

Glass L, ed. Occupational medicine practice guidelines: American College of Occupational and Environmental Medicine. Beverly Farms, MA: OEM Press, 2004.
This guide begins with general approaches to prevention, assessment, treatment, determination of work-relatedness, disability prevention, and management. It then is organized by presenting complaints, such as the neck, upper back, and shoulder problems. Each section includes the general approach, with initial assessment, medical history, examination, diagnostic criteria, work-relatedness, treatment, and follow-up.

National Research Council and Institute of Medicine Panel on Musculoskeletal Disorders and the Workplace. Musculoskeletal disorders and the workplace. Washington, DC: National Academies Press, 2001.
This report by U.S. researchers from a wide range of relevant scientific disciplines focuses on both back and upper extremity musculoskeletal disorders. The panel considered evidence from epidemiology, tissue mechanobiology, biomechanics, occupational stress, workplace interventions, and workplace trends. The report summarizes the patterns of evidence, conclusions, and recommendations and puts forth a research agenda.

Sluiter JK, Rest KM, Frings-Dresden MH. Criteria document for evaluating the work-relatedness of upper extremity musculoskeletal disorders. Scand J Work Environ Health 2001;27(Suppl 1):1–102.
This criteria document was developed in collaboration with researchers involved in work-related musculoskeletal epidemiology throughout Europe. It provides clear guidelines for case definitions, including pictures of how to conduct the physical examination. It is based on studies of different test methods and examples of work activities that could place a worker at low, medium, or high risk for various conditions.

CHAPTER 24

Cancer

Elizabeth M. Ward

Cancer encompasses a broad spectrum of diseases that arise in various organs and tissues throughout the body and have in common the uncontrolled growth of abnormal and potentially lethal cells that lose their differentiation and survive for abnormally long times. Cancer originates with changes in DNA, or gene expression, that may be triggered by endogenous products of metabolism or exogenous chemicals; physical agents, such as ionizing radiation; or biological agents, such as viruses, other microorganisms, or their products (such as aflatoxin). Inherited genetic factors play a role in susceptibility to cancer, often by influencing how the body responds to an environmental carcinogen (gene–environment interaction). The human health effects of many recognized environmental carcinogens were first documented through studies of occupational groups with heavy, prolonged exposure.

Cancer is a major public health problem. Each year, approximately 1.2 million Americans are diagnosed with invasive cancer, and just under half this number die of various cancers. Cancer accounts for almost one-third of all deaths, second only to heart disease. Among men, prostate cancer is the most common incident cancer, followed by lung cancer and colorectal cancer; among women, breast cancer is the most common incident cancer, followed by lung cancer and colorectal cancer. In both sexes, the three most common cancer sites account for more than half of new cases. Because survival rate is worse for lung cancer than for these other common types, lung cancer is the most common cause of cancer death among both men and women.

Cancer incidence and mortality patterns shifted dramatically during the 20th century. In the United States and most developed countries, lung cancer increased sharply after World War II, peaked in men in the early 1990s, but continued to rise in women until the year 2000. Cigarette smoking has been the predominant cause of lung cancer in the general population, although widespread exposure to occupational carcinogens, such as asbestos, also contributed. Stomach cancer incidence declined steadily during the 20th century, probably due to advances in food preservation, increased availability of fresh fruits and vegetables, and decline in the prevalence of *Helicobacter pylori* infection. Cervical and uterine cancer mortality has declined because of early detection and treatment; so has colorectal cancer mortality for both men and women. Death rates from all types of cancer combined have been decreasing in the United States since the early 1990s, after increasing for several decades.

Both inherited genes and environmental factors play a role in the development of cancer. A recent study of twins concluded that environmental factors are the principal cause of most cancers, with a significant role of heritable factors for prostate cancer (42 percent of the risk may be explained by inherited genes), colorectal cancer (35 percent), and breast cancer (27 percent).[1] In the public mind, the term *environmental factors* is limited to human-made chemical exposures, especially air and water pollution; most researchers, however, use this phrase to cover all external conditions that affect human cancer, including behavioral risk factors, such as cigarette smoking, diet, and alcohol consumption. Behavioral risk factors may account for as much as 60 percent of human cancers. However, in this chapter, the focus is on involuntary environmental exposures, such as occupational chemical and radiation exposure, ambient and indoor air pollution, and infectious agents, as causes of human cancer.

Patterns of cancer and associated environmental risk factors vary between developed and developing countries. In developed countries, cancers of the lung, colon and rectum, breast, and prostate are most common, whereas in developing countries, cancer of the liver, stomach, and cervix represent a greater part of the cancer burden. In the United States and other developed countries, the most important environmental causes of cancer are cigarette smoking, dietary patterns, and physical inactivity, with smaller roles for occupational factors, viruses and other biological agents, reproductive factors, alcohol, environmental pollution, and ionizing and ultraviolet radiation. A newly recognized hazard, especially in developed countries, is overweight and obesity, which are associated with increased mortality from several cancers. In developing countries, air pollution—especially indoor air pollution—plays a significant role in the causation of lung cancer, and infectious agents play a greater role than in developed countries in causation of cancer overall.

OCCUPATIONAL AND ENVIRONMENTAL CARCINOGENS

Historically, clinicians were the first group to recognize occupational and environmental cancers. In 1761, Dr. John Hill of London published the first modern clinical report of environmental carcinogenesis—a description of cancer of the nasal passages among tobacco snuff users. In 1775, another perceptive London physician, Dr. Percival Pott, became the first to recognize an occupational cancer—scrotal skin cancer among chimney sweeps heavily exposed to soot in their work. Lung cancer in uranium miners was first noted in 1879 and urinary bladder cancers were recognized in dye industry workers in 1895. Subsequently, early occupational cohort studies documented the association of β-naphthylamine and benzidine with bladder cancer, arsenic with lung and skin cancer, and asbestos with lung cancer and pleural and peritoneal mesothelioma.

In parallel with the development of methods to elucidate the relationships between chemical exposures and cancer in humans, the foundation for study of chemical carcinogenesis in animals was established early in the 20th century. In 1918, Katsusabura Yamagawa and Koichi Ichikawa demonstrated that chronic application of coal tar to the ears of rabbits could induce skin carcinomas, and, in 1933, James Cook described the successful extraction of a crystalline substance, benzo[*a*]pyrene (BAP), responsible for the carcinogenicity of coal tar on rabbit skin. In 1968, a formal bioassay program was established at the National Cancer Institute (NCI), and, by 1978, 356 chemicals had been entered into testing. Most animal carcinogenicity testing was transferred from NCI to the National Toxicology Program (NTP) in 1981. The development of experimental models for carcinogenesis and the passage of the Occupational Safety and Health Act in 1970 stimulated many occupational cancer investigations in the 1970s and 1980s. Studies initiated during this period documented the carcinogenicity of asbestos, benzene, beryllium, bischloromethyl ether (BCME), coke oven emissions, vinyl chloride, and other widely used chemicals and environmental contaminants.

In 1981, Richard Doll and Richard Peto estimated that 4 percent of all cancer deaths in the United States were due to occupational exposures. A more recent estimate is in the same range (2.4 to 4.8 percent).[2] Cancer sites most commonly associated with occupation as well as their causes and attributable fractions are listed in Table 24-1. These data do not include cancer sites, such as stomach and pancreas, for which occupational associations have been suggested by epidemiologic studies but not well established. The proportion of cancer deaths due to occupation is likely to vary in different countries at different stages of industrialization.

Associations have also been documented between environmental pollutants and cancer. Exposure to fine particulates, including sulfates in ambient air pollution in the urban environment, environmental tobacco smoke, and radon exposure in the indoor environment have been associated with lung cancer. In developing countries, burning of solid fuels, including coal and biomass (wood, charcoal, crop residues, and dung), for heating and cooking results in high levels of indoor air pollution. Indoor air pollution from burning of solid fuel has been associated with acute and chronic respiratory disease. Studies conducted in China have associated indoor burning of coal with lung cancer. An increased risk of mesothelioma has been detected among people exposed to asbestos in their

TABLE 24-1

Estimated Number of Occupationally Related Cancer Deaths, 1997 (Selected Cancers)

Cause of Death and Exposure	Number of U.S. Deaths Male (M); Female (F)	Estimated Number of Exposed	Estimated Percent Exposed	Relative risk	Estimated Percentage due to Occupational Exposures (Attributable Fraction)	Estimated Number Occupational Deaths
Lung cancer	91,289 (M); 61,877 (F)	n.a.[a]		n.a.[a]		9,677–19,901
Chemical exposures					6.3–13.0 (combined)	
					6.1–17.3 (M); 2 (F)	6,807–17,031
ETS (never smokers only, 10% of all lung cancer deaths)					0.6 (M+F)	870
Indoor radon at work					1.3 (M+F)	2,000
Bladder cancer	7,638 (M); 3,897 (F)	n.a.[a]		n.a.[a]	7–19 (M); 3–19 (F)	651–2,191
Mesothelioma	2,081 (M); 548 (F)	n.a.[a]		n.a.[a]	85–90 (M); 23–90 (F)	1,895–2,366
Leukemia	19,038 (M+F)				0.8–2.8 (combined)	152–533
Benzene		1,000,000	0.72	2–4	0.8–2.0	
Ethylene oxide		1,000,000	0.72	1.1–3.5	0–1.6	
Ionizing radiation (100+ mSv)		61,700	0.04	1.3–2.1	<0.05	
Ionizing radiation (50–100 mSV)		70,900	0.05	1.1–1.4	<0.05	
Laryngeal cancer	3,016 (M)				1.0–20.0 (combined)	30–603
Sulfuric acid		3,000,000	4.4	1.1–5.0	0.4–15.0	
Mineral oils		4,400,000	6.4	1.1–2.0	0.6–6.0	
Skin cancer	1,407 (M)				1.5–6.0 (combined)	21–84
PAHs		8,222,800	12.0	1.1–1.5	1.2–5.7	
Arsenic		240,000	0.36	2	0.1	
Sinonasal (SN) and nasopharynx (NP) cancer	303 (SN) (M) and 436 (NP) (M)				33.0–46.0 (SN) and 30.0–42.0 (NP)	231–322 (SN and NP)
Wood dust		4,515,200	6.8	3.1 (SN); 2.4 (NP)	12.5 (SN); 8.7 (NP)	
Nickel compounds		4,000,000	6.0	2.2	6.7 (SN and NP)	
Hexavalent chromium		3,400,000	52	5.2–10.8	18.0–33.8 (SN and NP)	
Kidney cancer	7.131					0–164
Coke production		520,000	0.76	2	0.0–2.3	
Liver cancer	7,283					29–80
Vinyl chloride		320,000	0.48	2.5	0.4–1.1	
Total occupationally related cancer deaths						12,086–26,244

[a] n.a: Not applicable because the attributable fraction was derived from the literature rather than estimated from the relative risk and estimated percent exposed.

homes. Bladder, skin, and lung cancer occur more frequently after consumption of water with high arsenic content. Studies evaluating the effects of other water contaminants, such as chlorination by-products, are inconclusive.

In general, cancers caused by occupational or environmental exposures are pathologically and clinically indistinguishable from other cancers. However, some cancers have a very high probability of being occupationally or environmentally related, such as angiosarcoma of the liver due to vinyl chloride and mesothelioma caused by occupational or environmental exposure to asbestos. Documentation that an occupational or environmental exposure causes cancer in humans relies heavily on evidence from epidemiological studies. Unfortunately, given the long latency period (time from first exposure to a carcinogen to clinical disease) for cancer to develop, by the time a cancer risk can be identified in epidemiologic studies, widespread human exposure may have already occurred. Although high-quality epidemiologic data provide a strong basis for hazard identification and risk assessment, in many circumstances, it is not possible to conduct definitive studies in humans. Thus, the prevention of occupational and environmental cancer must often rely on extrapolation of findings in toxicological studies to predict effects in humans and to establish limits for human exposure.

THE PROCESS OF CARCINOGENESIS

Carcinogenesis is a multistage process characterized by four stages: initiation, promotion, malignant transformation, and tumor progression. Initiation occurs when a carcinogen interacts with DNA, most often by forming an adduct between the chemical carcinogen or one of its functional groups and a nucleotide in DNA, or by producing a strand break. If the cell divides before the damage is repaired, an alteration can become permanently fixed as a heritable error that will be passed on to daughter cells. Such heritable changes in DNA structure are called *mutations*. Many mutations have no apparent effect on gene function. However, when mutations occur in critical areas of genes that regulate cell growth, cell death, or DNA repair, the mutation may predispose toward clonal expansion and the accumulation of further genetic damage. *Promoters* are substances or processes that contribute to clonal expansion by stimulating initiated cells to replicate,

forming benign tumors or hyperplastic lesions. Promotion is thought to be completely reversible. The process of promotion does not itself cause heritable alterations or mutations. Rather it stimulates cell turnover, so that mutated cells can exploit their selective growth advantage and proliferate, increasing the probability that a cell will acquire additional mutations and become malignant. Unlike promotion, the end result of malignant transformation is irreversible. Tumor progression involves the further steps of local invasion and/or metastasis.

Many carcinogens are able to form DNA adducts, either because they are intrinsically reactive or are activated to a DNA reactive form through metabolism. Classes of organic compounds associated with cancer include alkylating agents, arylalkylating agents, and arylhydroxylamines. *Alkylating agents* are chemicals that attach alkyl groups, such as methyl or ethyl groups, to nucleotides to form DNA adducts. Examples of carcinogens in this group include nitrosamines and aflatoxin B_1, a potent liver carcinogen that can contaminate food products. *Arylalkylating agents* can transfer aromatic or multiringed compounds to a nucleotide to form an adduct. Examples of such compounds include polycyclic aromatic hydrocarbons, such as benzo[*a*]pyrene. *Arylhydroxylamines* are chemicals that transfer aromatic amines to nucleotides to form adducts. Examples of such compounds include the aromatic amines 2-naphthylamine and benzidine, responsible for very high risks of bladder cancer among exposed workers. Certain inorganic metals and minerals show carcinogenic activity in humans or animals, including arsenic, nickel, chromium, and asbestos. The mechanisms for carcinogenicity of particles and fibers include both primary genotoxicity through generation of reactive oxygen species and secondary genotoxicity through particle-induced inflammation. Particles may also carry mutagens to the surface and/or inside of cells. Ionizing radiation is a classic cancer initiator. The mechanism of carcinogenesis from ionizing radiation is believed to involve formation of mutagenic oxygen free radicals in the shell of hydration surrounding DNA. Once formed, the reactive oxygen species, such as hydroxyl radicals and hydrogen peroxide, can induce strand breaks and more than 30 different DNA adducts as well as DNA–protein cross-links.[3] Unrepaired or misrepaired DNA double-strand breaks are thought to be the principal lesions responsible for induction of genetic damage by ionizing radiation in mammalian cells, whereas base damage is generally the predominant mechanism for the production of such damage by chemical carcinogens.[4]

Metabolic activation is necessary to convert some chemicals to forms that can bond with DNA. For some well-studied chemical carcinogens, the metabolic pathways leading to activation or deactivation influence both target organ specificity and individual susceptibility. Genetic polymorphisms in metabolic enzymes are likely to affect susceptibility to occupational and environmental carcinogens. Studies have examined variation in (a) genes, such as *CYP1A1,* that code for cytochrome P450s; (b) intracellular proteins involved in the metabolism of carcinogenic polycyclic aromatic hydrocarbons (PAHs) to epoxides; (c) *GSTM1,* which codes for a cytosolic enzyme glutathione-*S*-transferase M1, which can conjugate epoxides of polycyclic aromatic hydrocarbons and aflatoxin; and (d) *NAT2,* which codes for the N-acetylation phenotype associated with metabolism of some carcinogenic aromatic amines. After a carcinogen has reached and interacted with cellular DNA, the carcinogenic process may be arrested by DNA repair or promoted by factors that increase cell replication or that interfere with the programmed death of damaged cells (*apoptosis*). Thus, the outcome of a carcinogen-DNA interaction may be influenced by factors such as cell division, clonal expression, loss of tumor suppressor function, and other genetic and epigenetic factors.

Although many mutations probably have no effect on the cell, mutations occurring in genes that regulate cell growth are the first step in the evolution of a cancer cell. During the past 20 years, more than 100 genes have been identified that can convert normal rodent cells in tissue culture to a transformed phenotype with abnormal growth characteristics in cell culture and the ability to form tumors when explanted into immunocompromised rodents. These dominant transforming genes, called *oncogenes,* encode proteins involved in signal transduction or cell-cycle regulation. Mutations in these genes may trigger production of oncogenic proteins that increase the proliferation of cells that express them. A set of recessive tumor suppressor genes has recently been identified. Deletion, point mutation, or inactivation of both gene copies allows cells to proliferate unregulated or with reduced restraints.

An oncogene is an altered form of a normal cellular gene called a proto-oncogene. *Proto-oncogenes* encode proteins that participate in the regulation of growth and/or differentiation of normal cells and are involved at various levels in signaling from the extracellular compartment to the nucleus. One of the best-studied examples is the *ras* oncogene, which was first identified in rat sarcomas. The *ras* oncogene can be activated by PAHs, *N*-nitroso compounds, and ionizing radiation, and has been found in a wide variety of human cancers, including bladder cancer, lung cancer, and other cancers of occupational and environmental importance.

Tumor suppressor genes, or *antioncogenes,* are also important. Ordinarily these function to regulate cell growth and stimulate terminal differentiation or trigger apoptosis of damaged cells. When inactivated, they fail to perform these functions, allowing neoplastic transformation to proceed. A prominent example is the *p53* gene, located on chromosome 17. Mutations in the *p53* gene have been identified in many cancers, including those of the colon, lung, liver, esophagus, breast, and reticuloendothelial and hematopoietic tissues, and in the Li–Fraumeni syndrome of familial multiple cancer susceptibility. Carcinogenic exposures such as aflatoxin and hepatitis B virus (HBV) have been associated with specific mutations on the *p53* gene, suggesting that some carcinogens may leave a unique genomic "signature." Epigenetic mechanisms for deactivation of tumor suppressor genes include methylation of DNA in the gene promoter region, a characteristic that has been observed in many cancers. Abnormal promoter hypermethylation can have the same effect as a coding region mutation in inactivating a tumor suppressor gene.[5]

Once a cell is initiated, clonal expansion may take place through a variety of mechanisms. Initiated cells may be more responsive to growth stimulation or may be unable to terminally differentiate or become resistant to apoptosis. Clonal expansion increases the probability that cells with critical mutations will acquire additional genetic damage needed for malignant transformation.

The events involved in progression are less well understood than those involved in initiation or promotion. During progression, populations of tumor cells undergo further selection, and the genome becomes unstable, causing chromosomal alterations with increasing frequency. As the progression phase ends, tumor cells have converted to the neoplastic phenotype, characterized by autonomous growth and ability to erode normal tissue barriers.

Endogenous factors, such as hormones, inflammation, and the by-products of metabolism, are major sources of initiating and promoting events.[6] Oxygen reactive species, including superoxide, hydrogen peroxide, and hydroxyl radicals, and singlet oxygen, generated by normal cellular processes including respiration, inflammation, and phagocytosis, have the ability to induce mutations. Endogenous DNA lesions are genotoxic and induce mutations that are commonly observed in mutated oncogenes and tumor suppressor genes.[7] The levels of oxidative DNA damage reported in many tissues or in animal models of carcinogenesis exceed the levels of lesions induced by exposure to exogenous carcinogenic compounds. Although it seems likely that oxidative DNA damage is important in the etiology of many human cancers, we do not know the precise role that it plays in carcinogenesis and how it synergizes with other forms of genetic and epigenetic events to accelerate cell transformation and malignant transformation.[7] The association of cancer with chronic inflammatory diseases, such as gastritis, chronic hepatitis, ulcerative colitis, and pancreatitis, may result from generation of reactive oxygen species.[6]

Endogenous and exogenous hormones also play a role in the development of cancer. Although metabolites of estradiol and estrone are genotoxic, a major action of these hormones is to accelerate the accumulation of somatic genetic errors. Endogenous and exogenous hormones play a particularly important role in the development of cancers of the breast, endometrium, ovary, and prostate. Higher cumulative exposure to estrogen and many ovulating cycles (associated with earlier menarche, later menopause, and lower parity) increases breast cancer risk. Among atomic-bomb survivors, increased risk of breast cancer was greatest among women exposed during adolescence. The developmental period when the terminal ducts and lobules of the breast have not completed differentiation may be a time of increased susceptibility to exogenous carcinogens.[8] Hormonal medications may have opposing effects in different organs. Oral contraceptives cause a small increase in breast cancer, but a large decrease in ovarian cancer. Tamoxifen, a weak estrogen agonist, is effective in treatment of breast cancer and in the prevention of breast cancer for high-risk women but is considered a carcinogen because it increases risk of endometrial cancer.

Environmental and occupational health researchers have increasingly focused on the potential health effects of *environmental endocrine disrupters,* defined as exogenous agents that interfere with the synthesis, secretion, transport, binding, action, or elimination of natural hormones in the body. Environmental contaminants, such as polychlorinated biphenyls (PCBs), dioxins, furans, phthalates, and some pesticides may have both estrogenic and antiestrogenic effects. Despite widespread concern about whether exposure to these contaminants can influence the development of cancers, especially those of the male and female reproductive system, studies thus far have not yielded strong evidence of such effects. However, elevations in these cancer rates may be difficult to detect in general population studies where exposures are low-level and ubiquitous.

In summary, the development of cancer is a multistage process, involving the activation of oncogenes, deactivation of tumor suppressor genes, disruption of DNA processes, and progressive genetic deterioration. In most instances, the process of carcinogenesis involves a series of probabilistic events, in which both exogenous exposures and endogenous factors influence the outcome. Substances that have been formally classified as carcinogens are those in which the increase in cancer risk in humans or animals has been sufficiently large to be detected in toxicologic and epidemiologic studies.

IDENTIFICATION OF POTENTIAL CARCINOGENS

Predictions Based on Chemical Structure

Knowledge about the relationship of chemical structure and carcinogenic activity can be used to identify potential chemical carcinogens. Computerized databases of carcinogenic and noncarcinogenic chemicals have been developed to relate structure to carcinogenic activity. Using results of rodent bioassays of more than 300 chemicals, John Ashby and David Paton developed a list of chemical structures that correlate with tumorogeneticity in rodent tests. These characteristics, or *structural alerts,* indicate chemicals that should be tested extensively and monitored for evidence of carcinogenicity.[9] However, studies comparing the results of widely used computer programs with *in vitro* studies have found only limited concordance.[10]

Toxicologic Testing

Short-Term Tests

Various short-term tests have been developed to detect mutagenicity. Among these, the *Ames assay* has been the best studied and most extensively used. This test uses special strains of *Salmonella typhimurium* that are deficient in DNA repair and cannot grow in the absence of histidine. Cell cultures are treated with several dose levels of the substance being tested. The cells are then tested for growth in the absence of histidine, which indicates reversion to the histidine-positive phenotype. Homogenates of mammalian liver may be added to the incubation mixture to allow detection of carcinogens that require metabolic activation. *In vitro* mammalian cell mutation assays also exist, including the mouse lymphoma L5178Y (MOLY) assay and the Chinese hamster ovary (CHO) assay. Other short-term tests involve both *in vitro* and *in vivo* (in animals) induction of chromosome aberrations, sister chromatid exchanges (SCEs), and micronuclei. The concordance between short-term tests of mutagenicity and the results of chronic bioassays (animal tests) depends on the databases selected for comparison; in general, the concordance has declined over time as an increasing proportion of nongenotoxic carcinogens have been tested in rodent bioassays. A recent analysis of 59 chemicals classified by the International Agency for Research on Cancer (IARC) as human carcinogens or probable human carcinogens (Group 1 or 2A) that had been tested for mutagenicity by multiple methods found positive results on the *Salmonella* assay for 38 (67 percent) of the 57 chemicals tested. A total of 93 percent were mutagenic in mammalian tests *in vivo* or *in vitro*.[11] Based on the accumulated information, it has been recommended that screening protocols for genetic effects *in vitro* include tests for gene mutation in *Salmonella* and/or mammalian cells and for chromosome aberrations and numerical chromosome changes (aneuploidy) in mammalian cells.[12] Some carcinogens are not detected by mutagenicity assays, including hormonal carcinogens, some metals, agents that have a multiple-target-organ mode of action, and agents with a nongenotoxic mode of action.

Chronic 2-Year Bioassay

The "gold standard" for determining the potential carcinogenic activity of a chemical is the *2-year bioassay* in rodents. This assay involves test groups of 50 rats and 50 mice of both sexes and at two or three doses of the test agent. In the United States, the B6C3F1 mouse and the F344 rat are commonly used. At about 8 weeks of age, test animals are placed on the test agent (or placebo) for the remaining 96 weeks of their life span. The test agent may be administered in feed, by gavage, or by in-

halation. The maximum dose level used in a 2-year bioassay is determined by the estimated maximally tolerated dose (MTD), usually derived from a 90-day study. The MTD is defined by the Environmental Protection Agency (EPA) as "the highest dose that causes no more than a 10 percent weight decrement, as compared to appropriate control groups; and does not produce mortality, clinical signs of toxicity, or pathological lesions (other than those that may be related to a neoplastic response) that would be predicted to shorten the animal's natural lifespan." Controversy exists around the use of the MTD, with some scientists claiming that it is not high enough to elicit the anticipated effects, and others voicing concern that the MTD is too high, it may overwhelm host defenses against low exposure levels, and may induce cancer because of toxicity and abnormal cell proliferation. In any case, high exposure levels are necessary to provide meaningful results without requiring studies that are prohibitively large and costly.

Even with the use of high exposure levels, the high cost of 2-year bioassays, estimated to be more than $1 million per chemical, limits the number of tests that can be conducted. Genetically altered mice are being evaluated as possible replacements for, or adjuncts to, conventional rodents for bioassays of chemical carcinogenesis. Some researchers speculate that transgenic mice will be well suited to identifying human carcinogens because they already possess altered genes known to be involved in human cancer.[13] However, the results of transgenic carcinogenesis testing must be well validated against known and probable human carcinogens before they can be used for risk assessment. Currently, the 2-year bioassay remains the only widely accepted indicator of carcinogenic potential to humans by international and national health and regulatory agencies.

Many substances that are carcinogenic in rodent bioassays have not been adequately studied in humans, usually because an adequate study population has not been identified. Among the substances that have proved carcinogenic in animals, all have shown positive results in well-conducted 2-year bioassays. Moreover, between 25 and 30 percent of established human carcinogens were first identified through animal bioassays. Because animal tests necessarily use high-dose exposures, in most cases, human risk assessment requires extrapolating the exposure-response relationship observed in rodent bioassays at higher doses to predict effects in humans at lower doses. There are uncertainties in both high- and low-dose extrapolation from animal cancer bioassays to humans. Typically, regulatory agencies in the United States have adopted the default assumption that no threshold level of exposure exists for carcinogenesis. For some chemicals, mechanistic hypotheses have been advanced to suggest that there may be a threshold, but for most carcinogens, it is considered infeasible to generate empirical data on the exposure–response curves at low levels to confirm or refute these hypotheses.

Whereas the presence or absence of carcinogenicity is similar across many species, the target organ affected by cancer may vary largely because of differing metabolic pathways. Benzidine, for example, causes bladder cancer in humans, hepatomas in mice, and intestinal tumors in rats. One database in which the results of animal bioassays are tabulated is the Carcinogenic Potency Database, maintained by the Lawrence Berkeley Laboratory and the University of California, Berkeley. Results are published annually in the journal *Environmental Health Perspectives* and are available at the journal's Web site, <ehp.niehs.nih.gov>.

Studies in Humans

Cohort and Case-Control Studies

Two major epidemiologic study designs, cohort and case-control studies, have contributed substantially to understanding occupational and environmental cancer. (General aspects of the design and analysis of both types of studies are covered in Chapter 8 and in textbooks of epidemiology.) *Cohort studies* follow a defined group of people forward in time and compare disease incidence or mortality rates among exposed and unexposed persons. *Retrospective cohort studies* define the study population at some point in the past and follow the group forward to the present; *prospective cohort studies* define the population in the present and follow it for disease occurrence into the future. Cohort studies can be conducted in the general population if the exposures of interest are common, such as smoking or diet. Cohort studies of rare exposures are usually conducted in special populations selected based on their exposure history. Cohort studies often focus on a single exposure and multiple disease end-points; outcomes measured may be intermediate markers, incident disease, or death.

Occupational cohort studies have played a particularly important role in the understanding of cancers related to industrial chemicals because occupational exposures are often orders of magnitude higher than exposures in the general population. As early as the 1950s, occupational cohort studies documented the risk of cancer associated with occupational exposure to aromatic amines (beta-naphthylamine and benzidine) and asbestos. Many occupational cohort studies have used duration of employment in the occupation or industry under study as an index of cumulative exposure. The development of methods to measure air concentrations of chemicals in the workplace has enabled researchers to generate quantitative estimates of exposure and conduct exposure–response analyses. In some studies, exposure estimates are generated for multiple agents in a single population, with the goal of evaluating which agents are associated with cancer excesses. For example, in a study of the synthetic rubber industry, quantitative estimates of exposure to 1,3-butadiene, styrene, and benzene were developed to evaluate exposure–response relationships with leukemia.[14]

Prospective study cohorts may also be established to study the health effects of occupational exposures. These studies offer the advantage of obtaining and updating exposure information as the exposure occurs rather than estimating it retrospectively. In the United States, a large prospective cohort has been established of registered pesticide applicators in two states; early findings of this study include an association between methyl bromide (a fumigant that has been used in agriculture and structural fumigation) and prostate cancer.[15]

Cohort studies have also been conducted among individuals in selected groups of the population who experienced large, short-term exposure to a chemical or physical agent due to accidental or intentional release. For example, the study of atomic-bomb survivors in Hiroshima and Nagasaki has been central to studying the consequences of ionizing radiation. Other prospective study cohorts (or registries) have been established for individuals exposed to 2,3,7,8-tetrachlorodibenzo-*p*-dioxin (TCDD) after an accidental release in Seveso, Italy, in 1976, and persons exposed to radioactive isotopes after a nuclear reactor malfunctioned in Chernobyl, Ukraine, in the Soviet Union, in 1986.

Cohorts may also be assembled from the general population without regard to a specific exposure, and subsequently many different exposures can be studied. For example, a prospective mortality study (Cancer Prevention Study, or CPS II), of about 1.2 million U.S. men and women was begun by the American Cancer Society (ACS) in 1982. Data collected at baseline included personal identifiers, demographic characteristics, personal and family history of cancer and other diseases, reproductive history, and information on behavioral, environmental, occupational, and dietary exposures. Analyses from this study have examined the adverse health effects associated with occupational exposure to diesel exhaust, air pollution, and environmental tobacco smoke.

For many occupational and environmental chemicals of interest, it has not been possible to identify exposed cohorts for definitive epidemiologic studies. Minimum requirements for a cohort study to be informative are sufficient elapsed time from initial exposure for cancer to develop, adequate population size to detect an effect, and ability to exclude or control for other exposures that are present and may produce the same effects. In addition, mortality is a good outcome measure for cancers that have a high case-fatality rate, such as lung cancer, but a poor measure for cancers of the larynx and bladder, which have a low case-fatality rate. Inadequate data on historical exposures may produce false-negative results, especially when cohorts with widely diverse levels of exposure are studied and it not possible to differentiate those with higher and lower levels of exposure.

Case-control studies compare exposures of individuals with and without disease to potential risk factors. Case-control studies may be community-based or nested within cohorts. In *community-based case-control studies,* information about risk factors is usually obtained directly from study subjects; additional exposure measurements may be made in the environment or in biological tissues or environmental exposures, and supplemental information may be obtained from medical or other records. Case-control studies are particularly useful for studying rare diseases; they examine the relationship between a single outcome and multiple exposures.

The case-control design has played an important role in the understanding of lifestyle, infectious, and familial risk factors for cancer, and in generating and testing hypotheses about environmental and occupational causes. For example, the first evidence for a strong association between cigarette smoking and lung cancer was derived from five case-control studies published in 1950. Case-control studies have also been very useful in establishing attributable risks (proportion of cases associated with

a risk factor) for various occupations and exposures for cancers with a significant occupational component. Improvements in the methodology of case-control studies may increase their ability to generate risk estimates based on semiquantitative or quantitative exposure metrics.

Ecologic studies have also contributed to assessing the role of environmental (noninherited) causes of cancer. Geographic variation in cancer incidence worldwide and within the United States is considerable (Fig. 24-1); correlations between site-specific cancer incidence and dietary and other risk factors may lead to potential clues about cancer etiology. Studies looking at such correlations on a population level are termed *ecologic studies;* the unit of observation is a group and not an individual. Because many unmeasured factors also vary in addition to the exposure of interest, ecologic studies are more useful for hypothesis generation than hypothesis testing. Studies in migrants have been used to assess the contribution of environmental and heritable factors to variations in cancer rates in different parts of the world. Migrant studies compare (a) disease rates in migrants with rates in their country of origin (populations of similar genetic background but living in different environments) or (b) disease rates in migrants with rates in their host country (populations of different genetic background living in the same environment). For example, breast cancer incidence rates have historically been four to seven times higher in the United States than China or Japan; however, when Chinese or Japanese women migrate to the United States, breast cancer risk rises within a few generations and approaches that of U.S. whites, suggesting an important role for factors related to "Western lifestyle."

When interpreting data on associations between occupational or environmental exposures and risk of cancer, it is important to understand the principle that "absence of evidence (of risk) is not evidence of absence (of risk)."[16] Negative studies may fail to detect a true risk because of flaws in design or analysis or because of limitations in the study that could not be overcome, such as a small population exposed to the agent of interest. When epidemiologic study results do not demonstrate significant associations between a potentially carcinogenic exposure and increased risk of cancer, some important questions to ask are, Was the latency inadequate to observe an effect? What level of increased risk between the exposure and disease of interest could be detected, given the sample size? How was the exposure

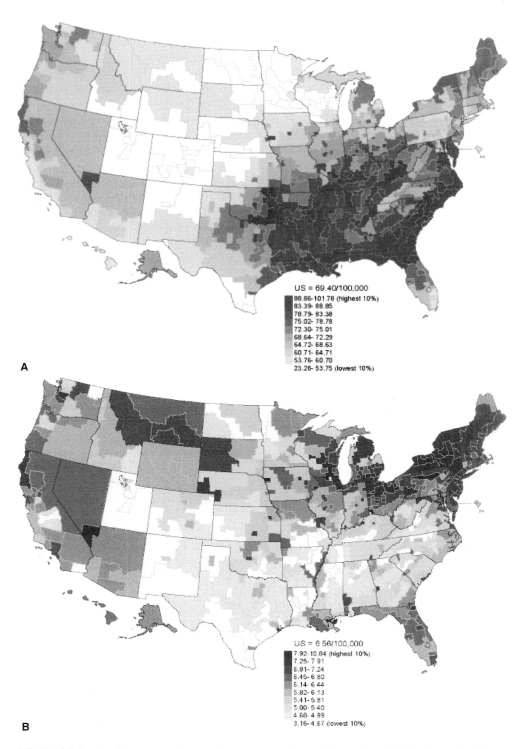

FIGURE 24-1 ● Cancer mortality rates by state economic area (age-adjusted 1970 U.S. population), white males, 1970–1994. (**A**) Cancer of the lung, trachea, bronchus, and pleura. (**B**) Bladder cancer. (From Devesa SS, Grauman DJ, Blot WJ, et al. Atlas of cancer mortality in the United States, 1950–94. [NIH Publication No. (NIH) 99-4564]. Washington, DC: US Government Printing Office; 1999. Available at: <http://www3.cancer.gov/atlasplus/>.) Examining geographic patterns can sometimes yield clues to occupational and environmental causes of cancer. (See Devesa SS, Grauman DJ, Blot WJ. Recent cancer patterns among men and women in the United States: Clues for occupational research. J Occup Med 1994;36:832–841.)

defined, and what was the level of exposure? Were adequate methods employed to detect the diseases and exposures of interest?

When positive epidemiologic study results are considered in the evaluation of a potential carcinogen, one of the most important questions is, Could the results be due to confounding? *Confounding* occurs when an extraneous factor distorts the apparent association between the exposure and outcome of interest and may suggest an association between and exposure and an outcome when in fact none exists. Confounding requires that the extraneous variable must be associated with both the exposure under study and the disease but not be in the pathway between exposure and disease. In occupational studies, concerns about confounding may relate to a higher prevalence of adverse lifestyle factors, such as cigarette smoking in the study population than the referent population, and also to the presence of confounding exposures in the work environment. It has been shown, however, that even for lung cancer, differences in smoking habits between an occupational group and the general population from which referent rates are derived are unlikely to result in a relative risk or standardized mortality ratio (SMR) greater than 1.2–1.4.[17] With regard to concomitant exposures in the work environment, it may or may not be possible to control for potential confounding. For example, in a study of bladder cancer incidence related to occupational exposure to *o*-toluidine and aniline, the presence of vinyl chloride would not be considered a confounding exposure, because vinyl chloride does not cause bladder cancer. In contrast, simultaneous exposure to aniline and *o*-toluidine could result in confounding, because both chemicals have evidence for carcinogenicity in animals and are aromatic amines, a class of chemicals likely to cause bladder cancer.

CLASSIFICATION OF CARCINOGENS

In 1969, IARC initiated its monograph program to evaluate the carcinogenic risk of chemicals to humans and to produce monographs on individual chemicals. (Information on the program can be obtained at <monographs.iarc.fr/>.) The program assembles international groups of experts to critically review and evaluate evidence on the carcinogenicity of a wide range of human exposures. Published data regarding an agent, mixture, or exposure circumstance are reviewed to determine the level of evidence for carcinogenicity in humans and experimental animals. The criteria for sufficient evidence of carcinogenicity are quite stringent. For humans, sufficient evidence for carcinogenicity requires that "…a positive relationship has been observed between the exposure and cancer in studies in which chance, bias and confounding could be ruled out with reasonable confidence." For animals, sufficient evidence for carcinogenicity requires "…an increased incidence of malignant neoplasms in (a) two or more species of animals or (b) in two or more independent studies in one species carried out at different times or in different laboratories or under different protocols. Rarely, a single study in one species may be considered to have sufficient evidence of carcinogenicity when malignant neoplasms occur to an unusual degree with regard to incidence, site, type of tumor, or age at onset." Based on separate evaluations of carcinogenicity in humans and experimental animals, the agent, mixture, or exposure circumstance is classified into one of five groups:

Group 1 - Carcinogenic to humans: This category is used primarily when sufficient evidence exists to demonstrate carcinogenicity in humans.

Group 2A - Probably carcinogenic to humans: This category is most often used when there is limited evidence of carcinogenicity in humans and sufficient evidence for carcinogenicity in animals.

Group 2B - Possibly carcinogenic to humans: This category denotes limited evidence of carcinogenicity in humans and less than sufficient evidence of carcinogenicity in animals, or inadequate evidence for carcinogenicity in humans, but sufficient evidence of carcinogenicity in animals.

Group 3 - Not classifiable as to its carcinogenicity in humans.

Group 4 - Probably not carcinogenic to humans.

IARC policy has been to recommend treating Group 2A and 2B chemicals as if they present a carcinogenic risk to humans. Using this classification, IARC has evaluated more than 885 chemicals, industrial processes, and personal habits. It has classified 88 agents, mixtures, and exposure circumstances in Group 1, 64 in Group 2A, 236 in Group 2B, 496 in Group 3, and 1 in Group 4. Tables 24-2 and 24-3 list agents, mixtures, and exposure circumstances (such as industrial processes) in Group 1 and Group 2A, for which exposures are predominantly occupational or environmental.

The National Toxicology Program (NTP) also has a systematic process for evaluating human

TABLE 24-2

Established Human Carcinogens (Group 1) with Potential for Occupational or Environmental Exposure (IARC Group 1): Chemicals and Mixtures[a]

Exposures	Examples of Occurrence	Primary Target Organs
Aflatoxins	Grains, peanuts (farm workers)	Liver
4-Aminobiphenyl	Dye and rubber industry	Bladder
Arsenic and its compounds	Insecticides	Lung, skin, hemangiosarcoma
Asbestos	Insulation, friction products	Lung, mesothelioma, respiratory tract, gastrointestinal system
Benzene	Chemical industry	Leukemia
Benzidine	Rubber and dye industries	Bladder
Beryllium and its compounds	Aerospace, nuclear, electric, and electronics industries	Lung
Bis(chloromethyl)ether and chloromethyl methyl ether	Chemical industry	Lung
Cadmium and its compounds	Metalworking industry, batteries, soldering, coatings	Prostate
Chromium (VI) compounds	Metal plating, pigments	Lung
Coal tar pitches	Coal distillation	Skin, scrotum, lung, bladder
Coal tars	Coal distillation	Skin, lung
Dioxin, 2,3,7,8-tetrachlorodibenzo-	Herbicide production and application	All sites combined, lung
Erionite	Environmental (Turkey)	Multiple (see asbestos)
Ethylene oxide	Sterilant in health care settings; chemical component	Lymphoma, leukemia
Hepatitis B and C viruses	Health care settings	Liver
HIV	Health care settings	Kaposi sarcoma, lymphoma
Mineral oils	Machining, jute processing	Skin
Mustard gas	Production, war gas	Lung
2-Naphthylamine	Rubber and dye industries	Bladder
Neutrons	Radiation workers	Unknown
Nickel compounds	Nickel refining and smelting	Nose, lung
Phosphorus-32, as phosphate	Phosphate mining and processing	Lung
Plutonium-239 and decay products, as aerosols	Plutonium production workers	Lung, liver, bone
Radon and its decay products	Indoor environments, mining	Lung
Radionuclides, alpha-emitting, internally deposited	Fallout from nuclear explosions and reactor accidents	Lung, bone, leukemia
Radionuclides, beta-emitting, internally deposited	Fallout from nuclear explosions and reactor accidents	Thyroid, bone
Radium 222, 224, 226, and 228 and decay products	Uranium mining and milling	Lung
Schistosoma hematobium infection	Farming and other outdoor work in endemic areas	Bladder
Shale oils	Energy production	Skin

(continued)

TABLE 24-2 (Continued)

Established Human Carcinogens with Potential for Occupational or Environmental Exposure (IARC Group 1): Chemicals and Mixtures[a]

Exposures	Examples of Occurrence	Primary Target Organs
Silica, crystalline	Hard rock mining, sandblasting, glass and porcelain manufacturing	Lung
Solar radiation	Outdoor work	Skin
Soots	Chimneys, furnaces	Skin, lung
Sulfuric acid-containing strong inorganic acid mists	Metal, fertilizer, battery, and petrochemical industries	Larynx, lung, ? nasal sinus
Talc (with asbestiform fibers)	Talc mining, pottery manufacturing	Multiple (see asbestos)
Vinyl chloride	Plastic industry	Hemangiosarcoma
X- and gamma radiation	Medical, nuclear fuel cycle	Leukemia, thyroid, breast
Wood dust	Wood and furniture industries	Nose, sinuses

Exposure circumstances (industrial processes)

Aluminum production
Auramine manufacturing
Boot and shoe manufacturing and repair
Coal gasification
Coke production
Furniture and cabinet making
Hematite mining (with radon exposure)
Inorganic acid mists, strong, containing sulfuric acid
Iron and steel founding
Isopropyl alcohol manufacturing (strong acid process)
Magenta manufacturing
Painter (occupational exposure as)
Rubber industry

[a] Other carcinogens, including medications (especially cancer chemotherapeutic agents, a risk for health care workers), foods, tobacco, and viruses, are classified in group 1 but are not listed here.
Source: Adapted and updated from Stellman JM, Stellman SD. Cancer and the workplace. CA Cancer J Clin 1996;46:70–92. Up-to-date IARC evaluation data can be found at the IARC Web site, <http://www.iarc.fr>, or more specifically at the Monographs Database Web page, <http://193.51.164.11/>.

carcinogens, which classifies agents, substance mixtures, or exposure circumstances as "Known to be Human Carcinogens" or "Reasonably Anticipated to be Human Carcinogens." The 10th Report on Carcinogens, issued in 2002, listed 52 substances as known to be human carcinogens and 176 as reasonably anticipated to be human carcinogens.

During the past decade, the interpretation of bioassay results by the IARC Monograph Program has been modified to consider potential species differences. For example, a workshop held at IARC in 1997 on "species differences in thyroid, kidney and urinary bladder carcinogenesis" concluded that the "carcinogenic activity detected only in the thyroid

TABLE 24-3

Probable Human Occupational Carcinogens (IARC Group 2A): Chemicals and Mixtures[a]

Exposures	Examples of Occurrence
Acrylamide	Polyacrylamide manufacturing
Benz[a]anthracene	Coal distillation
Benzidine-based dyes	Dye industry
Benzo[a]pyrene	Coal and petroleum-derived products
1,3-Butadiene	Polymer and latex production
Captafol	Fungicide
alpha-Chlorinated toluenes	Plastics industry
4-Chloro-ortho-toluidine	Dye and chlordimeform manufacture
Creosotes	Wood preservatives
Dibenz[a,h]anthracene	Coal distillation
Diesel engine exhaust	Motor vehicles
Diethyl sulfate	Petrochemical industry
Dimethylcarbamoyl chloride	Chemical manufacturing
1,2-Dimethylhydrazine	Rocket propellants and fuels, boiler water treatments, chemical reactants, medicines, cancer research
Dimethyl sulfate	Former war gas, now used in chemical industry
Epichlorhydrin	Resin manufacturing, solvent
Ethylene dibromide	Fumigant, gasoline additive
Formaldehyde	Chemical manufacturing; tissue preservative
Glycidol	Chemical intermediate, sterilant
4,4′-methylene bis(2-chloroaniline) (MOCA)	Resin manufacturing
N-nitrosodiethylamine	Solvent
N-nitrosodimethylamine	Solvent
Nonarsenical insecticides	Agriculture
Polychlorinated biphenyls (PCBs)	Electrical equipment
Styrene-7,8-oxide	Chemical industry
Tetrachlorethylene	Dry cleaning
ortho-Toluidine	Diazo dye manufacturing
Trichloroethylene	Metal degreasing
1,2,3-Trichloropropane	Pesticide; rubber manufacturing; solvent
Tris(2,3-dibromopropyl)phosphate	Flame retardant, polystyrene foam manufacturing
Ultraviolet radiation A, B, and C	Outdoor work
Vinyl bromide	Plastic industry
Vinyl fluoride	Chemical industry

Industrial processes

Art glass, glass containers, and pressed ware
   (manufacture of)

Hairdresser or barber (occupational exposure as a)

Petroleum refining (occupational exposures in)

[a] Other probable carcinogens, including medications (especially cancer chemotherapeutic agents, a risk for health care workers), infectious agents, and foods, are classified in group 2A but are not listed here.

Source: Adapted and updated from Stellman JM, Stellman SD. Cancer and the workplace. CA Cancer J Clin 1996;46:70–92. Up-to-date IARC evaluation data can be found at the IARC Web site, <http://www.iarc.fr>, or more specifically at the Monographs Database Web page, <http://193.51.164.11/>.

follicular epithelium in rodents in association with a defined hormonal mechanism, in the male rat renal cortex in the presence of alpha-2-microglobulin-induced nephropathy or in the urinary bladder in rodents in the presence of urinary precipitates or calculi" may not be predictive of cancer in humans. These criteria and some of the evaluations in which they have been applied have been controversial.[18]

CARCINOGENS AND PUBLIC HEALTH

Cancer Risk Assessment

Risk assessment is a procedure for characterizing and quantifying the amount of harm expected to result from an exposure. This process was developed in the 1970s as regulatory agencies attempted to set permissible levels of exposure, based on acceptable levels of risk, and to quantify the amount of benefit that would be expected from regulation at a particular level. Although risk assessment is a generic process that can be applied to any risk, including nonmalignant diseases, it is discussed in this chapter because it arose in the context of cancer risk.

Four basic components of risk assessment were described by the National Research Council in 1983:

- Hazard identification involves a review of the relevant biological and chemical information bearing on whether an agent may pose a carcinogenic hazard.
- Dose–response assessment involves quantifying a dosage and evaluating its relation to the incidence of adverse health effects.
- Exposure assessment involves making qualitative or quantitative estimates of the magnitude, duration, and route of exposure.
- Risk characterization is an integration and summary of all of the preceding elements, presented with assumptions and uncertainties. This final step provides an estimate of the risk to public health and a framework to define the significance of the risk.

In *risk characterization,* the exposure level that will lead to a particular magnitude of risk is estimated, using mathematical models. Different models, based on different biological assumptions, yield different results. Because risk assessment always involves some estimates, uncertainty factors are often used to introduce margins of safety. Physiolog-

ically based pharmacokinetic (PBPK) models have recently been used to refine the predictions made when extrapolating animal data to humans and to assess the human relevance of certain animal tumors.

Risk assessment offers a quantitative approach to assessing the risk of exposures. If the aim of public policy is to control rather than eliminate carcinogenic exposures, then risk assessment provides a framework for deciding how much exposure to permit—the basis of regulations. Risk assessment is transparent, in that the assumptions used are generally made explicit. However, critics point out that many of these assumptions, such as cross-species extrapolation and linear extrapolation to low doses, do not eliminate important scientific uncertainties. Moreover, risk assessment is typically performed on one substance at a time, whereas real exposures do not occur in isolation. Finally, risk assessment raises ethical concerns, as those who bear the risk are not those who profit from the manufacturing enterprise nor are they usually represented in the process of quantifying and allocating risk.

Cancer Clusters

A *cluster* refers to an unusual aggregation of health events that are grouped together in time and space. Although clusters may be identified through routine surveillance, more often suspected clusters are reported to public health agencies by concerned citizens. Responses to inquiries about perceived environmental clusters may consume substantial resources on the part of public health agencies yet rarely lead to the identification of etiologic agents. Those clusters that have identified previously unrecognized carcinogens have been clusters of extremely rare diseases and/or clusters of disease in well-defined populations. Historically, the investigation of occupational cancer clusters has led to the identification of several human carcinogens. For example, the association between vinyl chloride monomer and angiosarcoma of the liver and between bischloromethyl ether (BCME) and oat cell carcinoma of the lung were first suspected on recognizing a cluster of cases at a single company.

Occupational Cancer Clusters

Although investigations of occupational cancer clusters have sometimes led to identification of new hazards, more often concerns about clusters arise from misperceptions of normal patterns of cancer occurrence in working populations. Overall, 46 percent of U.S. men and 38 percent of U.S. women will be diagnosed with cancer at some time in their lifetime, thus the occurrence of multiple cancers in any given workforce is not an uncommon event. An approach taken by some larger corporations, which allows them to respond quickly to concerns about cancer clusters and to monitor and detect any unusual mortality patterns, is to develop mortality surveillance databases. Optimally, a file can be developed of all workers employed by a company in a given period of time, who can then be followed to determine vital status and causes of death. Surveillance systems based on death certificates alone (proportionate mortality ratio, or PMR, analyses) have also been used. Ideally, work history and exposure information should be included in surveillance databases, so that the mortality experience of workers with and without exposures of concern can be contrasted. However, if this is not feasible, nested case-control studies can be performed to evaluate job and exposure histories for cancers or other diseases that appear to be in excess.

When concern about a cancer cluster arises in a company with an ongoing surveillance program, it may be possible to determine fairly quickly if the number of cases or deaths exceeds the number that would be expected.

In the absence of a surveillance system, investigation of a cancer cluster in the workplace involves a number of steps. The first is to obtain a list of the cancer cases on which the suspicion is based, with as much work history and clinical information as possible. It is important, for example, to know the date of onset of each cancer and the date of hire at the plant of each cancer patient, because cancers diagnosed before or shortly after hire should be excluded from consideration. It is also important to discern whether the cancers are primary or secondary, especially for sites such as liver and brain, where metastatic lesions are common. A suspected cluster based on a variety of common cancer types arising at expected ages is less likely to be occupationally related than a cluster of one type of cancer, especially if the latter is at an uncommon anatomical site or of an uncommon histological type or is occurring at younger ages than expected. Similarly, a suspected cluster arising from individuals with diverse jobs and exposures is less likely to be occupationally associated than one arising among workers employed in a common department or with similar exposures. Often, occupational cancer clusters represent cases from current, former, and retired workers. It is very difficult to estimate the number of expected cases in the population at risk, which might include all workers employed at the facility from the time it opened. The number of expected deaths from any specific cancer in that population depends on the total number of workers, when they were hired, their age at hire, and gender and race distribution. It is difficult to estimate this number accurately without conducting a full cohort mortality study. In evaluating a potential cancer cluster, it is also important to develop information about the workplace exposures at present and in the past. In those workplaces with exposures to confirmed or suspected carcinogens, concern about the potential cluster should be heightened. It is wise to get advice from experts early in the process to ensure that planned investigations are well designed and likely to yield useful information. It is particularly important that this process be perceived as open, with involvement of management and nonmanagement personnel and experts who are considered to be objective and credible.

Community Cancer Clusters

Each year, state and local health departments in the United States respond to more than 1,000 inquiries about suspected cancer clusters. Most states have developed a stepwise approach to triage requests from the public, using established criteria to determine their response. Most of the inquiries about cancer clusters to state health departments are situations that are clearly not clusters and can be resolved by telephone. For the remainder, follow-up is needed, first to confirm the number of persons affected, their age, type of cancer, dates of diagnosis, and other factors, and then to compare cancer incidence in the affected population with background rates in state tumor registries.

Not all suspected cancer clusters can or should be investigated extensively. Increasingly, epidemiologic studies of the community are only conducted when the following conditions are met:

1. The observed number of cases of a specific type of cancer significantly exceeds the number expected.
2. Either the type of cancer or age at onset is highly unusual.
3. The population at risk can be defined.
4. Prolonged exposures to known or suspected carcinogens at levels that exceed environmental limits can be documented.

Rigorous documentation and investigation of a cancer cluster is generally an expensive, multiyear process, complicated by anxiety and pressure to generate information quickly. For example, in 1999, what appeared to be an excessive number of children diagnosed with leukemia while living in Churchill County, Nevada, was brought to the attention of the Nevada State Health Department. After an extensive case-finding effort, it was confirmed that between 1997 and 2002, 16 children who lived in the county at the time of, or prior to, diagnosis were known to have developed leukemia. Among the 16 children, 11 lived in the county at the time of diagnosis, whereas only one case in a child would have been expected. Statistical testing indicated that the likelihood that this cluster was a random event was very small. Although the number of childhood leukemia cases was unusual, the distribution of leukemia cell types was not. The Nevada State Health Department, in collaboration with the Centers for Disease Control and Prevention (CDC) and other agencies, conducted extensive sampling in the county, testing for heavy metals, persistent and nonpersistent pesticides, polychlorinated biphenyls (PCBs), and volatile organic compounds (VOCs). Environmental samples were tested for radon and other radioactive elements. Levels of most contaminants measured were not elevated compared with national referent data or existing environmental standards, and none of the measured contaminants were associated with the occurrence of childhood leukemia. Investigations were also made of records concerning historical exposures in the community and possible exposures from a nearby naval air station. Although the investigation documented elevated levels of arsenic and tungsten in the municipal water supply, an expert panel concluded that this was not a likely explanation for the childhood leukemia cluster, because arsenic does not seem to be related to childhood leukemia, and elevated levels of tungsten are found in many parts of Nevada. The incidence of leukemia among children in the county continues to be monitored, although no child has developed leukemia since 2001.

CDC provides recommendations for local and state health departments on the management and investigation of cancer and other disease clusters reported by the public. Perhaps the most important challenge for public health agencies is to communicate effectively with the public. Informed clinicians can play an important role by helping to educate patients and their families about cancer and by contributing to public debate and decision making.

Controlling Occupational Cancer

Eliminating or reducing exposure to known or potential carcinogens is central to the prevention of occupational cancer. As described in Chapters 7 and 9, the best approach to controlling exposure to hazardous substances in the workplace is to eliminate exposure altogether by substitution, or to minimize exposure by engineering controls, such as process enclosure and ventilation. For example, benzene, which causes leukemia, can be replaced by toluene in many uses. Exposure to vinyl chloride monomer was drastically reduced after documentation of its carcinogenicity by enclosing the processes where it was present. Less desirable, but necessary in some settings such as hazardous work cleanup activities, is the use of personal protective equipment. However, establishment of an adequate program using personal protective equipment (PPE) requires considerable expertise, training, and management commitment. Technical issues include the proper type of dermal and respiratory protection, requirements for fit-testing of respirators, training, maintenance, and monitoring of compliance. PPE is uncomfortable to wear, may allow an exposure hazard if it malfunctions, and may even present its own hazards, such as hyperthermia from working in whole-body protective clothing. Therefore, process changes and environmental controls are almost always preferable to controlling exposure through PPE.

Other aspects of the primary prevention are also important. These include worker training and product labeling to increase awareness of workplace hazards and training in how to minimize exposures. Well-designed environmental monitoring programs should be established in workplaces where potential carcinogens are present to ensure the effectiveness of exposure control. In settings where exposure to a potential carcinogen or other hazardous substance may occur through multiple routes, such as respiratory and dermal, biological monitoring should be considered to ensure adequate control of exposure.

Secondary prevention through cancer screening may be warranted for occupational groups with known or suspected cancer excesses. Screening tests for early detection of bladder cancer have been employed for workers exposed to carcinogenic aromatic amines, such as β-naphthylamine, benzidine, and 4-aminobiphenyl. The two methods most commonly used are urinalysis for microscopic hematuria and urine cytology. Hematuria is relatively sensitive in detecting both superficial and invasive bladder cancer, but its low specificity results in a high false-positive rate, requiring many invasive studies on healthy individuals. Urine cytology has good sensitivity and specificity for high-grade bladder cancer, but poor sensitivity for low-grade, papillary lesions. Early detection may not produce a survival advantage for patients whose disease is detected through such screening. However, highly effective treatment exists for both low-grade and high-grade lesions detected at an early stage. More advanced screening techniques, such as flow cytometry, quantitative fluorescence image analysis, and the use of the protein marker (urinary Nuclear Matrix Protein 22 [NMP22]), have been used in research settings. The most recent systematic guidance for bladder cancer screening in high-risk groups stems from an International Conference on Bladder Cancer Screening in High-Risk Groups in 1989, which recommended that urinalysis and cytology might be employed for early detection in high-risk groups, despite lack of evidence that early detection by these methods reduced mortality.

Historically, the only methods available for early detection of lung cancer were periodic chest radiography and/or sputum cytology. These approaches were evaluated in a series of trials at the Mayo Clinic, Johns Hopkins University, and the Memorial Sloan-Kettering Cancer Center in the 1970s. The combination of chest x-rays and sputum cytology tests three times a year yielded a significant increase in lung cancer detection in the study, as compared to a control group, members of which were advised to be tested once a year. However, no significant decrease in lung cancer mortality occurred. These results, in combination with other data, supported for many years the recommendation that no routine surveillance for lung cancer be offered, even to high-risk populations. Recently, studies have established that low-dose spiral computed tomography (spiral CT) can detect smaller pulmonary abnormalities than conventional chest x-rays. However, whether such screening actually improves survival in high-risk populations is not yet known. The balance of risks to benefits is especially problematic because many of the small nodules detected are not malignant and chest surgery entails

substantial risks. A population-based trial is now underway to compare the new methodology to use of standard chest x-rays among 50,000 current and former smokers.

Even if CT screening is found to be effective in reducing mortality from lung cancer among high-risk individuals in the general population, it may pose special challenges in individuals at elevated risk due to occupational exposures. A single study of spiral CT screening among 602 workers with asbestos-related occupational disease did not yield promising results.[19] Among 66 patients with suspicious nodules referred for further hospital examination, a total of 5 lung cancers were found, 3 of which were potentially operable. However, in one patient the lung cancer was initially misdiagnosed and one patient refused further investigation after an inadequate fine-needle aspiration biopsy; both patients ultimately presented with advanced cancer and a third patient succumbed to this disease despite surgery. A high proportion of false-positive lesions were expected because asbestos exposure is associated with interstitial fibrosis and pleural thickening.

Many people alive today remain at increased risk of lung and bladder cancer due to prior occupational exposures. Research on the potential applications of advances in radiology and molecular biology to the prevention and early detection of cancer in these individuals should be a high priority.

ENVIRONMENTAL CANCER

Environmental causes of cancer are highly diverse, including biological, radiologic, and chemical hazards. The four topics covered in detail below were selected based on the magnitude of effect on human cancer, as well as to illustrate a diversity of exposures and exposure circumstances.

Hepatitis Infection, Aflatoxin Exposure, and Hepatocellular Carcinoma

Hepatocellular carcinoma (HCC) is the fifth most common cancer in the world. Eighty percent of cases occur in developing countries, with incidence rates in males exceeding 40 per 100,000 in some parts of eastern Asia and sub-Saharan Africa. In the United States, the incidence rate in 1992–1999 for males was 8.1 per 100,000 and for females was 3.1 per 100,000, with considerable variation by race and ethnicity. Incidence and mortality from HCC has been increasing in the United States since 1973. The major risk factors for HCC worldwide are chronic infection with hepatitis B virus (HBV) or hepatitis C virus (HCV) and exposure to aflatoxins as food contaminants, with HBV accounting for 70 percent of cases in developing countries.[20]

The presence of the hepatitis B surface antigen (HB$_s$Ag) in the bloodstream for a period of 6 months or more is the definition of HBV *carriage*. The antigen is produced by replication of the virus in the hepatocyte. HBV carriage has been associated with a 50-fold increased risk of HCC.[20] The highest HBV carrier rates are observed in Africa, China, and Oceania (excluding Australia and New Zealand). The main determinant of carriage of HBV is age at infection, with infection *in utero* or during the first 5 years of life associated with much greater rates of carriage than infection later in life. Approximately 90 percent of infants infected *in utero* or around the time of birth and 25 percent of those infected during the first 5 years of life become carriers, whereas fewer than 5 percent of those infected past the age of 10 years become carriers. In contrast, around 80 percent of all infections with HCV result in carriage.[20] Direct transmission by blood contamination, usually though a needle, is the most important mode of transmission, resulting in a high prevalence among intravenous drug users and a predominantly adolescent and young adult age at infection in most of the world. A 20 percent prevalence of HCV has been detected in Egypt, probably due to transmission of the virus in the mass-injection treatment of schistosomiasis in the past.

The risk of HBV carriage is greatly diminished by HBV vaccination within 48 hours after birth. Risk is further diminished by administration of hyperimmune globulin to infants with highly infectious carrier mothers; however, because this is expensive to manufacture, public health programs in Asia and Africa use vaccine alone. Even so, only 1 percent of children in Africa currently have access to the vaccine.[20] It is unlikely that a vaccine against HCV will be developed in the near future because HCV is an RNA virus that shows marked genetic heterogeneity. Preventive measures include screening for HCV in donated blood and emphasis on clean, safe needle use.

There are currently 360 million HBV carriers worldwide. One way to decrease their risk of HCC is by reducing contamination of food supplies with aflatoxins. Aflatoxins are mycotoxins (toxic fungal metabolites) produced by *Aspergillis flavus* and *Aspergillus parasiticus*. Aflatoxin contamination of foods occurs predominantly in developing countries with hot, humid climates. It is found on a variety of oilseeds and cereal crops. Often the regions with high exposure are the same as those with high HBV infection rates. Aflatoxins are potent hepatocarcinogens and HBV and aflatoxin have a synergistic effect on HCC risk.[20]

A variety of measures are available for the reduction of aflatoxin contamination, including pre- and post-harvest crop management and dietary change. These measures are particularly important in parts of the world where there is a high prevalence of HBV and HCV carriers. Research is being performed on chemoprevention of aflatoxin-related hepatotoxicity. Treatment with interferon in patients with HCV-related cirrhosis or HBV-related chronic hepatitis may reduce the risk of hepatocellular carcinoma.[20]

Indoor Air Pollution from Burning of Solid Fuels in Developing Countries

In developed countries, tobacco smoking is the most important risk factor for lung cancer, with the vast majority of lung cancer cases occurring among smokers. In developing countries, however, nonsmokers, frequently women, form a much larger proportion of patients with lung cancer. For example, two-thirds of lung cancers among women in China, India, and Mexico occur among nonsmokers. Indoor air pollution from burning of coal for indoor cooking and heating has been shown to contribute to lung cancer among women in China. Other important sources of indoor air pollutants that may contribute to lung cancer among nonsmoking women include environmental tobacco smoke from other family members, radon in some geographical areas and types of housing, and high-temperature burning of cooking oils.

Globally, almost 3 billion people rely on solid fuels, including coal and biomass (fuel from wood, charcoal, crop residues, and dung), as their primary source of domestic energy. Most households in developing countries burn biomass fuels in open fireplaces or in poorly functioning earth or metal stoves. Combustion is incomplete and results in substantial emissions that contain particles, carbon monoxide, nitrous oxides, sulfur oxides (primarily from coal), formaldehyde, and polycyclic organic matter, including carcinogens such as benzo[*a*]pyrene. The best-documented health effects of emissions from burning solid fuels are childhood acute upper respiratory infections and chronic obstructive pulmonary disease, both associated with many types of solid fuel, and lung cancer, which is associated with use of coal. Estimates suggest that indoor air pollution is responsible for more than 2 million excess deaths per year worldwide, most of which are from acute and chronic respiratory disease. Indoor air pollution is a major public health hazard for many of the world's poorest, most vulnerable people. The development and evaluation of interventions must consider many aspects of household energy supply and utilization, including affordability and sustainability. Because those living in poverty rely more on polluting fuels, economic development should be placed at the core of efforts to achieve healthier household environments.

Radon Exposure

Environmental (indoor) radon exposure is second only to cigarette smoking as a leading cause of lung cancer.[21] Radon (radon-222) is a naturally occurring decay product of radium-226, the fifth daughter of uranium-238. Both uranium-238 and radium-226 are present in most soils and rocks, although concentrations vary widely. Radon exposure in homes and workplaces is largely a result of radon-contaminated gas arising from soil. Although radon is ubiquitous in indoor and outdoor air and also in the air of underground passages and mines, its concentration is increased by the presence of a rich source and by low ventilation of air in contact with the source. Two of the decay products of radon-222 emit alpha particles, which are highly effective at damaging tissues.

The relationship between exposure to radon among miners and increase in lung cancer risk has been extensively studied. In the most recent follow-up of a cohort of more than 3,000 white males who mined uranium in the Colorado plateau, the SMR for lung cancer was 5.8 (95% CI, 5.2–6.4).[22] Although the size of the radon-related increase in risk varies in studies of uranium miners conducted in different countries, studies consistently demonstrate a linear increase in risk of lung cancer with increasing cumulative exposure to radon. Results of epidemiologic studies have been combined and

used to model the relationship between exposure to radon and risk of lung cancer for all miners and separately for miners who are nonsmokers and smokers. Although the increase in relative risk per unit exposure is higher for never-smokers than smokers, the increase in absolute risk is higher for smokers, as they have much higher rates of lung cancer.

Average radon exposures among miners were about one order of magnitude (10-fold) greater than average indoor exposures. Therefore, the extrapolation of the risk assessments from studies in miners to the effects of residential radiation may be uncertain. In order to measure the relationship between residential radon exposure and lung cancer directly, a number of case-control studies in the general population were initiated in the 1980s. A meta-analysis of eight such studies, published in 1997, found that the exposure-response trend was significantly different from 0 and was similar to model-based extrapolations from miners and to relative risks computed directly from miners with low cumulative exposures.[23] In 1999, the BEIR VI Committee estimated that between 10 and 14 percent of lung cancer deaths in the United States could be attributed to radon among ever-smokers and never-smokers combined.[24] Most of the radon-related lung cancers occur among ever-smokers. However, an estimated 2,100 to 2,900 of the 11,000 deaths from lung cancer among nonsmokers in the United States each year are estimated to be radon-related. A recent meta-analysis of 14 studies completed as of 2001 gave similar results and estimated that radon is responsible for about 6 percent of total deaths from lung cancer in the United Kingdom.[25]

Unlike exposure to cigarette smoke, radon is naturally occurring and cannot be completely eliminated from homes and workplaces. Within buildings, radon levels are usually highest in the basement due to its proximity to the ground, from which radon-containing soil gas diffuses. Thus, people who spend much of their time in rooms in basements (at home or at work) could face a greater potential for exposure. EPA sets action levels for concentration of radon in homes and provides information about how it is measured and how levels can be reduced by, for example, installing ventilation. Approximately one-third of radon-induced lung cancer could be avoided if homes with radon concentrations exceeding the EPA action level of 4 picocuries/L in air could reduce radon concentrations below that level.

Environmental Tobacco Smoke (Passive or Involuntary Smoking)

Involuntary smoking consists of exposure to a complex mixture of chemicals generated during the burning of tobacco products. It contains sidestream smoke—the material emitted from smoldering tobacco products between puffs—as well as exhaled mainstream smoke. Compounds identified in tobacco smoke include recognized carcinogens, such as 4-aminobiphenyl, arsenic, and benzo[*a*]pyrene. A summary of environmental tobacco smoke (ETS) exposure from U.S. homes and workplaces, published in 1999, found that the mean nicotine concentrations in offices allowing smoking were generally between 2 and 6 μg/m^3, although some workplaces had higher mean levels. In homes of smokers, the mean nicotine concentrations were generally between 1 and 3 μg/m^3.[26]

Numerous studies and meta-analyses have documented increased risk from lung cancer among nonsmokers exposed to ETS in the occupational and home environment. For example, a meta-analysis of 35 case-control and 5 cohort studies providing quantitative estimates of the association between exposure to ETS and lung cancer found a relative risk of 1.20 (95% CI, 1.12–1.29) among nonsmoking women ever exposed to ETS from their husband's smoking and 1.16 (95% CI, 1.05–1.28) among nonsmokers exposed to ETS in the workplace.[27] ETS exposure is also associated with an increased risk of death from heart disease. Although children of smoking mothers have higher levels of cotinine and PAH-albumin adducts in their blood than children of nonsmoking mothers,[28] exposure to ETS in childhood has not been linked with increased risk of lung cancer.[29]

In response to the health effects associated with cigarette smoking and exposure to ETS, many states have established comprehensive tobacco control programs with the goals of preventing the initiation of tobacco use among young people, promoting quitting among young people and adults, and eliminating exposure of nonsmokers to environmental tobacco smoke. Smoke-free ordinances, which prohibit smoking in the workplace and other public places, exist at the federal, state, and local levels, with more than 1,600 U.S. municipalities having laws that restrict smoking. By the end of the 1990s, nearly 70 percent of all indoor workers in the United States were covered by smoke-free policies. However, blue-collar and service workers, particularly males, are less likely to be covered by a smoke-free policy than are white-collar workers, and only 43 percent of the nation's 6.6 million food preparation and service occupations workers are covered.[30]

Case Studies in Occupational and Environmental Cancer

A computer company has a site with 4,200 employees engaged in research and development, manufacturing, sales and service, and repairs. The human resources director is interested in cancer prevention. What are the most important steps an employer can take to prevent cancer?

The first priority of the employer is to ensure that any exposure to potential carcinogens in the workplace is minimized or eliminated. In addition to compliance with regulatory requirements, companies should ensure that appropriate experts review toxicological data on all chemicals used, select the least toxic products, and implement proper exposure controls and monitoring for all potentially toxic substances. It is prudent to treat substances with animal evidence of carcinogenicity as potentially carcinogenic to humans and to institute appropriate exposure monitoring and control, even if not required by current regulations. Engineering controls are generally preferred over PPE as a means of exposure control. Depending on the nature and extent of chemical exposures, consideration should be given to change rooms, on-site laundering of work clothing, and other precautions to minimize potential transport of hazardous substances outside the workplace. Health and safety committees, with representation of management and nonmanagement personnel, should be engaged to review workplace health and safety procedures, prioritize issues, and coordinate efforts to inform and educate the workforce.

Employers can reduce the risk of cancer among all employees by offering health insurance benefits that include coverage for smoking cessation treatment and all recommended types of cancer screening. If employees are thought to be at increased risk of cancer due to workplace exposure, the possibility of offering additional cancer screening should be considered.

Cigarette smoking and obesity are the two most important causes of cancer in the general population. Smoke-free workplaces reduce exposure of nonsmokers to ETS, encourage smokers to cut back or quit, and reduce the potential for exposure to workplace chemicals through hand-to-mouth contact while smoking. Transition to a smoke-free workplace should be accompanied by support to help smokers quit, including counseling services and pharmacotherapy. The workplace environment may also be used to promote healthy dietary patterns and physical activity. Provision of healthy food choices in workplace cafeterias may encourage healthy eating habits, while on-site exercise facilities or subsidies for health club memberships can encourage physical activity.

A 44-year-old flight attendant is concerned about breast cancer due to her occupation and residence in a high-risk area. What information and advice can you provide?

Several epidemiologic studies have found increased risks of breast cancer among flight attendants. Occupational exposures that might explain increased breast cancer risk among flight attendants are cosmic radiation exposure and circadian rhythm disruption. Although radiation exposures among flight crews are not routinely monitored, those who regularly fly long distance at high altitudes, or on flight routes near the North and South Poles, may have radiation exposures higher than the average U.S. radiation worker. Flight attendants who work during pregnancy may exceed the International Commission on Radiation Protection (ICRP) recommended limit of 1 mSv to the conceptus during pregnancy. Disruption of circadian rhythms may interfere with endocrine function, affecting melatonin production, and female menstrual cycles. Flight attendants who cross multiple time zones or staff overnight flights within time zones may be at greater risk. Although studies are ongoing to investigate whether flight attendants are at increased risk of breast cancer and what the mechanisms might be, there is no scientific consensus for an increased risk of breast cancer among flight attendants due to their occupation.

In the general population, important breast cancer risk factors include a family history of breast cancer in a parent or sibling, nulliparity or older age at first birth, earlier age at menarche and later age at menopause, use of hormone replacement therapy, and obesity. Screening mammography can increase incidence and shift the diagnosis of breast cancer toward earlier ages. Occupational studies of breast cancer risk should control for differences in these factors.

Despite widespread public concern that environmental exposure to pesticides or other pollutants may contribute to geographic variations in breast cancer incidence and mortality, much or all of this variation has been attributed to population differences in known risk factors. Studies in Long Island and elsewhere have provided little evidence for the role of environmental chemical exposures in breast cancer. However, evidence from animal studies shows that some carcinogens accumulate in mammary tissue and cause mammary cancer in rodents.[8] Research on the potential role of environmental pollutants in human breast cancer continues.

In addition to providing a perspective on potential environmental and occupational risks, the clinician should inform the patient about other behaviors that can decrease morbidity and mortality from breast cancer. These include maintenance of a healthy body weight, regular physical activity, the avoidance of long-term use of hormone replacement therapy, minimization of alcohol consumption, and age-appropriate screening. The American Cancer Society recommends that women of average risk begin annual clinical breast exam and mammography at age 40 and inform their physician promptly about any changes in their breasts between exams. The patient's personal risk profile for breast cancer should be determined based on family history and other factors. Additional options, such as tamoxifen prophylaxis, should be offered to high-risk women who meet established criteria.

A 67-year-old machinist is diagnosed with rectal cancer. He asks his surgeon if his workplace exposure to metalworking fluids could have caused his cancer. He wonders if his son, who now works as a machinist, is also at risk.

Millions of gallons of metalworking fluids are used each day in United States industry for cutting, milling, drilling, stamping, and grinding. NIOSH and OSHA have estimated that more than 1 million workers are engaged in these activities and are potentially exposed to metalworking fluids by inhalation and dermal contact. Metalworking fluids are a complex mixture of chemicals that are classified into three major types:

1. *Straight oils* are composed primarily of mineral oils (60 to 100 percent). Untreated and mildly treated mineral oils containing polycyclic aromatic hydrocarbons (PAHs) that were used in the past are recognized human carcinogens. Straight oils may contain elemental sulfur, sulfur compounds, and chlorinated compounds, such as chlorinated paraffins, some of which are carcinogenic. Before the 1940s, metalworking fluids were predominantly straight oils. Refined straight oils continue to be used in lower production operations and those requiring lubrication.

2. *Soluble oils* are emulsions of highly refined petrochemicals typically diluted with water for use.

3. *Synthetic oils* are composed of water with additives, including buffers, such as ethanolamines.

Exposures to metalworking fluids have been associated with increased risks of cancers of several sites, including stomach, esophagus, lung, prostate, brain, colon, rectum, and the hematopoietic system. The specific metal-working fluid constituents or contaminants responsible for the various site-specific cancer risks have not been determined.[31]

A comprehensive study of the health effects of exposure to metalworking fluids found a significant association between exposure to straight oils and rectal cancer, with a twofold increased risk among workers with a cumulative exposure of over 3 mg/m^3-years. Risk was greatest for those hired before 1970, perhaps reflecting either less carcinogenicity of more modern metalworking fluids or the relatively short follow-up of workers hired after 1970. Other studies also report an association between exposure to metalworking fluids and rectal cancer.

Although it is plausible that exposure to metalworking fluids may have contributed to the development of rectal cancer in this 67-year-old machinist, it is unclear whether his son will be at risk as a result of present-day metalworking fluid exposures. During the past several decades, substantial changes have been made in the metalworking industry, including changes in metalworking fluid composition, reduction of impurities, and reduction in exposure concentrations, which may decrease the risk of rectal cancer among more recent workers. Given that the specific constituent of metalworking

fluids responsible for the increased risk of rectal cancer is unknown, continued risk among workers who began exposure recently cannot be ruled out. Metalworking fluids have been nominated for toxicologic testing to the National Toxicology Program, with the goal of better understanding the carcinogenicity of formulations currently used in industry. (see <ntp-server.niehs.nih.gov/htdocs/liason/ICCEC010508FR.html>).

At a chemical manufacturing facility with 5,000 employees, it is reported that 10 current and former workers have developed brain cancer over the past 10 years. The union presses for an investigation and asks: Is some exposure in our plant causing brain cancer? What should we do about it?

The first step in a cancer cluster investigation in to identify and confirm all suspected cases. In this hypothetical cluster, this process identifies two additional cases, yielding a total of 12. Among these cases, no medical records are available for three. Five appear to have died with malignant brain tumors. And four appear to have been diagnosed with benign brain tumors. While efforts at case-confirmation are ongoing, a current worker is diagnosed with a malignant glioblastoma. The local newspaper interviews the wife of this worker and writes a story suggesting a conspiracy on the part of the company to cover-up a brain cancer epidemic. Concern begins to center around a plant department with historical exposure to nitrosamines, as well as many other types of chemicals.

Union and management agree to bring in outside consultants to review the case and exposure information. The consultants advise that it is unclear whether the observed cases represent an excess or not. The number of brain cancer deaths does not greatly exceed the number that might be expected from studies of other occupational cohorts. However, because the ascertainment of cases was not done in a systematic way, it is not known whether all brain cancer cases have been identified. Consultants agree that although brain cancer clusters have been reported in the chemical industry, limited evidence exists for an association between specific chemical exposures and brain cancer. They further agree that given the wide variety of chemical processes present at the manufacturing facility in question, retrospective exposure assessment would be an extremely time consuming and expensive process.

The best way to approach a possible brain cancer excess at the facility is to conduct a cohort mortality study. This can be done fairly quickly if the study is confined to employees working at the facility on or after January 1, 1978, as records containing employee work history and demographic information are already computerized and can be linked with records of the National Death Index, which can provide highly accurate information on deaths from 1978 to 2000. It is also agreed that a comprehensive industrial hygiene survey will be conducted, by an independent contractor, to ensure that current exposure protections are adequate.

It is agreed that the consultants will reconvene at the conclusion of the study to review the results. If the results of the study confirm excess mortality from brain cancer, further studies may be indicated to identify high-risk departments and processes. If not, it is recommended that the company continue to update the mortality experience of the cohort for surveillance purposes.

Challenges in the Prevention of Occupational and Environmental Cancer

Gaps Between Industrialized and Developing Countries

During the 20th century, tremendous strides were made in the development of methods to identify potential carcinogens and apply these findings to public health in most industrialized countries. Although delays in recognition and abatement of some hazards, including asbestos, resulted in countless deaths, public health measures were effective in reducing exposures to many known and potential carcinogens in the workplace and environment. For example, major companies routinely use *in vitro* and *in vivo* tests to screen-out chemicals likely to be mutagenic or carcinogenic early in the process of product development. Elimination of the widespread use of DDT and PCBs in the United States and other developed countries resulted in declines in their levels in the environment, accompanied by lower body burdens. Air and water pollution has also been greatly reduced due to environmental regulations. This progress has been the result of a dynamic interplay between social, political, and economic forces, in which public health, labor, and environmental activists have played important

roles. Even within the context of overall progress, some environmental and occupational hazards are inadequately regulated and some segments of society, such as industrial workers and those living in poverty, are more likely to be exposed to carcinogens and other hazardous substances than others. For example, urban air pollution has surfaced as an environmental justice concern because of the large proportion of minority and low-income residents living in urban environments with unhealthful air quality.

The situation of occupational and environmental health in many developing countries is starkly different than that in industrialized countries. A recent study of the 20 leading global risk factors and their contribution to the global burden of disease found that the major environmental risks were unsafe water, sanitation, and hygiene (3.7 percent); indoor smoke from solid fuels (2.7 percent); and elevated blood lead concentrations (0.9 percent).[32] More than 70 percent of the asbestos production worldwide is used in Eastern Europe, Latin America, and Asia. Due to economic pressures, lack of technology, and lack of public health expertise, current levels of exposure to known and suspected carcinogens in developing countries may be as high as they were in developed countries early in the 20th century. It is difficult to even begin to address these problems in the context of the enormous global inequality in economic resources present at the beginning of the 21st century, with an estimated 2.8 billion of the people worldwide living on less than $2 a day.

Research and Methods Development to Clarify Effects of Animal Carcinogens in Humans

A major challenge is to develop better data to evaluate the hazards of chemicals, mixtures, and exposure circumstances currently listed by IARC in groups 2A and 2B, as well as others with some evidence of carcinogenicity in animal or human studies. Historically, many of the recognized human carcinogens were identified in occupational cohorts where very high exposures resulted in very high relative risks. The changing nature of the workplace and increasing complexity of exposures have made such occupational epidemiology studies more difficult. As a result of regulatory and voluntary controls, exposure levels and the attendant risks are much lower than in the past. Many exposures are mixtures, and many occupations involve exposure to an ever-changing and diverse array of substances. These changes create the need for more sensitive measures to detect cancer risks in occupational populations. For example, studies may need to incorporate quantitative estimates of risk for multiple exposure agents, examine possible interaction between occupational and nonoccupational exposures, and consider the use of biomarkers to better define intermediate markers related to exposure and biological effects.

The potential for biomarkers to play a role in improving understanding of human cancer risks has been recognized but not fully exploited. Biomarkers can play an important role in understanding a number of stages in the process though which exogenous exposures result in cancer, including internal dose, biologically effective dose, early biological effect, altered structure/function, premalignant changes, and clinical disease. In two instances (ethylene oxide and TCDD), biomarker results have been used to support an IARC group 1 carcinogen classification in the absence of definitive evidence of increases in cancer incidence or mortality from epidemiologic studies. Incorporation of biomarkers of genetic susceptibility may play a role in studies of potential occupational and environmental carcinogens. However, scientific knowledge about genetic susceptibility to environmental and occupational cancer is currently too limited for clinical application.

Application of Advancing Knowledge to the Protection of Occupational and Environmental Health

Occupational and public health practitioners concerned with occupational and environmental cancer currently operate in a climate of scientific controversy and debate about the extrapolation of effects in animals to humans, particularly at low levels of human exposure. Particularly contentious debate currently centers on the strength of the evidence that certain mechanisms of action in rodents are not applicable in humans. These debates, though highly technical, have practical consequences for the classification and control of exposure for chemicals of public health importance. It is important that research conducted to clarify these issues is objective and supported, at least in part, by public and private institutions with no financial interest in the outcome. In addition, it is important that scientific and government agencies considering these issues ensure representation from all points of view, including the interests of labor and other affected communities.

In the face of scientific uncertainty about potential carcinogens, the Precautionary Principle has been advanced to provide a framework within which to consider public health actions. The key element is the justification for acting in the face of uncertain knowledge about risks from environmental exposures. Appropriate public health action should be taken in response to limited, but plausible and credible, evidence of likely and substantial harm. The Precautionary Principle is aimed at avoiding possible future harm associated with suspected, but not conclusive, environmental risks. The burden of proof is shifted from demonstrating the presence of risk to demonstrating the absence of risk.

Clinicians' Role

Clinicians' role in confronting occupational cancer is varied. They should maintain a high index of suspicion of workplace causes when treating cancer, especially lung, bladder, and brain cancers and leukemia. Clinicians should work to identify past exposures, using the patient's knowledge, toxicological resources, and consultants. In case of ongoing exposures, clinicians should assume a public health role, working to end these exposures. Finally, clinicians should educate patients, employee and employer groups, and communities about the hazards of carcinogenic exposures and ways to prevent them.

ACKNOWLEDGMENTS

The author acknowledges Dr. Howard Frumkin and Dr. Michael Thun, who authored the chapter on Carcinogens in the previous edition, for their thoughtful comments and Ms. Dama Laurie, who assisted with the literature review.

REFERENCES

1. Lichtenstein P, Holm NV, Verkasalo PK, et al. Environmental and heritable factors in the causation of cancer—Analyses of cohorts of twins from Sweden, Denmark, and Finland. N Engl J Med 2000;343:78–85.
2. Steenland K, Burnett C, Lalich N, et al. Dying for work: The magnitude of US mortality from selected causes of death associated with occupation. Am J Ind Med 2003;43:461–82.
3. Feig DI, Reid TM, Loeb LA. Reactive oxygen species in tumorigenesis. Cancer Res 1994;54(7 Suppl):1890s–1894s.
4. Little J. Ionizing Radiation. In: Holland J, Frei E, eds. Cancer medicine. Vol. 2. Hamilton, London: BC Decker Inc., 2003:289–301.

5. Herman JG, Baylin SB. Gene silencing in cancer in association with promoter hypermethylation. N Engl J Med 2003;349:2042–54.
6. Jackson AL, Loeb LA. The contribution of endogenous sources of DNA damage to the multiple mutations in cancer. Mutat Res 2001;477:7–21.
7. Marnett LJ. Oxyradicals and DNA damage. Carcinogenesis 2000;21:361–70.
8. Russo J, Hu YF, Yang X, et al. Developmental, cellular, and molecular basis of human breast cancer. J Natl Cancer Inst Monogr 2000;27:17–37.
9. Ashby J, Paton D. The influence of chemical structure on the extent and sites of carcinogenesis for 522 rodent carcinogens and 55 different human carcinogen exposures. Mutat Res 1993;286:3–74.
10. Cariello NF, Wilson JD, Britt BH, et al. Comparison of the computer programs DEREK and TOPKAT to predict bacterial mutagenicity. Deductive Estimate of Risk from Existing Knowledge. Toxicity Prediction by Komputer Assisted Technology. Mutagenesis 2002;17:321–29.
11. Waters MD, Stack HF, Jackson MA. Genetic toxicology data in the evaluation of potential human environmental carcinogens. Mutat Res 1999;437:21–49.
12. Ashby J, Waters MD, Preston J, et al. IPCS harmonization of methods for the prediction and quantification of human carcinogenic/mutagenic hazard, and for indicating the probable mechanism of action of carcinogens. Mutat Res 1996;352:153–7.
13. Tennant RW. Evaluation and validation issues in the development of transgenic mouse carcinogenicity bioassays. Environ Health Perspect 1998;106 (Suppl 2):473–6.
14. Macaluso M, Larson R, Delzell E, et al. Leukemia and cumulative exposure to butadiene, styrene and benzene among workers in the synthetic rubber industry. Toxicology 1996;113:190–202.
15. Alavanja MC, Samanic C, Dosemeci M, et al. Use of agricultural pesticides and prostate cancer risk in the Agricultural Health Study cohort. Am J Epidemiol 2003;157:800–14.
16. Alderson P. Absence of evidence is not evidence of absence. BMJ 2004;328:476–7.
17. Siemiatycki J, Wacholder S, Dewar R, et al. Degree of confounding bias related to smoking, ethnic group, and socioeconomic status in estimates of the associations between occupation and cancer. J Occup Med 1988;30:617–25.
18. Huff J. IARC monographs, industry influence, and upgrading, downgrading, and undergrading chemicals: A personal point of view. International Agency for Research on Cancer. Int J Occup Environ Health 2002;8:249–70.
19. Tiitola M, Kivisaari L, Huuskonen MS, et al. Computed tomography screening for lung cancer in asbestos-exposed workers. Lung Cancer 2002;35:17–22.
20. Wild CP, Hall AJ. Primary prevention of hepatocellular carcinoma in developing countries. Mutat Res 2000;462:381–93.
21. Frumkin H, Samet JM. Radon. CA Cancer J Clin 2001;51:337–44, 322; quiz 345–8.
22. Roscoe RJ. An update of mortality from all causes among white uranium miners from the Colorado Plateau Study Group. Am J Ind Med 1997;31:211–22.
23. Lubin JH, Boice JD. Lung cancer risk from residential radon: Meta-analysis of eight epidemiologic studies. J Natl Cancer Inst 1997;89:49–57.
24. Anomymous. Health effects of exposure to radon BEIR VI. Washington, DC: National Academy Press, 1999.
25. Darby S, Hill D, Doll R. Radon: A likely carcinogen at all exposures. Ann Oncol 2001;12:1341–51.
26. Jaakkola MS, Samet JM. Occupational exposure to environmental tobacco smoke and health risk assessment. Environ Health Perspect 1999;107(Suppl 6):829–35.
27. Zhong L, Goldberg MS, Parent ME, et al. Exposure to environmental tobacco smoke and the risk of lung cancer: A meta-analysis. Lung Cancer 2000;27:3–18.
28. Perera FP. Molecular epidemiology and prevention of cancer. Environ Health Perspect 1995;103(Suppl 8):233–6.
29. Boffetta P, Agudo A, Ahrens W, et al. Multicenter case-control study of exposure to environmental tobacco smoke and lung cancer in Europe. J Natl Cancer Inst 1998;90:1440–50.
30. Shopland DR, Anderson CM, Burns DM, et al. Disparities in smoke-free workplace policies among food service workers. J Occup Environ Med 2004;46:347–56.
31. Savitz DA. Epidemiologic evidence on the carcinogenicity of metalworking fluids. Appl Occup Environ Hyg 2003;18:913–20.
32. Ezzati M, Hoorn SV, Rodgers A, et al. Estimates of global and regional potential health gains from reducing multiple major risk factors. Lancet 2003;362:271–80.

BIBLIOGRAPHY

Ecobichon DJ. Mutagenesis-carcinogenesis. In: Ecobichon DJ, ed. The basis of toxicology testing. Montreal: CRC Press, 1997:157–90.

Ezzati M, Kammen DM. The health impacts of exposure to indoor air pollution from solid fuels in developing countries: Knowledge, gaps, and data needs. Environ Health Perspect 2002;110:1057–68.

Fung VA, Barrett JC, Huff J. The carcinogenesis bioassay in perspective: Application in identifying human cancer hazards. Environ Health Perspect 1995;103:680–83.

McKinnell RG, Parchment RE, Perantoni AO, et al. The biological basis of cancer. Cambridge: The Press Syndicate of the University of Cambridge, 1998.

Rothman KJ, Wacholder S, Caporaso NE, et al. Oncology corner: The use of common genetic polymorphisms to enhance the epidemiologic study of environmental carcinogens. Biochim Biophy Acta 2001;1471:C1–C10.

Rushton L. How much does the environment contribute to cancer? Occup Environ Med 2003;60:150–6.

Thun M, Sinks T. Understanding cancer clusters. CA Cancer J Clin 2004;54:273–80.

Tomatis L, Huff J, Hertz-Picciotto I, et al. Avoided and avoidable risks of cancer. Carcinogenesis 1997;18:97–105.
These are useful publications that provide more detail on cancer and its causation.

CHAPTER 25

Respiratory Disorders

Paul D. Boyce, David C. Christiani, and
David H. Wegman

A 60-year-old man, who had been a sandblaster for 23 years, was hospitalized for the third time in the past 4 months for shortness of breath. Three years ago, he began having respiratory problems, initially mild shortness of breath and increased heart rate when walking in snow and climbing steps as well as heavy exertion at work. These symptoms increased moderately over the next several months. He was seen by the company physician, who told him that he had "bad lungs," but gave him no treatment. Two years ago, he sought therapy at a community hospital due to increasing shortness of breath while walking at normal speed on the level ground for one to two blocks. He was hospitalized. Resting room-air arterial blood gases were normal with a $Pao_2 = 87$ mm Hg and $Paco_2 = 31$ mm Hg. A chest x-ray showed multiple interstitial nodules without evidence of hilar disease. Pulmonary function tests revealed a reduced forced vital capacity (FVC; 73 percent of predicted) with a normal diffusing capacity. Tuberculosis smear, culture, and cytology of bronchial washings were all negative. He was sent home without therapy and was told not to return to work. He has not worked since.

Seven months ago, he acquired a cough occasionally productive of thin, clear-to-grayish sputum. Three more hospital admissions for increasing shortness of breath occurred with no new findings reported. Since the last hospitalization, 1 month ago, he has been on oxygen continuously and stays in bed most of the day. He has also had dysuria and some trouble initiating his urinary stream, which seems to make his shortness of breath worse.

The patient had smoked one pack of cigarettes per day for 5 years, until he quit 20 years ago. He has no history of asthma, pneumonia, surgery, or allergies.

His occupational history consisted of a 23-year period of operating a sandblasting machine located in a basement room (20×40 feet). Dust escaped continuously through crevices of the sandblasting unit; every time he opened the door to remove and install a piece to be blasted, much fine dust escaped. The windows were closed and an exhaust fan in the wall did not seem to remove any dust. A room fan, installed to circulate the air in the room, was often out of order. The patient wore a helmet with a cloth apron on the bottom, covering his shoulders, and, when the room was especially dusty, a compressed air supply.

Physical examination revealed a thin man in moderate respiratory distress, sitting hunched over, gasping for breath, with grunting expirations. Pulse was 110 beats per minute, respiratory rate 40 per minute, blood pressure 110/80 mm Hg, and temperature 98°F. Pulmonary and cardiac examinations were normal, except for a systolic ejection murmur and an increased second heart sound over the pulmonic area. His extremities revealed clubbed fingernails and cyanosis. The rest of the examination was normal. Resting room-air arterial blood gases revealed significant hypoxia with a $Pao_2 = 39$ mm Hg and $Paco_2 = 38$ mm Hg. A chest x-ray showed diffuse, interstitial, small, rounded densities throughout both lung fields with hilar fullness. These were judged to be "q"-sized with a 2/2 profusion in all lung fields, using the International Labor Organization (ILO) nomenclature for chest radiographs.[1] The diagnosis of silicosis was made. He remained completely disabled and died 3 months later.*

This case is an example of a severe occupational respiratory disease—in this instance, pneumoconiosis. However, workplace exposure responsible for such chronic disabling lung disease occurs gradually over long periods of time; initially, exposures do not result in any obvious acute symptoms, but once symptoms do appear, often little can be done beyond making the worker comfortable. Unless discovered very early in their course, most work-related respiratory diseases are not curable. Disease prevention is therefore critically important.

Occupational lung disease is recorded in accounts of ancient history. Case reports exist in the writings of Hippocrates, and evidence of silicosis is present in pictographs from Egypt. Yet, some of those chronic diseases remain important problems for workers today. Estimates of the prevalence and incidence of occupational respiratory disease suggest that only a small fraction of chronic occupational respiratory disease is correctly identified as associated with work.

Pneumoconiosis and *occupational asthma* are two work-related respiratory diseases that often are not correctly diagnosed. For example, approximately 5 percent of Americans have what physicians diagnose as asthma, but a much larger proportion of people report either having asthma or episodes of wheezing; physicians who see workers who report wheezing should determine if a work-related bronchoconstrictive response is occurring.

Investigations into occupational lung diseases have resulted in a better understanding of the effect of air pollutants on respiratory illness. This resulted in the recognition of community air pollution as a contributor to pulmonary disease, starting with the first use of coal in the 14th century.[2] Recently numerous prospective studies have confirmed an association between increased mortality and elevated ambient air pollution.[3] These adverse effects of ambient air pollution span a wide range of outcomes, as evidenced by the acute morbidity and mortality seen in the severe pollution episodes in the 1940s and 1950s in Donora, Pennsylvania, and in London, and more recently after the September 11, 2001,

attacks in New York. In addition to history of air pollution effects due to the Industrial Revolution in developed countries, developing countries are now facing the adverse effects of rapidly increasing dependence on automobiles in places like Hong Kong, Mexico City, Delhi, and Beijing.

The public health impact of ambient air pollution has been tremendous, especially with regard to children.[4] Air pollution, both indoor and outdoor, appears to play a central role in (a) the increased rate of acute respiratory hospital admissions in children, (b) increased grade-school and kindergarten absences, (c) decrements in peak flow rates in otherwise normal children, and (d) increased medication use in children and adults with asthma.

EVALUATION OF INDIVIDUALS

Evaluations of pulmonary response to occupational and environmental exposures are important because both are frequently a contributory cause—and commonly a primary cause—of pulmonary disability. Usually performed in a physician's office, they include a minimum of four elements: (a) a complete history, including occupational (direct and indirect) and environmental exposures (including those at home and at recreational sites), a cigarette-smoking history, and a careful review of respiratory symptoms (see Chapter 6); (b) a physical examination, with special attention to breath sounds; (c) a chest x-ray with appropriate attention to parenchymal and pleural opacities; and (d) pulmonary function tests.

History

Review of symptoms should include questions on chronic cough, chronic sputum production, shortness of breath (dyspnea) on exertion compared with peers or usual level of activity, wheezing unrelated to respiratory infections, chest tightness, chest pain, and allergic or asthmatic responses to working or nonworking environments. For example, one peculiar characteristic of several types of occupational asthma and pulmonary edema is that symptoms may peak in intensity approximately 8 to 16 hours after exposure has ended. The symptoms often occur at night as shortness of breath or cough. In assessing acute airway disease, the clinician should question the patient about the principal symptoms: chest tightness, wheezing, dyspnea, and cough. Symptom periodicity or timing is critical. For example, respiratory symptoms (cough, wheeze, and chest

---

* *Case courtesy of Stephen Hessl, M.D., Daniel Hryhorczuk, M.D., and Peter Orris, M.D., Section on Occupational Medicine, Cook County Hospital, Chicago, Illinois.*

tightness) occurring on work days (or nights), with improvement on weekends or holidays, strongly suggest a workplace-induced condition. The temporal relationship for environmental exposures proves to be more difficult as these exposures can occur daily in the home environment. A formal survey questionnaire for systematic respiratory effect studies, the American Thoracic Society (ATS) Respiratory Symptom Questionnaire, is available.[5]

Physical Examination

The physical examination is helpful when the results are abnormal. The most remarkable finding in most patients with occupational and environmental lung diseases is the relative absence of physical signs; however, certain conditions are associated with physical signs, and the presence or absence of such abnormalities should be noted.

Auscultation can reveal important diagnostic clues. Fine rales at the bases, often at end-inspiration, are more common in asbestosis than in other interstitial lung diseases. Wheezes and their relationship to exposure are helpful in evaluating a suspected case of work-related asthma. A pleural rub can occur due to the pleural reaction caused by acute, chronic, or distant asbestos exposure.

Clubbing of the digits is a nonspecific sign that occurs rarely and usually in relatively advanced lung diseases, including asbestosis, and therefore usually appears after other evidence of the disease has become apparent. This finding is nonspecific and cannot be used as a reliable clinical indication for the diagnosis of asbestosis. It does not usually occur in other mineral pneumoconioses or in hypersensitivity pneumonitis. The most common nonoccupational causes of clubbing are bronchial carcinoma and idiopathic pulmonary fibrosis.

Examination of the heart is important because left ventricular failure can present as dyspnea alone, and right ventricular failure may indicate severe lung disease.

Chest Radiography

A chest x-ray should be taken and, in addition to a standard interpretation, it should, if possible, be interpreted according to the ILO system for pneumoconiosis by a trained reader (Fig. 25-1).[1] Although this classification was developed for epidemiologic studies and not for clinical evaluation per se, it may be an important function in the common posteroanterior chest x-ray interpretation. This scheme is not useful for evaluation of occupational asthma but is relevant for suspected pneumoconiosis. The standard technique permits semiquantitative interpretation of x-rays to identify early evidence and progression of parenchymal and pleural disease; it focuses on size, shape, concentration, and distribution of small parenchymal opacities as well as distribution and extent of pleural thickening or calcification. For example, rounded opacities in the upper lung fields are usually associated with silicosis, whereas linear (irregular) opacities in the lower lung fields are usually associated with asbestosis (Fig. 25-2). Deviations from these patterns are common; for example, silicosis and coal workers' pneumoconiosis (CWP) can be associated with irregular opacities. Moreover, workers exposed to mixed dusts, such as silica and asbestos, can present with mixed, rounded, irregular opacities in any or all lung fields. The ILO system has the advantage of using a standardized set of comparison radiographic films, which can be used to classify x-rays at one point in time or to follow an individual or a population for change over time. Even though chest x-rays present evidence of abnormality, they do not provide information on disability or impairment and do not necessarily correlate well with pulmonary function test findings. A person with severe obstructive disease may show little evidence of it on chest radiography. In contrast, a person exposed chronically to iron oxide or tin oxide may show a dramatically abnormal chest x-ray, though little, if any, pulmonary inflammatory reaction or lung function abnormality (Fig. 25-3). Additionally, conventional chest x-rays may prove to be insensitive to subtle lung abnormalities. The advent of high-resolution computed tomography (HRCT) scanning has improved dramatically physicians' ability to detect and classify subtle lung diseases that are not or only barely visible on conventional chest radiographs (Fig. 25-4). The present ILO classification system does include this recent imaging technique.

Pulmonary Function Tests

A critical element in determining respiratory status is an evaluation of pulmonary function. In a well-equipped pulmonary function laboratory, spirometry, lung volume determinations, gas exchange analyses, and exercise testing can be performed with relative ease. In a physician's office, only spirometry is readily and inexpensively performed; it does, however, provide a surprising amount of

I.   **Size and Shape of Small Opacities**

ROUNDED OPACITIES		IRREGULAR OPACITIES	
p	≤ 1.5 mm diameter	s	fine linear opacities > 1.5 mm width
q	1.6 - 3.0 mm diameter	t	medium opacities 1.6 - 3.0 mm width
r	3.1 - 10.0 mm diameter	u	coarse, blotchy opacities 3.1 - 10.0 mm width

<p style="text-align:center">* Size recorded by two letters to distinguish single type from mixed type. For example, q/q
if only q opacities are present, but q/t if q opacities predominate but t are also present.</p>

II.   **Concentration (Profusion) and Distribution**

SMALL OPACITIES

	Major Categories	Minor Divisons			Distribution*	
0	Small Opacities Absent or Less Than Category 1 Normal Lung Markings Visible	0/-	0/0	0/1	RU	LU
1	Small Opacities Present but Few Normal Lung Markings Usually Visible	1/0	1/1	1/2	RM	LM
2	Small Opacities Numerous Normal Lung Markings Partially Obscured	2/1	2/2	2/3	RL	LL
3	Small Opacities Very Numerous Normal Lung Markings Totally Obscured	3/2	3/3	3/+		

LARGE OPACITIES

A	One or More Opacities with Greatest Summed Diameter 1 - 5 cm
B	One or More Opacities Larger or More than Category A. Total Area < Equivalent of Right Upper Zone
C	One or More Opacities. Total Area Exceeds Equivalent of Right Upper Zone

<p>* Recorded by dividing lungs into 3 regions per side and checking all regions containing the designated small opacities</p>

III.   **Pleural Thickening**

	WIDTH*		EXTENT*		CALCIFICATION*
a	Maximum Up to 5 mm	1	Up to 1/4 Lateral Wall	1	One or Several Regions Summed Diameter ≤ 2 cm
b	Maximum 5 - 10 mm	2	1/4 - 1/2 Lateral Wall	2	One or Several Regions Summed Diameter 2 - 10 cm
c	Maximum > 10 mm	3	Exceeds 1/2 Lateral Wall	3	One or Several Regions Summed Diameter > 10 cm

<p>* **Width** estimated only if seen in profile. **Extent** estimated as maximum length of thickening (profile or face on).
Calcification site (diaphragm, wall, other) and extent are noted separately for two sides.</p>

FIGURE 25-1 ● Schematic of International Labor Organization classification system for chest x-rays. In addition to these scores, the reader is guided in scoring technical quality of the x-ray (good, acceptable, poor, unacceptable) and in identifying other relevant features (for example, bullae, cancer, abnormal cardiac size, emphysema, fractured rib, pneumothorax, tuberculosis).

information. Pulmonary function tests, required for medical surveillance by some Occupational Safety and Health Administration (OSHA) standards, are used commonly and are easy to perform, reliable, and reproducible. Most lung disease yields abnormal results or accelerated declines within the "normal" ranges before onset of clinical symptoms, especially if patients are followed at regular 1- to 3-year intervals. Although these tests may demonstrate several patterns of abnormalities, alone they are not capable of determining etiology. Hospital-based tests (lung-volume determinations, gas-exchange analyses, exercise tests, and bronchial-challenge tests) can contribute to a refined diagnostic evaluation once an abnormality is suspected.

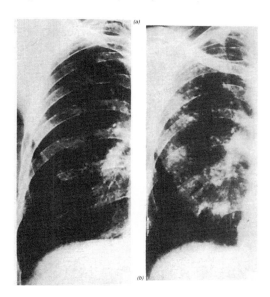

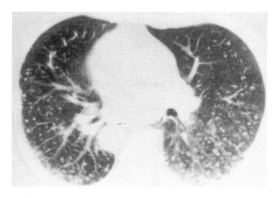

FIGURE 25-4 ● High-resolution CT scan (HRCT) of a 55-year-old construction worker diagnosed with silicosis. (From N Engl J Med 1995;333:1340–6, Weekly Clinicopathological Exercises. Copyright © 1995 Massachusetts Medical Society.)

FIGURE 25-2 ● Progression of discrete nodules of silicosis over 10 years in a slate quarry worker. (From Parkes WR. Occupational lung disorders. 3rd ed. Oxford: Butterworths-Heinemand, 1994.)

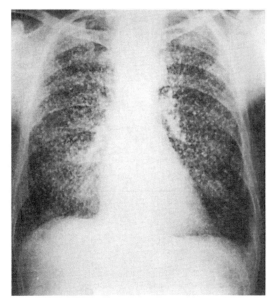

FIGURE 25-3 ● Chest x-ray demonstrating stannosis, the benign pneumoconiosis due to the inhalation of tin oxide, in a man who worked as a furnace charger in a smelting works for 42 years. (From Parkes WR. Occupational lung disorders. 3rd ed. Oxford: Butterworths-Heinemand, 1994.)

The basic tests of ventilatory function can be obtained with a simple portable spirometer. Test results are derived from the forced expiratory curve (Fig. 25-5). Many types of equipment are marketed to provide these tests, yet several have been inadequately standardized; the ATS has provided guidelines on the standardization of spirometry, including information on instrument reliability as well as test performance.[6] Although many measures can be derived from the forced expiratory curve, the simplest and generally the most useful ones for evaluating work-related respiratory disease are forced vital capacity (FVC), forced expiratory volume in the first second of a forced vital capacity maneuver (FEV_1), and the ratio of these two measurements (FEV_1/FVC). A simple scheme for the interpretation of these tests is shown in Table 25-1 and Fig. 25-5. Results are compared with expected values, derived from a normal population of nonsmoking adults, and are expressed as a percentage of the expected value. Criteria for the proper performance and evaluation of spirometry are based on ATS recommendations.[7–9]

Pneumoconioses, such as silicosis and asbestosis, are considered restrictive diseases because they result in reduction in total lung volume. In the absence of significant airways disease, flow rates are maintained and may be above normal because of decreased lung compliance with increased elastic recoil. CWP, on the other hand, is more often associated with an obstructive pattern, with decreased air-flow and normal or increased lung volumes. Occupational asthma is also considered an obstructive disease causing obstruction of airflow without

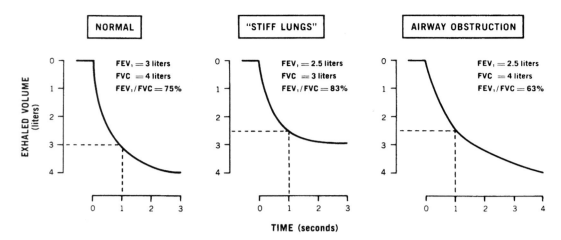

FIGURE 25-5 • Spirographic results in normal and disease states. (Adapted from Nadel JA. Pulmonary function testing. Basis of Respiratory Disease [American Thoracic Society] 1973;1:2.)

reduction in lung volume. With multiple environmental exposures (including tobacco smoking), a mixed condition is frequently present. Moreover, some mineral dusts, such as asbestos and coal, have been shown to cause abnormalities in both the airways and the interstitium. Nevertheless, the basic distribution of ventilatory function abnormalities is useful in considering the general characteristics of work-related and environmentally related respiratory disease (Table 25-1).

EVALUATION OF GROUPS

If the physician is able to examine several individuals from the same work environment and community, careful attention should be directed toward evaluation of the grouped results in addition to those of each person. For an individual, emphasis is on the work history, environment, and collection of information to explain specific symptoms and signs. The absence of basilar rales, however, does not exclude asbestosis; wheezes do not necessarily diagnose occupational asthma; opacities on chest radiography do not specify the underlying pathologic process; and pulmonary function tests may be falsely considered normal because of the wide variation in standard populations. It may not be until a group of individuals is evaluated that pulmonary disease can be recognized as associated with work or the environment.

TABLE 25-1

Spirometry Interpretation

| | Percentage Predicted[a] | | | Response to Inhaled |
Type of Response	FEV$_1$	FVC	FEV$_1$/FVC %	Bronchodilators
Normal	≥80%	≥80%	≥75%	—
Obstructive	<80%	≥80%[b]	<75%	±
Restrictive	≥80%	<80%	≥75%	—
Mixed	<80%	<80%	<75%	±

FEV$_1$, forced expiratory volume in 1 second; FVC, forced vital capacity.
[a] Predicted FEV$_1$ and FVC based on RJ Knudson, Lebowitz MD, Holberg CJ, et al. Changes in the normal maximal expiratory flow volume curve with growth and aging. Am Rev Respir Dis 1983;127:725.
[b] Severe obstruction can result in reduction of FVC also.

Group evaluations enable subdivision of results according to duration of work or types of exposure. Chest x-ray findings, pulmonary function tests, and symptom histories can be examined by subgroups to evaluate previously unrecognized work effects (see examples in Chapter 8). Furthermore, the average value of a group of tests has less variability than an individual test result. For example, individual measurements of FEV_1 and FVC that vary between 80 percent and 120 percent of the population standards are still considered normal; a group of 10 or 20 actively working people, however, should have a mean result much closer to the standard values (100 percent). If the average population difference is as little as 5 percent lower—that is, 95 percent of the predicted value—then an adverse health effect in that population should be seriously considered.[9]

Comparisons with baselines should be performed whenever possible to permit evaluation of change over time in individuals or a group compared to a known—not a predicted—value. Accelerated decrements in lung function, accelerated development of respiratory tract symptoms, or recognition of subtle chest x-ray abnormalities are far more significant when the comparison is based on earlier examinations rather than on expected population experience. Any worker potentially exposed to respiratory hazards at work should have a baseline ventilatory function test before being exposed.

More than 40 million Americans are uninsured. These individuals, a high proportion of who are children, use emergency departments (EDs) as their sole source of health care. The intrinsic aspects of the emergency department, with its association as a "first responder" and the sheer volume of patients, afford the investigator with an excellent opportunity to assess the impact of environmental precipitators of lung disease. It is known that ED visits for asthma and bronchitis acutely increase during times of high ozone, pollen, and smog levels. In addition, cases involving substantial indoor pollution exposures tend to cluster in socioeconomically deprived areas, which often include the same patient population served by most large inner-city EDs.

The major types of respiratory response to external agents discussed in this chapter are summarized in Tables 25-2 and 25-3. Occupational lung cancer is discussed in Chapter 24, and work-related infectious diseases of the respiratory tract are discussed in Chapter 15.

ACUTE IRRITANT RESPONSES

Irritation in the upper respiratory tract, in contrast to the lower airways, is frequently associated with symptoms. Acute symptoms are often due to regional inflammation, which a patient perceives as irritation. Nasal and paranasal sinus irritation can cause congestion that may result in violent frontal headaches, nasal obstruction, runny nose, sneezing, and nosebleeds. Throat inflammation is commonly reported as a dry cough. Laryngeal inflammation can cause hoarseness and, if severe, may result in laryngeal spasms associated with glottal edema, dramatic anxiety, shortness of breath, and cyanosis.

In the lower airways, the acute reaction is characteristically bronchospasm. The extreme case is asthma, which is histologically distinguished by a thickened basement membrane, increased number of goblet cells with secretions, mucus plugging, and increased smooth muscle at preterminal bronchioles. Asthma associated with work is being recognized with increasing frequency. Precipitating agents number over 250 and include isocyanates, detergent enzymes, and Western red cedar dust (Table 25-4). In addition to asthma caused by exposure to agents listed in this table, many irritant substances not usually associated with asthma can produce bronchial hyperreactivity when high levels of exposure have occurred. Single high-dose exposure and episodic low-dose exposure to irritants such as ammonia or chlorine can result in nonspecific bronchial reactivity, referred to by some authors as *reactive airways dysfunction syndrome* (RADS) or *irritant-induced asthma*, which may persist for months to years or may never fully resolve.[10]

Pulmonary edema and pneumonitis can occur after acute irritation of the deep respiratory tract. *Pulmonary edema* occurs after extravasation of fluid and cells from the pulmonary capillary bed into the alveoli. Primary pulmonary edema is due to direct toxic action on the capillary walls. For example, exposure to ozone or oxides of nitrogen, common in industrial settings, can cause pulmonary edema—either acutely when a trapped worker cannot escape exposure or in a more delayed fashion when overexposures are not too high. *Pneumonitis*, on the other hand, is an inflammation of the lung parenchyma in which cellular infiltration rather than fluid extravasation predominates. Beryllium and cadmium are metals that can cause acute pneumonitis.

TABLE 25-2

Major Types of Occupational Pulmonary Disease

Pathologic Function Process	Occupational Disease Example	Clinical History	Physical Examination	Chest x-Ray	Pulmonary Function Pattern
Fibrosis	Silicosis	Dyspnea on exertion, cyanosis, shortness of breath	Clubbing	Nodular opacities	Restrictive or mixed obstructive and restrictive
	Asbestosis	Dyspnea on exertion, cyanosis, shortness of breath	Clubbing, rales	Linear opacities, pleural plaques, calcifications	DLCO normal or decreased
Reversible airway obstruction (mucous plugging, asthma)	Byssinosis, isocyanate asthma, RADS	Cough, chest tightness, shortness of breath, asthma attacks	↑Respiratory rate, wheeze	Usually normal	Normal or obstructive with bronchodilator improvement
					Normal or high DLCO
Emphysema	Cadmium poisoning (chronic)	Cough, sputum, dyspnea	↑Respiratory rate, ↑ expiratory phase	Hyperaeration, bullae	Obstructive low DLCO
Granulomata	Beryllium disease	Cough, weight loss, shortness of breath	↑Respiratory rate	Small nodules	Usually restrictive with low DLCO
Bronchiolitis obliterans	Flavoring or flavoring ingredients	Cough, chest tightness, shortness of breath, fixed airway obstruction	↑Respiratory rate, ↑ expiratory phase	Usually normal	Obstructive without bronchodilator improvement DLCO normal
Pulmonary edema	Smoke inhalation	Frothy, bloody sputum production	Coarse, bubbly rales	Hazy, diffuse air-space disease	Usually restrictive with decreased DLCO Hypoxemia at rest

DLCO, diffusing capacity of lung for carbon monoxide; RADS, reactive airways dysfunction syndrome.

Factors Involved in Toxicity

The most widespread causes of acute responses are irritant gases. Water is a major constituent of the respiratory tract lining, and solubility of these gases in water is the most significant factor influencing their site of action. Gases with high solubility act on the upper respiratory tract within seconds. For example, fatal epiglottic edema has been associated with irritants of high solubility, such as ammonia, hydrogen chloride, and hydrogen fluoride. The moderately soluble gases act on both the upper and lower respiratory tract within minutes. Chlorine gas, fluorine gas, and sulfur dioxide are irritants of this type, producing upper respiratory irritation as well as symptoms of bronchoconstriction. The low-solubility irritants are most insidious. With few warning signs, they penetrate to the deep portions

TABLE 25-3

Common Environmental Pollutants with Respiratory Effects

Pollutant	Common Sources	Health Effects
Sulfur oxides	Coal and oil power plants Oil refineries, smelters Stoves burning wood, coal, kerosene Industrial chemical manufacture	Throat irritation Exacerbation of asthma, chronic bronchitis and other respiratory illnesses with significant airflow obstruction
Particulates	Motor vehicle exhaust Fossil-fuel power plants Heavy construction Natural sources such as volcanoes, bushfires, windblown dust, and oceans	Increased susceptibility to lung infections Exacerbation of asthma, chronic bronchitis and other respiratory illnesses with significant airflow obstruction
Oxides of nitrogen (NO_x)	Motor vehicle exhaust Fossil-fuel power plants Oil refineries	Throat irritation Lung injury Exacerbation of asthma and chronic obstructive pulmonary disease Increased susceptibility to lung infections
Ozone (O_3)	Motor vehicle exhaust Ozone generators Aircraft cabins Power plants	Same as NO_x
Carbon monoxide (CO)	Motor vehicle exhaust Fossil-fuel burning Kerosene space heaters Incinerators Industrial equipment	Hypoxia leading to heart and nervous system damage, death
Polycyclic aromatic hydrocarbons (PAHs)	Surface runoff from roads and land surfaces Sewage effluents Diesel exhaust Cigarette smoke Stove smoke	Lung cancer
Radon	Soil, rock, and groundwater	Lung cancer
Asbestos	Asbestos mines and mills Insulation Building materials	Mesothelioma Lung cancer Asbestosis
Arsenic	Copper smelters Cigarette smoke Pressure-treated wood Pesticides	Lung cancer

of the respiratory tract and act predominantly on the alveoli 6 to 24 hours after exposure. Because of this considerable delay in onset of symptoms, individuals can be exposed to large doses of these irritants without any symptoms to serve as warnings. Pulmonary edema is the major effect of overexposures to materials such as ozone, oxides of nitrogen, and phosgene.

Other factors influencing the site of action of an irritant gas are intensity and duration of exposure. The amount of exposure depends not only on air concentrations but also on work effort: A worker

TABLE 25-4

Selected Causes of Occupational Asthma[a]

Agents	Occupations
High-molecular-weight compounds	
Animal products: dander, excreta, serum, secretions, fish glue	Animal handlers, laboratory workers, veterinarians, bookbinders, postal workers
Plants: grain, dust, flour, tobacco, tea, hops, latex, cotton, coffee beans	Grain handlers, tea workers, textile workers, bakers and workers in natural oil manufacturing and in tobacco, food processing, and health care workers
Enzymes: *B. subtilis*, pancreatic extracts, papain	Bakers and workers in the detergent, pharmaceutical, trypsin, fungal amylase, and plastics industries
Dyes: anthraquinone, carmine, paraphenyl diamine, henna extract	Fabric and fur dyers, beauticians
Other: crab, prawn	Crab and prawn processors
Low-molecular-weight compounds	
Diisocyanates: toluene diisocyanate, methylene-diphenyldiisocyanate	Polyurethane industry workers, roofers, insulators, painters, plastics workers, workers using varnish, and foundry workers
Anhydrides: phthallic and trimellitic anhydrates	Epoxy resin and plastics workers
Wood dust: oak, mahogany, California redwood, Western red cedar	Carpenters, sawmill workers, and furniture makers
Metals: platinum, nickel, chromium, cobalt, vanadium, tungsten carbide	Platinum- and nickel-refining workers and hard-metal workers, platers, and welders
Soldering fluxes	Solderers
Drugs: penicillin, methyldopa, tetracyclines, cephalosporins, psyllium, organophosphates	Pharmaceutical and health care industry workers, and farm workers
Other organic chemicals: urea formaldehyde, dyes, formalin, azodicarbonamide, hexachlorophene, ethylene diamine, dimethyl ethanolamine, polyvinyl, chloride pyrolysates	Workers in chemical, plastics, and rubber industries; hospitals; laboratories; foam insulation, manufacture; food wrapping; and spray painting

[a] Mechanism believed to be IgE-mediated for high-molecular-weight compounds and for some low-molecular-weight compounds. The immunologic mechanism for asthma from many low-molecular-weight substances remains undefined.

Adapted from Chan-Yeung M, Lam S. Occupational asthma. Am Rev Respir Dis 1986;133:686–703.

with a sedentary job exposed to a given concentration of a respiratory irritant receives a much lower dose than one with an active job requiring rapid breathing and a high minute ventilation (tidal volume × respiratory rate).

A final element that influences the site of action is interaction—both *synergism* and *antagonism*. Sulfur dioxide and water droplets are synergistic; they combine to deliver a sulfuric acid–like vapor to the respiratory tract. Ammonia and sulfur dioxide, however, are antagonistic and together produce less response than either can individually. The presence of a carrier, such as an aerosol, may

increase the effect of an irritant gas: Sulfur dioxide may cause a moderate effect and a sodium chloride aerosol no effect on the respiratory tract, but the two combined may result in a marked effect because the aerosol delivers the sulfur dioxide more deeply into the lung.

Highly Soluble Irritants

Primary examples of highly soluble irritants are (a) ammonia, used as a soil fertilizer, in the manufacture of dyes, chemicals, plastics, and explosives, in tanning leather, and as a household cleaner;

(b) hydrogen chloride, or hydrochloric acid, used in chemical manufacturing, electroplating, and metal pickling; and (c) hydrogen fluoride, or hydrofluoric acid, used predominantly for etching and polishing of glass, as a chemical catalyst in the manufacture of plastics, as an insecticide, and for removal of sand from metal castings in foundry operations.

The primary physical effects of highly water-soluble irritants are first the odor and then eye and nose irritation; throat irritation is slightly less frequent. In high doses, the respiratory rate can increase and bronchospasm can occur. Lower respiratory tract effects, however, do not occur unless the person is severely overexposed or trapped in the environment. The irritant effects are powerful and usually provide adequate warning to prevent overexposure of people free to escape from exposure. The history and physical examination are the most important parts of irritant exposure evaluation. Pulmonary function tests may show significant flow limitation reflecting bronchospasm shortly after exposure. Chest x-rays are not helpful unless there is pulmonary edema.

Management of reactions to these irritants is immediate removal of the worker and, if breathing is labored or hypoxemia is present, administration of oxygen. If severe exposure or loss of consciousness occurs, observation in a hospital for development of pulmonary edema is advisable.

Prevention of exposures relies on proper industrial hygiene practices with local exhaust ventilation as an essential component. Respirators should be used only as a temporary control measure in an emergency. If respirators are required to prevent overexposure, workers must be trained in their proper use and maintenance.

A 25-year-old man came to the emergency room with acid burns. Before taking a job as an electroplater 5 weeks before admission, he was in perfect health. On the first day at this job, he developed itching. Subsequently, he developed sores, which healed with scars, at sites of splashes of workplace chemicals. After 4 days on this job, he had a runny nose, throat irritation, and a productive cough. He also noted some shortness of breath at work.

His work involved dipping metal parts into tanks containing chrome solutions and acid. He wore a paper mask disposable respirator, rubber gloves, and an apron, but no eye protection. Although heavy fumes were present in the 60 × 20 × 14-foot room,

no ventilation was provided. Apparently, none of the other eight workers in the room had similar medical problems.

Past history revealed three prior hospitalizations for pneumonia but not asthma or allergies. He smoked about four cigarettes per day.

From age 16 to 18 years, he worked as a sheetmetal punch-press operator for a tool and die company. At age 18 years, he worked as a drip-pan cleaner for a soup company. He was a student in an auto mechanics' school from age 19 to 21 years. From age 21 to 24 years, he occasionally worked as a gas station attendant.

Physical examination was normal, except for multiple areas of round, irregularly shaped, depigmented, 1-mm atrophic scars on both forearms and exposed areas of the anterior thorax and face; a 4-mm, rounded, punched-out ulcer, with a thickened, indurated, undermined border and an erythematous base on his left cheek; an erythematous pharynx; and bilateral conjunctivitis. The nasal septum was not perforated. Patch tests with dichromate, nickel, and cobalt were all negative. A chest x-ray was normal.

The diagnoses were irritation of the upper respiratory tract and an irritant contact dermatitis, both due to chromic acid mist. His symptoms resolved with removal from exposure. Periodic medical surveillance was advised to provide early diagnosis of a possible malignancy of the nasal passages for which he may be at risk as a result of the chromium exposure. Finally, a follow-up industrial hygiene survey of the workplace was initiated to control exposures for the other exposed workers.[*]

Many small electroplating firms have no local ventilation over open vats of chromic and other acids. Frequently, a high level of chrome or other metals in the fumes is liberated when metal parts that are being plated are immersed. Chrome and chromic acid mist are local irritants. Primarily in hexavalent forms, chromium is considered to be a carcinogen; epidemiologic studies have shown an elevated lung cancer risk among exposed workers.[11]

Moderately Soluble Irritants

The moderately soluble irritants commonly encountered in industrial settings are chlorine,

---

[*] *Case courtesy of Stephen Hessl, M.D., Daniel Hryhorczuk, M.D., and Peter Orris, M.D., Section of Occupational Medicine, Cook County Hospital, Chicago, Illinois.*

fluorine, and sulfur dioxide (SO_2). Chlorine is widely used in the chemical industry to synthesize various chlorinated hydrocarbons, whereas outside the chemical industry its major use is in water purification and as a bleach in the paper industry. Fluorine is used in the conversion of uranium tetrafluoride to uranium hexafluoride, in the development of fluorocarbons, and as an oxidizing agent. Fluoride is used in the electrolytic manufacture of aluminum, as a flux in smelting operations, in coatings of welding rods, and as an additive to drinking water. SO_2 is commonly used as a disinfectant, a fumigant, and a bleach for wood pulp and is formed as a by-product of coal burning, smelter processes, and the paper industry. SO_2 has proved to be an important environmental pollutant. It is a colorless, highly water-soluble gas, and hence it affects mostly the upper respiratory tract and has limited deposition in the lower airways. However during exercise, the resultant increased minute ventilation may result in greater lower airway deposition than what would be usually expected. When SO_2 is released in the atmosphere, it combines with water, metals, and other pollutants to form aerosols, most importantly sulfuric acid, metallic acids, and ammonium sulfates. It is these aerosols that have been shown to induce asthmatic responses in both adults and children.

Particulate air pollution is closely related to SO_2 and its acidic aerosols both in terms of sources and respiratory health effects (see Table 25-3). The term refers to particles suspended in the air after various forms of combustion or other industrial activity. Numerous studies have shown increased morbidity and mortality with increased particulate counts.[12] Recent interest in particulate air pollution has focused on particle size. Particles less than 2.5 μm in diameter ($PM_{2.5}$), in contrast to particles greater than 10 μm in diameter (PM_{10}), have been more recently investigated as it is believed that these particles are more likely to be deposited in the lower airways.[13]

These irritants, like the highly soluble ones, initially cause mucous membrane irritation, often manifested by a persistent cough. Acute symptoms are usually of short duration.[14] Low levels of continuous exposures, which are better tolerated than exposures to highly soluble irritants, may cause obstructive respiratory disease.

In addition to causing respiratory symptoms, these irritants lead to other health problems. Chlorine gas contributes to corrosion of the teeth, whereas fluorine is a significant cause of chemical skin burns. Chronic exposure to fluoride is associated with increased bone density, cartilage calcification, discoloration of teeth in the young, and possibly rheumatologic syndromes. Sulfur dioxide exposure, in particular, is associated with bronchospasm, especially in people with asthma; it may eventually lead to chronic obstructive pulmonary disease. Management and prevention are similar to those for highly soluble irritants. Pulmonary function tests, especially the FEV_1, are recommended in surveillance programs for individuals with chronic exposure.

Low-Solubility Irritants

Usually, the effects of irritants with low solubility are mild throat irritation and occasionally headache. Much more significant is pulmonary edema, which manifests itself 6 to 24 hours after exposure, preceded by symptoms of bronchospasm—chest tightness and wheezing (Fig. 25-6). Two of the most commonly produced industrial and urban pollutants are *ozone* (O_3) and *oxides of nitrogen* (NO_x), which are usually produced by the action of sunlight on the waste products of the internal combustion engine. Both are present in welding fumes and therefore are found in many work environments. Ozone is used as a disinfectant; as a bleach in the food, textile, and pulp and paper industries; and as an oxidizing agent. Oxides of nitrogen are used in chemical and fertilizer manufacture and in metal processing and cleaning operations.

The most concerning of these products are unburned hydrocarbons and nitrogen dioxide (NO_2). It is these pollutants that are the main constituents of smog, as commonly seen in cities such as Los Angeles, Mexico City, and Bangkok. Higher levels are found in the summertime when the sunlight is more intense and the temperatures are higher, levels usually lowest in the morning hours, highest at midday, and then taper off after sunset.

Both O_3 and NO_x are thought to be particularly damaging to the lung as they are both relatively water insoluble and will likely travel to more distant parts of the lungs as compared to gases such as SO_2. Chronic exposure to NO_x may result in bronchiolitis obliterans. An acute obstructive defect is revealed by spirometry. The chest x-ray may show early pulmonary edema and bilateral patchy

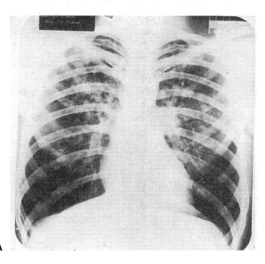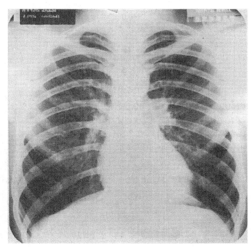

A **B**

FIGURE 25-6 ● Chest x-rays in a copper miner. **(A)** Twenty-four hours after overexposure to oxides of nitrogen, pulmonary edema is evident. **(B)** One week after exposure, there is resolution of pulmonary edema. (Courtesy of the late Benjamin G. Ferris, M.D., Harvard School of Public Health, Boston, Massachusetts.)

airspace opacities suggestive of bronchiolitis obliterans.

A specific syndrome associated with oxides of nitrogen is silo filler's disease, which results from exposures to this gas in the upper chambers of grain silos, where it forms in the anaerobic fermentation of green silage. The brownish color of NO_x is an important warning sign for farmers. Numerous instances of acute overexposure and death have resulted from inadequately ventilated silos.

Numerous animal and human studies have shown that exposure to ozone levels even below the U.S. National Air Quality Standard of 80 ppb for 8 hours have resulted in symptoms and changes in peak expiratory flow.[15] These exposure levels are less than those seen in cities such as Los Angeles and in the northeastern United States. NO_x have shown similar results in animal and human studies. The only difference was that NO_x levels shown to have adverse effects are above the levels noted in ambient air measurements. Individuals with significant respiratory illnesses are recommended to stay indoors, close car windows, and use air-conditioning as ways to protect against harmful ozone exposure.

Although management and prevention are similar to those for highly soluble irritants, overnight observation of patients is frequently necessary when excess exposure has occurred because of the insidious onset of pulmonary edema.

NONIRRITANT EXPOSURES

Carbon Monoxide

CO is emitted mainly from internal combustion engines used in motor vehicles. Other causes of exposure include incomplete combustion of coal, paper, wood, oil, gas, or any other carbonaceous material. The medical literature has numerous accounts of the medical complications and treatment of this commonly known asphyxiant. The effect of CO on the respiratory system is mainly limited to its direct effect on blood oxygenation. The affinity of CO for hemoglobin is 240 times more than oxygen, thus severely reducing the blood's ability to transport oxygen. Depending on the extent of the exposure, CO can cause significant hypoxia resulting in fatal neurological and cardiac consequences.

Indoor Air Pollution

Indoor air pollution, referring to homes and nonfactory public buildings such as office buildings, schools, and hospitals, has been associated with mucous membrane irritation, discomfort, illness, and even death. This is of particular concern in developing nations, due to the burning of biomass in homes.[16] The World Health Organization (WHO) estimates that 2 to 3 million deaths annually in developing countries are caused by exposure to severe indoor pollutants and that a disproportionate number occur in women and children. There are clearly strong associations between respiratory illnesses in children under the age of 5 and high levels of indoor air pollution. Indeed, residents of developed countries are also being exposed to high levels of indoor pollution due to tighter building constructions and the use of buildings materials with high levels of volatile organic compounds (VOCs).

In developing nations, the exposure of high levels of indoor pollution occurs during the burning of biomass in forms such as wood, crop residues, and animal dung. Homes that use biomass for cooking expose themselves to mean 24-hour CO levels estimated from 2 to 50 ppm, rising to 10 to 500 ppm during cooking—compared to the EPA's 8-hour standard of 9 ppm.[17]

OCCUPATIONAL ASTHMA

An 18-year-old woman arrived at an emergency department complaining of shortness of breath. Eight weeks previously, she had consulted her physician about daytime wheezing and cough productive of white phlegm. She was treated with antibiotics and an expectorant and remained at home for 3 days with significant improvement. A week later, a cough and shortness of breath again developed. Again, she was treated with antibiotics, an expectorant, and bed rest with significant improvement. She had an exacerbation of coughing, shortness of breath, and cyanosis of her fingertips the day before her visit.

Her occupational history revealed that she had begun working at a tool supply and manufacturing company 9 weeks previously, 1 week before her symptoms began. Her usual job was grinding carbide-steel drill bits. In her work, she used one of four machines that sharpened drill bits. Her machine generated much metal dust, often covering the machines and her face, hands, and clothes. There was no exhaust system to draw dust away from her breathing zone, and no respiratory protection was provided.

After being treated for the first time 8 weeks previously, she was temporarily assigned to cleaning drill bits in a solvent bath. On this job, she felt lightheaded but had no difficulty breathing. After a long holiday weekend, she was again assigned to drill-bit grinding and after several hours acquired a cough. The next day, the cough increased and she experienced shortness of breath, prompting a second visit to her physician. When she improved from that

episode, she returned to work again and experienced exacerbation of coughing and shortness of breath. This prompted her emergency department visit.

Past medical history revealed occasional seasonal rhinitis as a child but no asthma, eczema, or other allergies. There was no family history of allergies or asthma.

Physical examination revealed a pulse rate of 128 and a respiratory rate of 40. She had cyanosis of the lips and fingertips. Chest examination revealed diffuse bilateral wheezes and use of accessory muscles for breathing.

Arterial blood gases in room air at rest revealed a markedly low PaO_2 of 39 mm Hg. Spirometry showed a normal FVC, but a markedly abnormal FEV_1 (53 percent of predicted). A chest x-ray was normal. White blood cell count was elevated at 11,200 cells/mm^3, with an elevated percentage of eosinophils (10 percent).

She was treated with oxygen, bronchodilators, and steroids. She improved clinically; by the second day, her FEV_1 had improved to 82 percent of predicted.

A later call by her physician to the state occupational safety and health agency revealed that carbide-steel bit alloys contain nickel, cobalt, chromium, vanadium, molybdenum, and tungsten. Grinding such bits can produce cobalt and tungsten carbide dusts, which are recognized pulmonary sensitizers.

The diagnosis in this case was occupational asthma. No specific agent was proved responsible, but the presence of tungsten carbide and cobalt dusts suggest probable agents. Since changing jobs, she has felt well and has not had further bronchospasm.[*]

In 2001, it was estimated that about 31 million Americans, or 113 per 1,000, had been diagnosed with asthma by a health professional within their lifetime. From 6 to 21 percent of new-onset asthma can be attributed to occupational asthma. There is a significantly greater contribution of work to the burden of asthma when work exposures that exacerbate preexisting asthma are added to work-induced asthma.

Individual responses may be so clear and occur so early in a new job that those workers who respond adversely may leave quite soon after

---

[*] *Case courtesy of the late James Keogh, M.D., University of Maryland School of Medicine, Balitmore, Maryland (unpublished curriculum materials).*

being hired. Thus, population surveys may be biased due to the *healthy worker survivor effect*[18] hence underestimating the number of workers identified with immediate sensitivity because most of those who had experienced adverse effects had already left the job to avoid the asthma-producing exposure. A wide variety of materials and circumstances have been shown to cause occupational asthma (see Table 25-4).

Diagnosis of Occupational Asthma

Diagnosis of occupational asthma depends greatly on the occupational history. However clinical history has been shown to be more sensitive than specific.[19] Major or minor constituents of substances as well as accidental by-products can incite attacks. Many people with occupational asthma have a history of atopy, especially when the exposure is to high-molecular-weight compounds. However, those without such a history may become sensitized after exposure to specific environmental agents, such as diisocyanates. The latency period between onset of exposure and symptoms can be highly variable, from immediate up to 5 years in certain instances. Suspicion of this diagnosis should be aroused even when a worker has had no previous history of asthma. Often the worker reports wheezing, chest tightness, shortness of breath, or severe cough developing in the evening or at night with recovery overnight or over a weekend away from work. However, if exposure and its effects have been prolonged, the symptoms may persist at home or over the weekend. In addition, removal from exposure does not always lead to a cure. In fact, only one-fourth to one-half of cases experience improvement of symptoms after removal from exposure.[20,21] The physical examination of an acutely ill worker reveals wheezing and rhonchi.

A useful, but not particularly sensitive, test for bronchoconstriction of occupational origin is the FEV_1 before and after a work shift. A drop of at least 300 mL, or 10 percent, of the FEV_1 (measured as the mean of the two best of three acceptable results each time) between the beginning and end of the first shift of the work week suggests a work-related effect. However, this does not help to identify the inciting agent. An acute drop in FEV_1 as large as 1.8 L has been measured without the worker reporting symptoms. Serial measurements of peak flow, such as four times daily for at least 2 weeks, both on days at and days away from work, with a simple, inex-

pensive peak-flow meter can be extremely valuable in detecting work-associated declines in airflow.[22] Peak-flow monitoring has also become a mainstay of asthma management. Excessive eosinophils in the sputum or blood may help distinguish asthma from bronchitis, reflecting an allergic type of reaction. Reliance should not be placed on skin tests for diagnosing allergic reactions because skin and bronchial responses do not always correlate well. Many individuals will have positive results that may have no correlation with their respiratory symptoms. In addition, skin testing is limited by the unavailabity of a wide range of possible occupational reagents. However, a negative test essentially rules out the possibility that the tested antigen is responsible for the respiratory symptoms. Specific bronchoprovocation, performed at certain specialized centers, with suspected offending agents is usually not needed for diagnosis and can be dangerous.[23] Nonspecific bronchoprovocation testing is the most objective test used to confirm reversible airways disease. Because virtually any chemical substance can precipitate an asthma attack, physicians should rely heavily on the patient's medical and work histories even in the absence of a documented association between a given exposure and asthma. Clinical guidelines for diagnosis and management of occupational asthma have been formulated recently and published.[24,25]

Acute care of those with attacks of occupational asthma is the same as for any case of asthma. Long-term management, however, almost always requires removal from exposure, because after sensitization even very low levels of exposure can trigger an asthmatic response. Close monitoring of symptoms and lung function should be maintained for a person who must continue exposure to a suspected offending agent.[26]

An important and increasingly prevalent challenge is the recognition, management, and prevention of occupationally exacerbated asthma (workplace triggering of symptoms and airflow obstruction in a person with otherwise controlled asthma). All people with asthma are at risk, and the inciting conditions may be chemical, biological, or physical.[27] The diagnosis of asthma should not automatically prohibit an individual from certain occupations. The variability of severity, triggers, and comorbid conditions adds to the difficulty of establishing guidelines and should be approached on an individual basis. In difficult situations it may even involve specific bronchoprovocation testing as discussed above. Recommendations must take into consideration numerous factors including both adverse and beneficial factors. Actual site visits and trial periods may be required. In general if specific sensitization to a workplace agent is identified, employment should not be recommended. Identification of employment activities that may exacerbate symptoms may be difficult. It requires a thorough examination of the potential exposures and an objective assessment of what the consequences of these exposures will be, keeping in mind that early recognition and prompt control results in the best outcomes.

In the event that the physician is asked to assist in the control of a present worker, the clinician may recommend workplace modifications, exposure control, protection devices, and systematic monitoring of implemented changes. The primary goal is optimization of the patient's status as a productive and functional individual while minimizing any adverse health and economic effects. In addi-

tion, occupational physicians should be aware of the major laws, regulations, and agencies that pertain to the respiratory health of workers.

HYPERSENSITIVITY PNEUMONITIS

Hypersensitivity pneumonitis (HSP), also known as *extrinsic allergic alveolitis*, refers to reactions associated with the most picturesque of all occupational disease names (Table 25-5). This response results from organic materials, commonly fungi or thermophilic bacteria that are present in a surprising variety of settings. In contrast to asthma, this response is more focused in the lung parenchyma (respiratory bronchioles and alveoli). Characteristics of this kind of reaction include antibodies (precipitins) in serum, which are highly sensitive but not specific; and a lymphocytosis in bronchoalveolar specimens of greater than 20 percent. Activation of pulmonary macrophages with an increased number of T lymphocytes and probably a change in their function

TABLE 25-5

Examples of hypersensitivity pneumonitis

Disease	Antigenic Material	Antigen
Farmer's lung	Moldy hay or grain	Thermophilic actinomycetes
Bagassosis	Moldy sugar cane	
Mushroom worker's lung	Mushroom compost	
Humidifier fever	Dust from contaminated air conditioners or furnaces	
Maple bark disease	Moldy maple bark	*Cryptostroma* species
Sequoiosis	Redwood dust	*Graphium* species, Pallurlaria
Bird fancier's lung	Avian droppings or feathers	Avian proteins
Pituitary snuff taker's lung	Pituitary powder	Bovine or porcine proteins
Suberosis	Moldy cork dust	*Penicillium* species
Paprika splitter's lung	Paprika dust	*Mucor stolonifer*
Malt worker's lung	Malt dust	*Aspergillus clavatus* or *Aspergillus fumigatus*
Fishmeal worker's lung	Fishmeal	Fishmeal dust
Miller's lung	Infested wheat flour	*Sitophilus granarius* (wheat weevil)
Stipatosis	Esparto fibers	*Aspergillus fumigatus*
Metalworking fluid–associated HSP	Metalworking fluid (coolants)	*Mycobacterium chelonae* (?) *Pseudomonas nitroreducens*
Furrier's lung	Animal pelts	Animal fur dust
Coffee worker's lung	Coffee beans	Coffee bean dust
Chemical worker's lung	Urethane foam and finish	Isocyanates (such as toluene diisocyanate), anhydrides

appear to be the underlying cellular mechanisms. The end result can be fibrosis, yet the responses are much less dose-dependent than those for primary fibrosis due to inorganic dusts. Once hypersensitivity is established, small doses may trigger episodes of alveolitis. This disease is a complex inflammatory response, often due to bacterial or fungal material—neither an infection nor a true allergic response. Therefore, the commonly used clinical terms *hypersensitivity pneumonitis* or *extrinsic allergic alveolitis* are inaccurate. Research has focused on the etiologies, pathophysiology, treatment, and prevention of this condition.

Outbreaks of hypersensitivity pneumonitis have been described in numerous workers as shown in Table 25-5. Most recently, it has been seen in workers exposed to metalworking fluid (coolants) suggested to be due to inoculation of nontuberculous mycobacteria.[28,29]

The worker with hypersensitivity pneumonitis experiences shortness of breath and nonproductive cough. In contrast to asthma, wheezing is not a prominent component. In acute episodes, the sudden onset of the respiratory symptoms along with fever and chills is dramatic. Physical examination may show rapid breathing, fine basilar rales, and possibly hypoxemia. Pulmonary function tests can show marked reduction in lung volumes consistent with restrictive disease. The FEV_1 is reduced, but in proportion to the decreases in FVC and total lung capacity; in general, there is a normal or increased FEV_1/FVC ratio. Arterial blood gas measurements show an increased alveolar–arterial oxygen difference [$P(A-a)O_2$] and a reduced lung diffusing capacity for carbon monoxide (D_{LCO}). A chest x-ray, both conventional and HRCT, can be helpful in acute episodes by revealing patchy infiltrates or a diffuse, fine micronodular shadowing.

If the person is removed from exposure, symptoms and signs usually disappear in 1 to 2 weeks, but in certain instances it can take years to recover. In addition, in severe cases corticosteroid treatment is required. If repeated exposures are experienced, especially at levels low enough to result in only mild symptoms, a more chronic disease may ensue. The worker may be unaware of the work association because the low-level effects may appear symptomatically like a persistent or intermittent respiratory "flu." Over a period of months, however, there is a gradual onset of dyspnea, which can be accompanied by weight loss and lethargy. The physical examination is similar to that in the acute episode,

although the patient may appear less acutely ill and may demonstrate finger clubbing. The chest x-ray, however, is more suggestive of chronic interstitial fibrosis, and the pulmonary function tests show a restrictive defect. The disease may progress to severe dyspnea and the end result resembles, even histologically, idiopathic pulmonary fibrosis (IPF). Sometimes an asymptomatic patient without an episode of acute pneumonitis in the past acquires interstitial fibrosis.

Prevention rests on removal from exposure. This can be more readily accomplished than with asthma because environmental controls can focus on the elimination of conditions that foster bacterial or fungal growth. Process changes may also be necessary to prevent antigen production, and local exhaust ventilation, rather than personal protective equipment (masks), should be used.

BYSSINOSIS AND OTHER DISEASES CAUSED BY ORGANIC DUSTS

Some types of airway constriction are believed to be due not to sensitization but to direct toxic effects on the airways. This has been referred to as *pharmacologic bronchoconstriction*. For byssinosis, however, the pathogenesis is still poorly understood.

Byssinosis (meaning "white thread" in Greek) is associated with exposure to cotton, hemp, and flax processing. It has been popularly called *brown lung* (a misnomer because the lungs are not brown), by analogy to the popular term *black lung* used to describe CWP.

Byssinosis has been shown to develop in response to dust exposure in cotton processing but prevalence can range from 2 percent to 50 percent.[30,31] It is especially prevalent among cotton workers in the initial, very dusty operations where bales are broken open, blown (to separate impurities from fibers), and carded (to arrange the fibers into parallel threads). A lower prevalence of disease occurs in workers in the spinning, winding, and twisting areas, where dust levels are lower. The lowest prevalence of byssinosis has been found among weavers, who experience the lowest dust exposure. Processing of cloth is practically free of cotton dust, as in the manufacture of denim, which is washed during dyeing, before thread is spun. Byssinosis has also been described in other than textile sectors where cotton is processed, such as cottonseed oil mills, the cotton waste utilization industry, and the garneting, or bedding and batting, industry.

The same syndrome has been shown to occur in workers exposed in processing soft hemp, flax, and sisal.

Byssinosis is characterized by shortness of breath and chest tightness. These symptoms are most prominent on the first day of the work week or after being away from the factory over an extended period of time ("Monday morning tightness"). No previous exposure is necessary for symptoms to develop.

Symptoms are often associated with changes in pulmonary function. One characteristic of the acute pulmonary response to cotton dust exposure is a drop in the FEV_1 during the Monday work shift or the first day back at work after at least a 2-day layoff. Because workers do not normally lose lung function during a workday, an acute loss of at least 10 percent or 300 mL (whichever is greater) in an individual, or 3 percent or 75 mL (whichever is greater) in a group of 20 or more workers, can be considered significant enough to require further investigation. Over time, cotton dust workers have an accelerated decrement in FEV_1 consistent with fixed airflow obstruction and chronic obstructive lung disease. Diagnosis is based mainly on symptoms; no characteristic examination or chest radiographic findings are associated with byssinosis. Therefore, the patient should be questioned systematically about symptoms.

It is assumed that the disease progresses if duration of exposure to sufficiently high dust levels is prolonged. Mild byssinosis probably is reversible if exposure ceases, but long-standing disease is irreversible. People with severe byssinosis are rarely seen in an industrial survey because they are too disabled to be working. Byssinosis seems more severe when it is associated with chronic bronchitis. The end stage of the disease is fixed airway obstruction with hyperinflation and air trapping. Cigarette smokers are at increased risk of irreversible byssinosis.[32]

Much research has been done on possible etiologic mechanisms and effects. Extracts of cotton bract have been shown to release pharmacologic mediators, such as histamine, as well as prostaglandins. It seems likely that the mechanism of byssinosis involves stimulation of the same inflammatory receptors by endotoxin and by cotton dust. Gram-negative bacterial endotoxin contaminates cotton fiber, and aqueous extracts of endotoxin have produced acute symptoms and lung function declines.

Two other respiratory conditions are associated with work in the cotton industry:

1. *Mill fever*: This self-limited condition usually happens on first exposure to a cotton dust environment. It lasts for 2 or 3 days and has no known sequelae. It is characterized by headache, malaise, and fever. A flu-like illness, it has symptoms similar to metal fume fever and polymer fume fever. Mill fever is probably related to Gram-negative bacterial material in mill dust; it usually affects workers only once, but after prolonged absence from a mill, reexposure may trigger another attack.

2. *Weaver's cough*: Weavers have experienced outbreaks of acute respiratory illness characterized by a dry cough, although their dust exposure is comparatively low. It may result from sizing material or from mildewed yarn that is sometimes found in high-humidity weaving rooms.

Other organic/vegetable materials are associated with respiratory diseases, including flax (baker's asthma), swine confinement buildings (acute airflow obstruction), and wood dust (asthma, chronic airflow obstruction). Evidence is accumulating that chronic exposure to organic dusts can result in both acute and chronic lung disease.[33]

CHRONIC RESPIRATORY TRACT RESPONSES

Pneumoconiosis

Pulmonary fibrosis is a well documented environmental and work-related chronic pulmonary reaction. This condition, which varies according to inciting agent, intensity, and duration of exposure, is generally referred to as a pneumoconiosis. It is usually due to an inorganic dust or coal that must be of respirable size (<5 μm) to reach terminal bronchioles and alveoli; dust of this size is not visible and so its presence may not be recognized by a worker. There are two basic types of fibrosis: (a) localized and nodular, usually peribronchial fibrosis; and (b) diffuse interstitial fibrosis. Both usually lead to a restrictive lung disease pattern by spirometry. The clinical features of all pneumoconioses are similar: initial nonproductive cough, shortness of breath of increasing severity, and, in the later stages, productive cough, distant breath sounds, and signs of right heart failure. The pneumoconioses are often associated with obstructive airways disease caused by the same agents.

Silica-Related Disease

Crystalline silica (SiO_2) is a major component of the earth's crust. Therefore, exposure occurs in a wide variety of settings, such as mining, quarrying, and stone cutting; foundry operations; ceramics and vitreous enameling; and in use of fillers for paints and rubber.

WHO estimates that approximately 72 million workers are exposed to silica, and 10 percent are at risk for developing silicosis. In the United Kingdom, there were 1,164 reported new cases in 2002. In the United States, reports suggest that silicosis still accounts for around 5,000 new cases and 300 deaths yearly. No distinct clinical features can be cited beyond the ones already listed, but there is distinct pathologic process. Silicosis occurs more frequently in the upper rather than the lower lobes, with nodules varying in size from microscopic to 6 mm in diameter. In severe cases, nodules aggregate and become fibrotic masses several centimeters in diameter. Nodules are firm and intact with a whorled pattern, and rarely cavitate (Fig. 25-7). Microscopically, the nodules are hyalinized, with a well-organized circular pattern of fibers in a cellular capsule. The amount of fibrosis appears proportional to the free silica content and to the duration of exposure. One notable characteristic of this disease is that fibrosis progresses even after removal from exposure. Except in acute silicosis, symptoms

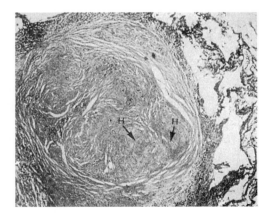

FIGURE 25-7 ● Microscopic section of a typical silicotic nodule showing the concentric (onion skin) arrangement of collagen fibers, some of which are hyalinized (H); lack of dust pigmentation; and peripheral cellularity. The lesion is clearly demarcated from adjacent lung tissue, which is substantially normal. (From Parkes WR. Occupational lung disorders. 3rd ed. Oxford: Butterworths-Heinemand, 1994.)

usually do not occur until 10 to 20 years after initiation of exposure. Evidence of pathologic response to silica exposure exists well before symptoms occur.

Evaluation of workers exposed to silica includes lung function tests (which may show reduced FVC or total lung capacity, or mixed obstructive and restrictive patterns), a chest x-ray (which may appear more abnormal than the lung function tests), and determination of (a reduced) hemoglobin oxygen saturation on exercise. As the disease progresses, there can be decreased oxygen saturation at rest and reduced total lung capacity. The chest x-ray usually shows rounded opacities, localized initially to the upper lung fields (see Fig. 25-2). The size and distribution of these opacities increase over time, and "eggshell" calcification of hilar lymph nodes occurs in a few cases.

Chronic silicosis is classified either as simple or complicated, although there is a continuum between these two forms of the disease. The simple form is noted on the chest film by the presence of multiple, small, round opacities, usually in the upper zones. The concentrations of these opacities are used in classifying simple silicosis (categories 1 to 3).[1] Although simple silicosis alone is not a common cause of disability, it can contribute to disability as well as progress to complicated silicosis. In progressive massive fibrosis (PMF), several of the simple nodules appear to aggregate and produce larger conglomerate lesions, which enlarge and encroach on the vascular bed and airways (ILO categories A, B, and C). The extent of lung function impairment appears directly related to the radiographic size of the lesions and is most severe in categories B and C.

An important complication of silicosis is tuberculosis (TB), which persists today as an added hazard peculiar to this pneumoconiosis. The association between silicosis and pulmonary TB has been known for decades. More recent publications also show an increased incidence of TB among workers in the mining, quarrying, and tunneling industries and in steel and iron foundries. Workers exposed to silica may be at increased risk of TB even in the absence of radiographic evidence for silicosis. Infections with atypical mycobacteria such as *Mycobacterium kansasii* and *Mycobacterium avium-intracellulare* can also occur and are related to the geographic distribution of these organisms. Treatment of such cases may require more vigorous drug treatment than TB without silicosis. No relationship has yet been shown between silicosis and cigarette smoking. Another potential complication of silica exposure is lung cancer. Epidemiologic studies have shown a link between silica exposure and lung cancer, and the International Agency for Research on Cancer (IARC) has classified silica as a group 1 carcinogen.

Prevention of silicosis focuses on reduction of exposure through wet processes, isolation of dusty work, and local exhaust ventilation. Annual TB screening by purified protein derivative (PPD) skin testing or, if the PPD is positive, chest radiography is essential in silica-exposed workers. There is an ongoing effort in the United States to eliminate silicosis in all sandblasting operations. Elimination of silicosis from each work practice would reduce the at-risk population substantially.

Acute silicosis, a distinct entity, is a devastating disease. It is due to extraordinarily high exposures to small silica particles (1 to 2 μm). These exposures occur in abrasive sandblasting and in the production and use of ground silica. Symptoms include dyspnea progressing rapidly over a few weeks, weight loss, productive cough, and sometimes pleuritic pain. Diminished resonance on percussion of the chest and rales on auscultation can be found. Lung function tests show a marked restrictive defect, with an impressive decrement in total lung capacity. The chest x-ray has a diffuse ground-glass, or miliary TB–like appearance, rather than the classic nodular silicosis. The pathologic process in this disease is characterized by a widespread fibrosis, with a diffuse interstitial, rather than nodular, macroscopic appearance, and a microscopic appearance and chemical constituency resembling pulmonary alveolar proteinosis, but with doubly-refractile particles of silica lying free within the alveolar exudate. Disease onset usually occurs 6 months to 2 years after initial exposure. Acute silicosis is often fatal, usually within 1 year of diagnosis.

Diatomaceous earth is an amorphous silica material mined predominantly in the western United States. It is used as a filler in paints and plastics, as a heat and acoustic insulator, as a filter for water and wine, and as an abrasive. In contrast to the various forms of crystalline silica, amorphous silica has relatively low pathogenicity. However, some processes using diatomaceous earth include heating (calcinating) it to remove organic material. This heating process can produce up to 60 percent crystalline silica as cristobalite, which is highly fibrogenic. Exposure to this form of diatomaceous earth,

therefore, must be treated the same as exposure to crystalline silica.

Silica appears in a wide variety of minerals in different combined forms known as *silicates*. Many of these silicates, such as asbestos, kaolin, and talc, also cause pneumoconiosis, but the forms they produce have features distinct from those of silicosis. Asbestos is the most widespread and best known of the silicates and is responsible for asbestosis as well as several types of cancers (see Chapter 24).

Asbestos appears in nature in four major types (chrysotile, crocidolite, amosite, and anthophyllite) that produce similar chronic respiratory reactions. All four types are characterized by being fibrous and are indestructible at temperatures as high as 800°C. Use and production of these materials has greatly increased in the past century; more than 3,000,000 tons of asbestos are produced in the world annually. More than 30 million tons have been used in construction and manufacture in the United States alone. Asbestos is used in a variety of applications: asbestos cement products (tiles, roofing, and drain pipes), floor tile, insulation and fireproofing (in construction and ship building), textiles (for heat resistance), asbestos paper (in insulating and gaskets), and friction materials (brake linings and clutch pads). Probably the most hazardous current exposures occur in repair and demolition of buildings and ships and in a variety of maintenance jobs where exposures may be unsuspected by the workers (Fig. 25-8). In the United States, the construction industry is the major source of asbestos exposure to workers, mainly from disrupting previously installed asbestos products. The effect of asbestos exposure in the community can be significant, as seen in Libby, Montana. Strip mining, transportation, and processing of vermiculite ore containing asbestiform minerals was conducted in the area from 1923 until 1990. As a result, asbestos-related lung diseases have been observed in Libby residents. Numerous potential exposure sources existed, which included work, community, actual material use at home, and inadvertent exposure to family members by the workers themselves.[34]

As with silicosis, the predominant symptoms of asbestosis are shortness of breath, which may be more severe than the appearance of the chest x-ray might indicate, and cough. Although not common, pleuritic pain or chest tightness may occur, and these are more frequent than in other pneumoconioses. In 20 percent of those affected, basilar rales are present, heard best at the end of inspiration

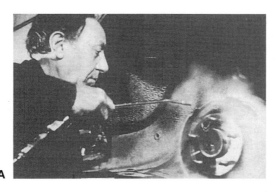

A

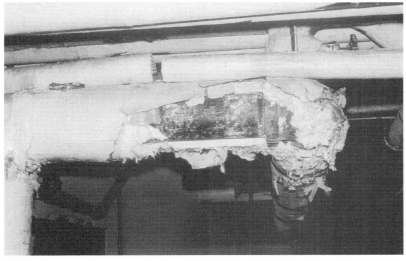

B

FIGURE 25-8 ● **(A)** Brake mechanic exposed to asbestos fibers while using compressed air to clean brake drum. (Photograph by Nick Kaufman.) **(B)** Exposed asbestos pipe insulation. (Photograph by Earl Dotter.)

or early expiration, and pleural rubs and pleural effusions can occur. Pleural effusion in a person with a history of asbestos exposure even many years earlier should be evaluated for mesothelioma, although benign asbestos effusions also occur.

Pathologically, the lung appears macroscopically as a small, pale, firm, and rubbery organ with fibrotic adherent pleura. The cut surface shows patchy to widespread fibrosis, and the lower lobes are more frequently affected than the upper. The microscopic appearance is characterized by interstitial fibrosis. Chest x-rays show widespread irregular (linear) opacities more common in the lower lung fields, in contrast to the round opacities seen in silicosis, which occur first in the upper lung fields.

Much attention has focused on asbestos (or ferruginous) bodies in sputum and lung tissue. These are dumbbell-shaped bodies 20 to 150 μm in length

that appear to be fibers covered by a mucopolysaccharide layer. Iron pigment (from hemoglobin breakdown) makes them golden-brown. They are not diagnostic of asbestos-related disease, but when present even in small numbers in sputum or tissue sections, they indicate substantial occupational exposure to airborne fibers. Most urban dwellers in industrialized countries have a measurable asbestos burden, but the concentrations of asbestos bodies in the nonoccupationally (or paraoccupationally) exposed populations are orders of magnitude lower than in those with known occupational exposures. Pathology studies have shown that in the "background" population of urban dwellers, 50 to 100 microscopic sections of lung would have to be searched to find a single asbestos body, whereas people with very early asbestosis have asbestos bodies in nearly every section, and those with more severe asbestosis have scores of asbestos bodies per section. Asbestos bodies may also be found in other parts of the body besides the lungs; they form round fibers that are transported by lung lymphatics into the circulation.

A particular feature of asbestos exposure, unlike other pneumoconioses, is the frequent presence of asbestos-induced circumscribed pleural fibrosis, known as *pleural plaques*, which are sometimes the only evidence of exposure. These plaques, which can calcify, may be bilateral, and are located more commonly in the parietal pleura. In fact, the evidence for prior asbestos exposure or the explanation of abnormal pulmonary function tests may sometimes be found because of the calcified pleural plaques seen on chest radiography (Fig. 25-9).

Pleural plaques are one manifestation of the rather marked pleural reaction to asbestos fibers. Other such evidence seen on the chest x-ray is a "shaggy"-appearing cardiac or diaphragmatic border. An early, nonspecific sign is a blunted costophrenic angle. Diffuse pleural thickening also occurs, probably less commonly than the more specific pleural plaques. Asbestos-induced diffuse visceral pleural fibrosis may also occur and may im-

pair lung function. Advanced pleural fibrosis may act like a cuirass, severely constricting breathing and leading to respiratory failure.

The evaluation of an individual suspected of having asbestosis includes determining if there has been a history of exposure; a physical examination to ascertain if rales are present; a chest x-ray, which may show irregular linear opacities and a variety of pleural reactions; and pulmonary function tests, which may show evidence of an interstitial type of abnormality—that is, restrictive disease and a diminished DLCO. In addition, the peribronchiolar fibrosis may have an obstructive component. Hence, in both nonsmokers and smokers with asbestosis (as with all pneumoconioses), a mixed restrictive–obstructive pattern may be seen.

Asbestosis, like silicosis, may progress after removal from exposure. Asbestos exposure even without asbestosis carries with it the added risk of cancers of the lung, pleura, and peritoneum (mesotheliomas), gastrointestinal tract, and other organs (see Chapter 24). Prevention focuses on substitution with materials such as fibrous glass, use of wet processes to reduce dust generation, local exhaust ventilation to capture the dust that is generated, and respiratory protection. Exposed patients

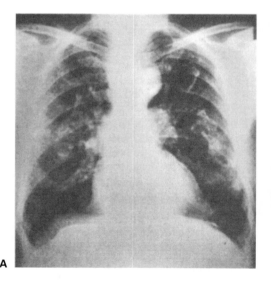
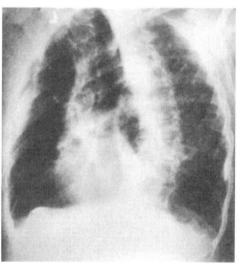

A

B

FIGURE 25-9 ● Bilateral calcified pleural plaques on chest walls and diaphragm. **(A)** Note irregular outline and variable density of the large lesion seen *en face* and the rim of calcification along the left cardiac border. The small, rounded lesions also represent calcification in plaques and are not intrapulmonary. **(B)** The large plaque in the right lung field on the posteroanterior film is seen end-on against the chest wall (left field). There is no evidence of diffuse interstitial pulmonary fibrosis in either film. The patient was an ex-insulation worker (1925 to 1932), 65 years of age. There were no crackles in the lungs, and lung function testing showed severe airflow obstruction and hyperinflation only. (From Parkes WR. Occupational lung disorders. 3rd ed. Oxford: Butterworths-Heinemand, 1994.)

who smoke should be advised to stop smoking for the rest of their lives.

Talc is a hydrated magnesium silicate that occurs in a variety of natural forms. The two major types are nonfibrous and fibrous. The nonfibrous forms, such as those found in Vermont, are free of both crystalline silica and fibrous asbestos tremolite; the fibrous forms, such as those found in New York State, can contain up to 70 percent fibrous material, including amphibole forms of asbestos. Talc exposures occur mainly during its use as an additive to paints and as a lubricant in the rubber industry, especially in innertubes. Evidence suggests that high doses of nonfibrous talc or moderate doses of fibrous talc accumulated over a long time result in chronic respiratory disease known as *talcosis*, with the same symptoms as other pneumoconioses.

Pathologically, the macroscopic appearance of the lung is characterized by poorly structured nodules, unlike the firm nodules of silicosis and the diffuse fibrosis of asbestosis. The microscopic appearance consists of ill-defined nodules with some diffuse interstitial fibrosis. Evaluation of people exposed to talc includes pulmonary function tests and a chest x-ray. The chest x-ray may show both nodular and linear opacities and also pleural plaques. Studies addressing the possibility of a cancer risk associated with fibrous talc exposure found a fourfold increased risk of lung cancer in New York State talc miners.

Kaolin (China clay) is a hydrated aluminum silicate found in the United States (in a band from Georgia to Missouri), India, and China. It is used in ceramics; as a filler in paper, rubber, paint, and plastic products; and as a mild soap abrasive. Kaolin is not particularly hazardous in the mining processes because it is usually a wet ore and mined by jet-water mining techniques.

The pneumoconiosis (kaolinosis) resulting from chronic exposures to kaolin dust produces no unique clinical features. Pathologically, the macroscopic appearance is one of immature silicotic nodules, although conglomerate nodules may appear. Pleural involvement occurs only if the lung is massively involved. The microscopic appearance consists of nodules with randomly distributed collagen.

Coal Workers' Pneumoconiosis

In the United States until the 1960s, coal workers' respiratory disease was considered a variant of silicosis and was often known an *anthracosilicosis*. It is now clear that CWP is an etiologically distinct entity that can be induced by both coal dust and pure carbon. CWP exists both in uncomplicated and complicated forms; the latter, known as *progressive massive fibrosis* (PMF), is the most severe form of the disease. Although exposure to coal dust occurs most commonly in underground mines, there is also some exposure in handling and transportation of coal. Significant exposure also occurs in the trimming or leveling of coal in ships when preparing material for transport.

Uncomplicated CWP increases the likelihood for future development of the complicated form, which is generally agreed to be a disabling condition. The diagnosis of CWP has relied primarily on the chest x-ray, which shows nodular opacities of less than 1 cm (mostly <3 mm) in diameter. PMF, in contrast, is seen on chest radiography as the development of conglomerations of these small opacities to sizes greater than 1 cm in diameter.

In the early stages, CWP is asymptomatic. The initial symptoms are dyspnea (breathlessness) on exertion with progressive reduction in exercise tolerance. As nodular conglomeration begins and PMF is diagnosed, symptoms become more severe, with marked exertional dyspnea, severe disability, or total incapacity. There is general agreement that PMF leads to premature disability and death. No such agreement, however, exists for the impact of simple CWP of grade 2 or less.

Coal dust also contributes independently to the disability observed in coal workers through the production of chronic bronchitis, airways obstruction, and emphysema. The bronchitis and pulmonary function loss is dose related to coal dust in both smokers and nonsmokers. The greater the intensity and duration of exposure (cumulative exposures), the more likely that a miner will get any of these diseases, as well as silicosis if the quartz content of the coal is high. Moreover, the diseases may present in any combination.

Pathologically, CWP appears as soft, black, indurated nodules. Microscopic observation shows dust in and around macrophages near respiratory bronchioles. Nodules show random collagen distribution, and the lung shows centrilobular emphysema. Chest x-rays show widely distributed, small, round opacities.

In PMF, the large conglomerate masses have variable shapes and do not respect the architecture of the lung. The surfaces are hard, rubbery, and black, and cavitation often occurs (Fig. 25-10).

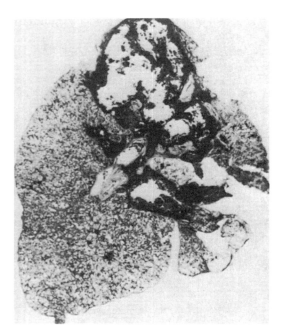

FIGURE 25-10 ● Gough section of lung of coal worker with 18 years of mining experience completed 20 years before death. It shows cavitation as well as centrilobular emphysema, which was present in both lungs. (Courtesy of J.C. Wagner, MRC Pneumoconiosis Unit, Llandough Hospital, Penarth, Wales, United Kingdom.)

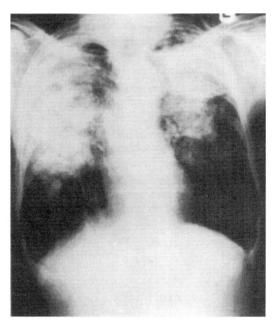

FIGURE 25-11 ● Chest x-ray of coal worker whose lung section appears in Fig. 25-10, taken 2 weeks before death. The appearance is classic for progressive massive fibrosis with larger conglomerate masses in both lung fields. (Courtesy of J.C. Wagner, MRC Pneumoconiosis Unit, Llandough Hospital, Penarth, Wales, United Kingdom.)

Copious, black sputum is often produced. Microscopically, the appearance is not distinct from the simple nodules. Chest radiography shows large conglomerate opacities (Fig. 25-11). A separate condition, called *Caplan syndrome*, or *rheumatoid CWP*, occurs when PMF is accompanied by rheumatoid arthritis. It has a different pathologic appearance, with alternate black and gray-white bands of material in the conglomerate masses. The conglomerate masses frequently cavitate or calcify. Whether there is a different clinical course for people with PMF accompanied by rheumatoid arthritis is not known.

Although evaluation for CWP is the same as for the other pneumoconioses, a particular feature affecting evaluation is the federal Mine Safety and Health Act of 1977, which prescribes what types of abnormalities make a person eligible for disability benefits. Because these are subject to continuous revision, consultation with the Mine Safety and Health Administration in the U.S. Department of Labor is advisable. Miners enjoy special rights to a low-dust environment with increased medical monitoring if they are found to have CWP, and they have the right to permanent removal from the high-

dust environment with wage retention. These rights are unique among American workers, although arguably such an approach should be applied in the prevention of all pneumoconioses.

Miscellaneous Inorganic Dusts

Fibrous glass and related products, referred to as *synthetic vitreous fibers* (SVF), *man-made vitreous fibers*, *man-made mineral fibers* (MMMFs), or *very fine vitreous fibers*, have been used for insulation purposes for more than 60 years. More recently, they have played an important role as an asbestos substitute. SVF are amorphous silicates with a length-to-diameter ratio of greater than 3:1. They are made mainly from rock, slag, glass, or kaolin clay and can be divided into three main groups: mineral wool, fibrous glass, and ceramic fiber.

Synthetic vitreous fibers can induce skin, eye, and upper respiratory tract irritant responses. There have been few case reports of pulmonary disease due to SVF exposure. Prevalence studies of chest radiographic findings, respiratory symptoms, and lung function in exposed workers have in general been negative. Limited studies of workers exposed to fine-diameter fibers have revealed evidence of irregular opacities consistent with pneumoconiosis. An excess of pleural changes, particularly pleural plaques, has consistently been demonstrated in the cohorts of workers in the United States and Europe involved in the production of refractory ceramic fibers. No abnormalities in lung function were reported in these studies. There is growing concern about the possible carcinogenicity of these very fine fibers. IARC has classified special-purpose glass fibers, such as E-glass and "475" glass fibers, and also ceramic fibers as possibly carcinogenic to humans; insulation glass wool, continuous glass filament, rock (stone) wool, and slag wool are not classifiable as to their carcinogenicity to humans. Results from the most recent cohort and nested case-control studies of U.S. workers exposed to glass wool and continuous glass filament and of European workers exposed to rock (stone) and slag wool have not provided consistent evidence of an association between exposure to fibers and risk for lung cancer or mesothelioma. There is limited epidemiological data to permit an adequate evaluation of the cancer risk associated with exposure to refractory ceramic fibers. In chronic inhalation studies, ceramic fibers produce an increase in the incidence of mesothelioma in hamsters and an increased incidence of lung tumors in rats. Because of persistent uncertainties, occupational exposures to SVF should be lowered as much as possible with engineering controls, proper worker training, and safe work practices.

Individual exposures to iron dusts, particularly those resulting from steel-grinding operations, welding, or foundry work, are common. The only clinical effect of pure iron oxide exposure is a reddish-brown coloring of the sputum. Lung function tests show no clinical abnormality, whereas the chest x-ray shows many small (0.5 to 2.0 mm) opacities without confluence (as with stannosis; see Fig. 25-3). Lung sections show macrophages laden with iron dust but without fibrosis or cellular reaction. With removal from further iron oxide dust exposure, the radiographic abnormalities slowly resolve. Similar results can be seen in exposures to tin, barium, and antimony.

Chronic Bronchitis

Probably the most common of the chronic responses of the respiratory tract is *chronic bronchitis*, which results from excessive mucus production in the bronchi. Diagnosis is made strictly on clinical grounds. Chronic bronchitis is a formally defined diagnosis that must meet ATS criteria: recurrent productive cough occurring four to six times a day at least 4 days of the week, for at least 3 months during the year, for at least 2 years. The definition of *simple bronchitis*—the production of phlegm on most days for as much as 3 months of the year—can be used to distinguish those with probably important symptoms from those without. The excess mucus production associated with bronchitis is often associated with airflow obstruction. Chronic bronchitis is not a unique occupational pulmonary response; it is frequently superimposed on other respiratory diseases due to occupational toxins and most often cigarette smoke. Occupational toxins that can cause chronic bronchitis include mineral dusts and fumes (such as from coal, fibrous glass, asbestos, metals, and oils), organic dusts, irritants (such as O_3 ozone and NO_x), plastic compounds (such as phenolics and isocyanates), acids, and smoke (such as experienced in firefighting).

Emphysema

Emphysema is a chronic response that depends more specifically on a pathologic description: it is the enlargement of air spaces distal to terminal (nonrespiratory) bronchioles that includes destruction of the alveolar walls and results in air trapping. Evidence suggests that fixed airway obstruction is the end stage of disease due to chronic coal dust or chronic cadmium exposure. Tobacco smoking is a well recognized cause of emphysema in long-term smokers.

Granulomatous Disease

Another type of chronic response not commonly described as work related is granuloma formation. In a *granuloma*, many cells responding to an inciting agent become surrounded by bundles of collagen. The foreign body granuloma in the skin is an analogous kind of tissue reaction. The best occupational example of pulmonary granulomas is chronic beryllium disease; workers who make metal alloys containing beryllium are exposed when dust control is poor. The disease appears as a restrictive pneumoconiosis, although the pulmonary reaction is out of proportion to the amount of metal dust in the lungs. It is very similar to sarcoid and can be impossible to distinguish without measuring tissue levels (in lung and lymph nodes) of beryllium. A more specific test, to determine cell-mediated immunity to the exposure in question, is the lymphocyte blast transformation test (LTT) on peripheral or lavaged lymphocytes. The LTT has been useful in the early diagnosis of beryllium disease. In this test, the proliferation of lymphocytes cultured in the presence of a beryllium salt is assessed by measuring the incorporation of radiolabeled thymidine. This *ex vivo* test is both highly specific and sensitive.

REFERENCES

1. International Labor Office. Guidelines for the use of the ILO international classification of pneumoconioses. Rev. ed. Geneva: International Labor Office, 2000.
2. Ayres SM, Evans RG, Buehler ME. Air pollution: A major public health problem. CRC Crit Rev Clin Lab Sci 1972;3:1–40.
3. Pope III CA, Thun MJ, Namboodiri MM, et al. Particulate air pollution as a predictor of mortality in a prospective study of U.S. adults. Am J Respir Crit Care Med 1995;151:669–74.
4. Leowski J. Mortality from acute respiratory infections in children under 5 years of age: Global estimates. World Health Stat Q 1986;39:138–44.
5. Ferris BG. Epidemiology Standardization Project (American Thoracic Society). Am Rev Respir Dis 1978; 118:1–120.
6. American Thoracic Society. Standardization of spirometry: 1994 update. Am J Respir Crit Care Med 1995;152: 1107–36.
7. Official American Thoracic Society statement. Screening for adult respiratory disease, March 1983. Am Rev Respir Dis 1983;128:768–74.
8. Gibson GJ. Standardised lung function testing. Eur Respir J 1993;6:155–7.
9. Hankinson JL, Odencrantz JR, Fedan KB. Spirometric reference values from a sample of the general U.S. population. Am J Respir Crit Care Med 1999;159: 179–87.
10. Piirila PL, Nordman H, Korhonen OS, et al. A thirteen-year follow-up of respiratory effects of acute exposure to sulfur dioxide. Scand J Work Environ Health 1996;22:191–6.
11. International Agency for Research on Cancer. Chromium, nickel and welding. In: IARC Monographs on the Evaluation of Carcinogenic Risks to Humans. Lyon, France: IARC, 1990.
12. Villeneuve PJ, Goldberg MS, Krewski D, et al. Fine particulate air pollution and all-cause mortality within the Harvard Six-Cities Study: Variations in risk by period of exposure. Ann Epidemiol 2002;12:568–76.
13. Schwartz J, Neas LM. Fine particles are more strongly associated than coarse particles with acute respiratory health effects in schoolchildren. Epidemiology 2000; 11:6–10.
14. Brevard TA, Calvert GM, Blondell JM, et al. Acute occupational disinfectant-related illness among youth, 1993-1998. Environ Health Perspect 2003;111: 1654–9.
15. Gold DR, Damokosh AI, Pope CA III, et al. Particulate and ozone pollutant effects on the respiratory function of children in southwest Mexico City. Epidemiology 1999;10:8–16.
16. World Health Organization. Epidemiological, social and technical aspects of indoor air pollution from biomass fuel. Geneva: World Health Organization, 1991.
17. Bruce N, Perez-Padilla R, Albalak R. Indoor air pollution in developing countries: A major environmental and public health challenge. Bull World Health Organ 2000;78:1078–92.
18. Arrighi HM, Hertz-Picciotto I. The evolving concept of the healthy worker survivor effect. Epidemiology 1994;5:189–96.
19. Malo JL, Ghezzo H, L'Archeveque J, et al. Is the clinical history a satisfactory means of diagnosing occupational asthma? Am Rev Respir Dis 1991;143:528–32.
20. Chan-Yeung MM, Malo JL. Natural history of occupational asthma. In: Bernstein IL, Chan-Yeung M, Malo JL, Bernstein DI, eds. Asthma in the workplace. New York: Marcel Dekker Inc, 1993:299–322.
21. Perfetti L, Cartier A, Ghezzo H, et al. Follow-up of occupational asthma after removal from or diminution of exposure to the responsible agent: Relevance of the length of the interval from cessation of exposure. Chest 1998;114:398–403.
22. Guidelines for diagnosis and management of asthma. Washington, DC: U.S. Department of Health and Human Services, Public Health Service, National Institutes of Health, 1991. (See also 2002 update)
23. Ortega HG, Weissman DN, Carter DL, et al. Use of specific inhalation challenge in the evaluation of workers at risk for occupational asthma: A survey of pulmonary, allergy, and occupational medicine residency training programs in the United States and Canada. Chest 2002;121:1323–8.
24. American Thoracic Society. Guidelines for assessing and managing asthma risk at work, school, and recreation. Am J Respir Crit Care Med 2004;169:873–81.
25. Chan-Yeung M. Assessment of asthma in the workplace. ACCP consensus statement. Am Coll Chest Phys. Chest 1995;108:1084–117.
26. Gassert TH, Hu H, Kelsey KT, et al. Long-term health and employment outcomes of occupational asthma and their determinants. J Occup Environ Med 1998;40: 481–91.
27. Milton DK, Solomon GF, Rosiello RA, et al. Risk and incidence of asthma attributable to occupational exposure among HMO members. Am J Ind Med 1998;33: 1–10.
28. Kreiss K, Cox-Ganser J. Metalworking fluid-associated hypersensitivity pneumonitis: A workshop summary. Am J Ind Med 1997;32:423–32.
29. Fox H, Anderson H, Moen T, et al. Metal working fluid-associated hypersensitivity pneumonitis: an outbreak investigation and case-control study. Am J Ind Med 1999; 35:58–67.
30. Zuskin E, Ivanokovic D, Schachter EN, et al. A ten-year follow-up study of cotton textile workers. Am Rev Respir Dis 1991;143:301–5.
31. Jiang CQ, Lam TH, Kong C, et al. Byssinosis in Guangzhou, China. Occup Environ Med 1995;52: 268–72.
32. Wang XR, Eisen EA, Zhang HX, et al. Respiratory symptoms and cotton dust exposure: Results of a 15-year follow up observation. Occup Environ Med 2003;60:935–41.
33. Christiani DC. Organic dust exposure and chronic airway disease. Am J Respir Crit Care Med 1996;154(4 Pt 1):833–4.
34. Whitehouse AC. Asbestos-related pleural disease due to tremolite associated with progressive loss of lung

function: Serial observations in 123 miners, family members, and residents of Libby, Montana. Am J Ind Med 2004;46:219–25.

BIBLIOGRAPHY

American Thoracic Society (ATS) Committee of the Scientific Assembly on Environmental and Occupational Health. Adverse effects of crystalline silica exposure. Am J Respir Crit Care Med 1997;155:761–8.
Expert committee review and statement.

Banks DE, Parker JE. Occupational lung disease: An international perspective. London: Chapman and Hall, 1998.
An excellent reference text. Up to date and global in perspective.

Harber P, Schenker M, Balmes J, eds. Occupational and environmental respiratory disease. St. Louis: Mosby-Year Book, 1996.
A well-written review of occupational and environmental respiratory diseases.

Parkes WR. Occupational lung disorders, 3rd ed. London: Butterworths, 1994.
Excellent, detailed summary of occupational respiratory disease. Includes clinical and pathologic details. Best used as a reference.

Rom WN, ed. Environmental and occupational medicine, 3rd ed. Boston: Little, Brown, 1998.
Excellent general reference text with strong chapters on occupational lung diseases.

Schenker M, Christiani DC, Husman K, et al. ATS Committee on the Scientific Assembly on Environmental and Occupational Health. Respiratory health hazards in agriculture: Conference Report. Am J Respir Crit Care Med 1998;158:S1–S76.
Excellent, in-depth review of the topic.

CHAPTER 26

Neurologic and Psychiatric Disorders

Edward L. Baker Jr. and Nancy L. Fiedler

A 29-year-old man was seen after 8 years of employment in a chloralkali plant, where he was primarily employed in maintenance and operation of the electrolytic cells. Four years after beginning work in the plant, he began to notice increased nervousness and irritability. His nervousness continued for 2 years; he then began to experience episodes of severe depression. At that time, he also experienced a tremor of the hands, bleeding gums, easy fatigability, increased salivation, and loss of appetite. He sustained an injury to his left Achilles' tendon and was away from work for 7 months, during which time most of his symptoms improved, but tremulousness, nervousness, and depression remained.

This man and his wife reported that before his employment at the plant he was outgoing, calm, and patient. He had been a military policeman in the U.S. Marines and did not experience emotional upsets during this tour of duty despite significant stress.

Urine mercury monitoring, which had been performed by his employer during the entire period of employment, had demonstrated numerous values over 500 μg/L, the highest of which was 736 μg/L in his fifth year of employment (normal range in the general population, 5 to 30 μg/L).

Physical examination performed at the end of the 7-month removal from work showed no evidence of tremor, a mild loss of pinprick sensation on the dorsal aspect of his arms, and an otherwise normal neurologic examination. Lines of increased pigmentation were observed at the gingival margins of several teeth.

Neuropsychological testing showed mild defects in his ability to perform mental calculations and in his immediate verbal and visual memory. Written spelling was particularly impaired, with an inability to copy simple sentences. He could not concentrate on various tasks and, as a result, his performance was erratic, with incorrect answers to simple questions and correct answers to more difficult ones. He was emotionally labile in the test situation, appearing anxious and depressed. He displayed average performance on tests of manual dexterity.

This patient's illness was manifested primarily by emotional disturbances and deficits on standardized tasks of psychological performance. He showed no particular deficits in memory, psychomotor performance, learning ability, or recall of current events. His most striking deficit was one of impaired concentration, which resulted in erratic performance on various tests. These effects were still detected months after he was removed from mercury exposure.

The occurrence of neurobehavioral and psychiatric disorders among workers in various occupations and among people exposed to neurotoxins in their communities is of increasing concern. The neurotoxic effects of chemicals such as lead or mercury are well-known, but as new substances are introduced into industry and commerce, neurologic and psychiatric disorders associated with them are being recognized. For example, in the 1970s, an industrial catalyst, dimethylaminopropionitrile (DMAPN), was found to cause an autonomic neuropathy affecting the bladder in workers producing polyurethane foam.[1] Another such discovery occurred when peripheral neuropathy was diagnosed in employees of a coated-fabrics plant and traced to the solvent methyl *n*-butyl ketone (MBK).[2] In some instances, as in the case above, specific chemical substances are responsible for characteristic pathologic processes within the nervous system However, in many other situations, workers have symptoms characteristic of both psychiatric and neurologic disease due to a combination of exposure to mixtures of chemicals and adverse psychosocial factors.

NEUROLOGIC DISORDERS

For more than 100 years, exposure to toxic substances has been known to affect behavior. During the past 50 years, quantitative methods applied to the study of behavioral abnormalities during and after toxin exposure have demonstrated a wide range of clinical and subclinical effects for numerous substances. Neuroimaging techniques, such as positron emission tomography (PET), single photon emission computed tomography (SPECT), and functional magnetic resonance imaging (MRI), are helping to improve our understanding of the impact of neurotoxic agents on the central nervous system (CNS), and nerve conduction studies are helping to quantify dysfunction of the peripheral nervous system (PNS). Many neurotoxic agents produce a dose-related spectrum of impairment, ranging from mild slowing of nerve conduction velocity or prolongation in reaction time to more serious neuropathy and encephalopathy.

Pathophysiology

Peripheral Nervous System Effects

Two basic forms of damage to peripheral nerves occur as a result of exposure to neurotoxins. *Segmental demyelination* results from primary destruction of the neuronal myelin sheath, with relative sparing of the axons. This process begins at the nodes of Ranvier and results in slowing of nerve conduction. Characteristically, there is no evidence of muscle denervation, although disuse atrophy may occur if paralysis is prolonged. As remyelination begins during the recovery phase, recovery is rapid and, except in severe cases, usually complete.

Axonal degeneration is associated with metabolic derangement of the entire neuron and is manifested by degeneration of the distal portion of the nerve fiber. Myelin sheath degeneration may occur secondarily. Nerve conduction rates are usually normal until the condition is relatively far advanced. Distal muscles show changes of denervation. Recovery may occur by axonal regeneration, but it is very slow and often incomplete.

In some instances, axonal degeneration and segmental demyelination coexist, presumably as a result of secondary effects derived from damage to each system. Therefore, although the classic descriptions of these syndromes hold in experimental models, the clinical manifestations of neuropathy in exposed individuals may represent a combination of both pathologic processes.

Further, it is not clearly understood at what dose or exposure duration these syndromes occur.

Central Nervous Systems Effects

Investigations of lead, chlordecone (Kepone), carbon monoxide, and other chemicals have shown significant disruption of neurotransmitter metabolism, affecting dopamine, norepinephrine, gamma-aminobutyric acid (GABA), and serotonin, which correlates with behavioral aberrations in experimental animals. Furthermore, many industrial solvents cause acute depression of CNS synaptic transmission, resulting in drowsiness and weakness. Such mechanisms may be responsible for the manifestations of CNS toxicity induced by neurotoxic substances.

Combined Peripheral and Central Nervous System Effects

Certain neurotoxins cause distal degeneration of axons in both the CNS and PNS. This form of axonal degeneration was originally described as *dying back neuropathy*. In view of the association of CNS and PNS degeneration, it has been suggested that this process be referred to as *central–peripheral distal axonopathy*. Substances associated with this effect include acrylamide, *n*-hexane, MBK, carbon disulfide, and organophosphorus compounds, most notably triorthocresyl phosphate (TOCP).

Characteristically, distal degeneration occurs within the long nerve fiber tracts of both the CNS and PNS. Once degeneration begins peripherally, it becomes more severe in the initially affected nerve segments while progressing centrally to involve more proximal segments of nerve fibers. Within the spinal cord, the long ascending and descending tracts (the spinocerebellar and corticospinal tracts) appear to be the most severely affected. Involved fiber tracts demonstrate axonal swellings, which are often focal and are associated with neurofilament accumulation within the axon. Although the length of the axon is a key determinant of fiber susceptibility, fiber diameter may also be important: large-diameter myelinated fibers are more frequently affected.

The precise locus of the metabolic derangement that is responsible for these manifestations of axonal damage is unknown. Chemical substances may bind to the inactive intra-axonal enzyme systems required for maintenance of normal axonal transport mechanisms. MRI may be useful in the clinical evaluation of individuals with combined central and peripheral effects of toxin exposure.

Manifestations

Peripheral Nervous System

Virtually all of the toxic substances that affect the PNS cause a mixed sensorimotor peripheral neuropathy. The initial manifestations of this disorder consist of intermittent numbness and tingling in the hands and feet; motor weakness in the feet or hands may develop somewhat later and progress to the development of an ataxic gait or an inability to grasp heavy objects. Although the distal portion of the extremities is involved initially and to a greater degree, severely affected patients may also have proximal muscle weakness and muscle atrophy. Nerve biopsies in affected persons have shown axonal swellings and paranodal myelin retraction. Extensor muscle groups usually manifest weakness before flexors do.

Although the manifestations are somewhat similar from one toxin to another, certain specific characteristics are unique to individual agents (Table 26-1). Painful limbs and increased sensitivity of the feet to touch are particularly characteristic of arsenical neuropathy. Sensory involvement predominates in the relatively rare neuropathy seen with alkyl

TABLE 26-1

Peripheral Nervous System Effects of Occupational Toxicants[a]

Effect	Toxic Agent	Comments
Motor neuropathy	Lead	Primarily wrist extensors
		Wrist drop and ankle drop rare
Mixed sensorimotor neuropathy	Acrylamide	Ataxia common
		Desquamation of hands and soles
		Sweating of palms
	Arsenic	Distal paresthesias earliest symptom
		Painful limbs (especially in calves)
		Hyperpathia of feet
		Weakness prominent in legs
	Carbon disulfide	Peripheral neuropathy (mild)
		CNS effects more important
	Carbon monoxide	Only seen after severe intoxication
	DDT	Only seen with ingestion
	n-Hexane	Distal paresthesias and motor weakness
		Weight loss, fatigue, and muscle cramps common
	Methyl *n*-butyl ketone	Distal paresthesias and motor weakness
		Weight loss, fatigue, and muscle cramps common
	Mercury	Predominantly distal sensory involvement
		More common with alkyl mercury exposure
	Organophosphate insecticides (selected agents)	Delayed onset following single exposure (usually nonoccupational)

[a] Includes most, but not all, of the neurotoxic substances associated with listed conditions.

mercury poisoning. Both motor and sensory disorders are observed in the neuropathies associated with exposure to *n*-hexane, MBK, and acrylamide.

The peripheral neuropathy associated with lead exposure is unusual because only the motor system is involved. The most characteristic early manifestation of lead neuropathy is wrist extensor weakness. Reports of involvement of the lower extremities resulting in ankle drop were made during the 1930s, when cabaret dancers consumed lead-contaminated illicit whiskey and developed lead neuropathy in the muscles that they used most actively. Overt wrist drop, which was a characteristic manifestation of lead neuropathy in reports of many years ago, is rare today. More common is the occurrence of significant exposure associated with electromyogram (EMG) changes.

The development of these syndromes is usually insidious. Very slow development of numbness and tingling of the fingers and toes occurs over several weeks and may then be followed by motor weakness. With several toxic substances, including acrylamide, *n*-hexane, and MBK, the neuropathy may progress even after the worker is removed from exposure. This deterioration may continue for 3 to 4 weeks; at that point, recovery may begin. The duration of the recovery process is proportional to the degree of severity of neuropathy: less severely affected patients may experience total resolution in 3 to 6 months, whereas those with advanced disease may continue to have signs and symptoms 1 to 2 years later.

Physical examination of affected workers shows a characteristic distribution of sensory loss, particularly to pain and temperature discrimination (Fig. 26-1). Frequently, vibration sensation is impaired and touch perception, particularly with acrylamide poisoning, is lost. Tremor of the hands is particularly common in several types of chemical intoxication; in most instances, it is a resting tremor that is not increased with movement. The tremor seen with chlordecone poisoning is a common manifestation of the disease and has characteristic features: it is irregular, it is nonpurposive, and it is most severe when the limb is static but unsupported against gravity. In contrast, the tremor seen with mercury poisoning has been described as a fine tremor that may effect the eyelids, tongue, and outstretched hands. Motor weakness in toxic neuropathies is often found in distal muscles of the arms and legs (see Fig. 26-1). Intrinsic muscles of the hands and feet are particularly affected in neuropathies caused by

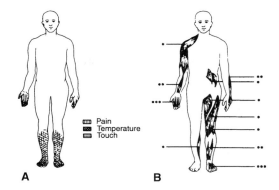

FIGURE 26-1 ● (**A**) Pattern of sensory loss in a severe case of MBK neuropathy. (**B**) Distribution of muscle weakness in MBK neuropathy. The degree of weakness is proportional to the number of asterisks shown. (From Allen N. Solvents and other industrial organic compounds. In: Vinken PK, Bruyn GW, eds. Handbook of clinical neurology: Intoxications of the nervous system, part I. Vol 36. Amsterdam: Elsevier North-Holland Biomedical Press, 1979.)

n-hexane, MBK, and acrylamide. Extensor weakness of the forearms is characteristic of lead neuropathy. Impaired coordination is often seen in persons with motor weakness in the extremities; cerebellar pathology need not be present for these manifestations to occur. In summary, distal sensory and motor impairment characterized by numbness and weakness of the hands and feet is followed by more proximal involvement as the toxic neuropathy develops.

Other Neurologic Manifestations

A wide variety of additional manifestations may be seen that are specific to individual toxicants (Table 26-2). Movement disorders that resemble Parkinson disease have been reported in persons exposed to carbon disulfide, carbon monoxide, and manganese[3]; hypotonia, dystonia, and other disorders of locomotion occur in persons with excessive exposure to these substances.

A characteristic abnormality of eye movements called *opsoclonus* can be caused by exposure to chlordecone. It consists of irregular bursts of involuntary, abrupt, rapid jerks of both eyes simultaneously; these movements usually are horizontal, but in severely affected persons they are multidirectional.

Seizures are often seen in workers with acute excessive exposure to industrial toxicants. Organochlorine insecticides, such as dichlorodiphenyltrichloroethane (DDT) and chlordane, have been

TABLE 26-2

Other Neurologic Manifestations of Occupational Toxicants[a]

Manifestation	Agent
Ataxic gait	Acrylamide
	Chlordane
	Chlordecone (Kepone)
	DDT
	n-Hexane
	Manganese
	Mercury (especially methyl mercury)
	Methyl n-butyl ketone
	Toluene
Bladder neuropathy	Dimethylaminopropionitrile
Constricted visual fields	Mercury
Cranial neuropathy	Carbon disulfide
	Trichloroethylene
Headache	Lead
	Carbon monoxide
Impaired visual acuity	n-Hexane
	Mercury
	Methanol
Increased intracranial pressure	Lead
	Organotin compounds
Myoclonus	Benzene hexachloride
	Mercury
Nystagmus	Mercury
Opsoclonus	Chlordecone (Kepone)
Paraplegia	Organotin compounds
Parkinsonism	Carbon disulfide
	Carbon monoxide
	Manganese
Seizures	Lead
	Organic mercurials
	Organochlorine insecticides
	Organotin compounds
Tremor	Carbon disulfide
	Chlordecone (Kepone)
	DDT
	Manganese
	Mercury

[a] Includes most, but not all, of the neurotoxic substances associated with listed conditions.

associated with seizures after acute ingestion of a large dose. Seizures are a rare manifestation of lead encephalopathy in adults.

Cranial nerve involvement is uncommon with peripheral neurotoxins. However, trichloroethylene has a predilection for the trigeminal nerves and has been associated with facial numbness and weakness. Carbon disulfide exposure is also associated with cranial neuropathies.

As noted above, an unusual manifestation of neurotoxicity was seen in a group of workers exposed to DMAPN.[1] This substance caused an autonomic neuropathy in the bladder, resulting in urinary retention, urinary hesitancy, and sexual dysfunction. Although symptoms and signs improved after cessation of exposure, some workers had persistent symptoms and signs for at least 2 years after cessation of exposure.

Diagnosis

Electrophysiologic tests that assess peripheral nerve function, including electromyograms (EMGs) and nerve conduction measurements, are important tools for assessing the extent and severity of neurologic disorders in workers exposed to industrial toxicants and are often useful in evaluating individual patients. Noninvasive techniques that measure sensory thresholds for vibration and temperature have been developed to monitor diabetic patients for the occurrence of sensory neuropathy; these are also efficient tools for reliable screening for individuals with significant exposure to neurotoxic agents or with early sensory symptoms. Because EMG and nerve conduction velocity testing assess only large fiber function, these tests of perception threshold, which assess small fiber function, may add value in individual diagnostic evaluations. In addition to detection of toxic neuropathy, these instruments may be useful in detection of compression neuropathies, such as carpal tunnel syndrome.

Electroencephalograms (EEGs) have also been used in the evaluation of workers exposed to neurotoxins, but these tests usually are not as useful as nerve conduction tests. The EEG may be of value as an adjunct in the assessment of altered states of consciousness of unknown cause. A more promising extension of EEG use is the measurement of cortical-evoked potentials after auditory or visual stimuli; for example, prolonged latency of visu-

ally evoked responses has been reported in workers chronically exposed to *n*-hexane.

BEHAVIORAL DISORDERS

Manifestations

Excessive exposure to industrial toxicants may result in behavioral effects ranging from mild symptoms of fatigue to persistent impairment of nervous system function. In view of the nonspecific nature of many behavioral manifestations of neurotoxin exposure, standardized psychometric testing has greatly facilitated the evaluation of these disorders. In general, neurotoxins particularly affect psychomotor performance by causing slowness in response time, impaired eye–hand coordination, and diminished concentration ability. Emotional effects are also seen, including irritability, depression, and, at times, emotional liability. Memory and attention may be impaired. Toxicants do not usually affect other aspects of cognitive functioning, such as remote memory and fund of general information.

Although few toxicants have unique behavioral effects, several substances deserve particular attention (Table 26-3). Carbon disulfide affects all levels of the CNS and may result in bizarre clinical syndromes including acute psychosis. Neurotoxins may cause both behavioral effects and peripheral neuropathy in the same person.

Most chlorinated hydrocarbon solvents in current use in industry cause a relatively brief "high" after exposure to significantly elevated concentrations in air. Intentional abuse of industrial solvents by individuals desiring these intoxicating effects can cause permanent damage to the PNS and CNS.

Diagnosis

Standardized psychometric testing, using measures of memory, intelligence, attention, dexterity, reaction time, personality, and general psychomotor function, is very useful in evaluating exposed individuals as well as groups of workers.[4] To facilitate reproducibility in testing of groups and to improve data-handling efficiency, these neurobehavioral tests have been adapted for computer administration. Computerized testing has been used in epidemiologic and clinical research to evaluate effects of neurotoxins. For accurate evaluation of the etiologic role of toxic exposure, interpretation of test results must consider confounding factors, such as age, education, alcohol consumption, and

TABLE 26-3

Behavioral Effects of Occupational Toxicants[a]

Manifestation	Agent
Acute psychosis or marked emotional instability	Carbon disulfide
	Manganese
	Toluene (rare)
Acute intoxication	Organic solvents
	Carbon monoxide
Chronic behavioral symptoms	Acrylamide
	Arsenic
	Lead
	Manganese
	Mercury
	Methyl *n*-butyl ketone
	Organotin compounds
Chronic toxic encephalopathy	Organic solvents
	Styrene
	Lead
	Carbon disulfide

[a] Includes most, but not all, of the neurotoxic substances associated with listed conditions.

preexisting neurologic disease. The most important feature of the diagnostic process is a carefully obtained occupational history that identifies specific neurotoxins and assesses the magnitude and duration of exposure to each. The work history is particularly important in evaluating behavioral disorders, because these conditions are often attributed to factors unrelated to work (see Chapter 6).

PSYCHIATRIC DISORDERS

There are few epidemiologic studies of the prevalence of psychiatric disorders in the workplace. One strategy has been to identify occupations with higher rates of admission to psychiatric treatment facilities.[5] For example, health care workers have higher rates of suicide and hospital and mental health center admissions, although this could be explained by demographic factors or increased awareness and acceptability of mental health problems. More rigorous studies have found that lawyers, teachers, counselors (except college counselors), and secretaries had elevated rates of

major depression[6] and that managers and construction laborers had increased rates of alcoholism when they were unemployed.[7]

Employees in low-status positions demonstrate higher rates of psychiatric disorders than those in high-status positions.[8] Workers in low-status positions often experience high job demands with little control over job decisions—characteristics associated with job strain.[9,10] Although high workload is perceived to be a risk factor for psychiatric illness, it is often difficult to separate workers' perceptions of job characteristics from their negative affective traits; for example, depressed employees may perceive their workload as heavier than healthier workers do. Furthermore, high workload is not consistently associated with increased risk for all psychiatric disorders (see Chapter 16).

Other psychosocial factors that may contribute to stress and psychiatric disorders among workers include conflicting demands and poor social support, both of which may exert a greater detrimental effect than high workload.[10,11] High social support at work (high levels of support from colleagues and supervisors coupled with clear and consistent information from supervisors) and skill discretion (job variety and the opportunity to use skills at work) have been shown to decrease absence due to psychiatric illness. Fair decision-making procedures at work may also contribute to a lower incidence of psychiatric disorders.[12]

Chemical Hazards

The causal relation between neurotoxic exposure and psychiatric symptoms is unclear. Although associations between neurotoxicant exposure and psychiatric symptoms have been reported, a major study did not find higher prevalence of depression among workers in occupations expected to have greater chemical exposures, such as construction laborers and metal workers.[6] Because cognitive deficits and various physical symptoms are also associated with exposure, it is possible that recognition of these impairments may lead to reactive depression. Alternatively, psychiatric responses may reflect CNS dysfunction within the frontal, temporal, and limbic regions that is a direct result of exposure. Brief reactive psychosis has been reported in cases where acute high-level exposures to solvents and some metals have occurred. More studies are needed to better understand the pathogenesis of psychiatric disorders, such as depression, that may result from work-related exposures to neurotoxicants.

Physical and Psychosocial Hazards

Exposure to physical agents in the workplace may lead to psychiatric symptoms. For example, factory workers exposed to high levels of noise have been found to have depressive symptoms, such as insomnia, anxiety, and weight loss.[13] Shift workers have reported lower subjective levels of physical health and well-being[14,15] and been found to have higher rates of alcohol and substance abuse[16] and high rates of neuroticism.[17] It is not clear if depression is increased in shift workers.

The proliferation of conditions characterized by nonspecific symptoms has expanded the range of potential mental health concerns within the workplace. The extent to which minor exposures produce symptoms varies widely.[18] Factors that may influence nonspecific symptom reporting, in addition to hazardous workplace exposures, include personality style, individual attitudes and belief systems, premorbid psychiatric status, and social pressures such as employees' perceptions of the competence of managers.[19]

Trauma in the Workplace

A range of traumatic events can occur in the workplace, including serious and fatal injuries and workplace violence, ranging from threats and harassment to murder.[20] These events often have significant economic and psychological consequences. Homicide is the second leading cause of occupational death, after work-related motor vehicle accidents. Certain workplace factors, such as exchanging money, interacting with the public, working at night or in the early morning, delivering goods, and working alone, place employees at high risk for violent attacks.[20]

Controlling the risk of psychological trauma in the workplace presents a challenge. Although there is no specific profile of a violence-prone employee, possible early warning signals include paranoid behavior, desperation over recent personal problems, an inability to accept criticism of job performance, blaming others for problems, and direct or subtle threats of harm.[21] The work environment may increase the risk of workplace violence. For example, a work environment in which the dignity of employees is not respected, such as one with frequent invasions of privacy or high levels of secrecy or an authoritarian management style, may play a role in leading a potentially violent employee to commit a violent act.

A potential consequence of trauma in the workplace is post-traumatic stress disorder (PTSD). PTSD occurs after exposure to a traumatic event involving threatened death or serious injury to self or others, such as witnessing the death of a co-worker. The individual's response to such an event involves feelings of intense fear, helplessness, and horror. Symptoms of PTSD include intrusive thoughts or dreams and recollections of the trauma, reexperiencing of the trauma, and avoidance of stimuli that arouse recollection of the trauma. PTSD, or more subtle forms of this diagnosis, may be involved in chronic pain or post-traumatic head injury syndromes. PTSD was first recognized among veterans of the Vietnam War, a unique occupational setting. The extreme traumas of war are not often seen on such a scale within nonmilitary workplaces, although workers in certain occupations, such as police, firefighters, and emergency medical technicians, are at high risk for psychological trauma as are those who have experienced significant workplace trauma, such as through explosions or assaults.[22]

EFFECTS OF SELECTED NEUROTOXICANTS

Lead

Lead is a commonly encountered workplace substance with clearly recognized neurotoxic effects (see also Chapters 13, 29, and 30). NIOSH has estimated that more than 1 million U.S. workers are daily exposed to lead (Fig. 26-2). Community lead exposure affects the health of millions more through exposure to lead in the air, drinking water, dust, and peeling paint.[23] The most common neurologic finding is impaired CNS function, manifested by symptoms of fatigue, irritability, difficulty in concentrating, and inability to perform tasks requiring sustained concentration. These symptoms are associated with abnormalities on standardized neuropsychological testing that indicate impairment of verbal intelligence, memory, and perceptual speed. Symptoms of arm weakness, characteristically affecting extensor muscle groups, are also seen in the early phases of lead toxicity. Often, weakness

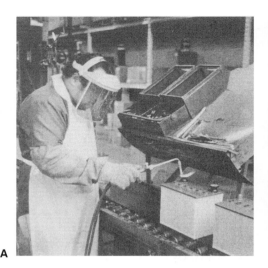
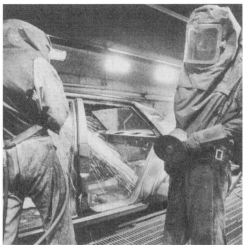

A   B

FIGURE 26-2 ● Current work practice rules require significant personal and environmental protection in situations of lead exposure. (**A**) Lead battery worker is protected mainly by local exhaust ventilation. (**B**) Automobile lead grinder is protected by air-supplied hood and floor exhaust ventilation. (Photographs by Earl Dotter.)

occurs before abnormalities are seen on nerve conduction testing. After removal from exposure, these symptoms and abnormalities resolve slowly over weeks to months, the duration depending on their initial intensity and other factors.[24] In children, lead exposure has been shown to have an adverse effect on cognitive function, even at relatively low levels of exposure (<10 ug/dL).[25]

Neurologic abnormalities caused by lead exposure usually occur after hematologic toxicity, as manifested by an elevated zinc protoporphyrin (ZPP) level and a reduced blood hemoglobin concentration. Permanent renal damage occurs much later than neurologic dysfunction and characteristically develops only after at least 5 years of lead exposure. In contrast, neurologic abnormalities may develop within 2 to 3 months after the onset of work in a lead-contaminated environment, particularly where exposure is relatively poorly controlled. Abnormalities of nerve conduction tend not to occur before at least 6 to 8 months of chronic exposure to lead.

Mercury

Although disease as striking as that experienced by Lewis Carroll's Mad Hatter no longer occurs in workplaces in the United States, behavioral effects of exposure to elemental mercury are still seen. Erethism, a set of behavioral symptoms classically associated with mercury toxicity, is characterized by unusual shyness, irritability, and other symptoms. A fine tremor of the hands is associated with mercury poisoning; and computer-assisted analysis of EMGs has shown a shift in the frequency of normal forearm tremor as an early manifestation of mercury toxicity. Peripheral neuropathy is not known to occur in elemental mercury poisoning. Measurement of mercury in urine and blood is a useful tool in the assessment of workplace exposure.

Organic mercurials, particularly alkyl mercury compounds such a methylmercury, have a strong affinity for the CNS, and severe neurologic and psychiatric effects have been associated with excessive exposure.[26] The best-described episode of organic mercury poisoning occurred in Minamata, Japan, due to ingestion of fish that had been contaminated by industrial pollution of Minamata Bay with inorganic mercury. Early symptoms of poisoning consisted of distal paresthesias, cerebellar disorders, visual impairment, deafness, and mental disturbances. Sensory deficits were seen, with loss of position sense and impaired two-point discrimination. Some affected individuals had constriction of their visual fields. Mental disturbances were characterized by agitation alternating with periods of stupor and mutism. The more severely affected patients exhibited dystonic flexion postures.

The devastating and usually irreversible neurologic effects of organic mercury poisoning should be prevented through restriction of the use of mercury. To that end, the practice of treating seed grain with organic mercurial fungicides has been curtailed by the U.S. Environmental Protection Agency (EPA), following outbreaks of neurologic disease in the United States and Iraq among people ingesting food that had been inadvertently contaminated with these fungicides.

Organophosphate Insecticides

Acute organophosphate insecticide poisoning is characterized by the inhibition of acetylcholinesterase, with resultant overactivity of cholinergic components of the autonomic nervous system, inhibition of conduction across myoneural junctions in skeletal muscle, and interference with CNS synaptic transmission. Manifestations of acute toxicity include meiosis (pinpoint pupils), blurring of vision, chest tightness, increased bronchial secretion, and wheezing. Gastrointestinal effects are also seen, including abdominal cramps, nausea, and vomiting. Increased sweating, salivation, and lacrimation are additional characteristic features.

Because organophosphate compounds bind irreversibly to cholinesterase, reactivation of the enzyme system occurs only through synthesis of additional cholinesterase molecules. Therefore, recovery of normal cholinesterase concentrations in red blood cells is slow, and repeated exposure may result in cumulative depression of cholinesterase stores. Recovery after an acute episode of poisoning is usually complete within 7 days unless anoxia has occurred during the acute phase of the episode. Measurement of red blood cell cholinesterase concentrations is valuable during the acute intoxication episode and for surveillance of occupationally exposed workers. Plasma cholinesterase concentrations are of less value in workers because they can be altered by many factors.

A syndrome of delayed neurotoxicity, which develops 8 to 35 days after exposure, has been reported with certain organophosphate compounds. Progressive weakness begins in the distal lower extremities, often with toe and foot drop, followed by finger weakness and wrist drop. Sensory loss is minimal. Deep tendon reflexes are frequently depressed. The disease may progress for 1 to 3 months after onset, and recovery is very slow. There may be psychomotor impairment and abnormal EEG findings.

Evaluation of patients exposed to organophosphate insecticides should include, in addition to evaluation of manifestations of autonomic nervous system dysfunction, measurement of the red blood cell cholinesterase concentration, which correlates reasonably well with manifestations of clinical toxicity. Migrant workers are at high risk for the acute and chronic effects of exposure to organophosphate insecticides used in agriculture. This population has not been adequately studied, and often migrant workers do not receive adequate protection from pesticide exposure.

Organic Solvents

Exposure to organic solvents occurs daily for more than 1 million U.S. workers.[27] The most frequently used solvents are toluene, xylene, trichloroethylene, ethanol, methylene chloride, and methyl chloroform (trichloroethane). Although chemically heterogeneous, these compounds are often discussed as a group because of toxicologically similar effects and the high frequency of exposure to various combinations of these substances (Fig. 26-3).

Acute intoxication, with symptoms of dizziness, lightheadedness, or feeling "high," occurs after exposure to excessive concentrations of solvent vapors. Exposure to very high concentrations of solvent vapors or fumes may lead to narcosis with

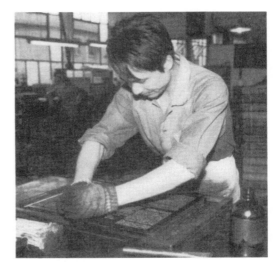

FIGURE 26-3 ● Letterpress printer washing plates with organic solvent, which is absorbed via the skin through permeable cloth gloves and inhaled via evaporation from the work surface and open bottle. (Photograph by Barry S. Levy.)

loss of consciousness. Certain psychiatric disorders have been reported after solvent exposure, including somatoform disorder, schizophrenia, and panic disorder.

To facilitate the characterization of persistent health effects of solvent exposure, a nomenclature has been developed by a World Health Organization (WHO) working group[28] and by a workshop of invited experts held in the United States.[29] The mildest form of effect, *organic affective syndrome (type 1 solvent health effect)*, which is typically reversible, is characterized by symptoms of irritability, fatigability, difficulty in concentrating, and loss of interest in daily events. In *mild chronic toxic encephalopathy* (type 2 effect), the symptoms are similar, but abnormalities on neurobehavioral testing are observed. Sustained personality or mood change *(type 2a effect)* and/or impairment in intellectual function (*type 2b effect*) may be seen. Type 2 effect may be reversible or may lead to permanent cognitive impairment. *Severe chronic toxic encephalopathy (type 3 effect)* is characterized by dementia with global deterioration of memory and other cognitive functions that are usually irreversible. Workers exposed to solvents may exhibit any of these three syndromes, depending on the intensity and duration of their exposure. Workers with prolonged exposure to solvents may develop decreases in reaction time, dexterity, speed, and memory. Relatively few abnormalities have been demonstrated in PNS function; nerve conduction abnormalities have been reported in mixed solvent exposure. Measurement of urinary metabolites, such as hippuric acid in toluene exposure, may be useful in monitoring exposed populations.

Clinical diagnosis of chronic toxic encephalopathy caused by exposure to organic solvents is made by obtaining a careful exposure and clinical history and by performance of standardized neurobehavioral testing.[27] Government agencies have concluded that workers exposed to solvent vapors at excessive levels—those sufficient to frequently cause acute intoxication—for more than 10 years are at increased risk of toxic encephalopathy.[28] Some studies have shown that workers excessively exposed to solvents for 5 to 10 years are at risk for toxic encephalopathy[29]; there is little epidemiologic evidence that exposure for less than 5 years is sufficient to place a worker at increased risk. Therefore, any worker with more than 5 years of excessive solvent exposure should be considered potentially at risk of solvent encephalopathy and provided a thorough medical and neurobehavioral assessment to determine whether symptoms or signs of neurobehavioral dysfunction are present.

Carbon Monoxide

Sources of carbon monoxide (CO) that may cause poisoning include exhaust fumes from motor vehicles, inhaled smoke, malfunctioning heating systems, and cleaner fuels, such as propane and methane. Psychological symptoms of CO poisoning include fatigue, apathy, emotional lability accompanied by lowered frustration tolerance, impulsivity, irritability, and, at times, psychosis. Psychological symptoms are often delayed, occurring between 3 and 240 days after recovery from acute intoxication; approximately 50 to 75 percent of exposed patients recover from this delayed syndrome within 1 year.[30]

Manganese

Excessive exposure to manganese has long been known to cause profound psychosis (*manganese madness*) and/or a movement disorder consistent with parkinsonism.[3] Prominent features of the movement disorder, referred to as *manganism*, include impairment of gait, decreased facial expression, tremor of the hands, and impaired speech. Some improvement has been noted after treatment; however, this benefit has been variable in other studies and is often transient.[31] Chronic lower level exposure in the workplace is associated with impairment of behavioral function as assessed by standardized neuropsychological tests.[32] Significant exposure to manganese occurs in various occupations, including welding; manganese in welding fume constitutes a significant neurotoxic risk if not properly controlled. Recent studies linking manganese exposure from welding and increased rates of parkinsonism deserve particular attention.

MANAGEMENT AND CONTROL OF NEUROLOGIC AND BEHAVIORAL DISORDERS

Management of toxic neurologic problems consists primarily of identification of the offending agent and removal from continued exposure. Medical management of signs and symptoms may also be of value over the long term. In some instances, removal of the offending agent from the workplace may prevent the development of new cases. Some workers with known exposure may develop mild, early symptoms of neurotoxicity; objective demonstration of functional impairment on standardized tests is essential in the management of individual cases. Workers with evidence of toxic symptoms or functional impairment should be removed from exposure until these deficits resolve and exposure in the workplace is terminated.

Prevention of occupationally induced neurologic disorders can be accomplished through workplace medical and environmental control programs. The goal of environmental control is to reduce concentrations of neurotoxic substances in the work environment by various manipulations. Medical strategies designed to reduce neurologic morbidity include preplacement evaluation and periodic medical monitoring. The goal of preplacement evaluation as it relates to neurologic disorders is to avoid placement of workers with preexisting disease, such as peripheral neuropathy, in jobs with exposures that might exacerbate these conditions. Conditions that might impair a worker's ability to perform a job, such as uncontrolled epilepsy in a person operating hazardous machinery, would be grounds for medical exclusion from such jobs.

Periodic medical monitoring programs are becoming more common in industries where neurotoxic substances are used. An important element of such programs is measurement of the neurotoxic agent in biological fluids. The most common such application occurs in industries where lead or mercury is used.

Periodic monitoring of lead-exposed workers should include occupational and medical histories; a physical examination with special attention to the nervous system; blood and urine studies to evaluate hematologic and renal effects of lead exposure; and, most importantly, determination of the blood lead level (BLL) and concentrations of zinc protoporphyrin (ZPP). The content of such examinations is mandated by the Occupational Safety and Health Administration (OSHA) standard on occupational exposure to lead, in which specific guidelines are provided for job transfer of workers with BLLs. The standard requires that employers make routine BLL monitoring available to all employees who are exposed to lead at concentrations greater than the action level regardless of whether respirators are worn. Specific actions must be taken depending on the results of BLL testing. Any worker removed from a job because of an elevated BLL is protected by the medical removal protection provision of the OSHA lead standard. This provision requires an employer to "maintain the worker's earnings, seniority, and other employment rights and benefits (as though the worker had not been removed) for a period of up to 18 months."

The evaluation of mercury-exposed workers is similar, except that determinations are made of mercury in urine and no enzymatic test, such as the Zinc protoporphyrin (ZPP) test, exists to measure the metabolic toxicity of mercury exposure.

Workers exposed to cadmium and arsenic should be monitored periodically with urinary determinations of these metals in addition to standard medical evaluations.

Workers chronically exposed to solvents should have periodic medical histories and examinations with attention to the nervous system. Measurement of urinary metabolites of solvents is sometimes helpful as an adjunct to other medical monitoring techniques.

Pesticide-exposed workers, particularly those using organophosphate insecticides, should be periodically evaluated, including red blood cell cholinesterase levels, to assess their degree of pesticide exposure. Nerve conduction testing is not suitable for routine monitoring of asymptomatic workers.

Treatment of occupational neurologic disease beyond removal of the worker from continued toxic exposure may consist of the administration of drugs designed to remove the offending agent or counteract its effects. Chelating drugs, such as ethylene diamine tetraacetic acid (EDTA), dimethylsuccinic acid (DMSA), and penicillamine, are given as treatment for symptomatic poisoning by lead and other heavy metals. These drugs should not be given prophylactically to lower blood levels of the metal; they have known toxicities, which may add to the toxic effects of the metal and also may increase gastrointestinal absorption of the metal. Individuals should be removed from exposure to the offending agent before initiation of drug therapy.

Atropine, a pharmacologic antagonist of organophosphates, is the drug of choice for treatment of the acute manifestations of organophosphate insecticide poisoning. Repeated doses are given to the point of atropinization, and subsequent doses of the drug may be required, as the duration of action of atropine is less than that of organophosphate insecticides. If patients are seen very soon after exposure, oximes can be given to regenerate inhibited cholinesterase enzyme.

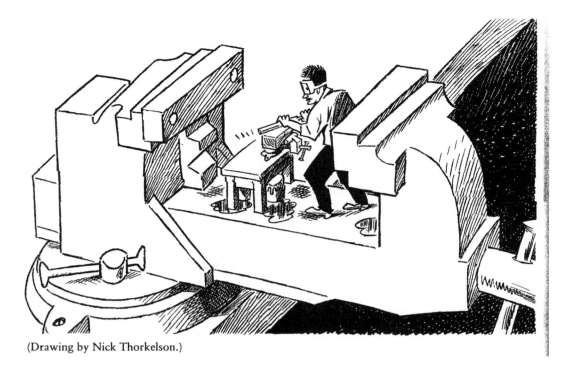

(Drawing by Nick Thorkelson.)

Evidence of lead-related cognitive impairment has resulted in major policy change that has dramatically reduced lead exposure in the United States, particularly for children, who are most vulnerable. This major public health success story represents a model for the use of sound science in shaping prudent public health policy. This model applies by extension to other environmental hazards.[24]

Ultimately, prevention of diseases of the nervous system caused by environmental neurotoxicants rests on adequate testing of chemicals before their introduction and on environmental measures designed to reduce exposure. The Toxic Substances Control Act (TSCA) addresses the issue of premarket testing, and EPA, which administers TSCA, has specified criteria for neurologic evaluation of chemical substances. Biological assays of organophosphate compounds have successfully predicted those substances that are neurotoxic to humans. Substances such as *n*-hexane and MBK, which produce an axonal neuropathy in exposed humans, have been shown to produce similar effects in animals, and the neurologic disorder associated with chlordecone toxicity was seen in experimental animals several years before it was reported

in exposed humans. Therefore, testing of industrial substances by administration of toxic agents to experimental animals is essential in the identification of substances with neurotoxic potential.

In rare instances, structural similarity alone has proved useful in predicting toxicity. *n*-Hexane and MBK are metabolized to 2,5-hexanedione, which is thought to be responsible for the neurotoxic manifestations of these two industrial chemicals. Investigation of structure–activity relationships therefore may be of value in identifying substances with potential neurotoxicity. In those instances in which neurotoxicity is suspected because of the chemical structure of the compound, animal tests are still required.

MANAGEMENT AND CONTROL OF PSYCHIATRIC DISORDERS

Employee Assistance Programs

Psychiatric disorders can result in increased absenteeism or disability days from work. In some cases, individuals with mental health problems are more likely to go to work but require greater effort to function, suffering from on-the-job impairment.[33,34]

Therefore, the effects of mental illness may have a more subtle effect on performance. In recognition of the impact that untreated psychiatric disorders have on productivity and morale in the workplace, more than 20,000 U.S. companies offer employee assistance programs (EAPs) to detect and treat employees with psychiatric disorders.[35] Initially, EAPs were developed in response to alcohol-related problems, but it became clear that personal problems beyond substance abuse could also interfere with work performance. Moreover, early detection, before recognition of impaired work performance by a supervisor, is preferable. Therefore, EAPs broadened their scope to include evaluation and referral services for personal problems, such as marital, individual psychiatric, and financial issues. Where broad-based programs are offered, employees are encouraged to seek services on their own or as self-referrals rather than waiting until their job performance suffers. Table 26-4 provides a description of the primary elements of EAPs.

Despite the proliferation of EAPs and widespread claims that EAPs are cost-effective, few data are available to address this issue. Evaluation of broad-based EAPs has demonstrated significant improvements in absenteeism, lost time, warnings given to employees, and supervisor ratings of performance after institution of counseling services.[36,37] As managed care has increased, EAP staff members are being asked not only to evaluate and refer troubled employees but also to act as case managers and gatekeepers for use of mental health benefits.

TABLE 26-4

Elements of Employee Assistance Programs (EAPs)

Program type
　Internal: EAP staff are company employees
　External: Outside consultant or organization provides EAP

Eligible participants
　Employees only
　Employees and eligible dependents

Referral to EAP
　Self-refer; voluntary
　Supervisor referral: Voluntary or involuntary based on documented poor job performance

Problem type
　Substance abuse or dependence
　"Broad brush": Substance abuse, psychological, marital, financial, elder care

Service type
　800-number telephone evaluation
　One to three evaluation sessions; referral recommendations; crisis intervention
　Short-term treatment (up to 10 sessions)

Supervisor training
　Documentation of work performance and referral procedures
　Prevention (stress-management skills)

Psychiatric Treatment and Productivity

From an organizational perspective, psychiatric disorders impair productivity in several ways, including reducing the number of workers, increasing absenteeism of existing workers, decreasing morale, and reducing quality of work. The annual economic impact of depression in the United States is at least $43.7 billion, including the costs of lost productivity and health care.[38] Although the economic burden of alcoholism is frequently cited, drinking behavior, such as coming to work hung over, in a random undiagnosed sample of employees was also associated with problems at work.[39] The costs of behavioral problems and psychiatric disorders affect not only workers and their families but also managers, employers, and insurance companies.

In sum, psychiatric disorders and associated behavioral problems, such as alcohol consumption, significantly affect productivity—regardless of their cause or their relation to workplace factors and stressors. It appears that when employed persons are treated, their work improves—an encouraging finding that supports the inclusion of psychiatric treatment in health insurance benefits.

Fitness for Duty

When an employee has been out of work because of treatment of a psychiatric disorder, such as depression or anxiety, or a question arises about the employee's ability to function on the job, a fitness-for-duty evaluation may be requested. Fitness for duty is defined as the ability of an individual to perform a job, based on the specific job requirements. A detailed understanding of the job duties is required—often a problem, because job descriptions are not necessarily informative or sufficiently behaviorally oriented. Ancillary information, such as interviews with workers in similar positions or with supervisors, may be needed to understand the essential behaviors expected on the job. Fitness for duty can never be based solely on a psychiatric diagnosis; rather, it must be based on a behavioral analysis of the employee's abilities. Past job performance is the best predictor of future job performance. Further, a global assessment of functioning can be useful as a behavioral guide for the individual's current level of functioning and ability to perform daily tasks related to work.[40] Overall, matching of an assessment of the employee's current behavioral functioning with the essential functions required to perform a job, along with consideration of the employee's premorbid level of function on the job, yields the best prediction of the employee's fitness for return to the job.

Accommodation in the Workplace

Since the American with Disabilities Act (ADA) was passed in 1990, employers have been under increasing pressure to hire and accommodate workers with disabilities, including psychiatric illness. The number of discrimination claims against employers based on emotional or psychiatric impairment has also increased since the passage of the ADA. For example, in 1997, the Equal Employment Opportunity Commission reported that 15 percent of discrimination claims were related to emotional or psychiatric impairment—the largest category of claims in that year. The need to properly evaluate an individual's ability to perform a job and the ability to make reasonable accommodations is a growing concern among employers in the United States.

The ADA prohibits discrimination based on disability and provides that employers must make "reasonable accommodations" to the disabilities of "qualified" applicants so long as this does not impose "undue hardship." "Qualified" means that the individual can perform the essential functions of the job, except for the disability. "Reasonable accommodation" refers to any modification or adjustment to a job or work environment that allows the qualified employee with the disability to perform the job functions. "Undue hardship" refers to "an action requiring significant difficulty or expense."[41]

Employers are not allowed to inquire about a disability before hiring, and the applicant does not have to reveal a psychiatric history at the time of hire. Moreover, if a long-term employee who was previously performing the job develops a psychiatric disorder, the employer is obligated to make accommodations.[42]

Individuals who are hospitalized for psychiatric diagnoses such as schizophrenia have low employment rates, often less than 20 percent.[42] For those who are chronically mentally ill, the best predictors of future work performance seem to be ratings of work adjustment in a sheltered job site, ability to function socially with others, and previous employment history.[43] Therefore, type of psychiatric diagnosis is not as predictive of work capacity as is assessment of objective behavioral performance. Although these findings apply specifically to the psychoses, the same guideline seems to be applicable for any physical or psychiatric illness.

Reasonable accommodations for persons with psychiatric disabilities include analysis of the individual employee's behavioral problems, such as anxiety or sensitivity to criticism, and development of accommodations based on individual needs.[44] For example, when a sensitive employee returns from a hospitalization, the supervisor needs to be trained to offer positive feedback, along with critiques of performance.

A significant number of workers have diagnosable psychiatric conditions, especially depression, and some occupations have higher rates of such disorders that may significantly affect productivity.[45,46] Some occupations appear to place workers at greater risk for traumas that result in psychiatric disorders, such as PTSD. Whatever the causes, psychiatric illness will continue to affect workers and the workplace and therefore must be recognized, treated, and accommodated—rather than dismissed or ignored.[47]

Acknowledgment

We thank Jonathan Rutchik, M.D., for reviewing this chapter.

REFERENCES

1. Keogh JP, Pestronk A, Wertheimer D, et al. An epidemic of urinary retention caused by dimethylaminopropionitrile. JAMA 1980;243:746–9.
2. Allen N, Mendell JR, Billmaier DJ, et al. Toxic polyneuropathy due to methyl n-butyl ketone. Arch Neurol 1975;32:209–12.

3. Levy BS, Nassetta WJ. Neurologic effects of manganese in humans: A review. Int J Occup Environ Health 2003;9:153–63.
4. White RF, Feldman RG, Proctor SP. Neurobehavioral effects of toxic exposure: Clinical symptoms in adult neuropsychology. In: White RF, ed. The practitioner's handbook. Amsterdam: Elsevier, 1992:1–51.
5. Colligan MJ, Smith MJ, Hurrell JJ Jr. Occupational incidence rates of mental health disorders. J Human Stress 1977;3:34–9.
6. Eaton WW, Anthony JC, Mandel W, et al. Occupations and the prevalence of major depressive disorder. J Occup Med 1990;23:1079–87.
7. Mandell W, Eaton WW, Anthony JC, et al. Alcoholism and occupations: a review and analysis of 104 occupations. Alcohol Clin Exp Res 1992;16:734–46.
8. Hotopf M, Wessely S. Stress in the workplace: Unfinished business. J Psychosom Res 1997;43:1–6.
9. Karasek RA. Job demands, job decision latitude, and mental strain: Implications for job redesign. Adm Sci Q 1979;24:285–308.
10. Stansfeld SA, Fuhrer R, Head J, et al. Work and psychiatric disorder in the Whitehall II Study. J Psychosom Res 1997;43:73–81.
11. Hammar N, Alfredsson L, Johnson JV. Job strain, social support at work, and incidence of myocardial infarction. Occup Environ Med 1998;55:548–53.
12. Kivimaki M, Elovainio M, Vahtera J, et al. Association between organization inequity and incidence of psychiatric disorders in female employees. Psychol Med 2003;33:319–26.
13. Bing-shuang H, Yue-lin Y, Ren-yi W, et al. Evaluation of depressive symptoms in workers exposed to industrial noise. Homeostasis in Health Disease 1997;38:123–5.
14. Akerstedt T. Psychological and psychophysiological effects of shift work. Scand J Work Environ Health 1990;16:67–73.
15. Frese M, Semmer N. Shiftwork, stress, and psychosomatic complaints: A comparison between workers in different shiftwork schedules, non-shiftworkers, and former shiftworkers. Ergonomics 1986;29:99–114.
16. Costa G, Apostali P, D'Andrea F, et al. Gastrointestinal and neurotic disorders in textile shift workers. In: Reinberg A, Vieux N, Andlauer P, eds. Night and shift work: Biological and social aspects. Oxford: Pergamon Press, 1981:187–96.
17. Harma M, Illmarinen J, Knauth P. Physical fitness and other individual factors relating to the shiftwork tolerance of women. Chronobiol Int 1988;5:417–24.
18. Arnetz BB, Wilhom C. Technological stress: Psychophysiological symptoms in modern offices. J Psychosom Res 1997;43:35–42.
19. Spurgeon A, Gompertz D, Harrington JM. Non-specific symptoms in response to hazard exposure in the workplace. J Psychosom Res 1997;43:43–9.
20. National Institute for Occupational Safety & Health. Violence in the workplace: Risk factors and prevention strategies. Current Intelligence Bulletin # 57. Washington, DC: NIOSH, 1996:1–22.
21. Trafford C, Gallichio E, Jones P. Managing violence in the workplace. In: Cotton P, ed. Psychological health in the workplace: Understanding and managing occupational stress. Carlton, Australia: The Australian Psychological Society, 1996:147–58.
22. Williams T. Trauma in the workplace. In: Wilson JP, Raphael B, et al., eds. International handbook of traumatic stress syndromes. New York: Plenum Press, 1993:925–33.
23. Landrigan PJ, Todd AC. Lead poisoning. West J Med 1994;161:153–9.
24. Baker EL, White RF, Pothier LJ, et al. Occupational lead neurotoxicity: Improvement in behavioral effects after exposure reduction. Br J Ind Med 1985;42:507–16.
25. Needleman HL, Landrigan PJ. Raising children toxic free. New York: Farrar, Straus & Giroux, 1994.
26. Maghazaji HI. Psychiatric aspects of methylmercury poisoning. J Neurol Neurosurg Psychiatry 1974;37:954–8.
27. Baker EL. A review of recent research on health effects of human occupational exposure to organic solvents: A critical review. J Occup Med 1994,36:1079–92.
28. World Health Organization and Nordic Council of Ministers. Chronic effects of organic solvents on the central nervous system and diagnostic criteria. Copenhagen: WHO Regional Office for Europe, 1985.
29. Cranmer JM, Goldberg L. Workshop on neurobehavioral effects of solvents. Neurotoxicology 1987;7:1–95.
30. NIOSH. Organic solvent neurotoxicity (Bulletin 48). Washington, DC: NIOSH, 1987.
31. Mikkelsen S, Jorgensen M, Browne E, et al. Mixed solvent exposure and organic brain damage. Acta Neurol Scand 1988;78(Suppl 118):1–96.
32. Ernst A, Zibrak JD. Carbon monoxide poisoning. N Engl J Med 1998;339:1603–8.
33. Koller WC, Lyons KE, Truly W. Effect of levodopa treatment for parkinsonism in welders. Neurology 2004;62:730–3.
34. Roels H, Lauwerys R, Buchet J-P, et al. Epidemiological survey among workers exposed to manganese. Am J Ind Med 1987;11:307–27.
35. Goetzel RZ, Ozminkowski RJ, Sederer LI, et al. The business case for quality mental health services: Why employers should care about the mental health and well-being of their employees. J Occup Environ Med 2002;44:320–30.
36. Dewa CS, Lin E. Chronic physical illness, psychiatric disorder and disability in the workplace. Soc Sci Med 2000;51:41–50.
37. Adamson DW, Gardner MD. Employee assistance programs and managed care: Merge and converge. In: SR Sauber, ed. Managed mental health care: Major diagnostic and treatment approaches. Bristol, PA: Brunner/Mazel, 1997:67–82.
38. Ramanathan CS. EAP's response to personal stress and productivity: Implications for occupational social work. Soc Work 1992;37:234–9.
39. Walsh DC, Hingson RW, Merrigan DM, et al. A randomized trial of treatment options for alcohol-abusing workers. N Engl J Med 1991;325:775–82.
40. Greenberg PE, Stiglin LE, Finkelstein SN, et al. The economic burden of depression in 1990. J Clin Psychiatry 1993;54:405–18.
41. Ames GM, Grube JW, Moore RS. The relationship of drinking and hangovers to workplace problems: an empirical study. J Stud Alcohol 1997;58:37–47.
42. Sperry L. Psychiatric consultation in the workplace. Washington, DC: American Psychiatric Press, 1993.
43. United States Department of Justice. The Americans with Disabilities Act: Questions and answers. Washington, DC: U.S. Department of Justice, Civil Rights Division, 1991.
44. Carling PJ. Reasonable accommodations in the workplace for individuals with psychiatric disabilities. Consult Psychol J 1993;45:46–62.
45. Massel HK, Liberman RP, Mintz J, et al. Evaluating the capacity to work of the mentally ill. Psychiatry 1990;53:31–43.

46. Mechanic, D. Cultural and organizational aspects of application of the Americans with Disabilities Act to persons with psychiatric disabilities. The Milbank Quarterly, 1998;76:5–23.
47. Ad Hoc Committee on Health Research Relating to Future Intervention Options (WHO). Investing in Health Research and Development. (Document TDR/GEN/96.1). Geneva: World Health Organization, 1996.

BIBLIOGRAPHY

Baker EL, Feldman RG, French JG. Environmentally related disorders of the nervous system. Med Clin North Am 1990; 74:325–45.
A review of neurologic disorders caused by clinical and physical factors encountered in the workplace or the general environment.

Carling P. Reasonable accommodations in the workplace for individuals with psychiatric disabilities. Consult Psychol J 1993;45:46–62.
This article reviews information related to accommodation for persons with psychiatric disabilities and the methods to assist employers and employees in complying with the Americans with Disabilities Act.

Feldman RG. Occupational and environmental neurotoxicology. Philadelphia: Lippincott-Raven Publishers, 1999.
A definitive, comprehensive textbook covering the wide range of neurotoxic disorders, authored by a distinguished pioneer in the field.

Kurland LT, Faro SN, Siedler H. Minamata disease. World Neurol 1960;1:370.
Extensive discussion of historic outbreak of methyl mercury poisoning.

Landrigan PJ. Current issues in the epidemiology and toxicology of occupational exposure to lead. Toxicol Ind Health 1991;7:9–14.
An authoritative update on health effects of occupational lead exposure.

Mental Health Law Project. Mental health consumers in the work place: How the Americans with Disabilities Act protects you against employment discrimination. Washington, DC: Mental Health Law Project, 1992.
This guide-book offers practical recommendation for workplace accommodations to serve individuals with mental health problems affecting their behavior at work.

Mintz J, Mintz L, Arruda M, et al. Treatments of depression and the functional capacity to work. Arch Gen Psychiatry 1992;49:761–8.
This review summarizes the literature on the effects of antidepressants and psychotherapy treatment on the functional capacity to work.

Sauter SL, Murphy LR, Hurrell JJ. Prevention of work-related psychological disorders. Am Psychol 1990;45:1146–58.
This article reviews the scientific literature regarding work stress and its impact on psychological and emotional well-being.

Schottenfeld RS. Psychological sequelae of chemical and hazardous materials exposures. In: JB Sullivan JB, Kreiger GR, eds. Hazardous materials toxicology: Clinical principles of environmental health. Baltimore: Williams & Wilkins, 1992.
This chapter provides an overview of the psychiatric issues that arise as a consequence of exposure to toxic substances.

Spencer PS, Schaumberg HH, eds. Experimental and clinical neurotoxicology. 2nd ed. New York: Oxford University Press, 2000.
In-depth discussion of the pathophysiology of neurotoxic-induced disease.

White RF, Proctor SP. Research and clinical criteria for development of neurobehavioral test batteries. J Occup Med 1992;34:140–8.
A comprehensive discussion of the issues related to the use of neurobehavioral testing in the evaluation of workers at risk for toxic encephalopathy.

CHAPTER 27

Hearing Disorders

Thais Catalani Morata

I n the United States, 10 million people suffer from irreversible noise-induced hearing loss, and 30 million more are exposed to dangerous levels of noise each day. Work-related hearing loss has been one of the most common occupational health conditions in the United States for more than 25 years.[1] Hearing loss can be a seriously disabling condition due to the integral role of hearing in human communication. People often avoid situations in which communication is difficult rather than struggle through. This tendency leads to isolation, difficulties at work, and can have adverse psychological consequences. The following scenarios illustrate difficulties associated with hearing loss:

- Going to restaurants, parties, or other gatherings becomes a chore, as background noise or music make conversation difficult, if not impossible.
- Watching television requires the volume to be set very loud, making it impossible for the rest of the family to join in.
- Working in a noisy job and wearing traditional hearing protectors may further "deafen" workers, making communication more difficult and increasing the risk of workplace injuries due to an inability to hear environmental sounds and warning signals.
- Dealing with tinnitus becomes an unexpected consequence for some, who understood that their hearing could one day worsen, but expected silence, not an ever-present ringing.

Greater attention and improved control strategies are needed for the prevention of these hearing disorders.

THE IMPACT OF HEARING DISORDERS

The impact of hearing disorders may range from slight to serious and debilitating consequences. At work, a hearing loss can increase the difficulties associated with the use of hearing protectors, interfering with communication and detection of warning signals. It is estimated that those with a severe hearing loss who are working are expected to earn only 50 to 70 percent of their non–hearing-impaired peers.[2]

Hearing loss can have a severe impact on social interaction and family life. Hearing disabilities may have a negative effect on self-image, causing a perception of oneself as abnormal, prematurely old, or as a burden, because of the need to keep asking people to repeat themselves. Several barriers to seeking help and using hearing aids exist including cost, denial, the stigma attached to deafness, and pride. People with hearing difficulty will often try to minimize or conceal its seriousness in order to cope with the risk of being marginalized and may avoid seeking help.

A survey of 2,300 hearing-impaired adults conducted by the National Council on Aging found that those with untreated hearing loss were more likely to report conditions like depression and anxiety and were less likely to participate in social activities compared to those who wear hearing aids.[3] Unfortunately, less than 20 percent of the estimated 28 million Americans who could benefit from hearing devices own them, and less than 20 percent of physicians include hearing testing in regular physician examinations.[4]

Noise-Induced Hearing Loss

At work, millions of people are exposed to excessive and potentially harmful levels of noise. Unfortunately, exposures to excessive levels of noise are not restricted to the work environment. Noise from recreational activities, such as music concerts, motor sports, traffic, and airports, often reaches levels that can constitute a health risk. Noise exposure from such activities may be associated with hypertension and ischemic heart disease, annoyance, sleep disturbance, and decreased school performance—the most studied health outcomes concerning environmental noise exposure. Hearing loss is the outcome most studied from occupational exposures, but it can also be caused by environmental sources.

Noise-induced hearing loss (NIHL) is a specific condition with established symptoms and objective findings. The Bureau of Labor Statistics identified it as a leading work-related condition.[1] The reported prevalence of work-related hearing loss varies considerably among occupational groups. With 10 or more years of noise exposure, it is estimated that 8 percent of the workers exposed to 85 dBA,[*] 22 percent of the workers exposed to 90 dBA, 38 percent of the workers exposed to 95 dBA, and 44 percent of those exposed to 100 dBA will develop hearing impairment.[5] NIHL loss is estimated to be among the most common causes of acquired hearing loss. The National Institutes of Health estimates that approximately one-third of all hearing losses can be attributed, at least in part, to noise exposure.[6]

Because noise is present in most occupational settings, the hearing disorders observed among workers are often attributed to noise exposure alone without considering the effects of other agents. The terms *occupational hearing loss* and *work-related hearing loss* came to be used as synonyms for *noise-induced hearing loss*. It is now clear that this is not always correct, as chemical agents have also been implicated in hearing loss. In several settings, noise coexists with other factors that are potentially dangerous for hearing, so caution should be taken before identifying a hearing loss as noise-induced. Moreover, when one considers the possibility that other environmental and occupational factors can affect hearing, current hearing-loss prevention initiatives need to be reexamined. These issues will be dealt with later on this chapter. Next, characteristics of NIHL and hearing losses from chemicals will be considered.

The following features characterize cases of NIHL:

1. Irreversible sensorineural hearing loss, with damage mainly to the cells in the peripheral auditory organ, which are responsible for transforming the sound waves into neural signals.
2. A history of long-term exposure to noise levels—exposure to continuous noise levels greater than 85 dBA for 8 hours a day or exposure to impact noise (a noise that arises as the result of the impact between two objects), even if for shorter periods, sufficient to cause the degree and pattern of hearing loss (HL) found in audiograms. *Audiograms* indicate an individual's hearing detection thresholds. Results are given in decibels, which indicate the intensity or loudness a sound has to be for the listener to be able to detect it. Thresholds below 25 dB HL are considered as normal. Several frequencies are tested. Frequency determines the pitch of a sound (see Box 27-1). NIHL usually is not a profound hearing loss but may reach up to 75 dB HL in the higher frequencies, such as 4 and 6 kHz, and up to 40 dB HL in the lower frequencies, such as 1 and 2 kHz.
3. Hearing loss develops gradually over a period of years, most rapidly during the first 6 to 10 years of exposure. The rate of loss decreases as hearing thresholds increase, in contrast to age-related loss.
4. NIHL usually starts at the high frequencies (high-pitched sounds) of the audiogram (the usual order is 6, 4, 8, 3, 2 or 4, 6, 8, 3, 2 kHz) and is bilaterally symmetric.
5. Speech discrimination scores are consistent with the high-frequency losses.

---

[*] *The human ear does not respond equally to all sound frequencies. It is much more sensitive to sounds in the frequency range of 1 kHz to 4 kHz (1,000 to 4,000 vibrations per second) than to very low or high frequency sounds. For this reason, sound meters are usually fitted with a filter whose response to frequency is similar to that of the human ear. When the "A-weighting filter" is used, the second pressure level is given in units of dBA or dB(A). Sound pressure level on the dBA scale, which is logarithmic, is widely used.*

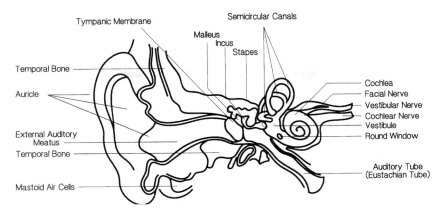

FIGURE 27-1 ● Schematic drawing of the ear.

6. NIHL does not continue to progress if the patient is removed from noise exposure.

Hearing loss resulting from hazardous long-term exposure to noise progresses in a fairly well-established, recognizable pattern. The noise-induced hearing loss at the frequencies maximally affected (4 and 6 kHz) indicates a rapid increase over the first 10 years of exposure; the development of the hearing loss then slows and tends to plateau. Hearing loss at frequencies below those maximally affected show hearing loss developing at a slower rate but continuously throughout the entire exposure period.

NIHL has a gradual onset. The affected individual might be unaware of any change. Permanent losses may be preceded by temporary ones. Remedial behaviors, such as turning up the radio or television volume or blaming others for not speaking clearly, may further conceal initial difficulties. The affected person may be unaware of any hearing problem even when the audiogram indicates abnormal hearing.

Traditionally, the mechanism underlying NIHL has been explained as physical trauma causing damage to the cochlea, which contains hair cells responsible for transforming the sound waves into neural signals that are transmitted to the auditory nerve and ultimately to the brain (Fig. 27-1). Hair cells are attached to the basilar membrane, and the stereocilia are in contact with the tectorial membrane. Sound waves lead the basilar membrane to vibrate up and down. The vibration creates a shearing force between the basilar membrane and the tectorial membrane, causing the hair-cell stereocilia to bend back and forth. This leads to internal changes within the

hair cells that create electrical signals. Auditory nerve fibers rest below the hair cells and pass these signals on to the brain. Therefore, hair cells respond to sounds by bending of the stereocilia.[7,8]

The most common morphological finding in noise-induced hearing loss is degeneration of the hair cells (mainly the outer ones), which are thought to be the most vulnerable structures of the organ of Corti. The damage of inner and especially outer hair cells is described as a disarrangement of hairs, fusion of stereocilia, the formation of giant hairs that exceed the normal stereocilia in length and thickness, and deformation of cuticular plates. The loss of the outer hair cells induces retrograde degeneration of the efferent fibers but has little effect on the afferent cochlear neurons. Therefore, if there were damage to the outer hair cells alone, the lesion would be less obvious, as only rather extensive damage to the inner hair cells causes substantial degeneration of the afferent nerve fibers.

Recently, metabolic processes involving oxidative stress have been shown to contribute to noise-induced hearing loss. The generation of reactive oxygen species (ROS), or free radicals, has been associated with cellular injury in different organ systems. Free radicals produce cell damage by binding to macromolecules and producing lipid peroxidation—a basic mechanism of toxicity that is thought to be part of the mechanism of acquired hearing loss.

Hearing Loss from Other Factors

The incidence and degree of hearing loss varies greatly among groups. The cause of this variability

BOX 27-1

Case of Noise-Induced Hearing Loss (NIHL) and Tinnitus

Peter M. Rabinowitz

A 55-year-old dockworker with tinnitus is evaluated. His job involves working in the hold of freighters, loading and unloading cargo, including steel girders and rods and crates of frozen produce. From a cab, he also operates a loading crane several hours a day. He reports exposure to frequent impact noise from metal striking metal. He notes that when he operates the crane, he has to shout to be able to communicate to a co-worker nearby. He does not wear hearing protection, saying that he needs to hear sounds, such as that of the overhead crane when he is loading and shouted communication when he is operating the crane. For 1 or 2 hours a day, he operates a forklift in a refrigerated warehouse, where noise from the refrigerating units are so loud that he must shout to communicate with a co-worker at arm's length. He does not wear hearing protection when he drives the forklift because of the need to hear warning signals and communication from co-workers.

He reports that he first noticed tinnitus 15 years ago, when after noisy work shifts his ears rang for several hours. Gradually, it became more frequent; it now interferes with his hearing when there is background noise. He reports that many times his hearing decreased after a work shift, then improved the following day; he noticed that when he turned on his car radio in the morning, it seemed excessively loud because he had turned up the volume the night before.

Recently, he has argued with his wife about the television volume. When she turns it down to a level that she prefers, he has difficulty hearing what people are saying, so he turns it up. He also notices that talking on the phone is difficult for him if there is background noise, and that having a conversation in a bar is also increasingly difficult. He admits that his friends have kidded him about being "in need of a hearing aid" and that the thought of having a hearing loss has led to some feelings of depression. On physical exam, his blood pressure is 140/88 and he has normal external auditory canals and tympanic membranes. His audiogram is illustrated in Fig. 27-2.

This case illustrates many of the clinical aspects of noise-induced hearing loss. The worker reports exposure to occupational noise at or above 85 dBA as indicated by the "shout test." In addition to sources of steady-state noise, such as refrigerator fans and crane motors, he

is also exposed to impact noise, such as crashes of metal on metal. Additionally, he gives a history of recurrent TTSs after work shifts, with loss of hearing acuity and tinnitus that would improve overnight. Over the years, however, such temporary changes have progressed to permanent hearing loss and tinnitus.

Although the symmetric nature of the hearing loss and the "notch" at high frequencies on his audiograms all point to the diagnosis of noise-induced hearing loss, he should be referred for a full audiological evaluation for other audiological disorders, such as otosclerosis. He may also be a candidate for a trial of amplification and for tinnitus treatment.

He needs to protect his hearing if he wishes to remain in a noisy area. Although noise reduction through engineering controls would be the ideal way to reduce his exposure, adequate noise reduction may be difficult given the nature of his work. Therefore, hearing protection may be necessary. Standard earplugs that preferentially attenuate at higher frequencies may worsen his problem of discriminating speech. Therefore, a "flat-attenuation" earplug may be more appropriate for him, given his preexisting high-frequency loss.

Another occupational issue facing this man is whether he can safely operate a forklift with his degree of hearing loss. His hearing, with and without amplification, can be compared to company policies regarding mobile-equipment operators, if such exist, and to the U.S. Department of Transportation guidelines. A workplace accommodation would be for him to have a radio-communication headset that could also provide earmuff hearing protection, in order to allow him both to protect his hearing and to communicate with others while operating the crane.

Finally, his hearing level according to American Academy of Otolaryngology-Head and Neck Surgery (AAO-HNS) criteria indicates that he has a degree of hearing impairment, which, more likely than not, is due to his occupational noise exposure—although his audiogram also suggests an element of aging. His history of not wearing hearing protection is not a reason to deny him workers' compensation for his hearing loss.

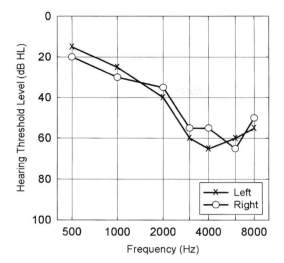

Hearing Loss from Chemical Exposures

Sensorineural hearing loss is increased in noise-exposed workers who are also exposed to organic solvents, due to the effects of solvents on the cochlea or brain. Toluene adversely affects the auditory system of experimental animals, even in the absence of excessive noise.[13] Exposure to solvents was implicated as a causative factor for hearing loss in a 20-year longitudinal study in a company where 23 percent of workers in the chemical division had compensable hearing loss compared to 5 to 8 percent of company workers not exposed to chemicals—an effect found despite the lower noise levels in the chemical division (80 to 90 dBA compared to 95 to 100 dBA elsewhere).[14]

At least four classes of industrial chemicals—metals, solvents, pesticides, and asphyxiants (such as carbon monoxide)—are ototoxic (Table 27-1). If workers are exposed to these chemicals at sufficiently high concentrations, their hearing may be impaired, even in the absence of exposure to loud noise. Work activities that involve exposure to these agents, often in combination with noise, include manufacturing of metal, leather, and petroleum products; painting; printing; woodworking; construction; furniture-making; fueling vehicles and aircraft; degreasing; and firefighting. Hearing loss may also occur after ingestion of fish or water contaminated with these substances.

Hearing loss is more common in workplaces where chemical exposures occur. Hearing loss from ototoxicity is often moderate to severe. The high-frequency "notch" on the audiogram is often present after long-term exposure to ototoxic chemicals,

FIGURE 27-2 ● Audiogram of a 55-year-old dockworker, illustrative of noise-induced hearing loss.

is poorly understood but is believed to be multifactorial. Some of the factors are endogenous, individual attributes that affect susceptibility. Factors include age, gender, race, blood pressure, and use of certain medications. It is important to gather information on these factors.

The effects of noise and age are challenging to differentiate but seem to be additive. Hearing may decline with aging, but the healthy individual who has not been exposed to ototraumatic agents may have normal hearing beyond the age of 65. The median hearing level across the frequencies of 1, 2, 3, and 4 kHz for 60-year-olds not exposed to noise is 17 dB HL for males and 12 dBHL for females.[9] Gender and race seem also to be associated with the susceptibility to hearing loss. Studies conducted of groups with similar jobs and exposures have shown that white males as a group have the highest rates of noise-induced hearing loss and African-American females the lowest.

External factors, such as loudness of noise and duration of exposure, also affect the outcome. Certain nonacoustic factors in the workplace, which may directly affect hearing or interact with noise, are considered possible contributors to variability in individual susceptibility to noise-induced hearing loss.[10,11] For example, workers with vibration-induced white finger (VWF) syndrome have a higher rate of hearing loss than workers exposed to similar noise levels but not vibration.[12] It is not known if whole-body vibration enhances risk for hearing loss.

TABLE 27-1

Priority Ototoxic Chemicals

- Solvents: toluene, styrene, xylene, *n*-hexane, ethyl benzene, white spirits/Stoddard solvents, carbon disulfide, fuels, and perchloroethylene
- Asphyxiants: carbon monoxide and hydrogen cyanide
- Metals: lead and mercury
- Pesticides and herbicides: Paraquat and organophosphates

Source: Morata TC. Chemical exposure as a risk factor for hearing loss. J Occup Environ Med 2003;45:678–82.

BOX 27-2

Case of Hearing Loss After Noise and Chemical Exposures

Peter M. Rabinowitz

A 41-year-old man comes to the occupational medicine clinic for his annual physical examination. He works in a company that makes specialized paints. His job in the paint mixing rooms is to open and mix the contents of large barrels of solvents, including xylene, toluene, and methyl ethyl ketone, in a specified manner with intermittent use of a loud mixing machine. He does not wear hearing protection because the results of an 8-hour dosimetry study during the previous year indicated that the 8-hour TWA of noise exposure was 84 dBA. The ventilation in the mixing room has not always been optimal, causing a usually strong solvent smell. He also notices that he often spills small amounts of solvents on his hands and arms that he wipes off with a rag. He has noticed that his hearing has been getting worse, and he is concerned about going deaf. He has no major medical problems and no family history of significant hearing loss.

His physical examination is normal, except for some defatting of his fingertips and apparent hearing difficulty. His audiogram shows a significant hearing loss at high frequencies bilaterally (Fig. 27-3). Compared to his baseline audiogram with the company, he has lost more than 10 dB (as an average over 2, 3, and 4 kHz), and also has an absolute loss greater than 25 dB at those frequencies. (Therefore, his loss is potentially recordable under OSHA record-keeping standards if it is thought to be due to

workplace exposures.) A full audiological evaluation reveals that his hearing loss is sensorineural and there is no other medical explanation for it.

The occupational medicine physician for this man is faced with several questions:

1. Given that the TWA noise measurements were not excessive, what are possible explanations for his degree of hearing loss?
2. Should his hearing loss be counted as a work-related medical condition?
3. What further steps in evaluation of his hearing loss and prevention of further hearing loss are warranted?

This man has been exposed to noise at work of an intermittent nature. His noise exposure, as an 8-hour TWA, is below the OSHA action level, but peak exposures from the mixing machine may be high enough to cause hearing loss over time, even if the 8-hour TWA is less than 85 dBA.

In addition, this worker has simultaneously been exposed to a variety of organic solvents, including xylene and toluene, which are both neurotoxic and ototoxic. These solvent exposures in this relatively young man may be potentiating the adverse effects of noise on cochlear hair-cell function and survival and/or having a direct independent ototoxic effect.

Reducing his exposures to both noise and solvents will be necessary to preserve his hearing.

---

although a wider range of frequencies may be affected; abnormal thresholds may even occur at 2 and 8 kHz.[15,16]

Ototoxicity of chemicals had been overlooked for a long time because (a) workers exposed to ototoxic chemicals are often also exposed to loud noise, and (b) audiograms do not identify the cause of hearing loss.

It is difficult to perform a differential diagnosis of hearing impairment and assign causation. The nature and severity of ototoxic damage varies according to type of chemical, chemical interactions, and level, duration, and pathway exposure—as well as exposure to excessive noise.

Hearing loss is bilaterally symmetrical and often irreversible. Onset is usually in the high-frequency

range (3 to 6 kHz)—reflected by a "notch" on the audiogram—and progresses at a rate determined by the risk factors listed above. It usually affects the cochlea (see Box 27-2).

NIOSH recommends that hearing loss prevention programs consider chemical exposures when monitoring for hazards, assessing hearing, and controlling exposures.[17,18] The American Conference of Governmental Industrial Hygienists recommends audiograms for workers exposed to toluene, lead, manganese, or *n*-butyl alcohol.[19]

Tinnitus

Tinnitus, the sensation of noise in the absence of acoustic stimuli, is a condition often associated with many forms of hearing loss. It is

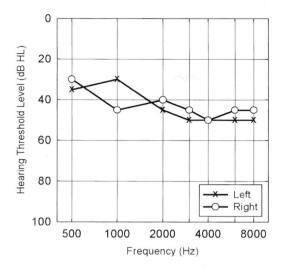

FIGURE 27-3 ● Audiogram of a 41-year-old man who works in paint manufacturing.

described usually as "ringing in the ears," but other forms of sound have been reported, such as buzzing, pulsing, hissing, knocking, roaring, whooshing, chirping, whistling, and clicking. Tinnitus can be intermittent—for minutes to a few hours at a time—or continuous. It can be a minor annoyance or a serious and nearly intolerable condition.

In severe cases, it may interfere with daily activities and sleep. Tinnitus is most commonly associated with noise exposure and also with more than 200 medications as well as dietary, nutritional, hormonal, immunological, and stress factors.

The reported prevalence of work-related tinnitus varies considerably among occupational groups, ranging from 17 to 60 percent of cases among noise-exposed workers.[20,21] However, it has attracted relatively little interest. For example, only 13 U.S. states as well as the United Kingdom, Canada, Australia, Germany, Denmark, and Sweden and provide workers' compensation for tinnitus.[21] It is likely that there are several mechanisms accounting for tinnitus. Studies suggest that it results from increases in the spontaneous neural activity in the auditory system. The first relay of the primary auditory pathway is in the cochlear nuclei in the brainstem, which tend to develop hyperactivity that might be relayed to higher levels in the brain. Alternatively, heightened activity of some descending pathway might explain the hyperactivity or other central mechanisms might operate.

GOVERNMENTAL REGULATION

Federal, state, and local governments set and enforce noise standards for aircraft, airports, interstate motor carriers, railroads, medium- and heavy-duty trucks, motorcycles, mopeds, and many commercial, industrial, and residential activities.

The Environmental Protection Agency (EPA) coordinated all federal noise-control activities until 1983. Then, responsibility of regulating noise was transferred to state and local governments. Although EPA no longer plays a prominent role in regulating noise, its past standards and regulations remain in effect, and other federal agencies continue to set and enforce noise standards for sources within their regulatory jurisdictions.

Workers in general industry who are exposed to noise levels above 85 dBA are required by the Occupational Safety and Health Administration (OSHA) to be in a hearing conservation program. This program for manufacturing and mining workers includes noise measurement, noise control, periodic audiometric testing, hearing protection, worker education, and recordkeeping.

In construction, noise exposures are required to be evaluated and controlled, and hearing protectors must be offered when exposures exceed 85 dBA. Apart from exposure limits, there is no mandatory hearing conservation program for construction workers. There is no hearing-loss prevention regulation for workers in agriculture, despite their high prevalence of hearing loss, or for workers in the service and public sectors.

OSHA's new recordkeeping rule, in effect since 2003, significantly altered the criteria for documenting what constitutes a reportable hearing threshold shift.[22] Work-related hearing loss in either ear is recordable when there is both:

1. An average shift in hearing threshold of 10 dB or greater at 2,000, 3,000, and 4,000 Hz (2, 3, and 4 kHz), relative to the audiometric baseline (called a standard threshold shift, or STS); and

2. The average hearing level in the same ear is 25 dB or greater at 2,000, 3,000 and 4,000 Hz.

The prior recording criteria required an average hearing threshold shift at 2,000, 3,000, and 4,000 Hz of 25 dB or greater to establish a significant change compared to audiometric baseline. It is likely that the number of recordable hearing loss cases will increase in most states,[23] which may lead to improved hearing-conservation and noise-control programs. In 2004, OSHA improved mandated employer recordkeeping for occupational hearing loss. The National Institue for Occupational Safety and Health (NIOSH) has published the *Practical Guide for Preventing Occupational Hearing Loss*, based on experiences in hearing conservation.[17] This guide presents attributes of successful hearing loss prevention programs and identifies responsibilities of management, those who implement the hearing-loss prevention programs, and workers affected by noise exposure.

STRATEGIES FOR IMPROVING HEARING-LOSS PREVENTION PROGRAMS IN THE WORKPLACE

In 2000, the participants in a conference on noise-induced hearing loss held in Wisconsin recognized that past measures failed to adequately promote noise control or noise-induced hearing loss and thus recommended new strategies and technologies.

Controlling Hazardous Exposures

Initial steps of hearing-loss prevention programs are hazard assessment and control. Federal regulations consider only noise as a risk factor for hearing loss. Required noise measurements serve as the basis for assessing noise-control alternatives. If noise exposure is controlled to levels below 85 dBA time-weighted average (TWA), a hearing conservation program is not legally required.

Occupational exposure to noise at the NIOSH REL for occupational noise exposure (85 dBA TWA)[18] for 40 years increases the risk of noise-induced hearing loss by 8 percent—considerably lower than the 25 percent increased risk at the current OSHA and Mine Safety and Health Administration (MSHA) permissible exposure level (PEL) of 90 dBA TWA.

NIOSH previously recommended an exchange rate of 5 dB for halving the exposure time in the calculation of TWA exposures to noise; that is, starting at the 85 dBA recommended exposure level (REL) for an 8-hour period, for each 5-dB increase in exposure, the permissible exposure was to be halved. However, since 1998, NIOSH has recommended a 3-dB exchange rate, which is more firmly supported by scientific evidence.[18] The 5-dB exchange rate is still used by OSHA and MSHA.

Whenever hazardous noise exists in the workplace, measures should be taken to reduce noise levels as much as possible to protect exposed workers and to monitor the effectiveness of these intervention processes.[24,25] The most effective way to prevent noise-induced hearing loss is to remove the noise source from the workplace, such as by engineering controls, or to remove the worker from hazardous noise.

Unfortunately, hearing protection devices (HPDs) are often adopted in lieu of controlling noise exposure. Although relatively inexpensive and easy to use, providing HPDs to control noise exposure is often problematic. In order to achieve the desired noise attenuation, workers must wear HPDs consistently during exposure to noise levels greater than 85 dBA, as a TWA. Workers often find it difficult to do so because HPDs can be uncomfortable and interfere with communication. Consequently, use of HPDs is inconsistent and varies widely. They are usually purchased on the basis of minimum cost and maximum attenuation, leading to use of devices that overprotect and interfere with communication. New electronic devices now exist that not only protect at appropriate levels but also facilitate communication. Recommendations to increase the use of HPDs include identifying devices that offer adequate attenuation and provide workers with better comfort.

The rating system developed by EPA is recognized as obsolete. The attenuation of HPDs determined in a laboratory is not predictive of how they function in the workplace. A new system of ratings is being evaluated to better reflect real-world performance. OSHA has instructed its compliance officers to de-rate the noise reduction rating (NRR) of HPDs by 50 percent in enforcing the engineering control provision of the OSHA noise standard. NIOSH recommends de-rating by subtracting from the NRR 25 percent for earmuffs, 50 percent for formable earplugs, and 70 percent for all other earplugs.[18] This variable de-rating scheme, as opposed to OSHA's straight de-rating scheme, distinguishes among the performance of different types of hearing protectors.

Eligibility for Hearing-Loss Prevention Programs

Preventive strategies that are used to protect workers from noise exposure will not protect workers from chemical exposure. When ototoxic chemicals are present in the workplace, hearing-loss prevention measures may be needed even where noise exposure does not exceed 85 dBA.

The American Conference of Governmental Industrial Hygienists (ACGIH) advises that workers exposed to ototoxic chemicals have periodic audiograms.[19] The U.S. Army requires that hearing conservation programs consider ototoxic chemical exposures, especially when noise exposure does not exceed permissible or recommended limits.[26] It recommends annual audiograms for workers whose airborne exposures are at 50 percent of the most stringent occupational exposure limits for toluene, xylene, *n*-hexane, organic tin, carbon disulfide, mercury, organic lead, hydrogen cyanide, diesel fuel, kerosene fuel, jet fuel, JP-8 fuel, organophosphate pesticides, or chemical-warfare nerve agents—regardless of the noise level. This 50 percent level, while somewhat arbitrary, ensures data collection from exposure situations below occupational exposure limits. When dermal exposures to these agents result in a systemic dose equivalent to 50 percent or more of the occupational exposure limit, annual audiograms are also recommended. For workers participating in hearing conservation programs because of excessive noise, reviewers of audiometric data should be alert to possible additive, potentiating, or synergistic effects between noise and ototoxic chemicals, and should, if necessary, initiate reduction of exposure to the noise and/or the chemicals.

Audiometric Monitoring

The OSHA criterion for the standard threshold shift (a change of 10 dB or more in the average of hearing thresholds at 2,000, 3,000, and 4,000 Hz) identifies hearing loss relatively infrequently. NIOSH recommends a better criterion for the calculation of significant threshold shift: an increase of 15 dB in the hearing threshold level at any of the test frequencies in either ear (at 500, 1,000, 2,000, 3,000, 4,000, or 6,000 Hz), as determined by two consecutive audiometric tests[18]—a new criterion that has both high sensitivity and high specificity.

NIOSH suggests that (a) monitoring audiometry be conducted on noise-exposed workers late in, or at the end of, their daily work shifts; and (b) audiometry be repeated immediately after any monitoring audiogram indicates a significant threshold shift.[18] Before conducting retests, workers should be reinstructed and headphones refitted. Those who

employ the retest strategy will find a significant reduction in the number of workers called back for a confirmation audiogram—because if the retest audiogram does not show the same shift as the initial audiogram, the retest audiogram becomes the test of record.

By testing workers during their work shifts, one may identify temporary threshold shifts (TTSs). Even though the relationship between permanent threshold shifts and TTSs is not completely understood, it is clear that workers with a TTS are being overexposed to noise. Discovering a TTS and taking action to prevent its increase will help protect workers from permanent hearing damage. If annual monitoring audiograms are performed before or at the beginning of workshifts, TTSs from noise exposure on the previous workshift will have been cleared so that any threshold shifts observed will represent permanent shifts in hearing.

Audiometry should be conducted again within 30 days of any monitoring or retest audiogram that continues to show a significant threshold shift. A minimum of 12 hours of quiet should precede the confirmation audiogram to determine whether the shift is a TTS or a permanent threshold shift. Hearing protectors should not be considered as a substitute for a quiet work environment.[18]

Age Correction

Although some people experience decrease in hearing acuity with age, others do not, and it is not possible to predict who will and who will not develop hearing loss as they age. The median hearing loss attributable to aging for a given age group cannot be generalized to all individuals in that age group. Thus, in calculating significant threshold shifts, age-correcting hearing thresholds will overestimate the expected hearing loss for some and underestimate it for others.

The adjustment of audiometric thresholds for aging has become a common practice in workers' compensation litigation. In this application, age corrections reduce the amount of hearing loss attributable to noise exposure, with a consequent reduction in the amount of compensation paid to workers for their hearing losses. "Age correcting" is still applied, but it is technically inappropriate to apply population statistics to an individual.

NIOSH states that age-correcting audiograms obtained in an occupational hearing-loss prevention program is not appropriate.[18] The purpose of the program is to prevent hearing loss. If an audiogram is age-corrected, regardless of the source of the correction values, the time required for a significant threshold shift to be identified will be prolonged.

Accommodating Workers with Hearing Loss

After a confirmation audiogram that indicates a permanent threshold shift, NIOSH recommends a written notification to the worker and a referral to the audiometric manager or professional supervisor for review and determination of probable etiology. This referral should explore all possible causes in addition to occupational noise, including ototoxic chemicals, age-related hearing loss, familial hearing loss, nonoccupational noise exposure, and medical conditions. Workers with a threshold shift due to causes other than noise should be counseled by audiometric managers and referred to their physicians for evaluation and treatment. Appropriate actions should be planned for workers showing a threshold shift that is determined by the audiometric manager to be likely due to occupational noise. Actions should, at a minimum, include reinstruction concerning, and refitting of, hearing protectors; additional training in worker responsibilities for effective hearing-loss prevention, and/or reassignment to a quieter work area. The "professional supervisor" should be responsible for making whatever decisions deemed necessary and for ensuring that they are implemented. According to OSHA's Hearing Conservation Amendment, the "professional supervisor" of the audiometric testing component of a hearing conservation program must be a licensed or certified audiologist or otolaryngologist, or other physician.

The main factors that enable workers with hearing loss to continue working are ability to cope with the hearing loss, support from management and co-workers, adequate work conditions, psychological support from patient organizations as well as family members and friends, support from medical professionals and programs, and financial and other benefits.[27] A set of guidelines can be used by health professionals for managing the work-related conditions.[27] Important to workers with hearing loss is knowledge about and availability of better hearing protectors and hearing aids, alternative means of obtaining and financing hearing aids, self-acceptance, a quiet work environment, deter-

mination and persistence to ask for needed accommodations at work, education of co-workers about hearing loss, and opportunities to communicate information and experiences with other affected workers.

Accommodating Workers with Tinnitus

The most important step in managing workers with tinnitus is to refer them to otolaryngologists or otologists (ear specialists). The specialist will try to determine the cause of tinnitus by assessing the auditory system, measuring blood pressure and kidney function, and assessing diet, allergies, and medications. The specialist will determine treatment, which may include maskers (electronic devices the size of hearing aids that use sound to make tinnitus less noticeable), support and counseling, surgery, drug therapy (such as tricyclic antidepressants), diet, psychotherapy, electrical/magnetic stimulation, acupuncture, biofeedback, and hypnosis. Specialists should explain to patients the pathophysiology of their tinnitus, make recommendations for hearing aids when appropriate, and provide periodic monitoring.[28]

ACKNOWLEDGMENT

This chapter is dedicated to the memory of Dr. Derek E. Dunn.

REFERENCES

1. Bureau of Labor Statistics, News Bureau of Labor Statistics USDL 02–687. Washington, DC: United States Department of Labor, 2002. Available at <http://www.bls.gov/iif/oshwc/osh/os/osnr0016.pdf>.
2. Mohr PE, Feldman JJ, Dunbar J et al. The societal costs of severe to profound hearing loss in the United States. Int J Technol Assess Health Care 2000;16:1120–35.
3. National Council on Aging. Untreated hearing loss linked to depression, anxiety, social isolation in seniors. NCOA News, May 26, 1999. Available at <www.ncoa.org>.
4. Kochkin S, Rogin CM. Quantifying the obvious: The impact of hearing instruments on quality of life. The Hearing Review 2000;7:6–34.
5. Prince MM, Stayner LT, Smith RJ, et al. A reexamination of risk estimates from the NIOSH Occupational Noise and Hearing Survey (ONHS). J Acoust Soc Am 1997;101:950–63.
6. National Institutes of Health. Noise and Hearing Loss. NIH Consensus Development Conference: Consensus Statement, Bethesda, MD: National Institutes of Health, 1990, p. 8.
7. Lim DJ, Dunn DE. Anatomical correlates of noise induced hearing loss. Otolaryngol Clin N Am 1979;12: 493–513.

8. Durrant JD, Lovrinic JH. Bases of hearing science. 3rd ed. Baltimore: Williams & Wilkins, 1995.

9. American National Standards Institute. American National Standard: Determination of occupational noise exposure and estimation of noise-induced hearing impairment. ANSI S3.44–1996. New York: ANSI, 1996.

10. Phaneuf R, Hetu, R. An epidemiological perspective of the causes of hearing loss among industrial workers. J Otolaryngol 1990;19:31–40.

11. Morata TC, Franks JR, Dunn DE. Unmet needs in occupational hearing conservation. Lancet 1994;344:479.

12. Palmer KT, Griffin MJ, Syddall HE, et al. Raynaud's phenomenon, vibration induced white finger, and difficulties in hearing. Occup Environ Med 2002;59:640–2.

13. Pryor GT, Rebert CS, Dickinson J, et al. Factors affecting toluene-induced ototoxicity in rats. Neurobehav Toxicol Teratol 1984;6:223–38.

14. Bergstrom B, Nystrom B. Development of hearing loss during long-term exposure to occupational noise: A 20-year follow-up study. Scand Audiol 1986;15:227–34.

15. Morata TC. Chemical exposure as a risk factor for hearing loss. J Occup Environ Med 2003;45:676–82.

16. Sliwinska-Kowalska M, Zamyslowska-Szmytke E, Szymczak W, et al. Ototoxic effects of occupational exposure to styrene and co-exposure to styrene and noise. J Occup Environ Med 2003;45:15–24.

17. Franks JR, Stephenson MR, Merry CJ. Preventing occupational hearing loss: A practical guide. Cincinnati: NIOSH, 1996. (Publication no. 96–110.)

18. NIOSH. Criteria for a recommended standard: Occupational exposure to noise (revised criteria). Cincinnati: NIOSH, 1998. (Publication no. 98–126.)

19. American Conference of Governmental Industrial Hygienists. Threshold Limit Values and Biological Exposure Indices for 1998–1999. Cincinnati: ACGIH, 1998.

20. Parving A, Hein HO, Suadicani P, et al. Epidemiology of hearing disorders: Some factors affecting hearing. The Copenhagen Male Study. Scand Audiol 1993;22:101–7.

21. Axelsson A, Coles R. Compensation for tinnitus in noise-induced hearing loss. In: Axelsson A, Borchgrevink HM, Hamernik RP, et al., eds. Scientific basis of noise-induced, hearing loss. New York: Thieme, 1996:423–9.

22. Megerson SC. Tracking work-related hearing loss. The ASHA Leader 2003;14:1–10. Available at <http://www.asha.org/about/publications/leader-online/>.

23. Rabinowitz PM, Slade M, Dixon-Ernst C, et al. Impact of OSHA final rule–recording hearing loss: An analysis of an industrial audiometric dataset. J Occup Environ Med 2003;45:1274–80.

24. Metz M. The failed hearing conservation paradigm. Audiology Today 2000;12:13–15.

25. Suter A. Council for Accreditation in Occupational Hearing Conservation. Hearing conservation manual. 4th ed. Milwaukee: CAOHC, 2003.

26. U.S. Army. Hearing Conservation Program. Department of the Army Pamphlet 40-501. Washington, DC: Headquarters, Department of the Army, 1998.

27. Detaille SI, Haafkens JA, van Dijk FJH. What employees with rheumatoid arthritis, diabetes mellitus and hearing loss need to cope at work. Scand J Work Environ Health 2003;29:134–42.

28. Dobie RA. A review of randomized clinical trials in tinnitus. Laryngoscope 1999;109:1202–11.

BIBLIOGRAPHY

Centre Régional d'Imagerie Cellulaire, Université Montpellier, Institute National de la Santé et de la Recherche Médicale [homepage on the Internet]. Montpellier: Université Montpellier, c1999–2003. Available from http://www.iurc.montp.inserm.fr/cric. Accessed August 17, 2005.
Describes the anatomy, physiology, and pathophysiology of the auditory system.

American Tinnitus Association, ATA [homepage on the Internet]. Portland, OR: American Tinnitus Association, c2001–2005. Available from http://www.ata.org. Accessed August 17, 2005.
The American Tinnitus Association (ATA) promotes tinnitus awareness, prevention, and treatment. It offers information on prevention programs in schools, urges governmental and private organizations to support hearing conservation, funds research, and facilitates self-help groups.

Dobie R. Estimation of occupational contribution to hearing handicap. In: Axelsson A, Borchgrevink HM, Hamernik RP, et al., eds. Scientific basis of noise-induced hearing loss. New York: Thieme, 1996:415–22.
For estimates on age-related and noise-induced threshold shifts.

Suter A. Hearing conservation manual. 4th ed. Council for Accreditation in Occupational Hearing Conservation, CAOHC. Milwaukee, WI: CAOHC, 2003.
The fourth edition of the Council for Accreditation in Occupational Hearing Conservation (CAOHC) Hearing Conservation Manual also covers all facets of developing a successful hearing-loss prevention program. CAOHC indicates that to achieve success in a hearing-loss prevention program, one should not be limited by legislative requirements, and this document discusses methods to accomplish hearing loss prevention.

United States Army Center for Health Promotion & Preventive Medicine [homepage on the Internet]. Aberdeen Proving Ground: United States Army, c2003–2005. Available from http://chppm-www.apgea.army.mil/documents/ FACT/51-002-0903.pdf. Accessed August 17, 2005.
This Web site contains a fact sheet regarding ototoxic chemical exposures and guidelines for hearing conservation developed by the U.S. Army.

The findings and conclusions in this chapter are those of the author and do not necessarily represent the views of the National Institute for Occupational Safety and Health.

CHAPTER 28

Skin Disorders

Boris D. Lushniak

T he skin plays an important role in providing a protective, living barrier between the external environment of the world around us and the internal environment of the human body. As a first-line protective barrier, the cutaneous surface is subjected to the hostile forces of the external environment and, as such, can be directly injured or damaged by these environmental forces.

In general, the causes of environmental skin disorders can be grouped into the following categories:

1. *Physical insults*: friction, pressure, trauma, vibration, heat, cold, variations in humidity, ultraviolet/visible/infrared radiation, ionizing radiation, and electric current.
2. *Biologic causes*: plants, bacteria, rickettsia, viruses, fungi, protozoa, parasites, and arthropods.
3. *Chemical insults*: water, inorganic acids, alkalis, salts of heavy metals, aliphatic acids, aldehydes, alcohols, esters, hydrocarbons, solvents, metallo-organic compounds, lipids, aromatic and polycyclic compounds, resin monomers, and proteins.

These insults are present everywhere in the environment, and the settings where they may threaten the skin include the home setting, during outdoor leisure activities, while involved in hobbies, and the work environment, which is likely to be the most

important setting where physical, biological, and chemical insults can affect the skin.

Occupational dermatology is the facet of dermatology that deals with skin diseases whose etiology or aggravation is related to some exposure in the workplace. By its nature, occupational dermatology is also related to occupational and preventive medicine. The ideal role of a medical practitioner involved in occupational dermatology is not only to diagnose and treat patients but also to determine the etiology of the occupational skin disease and to make recommendations for its prevention. Making the diagnosis and offering treatment, determining etiology, and recommending preventive measures can all be difficult undertakings.

Environmental and occupational skin diseases can manifest themselves in a variety of ways. This chapter will emphasize skin conditions caused by environmental agents that have a direct effect on the skin. These include irritant contact dermatitis, allergic contact dermatitis, contact urticaria, skin infections, skin cancers, and a large group of miscellaneous skin diseases. Certain common skin diseases, such as atopic dermatitis and psoriasis, are exacerbated by environmental factors, but their etiology remains unclear and they will not be covered here.

CONTACT DERMATITIS

Contact dermatitis is the most common occupational and environmental skin disease. Epidemiologic data show that contact dermatitis comprises 90 to 95 percent of all occupational skin diseases.[1] *Contact dermatitis*—both irritant and allergic—is an inflammatory skin condition caused by skin

---

This chapter has been updated from a published U.S. government work.

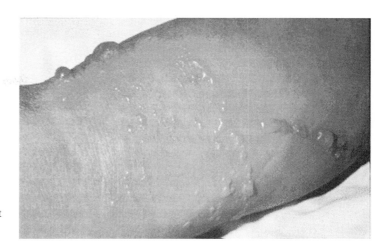

FIGURE 28-1 ● Acute contact dermatitis from exposure to the strong irritant ethylene oxide.

contact with an exogenous agent or agents, with or without a concurrent exposure to a contributory physical agent, such as ultraviolet light. Contact dermatitis can result from a nonimmunologic reaction to chemical irritants (irritant contact dermatitis) or from an immunologic reaction to allergens (allergic contact dermatitis). *Irritant contact dermatitis* is a cutaneous inflammation resulting from a direct cytotoxic effect of a chemical or physical agent, whereas *allergic contact dermatitis* is a type IV, delayed or cell-mediated, immune reaction. There are more than 57,000 chemicals reported to cause skin irritation, but only 3,000 chemicals are potential human allergens. These allergens are mostly confined to large-molecular-weight proteins and to small-molecular-weight chemicals that act as haptens, and usually only a small proportion of people are susceptible to them.

In contact dermatitis, the skin initially turns red and can develop small, oozing vesicles and papules. After several days, crusts and scales form. Stinging, burning, and itching may accompany the skin lesions. With no further contact with the etiologic agent, the dermatitis usually disappears in 1 to 3 weeks. With chronic exposure, deep fissures, scaling, and hyperpigmentation can occur. Exposed areas of the skin, such as hands and forearms, which have the greatest contact with irritants or allergens, are most commonly affected. If the agent gets on clothing, it can induce dermatitis at areas of greatest contact, such as thighs, upper back, armpits, and feet. Dusts can produce dermatitis at areas where the dust accumulates and is held in contact with the skin, such as under the collar and belt line, at the tops of socks or shoes, and in flexural areas, such as the antecubital and popliteal fossae. Mists can produce a dermatitis on the face and anterior neck. Irritants and allergens can be transferred to other areas of the body, such as the trunk or genitalia, by unwashed hands or from areas of accumulation, such as under rings or interdigital areas. It is often impossible to clinically distinguish irritant contact from allergic contact dermatitis, as both can have a similar appearance and both can be clinically evident as an acute, subacute, or chronic condition (Figs. 28-1 through 28-3).

Public Health Importance

Measures of the public health importance of a disease include the absolute number of cases, the incidence rate, the prevalence (rate), the economic impact of the disease, and the prognosis and preventability of the disease.[2]

Specific national data sources on contact dermatitis are limited. In the United States, data from the National Ambulatory Medical Care Survey, a national probability sample survey of nonfederal office-based physicians, showed that in 2002 skin rash was the principal reason for 11.8 million patient visits—1.3 percent of all visits for that year.[3] Based on previous surveys, it is estimated that approximately one-half of these visits would have had a diagnosis of contact dermatitis or other eczemas.

In 1988, the National Health Interview Survey (NHIS) included an Occupational Health Supplement, which included questions on dermatitis. The

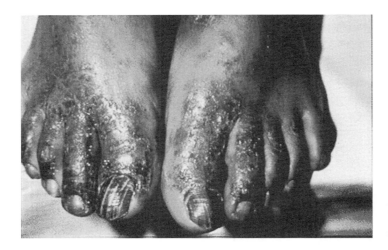

FIGURE 28-2 ● Subacute dermatitis from the rubber accelerator, mercaptobenzothiazole, from the rubber in a work boot.

survey consisted of personal interviews of people in randomly selected households. For 30,074 people participating in the NHIS, the period prevalence for all dermatitis was 11.2 percent and for contact dermatitis was 2.8 percent. Projecting these results to the U.S. working population resulted in an estimate of 13.7 million people with dermatitis and 3.1 million people with contact dermatitis.[4]

More information is available on the public health impact of occupational contact dermatitis. Specific national occupational disease and illness data are available from the U.S. Bureau of Labor Statistics (BLS), which conducts annual surveys of approximately 160,000 employers selected to represent all private industries in the United States.[5]

All occupational skin diseases or disorders, including contact dermatitis, are tabulated in this survey. BLS data show that occupational skin diseases accounted for a consistent 30 to 45 percent of all cases of occupational illnesses from the 1970s through the mid-1980s and in recent years accounted for 12 percent of all occupational illness.[5] A decline in this proportion may be partially related to an increase seen in disorders associated with repeated trauma.

BLS data for occupational skin diseases for 1973 to 2001 are shown in Fig. 28-4. In 2001, BLS estimated 38,900 cases of occupational skin diseases or disorders in the U.S. workforce.[5] However, because of BLS survey limitations, it has been estimated that the number of actual occupational

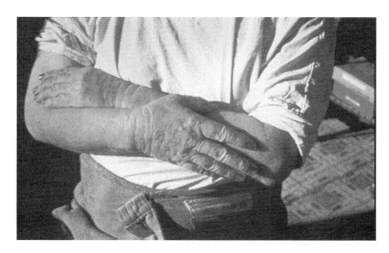

FIGURE 28-3 ● Chronic dermatitis from exposure to kerosene, a solvent that was used for cleaning the skin.

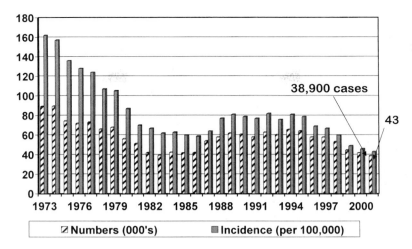

FIGURE 28-4 ● Annual incidence (number and rate) of occupational skin diseases per year, United States, 1973–2001. (Source: U.S. Bureau of Labor Statistics Annual Survey, 1973–2001.)

skin diseases may be of the order 10 to 50 times higher than that reported by the BLS[6]. This increase would potentially raise the number of occupational skin disease cases to between 400,000 and 2 million per year. In 2001, BLS data showed an annual incidence rate of 43 cases per 100,000 workers.[5]

In 1988, the Occupational Health Supplement of the NHIS indicated that the period prevalence for occupational contact dermatitis occurring in the preceding year was 1.7 percent. Projecting these results to the U.S. working population resulted in an estimate of 1.87 million people with occupational contact dermatitis and a 1-year period prevalence of 1,700 per 100,000 workers for the year.[4] The numbers and rates in the BLS and NHIS surveys are not directly comparable because they rely on different information sources with different ascertainment methods and different case definitions.

The economic impact of a disease can be measured by the direct costs of medical care and workers' compensation or disability payments and the indirect costs associated with lost workdays and loss of productivity. In 1984, the estimated annual direct and indirect costs of occupational skin diseases exceeded $22 million.[6] However, considering that the actual annual incidence may be 10 to 50 times greater than reported in the BLS data, the total annual cost of occupational skin diseases in 1984 may have ranged from $222 million to $1 billion.[6] (These estimates do not include costs of occupational retraining.)

A review of 1993 BLS data showed that of 60,200 cases of occupational skin diseases, 12,613 (21 percent) resulted in days away from work.[7] The mean time away from work was 3 days, but 17 percent of lost workday cases had more than 11 days away from work. Of those with days away from work, 70 percent had a diagnosis of dermatitis. In 2001, of the 38,900 skin disease cases, 6,051 (16 percent) resulted in days away from work, with a median of 3 days lost.[5] Of these, 78 percent had dermatitis. A study of 235 Canadian workers with occupational skin diseases showed that 35 percent had been away from work for greater than 1 month, 14 percent between 1 week and 1 month, 17 percent less than 1 week, and 33 percent did not lose workdays because of the skin condition.[8]

Studies on the prognosis of occupational contact dermatitis point out that primary prevention is very important. For example, of 555 patients completing a follow-up questionnaire 2 to 3 years after diagnosis, only 26 percent of the women with contact dermatitis had complete healing (22 percent had continual symptoms and 52 percent had recurring symptoms), and only 31 percent of the men had complete healing (29 percent had continual symptoms, 40 percent had recurring symptoms).[9] A telephone survey of 235 occupational skin disease patients, conducted a mean of 4 years after diagnosis, showed that 40 percent had continuing dermatitis, although of this group, 76 percent reported an improvement in their skin condition.[8] Outcomes may or may not be influenced by leaving the dermatitis-provoking job. In addition, many skin disorders, including contact dermatitis, have been shown to have a significant impact on quality of life.[10]

Over the years, there have been changes in the epidemiology of occupational skin diseases. A decrease in the absolute number of cases and the incidence rate in the BLS survey from the 1970s to the early 21st century may be attributable to several factors, including changes in industry and industrial practices, increased awareness and preventive measures, and possible underreporting, underrecognition, and misclassification. Still, occupational contact dermatitis remains a relatively common disease with a noteworthy public health impact. These factors, along with the potential chronicity of the disorder, its effect on an individual's vocational and avocational activities, and its preventability, make occupational contact dermatitis a disease of public health importance.

Population at Risk and Etiologic Agents

There is a myriad of occupations that have unique exposures resulting in occupational contact dermatitis. Total numbers and incidence rates of occupational dermatologic conditions, by major industry division, based on the BLS survey for 2001 are shown in Table 28-1.[5] The greatest number of cases of occupational skin diseases is seen in manufacturing, but the highest incidence rate is seen in agriculture/forestry/fishing.

In the NHIS, the occupational groups with the highest prevalence of self-reported occupational contact dermatitis included physicians, dentists, nurses, pharmacists, and dieticians (5.6 percent); public transport attendants, cosmetologists, and other personal service occupations (4.9 percent); health care therapists, technologists, technicians, and assistants (3.5 percent); and mechanics and repairers of vehicles, engines, heavy equipment, and machinery (3.5 percent).[4] Of all accepted workers' compensation claims for occupational contact dermatitis in Oregon, the most common occupations were laborers (14.2 percent), food service workers (13.8 percent), machine operators

TABLE 28-1

Number and Incidence Rate of Occupational Skin Diseases, by Industry Sector, 2001

	Number	Incidence Rate (per 100,000)
Agriculture/forestery/ fisheries	2,600	175
Manufacturing	16,100	93
Services	13,400	48
Transport/utilities	1,600	24
Construction	1,400	23
Wholesale and retail trade	3,200	14
Finance/insurance/real estate	600	9
Mining	<50	2
Total/Overall	38,900	43

(13.1 percent), agricultural workers (9.0 percent), health professionals (8.2 percent), and janitors/maids (6.4 percent), followed by production crafts workers, mechanics, construction workers, and hairdressers/cosmetologists.[11]

The most frequent causes of irritant contact dermatitis include soaps and detergents, fibrous glass and other particulate dusts, food products, cleaning agents, solvents, plastics and resins, petroleum products and lubricants, metals, and machine oils and coolants.[1] Causes of allergic contact dermatitis include plants (poison ivy, poison oak, and poison sumac), metallic salts, organic dyes, plastic resins, rubber additives, and germicides.[12] The most common skin patch test allergens found to be positive in patients along with potential sources of exposure are shown in Table 28-2.[13] In patients with occupational contact dermatitis who were skin patch tested, the common allergens included carba mix, thiuram mix, formaldehyde, epoxy resin, and nickel.[14]

Diagnosis

The environmental cause or work-relatedness of contact dermatitis may be difficult to prove. The accuracy of the diagnosis is related to the skill level, experience, and knowledge of the medical professional who makes the diagnosis and confirms

TABLE 28-2

North American Contact Dermatitis Group Patch-Test Results,[a] 1998 to 2000

Test Substance	Common Sources	Percent Positive
Nickel sulfate 2.5%	Metals, jewelry	16.2
Balsam of Peru 25%	Perfumes, creams	12.3
Neomycin	Creams, lotions	11.5
Fragrance mix 8%	Toiletries, scented products	10.9
Thimerosal 0.1%	Cosmetics, cleansers	10.8
Sodium gold thiosulfate 0.5%	Jewelry, dental products	10.5
Formaldehyde 1% aqueous	Fabrics, skincare products	9.2
Quaternium-15 2%	Cosmetics, sunscreens	9.2
Bacitracin 20%	Ointments, creams	9.2
Cobalt chloride 1%	Metals, jewelry	7.6
Methyldibromo glutaronitrile phenoxyethanol 2.5%	Biocides, skincare products	6.0
Potassium dichromate 0.25%	Cement, leather	5.8
Ethyleneurea melamine formaldehyde resin 5%	Textiles	5.0
p-Phenylenediamine 1%	Hair dyes, leather	4.9
Carba mix 30%	Rubber, pesticides	4.8
Thiuram 1%	Rubber, pesticides	4.7
Propylene glycol 30% aqueous	Cosmetics, topical meds	3.7
Cinnamic aldehyde 1%	Fragrances, flavorings	3.6
Methyldibromo glutaronitrile phenoxyethanol 0.4%	Biocides, skincare products	3.5
Amidoamine 0.1% aqueous	Shampoos, liquid soap	3.4

[a] Prevalence of 20 most common positive reactions (n varies from 5,770 to 5,835).
From Marks JG, Belsito DV, DeLeo VA, et al. North American Contact Dermatitis Group patch-test results, 1998 to 2000. Am J Contact Dermatitis 2003;14:59–62.

the relationship with environmental or workplace exposures. Guidelines are available for assessing the work-relatedness of dermatitis, but even with guidelines the diagnosis may be difficult.[15] The diagnosis is based on the medical and occupational histories and physical findings. The importance of the patient's history of exposures and disease onset is clear. Standardized questionnaires for surveying work-related skin diseases are available and can be helpful in the workplace.[16] In irritant contact dermatitis, there are no additional confirmatory tests. Patch tests or provocation tests are discouraged because of a high false-positive rate. In many instances, allergic contact dermatitis can be confirmed by skin patch tests using specific standardized allergens or, in some circumstances, by provocation tests with nonirritating dilutions of industrial contactants. Skin patch tests should only

be conducted by health care professionals trained in conducting and interpreting the tests. Skin patch tests should never be conducted with unknown substances.

The following questions can be used as criteria for determining work-relatedness:

1. Is the clinical appearance consistent with contact dermatitis?
2. Are there workplace exposures to potential cutaneous irritants or allergens?
3. Is the anatomic distribution of dermatitis consistent with cutaneous exposure in relation to the job task?
4. Is the temporal relationship between exposure and onset consistent with contact dermatitis?
5. Are nonoccupational exposures excluded as probable causes?

6. Does dermatitis improve away from the exposure to the suspected irritant or allergen?
7. Do patch tests or provocation tests identify a probable causal agent?[15]

Treatment and Prevention

Avoiding etiologic irritants and allergens is the first step in any treatment regimen. Dermatitis is treated according to its clinical stage. Acute dermatitis treatment options can include a short course of systemic steroids, topical steroids, and soothing compresses or baths. Antihistamine therapy or use of sedatives may be helpful to decrease pruritus. If secondary infection is present, topical or systemic antibiotics are indicated. Subacute dermatitis and chronic dermatitis are usually treated with topical steroid therapy and lubrication of the skin. Potential dangers of long-term use of topical steroids, especially high-potency steroids, include systemic effects and skin atrophy. In addition, contact dermatitis can be caused by ingredients found in topical agents, including antibiotics, fragrances, vehicles, or steroids.

Strategies for the prevention of occupational contact dermatitis include:

- identifying irritants and allergens;
- substituting chemicals that are less irritating or allergenic;
- establishing engineering controls to reduce exposure;
- using personal protective equipment (PPE), such as gloves and special clothing;
- emphasizing personal and occupational hygiene; and,
- establishing educational programs to increase awareness in the workplace.[17]

Chemical changes in industrial materials have proved to be beneficial. For example, the addition of ferrous sulfate to cement to reduce the hexavalent chromium content was effective in reducing occupational allergic contact dermatitis in Europe. The use of PPE must be considered carefully, as it may actually create problems by occluding irritants or allergens or by directly irritating the skin. Similarly, the excessive pursuit of personal hygiene in the workplace may actually lead to misuse of soaps and detergents and resulting irritant contact dermatitis. The effectiveness of gloves depends on the specific exposures and the types of gloves used. The effectiveness of barrier creams is controversial,

as there are limited data on the protective nature of these topical products during actual working conditions involving high-risk exposures. Other interventions, including providing advice on PPE and educating the workforce about skin care and exposures, are beneficial.[18]

CONTACT URTICARIA

Urticaria is defined as the transient appearance of elevated, erythematous pruritic wheals or serpiginous exanthem, usually surrounded by an area of erythema. In addition, areas of macular erythema or erythematous papules may also be present. These skin lesions appear and peak in minutes to hours after the etiologic exposure, and individual lesions usually disappear within 24 hours. Urticarial lesions usually involve the trunk and extremities, although they can involve any epidermal or mucosal surface. Large wheal formation, where the edema extends from the dermis into the subcutaneous tissue, is referred to as *angioedema*. This condition is more commonly seen in the more distensible tissues, such as the eyelids, lips, ear lobes, external genitalia, and mucous membranes.

Urticarial lesions can be classified in one or more of the following categories based on characteristic features:

1. Duration or chronicity: acute or chronic.
2. Clinical distribution of the lesions or the extradermal manifestation: localized, generalized, or systemic associated with rhinitis, conjunctivitis, asthma, or anaphylaxis.
3. Etiology: idiopathic or cause-specific.
4. Routes of exposure: direct contact, inhalation, or ingestion.
5. Mechanisms: nonimmunologic, immunologic, or idiopathic.

Acute urticaria ranges from a single episode to recurrences over a period of less than 6 weeks. Common causes of acute urticaria include insect bites or stings and food or drug allergies. Chronic urticaria occurs daily, or almost daily, over a period longer than 6 weeks. Food, drugs, and infections can also be causes of chronic urticaria. However, in the chronic form, the exact causative agents may never be identified. In most cases of urticaria, the cause is unknown.

Occupational urticaria is presumed or proved to be caused by exposure to one or more substances or physical agents in the workplace. Occupational urticaria may be acute or chronic, localized or generalized, or associated with systemic manifestations, such as asthma. In occupational settings, direct contact with substances, and possibly inhalation, may be the most common routes of exposure inducing urticaria. The pathologic mechanisms may be nonimmunologic, immunologic, or not known. Contact urticaria is defined as urticaria that occurs after direct skin contact with a substance. Urticarias that result from nonchemical exposures are commonly classified as physical urticarias. These include mechanical urticarias, caused by trauma, pressure, friction, and vibration; and urticaria resulting from local exposure to physical agents, such as cold, heat, solar radiation, and water.

Public Health Importance

Data specific for environmental and occupational urticaria are limited. In 2001, BLS estimated 38,900 cases of occupational skin diseases or disorders in the U.S. workforce.[5] Further information is available on the 6,051 cases that involved days away from work. Of this subgroup, 336 (5.5 percent) had urticaria/hives; their median time away from work was 3 days.

Population at Risk and Etiologic Agents

In general, risk factors for contact urticaria include a history of atopy; a compromise to the barrier function of intact skin, due to conditions such as eczema, abrasions, ulcers; and, in some cases, occupation. Based on reviews of epidemiologic studies, exposures, and patterns seen in case reports, several occupations may be at higher risk for the development of contact urticaria. These include food handlers, cooks, caterers, and bakers; general health care workers, dental professionals, and pharmaceutical industry workers; animal handlers, such as laboratory workers and veterinarians; and gardeners, florists, woodworkers, and agricultural workers.

For food handlers, cooks, caterers, and bakers, the following foods have been reported to induce contact urticaria: apples, beans, beer, caraway seeds, carrots, eggs, endives, fish, garlic, kiwi fruit, lettuce, meat (beef, chicken, lamb, liver, pork, and turkey), milk, peaches, potatoes, rice, shellfish, spices, and strawberries.[19,20] Bakers can de-

velop contact urticaria and other systemic symptoms after exposure to cereal flours, buckwheat flour, and additive flour enzymes such as alpha-amylase.

In health-care, dental, and pharmaceutical environments, exposure to a variety of medications or chemical disinfectants can put workers at risk. Exposures that can cause contact urticaria include aminothiazole, bacitracin, benzocaine gel, cephalosporins, chloramine, chloramphenicol, chlorhexidine, chlorocresol, ethylene oxide, gentamicin, neomycin, nitrogen mustard, penicillin, pentamidine isethionate, phenothiazines, rifamycin, and streptomycin.[19,20] Furthermore, natural rubber latex has been found to be an important cause of contact urticaria in health care professionals.[21] Natural rubber latex gloves were the most common source of exposure.

Contact urticaria has been found to be caused by animal hair, insects, dander, animal placenta, saliva, seminal fluid, and serum. Slaughterhouse workers can develop contact urticaria upon exposure to animal blood. Contact urticaria can be seen in veterinarians after exposure to cow's hairs and placenta, horse dander, and pig's bristles.

Certain woods and plants can cause contact urticaria. These include the larch, limba, obeche (African maple), and teak woods and plants, such as chrysanthemum, Ficus benjamina (weeping fig), lilies, *Limonium tataricum*, *Phoenix canariensis* (canary palm), *Spathiphyllum walisii* (spathe flower), tulips, and fungi (shiitake mushroooms). High-risk occupations include agricultural workers, carpenters, florists, gardeners, and woodworkers. Caterpillar hair, insect stings, and moths can also cause contact urticaria in outdoor workers. Agricultural workers may also be exposed to fertilizers and pesticides, some of which can cause contact urticaria.

A variety of industrial chemicals can cause contact urticaria, including acrylic monomers (plastics), aliphatic polyamines (epoxy resins), alkyl-phenol novolac resin, ammonia, castor bean (fertilizers), diethyltoluamide (DEET), formaldehyde (used in clothing, leather, fumigation, and resins), lindane (a parasiticide), paraphenylenediamine, phenylmercuric priopionate (an antibacterial fabric softener), plastic additives (such as butylhydroxytoluene and oleylamide), reactive dyes, sodium sulfide (used in photographs, dyes, and tanning), sulfur dioxide, vinyl pyrilidine, and xylene and other solvents.[19,20] Contact urticaria can occur with exposure to a variety of metal salts, including iridium, nickel, platinum, and rhodium.

Diagnosis and Treatment

The diagnosis of environmental or occupational urticaria is based on the medical and exposure history, physical findings, and *in vitro* or *in vivo* testing. Proving etiology or work-relatedness may be difficult. Suggested criteria include[22]:

1. Documentation of urticaria by physical examination;
2. Exposure to an agent known or presumed to cause urticaria;
3. A temporally consistent relationship between exposure and onset of urticaria (usually 30 to 60 minutes);
4. Associated medical symptoms and localization of urticaria consistent with the route of exposure;
5. Resolution of the urticaria away from the exposure;
6. Exclusion of nonenvironmental or nonoccupational causes; and
7. Medical testing results indicating allergy to a substance in the environment or workplace. Useful medical tests include the open or closed patch test, prick or scratch test, and tests demonstrating specific IgE to suspect occupational antigens, such as by radioallergosorbent (RAST) assays.

In cases of environmental or occupational urticaria where a specific causal agent can be identified, the initial treatment is avoidance of the offending agent. First-generation antihistamines, such as diphenhydramine or hydroxyzine, which block H1 receptors, can be employed initially, but they can cause sedation; this may present a safety issue for certain occupations, such as heavy-equipment operators. When sedation occurs or presents a safety concern, nonsedating, second-generation antihistamines may be employed. When H1 histamine blockers alone are not sufficient, they may be combined with H2 blockers or doxepin, a tricyclic antidepressant with potent H1 and H2 blocking activity. Doxepin is extremely sedating and should be used cautiously, if at all, when safety concerns arise on the job. Oral corticosteroid therapy may be employed for severe cases of chronic urticaria, especially those associated with angioedema.

Prevention

Strategies in the prevention of environmental and occupational urticaria overlap with those strategies used in the prevention of contact dermatitis and include:

- identifying allergens;
- substituting chemicals that are nonallergenic;
- establishing engineering controls to reduce exposure;
- using PPE, such as gloves and special clothing;
- emphasizing personal and occupational hygiene; and
- establishing educational programs to increase awareness in the workplace.

Recommendations for preventing allergic reactions to natural rubber latex in the workplace have been published by NIOSH.[23]

DERMATOLOGIC INFECTIOUS DISEASES

Environmental or occupational dermatologic infectious diseases are diseases that have a major manifestation on the skin surface and that result from exposure to an infectious agent found in the environment or workplace. (The very common secondarily-infected wounds will not be discussed here.) Many of the environmental and occupational dermatologic infectious diseases result not only in cutaneous signs and symptoms but also in systemic effects as well. The exposure can occur through direct skin contact (epicutaneous), inoculation (percutaneous), or through the respiratory system (inhalational).

Public Health Importance

Epidemiologic data specifically related to environmental or occupational dermatologic infectious diseases are very limited. Other than limited descriptions in case presentations, case studies, and epidemic investigation reports, little is known about the epidemiology of most of these diseases in the United States. For the infectious diseases that are nationally reportable, it is impossible to determine what proportion are due to occupational exposures. In 2001, BLS estimated 38,900 cases of occupational skin diseases or disorders in the U.S. workforce.[5] Further information is available on the 6,051 cases that involved days away from work. Of this subgroup, 710 (11.7 percent) had infections of the skin and subcutaneous tissue; their median time away from work was 5 days.

Population at Risk and Etiologic Agents

Environmental and occupational dermatologic infectious diseases can be grouped by etiologic agent into the following disease categories: bacterial, rickettsial, viral, superficial fungal, subcutaneous fungal, systemic fungal, and parasitic.[24] In general, risk of infection can be associated with individual susceptibility, which includes factors such as immune status and trauma to the skin breaching its protective barrier; the distribution of the pathogen in the environment; and exposure to the pathogen, considering its reservoir, mode of transmission, and conditions in which the pathogen thrives. Reservoirs and fomites of the pathogens include people, such as co-workers, clients, patients, or children; animals and animal products; soil and plant materials; ticks and insects; and water and marine life. Conditions in which pathogens can thrive and increase susceptibility include wet conditions, such as wet work, and hot and humid environments. The environmental and occupational dermatologic infectious diseases associated with these sources and conditions are listed in Table 28-3. In addition, laboratory personnel working directly with pathogens are at risk of infection. Recently, there has been concern over possible work-duty exposures for first responders and health care professionals as part of bioterrorist events, such as deliberate releases of anthrax or smallpox.

Diagnosis and Treatment

Specifics on diagnosis and treatment are disease-specific and are beyond the scope of this chapter. In many cases, it is often difficult to definitively prove the environmental or occupational relatedness of the disease process. The questions to be answered by the clinician include the following:

1. Is the patient's condition a dermatologic infectious disease?
2. Is the organism found in the patient's environment?
3. Was there an opportunity for the person/worker to become infected in the environment/workplace?
4. What other exposures, such as recreational activities, must be considered?

Prevention

The clinician should view each patient with a potential environmental or occupational dermatologic infectious disease from a broader public health perspective. A case of a dermatologic infectious disease should be viewed as a potential sentinel health event. This recognition and resultant action by the clinician, in appropriate consultation with public health authorities, could lead to potential disease prevention in other people. This can only occur with proper diagnosis, a high level of suspicion on the part of the clinician in suspecting environmental/workplace exposures, ultimate confirmation of the association to the exposures that caused the disease, and finally, steps taken to modify those exposures. If successful, this approach would lead to the prevention of relapses and of new cases of dermatologic infectious diseases.

SKIN CANCERS

As early as 1894, Dr. P.G. Unna in Germany drew attention to the association between chronic sun exposure and skin cancers in outdoor workers, such as farmers and sailors. Skin cancers include melanoma, basal cell carcinoma, and squamous cell carcinoma. Studies have shown an association between excessive sun exposure and premature skin aging, pre-skin cancers (actinic keratoses), and skin cancer. Non-ionizing ultraviolet radiation (UVR) from the sun is the primary cause of skin cancer, in general, and is also the primary cause of occupational skin cancer. In addition, a variety of chemical exposures may play a role in the etiology of skin cancers.

Public Health Importance

Melanoma is the least prevalent of the three skin cancers but has the greatest risk of fatality, accounting for 85 percent of skin cancer deaths. The American Cancer Society estimated that, in 2004, more than 55,000 Americans would be diagnosed with melanoma and 7,900 would die of this disease.[25] Melanoma is likely to be related to excessive sun exposure, although the relationship is complex; it seems to be associated with severe sunburns during childhood. Basal cell carcinoma and squamous cell carcinoma are more clearly related to sun exposure, probably as a result of cumulative, chronic exposure. Basal cell and squamous cell skin cancers are, by far, the most common cancers in the United

TABLE 28-3

Exposures Associated with Dermatologic Infectious Diseases

Other People, Patients, and Children	Animal and Animal Products	Soil and Plants
Tuberculosis (cutaneous)	Anthrax	Anthrax
Herpetic whitlow	Brucellosis	Dermatophytes (geophilic)
Warts	Cat scratch disease	Chromomycosis
Measles	Erysipeloid	Mycetoma
Rubella	Tuberculosis (cutaneous)	Sporotrichosis
Chickenpox	Tularemia	Blastomycosis
Herpes zoster (shingles)	Orf	Paracoccidioidomycosis
Hand-foot-mouth disease	Milker's nodules	Cutaneous larva migrans
Erythema infectiosum (fifth disease)	Cowpox	**Wet Work and Hot and Moist Environments**
Dermatophytes (anthropophilic)	Monkeypox	Candidiasis
	Warts	Dermatophytoses
Scabies	Dermatophytes (zoophilic)	*Tinea versicolor*
Ticks and Insects	**Water, Marine, Fish, and Shellfish Exposures**	
Lyme disease	Erysipeloid	
Tularemia	*Mycobacterium marinum* granuloma	
Spotted fevers (Rocky Mountain spotted fever)	Tularemia	
Typhus	*Vibrio vulnificus* infection	
Ehrlichiosis	*Aeromonas hydrophila* infection	
Leishmaniases	*Vibrio parahaemolyticus* infection	
	Pseudomonas aeruginosa infection	
	Warts	
	Cercarial dermatitis	

States with up to 1 million Americans affected each year and more than 2,000 deaths. Accurate data on the general prevalence of skin cancers related to occupational exposures are not available.

Population at Risk and Etiologic Agents

Implicated etiologies for skin cancers include non-ionizing radiation from sunlight exposure and other sources of UVR, ionizing radiation, and thermal and chemical stimuli. Outdoor workers may receive up to six to eight times the dose of UVR compared to indoor workers,[26] and rates for some skin cancers among outdoor workers have been associated with cumulative UVR exposure.[27] According to the BLS, in 2003, more than 6 percent of the workforce

(more than 8 million workers) were listed in the following potential outdoor occupations: construction, farm, and forestry workers; fishing workers; gardeners; groundskeepers; mail carriers; amusement/recreation attendants; and surveying and mapping workers. There are likely many more workers occupationally exposed to UVR from sunlight. In addition, workers exposed to chemical agents, such as polycyclic aromatic hydrocarbons, arsenic, alkylating agents, and nitrosamines, may be at increased risk. Arsenic intoxication, which can result from ingestion of contaminated well water, has resulted in hyperpigmentation, palmar and plantar arsenical keratoses, and superficial squamous cell and basal cell carcinomas. Other risk factors for skin cancers include Northern European or Celtic family origins and fair skin types.

Diagnosis and Treatment

Diagnosis is based on history, physical findings, and pathology results. Treatment of specific skin cancers, which is beyond the scope of this chapter, depends on the specific type of skin cancer, size, depth, and location of the lesion, and evidence of metastases.

Prevention

The strategies for prevention include preventing excessive UVR exposure by limiting exposure to sunlight, introducing changes in practices to limit sun exposure during peak UVR hours (10 a.m. to 4 p.m.), wearing UVR-protective clothing and wide-brimmed hats, using broad-spectrum sunscreens (blocking both UVA and UVB), and wearing UV-blocking sunglasses. Limiting skin exposure to chemicals known to play a role in skin cancers is also important.

In many areas, the National Weather Service, in cooperation with the Environmental Protection Agency, issues daily predictions for UVR exposure.

The daily UV Index, reported on a scale from 0 up to 11+ (11+ being extreme), is part of selected local weather broadcasts and can be used to warn outdoor workers and others of potential high-exposure days, when prevention strategies should be emphasized.

OTHER SKIN DISEASES

Many other skin diseases may be related to environmental and occupational exposures (Table 28-4). Other skin diseases may not be caused by occupational exposures but may be exacerbated by such exposures. Examples include lesions of psoriasis produced at sites of skin friction or injury, heat exacerbating rosacea, and wet work initiating dyshidrotic eczema.

CONCLUSION

Environmental and occupational skin diseases include allergic contact dermatitis, irritant contact dermatitis, contact urticaria, a variety of infectious diseases, skin cancers, and other diseases.

TABLE 28-4

Other Environmental and Occupational Skin Disorders and Examples of Associated Exposures

Disorder	Associated Exposures
Hyperkeratoses/calluses/fissuring/blistering	Mechanical trauma
Burns	Heat, electricity, radiation, acids, alkalis
Frostbite/immersion foot, chilblain	Cold, moist environments
Folliculitis/furuncles and acneform dermatoses	Oils, greases
Chloracne	Chlorinated hydrocarbons
Photodermatitis (phototoxic and photoallergic)	Plants, coal tar, creosote, fragrances
Depigmentation/leukoderma	Phenols, hydroquinones
Hyperpigmentation/occupational melanosis	Coal tar, pitch
Skin discolorations	Silver, gold
Occupational Raynaud disease/vibration white finger	Tools causing hand/arm vibration
Miliaria rubra/prickly heat	Hot, humid work environments
Asteatotic eczema/winter eczema	Cool, dry work environments
Granulomatous dermatoses	Beryllium, zirconium
Ulcerative lesions	Chromium, chemical burns
Connective tissue disorders such as scleroderma	Silica, vinyl chloride
Nail disorders	Mechanical trauma, contact dermatitis, infections
Alopecia	Chlorbutadine, dimethylamine

Thorough investigations of workers with occupational skin diseases can be difficult. Workers should be encouraged to report all potential work-related skin problems to their employers and to their physicians. Because the work-relatedness of skin diseases may be difficult to prove, each person with possible work-related skin problems needs to be fully evaluated by a physician, preferably one familiar with occupational/dermatological conditions. A complete evaluation would include a full medical and occupational history and a review of exposures; a medical examination; diagnostic tests, such as skin patch tests to detect causes of allergic contact dermatitis; and complete follow-up to note the progress of the affected worker. Individuals with occupational skin diseases should be protected from exposures to presumed causes or exacerbators of the disease. In some cases of allergic contact dermatitis and contact urticaria, workers may have to be reassigned to areas where exposure is minimized or nonexistent.

Environmental and occupational skin diseases as diseases have a major public health impact. They are common, often have a poor prognosis, and result in a noteworthy economic impact for both affected individuals and society as a whole, as they effect vocational and avocational activities. They are also diseases amenable to public health interventions. The U.S. Public Health Service goal for 2010, as stated in its *Healthy People 2010: National Health Promotion and Disease Prevention Objectives*, is to reduce national occupational skin disorders or diseases to an incidence of no more than 46 per 100,000 full-time workers.[28] Both irritant and allergic contact dermatitis are considered priority research areas, as outlined in the National Occupational Research Agenda, introduced in 1996 by NIOSH.[29] Increased knowledge and awareness of environmental and occupational skin diseases by health care professionals will assist in achieving the national public health goals.

ACKNOWLEDGMENT

David E. Cohen, MD, MPH, reviewed the manuscript of this chapter.

REFERENCES

1. Mathias CGT. Occupational dermatoses. J Am Acad Dermatol 1988;16:1107–14.
2. Lushniak BD. The importance of occupational skin diseases in the United States. Int Arch Occup Environ Health 2000;76:325–30.
3. Woodwell DA, Cherry DK. National ambulatory medical care survey: 2002 Summary. Advance Data from Vital and Health Statistics. Hyattsville, HD: National Center for Health Statistics, Number 346, August 26, 2004.
4. Behrens V, Seligman P, Cameron L, et al. The prevalence of back pain, hand discomfort, and dermatitis in the U.S. working population. Am J Public Health 1994;84:1780–85.
5. Bureau of Labor Statistics (BLS). Occupational Injuries and Illnesses in the United States. Washington, DC: U.S. Department of Labor. Available at http://www.bls.gov/iif.
6. Mathias CGT. The cost of occupational skin disease. Arch Dermatol 1985;121:332–4.
7. Burnett CA, Lushniak BD, McCarthy W, et al. Occupational dermatitis causing days away from work in US private industry. Am J Industr Med 1988;34:568–73.
8. Holness DL, Nethercott JR. Work outcome in workers with occupational skin disease. Am J Ind Med 1995;27:807–15.
9. Fregert S. Occupational dermatitis in a ten-year material [sic]. Contact Dermatitis 1975;1:96–107.
10. Kadyk DL, McCarter K, Achen F, et al. Quality of life in patients with allergic contact dermatitis. J Am Acad Dermatol 2003;49:1037–48.
11. Oregon Health Division. A new program to reduce occupational dermatitis in Oregon. CD Summary, Center for Disease Prevention and Epidemiology, Oregon Health Division: 42, No. 21, 1993.
12. Mathias CGT. Prevention of occupational contact dermatitis. J Am Acad Dermatol 1990;23:742–8.
13. Marks JG, Belsito DV, DeLeo VA, et al. North American Contact Dermatitis Group patch-test results, 1998 to 2000. Am J Contact Dermatitis 2003;14:59–62.
14. Rietschel RL, Mathias CG, Fowler JF, et al. Relationship of occupation to contact dermatitis: Evaluation in patients tested from 1998 to 2000. Am J Contact Dermatitis 2002;13:170–6.
15. Mathias CGT. Contact dermatitis and workers' compensation—Criteria for establishing occupational causation and aggravation. J Am Acad Dermatol 1989;20:842–8.
16. Susitaival P, Flyvholm MA, Meding B, et al. Nordic occupational skin questionnaire (NOSQ-2002): A new tool for surveying occupational skin diseases and exposure. Contact Dermatitis 2003;49:70–6.
17. NIOSH. Proposed national strategy for the prevention of leading work-related diseases and injuries—Dermatological conditions. Cincinnati: NIOSH, 1988. (DHHS publication no. [NIOSH] 89–136.)
18. Schwanitz HJ, Riehl U, Schlesinger T, et al. Skin care management: Educational aspects. Int Arch Occup Environ Health 2003;76:374–81.
19. Reitschel RL, Fowler JF. Contact urticaria. In: Reitschel RL, Fowler JF, eds. Fisher's contact dermatitis. 4th ed. Baltimore: Williams and Wilkins, 1995:778–807.
20. Taylor JS, Leow YH, Fisher AA. Contact urticaria. In: Adams RM, ed. Occupational skin disease. 3rd ed. Philadelphia: W.B. Saunders, 1999:111–34.
21. Turjanmaa K, Alenius H, Makinen-Kiljunen S, et al. Natural rubber latex allergy. Allergy 1996;51:593–602.
22. Lushniak BD, Mathias CGT. Occupational Urticaria. In: Bernstein IL, Chan-Yeung M, Malo JL, et al., eds. Asthma in the workplace. 2nd ed. New York: Marcel Decker, 1999:341–62.

23. NIOSH. NIOSH Alert—Preventing allergic reactions to natural rubber latex in the workplace. Cincinnati: NIOSH, 1997. (DHHS publication no. [NIOSH] 97–135.)

24. Lushniak, BD. Occupational infectious diseases with dermatologic features. In: Couturier AJ, ed. Occupational and environmental infectious diseases. Beverly Farms, MA: OEM Press, 2000:389–404.

25. American Cancer Society. Cancer facts and figures, 2004. Atlanta: ACS, 2004.

26. Holman CDJ, Gibson IM, Stephenson M, et al. Ultraviolet radiation of human body sites in relation to occupation and outdoor activity: Field studies using personal UVR dosimeters. Clin Exp Dermatol 1983;8:869–71.

27. Vitasa BC, Taylor HR, Strickland PT, et al. Association of nonmelanoma skin cancer and actinic keratosis with cumulative solar exposure in Maryland watermen. Cancer 1990;65:2811–17.

28. Department of Health and Human Services. Healthy people 2010: Understanding and improving health. 2nd ed. Washington, DC: U.S. Government Printing Office, 2000.

29. NIOSH. National Occupational Research Agenda (NORA). Cincinnati: NIOSH, 1996:96–115.

BIBLIOGRAPHY

Occupational Dermatoses—A Program for Physicians Slide Show Prepared Originally in 1981 By Shmunes E, Key MM, Lucas JB, Taylor JS, Updated by Lushniak, BD in 2001. NIOSH, Cincinnati, OH *NIOSH offers this occupational dermatoses photolibrary and program for physicians on its Internet Web site.* <http://www.cdc.gov/niosh/ocderm.html>.

Adams RM. Occupational skin disease. Philadelphia: W.B. Saunders, 1999.

Hogan DJ. Occupational skin disorders. New York: Igaku-Shoin, 1994.

Kanerva L, Elsner P, Wahlberg JE, et al. Handbook of occupational dermatology. Berlin: Springer, 2000.

Lushniak, BD. Occupational infectious diseases with dermatologic features. In: Couturier AJ, ed. Occupational and environmental infectious diseases. Beverly Farms, MA: OEM Press, 2000:389–404.

Lushniak BD, Mathias CGT. Occupational urticaria. In: Bernstein IL, Chan-Yeung M, Malo JL, et al., eds. Asthma in the workplace. 2nd ed. New York: Marcel Decker, 1999:341–62.

Marks JG, Elsner P, DeLeo VA. Contact and occupational dermatology. St. Louis: Mosby, 2002.

Marks R, Plewing G, eds. The environmental threat to the skin. London: Martin Dunitz, 1992.

Reitchel RL, Fowler JF. Fisher's contact dermatitis. Philadelphia: Williams and Wilkins, 2001.

Rycroft RJG, Menne T, Frosch PJ, et al., eds. Textbook of contact dermatitis. New York: Springer-Verlag, 1992.

Taylor JS, Leow YH, Fisher AA. Contact urticaria. In: Adams RM, ed. Occupational skin disease. 3rd ed. Philadelphia: W.B. Saunders, 1999:111–34.

The findings and conclusions in this chapter are those of the author and do not necessarily represent the views of the National Institute for Occupational Safety and Health.

CHAPTER 29

Reproductive and Developmental Disorders

Linda M. Frazier and Deborah Barkin Fromer

Hazardous exposures among men or women can adversely affect reproductive outcomes. The challenge is to determine when a particular couple may be at risk, as reproductive problems are common when no toxic exposure can be identified. In the United States, one in seven married couples is involuntarily infertile, and about 1 percent of all births are conceived using assisted reproductive technologies.[1] Between 10 and 20 percent of pregnancies end in clinically recognized spontaneous abortion, and rates of earlier, peri-implantation loss are even higher. Developmental problems among children range from structural birth defects to neurobehavioral problems. About 3 percent of newborns have major congenital malformations, and about 10 percent of school-age children have learning disabilities.[2]

In developed countries, the proportion of adverse reproductive outcomes that is attributable to known reproductive toxicants is thought to be relatively low. However, some subgroups of men and women in developed countries have substantial exposures to agents that are known or suspected reproductive toxicants. Some of these exposures occur in workplaces, and others occur at home through hobbies and household repairs. As research methods in reproductive toxicology and epidemiology have become more sensitive, adverse health effects have been noted at lower exposure levels than were previously implicated—and for additional agents. Biological monitoring has revealed elevated levels of persistent pollutants in fatty tissues and in breast milk, although it is often not known if these levels cause health problems.[3]

In developing countries, agents with higher toxicity and longer half-lives are often used because those hazardous agents and polluting technologies are cheaper than newer alternatives. Lack of protective equipment and absence of facilities for washing leads to higher risks for reproductive problems, such as infertility, birth defects, and congenital brain dysfunction.

Childbearing is not the only health outcome that may be harmed by reproductive toxicants. Reproductive hormones are involved in normal functioning of nonreproductive organ systems. Estrogen receptors are present in blood vessels, bone, brain, and heart in both men and women. Androgens influence hematopoiesis, hepatic enzyme function, and calcium exchange in the heart. The genes that regulate these physiologic processes are actively being investigated by reproductive toxicologists and epidemiologists. This research may provide insights into reproductive cancers, cardiovascular disease, menopause, osteoporosis, and age-related declines in cognitive function.

Historically, birth defects caused by pharmaceuticals taken during early pregnancy served to break the prevailing belief that the placenta acted as a protective barrier for the fetus. These drugs included thalidomide, which caused limb malformations and other anomalies, and diethylstilbestrol (DES), which caused uterine malformations and vaginal cancer in prenatally exposed women. Mercury and polyhalogenated-biphenyl exposures from contaminated food were shown to cause severe birth defects, even when the mothers were relatively asymptomatic. In addition, occupational exposure to dibromochloropropane (DBCP) has been shown to cause male infertility and alterations in the

BOX 29-1

DBCP: A Potent Male Reproductive Toxicant

In 1977, a small group of men in a northern California pesticide formulation plant noticed that few of them had recently fathered children. A strong association was found between decreased sperm count and exposure to dibromochloropropane (DBCP), a brominated organochlorine that had been used as a nematocide since the mid-1950s. Testicular biopsies showed the seminiferous tubules to be the site of action and spermatogonia to be the target cell. The relationship between reduced sperm count and exposure to DBCP, both in its manufacture and in its use, was confirmed in other studies in the United States and abroad. Follow-up of workers after cessation of exposure showed that spermatogenic function

eventually recovered in those less severely affected. However, many of the azoospermic men remained so for many years after cessation of exposure.

Much DBCP was exported by U.S.-based multinational corporations to developing countries. A substantial amount of this pesticide was exported even after DBCP was banned in the United States. Workers exposed to DBCP in developing countries were not informed of its hazards, trained in its use, or provided personal protective equipment to safeguard themselves adequately (Fig. 29-1). In one study of approximately 26,400 DBCP-exposed workers in developing countries who sued U.S. companies, 24 percent were azoospermic and 40 percent were oligospermic.[4]

---

sex ratio of offspring (see Box 29-1 and Fig. 29-1), demonstrating that reproductive toxicity could affect both women and men.[4]

PRECONCEPTION

Little reliable information exists to guide couples planning to have a child who are concerned about risk from a past exposure that has now ceased.

Most studies, whether in laboratory animals or reproductive epidemiological studies of workers, examine the effects of toxicant exposure that begins before conception and continues throughout gestation.

Preconception exposures can cause genotoxicity leading to adverse reproductive outcomes. Using bacterial assays, increased mutagenic activity has been detected in the urine of workers

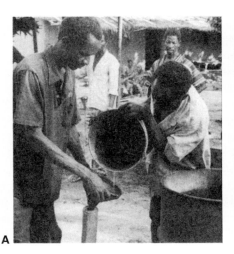 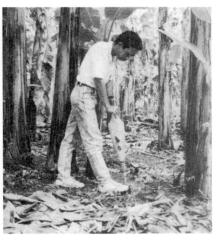

A   B

FIGURE 29-1 ● Many workers in developing countries became sterile from exposure to DBCP, even after it was banned in the United States. **(A)** Simulation of worker pouring DBCP solution, which he has mixed with a stick in a 55-gallon drum, into an applicator. **(B)** Simulation of worker injecting DBCP solution around the roots of a banana tree. (Photographs by Barry S. Levy.)

exposed to anesthetic gases, chemotherapeutic agents, or epichlorohydrin. Increased frequencies of chromosomal aberrations have been reported in radiation workers and in workers exposed to chemicals such as benzene, styrene, ethylene oxide, epichlorohydrin, arsenic, chromium, and cadmium. Although these assays are useful as biological markers of exposure to genotoxicants, they do not predict specific reproductive health effects in individuals.

Structural chromosomal abnormalities in the fetus may have no adverse effects or may be associated with birth defects, mental retardation, or other health problems. Numerical chromosomal abnormalities (*aneuploidy*) are a major cause of spontaneous abortion. For aneuploidies that are compatible with life, infants often suffer physi-

cal, behavioral, and intellectual impairments. Both structural and numerical chromosomal abnormalities may originate in either the male or female gamete.[5]

Men

The impact of a man's preconception exposure to toxic agents on pregnancy outcomes is an area of active research. Increased rates of pregnancy loss have been reported in the wives of men exposed to lead, inorganic mercury, organic solvents, pesticides, and other agents (Table 29-1). Male exposures can cause altered sex ratio in offspring, usually a deficit of male children.[6] Certain paternal occupations may pose an increased risk for congenital malformations, low birthweight, neurodevelopmental disorders, and childhood cancers.

TABLE 29-1

Selected Occupational Agents with Suspected Effects on Male Reproductive Function

Adverse Effects	Examples[a]
Decreased libido, hormonal alterations	Lead, mercury, manganese, carbon disulfide, estrogen agonists (such as, polychlorinated biphenyls, organohalide pesticides); workers manufacturing oral contraceptives
Spermatotoxicity	Dibromochloropropane (DBCP), lead, carbaryl, toluenediamine and dinitrotoluene, ethylene dibromide, plastic production (styrene and acetone), ethylene glycol monoethyl ether, welding, perchloroethylene, mercury, heat, military radar, Kepone, bromine, radiation (Chernobyl), carbon disulfide, 1,4-dichlorophenoxy acetic acid (2,4-D), possibly chlorination by-products
Spontaneous abortion in partner	Solvents, lead, mercury; workers in rubber and petroleum industries
Altered sex ratio in offspring	DBCP
Congenital malformations in offspring	Pesticides, chlorphenates, solvents; firefighters, painters, welders, auto mechanics, motor vehicle drivers, sawmill workers and workers in aircraft, electronics and forestry and logging industries
Low birthweight or preterm birth in offspring	Lead
Neurobehavioral disorders in offspring	Alcohols, cyclophosphamide, ethylene dibromide, lead, opiates
Childhood cancer in offspring	Solvents, paints, pesticides, petroleum products; welders, auto mechanics, motor vehicle drivers, machinists, and workers in aircraft and electronics industries.

[a] Some human evidence, albeit limited, is available for all examples listed except those associated with neurobehavioral disorders in offspring, for which animal evidence is available.

Modified from Paul M, Frazier L. Reproductive disorders. In: Levy BS, Wegman DH, eds. Occupational health: Recogizing and preventing work-related disease and injury. Fourth ed. Philadelphia: Lippincott Williams & Wilkins, 2000:589–603.

Workplace exposure can be taken into the home on a worker's skin, hair, or contaminated clothing or shoes, causing secondary exposure to spouses (and children). Mechanisms by which paternally mediated adverse pregnancy outcomes could occur include disruption of sperm production either directly (by injuring testicular cells) or indirectly (by interfering with the hormonal regulation of spermatogenesis). Sperm cells are vulnerable to genotoxic agents. As long as the stem cell precursors are spared, spermatogenic damage may be reversible over time.

Perhaps the best known spermatotoxicant is the pesticide DBCP, the first substance discovered to cause infertility in American workers (see Box 29-1). Another pesticide, ethylene dibromide, has been associated with post-testicular effects including decreased sperm velocity, motility, and viability. Occupational exposure verified by urine tests to the organophosphate pesticides ethyl parathion and methamidophos has resulted in aneuploidy in sperm cells, suggesting a genetic mechanism by which paternal exposure to these compounds could cause birth defects.[7] Increasingly sophisticated epidemiologic studies add plausibility to the paternal contribution to adverse reproductive outcomes from pesticide exposure. For example, in one study, measurement of dichlorodiphenyltrichloroethane (DDT) metabolites in body fat demonstrated a dose–response relationship with birth defects in offspring of men who applied this insecticide in a malaria-control program in Mexico.[8] Analysis of seasonality showed that miscarriages and birth defects were correlated with the spring spraying season.[6] In another study, spontaneous abortion risk was doubled if husbands applied herbicides but was increased fivefold if they did not wear protective equipment during application.[9]

Among toxic metals, lead has been most intensively studied. It may have a direct toxic effect on the gonads and may also act at the level of the hypothalamus and pituitary to impair endocrine function. Decreased libido has been associated with severe lead and manganese poisoning. In lead-exposed men, blood lead levels above 40 μg/dL have been associated with decreased sperm counts and aberrant sperm motility and morphology. Paternal lead exposure has been associated with low birthweight among offspring, mainly when the father's exposure level is high, of long duration, or combined with other exposures, such as solvents.[10]

The glycol ether 2-methoxyethanol (ethylene glycol monomethyl ether, or EGME) is an organic solvent that causes testicular atrophy and disruption of the seminiferous tubules; it has been associated with decreased sperm counts in exposed men. EGME and its acetate are metabolized in the body to methoxyacetic acid, which is responsible for their reproductive toxicity. The ethylene glycol ether 2-ethoxyethanol (ethylene glycol monoethyl ether, or EGEE) has a similar reproductive toxicity profile as EGME but requires about a 10-fold higher dose to cause these adverse effects.

In a study of rats, drinking water disinfection by-products adversely affected sperm motility. A mixture of chemicals (arsenic, chromium, lead, benzene, chloroform, phenol, and trichloroethylene) typically present in polluted groundwater near hazardous waste sites has been shown to alter sperm morphology and reproductive endocrine profiles of male rabbits.[11] These findings lend support to the biological plausibility of an epidemiologic study that found reductions in morphologically normal sperm in men who drank more than two glasses per day of tap water containing relatively high levels of trihalomethanes (80 μg/L).[12]

Some chemicals may disrupt endocrine function by binding to nuclear receptors for androgen, progesterone, or estrogen, or by interfering with receptor binding to DNA.[13] Polyhalogenated biphenyls and organohalide pesticides are structurally similar to the reproductive sex steroid hormones, raising the possibility that they could disrupt male reproduction. Several studies have suggested that birth defects of the male reproductive system have increased during the past several decades. More research is needed, however, to clarify the potential role of endocrine disrupting chemicals on male fertility and reproductive outcomes.

Women

Tobacco smoke can cause impaired fertility in the periconceptual period. For example, polycyclic aromatic hydrocarbons (PAHs)—components of tobacco smoke and products of fossil fuel combustion—cause oocyte destruction and ovarian failure in mice.[14] Another mechanism by which fertility may be impaired is through alterations in ovarian gene expression, which occurs among animals exposed to 2,3,7,8-tetrachlorodibenzo-*p*-dioxin (TCDD), a by-product of combustion and certain industrial processes.[15] Selected agents that

TABLE 29-2

Selected Occupational Agents with Suspected Effects on Female Reproductive Function

Adverse Effects	Examples[a]
Subfecundity	Certain herbicides, fungicides, and organic solvents, mercury, nitrous oxide; agricultural workers, hairdressers, semiconductor manufacture, woodworkers, dental assistants
Endometriosis	2,3,7,8-Tetrachlorodibenzo-p-dioxin (TCDD)
Menstrual dysfunction	Lead, mercury, shift work, antineoplastic drugs; hairdressers using chemicals, agricultural workers, athletes, dancers
Spontaneous abortion	Organic solvents (such as perchloroethylene, glycol ethers, toluene, xylene, formalin, chloroform), lead, mercury, nitrous oxide, ethylene oxide, antineoplastic drugs, certain pesticides, possibly chlorination by-products and arsenic in drinking water; semiconductor or shoe manufacture workers, laboratory workers, dental assistants, nurses, pharmacists, agricultural workers
Congenital malformations in offspring	Mixed organic solvents, trichloroethylene, halogenated aliphatic solvents, glycol ethers, aliphatic aldehydes or acids, lead, antineoplastic drugs, propellants, dyes, pigments, home pesticide application; agricultural workers, hairdressers, housekeepers
Hypertensive disorders of pregnancy	Organic solvents
Low birthweight	Lead, prolonged standing, frequent shift changes, PCBs. Possibly ethylene oxide, aromatic amines, chlorophenols, trihalomethanes in drinking water, air pollution
Infectious sequelae	Fetal carrier state (hepatitis B, human immunodeficiency virus), fetal morbidity/mortality (rubella, varicella-zoster, human parvovirus B19), serious maternal pneumonia (varicella-zoster)
Contamination of breast milk	Persistent organohalogen compounds such as DDT, PCBs, PBDEs, toxic metals, organic solvents, and others
Neurobehavioral disorders in offspring	Lead, mercury (including excessive fish consumption), PCBs, possibly organic solvents
Cancer in offspring	Diethylstilbestrol, possibly persistent organohalogen pesticides and other compounds
Earlier menopause	Ovotoxic agents such as PCBs and TCDD

[a] Some human evidence, albeit limited, is available for all examples listed, except for the compounds associated with earlier menopause.

affect reproductive function among women are shown in Table 29-2.

Women who work in agricultural occupations, especially if they mix and apply herbicides or fungicides, may develop fertility problems. Subfecundity has been identified among women who work intensively with organic solvents in semiconductor manufacture, woodworking occupations, and other settings. Dental assistants working with metallic mercury vapor or nitrous oxide without optimal in-

dustrial hygiene measures have been shown to have significantly reduced fertility.

In addition to acute effects from exposures at the time a woman is trying to conceive, fertility can be reduced by gynecologic disorders that have developed previously. Although toxicants are not thought to be the predominant cause of uterine fibroids or tubal disorders, organochlorines (such as the pesticides Kepone and endosulfan) stimulate rat leiomyoma cells, and polychlorinated biphenyls can cause changes in the fallopian tubes of rodents. Endometriosis can cause adhesions that reduce fertility. Endometriosis can be induced in monkeys by TCDD. Women who had been exposed to TCDD from an unintentional release in Seveso, Italy, had a doubled risk of endometriosis, although this risk was not statistically significant.

In adults, disturbances in ovulation can manifest clinically as menstrual dysfunction. In one workplace, substantial exposure to 2-bromopropane led to amenorrhea from primary ovarian failure confirmed histologically.[16] Menstrual disorders have been reported among women in various occupations, including athletes and dancers, agricultural workers, women employed in lead-battery plants or exposed to metallic mercury, hairdressers using chemicals, and shift workers. In a study that controlled for age, smoking, and work-related stress, menstrual dysfunction was over three times more common among nurses handling antineoplastic drugs than in nurses who did not handle these drugs.[17] Chlorination by-products in drinking water, as measured by total trihalomethanes, have been linked to reduced menstrual cycle length.

PREGNANCY

Working women have better pregnancy outcomes than unemployed women, especially in developed countries. This is likely a result of healthier behaviors by higher social class women, such as avoidance of smoking and alcohol during pregnancy; and the economic benefits derived from working, such as better nutrition and improved access to health care services. On the other hand, certain employment-related exposures increase the risk for adverse pregnancy outcomes (Table 29-2).

Fetal development is rapid during the first weeks of gestation, before a woman knows she is pregnant. The critical period for development of the heart, central nervous system, limbs, and kidneys begins at 3 to 4 weeks gestation. A hazardous exposure can disrupt the complex process of DNA transcription, protein synthesis, signal transduction, and cell division, differentiation, and migration. The second and third trimesters are marked by significant growth of the fetus and by the continued differentiation and maturation of some organ systems. Therefore, exposure to toxic agents after the first trimester can still cause problems. Certain occupational exposures may reduce fetal growth, result in functional or neurobehavioral abnormalities in offspring, or increase the risk of pregnancy complications, such as pre-eclampsia or preterm birth.

Miscarriage (Spontaneous Abortion)

Many types of hazardous exposures cause early fetal loss in laboratory animal studies. These exposures include solvents, such as chloroform, methyl alcohol, methylene chloride, and perchloroethylene (used as a dry cleaning agent and degreaser). Metals, such as lead and mercury, increase the rate of resorptions and decrease litter size. Anesthetic gases, such as enflurane, halothane, and nitrous oxide, are embryotoxic in rodents, causing fetal resorption and decreased litter size. A number of different classes of chemicals cause early fetal loss in laboratory animals, including certain pharmaceuticals (such as antineoplastic agents, pentamidine, ganciclovir, and ribavirin); pesticides (such as chlordecone, chlorpyrifos, and lindane); and polybrominated biphenyls (PBBs) and PAHs. Embryolethal effects have also been observed in pregnant mice exposed to continuous jet engine noise or to bursts of startling noises. Occupational exposure to solvents in dry cleaning facilities, semiconductor and shoe manufacturing workplaces, and laboratories have been associated with increased risk for miscarriage.

In women with low to moderate lead exposure, it was found that increasing blood lead levels were associated with increasing risk of spontaneous abortion (Fig. 29-2). Mercury exposure in chloralkaliplant workers, at levels that caused mild neurologic abnormalities, was associated with an increased rate of miscarriage, but the finding was not statistically significant.[18] Health care workers may be exposed to anesthetic gases, antineoplastic drugs, or the sterilizing agent ethylene oxide; poorly controlled exposure to each of these agents has been associated with increased miscarriage rates.

Women in agricultural families may have an increased risk for miscarriage, either from the toxic effect of pesticides on their husbands' sperm, take-home pesticide contamination on his clothing, or directly from application of pesticides. Although many of the highly toxic chlorinated hydrocarbon pesticides have been banned from use in the United States, these chemicals persist as environmental pollutants and are still applied widely in developing countries. Among textile workers in China who

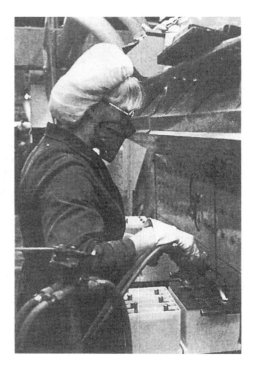

FIGURE 29-2 ● Adequate control of lead exposure for all workers requires a high level of engineering control and may also include the need for personal protective equipment. Because U.S. law prohibits exclusion of pregnant women from lead work, controls must be sufficient to protect the fetus as well. (From Zenz C. Occupational medicine: Principles and practical applications. Chicago: Year Book, 1975. Reproduced with permission.)

were exposed to DDT, higher serum levels of DDT metabolites correlated with higher rates of spontaneous abortion.[19]

Studies examining the effects of drinking water contaminants on the risk for miscarriage have conflicting results. However, several studies suggest that high levels of chlorination by-products (trihalomethanes) and pollutants, such as trichloroethylene or arsenic, increase the risk for spontaneous abortion.[20]

Birth Defects

Many of the same exposures that increase risk for miscarriage also increase risk for congenital anomalies. Organic solvent use at work increases risk for birth defects. Case-control studies suggest that women exposed to halogenated aliphatic solvents, glycol ethers, and trichloroethylene may be at special risk for development of orofacial clefts.[21]

Maternal lead exposure may increase the risk for neural tube defects, perhaps by interfering with folate metabolism. Agricultural work by pregnant women has been linked to risk of limb defects. Other maternal exposures that may increase risks for birth defects include aliphatic aldehydes and acids, antineoplastic drugs, propellants, dyes and pigments, working as a hairdresser or housekeeper, and professional application of pesticides in the home.

Ionizing radiation exposure may occur among health care workers or flight crews. The most sensitive window of vulnerability for induction of brain defects or mental retardation is at approximately 8 to 15 weeks of gestation. Substantially higher doses are required to induce birth defects than are received in most occupational settings. Selected health care workers may be at risk for acquiring infections in the workplace during pregnancy that can lead to congenital anomalies (Table 29-2). Environmental exposures from chlorination by-products in drinking water at the mother's residence have been associated with cardiac defects in some, but not all, studies.[22]

Low Birthweight

Low birthweight may occur as a result of fetal growth retardation and/or preterm birth. For many infants born with very low birthweight, early delivery was required because of pregnancy complications, such as placental abruption or eclampsia. Rodents do not experience preterm birth but do manifest fetal growth retardation when exposed to toxicants at sufficient doses.

Maternal exposure to organic solvents at work has been linked to preeclapsia as well as other causes of preterm birth. Exposure to high levels of aromatic amines or to moderate levels of chlorophenols has been associated with a statistically significant, sevenfold increase in fetal growth retardation.[23]

Women who work in occupations with lead exposure or who have blood lead levels above 5 to 10 μg/dL are at increased risk of delivering children with reduced birthweight. A study of placental membranes from births in a smelter community found that lead levels were higher in these tissues if the infant was preterm.[24] A blood lead level of 6.9 μg/dL or greater significantly increased the risk of hypertension during pregnancy in one study.[25] Occupational mercury exposure has been directly linked to fetal growth retardation. Occupational exposure to ethylene oxide has been linked to preterm birth in a study of 7,000 dental assistants.[26] Midwives' exposure to nitrous oxide has increased the risk of infants being small for gestational age.[27]

Performing physically demanding job tasks is associated with increased risk for preterm birth and gestational hypertension. Modest off-duty, voluntary exercise programs do not have this effect. Of all the factors that characterize physically intensive employment, standing for more than 6 hours per shift is a predominant correlate of preterm birth. Frequent shift changes may be a risk factor as well.

Contamination of drinking water with benzene or chlorinated solvents has been associated with low birthweight. Some studies show no relationship between trihalomethanes and low birthweight, whereas others suggest a possible association. A study of 80,938 birth certificates in New Jersey correlated carbon tetrachloride levels and trihalomethane levels in tap water at the mother's address, especially concentrations over 100 ppb, with fetal growth retardation.[28]

Air pollution has been linked to low birthweight in several countries. In a study of 74,671 births in Beijing, for example, the adjusted odds ratio for low birthweight increased 11 percent for each 100 μg/m^3 increase in sulfur dioxide and 10 pecent for each 100 μg/m^3 increase in total suspended particulates.[29] In the Czech Republic, among 108,173 births, preterm birth rates increased 18 percent for every 50 μg/m^3 increase in total suspended particulates and 27 percent for every 50 μg/m^3 increase in sulfur dioxide.[30] Maternal plasma levels of polychlorinated biphenyls (PCBs) have been associated with low birthweight in a Swedish fish-eating population and among Dutch infants exposed to PCBs.[31]

BREASTFEEDING

In 1951, DDT was discovered in breast milk. Since then, many other breast milk contaminants have been documented. Toxic metals, such as mercury, lead, cadmium, and arsenic, enter breast milk, as do organic solvents. Environmental chemicals with high lipid solubility and long half-lives are most likely to be found in breast milk. These include polyhalogenated compounds, such as PCBs, furans, and polychlorinated dibenzo-*p*-dioxins, such as TCDD. Organochlorine insecticides and fungicides are commonly present, including chlordane, dieldren, aldrin, DDT, heptachlor, hexachlorobenzene, and hexachlorocyclohexane. In addition, polybrominated diphenyl ethers (PBDEs) commonly contaminate breast milk; PBDEs are flame-retardants that have been added to plastics, textiles, polyurethane foam, rubber, paints, foam cushions, computer casings, fax machines, and even coffee makers. The chemical structure of the PBDEs closely resembles the structure of PCBs, dioxins, and furans.

During the past few decades, levels of these compounds have declined in breast milk in countries where they have been banned or regulated. In Europe, PBDE levels fell during the 1990s, but breast milk levels in the United States, where PBDEs have not been banned, remain 10 to 100 times higher than those in Europe.

LATENT EFFECTS

Less is known about latent effects of prenatal exposure on the developing child. There are, however, several well-documented examples of prenatal exposures that produce effects that are more prominent in childhood or adulthood than in early infancy.

Childhood

Neurobehavioral effects from prenatal toxicant exposures can be detected in newborns, but the more subtle effects may not be noticed until later in childhood. These effects include developmental delays, cognitive deficits, and problems in school. Lead exposure is the best documented risk factor for childhood neurobehavioral problems. Low-level lead exposure during brain development is associated with childhood problems in memory, learning, and behavior that may persist through adolescence. Assessing the biological contribution of isolated prenatal lead exposure can be somewhat difficult because exposure often begins *in utero* and continues throughout the first few years of life. Studies in laboratory animals demonstrate that gestational exposure is sufficient to cause persistent learning and memory deficits.[32]

Mercury is also a well-known developmental toxicant that results in neurobehavioral problems in children. Mercury bioaccumulates in fish, and as a result, health agencies in several countries have recommended that pregnant and lactating women limit their consumption of fish. Blood mercury levels in about 8 percent of women of childbearing age in the United States exceed the dose recommended by the Environmental Protection Agency (EPA).

Organic solvent exposure in the prenatal period has been associated with children's neurobehavioral performance, although this is less well documented than the effects of lead. For example, 3- to 7-year-old children of mothers who worked with organic solvents during pregnancy were shown, more often than controls, to score lower on tests of language and graphomotor skills and to be rated as having mild or severe problem behaviors. Deficits in color vision, which in adults has been linked with occupational exposure to organic solvents, are also more common among children whose mothers were exposed to organic solvents during pregnancy.

Environmental exposure to persistent organohalogen compounds have also been linked to later neurobehavioral problems. Studies from six different geographic locations have found that higher prenatal PCB exposures are associated with decreases in cognitive functioning during infancy or childhood.[33] Another study showed that prenatal DDT exposure was negatively associated with both mental and psychomotor development.[34]

Childhood cancer is another latent effect caused by prenatal toxicant exposures. The drug DES was the first major agent documented to cause transplacental carcinogenesis in humans. The National Toxicology Program (NTP) and the International Agency for Research on Cancer (IARC) have concluded that several pesticides banned from use in developing countries, such as mirex, heptachlor, hexachlorobenzene, and DDT, are carcinogenic. In addition, NTP and IARC are concerned that several pesticides that remain in common use such as ethylene dibromide and lindane may be carcinogenic to humans.

Prenatal exposure of both male and female laboratory animals to intensive radiation, certain antineoplastic drugs, nitrosourea compounds, and other agents has produced cancer in the offspring. A prospective study of 17,357 children found an elevated rate of childhood cancer when children from agricultural families were compared to the general public. The risk for childhood cancer nearly doubled if the father reported not using chemically resistant gloves when handling pesticides.[35]

Adulthood

Theoretically, certain prenatal exposures could increase risk for health problems of adulthood. Examples include functional disorders of reproductive organs, such as the prostate or breast, increased risk of reproductive cancers, or impact on other organ systems for which reproductive hormones play a physiologic role, such as bone and brain.[13] Few epidemiologic studies are available addressing these potential effects. One area of investigation is a woman's age at menopause. Laboratory animal studies of TCDD and PCBs have shown that when these ovotoxic agents are administered during pregnancy, the fertility of gestationally exposed females is diminished, and premature ovarian senescence occurs.[36] Among women, smoking causes ovarian toxicity and is associated with entering menopause several years earlier than nonsmokers. Studies of prenatal risk factors for menopause are difficult to conduct because of long latency and the need to measure exposures quantitatively.

EVALUATION AND CONTROL OF RISK

The evidence clearly shows that reproductive processes are vulnerable in both men and women. Even so, it is often difficult to determine the precise cause of a couple's subfecundity, a child's congenital anomaly, or other adverse reproductive events for several reasons: Precise assessment of exposures is difficult. There are other contributing health problems. And the research database is neither perfect nor complete. To evaluate a couple, four questions are relevant:

1. What is the agent? The names of chemicals can be found on product labels and material safety data sheets (MSDSs). Tracking these down is laborious, but necessary.
2. Is the person actually exposed to the agent(s), and if so, what are the timing and dose of exposure? Working with an agent is not necessarily the same as having an internal body exposure. A description of how the agent is handled, the protective equipment used, and workplace controls can give a sense of whether the exposure level is high, low, or negligible. Exposure levels can be quantitated by taking air samples in the workplace, although skin contact can cause high exposure levels to some compounds, even if air levels are low. Dosimetry badges can

measure workplace exposure levels for ionizing radiation. Timing of exposure is important. For example, a birth defect that occurs at gestational week 7 could not have been caused by an acute exposure that occurred only in the third trimester. The key period for genotoxic male exposures is thought to be about 2 to 3 months before conception, as spermatogenesis takes about 70 days to complete.

3. Is there evidence to suggest that this agent causes adverse reproductive or developmental effects? All pesticides or all solvents are not the same. The health information on MSDSs is often incomplete, so it is unwise to rely on them for information on reproductive health effects. In addition, new findings about reproductive toxicity are frequently published. A literature review or consultation with an expert in reproductive hazard assessment may be needed to answer this question.

4. Given the information collected, does the agent pose a reproductive or developmental risk? Reproductive health issues are intensely personal. Men or women who believe their workplace or neighborhood exposures may be contributing to the problem may feel anxious and vulnerable. The information available can usually be used to estimate whether there is some degree of risk, but often the risk is small and the health outcome is not severe. For example, small differences in neurobehavioral outcomes are important from a public health perspective, but a woman with a mildly elevated blood lead level during pregnancy needs to know that this will not cause severe mental retardation in her child. Uncertainties and limitations in the data must be clearly conveyed.

It is important to place the potential exposure in context, taking into account biological factors that may modify this risk. Reproductive risk factors other than hazardous exposures include parental age; family history of heritable syndromes; maternal metabolic conditions, such as poorly controlled diabetes mellitus; medications, such as certain antiepileptic, psychotropic, and anticoagulant drugs; and use or abuse of alcohol, tobacco, and certain recreational drugs. Context also includes balancing the benefits of employment with the magnitude of risk related to the potential exposure.

With regard to chemicals in breast milk, few data are available to correlate these exposures with developmental outcomes among children. The many studies of prenatal exposure to halogenated organic chemicals, metals, and solvents show a wide variety of adverse infant health outcomes, so lactational exposure is a concern. However, experts still recommend breast milk as the ideal food for infants. In one study where organochlorine exposures from breast milk were known to be present, neurodevelopment was best among the infants who were breastfed the longest.[34]

Existing data from animal and epidemiologic studies converge on certain occupational and environmental exposures that are associated with one or more adverse reproductive outcomes (Tables 29-1 and 29-2). Prominent examples of chemical agents that are reproductive hazards include toxic metals, antineoplastic drugs, organic solvents, persistent organohalogens, and certain pesticides. Exposures other than chemicals can also be hazardous. A precautionary approach is warranted, emphasizing use of less toxic alternatives, education about safe work practices, control of environmental pollution, and other methods of exposure reduction, beginning in the preconception period for both men and women. The following case illustrates this approach.

A 27-year-old man presented for medical evaluation because of inability to conceive with his wife for 13 months. In his job at an automobile repair shop, he disassembled radiators with an oxygen–acetylene torch and resoldered them with lead–tin solder. There was no special ventilation of his dusty work station, and his work overalls were laundered at home. His 25-year-old wife's infertility workup revealed no abnormalities. His semen analysis showed a low sperm count of 18 million sperm/mL, with mildly abnormal motility and morphology. He had a blood lead level of 63 μg/dL; his wife's level was 22 μg/dL.

This case involves lead poisoning due to inhalation of lead fumes during soldering and contamination of the work space with lead dust. Home laundering of work clothes laden with lead dust can result in exposure to family members and most likely accounts for the modestly elevated blood lead level in this worker's wife. Sometimes it is difficult to determine if a fertility problem has been caused by a toxicant exposure, although improvement in sperm indices after lead exposure is remediated suggests that lead may have contributed.

The husband is eligible for medical removal from the occupational exposure under the Occupational Safety and Health Administration (OSHA) lead standard. This action is triggered without loss of wages or benefits by blood lead levels of 60 μg/dL or higher. The man should be evaluated by a physician with expertise in treating lead poisoning. This couple should be counseled about the hazards of lead and ways to minimize exposures through safe work practices and personal hygiene measures. Reporting the case to OSHA should trigger a workplace inspection that would better assure control measures to protect all workers. Blood lead levels over 10 μg/dL before or during pregnancy should prompt action to identify and remove sources of exposure. Blood lead levels should be normalized in both the man and woman before conception. Although it may seem paradoxical to the couple, contraceptive counseling is important for the present time.

REFERENCES

1. Wright VC, Schieve LA, Reynolds MA, et al. Assisted reproductive technology surveillance—United States, 2001. MMWR 2004;53:1–20.
2. Msall ME, Avery RC, Tremont MR, et al. Functional disability and school activity limitations in 41,300 school age children: Relationship to medical impairments. Pediatrics 2003;111:548–53.
3. Schecter A, Pavuk M, Papke O, et al. Polybrominated diphenyl ethers (PBDEs) in U.S. mothers' milk. Environ Health Perspect 2003;111:1723–9.
4. Levy BS, Levin JL, Teitelbaum DT. DBCP-induced sterility and reduced fertility among men in developing countries: A case study of the export of a known hazard. Int J Occup Environ Health 1999;5:115.
5. Nicolaidis P, Petersen MB. Origin and mechanisms of non-disjunction in human autosomal trisomies. Hum Reprod 1998;13:313–19.
6. Garry VF, Harkins ME, Erickson LL, et al. Birth defects, season of conception, and sex of children born to pesticide applicators living in the Red River Valley of Minnesota, USA. Environ Health Perspect 2002;110(Suppl 3):441–9.
7. Padungtod C, Hassold TJ, Millie E, et al. Sperm aneuploidy among Chinese pesticide factory workers: Scoring by the FISH method. Am J Ind Med 1999;36:230.
8. Salazar-Garcia F, Gallardo-Diaz E, Ceron-Mireles P, et al. Reproductive effects of occupational DDT exposure among male malaria control workers. Environ Health Perspect 2004;112:542–7.
9. Arbuckle TE, Savitz DA, Mery LS, et al. Exposure to phenoxy herbicides and the risk of spontaneous abortion. Epidemiology 1999;10:752–60.
10. Lin S, Hwang SA, Marshall EG, Marion D. Does paternal occupational lead exposure increase the risks of low birth weight or prematurity? Am J Epidemiol 1998;148:173–81.
11. Veeramachaneni DN, Palmer JS, Amann RP. Long-term effects on male reproduction of early exposure to com-
mon chemical contaminants in drinking water. Hum Reprod 2001;16:979–97.
12. Fenster L, Waller K, Windham G, et al. Trihalomethane levels in home tap water and semen quality. Epidemiology 2003;14:650–8.
13. Hoyer P. Reproductive toxicology: Current and future directions. Biochem Pharmacol 2001;62:1557–64.
14. Matikainen T, Perez GI, Jurisicova A, et al. Aromatic hydrocarbon receptor-driven Bax gene expression is required for premature ovarian failure caused by biohazardous environmental chemicals. Nat Genet 2001;28:355–60.
15. Mizuyachi K, Sopn DS, Rozman KK, Terranova PF. Alteration in ovarian gene expression in response to 2,3,7,8-tetrachlorodibenzo-p-dioxin: Reduction of cyclooxygenase-2 in the blockage of ovulation. Reprod Toxicol 2002;16:299–307.
16. Koh KM, Kim CH, Hong SK, et al. Primary ovarian failure caused by a solvent containing 2-bromopropane. Eur J Endocrinol 1998;138:554–6.
17. Shortridge LA, Lemasters GK, Valanis B, et al. Menstrual cycles in nurses handling antineoplastic drugs. Cancer Nurs 1995;18:439–44.
18. Frumkin H, Letz R, Williams PL, et al. Health effects of long-term mercury exposure among chloralkali plant workers. Am J Ind Med 2001;39:1–18.
19. Korrick SA, Chen C, Damokosh AI, et al. Association of DDT with spontaneous abortion: A case-control study. Ann Epidemiol 2001;11:491–6.
20. Bove F, Shim Y, Zeitz P. Drinking water contaminants and adverse pregnancy outcomes: a review. Environ Health Perspect 2002;110:61–74.
21. Lorente C, Cordier S, Bergeret A, et al. Maternal occupational risk factors for oral clefts. Occupational Exposure and Congenital Malformation Working Group. Scand J Work Environ Health 2000;26:137–45.
22. Shaw GM, Ranatunga D, Quach T, et al. Trihalomethane exposures from municipal water supplies and selected congenital malformations. Epidemiology 2003;14:191–9.
23. Seidler A, Raum E, Arabin B, et al. Maternal occupational exposure to chemical substances and the risk of infants small-for-gestational age. Am J Ind Med 1999;36:213–22.
24. Baghurst PA, Robertson EF, Oldfield RK, et al. Lead in the placenta, membranes, and umbilical cord in relation to pregnancy outcome in a lead-smelter community. Environ Health Perspect 1991;90:315–20.
25. Rabinowitz M, Bellinger D, Leviton A, et al. Pregnancy hypertension, blood pressure during labor, and blood lead levels. Hypertension 1987;10:447–51.
26. Rowland AS, Baird DD, Shore DL, et al. Ethylene oxide exposure may increase the risk of spontaneous abortion, preterm birth, and postterm birth. Epidemiology 1996;7:363–8.
27. Bodin L, Axelsson G, Ahlborg G Jr. The association of shift work and nitrous oxide exposure in pregnancy with birth weight and gestational age. Epidemiology 1999;10:429–36.
28. Bove FJ, Fulcomer MC, Klotz JB, et al. Public drinking water contamination and birth outcomes. Am J Epidemiol 1995;141:850–62.
29. Wang X, Ding H, Ryan L, Xu X. Association between air pollution and low birth weight: A community-based study. Environ Health Perspect 1997;105:514–20.
30. Bobak M. Outdoor air pollution, low birth weight, and prematurity. Environ Health Perspect 2000;108:173–6.

31. Patandin S, Koopman-Esseboom C, de Ridder MA, et al. Effects of environmental exposure to polychlorinated biphenyls and dioxins on birth size and growth in Dutch children. Pediatr Res 1998;44:538–45.
32. Yang Y, Ma Y, Ni L, et al. Lead exposure through gestation-only caused long-term learning/memory deficits in young adult offspring. Exp Neurol 2003;184:489–95.
33. Schantz SL, Widholm JJ, Rice DC. Effects of PCB exposure on neuropsychological function in children. Environ Health Perspect 2003;111:357–76.
34. Ribas-Fito N, Cardo E, Sala M, et al. Breastfeeding, exposure to organochlorine compounds, and neurodevelopment in infants. Pediatrics 2003;111(5 Pt 1):e580–e585.
35. Flower KB, Hoppin JA, Lynch CF, et al. Cancer risk and parental pesticide application in children of agricultural health study participants. Environ Health Perspect 2004;112:631–5.
36. Pocar P, Brevini TAL, Fischer B, et al. The impact of endocrine disruptors on oocyte competence. Reproduction 2003;125:313–25.

BIBLIOGRAPHY

Agnesi R, Valentini F, Mastrangelo G. Risk of spontaneous abortion and maternal exposure to organic solvents in the shoe industry. Int Arch Occup Environ Health 1997;69:311–316.

In shoe manufacturing facilities that had mixed solvent exposures below the threshold limit values as documented by air samples, occupational histories conducted blindly were used to categorize women into no-, low-, or high-exposure groups. After controlling for confounders, such as smoking and age, women with spontaneous abortions were over three times more likely to have been in the higher exposure group.

Frazier LM, Hage ML, eds. Reproductive hazards of the workplace. New York: John Wiley & Sons, 1998.

This text provides practical strategies for assessing and managing occupational reproductive and developmental risks. Potential hazards from more than 100 commonly encountered chemicals are provided, including infectious and biological exposures, physical agents, radiation, shift work, job physical demands, travel, noise, electromagnetic fields, psychologic stressors, and others.

Garry VF, Harkins ME, Erickson LL, et al. Birth defects, season of conception, and sex of children born to pesticide applicators living in the Red River Valley of Minnesota, USA. Environ Health Perspect 2002;110(Suppl 3):441–9.

This study presents methods to determine correlations of reproductive outcomes with biologically plausible exposure periods among men and the effects of different kinds of pesticides.

Infante-Rivard C. Drinking water contaminants, gene polymorphisms, and fetal growth. Environ Health Perspect 2004;112:1213–16.

This genetic epidemiology study showed that among infants with the CYP2E1 gene, which causes chlorination by-products (trihalomethanes) to be metabolized into even more toxic products, exposure to trihalomethane levels over the 90th percentile had a more than 10 times greater rate of intrauterine growth restriction.

Shepard TH. Catalog of teratogenic agents. 10th ed. Baltimore: Johns Hopkins University Press, 2001.

A total of 3,073 agents are listed, including pharmaceuticals, chemicals, environmental pollutants, food additives, household products, viruses, and genes that cause heritable syndromes or congenital anomalies. Handy tables compare time periods of embryonic and fetal development in humans to those in laboratory animals.

CHAPTER 30

Cardiovascular, Renal, Hepatic, and Hematologic Disorders

Linda M. Frazier and Deborah Barkin Fromer

Occupational cardiovascular, renal and urinary tract, hepatic, and hematologic disorders comprise a wide range of problems. This chapter addresses these disorders and some of the workplace hazards causally associated with them.

Cardiovascular disease is the leading cause of death among both men and women in developed and developing countries. In 2002, it accounted for 17 million deaths worldwide. When an illness is very common, many cases will be attributable to hazardous exposures even if the relative risk for developing the illness from such exposures is small. For example, for individuals between the ages of 25 and 64 years, 5 to 10 percent of cardiovascular and cerebrovascular disorders are probably attributable to occupational factors, accounting each year for an estimated 41,550 to 87,400 cases and an estimated 5,092 to 10,185 deaths—leading to $4.7 billion in health care costs.[1]

Occupational exposures are thought to be responsible for at least 1 to 3 percent of the 22,957 deaths from renal disease in the United States each year, or at least 230 to 689 deaths.[1] About 21 to 27 percent of bladder cancer deaths among men are attributable to occupational exposures, or 1,496 to 1,923 deaths per year.[1] In the United States, 50 million adults have hypertension. Toxic exposures, such as lead and organic solvents, can increase the risk of hypertension and alter renal glomerular function. Of the 5 million people who have renal impairment in the United States, 280,000 have end-stage renal disease and 96,000 begin dialysis each year.

Chronic liver disease is the 12th leading cause of death in the United States, most frequently caused by alcohol consumption, hepatitis C virus (HCV), and hepatitis B virus (HBV). Two billion people have been infected with HBV worldwide, and approximately 320,000 die of HBV infection each year. Although HBV infections in adults primarily result from sexual transmission or intravenous drug use, occupational exposures to contaminated blood or body fluids account for many infections in health care workers, public safety officers, and others.

Anemia is the most widespread hematologic disorder. Iron deficiency anemia heightens vulnerability to environmental lead exposure by increasing the gastrointestinal absorption of lead. In developing countries, iron deficiency anemia affects up to half of all children and women. In the United States, iron deficiency anemia is present in 2 to 5 percent of children (700,000) and menstruating women (3.3 million). The proportion of risk for hematologic disorders that is attributable to toxic exposures is not known. In the United Kingdom during a recent 3-year period, 229 patients with occupational hematologic disorders were reported, most with malignancies or aplastic anemia.[2]

Hematologic malignancies in the United States each year include 55,800 new cases and 25,700 deaths from non-Hodgkin lymphoma, 30,200 new cases and 22,100 deaths from leukemia, and 13,700 new cases and 11,400 deaths from multiple myeloma. The proportion of these disorders attributable to hazardous exposures is not known.

CARDIOVASCULAR DISORDERS

Occupational hazards increase the risk for several cardiovascular disorders (Table 30-1). Several representative hazards are discussed below. Only

TABLE 30-1

Selected Agents Associated with Cardiovascular Disorders

Disorder or Risk Factor	Examples[a]
Myocardial ischemia	Carbon monoxide, methylene chloride metabolism to carbon monoxide, carbon disulfide
Coronary heart disease	Carbon monoxide, arsenic, trichloroethylene, drinking water contaminated with *Helicobacter pylori*
Worsened risk factors for ischemic heart disease	Carbon disulfide, job stress (lipid profile), metals such as lead and arsenic (hypertension), sedentary work (diabetes mellitus)
Arrhythmia	Carbon monoxide, trichloroethylene, trichloroethane, certain fluorocarbon solvents and propellants
Other	Cobalt (cardiomyopathy); drinking water contaminated with enteroviruses (myocarditis); nitroglycerin or aliphatic nitrates (rebound coronary vasospasm on days off work); vibration (occlusive arterial disease of extremities)

[a] Moderate to strong human evidence is available for all examples listed.

limited information is available on the mechanisms by which hazardous exposures may cause cardiovascular disorders. Inflammation is an important mechanism by which the risk for myocardial infarction and stroke is increased. The toxicants in cigarette smoke, for example, promote inflammatory processes that give rise to fatty–fibrous lesions in arteries, thrombosis, and oxidation of low-density lipoprotein (LDL). Blood levels of inflammatory markers, such as C-reactive protein and fibrinogen, are elevated in smokers, and certain genetic polymorphisms increase vulnerability to these effects.

Chemicals

Carbon Monoxide

Carbon monoxide (CO) is a product of incomplete combustion, and exposure to this chemical is widespread. When inhaled, CO combines with hemoglobin to form carboxyhemoglobin (COHb). CO displaces oxygen so COHb cannot carry it, depriving tissues of oxygen. The heart and brain are particularly sensitive to hypoxemia. Among individuals with heart problems, relative oxygen depletion can precipitate angina, congestive heart failure, arrhythmias, or myocardial infarction. Low-level CO exposure results in nonspecific flu-like symptoms; so when this occurs, the role of CO may not be appreciated.

Cigarette smoking is a major source of CO exposure, resulting in COHb levels as high as 12 percent of total hemoglobin. A study of 3,000 children in the United States showed that 23 percent had blood COHb levels higher than the recommended level of 3 percent; and these exposures occurred primarily from unvented fuel-burning appliances and passive smoking. In developing countries, CO reaches high indoor levels from cooking fires inside dwellings. Unintentional carbon monoxide exposure kills more than 500 people per year in the United States, often because exhaust from electrical generators is not vented properly during weather-related power outages. CO contamination of indoor air often affects more than one person and the diagnosis may be delayed, as illustrated by the following case.[3]

A 60-year-old man was found dead on the floor of his motel room. His comatose wife was taken to a hospital where the differential diagnosis included botulism, drug or alcohol overdose, and cyanide poisoning. CO intoxication was considered unlikely after initial inspection of the room showed no apparent source of CO. Meanwhile in an adjacent motel room, a couple slept through the day instead of checking out as planned. The woman was able to call for help at 7 p.m., and the couple was taken to hospital. At about the same time, the negative results from the drug and alcohol screen on the first woman became available, and the autopsy on the first man suggested CO poisoning. A blood sample collected on admission from the first woman was then analyzed, revealing a CO level of 35 percent. A systematic search of the motel located a fifth individual who was comatose. The source of CO was a gas-burning swimming pool heater in a mechanical room that was adjacent to all three rooms where guests had been poisoned. Negative pressure from room air conditioners had pulled CO through structural wall defects into the victims' rooms.[3]

A study of almost 1,000 foundry workers found that blood COHb levels exceeded 6 percent in three-quarters of the smokers and in one-quarter of the nonsmokers.[4] The prevalence of angina increased with higher CO exposure in a dose–response pattern. Coronary heart disease mortality was 4.4 times greater among smokers with occupational CO exposure compared with unexposed non-smokers.

Vehicle exhaust contributes to environmental exposure to CO in urban areas. For example, in a large study of health effects of air pollution in Southern California, every 1 ppm increase in 8-hour average CO exposure from air pollution resulted in a three-fold increase in same-day admissions among the sensitive subgroups of patients with congestive heart failure or arrhythmia.[5]

Metals

Occupational exposure to metals, such as lead, arsenic, mercury, cadmium, chromium, and uranium, are toxic to the kidney and increase the risk for hypertension and cardiovascular disease. Chronic arsenic exposure from drinking water is endemic in some countries, such as Taiwan, Argentina, and Bangladesh, and from burning high-arsenate-containing coal in certain regions of China. There is a dose–response relationship between arsenic exposure level and development of hypertension, cardiovascular disease, and cerebrovascular disease. The extent of carotid atherosclerosis is associated with consumption of arsenic-contaminated drinking water.

Cobalt exposure can lead to cardiomyopathy. There was an outbreak of cardiomyopathy in Quebec City, Canada, in 1966 from cobalt-contaminated beer, and a case has been reported from handling the powdered metal at work.

Drinking Water Hardness

Cardiovascular disease mortality varies substantially by geographic region. It has been hypothesized that water hardness, as measured by increased calcium and magnesium levels, may exert a protective effect.

Carbon Disulfide

Carbon disulfide (CS_2) is used to manufacture viscose rayon—spinners are typically the most highly exposed workers (Fig. 30-1). It is toxic to the nervous system, causes heart disease, increases diastolic blood pressure, and increases total cholesterol and decreases high-density lipoprotein (HDL) cholesterol. A reversible, direct cardiotoxic or thrombotic effect may also occur.

Other Solvents and Propellants

Methylene chloride (dichloromethane) is metabolized to CO, which leads to elevated COHb levels. Workers exposed to trichloroethylene and other organic solvents may have small increases in risk for ischemic heart disease and specifically for myocardial infarction.[6] Occupational benzene or xylene exposure may also cause conduction disturbances and hypertension. In addition, occupational exposure to organic solvents may

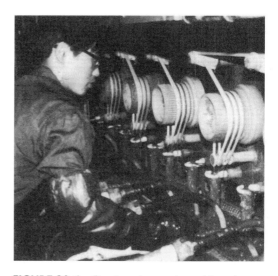

FIGURE 30-1 ● A worker tends machines that spool rayon thread from carbon disulfide. Worker exposure to carbon disulfide was high until this process was enclosed, which reduced worker exposure and, by recycling of the carbon disulfide, saved the company a substantial amount of money (Liang YX, Qu DZ. Cost benefit analysis of the recovery of carbon disulfide in the manufacturing of viscose rayon. Scand J Work Environ Health 1985;11(Suppl. 4):60–3. Photograph by Barry S. Levy.)

increase the risk of hypertensive disorders during pregnancy.

Chlorinated hydrocarbon compounds, such as 1,1,1-trichloroethane or trichloroethylene (TCE), are used as solvents or aerosol propellants. Workplace exposure or inhalational abuse of these agents may lead to atrial or ventricular arrhythmias—believed to be due to increased cardiac sensitization to catecholamines—that may be fatal.[7]

A healthy 24-year-old man was assigned to apply TCE by spray gun to clean a booth measuring 48 by 66 by 81 inches. The booth had an exhaust fan as did the room in which the booth was located. Excess TCE dripped down the walls and accumulated on the floor. He worked alone, and co-workers gave conflicting reports about whether he wore a paper dust mask. No other personal protective equipment was used. He was found unresponsive and could not be resuscitated. The TCE concentration in his breathing zone was later estimated to have been greater than 7,500 ppm. According to the OSHA Respiratory Protection Standard (29 CFR 1910.134), this task required use of a self-contained breathing apparatus and continuous presence of a co-worker.[7]

Biological Agents

Transmission of certain infectious agents particularly through drinking water may cause cardiovascular disease. Coxsackie B viruses found in drinking water in Egypt may have been responsible for an outbreak of acute myocarditis. Gastrointestinal infection with *Helicobacter pylori* found in well water may increase the risk of coronary heart disease, perhaps by raising systemic fibrinogen levels or otherwise provoking inflammatory processes in the coronary arteries.

Physical Agents

Intensive noise exposure may increase the risk for cardiovascular disease by increasing catecholamine secretion and promoting hypertension, although these associations are relatively weak. Occlusive arterial disease of the extremities can be caused by prolonged exposure to intensive vibration from tools such as drills, hammers, metal grinders, and chain saws. Alice Hamilton first described vibration white finger syndrome in 1917 in a group of stonecutters who used hammers powered by compressed air that delivered 3,000 to 3,400 strokes per minute: "The first man I saw came in from the bitter-cold morning air with the four fingers of his left hand a dead greenish white, quite without sensation and distressingly numb and cold. As he rubbed his hand and swung his arm about to restore the circulation the contrast between fingers and hand became startling, for the purplish and somewhat swollen hand met the white shrunken fingers abruptly, without any intermediate zone."[8] (See Chapters 14A and 14B.)

Stress and Other Factors

Psychological stress at work increases risk for heart disease (see Chapter 16). *High-strain* jobs, with high demands and low control, are thought to be the most stressful. Intermediate stress theoretically ensues from *low-strain* jobs that have high control with low demands, or from *passive* jobs that have low control but low job demands. Workers with high job demands and low decision latitude have increased carotid atherosclerosis and increased risk for cardiovascular mortality. Those who feel there is a large imbalance between their job effort and reward also have an increased risk for cardiovascular mortality.[9] Psychosocial characteristics of a job may affect women and men differently. In men, high occupational prestige at baseline significantly reduces heart disease risk, but in women this has no effect. High job demands with high decision latitude have been associated with an increase in heart disease risk among women, but not in men.[10]

Shift work has been linked to heart disease. The mechanisms by which heart disease risk may be increased in shift workers include altered circadian rhythms, increased family stress, and unhealthy coping mechanisms, such as smoking, poor diet, and lack of exercise. The metabolic syndrome is more common among shift workers than those working exclusively during the daytime.

Lack of leisure-time physical activity and other unhealthy behaviors have a stronger influence on heart disease risk factors than sedentary work. Physical activity at work can add to the health benefits of home exercise. In one study, each hour of daily brisk walking, either at home or at work, was associated with a 24 percent reduction in obesity and a 34 percent reduction in diabetes.

RENAL AND BLADDER DISORDERS

Toxicants adversely affect the kidney and urinary bladder (Table 30-2). The kidney has a large blood flow causing substantial renal exposure to

TABLE 30-2

Selected Agents Associated with Renal or Urinary Tract Disorders

Effect or Disorder	Examples[a]
Proximal tubule dysfunction or damage	Mercury, lead, cadmium, arsenic, chromium, uranium, mixed organic solvent exposure, trichloroethylene, ethylene glycol, carbon tetrachloride, bromobenzene, paraquat, diquat
Nephrolithiasis	Ethylene glycol, ethylene glycol ethers
Immune-mediated nephropathy or glomerulonephritis	Mercury, gold, organic solvents, silica, hepatitis A virus, hepatitis B virus, human immunodeficiency virus
Renal failure	Mercury, lead, organic solvents, silica, acute massive release of hemoglobin because of toxicant-induced hemolytic anemia (see Table 30-4)
Renal cell cancer	Organic solvents (especially if chlorinated), metals (such as cadmium), asbestos
Bladder cancer	Aniline derivatives used for dyestuffs or rubber manufacture, 4-aminobiphenyl, 2-naphthylamine, benzidine, *o*-toluidine; polycyclic aromatic hydrocarbons (such as coal tar, pitch, or products of combustion from furnaces, foundries, smelters and possibly vehicle exhaust); possibly metalworking or plastics manufacture

[a] Moderate to strong human evidence is available for all examples listed.

carcinogens and poisons in the blood. Some toxicants, such as cadmium, selectively accumulate in the renal parenchyma. The kidney metabolizes certain compounds, such as halogenated solvents, to produce more toxic products. It concentrates solutes, delivering a high dose to distal renal structures and the bladder. Several representative disorders and associated agents are discussed below.

Nonmalignant Disorders

A variety of mechanisms cause nonmalignant renal diseases, including necrosis, creation of reactive oxygen metabolites, induction of apoptosis, autoimmunity, and deposition of crystals in the tubules, collecting ducts, and ureters. Glomerulonephritis is associated with leaky glomerular capillaries that cause increases in urinary albumin levels and red blood cell casts. Tubulointerstitial disease is characterized by excretion of low-molecular-weight proteins, such as N-acetyl-β-D-glucosaminidase (NAG) and β_2-microglobulin, the presence of white blood cell casts in the urine, and electrolyte abnormalities. Ultrasonography and radiographic tests may demonstrate tumors, calculi, and disorders unrelated to toxicants. Renal biopsies can be helpful in determining the anatomic sites involved and specific pathologic changes, such as glomerular basement membrane thickening and deposits of immunoglobulins.

Mercury

Environmental exposure to mercury occurs in gold-mining areas of developing countries when elemental mercury is used to extract the gold from ore. Household mercury exposure has occurred among people exposed to an imported beauty cream that contained up to 10 percent mercurous chloride. Environmental exposure to organic mercury has occurred among people eating contaminated fish.

A variety of workers may be occupationally exposed, from dentists and dental nurses to chloralkali factory workers. Although mercury exposure is not a frequent cause of autoimmune disease, mercury can cause immune deposits in glomerular basement membrane and produce autoantibodies.[11]

Lead

Acute lead exposure primarily damages the proximal renal tubules. Chronic high-level exposure causes both glomerular and tubulointerstitial changes, leading to hypertension, interstitial fibrosis, and eventually renal failure. Over the past 40 years, much more evidence has accumulated to show that low-level lead exposure is harmful.

Environmental lead exposure increases the risk of hypertension, even when exposure levels are modest. As blood lead levels increase from 2 to 6 μg/dL, there is an associated increase in the rate of hypertension from 20 to 28 percent. Women not

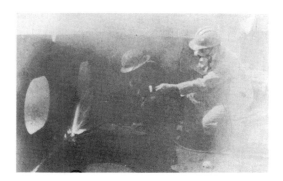

FIGURE 30-2 ● The worker at left is exposed to lead as he cuts apart a ship. The man at right is obtaining an air sample for lead determination. (Photograph courtesy of NIOSH.)

taking antihypertensives are about 50 percent more likely to have systolic hypertension and three times more likely to have diastolic hypertension if their blood lead level is over 4 μg/dL. Postmenopausal women are particularly affected due to increased mobilization of lead stores caused by bone demineralization.

Occupational lead exposure at levels permitted by the Occupational Safety and Health Administration (OSHA) is associated with adverse renal effects (Fig. 30-2). One study found that older workers are most vulnerable to worsening of renal function from lead exposure. The workers were employed in lead battery, lead oxide, lead crystal, and radiator manufacture, or lead smelting industries. They had an average blood lead level of 32 μg/dL and increased body burdens of lead.[12]

Cadmium

Cadmium accumulates in the renal cortex with a half-life of 10 to 30 years and initially causes proximal tubular dysfunction.[13] Renal disease may be progressive, and low-level exposure from environmental sources increases the risk for end-stage renal disease. Cadmium exposure may also occur from smoking. Cadmium is notable for inducing calcium excretion, which, together with its direct toxic effect on bone, can increase the risk for osteoporosis. In Japan after World War II, dietary cadmium exposure from rice grown in cadmium-polluted water induced *itai-itai* disease, a neurologic disorder accompanied by osteomalacia. Women were at greater risk than men because they absorb more cadmium from dietary sources, probably because they are more iron deficient. Occupational exposures may occur during cadmium battery produc-

tion, metal plating, smelting, and manufacturing of plastics. Exposure from metalworking is illustrated by the following case.[14]

A 28-year-old woman presented for evaluation of left flank pain and polyuria after having worked for approximately 3 years in a metals shop that produced materials used for jewelry manufacturing. She mixed gold and other precious metals with solid cadmium, melted the mixture, and then blasted the alloy with liquid nitrogen. The final product was a powder. She wore eye protection but no respiratory protection or gloves, and her clothes became contaminated. A proximal renal tubular effect was confirmed by presence of β_2-microglobulin in her urine. Her blood cadmium level was 19.2 μg/L, exceeding the criterion for mandatory medical removal (10 μg/L). She was provided alternate duty at work, but left the job about 5 months later. Her blood cadmium levels fell over a 6-month period, ultimately approaching 1 μg/L.

Solvents

Toluene abuse causes renal tubular dysfunction. Ethylene glycol is metabolized to oxalic acid, which increases the risk for producing crystals that can damage the renal interstitium, tubules, and glomeruli. Eventually this process can result in kidney stones. Increased oxalic acid excretion has been demonstrated in car mechanics exposed to ethylene glycol antifreeze. Silkscreen printers using ethylene glycol ethers (which are metabolized to ethylene glycol) are at increased risk of forming urinary stones.

TCE exposure adversely affects renal tubular and glomerular function in exposed workers, with increased urinary levels of NAG and albumin. Variations in sensitivity to TCE may be related to the three- to eightfold interindividual differences in activity of the glutathione conjugation bioactivation pathway.

Diverse scientific studies support the association between renal failure and solvent exposure including experimental studies among laboratory animals, prospective cohort studies of exposed workers, and improvement of renal function when solvent exposure is discontinued.[15] The mechanism by which renal failure occurs in solvent-exposed workers may be a combination of tubulointerstitial damage and glomerulonephritis. Worker susceptibility may vary based on comorbidities that affect renal function, such as hypertension or diabetes, or interindividual differences in efficiency of solvent metabolism.

Silica

Silica particles accumulate in the kidney, where they serve as an adjuvant to enhance the immune response, stimulate macrophages, and induce apoptosis. Silica exposure increases mortality from acute and chronic renal disease and increases the incidence of end-stage renal disease. Approximately 2 million people are occupationally exposed to silica in the United States—100,000 of them at more than twice the National Institute for Occupational Safety and Health (NIOSH) recommended exposure limit (REL) of 0.05 mg/m^3.[16]

Infections

Although most blood-borne infections are not contracted in the workplace, immune-mediated nephropathy may be caused by infection with hepatitis A virus (HAV), hepatitis B virus (HBV), and human immunodeficiency virus (HIV).

Malignant Disorders

Renal Cell Carcinoma

Most malignancies of the kidney are renal cell carcinomas. Individuals with renal cell cancer are more likely than controls to have been exposed to organic solvents; metals, such as cadmium; asbestos; and possibly pesticides. The risk of developing renal cell carcinoma is greater in women than men exposed to chlorinated aliphatic hydrocarbons, possibly due to women's higher body fat content, which provides a reservoir for lipophilic toxicants that increases the duration of internal exposure. Susceptibility to renal cell carcinoma may also vary among individuals because of genetic polymorphisms. For TCE exposure, risk-modifying genetic factors include absence of the von Hippel–Lindau tumor suppressor gene and presence of genes coding for bioactivation pathways involving glutathione conjugation.

Bladder Cancer

Smoking is a well-known risk factor for bladder cancer. Carcinogenic aromatic amines present in tobacco smoke include 4-aminobiphenyl, 2-naphthylamine, and benzidine. Workers exposed to these aromatic amines during manufacture of rubber or aniline dyes have had increased rates of bladder cancer. Cohorts of workers previously ex-

posed to these chemicals have been screened to try to detect bladder cancer at an early treatable stage. Manufacture of these compounds for industrial use has been banned in the United States. An alternative chemical used to manufacture rubber, *o*-toluidine, is thought to be responsible for a 1991 outbreak of bladder cancer in the United States.[17] This chemical and possibly phenyl-β-naphthylamine have been linked to bladder cancer at a facility manufacturing chemicals for the rubber industry in Wales.[18]

Polycyclic aromatic hydrocarbons (PAHs) comprise another group of carcinogenic chemicals found in tobacco smoke. Increased risk for bladder cancer associated with workplace exposure to these chemicals has been found among men who work with coal tar or pitch, and furnaces, foundries, or smelters. Similarly, presence of these substances in vehicle exhaust might account for increased risk in truck and equipment drivers.

Male nursery workers or gardeners have a higher bladder cancer risk, which may result from their exposure to aniline compounds used in the manufacture of some fungicides. Other occupations linked to increased risk for bladder cancer among men include workers in chemical or plastics manufacturing, operators of metal- or plastic-working machines, miners, workers in cafés and bars, and painters and dry cleaners. Some of these risks have also been documented in women workers in metalworking, textile manufacturing, field crop and vegetable work, and laundry and dry cleaning. Metalworking fluids may contribute to increased bladder cancer risk in metalworking occupations.

Aromatic amines and their hemoglobin adducts have been found among nonsmokers with no occupational source of exposure, suggesting that environmental pollutants may be responsible for some proportion of bladder cancers. Environmental exposure to PAHs from pyrolysis products of cooking oils, wood-burning stoves or unvented heaters, and other sources of combustion-related air pollution may be associated with increased bladder cancer risk.

HEPATIC DISORDERS

The liver is especially susceptible to adverse effects from hazardous exposures. It removes toxicants from the blood, subjecting it to higher doses than other organs. Sometimes when the liver metabolizes foreign compounds, more toxic products are produced. The liver has a remarkable capacity for self-repairing, which can be overwhelmed or damaged, resulting in various disorders.

Nonmalignant Disorders

Examples of hepatic disorders caused by hazardous exposures are shown in Table 30-3. Several representative agents are discussed below. In some cases, a hazardous exposure causes an isolated disorder of the liver, while in others liver pathology is part of multisystem toxicity. Rarely, toxicant-induced hepatic injury may be idiosyncratic, causing a rare sporadic injury, such as halothane hepatitis in an anesthesiologist. Usually, liver toxicity is a predictable outcome related to the dose of exposure. Inflammatory processes are involved in toxicant-related injuries to the liver.

Acute hepatic injuries may be cholestatic and/or cytotoxic. Cholestatic hepatitis is marked by elevated bilirubin, alkaline phosphatase, and γ-glutamyl transpeptidase. In cytotoxic hepatitis, elevated transaminase levels predominate. These measures are relatively insensitive, so new tests, such as hepatic detoxification capacity or production of reactive oxygen species, are being evaluated. Subacute or chronic liver disorders from hazardous exposures are diagnosed by liver biopsy and include fatty liver (steatosis), granulomatous disease, hepatoportal sclerosis or fibrosis, and cirrhosis.

Solvents

Intensive exposure to organic solvents causes transaminase changes or fatty liver disease. Of particular concern are chlorinated solvents including carbon tetrachloride, TCE, tetrachloroethylene (or perchloroethylene, PCE), and 1,1,1-trichloroethene as well as chlorinated naphthalenes.[19] At higher exposure levels, styrene induces transaminase elevations; at lower exposure levels, it causes mild cholestasis and less severe (but dose-related)

TABLE 30-3

Selected Agents Associated with Hepatic Disorders

Effect or Disorder	Examples[a]
Acute hepatocellular injury	Organic solvents, especially halogenated hydrocarbons (such as carbon tetrachloride, trichloroethylene, tetrachloroethylene, 1,1,1-trichloroethene), chlorinated naphthalenes, 2-nitropropane, dimethylformamide, and styrene; polychlorinated biphenyls, dioxin, chlorinated pesticides (such as hexachlorobenzene); nitrosamines (such as *N*-nitrosodimethylamine); aromatic nitro compounds (such as trinitrotoluene, 5-nitro-*o*-toluidine); metals (such as arsenic); hepatitis viruses; halothane; ionizing radiation; possibly polycyclic aromatic hydrocarbons
Acute cholestatic injury	Styrene, 5-nitro-*o*-toluidine, methylene dianiline
Fatty liver (steatosis)	Vinyl chloride, organic solvents, or volatile petrochemicals; dioxin
Hepatoportal sclerosis or fibrosis	Vinyl chloride; arsenic; dioxin
Cirrhosis	Metals (such as arsenic, copper); possibly chlorinated organic solvents, chlorinated naphthalenes and polychlorinated biphenyls; nitrosamines (such as *N*-nitrosodimethylamine)
Granulomatous liver disease	Beryllium, copper
Porphyria cutanea tarda	Chlorinated pesticides (such as hexachlorobenzene, pentachlorophenol); polychlorinated biphenyls, dioxin, vinyl chloride, possibly lead and arsenic
Hepatic angiosarcoma	Vinyl chloride, arsenic
Hepatocellular carcinoma	Vinyl chloride, arsenic, hepatitis B or C virus, aflatoxins
Other	Chronic infectious hepatitis (hepatitis B or C virus), hepatic failure (severe exertional heatstroke, massive radiation exposure, high doses of certain chemicals that cause hepatocellular injury)

[a] Moderate to strong human evidence is available for all examples listed.

hepatocellular injury.[20] Evidence for increased rates of cirrhosis among printers, painters, maintenance workers, and others with mixed solvent exposure is inconsistent; and alcohol intake may be a contributing factor.

Dimethylformamide (DMF) can cause disulfiram-like symptoms as well as elevations in transaminases and clinical hepatitis. With significant exposures, alcohol use or HBV carriage can have a synergistic effect. Like many solvents, DMF is well-absorbed through the skin. Hepatocellular injury can occur when air concentrations are at or below recommended levels, as illustrated by the following case.[21]

After working with *N,N*-dimethylformamide in the synthetics resins industry for 5 months, a 19-year-old man without previous liver disease was found to have an enlarged liver with a serum aspartate aminotransferase (AST) level of 578 IU/L (normal ≤40 IU/L), an alanine aminotransferase (ALT) level of 1,193 IU/L (normal ≤40 IU/L), a γ-glutamyl transpeptidase (GGT) level of 107 IU/L (normal ≤40 IU/L), and negative studies for hepatitis viruses. His urinary *N*-methylformamide level was 42.8 mg/L, consistent with exposure to DMF in air at 10 to 30 ppm. After recovering while removed from exposure, he returned to work in an area with less DMF exposure. On the 18th day after his reinstatement, his liver function tests again became elevated. After recovering, he was placed in a job without exposure.[21]

Halogenated Chemicals

In addition to the chlorinated solvents, other halogenated chemicals may result in liver disorders. Polychlorinated biphenyls (PCBs) have been linked to acute hepatocellular injury, cirrhosis, and subclinical porphyria.[22] 2,3,7,8-Tetrachlorodibenzo-*p*-dioxin (TCDD) may cause elevated transaminase levels, subclinical or clinical porphyria, and eventually steatosis or periportal fibrosis. Hexachlorobenzene, a fungicide, and pentachlorophenol, a wood preservative, can also disrupt hepatic porphyrin metabolism. An outbreak of hepatocellular injury was reported in nine workers exposed to hydrochlorofluoro-carbons used as ozone-sparing substitutes for chlorofluorocarbons. Vinyl chloride produces subclinical porphyria. The risk for periportal fibrosis is increased among vinyl chloride

workers with maximum yearly average exposure of 200 ppm or more and among workers with cumulative exposures of 1000 ppm-years or more.[23]

Nitrosamines and Aromatic Nitro Compounds

N-nitrosodimethylamine can cause hepatocellular toxicity, from both workplace exposure or contaminated foods. Rubber workers exposed to this and related nitrosamines during curing and vulcanization of technical rubber goods have increased mortality from cirrhosis. Trinitrotoluene exposure increases the risk for acute hepatitis and chronic liver impairment; alcohol intake further elevates this risk. A chemical intermediate in the production of azo dyes, 5-nitro-*o*-toluidine, causes severe mixed hepatocellular and cholestatic liver injury.

Metals

Arsenic exposure can occur from drinking contaminated water and from working in such occupations as smelting or pesticide application. It selectively accumulates in the liver, leading to acute hepatocellular injury, hepatoportal sclerosis or fibrosis, and cirrhosis.[24] Among children with a genetic predisposition to hepatic copper accumulation, elevated copper levels in drinking water may lead to cirrhosis. An excess of cirrhosis has been observed in a study of shipyard plumbers or coppersmiths.

Other Agents

Methylene dianiline can cause acute hepatic illness after occupational exposure; it caused a cholestatic liver injury in those who ate contaminated bread in an outbreak in the 1960s (Epping jaundice). Coke oven emissions, which contain PAHs, benzene, and other volatile organic compounds, are associated with transaminase elevations, especially among workers stationed closer to fumes. Granulomatous liver disease has been reported in workers exposed to beryllium, silica, copper sulfate, and cement and mica dust. Viral hepatitis is an occupational hazard not only of health care workers but also of emergency responders, morticians, and others (see Chapter 15). Mild transaminase elevations may be seen among workers with heat exhaustion; hepatic failure may rarely ensue.

Malignant Disorders

Hepatocellular carcinoma results from chronic HBV or HCV infection. Organic solvents, especially TCE, have been inconsistently linked to development of liver or biliary system neoplasms. Overexposure to the following chemicals increases the risk for liver cancer.

Vinyl Chloride

Vinyl chloride and its metabolites are human carcinogens. A cohort study among 12,700 exposed men in four European countries observed 18 incident cases and 53 deaths from primary liver cancer.[25] Of these, 37 were hepatic angiosarcomas, 10 were hepatocellular carcinomas, and 24 were liver cancers of other or unknown histology. There was an exposure–response trend among workers who had cumulative exposures greater than 1,500 ppm-years.

Arsenic

Inorganic arsenic exposure has been associated with both hepatocellular carcinoma and angiosarcoma, with latency periods of 13 to 29 years. These cancers have also been attributed to arsenic contaminated drinking water.

Aflatoxins

Aflatoxins are a family of mycotoxins that taint grains, nuts, and other crops and may enter eggs, milk, and other animal products through livestock feed. Aflatoxin contaminates harvests in both developed and developing countries, although poorer countries are less able to exclude affected crops from the food supply. These compounds, especially aflatoxin B1, cause liver cancer in laboratory animals. In a prospective cohort study of 18,244 people in Shanghai, urinary biomarkers of aflatoxin B1 exposure increased the risk for hepatocellular carcinoma more than threefold.[26] Among participants who were also hepatitis B surface antigen–positive, there was a striking synergistic effect, with a 59-fold increase in risk for hepatocellular cancer.

HEMATOLOGIC DISORDERS

Hazardous exposures may affect red blood cells, white blood cells, or platelets. Hematologic disorders may be marked by decreased production of these cells in bone marrow and/or decreased cell survival in peripheral blood. Hazardous exposures may also interfere with the functions of hematopoietic cells, such as carrying oxygen or preventing hemorrhage. Nonmalignant blood system disorders caused by certain occupational exposures increase the risk that a later hematologic malignancy may develop. Examples of hematologic disorders related

to hazardous exposures are shown in Table 30-4. Several representative hazards are discussed below.

Nonmalignant Disorders

Anemia

Anemia is a widespread disorder that has nonoccupational causes ranging from dietary iron deficiency to chronic diseases, such as rheumatoid arthritis or inflammatory bowel disease. Hazardous exposures can cause anemia by reducing production and/or survival of red blood cells.

Toxic metals that may induce anemia at relatively high exposures include lead, cadmium, arsenic, and chromium. A prototypical metal that produces anemia is lead, which interferes with the production of heme in the bone marrow by inhibiting several enzymes in the heme synthesis pathway. Lead adversely affects red blood cell membranes, which increases hemolysis. High levels of lead exposure are also directly toxic to human erythroid precursor cells in the bone marrow and impair renal production of erythropoietin in response to blood loss.[27]

Severe intravascular hemolysis can be induced by arsine gas, which is produced when a strong acid contacts a crude metal containing arsenic impurities. Arsine gas is also released when arsenic trioxide is mixed with an acid in the presence of zinc, or when a drain cleaner containing sodium hydroxide and aluminum chips is mixed with arsenical herbicides.

Reduced Oxygen-Carrying Capacity of Red Blood Cells

When CO forms COHb, the oxygen-carrying capacity of red blood cells is reduced. Other chemicals can impair oxygen-carrying capacity by altering the charge of iron molecules in hemoglobin, from Fe^{2+} to Fe^{3+}, producing methemoglobinemia. Cyanosis that fails to improve with administration of 100 percent oxygen is a sentinel finding in cases of methemoglobinemia. People are exposed to nitrites, potent inducers of methemoglobinemia, by eating improperly cured meats.

Nitrate is converted in the body to nitrite. Methemoglobinemia can occur from nitrate in drinking water polluted with runoff from manure, sewage, or fertilizer.[28] Contaminated wells may have nitrate levels (measured as nitrogen) substantially above the Environmental Protection Agency (EPA) recommended limit of 10 mg/L. Boiling water from

TABLE 30-4

Selected Agents Associated with Hematologic Disorders

Effect or Disorder	Examples[a]
Reduced red blood cell production	Reduced heme synthesis (lead), reduced proliferation of erythrocyte progenitor cells (lead, benzene), reduced release of erythropoietin by the kidney (lead); other mechanisms (ethylene glycol ethers)
Reduced red blood cell survival	Hemolysis (lead, arsine gas, intensive physical exertion)
Reduced oxygen-carrying capacity of red blood cells	Displacement of oxygen on hemoglobin (carbon monoxide, methylene chloride metabolism to carbon monoxide); methemoglobinemia (nitrites, nitrates in drinking water or foods, aniline dyes, nitrobenzenes, phenylenediamine, nitrogen dioxide, copper compounds, chlorite or chlorate compounds, and others)
Bleeding disorders	Reduced platelet counts (bone marrow toxicants); reduced synthesis of vitamin K–dependent clotting factors (liver toxicants [see Table 30-3], coumarin, or inandione rodenticides)
Nonmalignant disorders of white blood cells	Leukocytosis (intensive physical exertion); leukopenia (benzene, possibly ethylene glycol ethers); change in white blood cell subtype distribution (toluene diisocyanate, styrene, and other chemicals)
Premalignant syndromes	Bone marrow dysplasia, aplastic anemia, or myelodysplastic syndrome (ionizing radiation, benzene, alkylating drugs)
Leukemia	Acute myelogenous leukemia (ionizing radiation, benzene, alkylating drugs); other leukemias (ionizing radiation, benzene)
Other hematopoietic cancers	Non-Hodgkin lymphoma (agricultural work, possibly benzene); lymphoma (possibly ionizing radiation)

[a] Some human evidence, albeit limited, is available for all examples listed.

bacteria-contaminated wells further concentrates nitrate. Infants less than 6 months of age are particularly vulnerable because they have low amounts of methemoglobin reductase, the enzyme that converts methemoglobin back to hemoglobin. Infants may also be at risk from vegetables such as silver beets, spinach, or carrots, that naturally contain high amounts of nitrate—although levels vary by where the crop was grown and by adequacy of storage prior to consumption.

Occupational methemoglobinemia may occur after intensive exposure to aniline dyes, nitrobenzene, dinitrobenzene, phenylenediamine, or other compounds (Table 30-4).[29]

Bleeding Disorders

Agents that cause major bone marrow depression may induce bleeding because of low platelet counts. Severe-toxicant–induced liver dysfunction (Table 30-3) may be accompanied by bleeding from reduced synthesis of clotting factors. The following

case illustrates impairment of clotting after a single occupational exposure to a concentrated toxicant and the risks from dermal absorption.[30]

An 18-year-old pest exterminator spilled a concentrated liquid preparation of the inandione rodenticide, diphacinone, into his boot. He did not remove the boot or wash the area for 6 to 8 hours. He presented to an emergency department 7 days later with flank pain, hematuria, and nosebleeds. His platelet count was 273,000, and his prothrombin time and partial thromboplastin time were abnormal. Vitamin K therapy was given for 60 days. There were no permanent sequelae.[30]

White Blood Cell Disorders

Intensive physical exertion can induce transient leukocytosis. Workplace exposures can cause changes in the distribution of white blood cell subtypes. For example, sensitizing compounds, such as toluene diisocyanate, can cause eosinophilia. High levels of styrene exposure have been associated with an increase in peripheral monocytes, decreased proliferative activity of lymphocytes to mitogens, and an increased C4 component of complement.

Reduced white blood cell counts have been seen in shipyard painters and semiconductor manufacturing workers who perform photolithography or implantation tasks. Suspected causes of this leukopenia include ethylene glycol ethers and other solvents. Reduced white blood cell counts accompanying benzene-induced anemia may represent premalignant effects on myeloid progenitor cells.

Premalignant and Malignant Disorders

Ionizing Radiation

Ionizing radiation damages hematopoietic progenitor cells and stromal cells in the bone marrow. Disorders resulting from this exposure include aplastic anemia, myelodysplasia, and leukemia. Among Japanese atomic-bomb survivors, the risk for developing acute lymphocytic leukemia was 9.1 times higher among those exposed to 1 Sv of radiation compared to those without this exposure; for acute myelogenous leukemia, risk increased 3.3-fold; and chronic myelocytic leukemia, 6.2-fold.[31] Studies of nuclear power industry workers have shown that risk for leukemia is increased at a cumulative dose of 100 mSv and possibly at doses of 10 to 50 mSv. Radiation may possibly increase the risk for multiple myeloma and lymphoma, although studies are inconsistent.

Benzene

Benzene is radiomimetic; that is, exposure induces effects in the bone marrow that are similar to those of ionizing radiation. Its toxicity occurs through phenolic and ring-opened chemicals that are produced when benzene is metabolized in the liver. These compounds are clastogenic, producing micronuclei, DNA strand breaks, sister chromatid exchanges, and chromosome aberrations. Benzene-exposed individuals may pass through a premalignant phase, such as aplastic anemia, before developing acute leukemia; alternatively, leukemia may be the first disorder recognized.

Multiple large studies of benzene-exposed workers have analyzed workplace industrial hygiene monitoring data and have found increased risk for premalignant and malignant hematologic

disorders.[32,33] Industries studied have included rubber manufacturing, chemical manufacturing, and petroleum production and transport. These studies have shown increases in risk for acute leukemia that correlate with increasing benzene dose. The most common leukemias that develop are acute myelogenous leukemia and related conditions. The latency period for developing acute leukemia is often 10 or fewer years. The relative risk for leukemia is increased, even if exposure has occurred for 5 or fewer years. After cessation of exposure, risk decreases with time.

Outside of the workplace, exposure to benzene in gasoline or vehicle exhaust occurs when refueling, riding in vehicles, and from indoor air, especially in homes with attached garages. Benzene exposures from these sources are typically at least an order of magnitude lower than the lowest occupational exposures associated with leukemia.

Other Chemicals

Cancer patients treated with alkylating drugs have developed second malignancies of the same types that are caused by ionizing radiation and benzene. Cyclophosphamide, a chemotherapeutic drug, has been found in the urine of exposed health care workers, emphasizing the need for safer work practices.

Agricultural workers are at an increased risk for lymphoma. Non-Hodgkin lymphoma is associated with adult exposure to certain insecticides and herbicides as well as childhood exposure to professional extermination in the home.[34,35] Children in agricultural families have an increased risk of lymphoma, particularly if their fathers did not use chemically resistant gloves when handling pesticides.[36]

EVALUATION AND CONTROL OF RISK

Many workplaces provide wellness programs to assist employees to reduce medical and lifestyle-related risk factors for future illnesses. Although these programs can be quite good, attention to nonoccupational risk factors is no substitute for hazard communication and exposure control in the workplace. In addition, screening for medical risk factors should not supplant workplace safety. For example, individuals who have glucose-6-phosphate dehydrogenase (G6PD) deficiency are at increased risk for hemolysis if they take the antimalarial drug primaquine. Therefore, when individuals with this enzyme deficiency require prophylaxis, they must use other antimalarial drugs. Because hemolysis can also be caused by lead poisoning, some might think that people with G6PD deficiency should be excluded from working with lead. However, this is a discriminatory policy without basis in fact. Instead, work practices should be optimized and exposure levels should be lowered to safe levels based on up-to-date scientific information.

Monitoring for workplace exposure levels is indicated for a number of the hazardous agents described in this chapter. Physiologic parameters, such as serum cholesterol, urinary NAG, liver transaminases, hematologic indices, and markers of genetic damage, may be altered by certain chemicals. However, these tests may be influenced by factors other than toxicant exposures and may not exhibit changes until exposures have substantially exceeded recommended limits. Occupational and environmental health programs need to follow established principles for anticipating, recognizing, evaluating, and controlling hazards associated with disease.

REFERENCES

1. Leigh JP, Markowitz SB, Fahs M, et al. Occupational injury and illness in the United States: Estimates of costs, morbidity and mortality. Arch Intern Med 1997;157:1557–68.
2. Jacobs A, Geary C, Soman J. Haematological disorders and occupational hazards: A British Society for Haematology/Health and Safety Executive study. Br J Haematol 1993;84:442–3.
3. Wharton M, Bistowish JM, Hutcheson RH, et al. Fatal carbon monoxide poisoning at a motel. JAMA 1989;261:1177–8.
4. Koskela R-S, Mutanen P, Sorsa J-A, et al. Factors predictive of ischemic heart disease mortality in foundry workers exposed to carbon monoxide. Am J Epidemiol 2000;152:628–32.
5. Mann JK, Tager IB, Lurmann F, et al. Air pollution and hospital admissions for ischemic heart disease in persons with congestive heart failure or arrhythmia. Environ Health Perspect 2002:110:1247–52.
6. Blair A, Hartge P, Stewart PA, et al. Mortality and cancer incidence of aircraft maintenance workers exposed to trichloroethylene and other organic solvents and chemicals: extended follow up. Occup Environ Med 1998;55:161–71.
7. Ford ES, Rhodes S, McDiarmid M, et al. Deaths from acute exposure to trichloroethylene. J Occup Environ Med 1995;37:749–54.
8. Hamilton A. Exploring the dangerous trades: The autobiography of Alice Hamilton, MD, 1943. Beverly, MA: OEM Press, 1995.
9. Kivimaki M, Leino-Arjas P, Luukkonen R, et al. Work stress and risk of cardiovascular mortality: Prospective cohort study of industrial employees. Br Med J 2002;325:857.
10. Eaker ED, Sullivan LM, Kelly-Hayes M, et al. Does job strain increase the risk for coronary heart disease or death in men and women? Am J Epidemiol 2004;159:950–8.
11. Bigazzi PE. Metals and kidney autoimmunity. Environ Health Perspect 1999;107(Suppl 5):753–65.
12. Weaver VM, Lee G-K, Ahn K-D, et al. Associations of lead biomarkers with renal function in Korean lead workers. Occup Environ Med 2003;60:551–62.
13. Van Vleet TR, Schnellmann RG. Toxic nephropathy: Environmental chemicals. Sem Nephrol 2003;23:500–8.
14. Wittman R, Hu H. Cadmium exposure and nephropathy in a 28-year old female metals worker. Environ Health Perspect 2002;110:1261–6.
15. Ravnskov U. Hydrocarbon exposure may cause glomerulonephritis and worsen renal function: Evidence based on Hill's criteria for causality. Q J Med 2000;93:551–6.
16. Steenland K, Sanderson W, Calvert GM. Kidney disease and arthritis in a cohort study of workers exposed to silica. Epidemiology 2001;12:405–12.
17. Markowitz SB, Levin K. Continued epidemic of bladder cancer in workers exposed to ortho-toluidine in a chemical factory. J Occup Environ Med 2004;46:154–60.
18. Sorahan T, Hamilton L, Jackson JR. A further cohort study of workers employed at a factory manufacturing chemicals for the rubber industry, with special reference to the chemicals 2-mercaptobenzotiazole (MBT), aniline, phenyl-β-naphthylamine and o-toluidine. Occup Environ Med 2000;57:106–15.
19. Weber LW, Boll M, Stampfl A. Hepatotoxicity and mechanism of action of haloalkanes: Carbon tetrachloride as a toxicological model. Crit Rev Toxicol 2003;33:105–35.
20. Brodkin CA, Moon JD, Camp J, et al. Serum hepatic biochemical activity in two populations of workers exposed to styrene. Occup Environ Med 2001;58:95–102.
21. Nomiyama T, Uehara M, Miyauchi H, et al. Causal relationship between a case of severe hepatic dysfunction and low exposure concentrations of N,N-dimethylformamide in the synthetics industry. Ind Health 2001;39:33–6.
22. Sala M, Sunyer J, Herrero C, et al. Association between serum concentrations of hexachlorobenzene and polychlorobiphenyls with thyroid hormone and liver enzymes in a sample of the general population. Occup Environ Med 2001;58:172–7.
23. Maroni M, Mocci F, Visentin S, et al. Periportal fibrosis and other liver ultrasonography findings in vinyl chloride workers. Occup Environ Med 2003;60:60–5.
24. Centeno JA, Mullick FG, Martinez L, et al. Pathology related to chronic arsenic exposure. Environ Health Perspect 2002;110(Suppl 5):883–6.
25. Ward E, Boffetta P, Andersen A, et al. Update on the follow-up of mortality and cancer incidence among European workers employed in the vinyl chloride industry. Epidemiology 2001;12:710–18.
26. Ross RK, Yuan JM, Yu MC, et al. Urinary aflatoxin biomarkers and risk of hepatocellular carcinoma. Lancet 1992;339:943–6.
27. Osterode W, Barnas U, Geissler K. Dose dependent reduction of erythroid progenitor cells and inappropriate erythropoetin response in exposure to lead: new aspects of anaemia induced by lead. Occup Environ Med 1999;56:106–9.
28. Knobeloch L, Salna B, Hogan A, et al. Blue babies and nitrate-contaminated well water. Environ Health Perspect 2000;108:675–8.

29. French CL, Yaun SS, Baldwin LA, et al. Potency ranking of methemoglobin-forming agents. J Appl Toxicol 1995; 15:167–74.

30. Spiller HA, Gallenstein GL, Murphy MJ. Dermal absorption of a liquid diphacinone rodenticide causing coagulaopathy. Vet Hum Toxicol 2003;45:313–14.

31. Preston DL, Kusumi S, Tomonaga M, et al. Cancer incidence in atomic bomb survivors. Part III. Leukemia, lymphoma and multiple myeloma, 1950–1987. Radiat Res 1994;137(2 Suppl):S68–S97.

32. Rinsky RA, Hornung RW, Silver SR, et al. Benzene exposure and hematopoietic mortality: A long-term epidemiologic risk assessment. Am J Ind Med 2002;42:474–80.

33. Hayes RB, Yin S-N, Dosemeci M, et al. Benzene and the dose-related incidence of hematologic neoplasms in China. J Natl Cancer Inst 1997;89:1065–71.

34. De Roos AJ, Zahm SH, Cantor KP, et al. Integrative assessment of multiple pesticides as risk factors for non-Hodgkin's lymphoma among men. Occup Environ Med 2003;60:e11. Available at <http://www.occenvmed.com/cgi/content/full/60/9/e11>.

35. Buckley JD, Meadows AT, Kadin ME, et al. Pesticide exposures in children with non-Hodgkin lymphoma. Cancer 2000;89:2315–21.

36. Flower KB, Hoppin JA, Lynch CF, et al. Cancer risk and parental pesticide application in children of agricultural health study participants. Environ Health Perspect 2004;112:631–5.

BIBLIOGRAPHY

Kivimaki M, Lieno-Arjas P, Luukkonen R, et al. Work stress and risk of cardiovascular mortality: Prospective cohort study of industrial employees. Br Med J 2002;325:857.
This paper reviews methods of measuring psychosocial stresses in the workplace and, in a prospective cohort study that controlled for medical risk factors for ischemic heart disease, found that certain work stressors doubled cardiovascular mortality.

Knobeloch L, Salna B, Hogan A, et al. Blue babies and nitrate-contaminated well water. Environ Health Perspect 2000;108:675–8.
This paper describes typical cases of infant methemoglobinemia that continue to occur in the United States because approximately 2 million families drink water from private wells that are contaminated with nitrates at levels above recommended limits.

Maroni M, Mocci F, Visentin S, et al. Periportal fibrosis and other liver ultrasonography findings in vinyl chloride workers. Occup Environ Med 2003;60:60–5.
After vinyl chloride was conclusively linked to liver angiosarcomas in the 1970s, workplace exposure levels were lowered. This study among present-day workers shows how an exposure history can be assessed in several ways and how research on medical surveillance methods can control for nonoccupational hepatic risk factors, such as alcohol intake, obesity, and infectious hepatitis.

Steenland K, Burnett C, Lalich N, et al. Dying for work: The magnitude of US mortality from selected causes of death associated with occupation. Am J Ind Med 2003;43: 461–82.
This analysis provides estimates of the impact on total annual mortality in the United States of selected malignant and nonmalignant occupational cardiovascular, renal, hepatic, and hematologic disorders and conservatively concludes that occupation is the eighth leading cause of death in the United States.

Van Vleet TR, Schnellmann RG. Toxic nephropathy: environmental chemicals. Sem Nephrol 2003;23:500–8.
This paper provides an interesting review of biotransformation and other mechanisms by which proximal tubular injury is induced by heavy metals, halogenated hydrocarbons, herbicides, organic solvents, and herbal remedies.

An Integrated Approach to Prevention

CHAPTER 31

Disparities in Occupational and Environmental Exposures and Health

Sherry L. Baron and Joseph W. Dorsey

Case 1

A 25-year-old single mother of two elementary school-age children recently lost her welfare benefits but found a job in a small manufacturing plant 10 miles from her home. In order to arrive at her job on time, she has to catch a 7:30 a.m. city bus, but because her children's school bus comes at 7:45, she leaves them every morning alone at the school bus stop. Her job requires her to pass thin sheets of metal through a press that cuts seven screw holes. She repeats this same task every 10 seconds. At the end of her workday, her wrists and fingers ache so much that she has difficulty turning her key in the front door lock. On many days at the end of her 8-hour shift, she is told that her line is running 1 hour of mandatory overtime. As she leaves work, with aching arms and overwhelming anxiety as to whether her children ever made it onto the school bus safely, she runs three blocks to pick them up just as the YMCA after-school program is closing.

Case 2

A young woman loses her job because the factory where she worked downsized, laying off almost half of the workers. Unable to find work, she moves into an apartment with her sister in a low-income neighborhood in a nearby city. Her 10-year-old son begins to cough and wheeze and, as a result, misses many days of school. As the mother is waiting outside the principal's office to explain her son's frequent absences, she begins talking with several other mothers who have children with the same

medical problems. They tell her about a community meeting they had recently attended where a doctor from the hospital was discussing the high rates of asthma in their community. He also had several maps that showed the ring of chemical factories and hazardous waste sites surrounding their neighborhood, which he thought explained, in part, why their children were all so sick.

Although all workers and communities may potentially face one or more of the hazards discussed in this book, certain populations—because of their age, race, ethnicity, or economic position—are more likely to be employed in the most dangerous occupations and workplaces or live in the most polluted neighborhoods. Many of these same populations also represent a disproportionate share of those who (a) lack health insurance, (b) cannot afford decent childcare services, and (c) have insufficient political and economic influence to obtain adequate services and economic investment for their neighborhoods. This chapter will describe some of these inequities and explain how differential patterns of work-related injuries and illness have resulted and how many low-income and minority communities have become polluted by the disproportionate siting of hazardous industrial and waste facilities in their communities.

OCCUPATIONAL HEALTH DISPARITIES

Sherry Baron

During the last half of the 20th century, the size of the working population in the United States doubled, increasing by 79 million workers between 1950 and 2000. The composition of this new workforce has reflected the changing social, political, and demographic characteristics of the country.[1] Many more women and immigrant workers have entered the workforce, and the aging of the "baby boom" generation has increased the median age of the workforce. At the same time, the economy of the United States has been transformed as traditional permanent, full-time, often unionized manufacturing jobs have been eliminated or have moved to Latin America and Asia. These jobs have been replaced by an expanding service sector, and many of the new jobs created are non-union and may be temporary. Although there have been many significant advances in civil rights, African Americans and other racial and ethnic minority populations are still disproportionately employed in high-hazard jobs, while racism and other forms of discrimination—both in the community and the workplace—contribute to additional health risks.[2]

Innovative intervention programs in the workplace and society have not kept pace with the demands of this changing workforce, leaving many workers increasingly vulnerable to occupational injuries and illnesses, including work stress.

Women Workers

During the second half of the 20th century, the role of women in the U.S. economy dramatically changed, increasing by 2.6-fold between 1950 and 2000. About half of the workforce is now female, resulting in substantial new opportunities for women to have rewarding careers. However, much of the gain in women's income has occurred among college-educated women who have entered administrative and professional jobs. More than half (59 percent) of women still earn a wage that places a family of four below the poverty level.[3] For one out of six women, her family's total income is less than $25,000. Not surprisingly, low-wage women workers are also more likely to be single mothers, have less than a high school education, and be either Hispanic or African American.

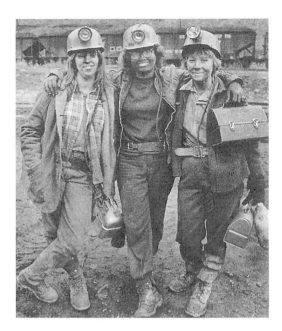

FIGURE 31-1 ● Many women now work in jobs that were traditionally held only by men. (Photograph by Earl Dotter.)

Although the number of women workers has increased, the job market remains highly segregated by gender (Fig. 31-1). For example, 90 percent of health care support workers are female, while more than 90 percent of construction workers are men. When women get jobs in traditionally male occupations, they can face discrimination and harassment (Box 31-1). In 2000, more than half of all women worked in just three occupational categories: administrative support, such as secretaries and other clerical support jobs (24 percent); professional specialty jobs, such as nurses and primary and secondary school teachers (20 percent); and service workers, such as restaurant workers, hairdressers, and cleaning workers (12 percent). Although overall, women are underrepresented in the manufacturing sector, they represent most workers in certain particularly hand-intensive industries, such as textile and garment manufacturing.

Not surprisingly, work-related injuries and illnesses in women occur most commonly in those industries where women are concentrated. In 2002, almost half of all injuries and illness involving lost workdays among women workers occurred in the service sector (47 percent). Of all male and female private industry workers in the United States, the occupation with the second highest number of lost

BOX 31-1

Women Construction Workers: An Example of Sexual Harassment in the Workplace

Sexual harassment of women workers, in the form of gender stereotyping, sexist jokes, and demeaning behavior, remains a problem and has been associated with both mental health problems, such as depression and anxiety, and physical health problems, such as high blood pressure. Although present in many sectors of the economy, some very clear examples have been documented in traditionally male-dominated occupations, such as construction. Researchers found the following comments in focus groups with women construction workers.

Regarding personal protective equipment:
"They gave me a welding leather jacket that was a foot longer than my hand . . . and they said they couldn't order anything smaller. They gave me gloves, humongous, I couldn't even pick anything up."

Regarding the need to prove themselves: ". . . a lot of times, I feel like I've got to do this because I'm a girl because if I don't they're going to say, 'See, whad I tell ya, she's a girl, she can't lift it'."

Regarding issues related to misperceptions about sexual interactions: "(The foreman) hired her very quickly. Until the wife showed up. And then it changes . . . she got every dirty job that was there. He more or less forced her to quit."

Adapted from Goldenhar L, Sweeney MH. Tradewomen's perspectives on occupational safety and health: A qualitative investigation Am J Ind Med 1996;29:516–20.

workday cases (79,000) in 2002 was nurse's aides, orderlies, and attendants—and 91 percent of cases occurred in women workers. The most common type of injury was sprains and strains to the back from lifting and moving patients.[4]

An important question for policymakers and researchers is the relative roles of biological factors and occupational exposures in explaining different rates of some occupational injuries and illness between male and female workers.[5] For example, based on some studies of work-related musculoskeletal disorders, some researchers have argued that women are more susceptible to carpal tunnel syndrome than men. There *are* documented physiological differences between the sexes, such as differences in reproductive hormones and in fat metabolism, that could theoretically affect occupational exposures and/or occurrence of occupational injury or disease. For example, toxins that bioaccummulate in fat tissues could act differently, given the differences in male and female fat metabolism. However, the relative importance of these physiological differences, in comparison to differences in workplace exposure levels, has been inadequately studied. Most studies have not rigorously collected sufficient exposure information to adequately measure the differences in exposure between genders, so misleading conclusions may have been drawn.

For example, in comparing rates of musculoskeletal disorders (MSDs) between male and female workers, those classified under the same broad job category may actually have different job tasks; women are often assigned to more hand-intensive tasks. Also, the design of a work station may be ergonomically optimal for the average male stature but require significant reaching and awkward postures for a female worker of a smaller stature, causing her to have greater ergonomic stresses and an increased injury risk.

In addition to the workplace-based hazards women workers face, they and their spouses experience stress due to conflicts between work and family responsibilities. Up to 40 percent of employed parents report conflicts in balancing work and family demands. For low-wage women workers, many of whom are single mothers, the struggle to balance their role as wage-earners and mothers is especially stressful. Many work nontraditional hours, which makes the search for safe and adequate childcare even more difficult. One out of five single mothers works evening, night, or rotating shifts, and one in three works weekends.[6] More than two-thirds of low-wage women workers do not receive health insurance coverage through their work, so that when a child is sick these stresses become even more acute.

African-American Workers

Case 3

In 1930, a subsidiary of Union Carbide Corporation contracted with a construction firm to dig a 3-mile tunnel through a stone mountain in West Virginia. The goal was to divert the New River to create a hydroelectric energy plant to power the operations of its Electro-Metallurgical Company. This massive project employed thousands of workers, of whom at least 75 percent were black, while the population of Fayette County, where the project was located, was 85 percent white. Many of these workers came from Alabama, Virginia, and the Carolinas, where work was hard to find during the Great Depression and to whom the $0.30 to $0.60 per hour seemed like good pay. The rock through which they drilled had some of the highest known content of silica, and, in order to complete the job quickly, they chose to use minimal water to suppress the dust levels. About 1 year after the project began, the local newspaper published a story commenting on "the unusually large number of deaths among the colored laborers. . . . The deaths total about 37 in the past two weeks." Although the initial deaths were attributed to the poor nutritional habits and unusual susceptibility to pneumonia of blacks, it soon became clear that they were dying of acute silicosis. Although it is hard to know the total number who died as a result of this incident, one author has estimated that as many as 581 of the 922 blacks who worked in the tunnels for at least 2 months of the 24-month project may have died.[7]

Although this case happened many years ago, and such blatant forms of discrimination against African-American workers are less common today, many economic and social disparities still exist. African Americans and other minorities are still concentrated in some of the more dangerous jobs. Residential segregation is still common in the United States as most African Americans still live in the South and more than half live in the center city of large metropolitan areas, compared to only 21 percent of non-Hispanic whites. These residential patterns also create disparities in educational and economic opportunities. Achievement levels in inner-city schools lag behind the national standards. Public transportation is often inadequate to provide access to jobs in the new industrial and office parks being developed in the corridors surrounding many major cities. Consequently, twice as many African Americans over age 25 have not completed a high school education (21 percent for both males and females) compared to non-Hispanic whites. Twenty-three percent of the African Americans live below the poverty level, three times the rate for non-Hispanic whites.

African Americans are disproportionately employed in some of the most dangerous occupations. Among men, African Americans are twice as likely as non-Hispanic whites to work in service occupations and as laborers, fabricators, and operators, yet they are half as likely to be in managerial or professional specialty occupations. As a result, for both men and women, the African-American occupational injury rate is about one-third higher than that of non-Hispanic whites (Fig. 31-2).

African Americans bear a disproportionate burden of such diseases as cancer, cardiovascular disease, and asthma. In 2000, blacks had an overall mortality rate 30 percent higher than that of whites and an infant mortality rate 2.5 times that of whites. Scientists have attempted to understand the many factors potentially contributing to these disparities, including access to health care, nutritional factors, environmental exposures, and genetic factors. Another pathway by which racism may contribute to increased mortality is through the disproportionate placement of minorities in the most dangerous industries.[8] For both male and female workers, those occupations that have a disproportionate share of black workers are also those occupations with the highest rate of work-related injuries (Fig. 31-3). In addition, within individual workplaces, African-American workers may experience the stress caused by a racist work climate. Although few studies have systematically studied the nature and magnitude of racism in the workplace, in a recent poll by the National Urban League, 39 percent of African Americans felt that race and gender discrimination is widely practiced at their workplaces.[9] In recognition of this potential problem, many workplaces have introduced diversity education programs. However, much more research is needed to better define the nature and extent of racism within workplaces and the efficacy of intervention programs to address it.

African Americans are also disproportionately affected by economic recession. Much of the rising social and economic status of the African-American population could be attributed to increases in employment in the relatively well-paid manufacturing sector between 1939 and 1959. As the economy

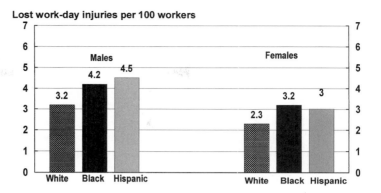

FIGURE 31-2 ● Lost workday injury rates, 1998–2000. "Black" and "white" designations exclude persons of Hispanic origin; persons of Hispanic origin may be of any race. (Source: Bureau of Labor Statistics. Derived from statistics presented in: National Research Council. Safety is Seguridad. Washington, DC: National Academies Press, 2003.)

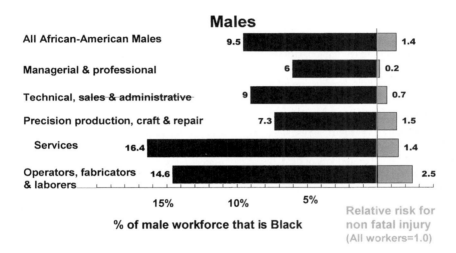

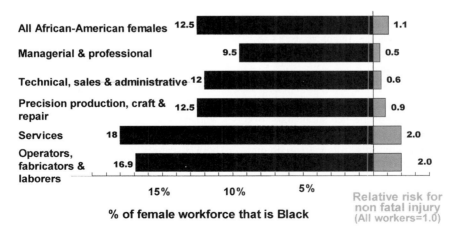

Source: Bureau of Labor Statistics, US Department of Labor

FIGURE 31-3 ● Work-related non-fatal injuries among African Americans, 1998–2000. (Source: Bureau of Labor Statistics. Derived from statistics presented in: National Research Council. Safety is Seguridad. Washington, DC: National Academies Press, 2003.)

was restructured from manufacturing to service, especially since 1970, African Americans have suffered a disproportionate share of the rise in unemployment; between 2001 and 2003, the increase in the African-American unemployment rate was twice that of whites. Unemployment has adverse economic effects as well as effects on health and well-being associated with the stress of unemployment. The unemployment rate is especially high for African-American youth, which may have long-term social and economic impacts as they become disillusioned and leave the job market.

Hispanic and Immigrant Workers

Case 4

A young Mexican man, in search of a job, crossed the border to the United States. He had a cousin living in Los Angeles, who told him that construction jobs were easy to obtain. Once he arrived, he found a job working as a sandblaster for a small construction company that was happy to pay him "under the table" and did not ask for any official documents. Although the sandblasting created lots of dust, his employer gave him no respiratory protection. To avoid breathing too much dust, he would tie bandanas around his face, much the way the farm workers in his small rural town in Mexico had done when they sprayed pesticides. He was able to earn a good income and send money back regularly to his family. However, after a few years doing this job, he began to develop a cough and wheezing. When he hardly had enough energy to make it through the workday, he finally saw a doctor who diagnosed him with a severe case of silicosis. Unable to work and without medical insurance, he returned to Mexico and died a few years later.

In the 2000 census, there were 35.8 million Hispanics in the United States, a 58-percent increase over 1990. This dramatic increase in the Hispanic population has resulted primarily from increased immigration. During the 1990s, more immigrants entered the United States than during any other period of history—with close to 1 million immigrants arriving each year. Foreign-born workers now make up 14 percent of the entire workforce. They accounted for about 50 percent of the net increase in the labor force during the second half of the 1990s.[10] About half of all those born abroad are originally from Latin America, and an even greater percent-

age of those who immigrated since 1990 are from Latin America. In 1999, the median earnings for all foreign-born workers with less than 10 years in the United States were $21,600. The median earnings for Mexican and Central American women were less than $16,000 and for Mexican males was only slightly more than $19,000.[11]

As with African Americans, Hispanics—and especially foreign-born Hispanic workers—are more likely to work in service occupations and as operators, fabricators, and laborers as compared to native-born workers and also are twice as likely to work in farming, forestry, and fishing. Central Americans and Mexicans, especially those with less than 10 years in the United States who are not citizens, are especially likely to work in these sectors.

Because foreign-born workers, particularly new immigrants, often have few geographic ties in this country, they may travel in search of jobs. This dispersion of new immigrants has led to a rapid shift in the demographics of the workforce in certain parts of the United States. Although states such as California, Texas, New York, and Florida continue to have the most Hispanic workers, during the 1990s many states, especially in the South and Midwest, have more than doubled their Hispanic population. This movement was initially fueled by employment in the low-wage, high-hazard meat and poultry processing industry and in agriculture. However, once immigrants began to settle in these areas, they not only found that jobs were available, but many found the lifestyle preferable to the congestion, high cost, and crime of the traditional inner-city immigrant communities, such as Los Angeles. Employment opportunities soon expanded to include construction, services, and other manufacturing jobs.

Hispanic workers, especially foreign-born Hispanics, have a higher occupational fatality rate than other workers.[12] Between 1995 and 2000, the occupational fatality rate for all foreign-born Hispanic workers was 50 percent higher (6.1 per 100,000 workers) than the rate for all workers and for native-born Hispanic workers (Fig. 31-4). The cause of this disparity is, in large part, due to the disproportionate distribution of Hispanic foreign-born workers in high-risk industries, such as construction, agriculture, and manufacturing. Even within high-risk industries, foreign-born workers may face the highest risk for injury. For example, a recent analysis found that Hispanic construction workers had an 80 percent greater fatality rate compared to non-Hispanic construction workers.[13]

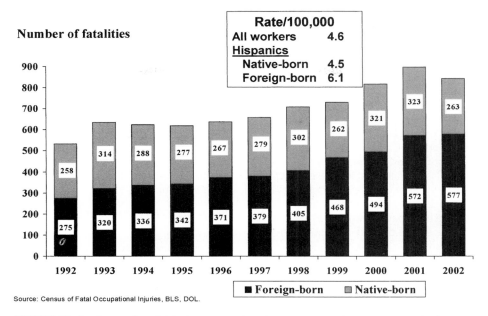

FIGURE 31-4 ● Fatal work injuries among Hispanics, 1995–2000. (Source: Bureau of Labor Statistics. Census of Fatal Occupational Injury Data.)

Concerns have also been raised regarding many of the linguistic, cultural, and legal barriers that foreign-born workers face. Most foreign-born Hispanic workers, especially from Mexico and Central America, have less than a high school education. For many raised in rural indigenous communities, Spanish is not their first language. Immigrants, especially new immigrants, may be unfamiliar with local laws regarding safety and health protection or workers' compensation. Recent estimates have placed the size of the undocumented immigrant worker population in the United States at approximately 8 million workers.[14] In the agricultural industry, over half of the approximately 1.8 million crop farm workers are undocumented. Systemic programs to improve the safety and health conditions for foreign-born workers must (a) address industry- and occupation-specific hazards, (b) develop linguistically and culturally appropriate training and education programs, and (c) address the legal barriers resulting from their immigration status.

Young Workers

Whereas in many parts of the world children work in dangerous conditions (Box 31-2), since the passage of strong federal child labor laws in the 1930s, exploitative child labor is rare in the United States. Youth employment, however, is extremely com-

mon, with the Department of Labor estimating that 44 percent of 16- and 17-year-olds work sometime during the school year and surveys showing that up to 80 percent of teenagers work at some time during their high school years.[15]

Although male and female youth are equally likely to work, youth in higher income families are more likely to work than those in lower income families, and white youth are almost twice as likely as black and Hispanic youth to work. This pattern may be due to greater availability of jobs in higher income communities and increased access there to transportation to find jobs outside of these communities. It also may be due to lower income youth needing to provide more assistance at home, including child care for younger siblings.

Young workers are largely low-wage workers, most earning less than $7 per hour. More than 50 percent of 16- to 19-year-old workers are employed in retail trade, most commonly in eating and drinking establishments. Although employment provides many benefits to youth, including increased self-confidence, job skills, and income, it also poses potential hazards.

Case 5

A 16-year-old boy was anxious, but excited, as he began his first job at a neighborhood hamburger

BOX 31-2

International Child Labor: The Impact of Economic Exploitation on the Health and Welfare of Children

Social policy questions concerning child labor are neither unique to the current era nor the Western world. Perhaps the earliest regulation of child labor dates to 1284, when a statute of Venetian glass makers forbade the employment of children in certain dangerous aspects of the glass trade. Efforts at reform have been and continue to be impaired by a lack of substantive data on the effects of child labor on health and development.

In 1919, the first meeting of the International Labor Organization (ILO) fixed a minimum age for the employment of children at 14 years. Subsequently, many international conventions and regulations have been adopted by the ILO, and most nations have set a minimum age for employment. However, as judged by educational data, a substantial number of nations report large numbers of children leaving school below the nation's specified minimum age.

The right of children to an education and freedom from exploitation are clearly stated in the Convention on the Rights of the Child adopted by the United Nations General Assembly in 1989 and in other international instruments. The passage of the 1989 convention represents a commitment on the part of member nations to work toward a future in which the rights of all children are respected. International law also provides a clear and generally accepted consensus on the nature and definition of child labor. In 1999, the ILO passed Convention 182 on the most hazardous forms of child labor. Ratifying nations obligate themselves to work toward the elimination of the most serious child labor abuses such as forced and bonded labor, prostitution, and child soldiers.

The Magnitude of Child Labor

In the 1970s, the ILO estimated that there were approximately 150 million working children in the world; more recently, the ILO has estimated that the number may be as high as 320 million. Even the latter estimate may be low. There are an approximately 1.1 billion children between 5 and 16 years of age in developing and the least developed nations in the world. In many nations, fewer than 50 percent of children complete primary school. If most of these children work, the number of working children may be closer to 500 million. In spite of the lack of comprehensive data, it is clear that children in developing nations spend long hours at work and often have little or no time away from the workplace (Figure 31-5).

The Health Effects of Child Labor

The impact of child labor should be seen in four parts: the effect of work on growth and development; job-specific hazards as they relate to injury and illness morbidity; the effect of latency on the future health of children; and sexual and emotional abuse.

Perhaps the most obvious impact of child labor is on intellectual development, and child labor has been frequently associated with adult illiteracy. In one study in Bangladesh, children of women with no education had a four- to fivefold risk of severe malnutrition compared with children of mothers with a university education.[1]

It is not surprising that there are few studies on the impact of specific work-related exposures on the health of children. First, children are often working illegally. Second, children are rarely the beneficiaries of any type of labor contract. Third, such studies are expensive and difficult to conduct. What is known is that working children can be found around the world cutting rock in stone quarries, working in heavy construction, tanning leather, electroplating metals, scavenging garbage for food, tending goats and sheep, and any of hundreds of menial tasks. Too often, work in developing nations is performed without adequate protections and, when available, personal protective equipment has been designed for use by adults and is virtually useless for a child.

Young workers in many developing nations are at substantial risk of developing both work-related and non–work-related illness. Most data indicate that the health status of young workers is poor. These health problems are compounded by the all-too-often intolerable work conditions. Although data on the toxic effects of occupational exposures to

(continued)

BOX 31-2

International Child Labor: The Impact of Economic Exploitation on the Health and Welfare of Children (Continued)

children are limited, existing disease models amply support the hypothesis that children are likely to acquire disease at an early age as a result of hazardous work. For example, young children are known to be more

susceptible than adults to the adverse health effects of lead.

Reference

1. Islam MA, Rahem MM, Mahalanabis D. Maternal and socioeconomic factors and the risk of severe malnutrition in a child: a case control study. Euro J Clin Nutr 1995;48:416–24.

---

joint. His job was to clear tables, wash dishes, and clean up the counter. He hoped that by the end of the school year he would have learned enough to become a fry cook and earn an extra dollar per hour. One Saturday, one of the cooks had to leave early and he eagerly volunteered to help close up the grill. He had watched the cook do these tasks for months and felt confident he knew what to do. One task was to empty the grease from the deep fryer. He grabbed a container—not realizing it was the refuse container for the meat scraps and would melt when filled with hot grease—and emptied the fryer. As he walked out to the dumpster, the hot grease burned a hole in the bottom of the container and fell onto his legs, causing severe burns.

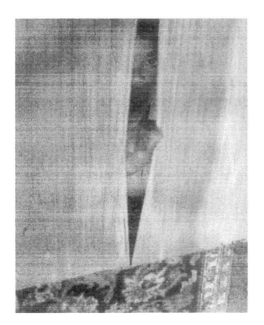

FIGURE 31-5 ● Child carpet weaver in India. (Photograph by David Parker.)

This case demonstrates some characteristics of young workers that raise concerns about their safety and health. Like all new workers, young workers are at increased risk for injury. In many surveys of working youth, almost half report they did not receive health and safety training on the job. Because the level of physical and cognitive development in teens is variable, developmental characteristics may also place youth at risk. Shorter teens may have a harder time reaching machines and may not have the physical strength required for certain tasks. Even when youth have reached adult stature, their psychological and cognitive maturity may lag behind in conventional wisdom or ability. Employers may assign them tasks to which they are not yet cognitively prepared. Their enthusiasm and desire to do well, although very positive attributes, may make them uncomfortable asking questions or expressing concerns about their ability to perform a challenging task.

In addition to the specific hazards youth may face at work, there may also be unintended consequences affecting their ability to function and succeed in their school and social lives. Using a relatively arbitrary cutoff, policymakers and researchers divide youth labor into high-intensity labor (more than 20 hours per week) and low-intensity labor. Whereas low-intensity labor is positively associated with future postsecondary education, high-intensity labor has been found to be associated with substance abuse, inadequate sleep, and decreased eventual educational attainment.

In 2002, there were 41 occupational fatalities to children under age 17. Among occupational fatalities in youth over the past 10 years, the most common industries of employment were agriculture (43 percent), retail trade (19 percent), and construction (16 percent). Twenty-eight percent of youth occupational fatalities occur in children less than 15, and 30 percent to those working in a family business, mostly agriculture. (For a more in-depth discussion of issues related to youth labor in agriculture, see Chapter 32.) Among fatalities in youth working in the retail sector, two-thirds were homicides—many occurring as a result of robberies.

In 2001, among 16- to 19-year-olds, there were 44,259 reported cases of occupational injuries and illness involving lost workdays, 46 percent in the retail sector. These data likely undercount many injuries to youth workers who never inform their employers of these injuries or work for small employers, such as in gardening and construction work. According to the National Electronic Injury Survey (NEISS), about 5 percent of working youth, age 15 to 17, were seen in emergency departments for a work-related condition in 1999. The full cost of these injuries to society can be considerable given the severity of the injury, medical care expenses, and missed school days and parents' missed workdays.

The primary focus of prevention programs for work-related injuries and illness in youth has been on protective legislation through the Fair Labor Standards Act of 1938. The act empowers the U.S. Department of Labor to establish (a) specific rules pertaining to child labor, which include limits on the hours of work for children under age 16, and (b) documents called *hazardous orders* that identify certain tasks, such as operating power-driven woodworking equipment, that cannot be performed by youth under age 18 in nonagricultural work (and under age 16 in agricultural work).

A more recent focus of prevention activities has been the establishment of many innovative occupational safety and health training programs targeting youth in communities and schools. Innovative curricula, peer counseling, role-playing activities, and public service announcements targeted to high-risk communities have helped increase awareness about occupational hazards.

Older Workers

Dominant factors affecting demographics in the United States have been the "baby boom" of about 80 million people born between 1946 and 1964, continually increasing life expectancy, and the decreasing fertility rate. These factors have together dramatically changed the shape of the population pyramid, such that between 1990 and 2000 the number of workers 25 to 44 years old did not change,

whereas the number 45 to 65 increased by more than 12 million.

A factor increasing the number of older workers is changing retirement patterns. After a decades-long trend toward earlier retirement, the workforce participation rate of those in their 60s began increasing in the 1990s such that in 2001 more than one-third of men were working past age 65 and one-quarter past age 70. This trend may be due to a combination of (a) changing policies regarding Social Security and the restructuring of many pension programs, which has caused workers to delay their retirement; and (b) the return of some retired individuals to part-time employment. Workers over age 65 are more likely to be employed in nonstandard employment, such as temporary work and independent contracting.

As health researchers and policy experts explore the issues raised by the increasing age of the population, two major issues have been the impact of aging on health and working capacity and the impact of working on the aging process. Although these issues may, in part, be job-dependent, important questions have been raised regarding the relative importance of (a) physiological and cognitive deterioration associated with the aging process (Fig. 31-6) and (b) positive attributes of experience and expertise. A recent report by the National Academy of Sciences reviewed these issues and made several recommendations for improving surveillance, etiological research, and assessing intervention effectiveness for the older worker population.[16]

Nonfatal occupational injury rates decrease with age, possibly due to job selection factors, improved vigilance and work experience, and/or changes in injury reporting patterns. However, when injuries occur in older workers, they are more severe than in younger workers, as measured in the number of lost workdays. In addition, the fatal occupational injury rate is higher in older workers.

The health of older workers results from their accumulated work-related and non–work-related exposures and life experiences. Work experiences become powerful predictors of occupational exposures and many factors associated with socioeconomic position, such as access to health care, rates of smoking and alcoholism, nutritional status, and communities in which workers live. A social gradient in health exists, with those employed in lower-level jobs suffering increased morbidity and mortality even after retirement.

Older workers who are members of racial and ethnic minority groups may experience age, racial,

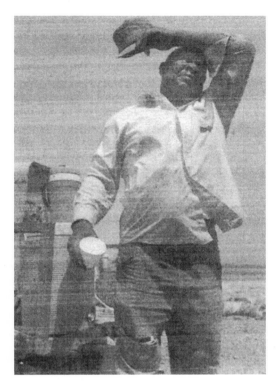

FIGURE 31-6 ● A heat-stressed farmworker in Mississippi takes a water break with the temperature approaching 105°F. The changed physiology of older workers places them closer to maximum tolerance when working in conditions such as extremes of temperature. (Photograph by Earl Dotter.)

and ethnic discrimination. Two-thirds of workers over 45 years of age experience age discrimination at work, which may impact their job advancement and their ability to find new work after job loss.[17]

Finally, as life expectancy increases and many families try to keep older individuals out of institutional care settings, many older individuals, especially women, are providing home care services for their friends and family—either as paid or unpaid workers. As older workers, these individuals may experience similar work–family conflicts as they did as parents.[18]

DISPARITIES IN ENVIRONMENTAL EXPOSURES

Joseph Dorsey

Industrial and hazardous waste facilities produce hundreds of toxic pollutants, occurring in literally thousands of combinations. These facilities are located disproportionately in low-income areas and communities of color. Children living in these communities may be particularly susceptible to the toxic

effects of these exposures (Box 31-3). In addition to increasing the burden of diseases such as childhood asthma and lead poisoning, long-term environmental exposures can affect communities by polluting groundwater and waterways, destroying green spaces, and contributing to the deterioration of homes and schools (Fig. 31-7). In response, community activists along with researchers and public health practitioners have created an international environmental justice movement to fight for greater environmental equity.[19] This section will provide a historical account of the rise of a social movement to address localized environmental inequalities. A case study is included to illustrate the challenges these communities face in attempting to influence decisions about the placement of hazardous waste facilities.

The environmental justice movement began to emerge in the United States in the late 1970s as part of the national civil rights movement. More specifically, the environmental justice movement evolved from emergent public concerns about the apparent inequities about where hazardous waste facilities were located and concerns about the resulting societal consequences and environmental impacts. The consequences and impacts may include chemical contamination, damaged ecosystems, visual blight, noise, offensive smells, public health problems, diminished property and land values, social stigma, and other factors affecting the quality of life of residents.

In 1976, the United Auto Workers (UAW) union held a conference at Black Lake, Michigan, called "Working for Environmental and Economic Justice and Jobs." The UAW conference, which included union members, farmers, environmentalists, and people of color, was perhaps the first of its kind to acknowledge the linkages between hazardous environments, economic inequities, and social injustice. By 1978, the federal government produced a brochure on the disproportionate impact of pollution on people of color, entitled *Our Common Concern*, which published comments on the special importance of environmental issues to blacks from civil rights activists such as Vernon Jordan, Coretta Scott King, and Bayard Rustin. The next year, the National Urban League and the Sierra Club jointly sponsored the 1979 City Care conference in Detroit. This conference broadened the definition of environment beyond wilderness and wildlife issues and brought together two organizations with divergent interests—one focused on civil rights, the other on environmental issues.

Children as a Special Population at Risk for Environmental Hazards

Adam Spanier

One summer afternoon, a frantic mother brought her 5-year-old son to an emergency department for evaluation. "He was just out playing in the barn," she told a physician there. "When I went to check on him, he was sweating, confused, vomiting, having difficulty breathing, and had wet himself." The physician noted a decreased heart rate, decreased blood pressure, and excessive tearing of the eyes. He learned that the child lived on a farm and was exposed to an organophosphate pesticide. He removed the child's clothing to decrease any continued exposure, asked the nurse to bathe him while wearing gloves, and treated him with pralidoxime (2-PAM) and atropine.

This case helps demonstrate that children are not just small adults. There are many reasons why a child's risk of environmental exposure differs greatly from that of an adult. Children may be particularly vulnerable to a specific chemical. For example, in the above case the likelihood of unintentional exposure to pesticides is higher in children, and the dose needed to produce equivalent symptoms is lower in children. Each of the stages of child development holds unique health risks from various environmental exposures.

Anything that may interfere with development of the fetus, which is undergoing rapid growth and organogenesis, can cause serious long-term effects. Low-molecular-weight compounds (such as carbon monoxide), fat-soluble compounds (such as ethanol and polycyclic aromatic hydrocarbons), and some heavy metals (such as lead and mercury) can cross the placental barrier. During fetal development, there are specific periods of elevated risk during which organs are developing. Some environmental exposures, medicines, and use of tobacco, alcohol, and recreational drugs during these periods can lead to devastating results. For example, thalidomide can cause severe birth defects of the limbs, ethanol can impair brain development, and diethylstilbestrol can later cause vaginal cancer and other reproductive system effects.

After birth, a child may face numerous other environmental risks. A breastfed child may be exposed to toxic chemicals in milk, such as pesticides, lead, mercury, nicotine (and its metabolites), and polychlorinated biphenyls (PCBs), as well as medicines that a nursing mother has taken. In addition, infant formula mixed with tap water may contain toxins present in the tap water.

Toddlers with increasing mobility and persistence of mouthing behaviors may ingest toxins in their environment, such as pesticides, lead (in house dust), and arsenic (in treated wood). Because they are close to the ground, they are more likely to breathe heavier airborne particles, such as some airborne allergens and mercury. In addition, children generally have more rapid respiratory rates than adults and are therefore exposed to more airborne toxins, such as environmental tobacco smoke. Because children ingest more water and food than adults per body weight, they are at increased risk of ingesting contaminants of water and food, such as pesticides.

Children also have a larger body surface-to-mass ratio than adults, so dermal exposures to hazardous substances that are absorbed throughout the skin, such as organophosphate pesticides, may pose proportionately more risks for children than for adults.

Children are at increased risk of physical injury from a variety of hazards, including open windows, swimming pools, pots of boiling liquid on stove-tops, stairs, and roads.

School may present new hazards for children. For example, some schools are built on property that is less than desirable. In Cincinnati, a school was built on a former shooting range and the schoolyard was found to have elevated soil lead levels, likely due to use of lead shot. As another example, most schools use pesticides, most of which have not been tested for adverse neurodevelopmental effects.

Adolescents are at increased risk of motor-vehicle, gun-related, and other injuries, and exposure to environmental toxins, such as cigarette smoke. Adolescents who work are at increased risk of occupational injuries.

The Association of Occupational and Environmental Clinics (www.aoec.org) has established a network of Pediatric Environmental Health Specialty Units throughout North America to provide education and consultation for health professionals concerning the impact of the environment on children's health.

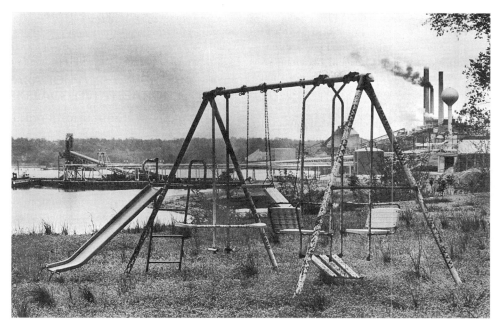

FIGURE 31-7 ● This children's play area located near a large industrial facility in Virginia is an example of how the siting of polluting industries can adversely impact the quality of life in neighboring communities. (Photograph by Earl Dotter.)

Long before the phenomenon known as "NIMBYism" (not in my back yard) was identified, middle-class whites skillfully used zoning laws, legal challenges, and every other means available to them to control and maintain the integrity of the communities in which they lived. By the 1980s, working-class white communities recognized that the path of solid-waste and industrial pollution went through their communities as well. As working-class communities organized to stop the placement of locally undesirable land uses (LULUs) in their neighborhoods, industry quickly adjusted to the new political reality. The path of least resistance increasingly led to vulnerable communities of color. By the 1990s, communities of color were characterized by declining air and water quality, increasing toxic contamination, and resultant health problems and declining quality of life.

For many years, minority residents of contaminated communities accepted the links between economic development and toxic exposure as an inevitable part of coexisting with America's chemical–industrial complex. Industrialization meant progress, and everyone benefited with increased goods and services. Employers often convinced workers in polluting industrial facilities that community environmental protests and demands were against their own interests, forcing workers to choose between their job and their community's health and impeding the creation of strong environmental coalitions among workers and community residents.

Low-income residents and people of color seem to have borne a greater proportion of these health and environmental risks than others. Because white race and income are highly correlated in most urban settings, a disproportionate number of black and Hispanic communities are sites for waste management facilities. Most times, industries site in locations where there is a preexisting physical infrastructure, with electrical power lines, underground water pipes, and transportation and communication links. Many companies site their facilities in locations where land is cheap or property values are low. Those who reside in such communities may find themselves unable to move to better neighborhoods, as they may lack the economic resources required to live in less polluted neighborhoods.

Targeted or inequitable exposure to these hazards, based on class or race, has become known as *environmental discrimination* or *environmental racism*. It is difficult to prove environmental discrimination and racism in court, because it depends on demonstrating intent to do harm to specific populations. But those experiencing it find it as real as the discrimination and racism found in housing, employment, education, and voting. And, a lack of intent does not lessen the effects of discrimination and racism.

In 1983, environmental sociologist Robert Bullard published a study indicating that lower income and minority neighborhoods in many urban areas are often less well served by municipal governments than high-income neighborhoods.[20] He studied solid waste sites in the black communities in Houston. He found that the land use pattern in Houston, one of the largest American cities without zoning, was erratic, but that incinerators and landfills were more likely to be located in black than non-black neighborhoods. Four of the five city-owned incinerators were located in black neighborhoods; the other incinerator was located in a Hispanic neighborhood.

Over time, collective protests and legal actions made it difficult for companies and public administrators to site facilities in low-income and minority neighborhoods. The first national protest by blacks concerning hazardous waste occurred in 1982. Demonstrations were triggered after Warren County, North Carolina, was selected as the burial site for more than 32,000 cubic yards of soil contaminated with highly toxic polychlorinated biphenyls (PCBs). The soil had been illegally dumped in 1978 along roads in 14 North Carolina counties. Civil rights leaders from around the country joined local organizers to protest the governor's proposal to dump the PCB-contaminated dirt near the town of Afton. Warren County had less-than-ideal geophysical features for a toxic waste landfill, with a water table just 5 feet below ground at some points and most local residents drinking well water. In addition, Warren County, one of the poorest counties in North Carolina, had the highest percentage of blacks in the state.

The Warren County protests provided the impetus for a 1983 U.S. General Accounting Office study, *Siting of Hazardous Waste Landfills and Their Correlation with Racial and Economic Status of Surrounding Communities.* That study revealed that three of the four off-site, commercial hazardous waste landfills in Region IV (which comprises eight states in the South) happened to be located in predominantly African-American communities. However, African Americans composed only 20 percent of the region's population. In all four communities,

at least 26 percent of the population lived below the poverty level, a rate more than double that for the United States as a whole.

In 1987, the United Church of Christ's Commission for Racial Justice (UCC/CRJ) published the first national study of the correlation between hazardous waste sites and community demographics. This seminal report, *Toxic Wastes and Race in the United States,* concluded that race was the most significant variable tested that was associated with the location of commercial hazardous waste facilities. Communities with the most commercial hazardous waste facilities had the highest composition of racial and ethnic residents (three times more likely than whites). In communities with one commercial hazardous waste facility, the average percentage of minorities in the population was twice that in communities without such facilities. Income levels and home values in the 369 communities with commercial hazardous waste facilities were significantly lower, and estimated numbers of hazardous waste generation sites and uncontrolled waste sites were significantly higher than in the surrounding counties. Although socioeconomic status appeared to play an important role in the location of commercial hazardous waste facilities, race was more significant than any other factor examined.

For example, in 1992, Alabama had the nation's largest hazardous waste landfill, located near the small town of Emelle in Sumter County—best described as black, rural, and poor. The whites in the county were mainly in two towns in the southern part, while Emelle is in the predominantly black northern half.

As another example, at the same time, Alsen in central Louisiana was being sited for a landfill that eventually became a hazardous waste incinerator site. This semirural community of about 2,000 people was 98 percent black and middle class. Its average annual income was more than $15,000, and nearly 80 percent of the population had at least some college education. From 1971 through 1986, however, Alsen experienced many environmental complications and filed numerous lawsuits.

In 1993, geographer Lauretta Burke used geographic information systems (GISs) to confirm a significant relationship between (a) census tracts in Los Angeles County with low income and high percentages of minorities and (b) number of EPA's Toxic Release Inventory (TRI) facilities. At a given income level, Hispanics and African Americans were more likely to be living near TRI facilities than whites or Asians.[21]

In addition, there has been more environmental justice activism. For example, in 1989, the Gulf Coast Tenants Organization organized a nationally publicized event—the Great Louisiana Toxics March through Cancer Alley—from Baton Rouge to New Orleans. By then, community-based organizations had matured into networks, sharing information, developing common strategies, and taking joint actions against industrial pollution and the inaction of state and federal agencies.

Grassroots organizations were initially isolated from the mainstream environmental movement because its main focus was on the earth's ecosystems—not on social injustice. Grassroots organizations arose to meet specific needs within affected minority communities that mainstream environmental organizations had ignored. Grassroots environmentalists have been concerned primarily with the urban, industrial environment. They are more racially and ethnically diverse and focus on issues relevant to minority and poor populations. They rely on certain common ideals to attract and retain members. Unlike the mainstream environmental organizations, such as the Sierra Club and the National Audubon Society, grassroots organizations have been able to attract and maintain the support of people of color and the poor because they are structurally flexible. After decades of environmental abuse, exploitation, and neglect, low-income and minority communities have begun to address environmental quality as a matter of social justice.

Frequent community protests as well as scholarly studies and publications have made environmental justice a prominent part of the national dialogue concerning citizen empowerment, social justice, and environmental quality. Much of this dialogue has focused on the number of hazardous waste sites in a given community, the frequency of sitings in minority communities, and if temporal, spatial, and/or market forces determine the location of hazardous waste sites.

Political pressure from the environmental justice movement has led to the establishment of EPA's Office of Environmental Justice and specific policy changes. For example, in response to growing concern over the government's role in protecting vulnerable populations from hazardous waste and toxic pollution, President Bill Clinton, in 1994, issued Executive Order 12898, entitled "Federal Actions to Address Environmental Justice in Minority Populations and Low-Income Populations." This order addressed environmental injustice within existing federal laws and regulations. It reinforced the 30-year old Civil Rights Act of 1964 (Title VI), which prohibits discriminatory practices in programs receiving federal funds. It also focused attention on the National Environmental Policy Act (NEPA), a 25-year-old law that set policy goals for the protection, maintenance, and enhancement of the environment. NEPA requires federal agencies to prepare a detailed statement on the environmental effects of proposed federal actions that significantly affect the quality of human health. In addition, the executive order called for improved methodologies for (a) assessing and mitigating health effects from multiple and cumulative exposure; (b) assessing and mitigating impacts on subsistence fishers and wildlife consumers; and (c) collecting data on low-income and minority populations who may be disproportionately at risk. It also encouraged participation of affected populations in various phases of assessment, including data gathering, analysis, mitigation (including identifying alternative solutions), and monitoring.

The magnitude of the vulnerability of the poor and people of color to concentrated hazards has made pollution a civil rights issue. Social injustice has become the focus of many environmental issues. The nature of hazardous exposures and related health risks has changed the focus of the environmental justice movement from recognition of minority civil rights to the realm of human rights—the right to a healthy and clean environment. As a grassroots movement, it has brought environmental concerns and action to the working class and racial and ethnic minorities by linking public health and ecological issues with social justice and equity.

A Case Study in Environmental Justice: The Siting of a Waste-to-Energy Facility in Flint/Genesee County, Michigan

The Michigan legislature passed the Waste to Energy Act in 1989. It provides a tax credit to energy companies that use waste as a power source. In August 1991, the Genesee Power Station Limited Partnership (GPSLP) applied for a permit to construct and operate a wood burning incinerator/generator through the Michigan Air

Pollution Control Commission (MAPCC). This proposed waste-to-energy facility (WTE) was to be sited in Genesee Township's Dort-Carpenter Industrial Park located in Genesee County, just north of Flint, Michigan The power plant would generate electricity to be sold to Consumer's Power, Inc., generating $1.8 million per year in revenues for the Genesee Economic Development Commission (GEDC), including $75,000 a year for the township's general fund and about $165,000 for the county general fund.

Facilities at the plant site would include a truck dumping facility, a cooling tower, an ash storage and load-out facility. The facility would be designed to use lower value fuels such as wood waste from demolition because no other power plant facility was currently using fuel in this area. In addition, the facility would use wood waste from pallet manufacturers, waste pallets and dunnage from automobile manufacturers and suppliers, sawdust and trimmings from furniture manufacturers, waste lumber from construction, and tree trimmings from tree service companies, municipalities, and utilities.

The demolition waste was considered the "dirtiest" and most controversial. It contained unpainted wood in old homes, found in boards inside walls, in roofing, and in floor joists. Building inspectors from some southeast Michigan cities estimated that between 5 to 50 percent of the wood in an old home was unpainted and untreated. The rest could be treated with lead-based paint or other chemicals. The Genesee Power Station Limited Partnership (GPSLP) assured the commission and community that the plant would not burn wood painted or treated with arsenic, creosote, or other chemicals.

In response, local residents organized the community-based group Flint-Genesee United for Action, Justice, and Environmental Safety (United for Action) and started a campaign to stop the placement of the proposed 35-megawatt demolition wood waste-to-energy incinerator (Genesee Power Station) in its collective backyard. This group and other concerned citizens considered the waste management facility siting efforts by the industry and the collaboration of local government bodies to be a form of environmental abuse and exploitation where social equity and environmental quality are neglected.

Protest in the community was partially based on the fact that in the area where they lived, there were already many other toxic exposures and hazardous conditions affecting the quality of the environment, therefore, the establishment of the incinerator would compound their environmental burdens. There were numerous junkyards that burned unregulated trash and tires all year around. There were bulk-storage gas tanks in the area. An asphalt company and a cement factory nearby contributed to noise and air pollution in the area. Community leaders feared that the constant onslaught of environmental pollutants and waste dumping was making the region potentially hazardous to all residents in the immediate area. The air and water quality of the region was deteriorating, and many in the community were concerned about risks to their health and declining property values.

Plus, there was a fenced-off holding pond that contained sludge and other liquid waste northwest of the industrial park that may have had negative effects on the local ground water. Many of the neighboring residents relied on wells for their water, and there was farmland immediately adjacent to the toxic pond. The Flint River was considered one of the most polluted rivers in Michigan. It ran close to the area, so the water table was relatively high. In addition, two streams that ran through the park to the river passed near residential sites. And, there was a fresh water reservoir a mile away.

Although these environmental factors could create a health risk for those living in the area, Genesee County was heavily residential and recreational, with many single-family dwellings. There were two apartment complexes in the area, several trailer home parks, and farms. There was an elementary school just across the road from the industrial park on the Flint side of Carpenter Road, a high school 1.2-miles away, and Mott Children's Farm in the vicinity. Much of the area was used for recreational purposes. With the Flint River nearby, boating and fishing were common activities, as well as swimming at Blue Bell Beach for children. The recreational aspect of the area made it ideal for some tourism and an outlet for children of all ages to learn, explore, and have fun.

Community activists were concerned about the fact that the waste wood to be burned at the facility would include construction and demolition debris and possibly virgin wood. Because a number of toxic chemicals such as sealants, paints, and stains are on demolition wood, the Genesee County Medical Society felt that burning of demolition wood may lead to the release of many toxic chemicals. Even though the plans were to remove painted and treated wood from the fuel supply, experts believed that it was not possible to remove all of the toxic or hazardous materials from the waste stream. The plant would burn wood chips at a temperature of more than 2,000°F, 24 hours a day, 7 days a week, for at least 35 years. Up to 175,000 tons of recycled wood chips would be burned yearly.

The representatives of the power industry stated that they had selected the area because of its convenience. It had an infrastructure in the industrial park, so there was already highway access, an existing road of entry, rail tracks nearby, water and gas pipes, electric power lines, sewage systems, and plenty of space for facility structures. They also stated that the technology to be used was the state-of-the-art and would have minimal environmental impacts on the ambient surroundings.

However, those opposed to the facility did not find the arguments of industry to be convincing enough to accept the siting in their neighborhood. United for Action held the belief that the facility would represent an environmental threat to their community's health and quality of life. There had long been dumping and burning of waste in the area. Public health in the region was poor, and Genesee County had one of the highest infant mortality rates in the whole state. At least 17 percent of the children in Flint had dangerously high blood lead levels, as confirmed by the Genesee County Department of Health. Cancer cases were on the rise, and there were many residents in the area with respiratory problems. Tire burning was unregulated in the area, so an incinerator would (in the minds of the people) compound the problem.

Moreover, many residents in the area considered the facility siting an issue of environmental injustice, as there were pockets of low-income and minority populations residing in the immediate vicinity of the site. This claim of siting inequity is partially supported by the fact that Genesee County has a minority population of 22 percent while Flint has a minority population of 52 percent, and the wood waste facility site was just a half-mile outside the Flint city limits.

The Ridge Crest Village and Housing and Urban Development (HUD)-run River Park Apartments both had resident populations at up to 90 percent ethnic minorities. African-American families occupied many of the single-family houses, and the portion of the city of Flint nearest to the proposed facility was mostly African American. Coincidence or not, it appeared that African-American residents would be the most affected group in the area. The white residents in the area were mostly lower income and retired, so they could be considered "victims of class and age" in their location to the incinerator siting. All in all, the community was socially, politically, and economically disadvantaged. Because the actual site for the proposed waste-to-energy facility was in Genesee County, the residents of Flint had no say, because it was out of their jurisdiction. Genesee Township is more than five miles away, so the proximal effects of the facility were not an issue to those residents. They favored the Genesee Power Station (GPS). But to the residents of Genesee County in the immediate vicinity and Flint's northern side, it was an incinerator that would pollute the ambient air and land. The siting seemed strategic to get the least community resistance to implementation. Those on the Flint side of Carpenter Road were closest to the facility but were relatively powerless to do anything legally and would be more immediately affected environmentally than those in Genesee Township.

The coalition's biggest fear was that if the permit for the GPS facility went through, it would make it easier for other similar facilities to be sited there. There was already a proposal for a biomedical waste incinerator to be placed in the industrial park, and there was some talk of a tar-burning facility to be sited at that location as well. This was a community at extreme environmental risk; already dealing with existing pollution, their neighborhoods were being singled-out for additional dumping. It might have been circumstantial evidence, but it appeared to be systematic exploitation of a vulnerable, target community. The community on the Flint side of Carpenter Road basically lacked financial resources, political clout, and regional solidarity. But the residents of this "environmental war zone" were determined to fight this and any other attempts to further degrade and damage their living space.

The president of the local chapter of the National Association for the Advancement of Colored People (NAACP) said she represented a community seeking "environmental justice." She argued that "environmental racism" was a prime mover in decisions to place hazardous substances and materials recovery facilities disproportionately in low-income and minority neighborhoods. She further elaborated, "Although we support the struggles of the environmental movement . . . it has become shockingly clear that the real and most endangered species is the people and communities of color!" She felt that this facility "seems to be a deliberate act of genocide to further poison this community!" She cited the United Church of Christ's 1987 *Report on Toxic Waste and Race* and stated that there were three criteria that determine the incidence of siting: economic status, level of education of residents, and race. She proposed that several questions be asked when looking for environmental equity in incinerator siting: Who is behind this incinerator? What type of waste will be incinerated? What types of fumes will be emitted? What will happen to it? Why was the north end of Flint chosen? How many proposed incinerators are there for the other areas of the county?

In the meantime, the Genesee County Medical Society and the Mackinac Chapter of the Sierra Club sent letters to the commission seeking a delay in any decision on the permit until certain questions were answered. The Sierra Club chapter president suggested that the GPSLP should be forced to consider another system, called a dry scrubber baghouse system, to remove mercury and acidic gases from the furnace's emissions. He believed that system (which captures particles in a large, coated bag), though more expensive, would be more efficient than an electrostatic precipitator.

The chairman of the Environmental Health Committee met with community representatives to discuss the health implications to the community. He issued a press release against the development. Representatives of the Genesee County Health Department wrote letters of concern for the potential health hazards. In addition, the deputy director of environment and occupational health at the American Lung Association of Michigan (ALAM) hand delivered a letter to the Michigan Air Pollution Control Commission (MAPCC) and the Michigan Department of Natural Resources (MDNR) regarding the proposed air discharge. The ALAM opposed issuance of the permit until after the U.S. Environmental Protection Agency, Region V, could conduct a complete review of the proposed facility and its proposed permit and until the EPA could review public comments of ALAM and others offered during the commission hearings.

After much debate, probing, and cross-examination, the MAPCC decided to grant the air use permit to the Genesee Power Station Limited Partnership by a vote of six to one. The vote came at 12:45 a.m. at the end of a 15-hour meet-

ing. The commission's approval gave developers of the Genesee Power Station the legal collateral they needed to complete the financing arrangement and begin building the plant. The partnership was successful in convincing the commission that their operation would have minimal impact on the social and physical environment of the Genesee/Flint area. The commission seemed swayed by the economic and technical arguments in favor of GPS. The prospect of new jobs for the region, increased revenues for local businesses, and a better tax base for the county were influential factors. Even though there could have been other sites in the county, this site did have the best infrastructure; it was cheaper and more convenient for industry to be there. The public health and environmental concerns were taken into consideration, but a review of the proposal by MDNR staff concluded that the plant's air emissions would meet state regulations. This was a significant finding that greatly influenced the commission's decision.

The reaction to the decision from community organizers was expectantly emotional and resentful, but not defeatist. Almost immediately, opponents of GPS asked EPA to review the decision. The Michigan Air Pollution Control Commission received petitions from the American Lung Association–Michigan, Flint Neighborhood Coalition (FNC), Society of African American People, and the National Association for the Advancement of Colored People. The Michigan Department of Natural Resources reviewed the petitions.

In their response to the petitions, the MDNR submitted that the commission had properly issued the Prevention of Significant Deterioration (PSD) permit in accordance with the requirements of state and federal air quality regulations, and that the petitioners had failed to demonstrate that the final PSD permit determination had been based on erroneous findings of fact or conclusion of the law. The MDNR further stated that all petitioners failed to establish an important matter of policy or exercise of discretion that warrants review, and that the petitioners had utterly failed to carry their burden of proof in the case. Therefore, MDNR declared that all of the petitions for review were to be denied.

By July 1995, members of Flint-Genesee United for Action, Justice, and Environmental Safety (plaintiffs) filed a complaint in the Genesee Circuit Court alleging that the permit to operate the waste-to-energy plant violated Title VI of the Civil Rights Act, the equal protection clause of the Michigan

Constitution, and the Michigan Environmental Protection Act. The plaintiffs' complaint also alleged a violation of the provision for equal enjoyment of public services under Michigan's Elliott–Larsen Civil Rights Act and sought broad equitable relief to enjoin the incinerator's operation and required the MDEQ to alter the permit.

In October 1995, the federal court dismissed the Title VI claim allowing the Genesee Power Station to begin operation in November 1995. Still, in 1996, the Lawyers Guild/Sugar Law Center secured a landmark consent judgment against the power plant that severely limited the amount of lead-tainted demolition wood that the facility could burn.

Representing the National Association for the Advancement of Colored People (NAACP) and the community organization, Flint-Genesee United for Action, Justice, and Environmental Safety, the Lawyers Guild/Sugar Law Center continued to appeal the case without success. However, on May 29, 1997, a circuit court judge enjoined the Michigan Department of Environmental Quality (MDEQ) from granting permits to major polluting facilities seeking to operate in Genesee County until there was a risk assessment analysis paid for by the industry. The judge stated that although the plaintiff failed to demonstrate intended "environmental racism," the MDEQ was negligent by granting operating permits to a potentially major polluter industry without assessing the cumulative risk factors affecting the local population. The ruling suggests that the plaintiffs need only prove that a state's permit policies resulted in a disparate impact on people of color and not discriminatory intent. This ruling is the first under a state constitution. This case encompasses the essence of the environmental justice movement and is a piece of a larger national effort.

In a final appeal by the defendants, the Michigan Court of Appeals vacated the injunction, ruling that the trial court had no authority to issue an injunction of its own based on a claim that the parties had neither pleaded nor litigated. The community chose not to appeal that decision to the Michigan Supreme Court. This case, while clearly showing how the environmental justice movement has led to new coalitions of civil rights organizations, health advocates, and environmentalists, also demonstrates how difficult it is for communities to use existing legislation to change hazardous waste siting decisions.

The emergence of environmental justice as a social movement has established an ideology that challenges the traditional apathy of many communities. The sheer existence of its symbolic call for justice has empowered many local activists across the country to confront corporations and community institutions and question business and policy decisions that affect the environment. With the collective cause being the protection of public health, environmental conditions, and the quality of life, public health practitioners along with community activists are supporting the development of policies to reduce, reuse, and recycle the waste stream and to promote greater environmental equity.

REFERENCES

1. Toossi M. A century of change: The U.S. labor force, 1950–2050 Monthly Labor Review 2002;125:15–28.
2. Murray LR. Sick and tired of being sick and tired. Am J Public Health 2003;93:221–6.
3. Kim M. Women paid low wages, who they are and where they work. Monthly Labor Review 2000;123:26–30.
4. Bureau of Labor Statistics. Lost-worktime injuries and illnesses: Characteristics and resulting days away from work, USDOL release 04-260, 2004. Available at <www.bls.gov/iif/home.htm>.
5. Messing K, Punnett L, Bond M, et al. Be the fairest of them all: Challenges and recommendations for the treatment of gender in occupational health research. Am J Ind Med 2003;43:618–29.
6. Presser H. Working in a 24/7 economy: Challenges for American families. New York: Russell Sage Foundation, 2003.
7. Cherniack, M. The Hawk's Nest incident: America's worst industrial disaster. New Haven, CT: Yale University Press, 1986.
8. Williams DR, Neighbors HW, Jackson JS. Racial ethnic discrimination and health: Findings from community studies. Am J Public Health 2003;93:200–8.
9. National Urban League. The state of black America. Washington, DC: National Urban League, 2004.
10. Sum A, Fogg N, Harrington P. Immigrant workers and the great American job machine: The contributions of new foreign immigration to national and regional labor force growth in the 1990s. Boston: Northeastern University, Center for Labor Market Studies, 2002.
11. U.S. Census Bureau. Population Profile of the United States: 2000. Available at <http://www.census.gov/population/www/pop-profile/profile2000.html>.
12. Loh K, Richardson S. Foreign-born workers: Trends in fatal occupational injuries, 1996–2001. Monthly Labor Review 2004;127:42–53.
13. Dong X, Platner J. Occupational fatalities of Hispanic construction workers from 1992 to 2000. Am J Ind Med 2004;45:45–54.
14. Passel J, Capps R, Fix M. Undocumented immigrants: Facts and figures. Washington, D.C. Urban Institute, 2004. Available at <http://www.urban.org>.
15. National Research Council. Protecting youth at work. Washington DC: National Academies Press, 1998.
16. Committee on the Health and Safety of Older Workers, Institute of Medicine, National Research Council. Health and safety needs of older workers. Washington, DC: National Academies Press, 2004.

17. American Association of Retired People. Staying ahead of the curve: The AARP work and career study. Washington, DC: AARP, 2002. Available at <http://research.aarp.org/econ/multiwork.html>.

18. Moen P, Robison J, Dempster-McClain D. Caregiving and women's well-being: A life course approach. J Health Soc Behav 1995;36:259–73.

19. Northridge ME, Stover GN Rosenthal JE, et al. Environmental equity and health: Understanding complexity and moving forward. Am J Pub Health 2003;93: 209–13.

20. Bullard RD. Solid waste sites and the Black Houston community. Sociological Inquiry 1983;53:273–88.

21. Burke LM. Race and environmental equity: A geographic analysis in Los Angeles. Geo Info Systems 1993;3:44–50.

BIBLIOGRAPHY

Bullard RD. Dumping in Dixie: Race, class and environmental quality. Boulder, CO: Westview Press, 1990.

Bullard RD, ed. Confronting environmental racism: Voices from the grassroots. Boston: South End Press, 1993.
Robert Bullard has been one of the most prominent voices in the environmental justice movement. The first book was one of the most important initial voices for the environmental justice movement. The second is an excellent collection of essays covering a broad range of environmental justice struggles.

Frumkin H, Pransky G, eds. Special populations. Occupational Medicine: State of the Art Reviews 1999;14:479–705.
This special issue provides an excellent overview of the issue with in-depth chapters focusing on specific populations including minorities, women, children, disabled, and contingent workers.

National Institute for Occupational Safety and Health. Worker health chartbook, 2004. Washington, DC: NIOSH, 2004. (NIOSH publication no. 2004-146.) Available at <http://www.cdc.gov/niosh/docs/chartbook/>.
This contains up-to-date statistics on occupational injuries and illnesses with sections on older and younger workers as well as racial and ethnic minorities.

National Research Council. Protecting youth at work. Washington, DC: National Academies Press, 1998.
A very complete analysis of safety and health for youth workers based on a multi-year review of the information by a national panel of experts. Includes detailed recommendations.

National Research Council. Safety is seguridad. Washington, DC: National Academies Press, 2003.
This book contains an overview of the most important issues concerning the improved dissemination of safety and health materials for the Hispanic working population. It also includes five white papers developed for a NRC workshop covering issues related to the statistics on injuries and deaths, availability of Spanish-language materials, and the considerations in developing culturally and linguistically appropriate safety and health materials.

U.S. Census Bureau. Population profile of the United States: 2000. Available at <http://www.census.gov/population/www/pop-profile/profile2000.html>.
This Web site contains detailed profiles of various population groups with statistics from the 2000 Census.

United Church of Christ, Commission for Racial Justice. Toxic waste and race in the United States: A national report on the racial and socio-economic characteristics of communities and hazardous waste sites. New York: Public Data Access, Inc., 1987.

United Church of Christ, Commission for Racial Justice. Toxic waste and race revisited. Washington, DC: Center for Policy Alternatives, 1994.
These two documents are landmark reports that documented the inequalities in the location of hazardous wastes sites. They had a major impact on the evolution of the environmental justice movement.

U.S. Department of Labor. Report on the youth labor force. Washington, DC: U.S. Department of Labor, 2000. Available at <http://www.bls.gov/opub/rylf/rylfhome.htm>.
Very complete statistics on the number and composition of young workers.

The findings and conclusions in this chapter are those of the authors and do not necessarily represent the views of the National Institute for Occupational Safety and Health.

CHAPTER 32

Addressing Health and Safety Hazards in Specific Industries: Agriculture, Construction, and Health Care

Sherry L. Baron, Laura S. Welch, and Jane A. Lipscomb

A 20-year-old immigrant farmworker was asked to place soil around the perimeter of a tarp covering a field that had been fumigated by injecting methyl bromide gas into the soil. The field was to be used to plant strawberries. It was his first day of work, and he was eager to prove that he was a good worker. It was 104°F, and after about 4 hours of this work he began to feel nauseous and dizzy. A co-worker told him to drink more water and to take a rest, but he continued to work because he was afraid he would not finish the task. After another hour, he was too dizzy to continue working. He was taken to the clinic in town, where the physician asked the worker's supervisor some questions and, after looking up the toxicity of methyl bromide, learned that heat would hasten the volatilization of the gas from the soil. Except for a slightly increased heart rate, the worker's physical examination was normal. Blood tests showed slight electrolyte abnormalities. The doctor diagnosed the worker as having either mild methyl bromide poisoning or heat exhaustion. The doctor called the closest major laboratory several hours away and found that it would take at least a week to obtain the results of a blood sample for methyl bromide levels. He called the regional poison control center, which told him that there was no specific treatment for mild methyl bromide intoxication. He decided to treat the worker for mild heat exhaustion and had the health educator explain to the worker, in Spanish, the need for frequent rest breaks and good

hydration when working in extreme heat and about ways of recognizing and preventing pesticide exposure.*

Some industries pose especially complex challenges for occupational and environmental health professionals due to the variability of exposures and the high mobility of the workforce. In these industries, where workers perform a variety of tasks as they are exposed to many different hazards, it can be difficult to determine which exposure, if any, is responsible for a worker's health complaint. Sometimes, as in the above case, multiple exposures may interact, making diagnosis, treatment, and prevention especially difficult. Although knowledge of the health effects of individual hazards is important, occupational and environmental health professionals need to appreciate the complex ways in which workers experience these hazards and how the dynamic characteristics of industry can challenge their ability to control exposures and resultant health effects. In this chapter, we describe three important industries where workers face many hazards and where job mobility and task variability make assessment and control of hazards challenging.

Although fictitious, this case was derived from the experience of Dr. Rupali Das, Director of the Pesticide Illness Surveillance Program at the Occupational Health Branch of the California Department of Health Services.

AGRICULTURAL WORKERS

Sherry L. Baron

Worldwide, more people work in agriculture than in any other industry, with most engaged in labor-intensive, small-scale subsistence farming. In the United States, although agriculture is dominated by larger and more mechanized production, farm work remains one of the most labor-intensive and lowest paid occupations. The broad occupational category of farmworker includes both family farmers who work on their own farms and hired farmworkers. Although this chapter focuses on the approximately 2 million hired farmworkers, family farm owners face many of the same classes and combinations of hazards.

In the United States, 84 percent of hired farmworkers are Hispanic and 79 percent were born in Mexico.[1] One-third of the foreign-born workers are recent immigrants who have worked in the United States for 2 years or less; many are living apart from their families and experiencing social isolation that creates additional stress. Farmworkers are younger (average age of 31) than the general workforce and most (79 percent) are men. Most have a very low literacy level, which can have significant impact on their ability to read warning labels or understand safety instructions. Only 22 percent of workers can read and write English well and more than half have less than an eighth grade education. For the many who come from rural areas of Mexico, where an indigenous language is spoken, Spanish is their second and English would be their third language.

Forty-two percent of farmworkers face additional stress because of their needs to migrate for work and live temporarily away from their homes, often in crowded and inadequate housing. Hired farmworkers, on average, only work in agriculture about 8 months of the year. Due to low wages and extended periods of unemployment, for more than half of hired farmworkers family income is less than $15,000 per year. Fifty-three percent are not legally authorized to work in the United States; therefore, they may be vulnerable to abuse and are unlikely to report mistreatment.

Occupational Exposures

In 1960, Edward R. Murrow's classic documentary, *Harvest of Shame*, shocked viewers by depicting the deplorable working conditions of farmworkers in the United States. Nonetheless, little attention was paid toward improving safety and health conditions for agricultural workers until relatively recently. In 1991, the Surgeon General convened a national meeting on the health of agricultural workers, and subsequently the National Institute for Occupational Safety and Health (NIOSH) established a network of research centers to improve health and safety of family farmers and hired farmworkers. In 1995, NIOSH convened a special panel to make recommendations on the priority occupational health problems for hired farmworkers.[2] This panel selected nine priority health outcomes as a focus for future research and intervention (Table 32-1). The most common of these occupational health problems are discussed in more detail below.

Musculoskeletal Conditions

From strawberry pickers harvesting crops in a sustained stooped posture to citrus pickers carrying heavy sacks up ladders while reaching for the next orange, farm work is associated with a variety of musculoskeletal disorders (Fig. 32-1). In addition, because one-fifth of farmworkers are paid based on the quantity of crops harvested (piece rate), in many work settings there are economic incentives for them to maintain a rapid, sustained work pace. About one-half of all agricultural injuries requiring time away from work are musculoskeletal injuries, such as sprains, strains, and injuries causing low back pain. To prevent such injuries, some research centers are developing innovative, low-cost methods of improving the ergonomic design of farm work, such as a redesigned tool to carry potted plants (Fig. 32-2).

Pesticide-Related Illness

Pesticide-related illness refers to a broad group of health outcomes, including dermatitis, cancer, eye injuries, and respiratory diseases. Although many research studies have been conducted on the toxicology and health effects of pesticides, few of these studies have been directed at the hired farmworker population. There is no national surveillance system to accurately record the national incidence or prevalence of pesticide-related illnesses that occur in the farm sector. California, which employs about one-third of all farmworkers in the United States, is one of the few states with a mandatory reporting system for occupational pesticide intoxications. Its data provide useful information on the nature of

TABLE 32-1

Selected Hazards, Health Effects, and Control Strategies in Agriculture

Health Effect	Hazard	Control Strategy
Musculoskeletal disorders	Prolonged stooping, heavy lifting, repetitive movements of the upper extremities during planting, pruning, and harvesting	Ergonomic reengineering of tools and workplace; decrease of weight of the loads; job rotation among repetitive and nonrepetitive tasks
Pesticide-related conditions	Mixing, loading, and applying pesticides; working in fields recently sprayed with pesticides; aerial drift of pesticides from adjacent fields; exposure to pesticides in living quarters	Substitution of less toxic substances; adequate protective equipment; training on prevention of pesticide exposures; administrative restrictions on working in fields where exposure may occur
Traumatic injuries	Work-related incidents with tractors and other farm equipment; motor vehicle crashes during transport to and from the fields; lacerations from sharp tools for cutting and pruning	Use of roll-over protection systems in tractors; training and enforcement of safe use of equipment; transportation vehicles equipped with personal restraint systems; safe cutting tools
Respiratory conditions	Airborne exposure to allergic and irritant substances, either naturally occurring in the soil and crops or due to chemical substances	Substitution of less toxic materials; use of respirators, if indicated; administrative controls to remove sensitized workers from exposure
Dermatitis	Skin contact with allergic and irritant substances, either naturally occurring in the soil and crops or in fertilizers and pesticides	Substitution of less toxic materials; use of gloves and sleeves, if indicated; administrative controls to remove sensitized workers from exposure
Infectious diseases	Inadequate sanitation facilities; exposure to tuberculosis, sexually transmitted diseases, and other infectious diseases due to living arrangements of migrant workers	Improved sanitation facilities; improved housing facilities; improved health care screening and treatment services
Cancer	Exposure to chemical substances in pesticides and other agricultural products; prolonged sun exposure	Substitution for less hazardous substances; protective clothing and sunscreen; administrative controls to limit exposure
Eye conditions	Exposure to dusty conditions; foreign bodies from plant material penetrating the eye	Use of protective eye wear; dust control
Mental disorders	Long working hours; inadequate pay; social isolation from family and friends	Improved working and housing conditions; availability of mental health services

farmworkers' exposures to pesticides (Table 32-2). Most overexposures do not occur in those who are applying pesticides but instead to workers who are inadvertently exposed to pesticides while performing routine farm tasks, such as harvesting and weeding. These overexposures commonly occur when pesticides being sprayed on one field drift into the breathing zone of farmworkers in nearby fields or when workers handle crops covered with pesticide residues.[3] Although less than one-third of pesticide poisoning cases lead to lost time from work, given the economic insecurity of most farmworkers, it is difficult to determine if this reflects the affected workers' need to continue working rather than the mild severity of most cases.

Traumatic Injuries

Agriculture is considered one of the most hazardous industries for occupational injuries and deaths.

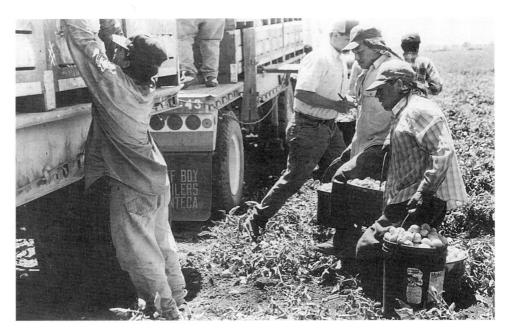

FIGURE 32-1 ● Farmworkers carrying buckets of tomatoes to be counted. These workers are paid based on the numbers of tomatoes they pick, which encourages them to work fast and carry very heavy loads. Bending and carrying heavy loads can cause musculoskeletal disorders. (Photograph by David Bacon.)

Agriculture has an occupational fatality rate comparable to the mining industry with close to 23 fatalities per 100,000 workers. In 2003, the fatality rate in agriculture was almost twice the rate in both the construction and transportation industries.

About one-half of all agricultural fatalities occur as a result of transportation accidents, primarily related to tractors. The use of new roll-over protective structures on tractors has helped to prevent these fatalities.

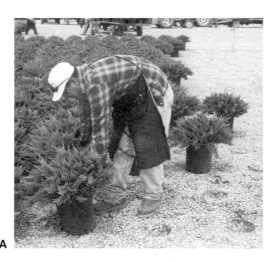

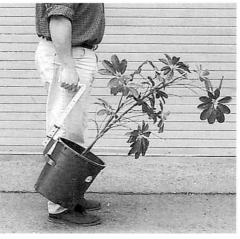

A   B

FIGURE 32-2 ● **(A)** Picking up and carrying large potted plants in this manner increases the risk of low back and upper extremity injuries. **(B)** This device, used as an ergonomic intervention for nursery workers, reduces the need to bend in order to pick up potted plants; it also has a handle designed to decrease stress on the upper extremities. (Courtesy of University of California Davis.)

TABLE 32-2

Characteristics of 486 Farmworker Pesticide Illness Cases Reported to the California Department of Health Services Pesticide Illness Surveillance System during 1998–1999

Characteristics	Number (Percent)
Demographic characteristics	
Hispanic surname	413 (85)
Male	387 (80)
Age, years: mean (range)	35 (13–73)
Organ system affected	
Dermatologic	215 (44)
Ocular	158 (33)
Nervous system	188 (39)
Gastrointestinal	185 (38)
Respiratory	115 (24)
Other	99 (20)
Time lost from work	
Yes	142 (29)
No	235 (48)
Not documented	109 (22)
Activity when illness occurred	
Applying pesticides	116 (24)
Mixing or loading pesticides	23 (5)
Routine activity, primarily field work	313 (64)
Other	12 (3)
Unknown	22 (5)

Adapted from Das R, Steege A, Baron S, et al. Pesticide-related illness among migrant farmworkers in the United States. Int J Occup Environ Health 2001;7:303–12.

The nonfatal occupational injury rate in farmworkers is about 7.5 injuries per 100 workers per year. Because of the lack of mandatory workers' compensation coverage for many agricultural workers and their fear of lost wages, there is probably significant underreporting of work-related injuries. For example, a study in North Carolina, a state that does not have comprehensive workers' compensation for farmworkers, found that 24 (8.4 percent) of 287 workers reported an injury at work in the previous 3 years. Of the 17 injured workers who considered medical attention necessary, 41 percent did not receive it within 24 hours, and 24 percent never received it. The most common reason why workers did not receive medical attention was refusal by their supervisors for them to leave work or lack of transportation. Medical expenses were paid for by employers for only 38 percent of injuries.[4]

Dermatitis

Dermatitis among agricultural workers has been associated with exposures to (a) a variety of chemical agents including pesticides; (b) sensitivity to plant materials, such as poison ivy and poison oak; and (c) infectious agents. In 2002, agricultural workers had the highest reported incidence rate of cases of dermatitis—more than twice that of manufacturing workers. Dermatitis is one of the major health problems associated with pesticide exposure (Table 32-2). A study at four clinics located along the Midwest migrant stream found that for men ages 20 to 29, dermatitis was the primary cause of clinic visits and, for men ages 30 to 44, dermatitis was second only to hypertension-related visits. The rate of dermatitis among these farmworkers was 2.5 times that of the general population.[5]

Children in Agriculture

Agricultural work is one of the most common forms and also the most dangerous form of child labor. In the United States, more than 2 million youths under age 20 are potentially exposed to agricultural hazards each year including farm residents, farmworkers, children of migrant or seasonal workers, and farm visitors (Fig. 32-3).[6] Although many of these youths are paid or unpaid children of family farmers, an increasingly important group of hired farmworkers are self-emancipated minors, who are primarily unauthorized recent immigrants living and working away from their families. These workers are especially vulnerable to injury because of their age, their undocumented legal status, and their social isolation from friends and family (see Chapter 31).

In 1998, there were about 33,000 injuries to children on farms in the United States. The primary causes of injury were falls and incidents involving animals and farm vehicles. Between 1982 and 1996, there were more than 2,000 farm deaths in children under age 20—almost half in children under age 10. The most common causes of deaths were machinery accidents, such as from tractors, and drowning.

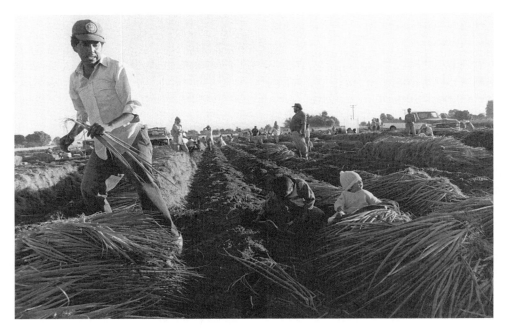

FIGURE 32-3 ● Toddlers play in the rows of a field of green onions while their parents work. (Photograph by David Bacon.)

Federal child labor laws, which regulate working conditions for minors, have many dual standards that provide lesser protection for children employed in agriculture than children employed in other industries, including:

- The minimum permissible work age is 14 in agriculture and 16 in other industries.
- Children ages 12 or 13 may work in agriculture with the consent of their parents.
- Work tasks that have been designated as hazardous by the federal government can be done at age 16 in agriculture but not until age 18 in other industries.

In 1996, a national coalition of organizations issued a National Action Plan entitled "Children and Agriculture: Opportunities for Safety and Health," which led to special congressional funding to improve research and prevention of child agricultural injuries. One of the major accomplishments of this initiative has been the creation of the North American Guidelines for Children's Agricultural Tasks, which, in the absence of laws to restrict hazardous work tasks for youth, created voluntary guidelines to assist adults in assigning age-appropriate tasks to children ages 7 to 16. These guidelines primarily focus on educating family farmers and influencing their decisions about which farm tasks their children can safely perform.[7]

Federal Regulations and Health Services Programs for Farmworkers

Most federal occupational health laws are less protective of agricultural workers than other industrial workers. Many Occupational Safety and Health Administration (OSHA) standards, such as the Hazard Communication Standard and protections against electrocutions and unguarded machinery, explicitly exclude agricultural workers. In addition, OSHA is prohibited from regulating farms with fewer than 11 employees. The OSHA regulations targeting agriculture include the Field Sanitation Standard, which requires drinking water, handwashing water, and toilets in the fields; regulations that require roll-over protective structures (ROPS) in tractors manufactured after 1976; and regulations concerning housing conditions in temporary labor camps operated by agricultural employers.

Occupational pesticide exposure is unique in that it is the only occupational exposure that is entirely regulated by the Environmental Protection Agency (EPA). In 1992, under the Federal Insecticide, Fungicide and Rodenticide Act (FIFRA),

EPA promulgated the Worker Protection Standard. This federal regulation governs the use of agricultural pesticides used for commercial production purposes. Its worker health and safety provisions require mandatory training programs, enforcement of pesticide reentry intervals, and provision of decontamination washing facilities. The enforcement of this standard, which is implemented by cooperative agreements between EPA and state agencies, has been criticized as being inadequate, in part because of the limitation of FIFRA to impose penalties against employers.

Under the Migrant Health Act of 1962, the federal government provides support to more than 120 community-based and state organizations that offer comprehensive primary care services to address the unique needs of hired farmworkers. As a result of this program, a network of migrant health clinics has been created that improves the provision of health care services for this unique worker population. However, significant obstacles still exist due to cultural, linguistic, and logistical barriers that result in many farmworkers lacking adequate health coverage (Box 32-1).

BOX 32-1

Farmworker Health in a Binational Context

Rick Mines

We walked up to the second story of a paint-deprived wooden apartment building on the outskirts of Salinas, California. The flat had two small bedrooms and a living room/kitchen combination. Furniture was scarce but clean. Cesar, 29, lived there with his wife and three small children. Cesar had come from a small town in southern Zacatecas for the first time about 10 years before. In the town, he had finished primary school and then worked helping his father plant corn, beans, and squash. He also had worked as a sharecropper for a neighbor planting hot chilis on irrigated land and worked tending cattle. But, like most young people from the town, he decided to follow his relatives and friends north to the Salinas area. He had come and gone from his hometown many times in the early years during the 10 years, working mostly in the lettuce and cabbage fields. His wife came across the border 4 years ago; two of his three children were born in Salinas. Cesar is lucky; he has a work permit and is waiting for his green card.

Cesar feels like he is doing pretty well. He gets about 8 months a year of work in the fields and earns about $15,000 a year. However, when the topic turned to the asthmatic condition of his son Salvador, his mood changed abruptly. He launched into an angry condemnation of the medical system in California. He had taken Salvador to many doctors, but no one really helped. They went to the clinic where they waited a long time to be seen. Finally, the doctor saw them. But, he did not speak Spanish well enough to communicate so they did not understand what he said. But, the worst part is that he did not give them any medicine to cure Salvador. They went

back several times to see the doctor who asked for several laboratory tests, all of which were very expensive. Finally, after many visits, he was given some medicine that did not work. Cesar is sure that the doctor is just trying to make money by delaying treatment, calling for tests, and charging money for everything. Cesar is now saddled with medical debt because of his interaction with this doctor. Cesar ended up taking his son back to Mexico where he got medicine that works. Cesar is furious and is convinced that the U.S. doctors are just a bunch of charlatans making money off poor Mexican immigrants.

The Binational Farmworker Health Survey (BFHS)

Why are Cesar and so many other farmworkers so angry about the treatment they get in our medical system? What is it about the system or about them that makes the relationship such a difficult one? To answer that question, we carried out a binational survey that took place partly in rural Zacatecas and partly in various settlement communities in the United States. By going to the place of origin, we hoped to get some insight into this challenging conflict.

It was found that the experience of the farmworker immigrant population with health care is extremely different in their home areas. Almost all farmworkers come to the United States after already having been raised in rural or small town Mexico. This very contrasting formative experience makes for a very difficult adaptation to institutions in the United States. In the farmworkers' hometowns, medical practitioners ("medicos") do not have doctoral

(continued)

BOX 32-1

Farmworker Health in a Binational Context (Continued)

degrees. They go straight from high school to medical school and begin practicing after getting a bachelor's degree. In the small towns, several of them set up consultation offices directly connected to pharmacies. The incentive for these medicos/pharmacists is to sell medicine as a useful source of income. The medicos keep no or few records about patients, give quick service, and usually provide quick treatment in the form of shots and pills. There are few laboratory tests done and diagnosis is done on the spot. However, the medicos have excellent rapport with their patients. Many are known as being extremely skilled—if a bit intuitive—diagnosticians. They are willing to allow a mix of traditional healing practices with their modern medical techniques. And they

speak the same language of the people and share their sense of humor and cultural approach to solving problems.

When the Mexicans come north, they are faced with a totally different environment. The paperwork—a totally new experience—is overwhelming for a poorly educated group. The long waits, their treatment by intake staff (who may feel contemptuous of the workers even if they speak some Spanish), frequent testing, and, above all, the relative timidity of U.S. physicians about prescribing strong medicines leaves the farmworkers extremely confused and often angry.

The solution to this deep cultural clash probably does not lie in spending much money on extra care for the immigrants; it lies in designing institutions that provide immigrant farmworkers with alternatives more similar to their formative experience.

CONSTRUCTION WORKERS

Laura S. Welch

Construction workers build, repair, renovate, modify, and demolish structures: houses, office buildings, temples, factories, hospitals, roads, bridges, tunnels, stadiums, docks, airports, and more. Construction work is composed of many different tasks undertaken by many different trades. To understand the risk for injury and illness, one must understand the work of specific trades and their characteristic tasks (Table 32-3).

Construction often must be done in extreme heat or cold; in windy, rainy, snowy, or foggy weather; or at night. Intermittent and seasonal work adds to the health risks and stress of job insecurity. Episodic employment, frequent changes of employer, and continuous changes in worksite exposures and ambient conditions make it difficult to document workers' jobs and hazardous exposures. Because of these factors, some of which are unique to construction, data on the extent or effect of toxic exposures in the construction industry is limited.

In industrialized nations, construction is consistently ranked among the most dangerous occupations. In the United States, 19 percent of all fatal on-the-job injuries occur in construction—about three

times its 6 percent share of the total employment. One-half of all fatal falls occur in construction. For nonfatal injuries, in 2001 there were 4 lost work-day cases per 100 full-time equivalent construction workers, a rate exceeding all other sectors. Leading causes of injuries with days away from work among construction workers in 2001 were contact with objects (34 percent), falls (21 percent), and overexertion (20 percent). Leading specific diagnoses were strains and sprains (38 percent), cuts and lacerations (12 percent), fractures (11 percent), and bruises and contusions (7 percent).[8]

The annual costs of occupational injuries in all industries in the United States is an estimated $40 billion in direct costs and $131 to $145 billion when indirect costs are included. (Few of the costs for occupational diseases are included in these estimates.) Construction injuries comprise a disproportionate share of the total. In 2000, the average level of workers' compensation injury payments for construction was $7,542—nearly double the level for all industries. In 2002 in Washington State, 27 percent of all costs to the state's workers' compensation fund were from injured construction workers, although construction represented only 6 percent of the workforce. As an indicator of costs, workers' compensation premiums had a median cost of

TABLE 32-3

Construction Occupations and Tasks

Boilermakers	Construct, assemble, maintain, and repair stationary steam boilers and boiler house auxiliaries. Work involves use of hand and power tools, plumb bobs, levels, wedges, dogs, or turnbuckles. Assist in testing assembled vessels. Direct cleaning of boilers and boiler furnaces. Inspect and repair boiler fittings, such as safety valves, regulators, automatic-control mechanisms, water columns, and auxiliary machines.
Brickmasons	Lay and bind building materials, such as brick, structural tile, concrete block, cinder block, glass block, and terra-cotta block, with mortar and other substances to construct or repair walls, partitions, arches, sewers, and other structures.
Carpenters	Construct, erect, install, or repair structures and fixtures made of wood, such as concrete forms; building frameworks, including partitions, joists, studding, and rafters; wood stairways, window and door frames, and hardwood floors. May also install cabinets, siding, drywall, and batt or roll insulation
Carpet installers	Lay and install carpet from rolls or blocks on floors. Install padding and trim flooring materials.
Cement masons and concrete finishers	Smooth and finish surfaces of poured concrete, such as floors, walks, sidewalks, roads, or curbs using a variety of hand and power tools. Align forms for sidewalks, curbs, or gutters; patch voids; use saws to cut expansion joints.
Construction laborers	Perform tasks involving physical labor at building, highway, and heavy construction projects, tunnel and shaft excavations, and demolition sites. May operate hand and power tools of all types: air hammers, earth tampers, cement mixers, small mechanical hoists, surveying and measuring equipment, and a variety of other equipment and instruments. May clean and prepare sites, dig trenches, set braces to support the sides of excavations, erect scaffolding, clean up rubble and debris, and remove asbestos, lead, and other hazardous waste materials.
Drywall and ceiling tile installers	Apply plasterboard or other wallboard to ceilings or interior walls of buildings. Apply or mount acoustical tiles or blocks, strips, or sheets of shock-absorbing materials to ceilings and walls of buildings to reduce or reflect sound. Materials may be of decorative quality. Include lathers who fasten wooden, metal, or rockboard lath to walls, ceilings or partitions of buildings to provide support base for plaster, fire-proofing, or acoustical material.
Electricians	Install, maintain, and repair electrical wiring, equipment, and fixtures. Ensure that work is in accordance with relevant codes. May install or service street lights, intercom systems, or electrical control systems
Insulation workers	Apply insulating materials to pipes or ductwork or other mechanical systems in order to help control and maintain temperature. Also line and cover structures with insulating materials. May work with batt, roll, or blown insulation materials
Operating engineers	Operate one or several types of power construction equipment, such as motor graders, bulldozers, scrapers, compressors, pumps, derricks, shovels, tractors, or front-end loaders to excavate, move, and grade earth, erect structures, or pour concrete or other hard surface pavement. May repair and maintain equipment in addition to other duties.
Painters	Paint walls, equipment, buildings, bridges, and other structural surfaces, using brushes, rollers, and spray guns. May remove old paint to prepare surface prior to painting. May mix colors or oils to obtain desired color or consistency.
Paperhangers	Cover interior walls and ceilings of rooms with decorative wallpaper or fabric, or attach advertising posters on surfaces, such as walls and billboards. Duties include removing old materials from surface to be papered.

(continued)

TABLE 32-3 Continued

Construction Occupations and Tasks

Plumbers, pipefitters, and steamfitters	Assemble, install, alter, and repair pipelines or pipe systems that carry water, steam, air, or other liquids or gases. May install heating and cooling equipment and mechanical control systems.
Plasterers and stucco masons	Apply interior or exterior plaster, cement, stucco, or similar materials. May also set ornamental plaster.
Reinforcing iron and rebar workers	Position and secure steel bars or mesh in concrete forms in order to reinforce concrete. Use a variety of fasteners, rod-bending machines, blowtorches, and hand tools. Includes rod busters.
Roofers	Cover roofs of structures with shingles, slate, asphalt, aluminum, wood, and related materials. May spray roofs, sidings, and walls with material to bind, seal, insulate, or soundproof sections of structures.
Sheet-metal workers	Fabricate, assemble, install, and repair sheet-metal products and equipment, such as ducts, control boxes, drainpipes, and furnace casings. Work may involve any of the following: setting up and operating fabricating machines to cut, bend, and straighten sheet metal; shaping metal over anvils, blocks, or forms using hammer; operating soldering and welding equipment to join sheet-metal parts; inspecting, assembling, and smoothing seams and joints of burred surfaces. Includes sheet-metal duct installers who install prefabricated sheet-metal ducts used for heating, air conditioning, or other purposes.
Stonemasons	Build stone structures, such as piers, walls, and abutments. Lay walks, curbstones, or special types of masonry for vats, tanks, and floors.
Structural iron and steel workers	Raise, place, and unite iron or steel girders, columns, and other structural members to form completed structures or structural frameworks. May erect metal storage tanks and assemble prefabricated metal buildings.
Terrazzo workers and finishers	Apply a mixture of cement, sand, pigment, or marble chips to floors, stairways, and cabinet fixtures to fashion durable and decorative surfaces
Tile and marble setters	Apply hard tile, marble, and wood tile to walls, floors, ceilings, and roof decks.

Source: Bureau of Labor Statistics, Standard occupational classification manual, 1998 revision. Available at <http://stats.bls.gov/soc/socguide.htm>.

more than $30 per hour worked for ironworkers and roofers. In addition to worker's compensation, there are liability insurance premiums and other indirect costs, including (a) reduced work crew efficiency; (b) clean-up costs, such as from a cave-in or collapse; and (c) overtime costs necessitated by an injury.[9]

Occupational diseases are also an important cause of morbidity in construction workers. Table 32-4 summarizes sentinel health events that may occur in construction workers and specific exposures that can lead to these diseases. These hazardous exposures include air contaminants such as wood dust, abrasive blasting dust, gypsum and alkaline dusts, silica, asbestos, lead, diesel exhaust, and welding fumes.

Lead

Lead exposure and lead toxicity are particularly important problems in the construction industry. Excessive lead exposures are associated with several construction tasks.[10] Nearly 1 million U.S. construction workers are exposed to lead on the job; more than 80 percent of these workers are involved in commercial or residential remodeling. However, before 1993, the OSHA lead standard applied only to general industry, not to construction. In 1992, blood lead levels (BLLs) in bridge construction workers ranged from 51 to 160 μg/dL, with 62 percent of elevated BLLs involving work in a containment structure. High-risk activities associated with lead dust and

TABLE 32-4

Sentinel Health Events in Construction and Illustrative Examples

Condition	Industry/Process/Occupation	Agent
Asbestosis	Asbestos industries and users	Asbestos
Bronchitis (acute), pneumonitis, and pulmonary edema due to fumes and vapors	Arc welders, boilermakers	Nitrogen oxides Vanadium pentoxide
Chronic or acute renal failure	Plumbers	Inorganic lead
Contact and allergic dermatitis	Cement masons and finishers, carpenters, floorlayers	Adhesives and sealants, irritants (such as cutting oils, phenol, solvents, acids, alkalis, detergents); allergens (such as nickel, chromates, formaldehyde, dyes, rubber products).
Extrinsic asthma	Wood workers, furniture makers	Red cedar (plicatic acid) and other wood dusts
Histoplasmosis	Bridge maintenance workers	*Histoplasma capsulatum*
Inflammatory and toxic neuropathy	Furniture refinishers, degreasing operations	Hexane
Malignant neoplasm of scrotum	Chimney sweeps	Mineral oil, pitch, tar
Malignant neoplasm of nasal cavities	Wood workers, cabinet and furniture makers, carpenters	Hardwood and softwood dusts Chlorophenols
Malignant neoplasm of trachea, bronchus, and lung	Asbestos industries and users	Asbestos
Malignant neoplasm of nasopharynx	Carpenters, cabinetmakers	Chlorophenols
Malignant neoplasm of larynx	Asbestos industries and users	Asbestos
Mesothelioma (malignancy of peritoneum and pleura)	Asbestos industries and users	Asbestos
Noise effects on inner ear	Occupations with exposure to excessive noise	Excessive noise
Raynaud's phenomenon (secondary)	Jackhammer operators, riveters	Whole body or segmental vibration
Sequoiosis	Red cedar mill workers, wood workers	Redwood sawdust
Silicosis	Sandblasters	Silica
Silicotuberculosis	Sandblasters	Silica + *Mycobacterium tuberculosis*
Toxic encephalitis	Lead paint removal	Lead
Toxic hepatitis	Fumigators	Methyl bromide

Adapted from Mullan R, Murthy L. Occupational sentinel health events: An up-dated list for physician recognition and public health surveillance. Am J Ind Med 1991;19:775–99.

fumes among bridge and structural steel workers include abrasive blasting, sanding, burning, cutting or welding on steel structures coated with lead paint, and using containment enclosures. The 1993 OSHA lead standard incorporates a presumption of exposure during specific high-risk tasks and requires specific protections during these tasks, unless air monitoring demonstrates exposure below the permissible exposure limit (PEL). However, the OSHA standard may not fully protect construction workers from lead toxicity. The standard requires monitoring every 2 months, but some tasks, such as burning lead-coated steel, can cause a rapid rise in BLL. Thus, more frequent monitoring and a lower threshold for mandated industrial hygiene inspection or medical removal has been recommended in some circumstances.

Noise

Construction workers generally have excessive noise exposures and high rates of noise-induced hearing loss. More than 500,000 construction workers are exposed to potentially hazardous levels of noise. The United States has a different standard for regulation of noise exposure in construction than in general industry; in the construction standard, there is no action level above which a hearing conservation program is required, and there are no detailed requirements for training or record keeping. Yet the work is very noisy. For example, a laborer using a heavy-duty bulldozer is exposed to 91 to 107 dBA, with a mean of 99 dBA. Exposure in crane cabs ranges from a mean of 81 dBA in insulated cabs to 97 dBA in those without insulation, but there is little to no medical monitoring. Models for improvement exist. British Columbia implemented a specific hearing conservation program in construction in 1987. Since that time, reported use of hearing protection has increased from 55 to 85 percent of workers surveyed, and the proportion of construction workers age 50 to 59 with a hearing handicap has dropped from 36 to 25 percent. This program clearly demonstrates the feasibility and efficacy of a hearing conservation program.[11]

Musculoskeletal Disorders

Soft-tissue musculoskeletal injuries make up a high proportion of all work-related injuries in construction[12] (Fig. 32-4). In 2001, there were in the United States an estimated 185,700 injuries and illnesses with lost workdays in construction; 21 percent of these injuries were attributable to overexertion and 21 percent were injuries to the low back. The rates for these injuries are considerably higher in construction than in all private industry combined.[13] Construction workers retire 2 years earlier than the average worker, often because of musculoskeletal conditions, such as arthritis and degenerative disc disease.

Construction workers have a high prevalence of chronic musculoskeletal complaints, such as pain, aches, and discomfort. For example, about half of the electricians in one study had back and hand or wrist symptoms; more than 80 percent had symptoms in the prior year that lasted more than a week or recurred at least three times, and more than 60 percent reported symptoms in two or more body areas.

In 1998, 10 percent of construction workers in the United States reported back pain due to repeated injury at work—twice the rate of all workers. Severe hand discomfort was present in almost 16 percent of construction workers compared to 11 percent of all workers. Strains and sprains are the leading compensable injury for construction workers. (See also Chapter 23).

Respiratory Diseases

Construction workers are exposed to a variety of respiratory hazards, including asbestos, silica, synthetic vitreous fibers, cadmium, chromates, formaldehyde, resin adhesives, cobalt, metal fumes, creosote, gasoline, oils, diesel fumes, paint fumes and dusts, pitch, sealers, solvents, wood dusts and wood preservatives, and excessive cold.[14]

Surveillance data on occupational respiratory disease among construction workers are limited. In the United States, respiratory conditions account for 14 percent of the approximately 7,000 reported occupational illness cases among construction workers each year. Their relative risk for both lung cancer and emphysema is 1.3, suggesting a 30 percent excess due to occupational exposures.

Asbestosis

Asbestos has been recognized as a respiratory hazard for several construction trades. Occupational exposure to asbestos with resultant asbestosis occurs in many construction workers, especially insulators, plumbers and pipefitters, electricians, and

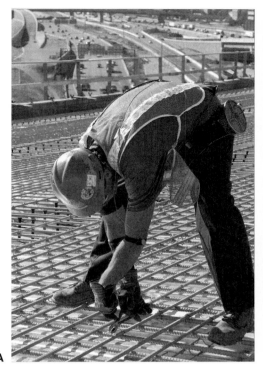 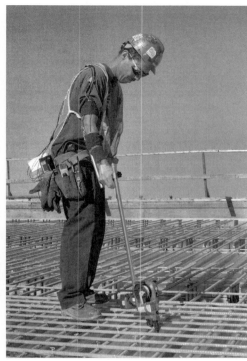

A B

FIGURE 32-4 ● **(A)** Construction workers are at increased risk of upper extremity and back strain. **(B)** An ergonomically designed device decreases the upper extremity and back strain on construction workers who are tying rebar. (Photographs by Earl Dotter.)

sheet-metal workers. Any construction worker may be at risk for asbestos-induced disease resulting from exposure associated with working near insulation. Although asbestos is no longer used in new residential or heavy construction, workers may continue to be exposed to previously installed asbestos during maintenance, renovation, addition, or demolition activities.

Silicosis

Occupational exposure to silica can occur among various types of construction workers, including those employed in concrete removal and demolition work, bridge and road construction, tunnel construction, and concrete or granite cutting, sanding, and grinding. Sandblasters are at increased risk from exposure to crystalline silica. Those working nearby on the same construction site may also be at risk from silica-related disease. In the United States, sand containing crystalline silica is still used in abrasive blasting operations for maintenance of structures, preparing surfaces for paint-

ing, and in forming decorative patterns during installation of building materials; these uses of sand have been banned in many other countries. Silica exposures in the construction industry in the United States continue to exceed recommended limits. Silicosis continues to occur in construction workers worldwide.

Chronic Obstructive Pulmonary Disease and Asthma

Chronic obstructive pulmonary disease (COPD) has been reported among construction workers exposed to asbestos, synthetic vitreous fibers, and welding fumes. Occupations at risk are spray painters, welders, tunnel construction workers, construction painters, and sheet-metal workers. Chronic nonspecific lung disease symptoms are increased among construction workers, woodworkers, and painters even after adjusting for smoking and age. Specific exposures associated with excess risk of chronic nonspecific lung disease include heavy metals, mineral dust, and adhesives. Construction workers can be exposed to many agents that can cause asthma and to cold, various particulates, dusts, fumes, and irritants, all of which can exacerbate underlying asthma. (See also Chapter 25).

Dermatitis

Construction workers are exposed to many chemicals that cause irritant or allergic dermatitis. Portland cement, found in plaster and in concrete mixes, is extremely alkaline. Wet plaster also contains slaked lime, or calcium hydroxide, which is even more caustic. In addition, Portland cement contains trace amounts of hexavalent chromium, a strong sensitizing agent responsible for allergic contact dermatitis in cement workers. Other sensitizing agents include epoxy adhesives, sealants, and chemicals mixed within cement and plaster. Rubber gloves also may cause allergic dermatitis.

One way to prevent allergic contact dermatitis in cement workers is to add ferrous sulfate. When ferrous sulfate is combined with hexavalent chromium in cement, it forms an insoluble trivalent compound when water is added; trivalent chromium is not easily absorbed by skin. In several Scandinavian countries where this is required by law, allergic contact dermatitis has been prevented in cement workers.

Cancer

Construction workers are exposed to many carcinogens (Table 32-5). Insulators, painters and plasterers, sheet-metal workers, and other construction workers are at increased risk of lung cancer. Woodworkers, cabinetmakers, and furniture makers as well as carpenters and joiners have an increased risk of nasal cancer. Excess rates of mesothelioma have been well documented in many trades after widespread exposure to asbestos from 1940 to 1980. Given the long latency period for mesothelioma, asbestos-related cases are likely to occur for many years to come.

REGULATIONS AND HEALTH SERVICES FOR CONSTRUCTION WORKERS

Construction workers are often not covered by the OSHA regulations that cover manufacturing and service sectors. For example, the standard for noise exposure for the construction industry has no action level above which a hearing conservation pro-

TABLE 32-5

Epidemiology of Lung Cancer in Construction Workers

Trade	Known Lung Carcinogens
Insulators	Asbestos
Painters and plasterers	Chromium, cadmium, asbestos
Sheet-metal workers	Asbestos, welding fume
Welders	Welding fume, asbestos, hexavalent chromium
Masons	Asbestos, hexavalent chromium, silica
Electricians	Asbestos
Plumbers and pipefitters	Asbestos, welding fume
Roofers	Coal tar, bitumen, PAHs
Carpenters	Wood dust

gram is required and no detailed requirements for training or record keeping. The OSHA lead standard did not apply to the construction industry until 1993, although many lead poisoning cases in the state lead registries were in construction workers. The rationale for separate OSHA standards for construction was that controls that work in general industry may not work in construction, and therefore feasibility of a standard had to be demonstrated specifically in construction before the standard was applied to the construction sector. Although this is a reasonable consideration, leaving construction out of a standard until feasibility was demonstrated led to decades of hazardous exposure for construction workers. Underreporting of injury and illness is prevalent in construction because the construction industry is composed mainly of small employers. A requirement to report injury by construction project, which may include many small employers, could help to better elucidate and focus more attention on these problems.

In the United States, intermittent employment and the high cost of health insurance can leave construction workers and their families without health care coverage. Even when construction workers work the 30 or 60 days frequently needed on a job to qualify for health insurance coverage, the high cost of coverage leaves many uninsured. Because construction is a complex industry, there are proportionately fewer research and prevention activities in construction than in general industry. All of these circumstances leave the construction industry in great need for improvement in health and safety.

HEALTH CARE WORKERS
Jane A. Lipscomb

More than 10 percent of workers in the United States are health care workers. Characterized as people committed to promoting health through treatment and care for the sick and injured, health care workers, ironically, confront perhaps a greater range of significant workplace hazards than workers in any other sector. Hazards facing health care workers include:

- Biological hazards associated with airborne contact and blood-borne exposures to infectious agents (Fig. 32-5);

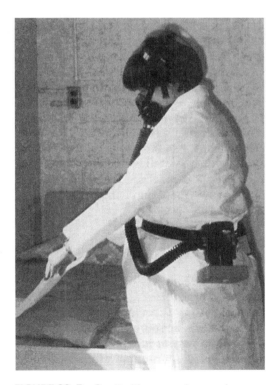

FIGURE 32-5 ● Health care workers can be protected from tuberculosis by proper isolation treatment of patients, use of enclosures, exhaust ventilation, and germicidal lamps. The last line of defense is the use of personal respiratory protection, one example of which (a powered air-purifying respirator) is illustrated above. (Courtesy of the National Institute for Occupational Safety and Health.)

- Chemical hazards, especially those found in hospitals, including waste anesthetic and sterilant gases, hazardous drugs (such as antineoplastic medications) and other therapeutic agents, mercury, and industrial-strength disinfectants and cleaning compounds;
- Physical hazards, including ionizing and nonionizing radiation;
- Safety and ergonomic hazards that can lead to a variety of acute and chronic musculoskeletal problems;
- Violence;
- Psychosocial and organizational factors, including psychologic stress and shift work; and
- The many health consequences associated with changes in the organization and financing of health care (Table 32-6).

In 2002, the Bureau of Labor Statistics (BLS) injury and illness rate among hospital workers (9.7 per 100 workers) was nearly double that of the overall private sector rate (5.3) and higher than rates for workers employed in mining (4.0), manufacturing (7.2), and construction (7.1). Although injury and illness rates have been declining among all private sector workers, the ratio of hospital worker injuries to the overall private sector rate has increased over the past 6 years.

The nursing home segment of the health care industry has consistently reported injury and illness rates significantly higher than those for the most hazardous industries—as high as 12.6 per 100 full-time workers in 2002. In health care, workers as well as patients are affected when occupational safety and health threats are not adequately identified and addressed. Nonetheless, the health care industry is a decade or more behind other high-risk industries in ensuring safety.

The generation and disposal of biological chemical, and radiologic wastes also pose risks to the communities surrounding health care facilities and beyond, especially if these facilities incinerate their waste on site. The widespread use and resulting incineration of plastics containing chloride compounds, such as polyvinyl chloride, have the potential to create and release into the atmosphere dioxins, which are highly toxic. Community organizations have successfully advocated for changes, such as the phasing out of products that contain mercury within the health care setting and a reduction in the incineration of mercury-containing products. In 1998, the American Hospital Association

TABLE 32-6

Selected Hazards, Health Effects, and Control Strategies in Health Care

Hazards	Health Effects	Control Strategies
Biological		
Viral (hepatitis B virus, hepatitis C virus)	Acute febrile illness, liver disease, death	Safer needle devices, hepatitis B vaccine
Bacteria (*Mycobacterium tuberculosis*)	TB infection and active disease, multiple drug resistance, death	Isolation of suspect patients, respirators, ultraviolet light, negative pressure rooms
Natural rubber latex proteins (and rubber chemical additives)	Type I and type IV immunologic responses; type I immediate hypersensitivity includes anaphylactic shock	Substitution with low–latex protein, powderless gloves or nonlatex gloves and supplies
Chemical		
Ethylene oxide	Peripheral neuropathy, cancer, reproductive effects	Substitution, enclosed systems, aeration rooms
Formaldehyde	Allergy, nasal cancer	Subsitution, local ventilation
Glutaradehyde	Mucous membrane irritation, sensitization, reproductive effects	Substitution, local ventilation
Antineoplastic drugs	Cancer, mutagenicity, reproductive effects	Class 1 ventilation hoods, isolation of patient excreta
Waste anesthetic gases	Hepatic toxicity, neurologic effects, reproductive effects	Scavenging systems, isolation of off-gassing patients
Mercury	Neurologic effects, birth defects	Substitution with electronic thermometers
Physical		
Patient handling	Back pain, injury	Patient handling devices, lifting teams, training
Static postures	Musculoskeletal pain and injury	Rest breaks, exercise, support hose and shoes
Ionizing radiation	Cancer, reproductive effects	Isolation of patients, shielding and maintenance of equipment
Lasers	Eye and skin burns, inhalation of toxic chemical and pathogens, fires	Local exhaust ventilation, equipment maintenance, respirators and face shields
Physical assault	Traumatic injuries, death	Alarm systems, security personnel, training
Psychosocial/Organizational		
Violence threat and physical assault	Traumatic injury, death, post-traumatic stress disorder	Training, postassault debriefing
Restructuring	Mental health disorders, exacerbation of musculoskeletal injuries, traumatic injuries, burn-out	Acuity-based staffing, employee involvement in restructuring activities
Additional work stress	Mental health disorders, burn-out	Stress prevention and management programs
Shift work	Gastrointestinal disorders, sleep disorders	Forward, stable, and predictable shift rotation

and EPA signed a memorandum of understanding to prevent the release of persistent, bioacculumative toxic chemicals by the industry.

Musculoskeletal Disorders

The highest proportion of musculoskeletal disorders (MSDs), which rank second among all work-related injuries, occur among health care workers. Exposures include the requirements to lift, pull, slide, turn, and transfer patients; move equipment; and stand for long periods of time. Among all occupations, hospital and nursing home workers experience the highest number of occupational injuries and illnesses involving lost workdays due to back injuries. In 2002, nursing home workers experienced a rate of back injuries of 25.9 per 10,000 workers—a rate nearly five times the rate of 5.3 per 10,000 reported among all private-sector industries. Nurses' aides, orderlies, and attendants reported the greatest number of cases of MSDs involving days away from work (44,400).

In a recent survey of nearly 1,200 registered nurses employed in various health care practice settings, nurses reporting highly physically-demanding jobs were five to six times more likely to report a neck, shoulder, or back MSD as compared with those with less physically-demanding jobs. Lifting teams and mechanical devices in the workplace have been associated with significantly lower risk of back MSDs.[15] However, only 10 percent of nurses reported having lifting teams in their workplace and only 50 percent had mechanical lifting devices. The risk for MSDs is also increased when nurses work shifts longer than 12 hours and on evenings, nights, and weekends.[16]

The nursing home industry spends more than $1 billion each year in workers' compensation premiums, even though there is strong evidence that reducing low back load by implementing engineering and administrative controls, such as by safe staffing levels, lifting teams, and use of newer mechanical patient handling devices, reduces the risk of injury to both patients and workers.

MSDs among other occupational groups within the health care industry are less well understood. Laboratory workers are at increased risk for cumulative trauma disorders of the hand and wrist related to repetitive work, such as pipetting. Operating-room workers who must maintain static postures for long periods of time and those involved in overhead work, such as holding instruments overhead during lengthy operations, experience neck and shoulder pain and injury.

Workplace Violence

The health care sector also leads all other industry sectors in the incidence of nonfatal workplace assaults. Of all nonfatal assaults against workers resulting in lost workdays in the United States, 32 percent occurred in the health care sector. In 51 percent of nonfatal assault injuries, the perpetrator of the violent act is a patient. In 2002, the BLS rate of nonfatal assaults among workers in "nursing and personal care facilities" was 18 per 10,000, compared to 3 per 10,000 in the private sector as a whole. Among these assault victims, 30 percent were government employees, even though they make up only 18 percent of the workforce.

In each year from 1993 to 1999, 1.7 million incidents of violence occurred in workplaces in the United States. Twelve percent of all victims reported physical injuries. Six percent of workplace crimes resulted in injury that required medical treatment. Only 46 percent of all incidents were reported to the police. Mental health professionals had an incidence rate of 68 per 1,000 workers compared with an overall rate of 12 per 1,000 workers. Nurses had an incidence rate of 22 per 1,000 workers, the highest rate in the "medical" category.[17] In a Washington State psychiatric facility, 73 percent of staff members surveyed had reported at least a minor injury related to an assault by a patient during the past year; only 43 percent of those reporting moderate, severe, or disabling injuries related to such assaults had filed for workers' compensation. The survey found an assault incidence rate of 437 per 100 employees per year, whereas the reported incidence rate for the hospital was only 35 per 100.[18]

Emergency department personnel face a significant risk of injuries from assaults by patients or their families. Weapon-carrying in emergency departments creates the opportunity for severe or fatal injuries. California and Washington State have enacted standards requiring safeguards for emergency department workers. Because no department in a health care setting is immune from workplace violence, all departments should have violence prevention programs.

Environmental and organizational factors have been associated with patient assaults; including understaffing (especially during times of increased activity such as meal times), poor workplace security, unrestricted movement by the public around the facility, and transporting patients. A study found that the presence of security personnel reduces the rate of assault; the rate of assault is increased when administrators consider assault to be part of the job, there is a high patient-to-personnel ratio, and work is primarily with mental health patients, or with patients who have long hospital stays.[18a]

Many psychiatric settings now require that all care providers receive annual training in the management of aggressive patients, but few studies have examined the effectiveness of such training. Those that have done so have generally found improvement in nurses' knowledge, confidence, and safety after taking an aggressive behavior management program.

The health care workplace must be made safe for all workers through the use of currently available engineering and administrative controls, such as security alarm systems, adequate staffing, and training.

Needlestick Injuries

The most prevalent, least reported, and largely preventable serious risk health care workers face comes from the continuing use of inherently dangerous conventional needles and sharps devices that lack an engineered injury protection feature. Such unsafe needles transmit blood-borne infections to health care workers employed in a wide variety of occupations. Elimination of unnecessary sharps and the use of sharps devices with engineered injury protection features can dramatically reduce injuries. (See Chapter 15.)

Percutaneous injuries continue to occur in unacceptably high numbers in health care despite the promulgation of the OSHA Bloodborne Pathogen (BBP) Standard of 1991. The physical and mental health consequences of transmission of a potentially fatal blood-borne infection have also remained unacceptable over this period. The requirement under the BBP Standard that hepatitis B vaccine be made available free of charge to health care workers has greatly reduced the consequences of exposure to this pathogen. The advances in the treatment of HIV infection with postexposure prophylaxis has improved the prognosis for those health care workers infected with HIV-contaminated blood. Tragically, there is no vaccine or treatment for hepatitis C virus (HCV), and, therefore, health care workers continue to suffer life-threatening illness after exposure to HCV-contaminated blood. As such, all health care workers, not only those working in the acute care setting or those who traditionally handle needles on a regular basis, should receive every available protection from occupational exposure to blood and body fluids.

After a needlestick injury, the risk of developing occupationally acquired hepatitis B virus (HBV) infection for the nonimmune health care worker ranges from 2 to 40 percent, depending on the hepatitis B antigen status of the source patient. The risk of transmission from a positive source for HCV is between 3 and 10 percent,[19] and the average risk of transmission of HIV is 0.3 percent.[20] However, the risk of transmission increases if the injury is caused by a device visibly contaminated with blood, if the device is used to puncture the vascular system, or if the stick causes a deep injury. All of these diseases are associated with significant morbidity and mortality, and only hepatitis B can be prevented by vaccine. Health care, laundry, and housekeeping workers are all too often engaged in duties that create an environment for these high-risk needlestick injuries.

An estimated 600,000 to 800,000 needlestick injuries occur annually, about half of which go unreported. It is estimated that each year more than 1,000 health care workers will contract a serious infection, such as with HBV, HCV, or HIV from one of these needlestick injuries. Most will become infected due to the growing spread of HCV, which infects 560 to 1,120 health care workers in the United States each year, with 85 percent becoming chronic carriers. At an average hospital, workers incur approximately 30 needlestick injuries per 100 beds per year. Fifty-four percent of reported needlestick and sharp-object injuries involve nurses.[21]

National case surveillance data for 20 years of the HIV epidemic in the United States include 57 health care workers with documented occupationally acquired HIV infection. Eighty-eight percent of health care workers' infections have resulted from percutaneous injuries—41 percent occurring after the procedure, 35 percent during a procedure, and 20 percent during disposal. Unexpected circumstances occurring during or after the procedure accounted for 20 percent of injuries. The national case surveillance system grossly underestimates the number of actual occupationally acquired HIV infections due to reporting difficulties.

There are numerous narrative accounts in the literature concerning the tremendous emotional impact to health care workers after a needlestick event.

The drug treatment regimen is extremely exhausting and debilitating. The emotional threat of having incurred what might be a fatal injury has a profound impact on the daily life of health care workers and their ability to perform their jobs, maintain stable relationships with their co-workers and family members, and have emotional balance. These emotional reactions may be manifest as symptoms of anxiety or even post-traumatic stress disorder.

Use of conventional sharps in the health care environment today has been compared with the use of unguarded machinery decades ago in the industrial workplace. Safer sharps devices have integrated safety features built into the product that prevent needlestick injuries. The term *safer needle device* is broad and includes many different devices, from those that have a protective shield over the needle to those that do not use needles at all. Needles with integrated safety features are categorized as more passive or more active. Passive devices offer the greatest protection because the safety feature is automatically engaged after use, without the need for health care workers to take any additional steps. An example of a passive device is a spring-loaded retractable syringe or self-blunting blood collection device. An example of an active safety mechanism is a sheathing needle that requires the worker to manually engage the safety sheath, frequently using the other hand and potentially resulting in more injuries.

The passage of the federal Needlestick Safety and Prevention Act in 2000 has afforded health care workers better protection from this unnecessary and potentially fatal hazard. Not only does the act amend the 1991 BBP Standard to require that safer needles be made available, but it requires employers to solicit the input of frontline health care workers when making safe needle purchasing decisions. Although there has been widespread conversion to safety in some device categories (such as phlebotomy needles and intravenous catheters), in others (such as laboratory equipment and surgical instruments), relatively few safety devices are in use. A comparison of 1993 and 2001 percutaneous injury rates for nurses documented a 51 percent reduction in needlestick injuries, supporting the use of new technology in reducing percutaneous injury risk.[22]

Latex Allergy

Despite the success of the BBP Standard and related guidance from the Centers for Disease Control and Prevention (CDC) and professional associations, a very significant health problem has emerged that can be attributed, in part, to the increased use of examination and surgical gloves required by the standard. The prevalence of latex allergy among health care workers is estimated to be between 5 and 18 percent, with atopic workers at even greater risk. Individuals with latex allergy are also more likely to develop sensitivity to other allergens, particularly food.

Three types of reactions can occur in persons using latex products: irritant contact dermatitis, allergic contact dermatitis (delayed hypersensitivity), and latex allergy. The most common reaction to latex products is *irritant contact dermatitis*—the development of dry, itchy, irritated areas on the skin, usually the hands. This reaction is caused by skin irritation from using gloves and possibly by exposure to other workplace products and chemicals. Irritant contact dermatitis is not a true allergy. *Allergic contact dermatitis (delayed hypersensitivity dermatitis)* results from exposure to chemicals added to latex during harvesting, processing, or manufacturing. These chemicals can cause skin reactions similar to those caused by poison ivy.

Latex allergy (immediate hypersensitivity) can be a more serious reaction to latex than irritant contact dermatitis or allergic contact dermatitis. Certain proteins in latex may cause sensitization. Although the amount of exposure needed to cause sensitization or symptoms is not known, exposures at even very low levels can trigger allergic reactions in some sensitized individuals. Mild reactions to latex involve skin redness, hives, or itching. More severe reactions may involve respiratory problems, such as runny nose, sneezing, itchy eyes, scratchy throat, and asthma, and anaphylaxis.

In 1997, NIOSH recommended the use of latex gloves only when protection from infectious agents is needed. Most importantly, NIOSH recommended that when latex gloves are used as protection when handling infectious materials, the use of powderless, low-protein latex gloves should be used for protection from blood-borne pathogens in health care and other settings. Substituting nonlatex or powder-free natural rubber latex for powdered gloves has been found to be an effective prevention strategy that reduces the incidence of suspected latex allergy and specifically latex-related occupational asthma. Hospitals with programs or policies to reduce employee exposure to latex reported a 40 percent decrease in latex-related symptoms, with those hospitals with programs in place for greater than 2 years having a greater decrease in symptoms than hospitals with recently implemented programs.

Chemical Hazards

Health care workers are exposed to a wide range of chemical disinfectants, anesthetic waste gases, and hazardous drugs (such as chemotherapetic medications) that are known to cause adverse health effects and others for which there has been inadequate testing or none at all. NIOSH estimates that the average hospital contains 300 chemicals—twice the number of the average manufacturing facility. Among disinfectants, formaldehyde is a probable human carcinogen and has been linked to occupational asthma in hospitals. Glutaraldehyde (Cidex), a widely used cold-sterilization solution for disinfecting and cleaning heat-sensitive instruments, such as endoscopes, and for fixing tissues in histology and pathology labs, is a respiratory irritant and sensitizer. Ethylene oxide (EtO), a gas sterilant, is a neurotoxin, carcinogen, and reproductive health hazard. EtO has also been associated with lens opacities among workers responsible for changing EtO cylinders. Thousands of health care workers were exposed to harmful levels of this gas before the 1984 OSHA standard for ethylene oxide was issued. It continues to be of concern to central supply hospital workers because of leaks from distribution lines, especially when gas cylinders are being changed. Of particular concern is the fact that the odor threshold for EtO (260 ppm) is well above the OSHA permissible exposure limit (PEL, 1.0 ppm) and the NIOSH recommended exposure limit (REL, 0.1 ppm) and approaches the immediately dangerous to life and health (IDLH) concentration level. In addition, it is highly flammable and therefore poses a dangerous fire and explosion risk.

Anesthetic agents, used in large amounts in hospitals, pose a threat to health care workers when operating room scavenging systems are poorly maintained. Health care workers are also exposed when patients are transferred to the recovery room and exhale anesthesia gases. Specially designed nonrecirculating general ventilation systems with adequate room-air exchanges are necessary in these areas.

Therapeutic agents associated with adverse health effects among workers who handle and administer them include hazardous drugs, such as antineoplastic agents, which are known to cause reproductive effects, cancer, and other adverse effects.

Safe handling guidelines were first published in the mid-1980s by the National Institutes of Health, and later by OSHA, to control dermal and inhalation exposures associated with the mixing and administration of these drugs. The guidelines state that these drugs should be prepared in a centralized area by trained individuals under a Class II (B) or III Biological Safety Cabinet. Use of proper glove material that is labeled for use with hazardous drugs is critical, because most of these substances easily penetrate regular latex gloves. Aerosolized medications pose unique threats because of how these drugs are administered. One aerosolized drug, ribavirin, is of particular concern as it is a potential human teratogen. Use of aerosolized medication requires the use of engineering controls, such as specially designed booths and worker respiratory protection, including compliance with all elements of OSHA's respiratory protection standard.

Organization of Work

Organization of work refers to management and supervisory practices as well as production processes and their influence on the way work is performed. Perhaps no other single factor influences worker injury and illness rates more than the manner in which work is organized and staffing decisions are made (Fig. 32-6). Few industries in the United States have undergone more sweeping changes over the past decade than the health care industry. Macro-level changes in the organization of the work of health care delivery have included organizational mergers, downsizing, changes in employment arrangements (such as contract work), job restructuring and redesign, and changes in worker–management relations. Many of these changes have accompanied the emergence of managed care, the priority given to cost containment, and conversions from nonprofit to for-profit health care institutions.

The widespread concern regarding inadequate nursing staffing levels in health care facilities and its impact on health care errors led to a 2003 Institute of Medicine study, which concluded that the work environment of nurses needs to be substantially transformed to better protect patients from health care errors. The report recommended changes in how nurse staffing levels are established, mandatory limits on nurses' work hours, involvement of nurse leaders in all levels of management, and nursing staff input on decisions about work design and implementation. An earlier IOM report (*To Err is*

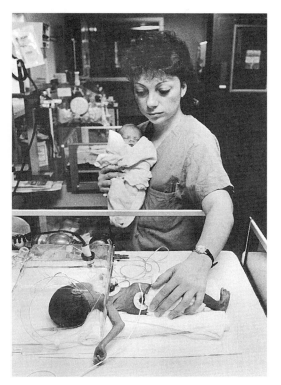

FIGURE 32-6 ● A nurse working in the neonatal intensive care unit carries one infant while attending to another. Inadequate staffing can increase nurses' occupational stress. (Photograph by Earl Dotter.)

Human, 1999) concluded that most medical errors result from basic flaws in the way the health system is organized and recommended that health care organizations create environments in which safety is a top priority and a feature of job design and work conditions.

Despite the increased focus on patient care and nurse staffing, few studies have examined the relationship between organization of work and worker injury and illness. A Minnesota Nurses Association study examined OSHA-200 worker injury and illness logs at 86 Minnesota hospitals over a 4-year period; it found that when nursing staff was reduced by 9 percent, a 65 increase in reported injuries and illnesses occurred. Needlestick and back injuries contributed most to the increase in reported injuries and illnesses.[23]

LEGISLATIVE AND REGULATORY ACTIONS TO PROTECT HEALTH CARE WORKERS

Legislation, regulations, and voluntary guidelines to protect health care workers have been slow in coming and inadequate in their coverage. In 1958, the American Medical Association and American Hospital Association issued a joint statement in support of worker health programs in hospitals. In 1977, NIOSH published criteria for effective hospital occupational health programs. In 1982, CDC published the *Guideline for Infection Control in Hospital Personnel*, which focused on infections transmitted between patient care personnel and patients, not exclusively on health care workers' risks of contracting infectious diseases. CDC guidelines for Blood and Body Fluid Precautions (1982) and Universal Precautions (1987) were published to provide guidance to health care workers. In 1984, OSHA promulgated its first health care worker–specific standard, covering the use of EtO, which was followed by the BBP standard in 1991 and its revision in 2000. OSHA standards addressing tuberculosis and ergonomics were completed but reversed. In 2004, Connecticut became the 10th state to enact nurse-staffing legislation to both protect patients and workers. Despite claims that the nursing shortage has prevented employers from finding nurses, the California nursing-staffing law has had the opposite impact. The wait time for nurses in California to obtain or renew a license increased from weeks to months—evidence that nurses are reentering the field of nursing in response to a more human and patient-friendly environment. Despite progress in efforts to decrease exposure to blood-borne infections, it is unlikely that the higher rates of occupational injuries and illnesses among health care workers will be reversed in the absence of adoption and strong enforcement of new federal regulations covering the leading unaddressed hazards facing health care workers.

REFERENCES

1. United States Department of Labor. Findings from the national agricultural workers survey (NAWS) 2001–2002. Office of the Assistant Secretary of Policy, Research report no. 9, 2005. Available at <http://www.dol.gov/asp/programs/agworker/report9/toc.htm>.
2. National Insititute for Occupational Safety and Health. New directions in the surveillance of hired farm worker health and occupational safety: A report of the work group convened by NIOSH, May 5, 1995, to identify priorities for hired farm worker occupational health surveillance and research. Available at <http://www.cdc.gov/ niosh/hfw-index.html>.
3. Reeves M, Katten A, Guzman M. Fields of Poison 2002: California Farmworkers and Pesticides. A Report by Californians for Pesticide Reform. 2002. Available at <www.panna.org/campaigns/docsWorkers?CPRreport.pdf>.

4. Ciesielski S, Hall SP, Sweeney M. Occupational injuries among North Carolina migrant farmworkers. Am J Pub Health 1991;81:926–7.

5. Dever GEA. Migrant health status: Profile of a population with complex health problems. Migrant Clinician's Network Monograph Series. Austin, TX: Migrant Clinician's Network, 1991.

6. National Institute for Occupational Safety and Health. Injuries among youth on farms in the United States, 1998. Washington, DC: NIOSH, 2001. (NIOSH [DHHS] Publication No. 2001-154.)

7. National Children's Center for Rural and Agricultural Health and Safety. North American guidelines for children's agricultural tasks. Marshfield, WI: National Children's Center for Rural and Agricultural Health and Safety, 2001. Available at <www.NAGCAT.org>.

8. Bureau of Labor Statistics. Workplace injuries and illnesses in 2001. Washington, DC: Bureau of Labor Statistics, 2001. Available at <http://www.bls.gov/iif/home/html>.

9. Center to Protect Workers' Rights (CPWR). The construction chart book: The US construction industry and its workers. 3rd ed. Silver Spring, MD: CPWR, 2002. Available at <http://www.cpwr.com/pulications/page%2049.pdf>.

10. Goldberg M, Levin SM, Doucette JT, et al. A task-based approach to assessing lead exposure among iron workers engaged in bridge rehabilitation. Am J Ind Med 1997;31:310–18.

11. Worker's Compensation Board of British Columbia. Engineering section report: Construction noise (ARCS reference no. 0135-20). Vancouver, BC: Worker's Compensation Board of British Columbia, 2000. Available at <http://www.nonoise.org/resource/construc/bc.htm>.

12. Schneider SP. Musculoskeletal injuries in construction: A review of the literature. Appl. Occup Environ Hyg 2001;16:1056–64.

13. Bureau of Labor Statistics, US Department of Labor. Workplace injuries and illnesses in 2001. Available at <www.bls.gov/iif/home/html>.

14. Sullivan PA, Bang KM, Hearl FK, et al. Respiratory disease risks in the construction industry. In: Ringen K, Englund A, Welch LS, et al., eds. Health and safety in construction. State of the Art Reviews in Occupational Medicine 1995;10:313–34.

15. Trinkoff AM, Lipscomb JA, Brady B, et al. Physical demands and neck, shoulder and back injuries in registered nurses. Am J Prev Med 2003;24:270–5.

16. Lipscomb J, Trinkoff A, Geiger-Brown J, et al. Work schedule characteristics and reported musculoskeletal disorders in registered nurses. Scand J Work Environ Health 2002;28:386–93.

17. Duhart D. Violence in the workplace, 1993–1996: Special Report Bureau of Justice Statistics National Crime Victimization Survey (NCJ 190076). Washington, DC: Bureau of Justice, 2001.

18. Bensley L, Nelson N, Kaufman J, et al. Injuries due to assaults on psychiatric hospital employees in Washington State. Am J Ind Med 1997;31:92–9.

18a. Lee SS, Gerberich SG, Waller LA, et al. Work-related assault injuries among nurses. Epidemiology 1999;10:685–91.

19. Gerberding JL. Prophylaxis for occupational exposures to bloodborne viruses. N Engl J Med 1995;332:444–55.

20. Centers for Disease Control and Prevention. Recommendations for preventing transmission of human immunodeficiency virus and hepatitis B virus to patients during exposure-prone invasive procedures. MMWR 1991;40:1–9.

21. EpiNet. Available at <www.healthsystem.virginia.edu/internet/epinet>.

22. Jagger J, Perry J. Comparison of EPINet data for 1993 and 2001 shows marked decline in needlestick injury rates. Advances in Exposure Prevention 2003;6:25–27.

23. Shogren E. Restructuring may be hazardous to your health. Am J Nurs 1996;96:64–6.

BIBLIOGRAPHY

American Nurses Association (ANA) Web site. Available at <www.nursingworld.org.dlwa/osh/>.
This Web site offers information on cutting-edge issues of primary concern to U.S. nurses. It contains ANA informational brochures on such topics as latex allergy, workplace violence, and pollution prevention in health care. It provides links to relevant Web sites.

Center to Protect Workers' Rights (CPWR). The construction chart book: The U.S. construction industry and its workers. 3rd ed. Silver Spring, MD: CPWR. Available at <http://www.cpwr.com/pulications/page%2049.pdf>.
An excellent compendium of statistics related to the safety and health of construction workers.

International Health Care Worker Safety Center, Charlottesville, Virginia. Available at <www.healthsystem.virginia.edu/internet/epinet>.
The center's Web site contains up-to-date information from their national needlestick injury surveillance program.

National Institute for Occupational Safety and Health (NIOSH) Web site. Available at <http://www.cdc.gov/niosh/homepage.html>.
The NIOSH Web site has special sections for health care, agricultural, and construction workers. Especially useful documents on health care include: Violence: Occupational Hazard in Hospitals at <www.cdc.gov/niosh/2002-101-html>; Latex Allergy: A Prevention Guide at <www.cdc.gov/niosh/93-113.html>; <www.cdc.gov/niosh/02-116 pd.html>. For agricultural workers and construction workers, there are electronic databases of available materials, which are periodically updated: The National Agricultural Safety Database at <www.cdc.gov/niosh/nasd.html> and the Electronic Library of Construction Safety and Health at <www.cdc.gov/niosh/elcosh.html>.

Occupational Safety and Health Administration. Guidelines for preventing workplace violence for health care and social service workers. Washington, DC: OSHA, 1996. Available at <http://www.osha.gov>.
This document provides a succinct discussion of the background of the problem and a detailed description of the critical elements of a violence prevention program. The documents provide excellent examples of how to respond to these performance-based guidelines, including a staff assault survey, checklists, and forms.

CHAPTER 33

Conducting Workplace Investigations

Bruce P. Bernard

The owner of a small neon sign shop that manufactured and repaired neon tubes for commercial signs or artwork was concerned about possible health effects related to his work exposures. The glass tubing contained lead to aid in softening the glass when heated; the inert gas within the tube had mercury added to create a more intense color; and the interior coating of the tubes contained cadmium compounds to produce a range of colors.

A floor manager noticed that employees emptying tomatoes out of the cardboard boxes had developed more skin rashes during the past year than the year before. He sought treatment advice from the contracted physician but did not know what steps to take to prevent these rashes.

A construction crew was using saws to cut cement tiles for the roof of a home that generated noise and much dust. Some workers were concerned that the dust, which was getting into their paper masks, was bad for their lungs and that no hearing protection was provided—and wanted these problems checked out.

A workers' compensation case worker noted that the OSHA 200 and 300 disease and injury report logs showed that cases of tendonitis and low-back pain had increased over the past 2 years. Was it time to find the reason for these increases?

RECOGNITION OF POTENTIAL HAZARDS

There are a variety of reasons to conduct a workplace investigation. Most workers are employed in workplaces that have fewer than 100 employees, that do not have on-site occupational safety and health specialists, and that rely on external consultants for assistance with occupational health and safety. Workers' illnesses or injuries may trigger on-site workplace investigations to determine the causes of these problems. These investigations are requested by employers or employees who are concerned about workplace hazards, government officials, and/or workers' compensation or other insurance carriers of workplaces where work-related illness or injury claims have increased.

Other common reasons for workplace investigations include:

- Trade publications, employee insurance communications, or reports in public media indicating that certain occupational injuries or illnesses are associated with one's job;
- Identification of similar cases of injury or illness in an industry, occupation, or workplace;
- Case reports on occupational safety and health listservs or from clinics or professional associations;
- Case reports from other sources, such as government agencies and medical journals;
- Communication with workers exposed to occupational safety and health hazards; and
- Reports from workers with persistent new symptoms after changes in work processes or job tasks.

This chapter is primarily aimed at occupational safety and health professionals to whom concern has been raised about safety or health hazards or increased injuries or illnesses at a particular work site. It outlines some of the workplace investigation techniques that have been used by the National Institute for Occupational Safety and Health (NIOSH) Health Hazard Evaluation Program and can be adapted for use at most workplaces.

It describes the general principles of workplace investigations to recognize potential hazards, prepare for and conduct these investigations, make useful and practical recommendations, and proactively intervene to implement preventive measures. After identification of uncontrolled hazards, exposures, or work conditions, the objectives are (a) to control, eliminate, or reduce them to acceptable risk levels, and then (b) to ensure that periodic reevaluation of the implemented controls is routinely performed.

A systematic approach to workplace problems is important, but equally important is to reassess the need to go further at each step of a workplace evaluation. Not every hazard, working condition, or workplace concern will require an in-depth investigation; most will not require special tools or monitoring. This chapter, however, attempts to give a method to systematically approach workplace problems in general and offers techniques that can be adapted to the particular work site.

IMPORTANCE OF WORKPLACE OBSERVATION

There is no substitute for being on-site, witnessing work processes, and seeing these processes being carried out in real-time. Observation of work tasks leads to a better understanding of workplace exposures and work conditions and then assists in developing better strategies for workplace intervention. It helps with the formulation of recommendations for specific engineering controls, such as local ventilation, and administrative controls, such as rotation of workers. On-site observation of tasks facilitates recognition or identification of hazards and conditions that may go unnoticed by workers for whom work tasks have become routine.

Evaluating the occupational environment often requires a multidisciplinary approach. Input by workers and supervisors, physicians, engineers, chemists, health physicists, social scientists, and others may be needed to successfully reduce or eliminate hazards and harmful work conditions. The most successful approaches coordinate multiple disciplines and incorporate effective communication between the employers and employees for the recognition, evaluation, and control of potential hazards. Although this multidisciplinary approach is not practical for many workplace situations, each person evaluating the work environment should be aware of the potential contributions of many disciplines in addressing specific problems. For example, the physician investigating chemical hazards in a workplace should have not only knowledge of the health effects of specific chemical exposures but also a basic understanding of chemistry, chemical-sampling techniques, and engineering requirements for control of these hazards.

The recognition of potential hazards at a workplace includes (a) becoming familiar with work processes, (b) obtaining or developing an inventory of chemical, physical, and biological agents potentially used there, (c) reviewing job activities of workers in the work areas of interest, and (d) reviewing existing control measures for the exposures and other hazards one expects to encounter.

Preparing for workplace investigations includes determining how management responds to workers' reports of symptoms, which is critical for preventive occupational public health. Managers' willingness to follow up on early reports of symptoms and investigate certain elements of the job will give clues on how they approach workplace problems and how willing they are to think about and implement preventive measures. Employee symptom reports usually indicate a need to evaluate jobs to identify which exposures may be causing adverse health effects.

The NIOSH Health Hazard Evaluation Program

A health hazard evaluation (HHE) is an investigation of a workplace performed to assess whether workers are exposed to hazards or to harmful conditions. The NIOSH Health Hazard Evaluation Program responds to requests for workplace evaluations from employees, unions, employers, and other governmental agencies. It has traditionally used an investigative team composed of an industrial hygienist and an occupational medicine physician with training in epidemiology—a combination of expertise that has worked well in conducting more than 400 investigations annually. Through the program, NIOSH identifies current hazards and harmful conditions and recommends practical, scientifically valid solutions for reducing them and preventing disease, injury, and disability. The NIOSH workplace investigation can be adapted by other agencies or organizations that are investigating workplace health and safety problems.

PREPARATION FOR A WORKPLACE INVESTIGATION

Gathering Information

Planning is necessary to determine the best method to conduct a workplace investigation. Collaboratively, the investigators should review initial plans, determine specific questions to be answered, and finalize the investigative strategy. An initial telephone call should be made to the originator of the request, employees, employer, and other relevant individuals to obtain the following information about the workplace problems or concerns:

- the operations of the plant, office, or other workplace;
- chemicals and other materials used, hazards present;
- current safety and health measures;
- duration and the time sequence of the problems or concerns;
- previous actions to address these problems or concerns;
- any recent process or materials changes; and
- the urgency of the situation.

Emergency situations—those involving immediate hazards to life or health— should be communicated immediately to the Occupational Safety and Health Administration (OSHA). Investigators need to determine whether managers are aware of these problems and concerns and to determine if there are labor unions at the workplace that would represent workers who may be exposed or adversely affected. If the workers are members of a labor union, investigators can contact the unions to inform them about the investigation and obtain important information. Many unions maintain data on their members' work cycles, work hours, health problems, and medical care (see Chapter 34). The initial telephone call should also review what health and safety hazards might be encountered at the workplace, and what personal protective equipment the investigators might need. (If respirators are required at the workplace, only personnel who have been medically cleared, trained, and fit-tested can use them.)

During the initial telephone call, the investigators should ideally determine who needs to be included in the investigation, such as employers, employees and their representatives (local and na-

tional unions), health care providers, local and state health department personnel, and others. From the start, involvement of employees or employee representatives, such as a union steward, along with management representatives is critically important. Because employees have a unique understanding of their jobs and workplaces, the information gained from them is valuable for determining whether hazards exist and assessing them. Involving employees from the start helps to minimize oversights, ensure a quality investigation, and obtain workers' support for the investigation.

With little background investigation, clues can usually be identified that indicate the scope of effort that may be required for a workplace investigation. For example, signs implicating multiple jobs in various departments and involving a large percentage of the workforce may indicate the need for a full-scale, workplace- or company-wide investigation; alternately, signs that the suspected problems are confined to isolated tasks and/or relatively few workers may suggest starting with a more limited, focused activity.

Roles of the Investigative Team

For the industrial hygienist, preparation for a field investigation begins with identifying exposures of concern, determining if there are appropriate sampling and analytical procedures that will need to be performed, assessing if analytical chemistry or microbiological services will be needed, determining proper instruments to be selected, and then making an industrial hygiene equipment list. It also involves determining which contract or consultant services may be needed. If sampling is to be performed, one must arrange for sampling equipment, supplies, and analytical services and learn about any hazardous-materials shipping requirements. Determining appropriate sampling usually requires one to be on-site or have enough information to know exactly what needs to be sampled, where, when, and why. Rushing to perform sampling and to obtain unneeded data points because "it may be the only opportunity to sample" is rarely fruitful.

For the occupational medicine physician, preparation involves performing medical literature searches, reviewing medical records, and considering differential diagnoses and methods to determine work-relatedness of problems. Responsibilities of medical staff can include study designing and organizing the investigative protocol; obtaining necessary approval from a human subjects review board; preparing consent forms and questionnaires and other data-collection forms; and arranging for field-study materials, personnel, and medical tests.

If biological testing is to be conducted, arrangements need to be made for clerical support and supplies, data collection forms, and collection and analysis of blood, urine, or other biological samples. Arrangements also need to be made for the request forms and analytic chemistry services, immunologic studies, and biological analyses not usually performed by clinical laboratories, such as for metals, pesticides, volatile organic compounds, polychlorinated biphenyls, furans, dioxins, polycyclic aromatic hydrocarbons, and phthalates. If needed, special studies, such as pulmonary function tests, chest x-rays, and neurobehavioral and other tests may require the help of consultants.

Obtaining Needed Information Before the Site Visit

Many manufacturers have information on their Web sites concerning product lines, work processes and technology, financial status, and the managerial system. Major unions also have useful information on their Web sites. Web-based scientific information is often available on relevant general and specific topics, such as previous research, available technical experts, and survey instruments.

If the workplace is a manufacturing facility, the investigators must learn about the goods produced, the chemicals or substances used, and any intermediate that might be formed in the process. Much of this information can be gathered prior to the site investigation through discussions with employees, employers, and a technical expert, and from Web sites.

Prior to the site visit, investigators should request copies of any workplace documents that would be helpful in the investigation. Managers of manufacturing workplaces should be asked about the availability of exposure monitoring records, purchasing and production records, health- and safety-related policies, and operating procedures—all of which can help determine the hazards of most concern. Employee rosters, staffing lists, employee turnover rates, and floor plans may also provide useful information. Reviewing these documents prior to the site visit will help the team understand the potential for hazards and the measures present to respond to them. The site visit will help to determine if these measures have been implemented. Manufacturing

plants are required by the OSHA Hazard Communication Standard to have material safety data sheets (MSDSs) on hazardous substances used at the plant, which can be requested from the management. Nonmanufacturing workplaces will generally not have MSDSs; however, containers of hazardous substances that they may use, such as cleaning products and insecticides, are required to have hazard warning labels, which provide general information about toxicity of ingredients. Once background information is obtained, it is the responsibility of the investigation project officer to assemble an investigative team.

OSHA Logs and Other Existing Records

Requests should be made to obtain the logs of injuries and illnesses that are required by OSHA. Medical records at the plant may yield information about the nature of the injuries and illnesses, as can workers' compensation claims, insurance claims, absentee records, and job transfer applications. If workers in certain departments or operations have more health problems than others, especially if they exhibit the same type of injuries or illnesses, this would suggest some immediate areas for further investigation of possible exposures. Jobs with elevated rates of certain types of symptoms often also have higher risks for acute injuries due to other safety hazards.

In 2004, OSHA mandated that illness and injury summaries be accessible at every workplace. As a result, this information can be easily collected during a workplace investigation. OSHA now requires that every employer post, in a common area where employee notices are usually posted, a summary of the total number of job-related injuries and illnesses that occurred, beginning in 2003. Fortunately for investigators, OSHA also required the posting of the annual average number of employees and the total hours worked during the calendar year, so that workplace injury and illness incidence rates can be calculated. Companies with no recordable injuries or illnesses must still post the form, indicating that none have occurred. All summaries must be certified by a company executive. OSHA also requires employers to make a copy of the summary available to employees who move from one workplace to another, such as construction workers and other employees who do not regularly work at the same workplace.

BOX 33-1

Ultraviolet Radiation Causing Eye Problems at an Airport

Shortly after moving into a newly renovated space at an international airport, 9 of 12 Immigration and Naturalization Service (INS) inspectors reported eye irritation, itching, burning, and redness. Some also reported skin rash. NIOSH was asked to evaluate potential ultraviolet (UV) radiation exposures to the inspectors, who routinely use UV lamps to verify the authenticity of documents submitted by international passengers. Lamps were found to contain two tubes: one UV-A tube and one UV-C tube. NIOSH visited the facility and measured UV-C irradiance levels at one of the booths where the lamps were used. At 254 nanometers (nm), the predominant UV wavelength emitted by the UV-C lamp, irradiance levels exceeded 465 microwatts per square centimeter (μW/cm^2) at 10 inches from the lamp. This irradiance level results in a permissible exposure time of less than 15 seconds for workers with unprotected eyes and skin. At 18 inches from the lamp and a height of 56 inches above the floor (approximating the potential exposure to the eyes), the measured irradiance was around 5 μW/cm^2, corresponding with a permissible exposure time of approximately 20 minutes. Thus, under typical conditions of use, employees could be overexposed to UV-C radiation in seconds to minutes depending on the actual distance of the unprotected eyes or skin to the lamp. A review of medical information for the affected employees revealed that three of nine

inspectors with eye symptoms also reported rash associated with itching, irritation, and reddening of the skin, primarily on the face, neck, and forearms. Eye symptoms reported by employees included blurred vision, burning eyes, intense pain, watery eyes, swollen eyes, and temporary loss of vision. Six employees filed notification of work-related illness or injury claims, and all six were diagnosed and treated for conjunctivitis; three employees were also diagnosed with "allergic dermatitis." Three of the nine symptomatic inspectors did not file claim reports but sought private medical attention. All three reported that they had been diagnosed with conjunctivitis by their physicians. Most workers' symptoms reportedly resolved within 3 to 6 days. Two of the three inspectors who did not report any eye or skin symptoms indicated that they had not used the lamps. After UV-C tubes were removed from the lamps, there were no further symptoms. The environmental measurements indicate that the UV lamps used by INS inspectors at the airport emitted high levels of UV-C radiation, representing a health hazard to those with close and direct contact with the lamps. The inspectors' symptoms and signs were consistent with occupationally induced photokeratitis and conjunctivitis due to UV-C overexposure. Recommendations were made to prevent future problems resulting from the use of UV lamps for document verification.

From National Institute for Occupational Safety and Health. Health hazard evaluation report, HETA-2001-0483-2884, Immigration and Naturalization Service, San Diego, California. Washington, DC: NIOSH, 2001.

Medical and First-Aid Records

Investigations should include, if possible, examination of first-aid and medical records to understand the magnitude and seriousness of problems (Box 33-1). The Health Insurance Portability and Accountability Act (HIPAA) requires specific medical-release authorization from individual workers and requires that employers and on-site health care providers comply with certain requirements to protect individual health data. Exempted from HIPPA are public health officials who are authorized by law to have access to individual

health information for preventing disease, injury, or disability—including for investigations and interventions. Examination of employee first-aid and health records may offer leads to jobs or operations that may cause or contribute to other work-related problems.

SPECIFIC ASPECTS OF A WORKPLACE INVESTIGATION

The Initial Workplace Visit

The primary purpose of the workplace visit is to determine, while on-site, the severity and extent of the

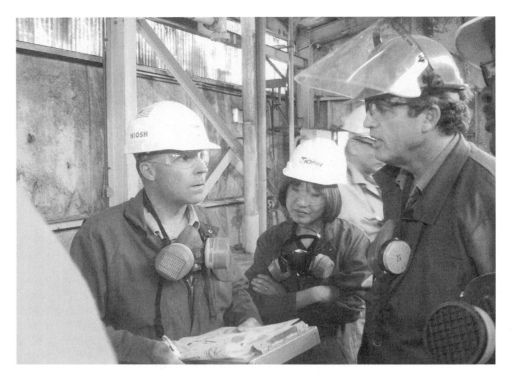

FIGURE 33-1 ● An industrial hygienist and an occupational physician pausing for questions during a workplace walk-through survey. (Courtesy of the National Institute for Occupational Safety and Health.)

problem, possible causes, possible solutions, and if further assessment is needed. The initial site visit can usually be completed in 1 or 2 days; it may be longer if the investigation needs to be completed without a follow-up visit.

Often it is best to begin with a meeting at the workplace among all those involved, including the manager of the workplace, the chief local union official, (or other appropriate worker representative if the employees are not represented by a union), medical and other health personnel, engineering or maintenance personnel who are familiar with the workplace, and consultants who have addressed the suspected problem.

In addition to discussing the suspected problem at the opening meeting, those involved should discuss the plan for confidentiality of information to be obtained in worker interviews and medical and personnel records. Procedures for videotaping, photographing, and making audio recordings should also be discussed. Finally, personal protective equipment requirements and any unusual safety hazards or procedures at the workplace should be reviewed.

Walk-through Observational Surveys of Workplaces

The walk-through survey can be the most important part of the workplace investigation (Fig. 33-1). It should include managers, employees, and union representatives (if there is a union), and the person who requested the workplace investigation (unless he or she has requested confidentiality or declines to participate). The purpose of the walk-through survey is to observe facility operations, note potential hazards, and talk informally to employees about the specific problem or others that may be recognized. The walk-through survey enables observation of workers performing job tasks, use of personal protective equipment or clothing, placement of materials and tools, physical layout of the workplace, and the organizational climate of the workplace. Many potentially hazardous operations can be detected by visual observation during the walk-through survey. Previously obtained lists of raw materials, chemicals, products, and by-products of the workplace will assist in investigating possible airborne and skin contaminants.

For burning operations, knowledge of fuels used will assist in determining which air contaminants are generated. Observation of exhaust ventilation systems may help to determine what controls are needed.

The walk-through survey can assist the investigator in understanding specific job and hazardous job tasks, so that he or she can better understand findings in OSHA logs or first-aid or medical records. During a walk-through survey, one can determine which areas may need industrial-hygiene sampling and which workers may need to have private interviews and medical testing.

The dirtiest, dustiest operations many not necessarily be the most hazardous. For example, dust particles that cannot be seen by the unaided eye can be the most hazardous because they are of respirable size. The absence of a visible dust cloud does not necessarily indicate a dust-free atmosphere. Noticeable odors may not be reliable indicators of exposure. Concentrations of various vapors and gases may be present considerably in excess of the permissible level, but their odors may not be detected. Olfactory fatigue may occur, so that perception of odors may quickly diminish even though excessive concentrations may still be present.

Workers' Job Tasks

Investigators should obtain a list of workers' routine job tasks and requirements in areas of the workplace being investigated. Changes in job requirements or modifications of techniques to accomplish work may have had profound effect on exposure to health hazards. Shift work or overtime work requirements may contribute to prolonged exposure of workers, which might not occur on a regular 8-hour daytime work schedule.

The task of most jobs can be described in terms of (a) the tools, equipment, and materials used to perform the job; (b) the work station layout and physical environment; (c) the task demands; and (d) the organizational climate in which the work is performed. More definitive procedures for collecting information on job tasks may include:

- Videotaping workers performing tasks for time-activity analyses;
- Photographing work station layout, tools, and chemicals and other materials used;
- Recording work station measurements and characteristics of work surfaces, including heights of

work surfaces, surface edges, reach distances, and slip resistance; and
- Determining subjective ratings of perceived exertion.

Although screening tools, such as checklists, have been widely used in many investigations, most have not been scientifically validated. Combining checklist observations with data on workers' symptoms may help overcome some uncertainty.

Focusing on Jobs

Jobs associated with increased occurrence of occupational illnesses and injuries deserve highest consideration in order to identify risk factors and implement control actions (Box 33-2). Jobs with current or very recent illnesses or injuries should receive immediate attention, followed by previous ones—even if there have been no current or recent cases. Priority for job analysis and intervention should be given to those jobs in which workers adversely are affected or process changes are scheduled to occur. Jobs associated with worker complaints of fatigue and/or discomfort should be ranked next in order of priority. Finally, where screening suggests significant risk factors or hazardous exposures, more detailed job analyses should be performed to assess the potential for problems. Higher levels of hazardous exposure or multiple risk factors, especially in combination, may indicate the need for immediate or short-term control measures.

Selection of Instruments to Evaluate the Workplace

Industrial hygiene sampling (Fig. 33-2) is sometimes necessary on the initial site visit to determine the range of exposures in order to begin planning for definitive sampling (see Chapter 9). Direct reading instruments and/or detector tubes are generally used for this purpose because of their portability and ease of use. Detailed quantitative air sampling is generally not performed during the initial workplace visit but may be performed during follow-up visits (Box 33-3).

Interviewing

The lead investigator should work with managers and employee representatives to set up an interview schedule. Interviews should involve:

- management representatives and other company personnel;

BOX 33-2

Use of OSHA Records at a Fibrous Glass Manufacturing Plant

NIOSH conducted a site visit in response to a confidential request from employees at a fibrous glass manufacturing plant. The request was prompted by concerns regarding the causes for injuries and symptoms in the back, shoulders, elbows, and wrists among employees in specific areas of the plant. The requesters were also concerned about repetitive work, shift work, production standards, and the working environment at the plant. During the visit, the team reviewed the Occupational Safety and Health Log and Summary of Occupational Injuries and Illnesses (OSHA 200 Log) to determine the extent of the recorded injuries and lost time, observed work practices of evaluated jobs to determine the physical demands on the upper extremities and the manual materials-handling activities, and interviewed 59 workers on two shifts who perform the selected jobs to determine the workers' perception of physical workload and symptoms of musculoskeletal disorders (MSDs).

Employees reported high prevalences of back, shoulder, hand, and wrist symptoms. During the previous $2^3/_4$- year period, there were 262 reported work-related MSDs in the entire 800-employee facility, which resulted in 2,772 lost workdays and 3,850 restricted workdays. Of all the entries, 170 (38 percent) involved the upper extremities and 92 (21 percent) involved the back. The incidence rates of MSDs in the specifically targeted jobs were much higher (up to 24.5 MSDs per 200,000 person-hours) compared to the overall rate of illness— including MSDs—in the pressed and blown glass industry (8.9 per 200,000 person-hours), based on Bureau of Labor Statistics data for that year. After analyzing OSHA records, NIOSH investigators determined that work in the targeted jobs at the fibrous glass plant was associated with high incidence and prevalence of MSDs, including those of the shoulder, hand/wrist, and back.

From National Institute for Occupational Safety and Health. Health Hazard Evaluation Report, HETA-97-0276-2724, Owens Corning, Amarillo, Texas. Washington, DC: NIOSH, 1997.

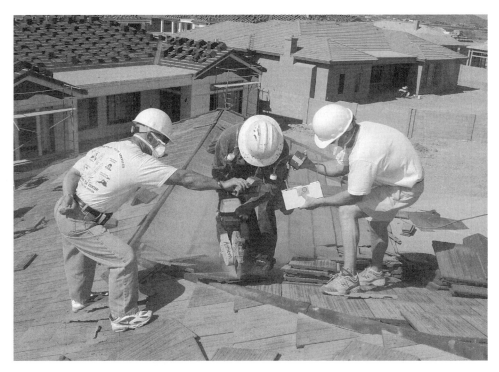

FIGURE 33-2 ● Industrial hygienists collecting follow-up samples for silica exposure among roofers. (Courtesy of the National Institute for Occupational Safety and Health.)

BOX 33-3

Investigation of Pesticide Exposures Among Aerial Applicators

The management at an aerial pesticide application firm requested a workplace evaluation of employee exposures to various pesticides during mixing, loading, and aerial application on rice or cotton. The request indicated that employees had not reported any adverse health problems. NIOSH investigators collected personal breathing-zone (PBZ) air samples to assess the ground crews' (mixer-loaders') and the aerial applicators' exposures to several pesticides, including methyl parathion. On the initial site visit, the potential for hand exposure with these pesticides was assessed for the three mixer-loaders, who wore cotton glove monitors underneath their protective gloves. Surface wipe samples were collected to evaluate pesticide contamination inside the cockpits and on exterior surfaces of three aircraft.

During a follow-up site visit, PBZ, cotton glove, and patch monitoring was conducted to evaluate mixer-loader and aerial applicator exposures to the pesticides. Methyl parathion was the only compound monitored that had a NIOSH recommended exposure limit (REL). All air sampling results were well below the 200 μg/m^3 REL. However, glove monitoring indicated that skin exposure to pesticides was occurring, even though protective gloves were worn. The monitoring suggested that the workers protective gloves were becoming contaminated and, when reused, resulted in additional skin exposure. Exposure standards have not been established for pesticides on skin or work clothes. Very low amounts of residual pesticide were detected on the surface samples collected from the aircraft. Detectable pesticide was found on patches worn on the outside of the mixer-loader's clothing, primarily on the worker's extremities.

The findings of this investigation led to changes in the EPA Worker Protection Standard regarding the use of glove liners and the requirement for agricultural applicator pilots to wear chemical protective clothing while operating aircraft. NIOSH found that mixer-loader skin exposure to pesticides occurred even with the use of protective gloves, and that the potential for pilot exposure was minimal. Additionally, contaminated PPE was being reused without proper decontamination, resulting in additional exposure and a false sense of protection. Recommendations were made for improving safety during the use of pesticides and for the implementation of a medical monitoring program for pesticides.

From National Institute for Occupational Safety and Health. Health Hazard Evaluation Report, HETA-95-0248-2562, Dirty Bird, Inc., Grady, Arkansas. Washington, DC: NIOSH, 1995.

- individual workers[*];
- union representatives;
- medical and other health and safety personnel; and
- human resources representatives.

Conducting Symptom Surveys

Symptoms surveys to gather information can assist in providing screening information to investi-

gators to focus on specific concerns of workers in an area (Box 33-4). Surveys have also been used to identify possible work-related disorders that might otherwise go unnoticed. These surveys need not be used for specific epidemiologic purposes but to provide the investigators with information to narrow the focus of investigation. In addition to questions about the type, onset, and duration of symptoms, and job title or job duties, survey forms may include a body map on which respondents are asked to locate and rate the level of discomfort experienced in different areas of their bodies. The Standardized Nordic Questionnaire (SNQ) is an example of a standardized body map. The SNQ was created by a team of Nordic researchers to study musculoskeletal disorders, but it has been adapted for use in other workplace investigations. Compared with a review of OSHA logs, symptom surveys provide a more sensitive way to determine who has symptoms and

---

[*]*Although it is reasonable to interview specific workers at their own request or at the request of the union or management representatives, the lead investigators are responsible for determining the selection strategy and number of workers interviewed. It is important to get a cross section of workers to interview to ensure that the focus of reported symptoms can be put into a broader perspective on what is happening in the workplace with regard to the suspected problem. When appropriate, the lead investigators may conduct group interviews in addition to individual interviews.*

BOX 33-4

Use of a Questionnaire

NIOSH received a request to evaluate specific exposures at a paper mill to determine the source of worker dermatitis. To assess workers' exposures, bulk samples of pulp, paper, and white water were collected from various locations throughout the paper manufacturing process. Samples were analyzed for various chemicals (biocides and naturally occurring compounds), metals, and biological organisms (mold/fungi and bacteria) that could possibly account for the rash. A self-administered questionnaire was used to obtain data on demographic information, skin problems, job tasks, work history, and the work environment for all employees. Workers who indicated they had a rash on the day they completed the questionnaire and agreed to have their skin examined were seen by a physician. Out of 407 employees, 354 (89 percent) completed the questionnaire. Forty-three workers fit a previously defined case definition of chronic rash. Forty workers fit the case definition of having work-related current rashes, which were clinically consistent with either dermatitis and/or folliculitis. The questionnaires and skin examinations revealed a variety of skin problems. Analysis of questionnaire data

showed a statistically significant association between chronic rash and "not laundering work clothes" (prevalence ratio [PR] = 2.0; confidence interval [CI], 1.1–3.8) and washing hands more than four times per day (PR = 1.9; CI, 1.1–3.2). There was a statistically significant association between a previous history of eczema and chronic rash (PR = 4.4; CI, 2.5–7.9). Chemical and metal analysis of the bulk materials did not identify any single compound in any substantial amount that could account for the skin disorders. Approximately 11 percent of the workers had dermatitis or folliculitis. A single definitive etiologic agent was not identified. However, exposure to pulp, white water, and/or finished paper alone or in combination with resin acids, dust, biocides, glass fibers, and heat may play a role in the skin problems. Based on the information gathered during multiple site visits, decreasing workers' exposures to the pulp and white water was recommended. Controls, such as elimination of potential sources of pathogens, administrative changes, and personal protective equipment, were also recommended.

From National Institute for Occupational Safety and Health. Health hazard evaluation report, HETA 2001-0381-2932, Smurfit-Stone Container Corporation, Missoula, Montana. Washington, DC: NIOSH, 2001.

who does not. A disadvantage of symptom questionnaires is their reliance on self-reports. Other factors besides the presence or absence of work-related injuries may influence reporting of symptoms, and analysis and interpretation of questionnaire data can be complex. It often is useful to consult with an epidemiologist concerning questionnaire design and analysis.

Using Medical Examinations

A disadvantage of using OSHA logs or company medical information to identify possible cases of work-related injury or illness is the lack of specific or uniform medical information. This limitation may make the identification of work-related illness or injury difficult. In the NIOSH HHE program, investigations have included directed, limited physical examinations, which focus on specific

signs and symptoms. These examinations are administered to workers to establish the prevalence of a work-related condition and to establish whether any evidence of excessive numbers of cases might be related to certain working conditions or exposures. Depending on the investigation, there can be a comparison group, involving an unexposed or lesser exposed group of workers to provide background prevalences (Box 33-5).

A few workplaces offer a periodic standardized physical examination for their workforce. Such an examination program can give valuable clues to workplace problems but is generally not set up for continued workplace surveillance, so reviewing these records to obtain specific needed information can be challenging. HIPAA requires that employers and on-site health care providers comply with certain requirements to protect individual health data.

BOX 33-5

Visual Changes at a Label-Making Plant

NIOSH received a request for a HHE from the management of one of the largest flexographic printing operations for product labeling in the United States. Many employees in the plant had been experiencing intermittent blurred vision, described as looking through "a fog" or "a mist." The plant had already been evaluated by industrial hygienists from the state bureau of workers' compensation and a private contractor, and some of the employees had already been examined by an ophthalmologist. None of them could determine what was causing the blurred vision. NIOSH officers performed a detailed walk-through of the facility and developed the hypothesis that the most likely culprit was one or both of two tertiary amine compounds used in the inks. There have previously been case reports in the medical literature of blurry, halo, and/or blue-gray vision in workers exposed to a variety of amines. However, industrial studies had failed to document the mechanism of the visual disturbances or to associate them with exposures—probably due to limitations in study design and/or sampling methods. The amines in the plant had never been reported to cause visual disturbances. Full-shift personal breathing-zone air samples for the two amines were collected. A questionnaire survey inquiring about work practices and symptoms and eye examinations were performed daily for 2 weeks at the beginning and end of both shifts. The exams were conducted by a contracted ophthalmologist and consisted of visual acuity, contrast sensitivity (at 2.5 percent and 1.2 percent contrast) ultrasonic pachymetry to determine corneal thickness, and a slit-lamp examination to determine the presence of corneal opacity. A significant association was found between time-weighted average exposure to the tertiary amines and symptoms of blurry, halo, and blue-gray vision; corneal opacity; decrements in visual acuity; and contrast sensitivity (at 2.5 percent contrast). The NIOSH officers informed the plant management, who diluted the pH adjuster with water, which immediately resolved the visual complaints. NIOSH investigators confirmed this by performing follow-up interviews and sampling, documenting both the absence of visual disturbances and a significant decline in amine levels. The mechanism of action of the corneal opacity was found to be direct deposition of dimethylisopropanol amine (DMIPA) a componant of an additive used to thin ink, into the corneal epithelium without significant cellular dysfunction or toxicity. In recent years, solvent-based inks have frequently been replaced by water-based inks containing amines, substantially increasing the number of workers exposed. As a direct result of this study, these compounds are now included in the NIOSH/Bureau of Labor Statistics Disease Agent Survey, which is designed to assess nationwide exposure to important disease-causing chemicals.

From National Institute for Occupational Safety and Health. Health Hazard Evaluation Report, HETA-2001-0144-2867, Superior Label Systems, Mason, Ohio. Washington, DC: NIOSH, 2001.

Integrating Gathered Data

It is necessary for all those involved in the investigation to meet on-site to discuss together their findings. The team approach must integrate what has been found and determine whether information leads the team to clear conclusions.

Summarizing On-site Information and Holding a Closing Conference

It is useful to hold a closing conference before the initial workplace visit is completed to discuss what was accomplished during the visit. All of those who were present at the initial opening conference, in addition to other key employees and managers identified during the visit, should attend. Investigators should review what has been accomplished up to that point. Investigators should present any preliminary recommendations that can be made or previous ones that can be further supported or modified by the investigation findings or observations during their visit. Discussion should occur on future activities and what reports will be issued. Confidentiality and impartiality policies should again be mentioned.

Performing Post–Site Visit Tasks

The industrial hygiene team should collect all notes, records, and forms from the site visit and keep them in a locked file. All sampling equipment used should be checked and decontaminated, packed, and labeled as appropriate. Analysis of collected samples should be arranged at the appropriate analytical laboratories. Analytical results should be reviewed and checked for reliability and concentrations should be calculated, as appropriate.

The medical team should collect all surveys, data forms, consent forms, and records and keep them in a locked file. Arrangements for coding, data entry, data analysis, and statistical consultation should be made.

Communicating After the Visit

A letter, written within a few days after the initial site visit, while it is fresh in the minds of the investigators, to summarize activities from the site visit is valuable. It provides written feedback to managers, union representatives, and employee representatives. The letter should be written using simple terminology and in a style that allows employers and employees to know and understand the potential effects associated with workplace hazards.

A telephone conference call can also be valuable to report the absence of a health hazard in order to alleviate misunderstandings or heightened concerns that may have been fueled by publicity. A conference call can also facilitate timely implementation of control measures. Any results and recommendations reported by telephone should be included in a subsequent written report. Preparation of the final report to employers and employees should integrate the industrial hygiene/environmental and medical/epidemiological components of the investigation.

CONSIDERING RECOMMENDATIONS FROM A WORKPLACE INVESTIGATION

The occupational health and safety three-tier hierarchy of controls, widely accepted as an intervention strategy for controlling workplace hazards, is useful in outlining report recommendations. The three tiers are

1. Reducing or eliminating potentially hazardous conditions using engineering controls;

2. Changing work practices and management policies (administrative controls); and

3. Using personal protective equipment.

These are described in detail below.

Engineering Controls

Recommendations should begin with examination of existing engineering control strategies, including whether:

- the work is set up to reduce worker exposures or minimize worker contact;
- substitution has been attempted to reduce harmful material exposure;
- work operations are isolated or enclosed to reduce the number of workers exposed;
- wet methods are being used to reduce generation of dusts;
- local exhaust and general ventilation are adequate;
- shielding from radiant heat, ultraviolet light, radiation, or other forms of energy is used;
- modifying the presentation of parts on assembly lines has been attempted;
- there is height-adjustable equipment, adequate location of tools (suspended or within short reaching distances), and reduction of weight of objects handled; and
- procedures have been implemented for general housekeeping, waste disposal, and eating, washing, and toilet facilities.

Administrative Controls

Recommendations for administrative controls are usually directed to management because they concern work policies that reduce or prevent exposures. They address:

- scheduling shifts and rest breaks;
- rotating of workers in and out of specific jobs (because of chemical or biological exposures or physical or mental aspects of the job);
- evaluating production quotas and performance standards with regard to impact on workplace stress, work pace, and worker control;
- providing meaningful light-duty jobs to allow workers recovering from an illness or injury to maintain contact with fellow employees and gradually return to normal activities while providing for specific medical accommodations;

- providing periodic training of employees about risk factors at work and record keeping;
- performing medical management and workplace medical surveillance; and
- implementing workplace policies, such as eating and smoking.

Most administrative recommendations should be seen as temporary measures until engineering controls can be implemented or as measures used only when engineering controls are not technically feasible. Managers should be reminded in writing that because administrative controls do not eliminate hazards, they must ensure that other health and safety practices and policies are fully implemented.

Personal Protective Equipment

Use of personal protective equipment (PPE) is not a substitute for good engineering or administrative controls or good work practices. Recommendations regarding PPE should only be given together with the assurance that these other controls have already been addressed. When PPE is determined to be required—that its use will decrease the likelihood of occupational injury and/or illness—recommendations must address the need for appropriate training regarding proper use and maintenance of the equipment.

Implementing controls normally consists of (a) performing trials or tests of the selected solutions, (b) making modifications or revisions, (c) undertaking full-scale implementation of controls, and (d) evaluating their effectiveness. Testing and evaluation verify that the proposed solution actually works and identifies any additional enhancements or modifications that may be needed. Employees who perform the job can provide valuable input into the testing and evaluation process. Worker acceptance of the controls is critical to their success. After the initial testing period, the proposed solution may need to be modified. If so, further testing should be conducted to ensure that the correct changes have been made, followed by full-scale implementation. Elements of the planning needed to ensure the timely implementation of controls include designating responsible personnel, creating a timetable, and considering the logistics necessary for implementation.

Ideally, implementation of workplace control measures starts on a small scale, targeting those problem conditions that have been identified by the workplace investigation. In addition, the initial control measures can be directed to those conditions that appear easiest to modify. Early successes can build the confidence and experience needed for later attempts to resolve more complex problems.

Evaluating Control Effectiveness

There should be periodic evaluation of the implemented controls to determine whether they have resulted in reducing the hazards and/or decreasing injuries or illnesses and not introduced to new risk factors. This follow-up evaluation should use the same methods that first documented the presence of risk factors. If the hazards are not substantially reduced or eliminated, the problem-solving process is not completed.

The follow-up may also include a symptom survey, which can be performed with a risk-factor checklist or other job analysis method. Results of the follow-up symptom survey can then be compared with results of the initial symptom survey to determine the effectiveness of the implemented solutions in reducing symptoms. Many times follow-up surveys will find the intensity of symptoms has lessened after controls are implemented. However, nonirritant symptoms may not have improved due to chronicity. For some, ergonomic changes in work methods, which require workers to use different muscle groups, may actually make employees feel sore or tired for a break-in period. Follow-up should generally occur no sooner than 6 weeks after implementation to avoid discarding a solution that takes some time to demonstrate success.

Proactive versus Reactive Approaches

Topics discussed thus far in this chapter have represented reactive approaches to dealing with workplace investigation. The steps have offered a plan for investigating problems and related exposures. In contrast, proactive approaches are geared to preventing these kinds of problems before they develop. Proactive solutions emphasize measures to design work processes that avoid risk factors that cause occupational illness and injury, including the design of operations that ensure proper selection and use of tools, job methods, work station layouts, and materials that impose no undue harm on the worker.

ESSENTIAL CONSIDERATIONS

Ideally, workplace problems are identified and re-solved in the planning process. In addition, general occupational health and safety knowledge, learned from an ongoing health and safety program, can be used to build a more prevention-oriented approach. Management commitment and employee involvement in the planning activity are essential. For example, management can set policy to require health and safety considerations for any equipment to be purchased, and production employees can offer ideas on the basis of their past experiences for alleviating potential problems.

Decision-makers planning new work processes, especially those involved in the design of job tasks, equipment, and workplace layout, must become more aware of health and safety factors and principles. Designers must have appropriate information and guidelines about risk factors for occupational illness and injuries and ways to control them. Studying past designs of jobs can offer useful input into determining what improvements are needed.

Design strategies attempt to target the causes of potential occupational illness and injury problems. For this reason, engineering approaches are pre-ferred over administrative ones because they eliminate the risk factors as opposed to simply reducing exposure to them. Administrative controls, such as worker rotation or allowing more rest breaks, are stop-gap measures—not permanent solutions.

BIBLIOGRAPHY

<http://www.cdc.gov/niosh/hhe/HHEprogram.html>
This site provides the complete guide to the nuts and bolts of the NIOSH Health Hazard Evaluation Program.
<http://www.bctransit.com/conference/2004_whi/workplace_investigations.pdf>
A guide developed by the British Columbia Transit Company describing, from the employer point of view, how to conduct employee interviews. It provides insight on the thinking behind the questioning—valuable to employees, unions, and managers.
<http://www.osha-slc.gov/comp-links.html>
A general resource for all of OSHA's regulations and interpretation letters about hazardous exposures.
<http://www.dir.ca.gov/dosh/dosh_publications/iipp.html>
A CAL/OSHA Consultation Service guide to a workplace injury and illness prevention program—includes elements covered in this chapter.

The findings and conclusions in this chapter are those of the author and do not necessarily represent the views of the National Institute for Occupational Safety and Health.

CHAPTER 34

Labor Unions: Their Role in Occupational and Environmental Health

Robin Baker and Laura Stock

All those who work in the environmental and/or occupational health fields are affected by labor unions. Some may work directly with a unionized workforce. Others may work in government agencies where labor unions are an important "stakeholder." Some may work on social justice or environmental campaigns that need labor support to succeed. Others may conduct research that requires labor participation. The labor movement will influence even those whose work never brings them in direct contact with a union because of labor's significant political and practical effects on the public health field.

Unions have been the most important force in the United States promoting safety protection and decent working conditions for all American workers, not just their own members. Throughout the 20th century, unions lobbied in the political arena for health and safety protection, the minimum wage, and child-labor laws. Without the labor movement, it is unlikely that we would have the Occupational Safety and Health Administration (OSHA), jobs for occupational health professionals, or any organized voice to effectively promote workers' rights.

Unions also have played an important role in environmental health. In the 1960s, the labor movement supported environmental protection efforts as well as other emerging movements, including the civil rights, women's rights, and antiwar movements.[1] Later, conflict between some unions and environmentalists led to a general perception of hostility between the two groups. Yet increasingly, workers and environmentalists have collaborated through activities called *blue-green alliances* because they bring together the "blue-collar" working class and "green" environmentalists.

Because of the important historical and current role of unions, it is important to understand how unions work, the structure and functions of the labor movement, how unions promote health and safety in the workplace and the community, and how to build effective collaborative relationships with labor unions on occupational and environmental issues.

AN INTRODUCTION TO LABOR UNIONS

The role of unions is to represent and pursue the collective interests of workers. These include wages, hours, benefits, and conditions of employment, including health and safety. In addition to these traditional issues related to the job and the workplace, many unions also consider building a better society as part of their mission. Thus, they address issues that extend beyond the workplace, such as peace, justice, and the quality of life.

Approximately 15 million Americans belong to a union, representing approximately 13 percent of the total U.S. labor force. The number of workers in unions has remained relatively stable, but the percent of U.S. workers represented by unions has dropped considerably, from a peak of 33 percent in 1955. As the economy has changed dramatically, jobs have been lost in sectors that were well organized and have been replaced by jobs in areas where union organizing has been more difficult. Service occupations are becoming more prominent than traditional manufacturing jobs. Part-time and contract work are growing. Only 1 in 10 new U.S. jobs is unionized. The degree of unionization varies significantly from sector to sector. Today, the highest levels of unionization are in education (35 percent) and government (32 percent) and the lowest are in finance and insurance, private services, and agriculture (all 3 percent or less).[2]

The core work of labor is typically carried out at the level of the local union. Local unions represent workers in a single workplace or group of workplaces and can include members in a specific trade or in a range of occupations. Locals are often responsible for negotiating collective bargaining agreements (union contracts) with employers and enforcing those contracts through the grievance procedure. Locals are democratic institutions governed by officers who are elected by the union members. Some members serve as shop stewards,

who represent their co-workers and help enforce the union contract. Many local unions also hire staff to help enforce the contract (*union representatives, business agents*) or to expand membership (*organizers*). Local unions may belong to an *international union*, which is made up of many locals of the same union (see Box 34-1).

The American Federation of Labor-Congress of Industrial Organizations (AFL-CIO) is a voluntary confederation of more than 60 international unions. More than 13 million U.S union members belong to unions affiliated with the AFL-CIO. The AFL-CIO engages in political action, lobbying, education, and organizing on behalf of the labor movement as a whole. It brings different unions together not just on the national level but also within states and local communities (see Box 34-2).

BOX 34-1
Glossary of Key Labor Terms

Term	Definition
Affiliate	A union that is a member of a central labor body or federation of unions.
Agency shop	A provision in a contract that requires all non-union members in a bargaining unit, as a condition of employment, to pay the union a fixed amount for services rendered, such as representation.
American Federation of Labor-Congress of Industrial Organizations (AFL-CIO)	A confederation of international unions in the United States, formed in 1955 in a merger of the AFL and the CIO. It engages in political action, education, lobbying, and organizing.
Bargaining unit	A group of employees recognized by the employer or designated by an authorized government agency for purposes of collective bargaining.
Building and Construction Trades Council	Unions that represent the construction trades are typically affiliated with the AFL-CIO's Building and Construction Trades Department. There are state and local councils (parallel to the CLCs).
Central Labor Council (CLC)	An organization made up of most local unions in a geographical area, often a county. CLC member locals represent many different trades and international unions. CLCs engage in political action, education, lobbying, and organizing on a local level.
Certification election (Representation election)	An election, usually conducted by the National Labor Relations Board or a state board, in which employees in a bargaining unit vote for or against representation by a union. ("Card check" is another way that employees join unions—if a majority sign union cards and the employer recognizes the union, they do not have to go through the often drawn-out and difficult election process.)
Closed shop (union shop)	A provision in a contract that requires the employer to employ only union members.

(continued)

BOX 34-1

Glossary of Key Labor Terms (Continued)

Term	Definition
Collective bargaining agreement/contract	A written agreement between a union and an employer. Both parties make offers and counteroffers on the conditions of employment for the purpose of reaching agreement. The process is called collective bargaining and the resulting agreement, signed by both parties, is the collective bargaining agreement or "union contract." The contract addresses matters such as wages, hours, working conditions, and procedures for settling disputes. A contract usually must be ratified by a vote of the union membership.
District council	An organization made up of local unions in a geographical area that belong to the same international union. This council may coordinate bargaining with different employers in the area or bargaining involving scattered locals having the same employer.
Executive board	The officers who run a local union, district council, or other labor body. On the local level, the executive board is normally elected by the membership. The board typically includes a president, vice president, secretary, treasurer, and trustees.
Grievance	A written complaint by employees or the union that the employer has violated the contract. Grievances are processed through the grievance procedure. The last step of the grievance procedure is usually arbitration, where a neutral party makes a binding decision.
International union	A large national organization made up of affiliated local unions in a given industry or in a certain kind of occupation. Most unions in the United States are called "international" because they may also represent workers in Canada.
Local union	The basic unit of union organization. A local union has its own bylaws and elected officials. Its jurisdiction may be just one workplace or hundreds, one occupation or many. Local unions may also be called "chapters" or "lodges." Most are affiliated with one of the large international unions.
National Labor Relations Board (NLRB)	An agency of the U.S. government that enforces the Wagner and Taft-Hartley Acts, which are the basic federal labor relations laws. The Wagner Act is often called the National Labor Relations Act. The NLRB conducts most private sector certification elections. It decides unfair labor practice charges, including safety-related discharges, failure to provide information, and other safety issues.
Organizer	Organizers may be rank-and-file members or paid union staff members. They work to expand membership in the union.
Steward	The first-line officer of a local union. Stewards are usually rank-and-file workers, elected by union members in a workplace. When workers have complaints or grievances, they usually go first to the steward. In most locals there is a chief steward, and the stewards may constitute a stewards' council.
Unfair labor practice	Action by either an employer or union that violates certain provisions of the labor relations laws, such as refusal to bargain in good faith or retaliation against a worker for union activity.
Union representative (Business agent)	Many local unions and councils have their own paid staff. These union representatives or business agents carry out the day-to-day activities of the union, represent members, and help enforce the contract.

BOX 34-2

Names of Unions

Unions are generally known by their initials. These can appear to be an overwhelming alphabet soup. However, nearly two-thirds of all U.S. union members belong to 1 of the 10 largest international unions, listed below in order of size:

SEIU: Service Employees International Union

AFSCME: American Federation of State, County, and Municipal Employees

IBT: International Brotherhood of Teamsters

UFCW: United Food and Commercial Workers

AFT: American Federation of Teachers

UAW: United Automobile, Aerospace, and Agricultural Implement Workers of America

IBEW: International Brotherhood of Electrical Workers

CWA: Communications Workers of America

IAM: International Association of Machinists and Aerospace Workers

USWA: United Steelworkers of America

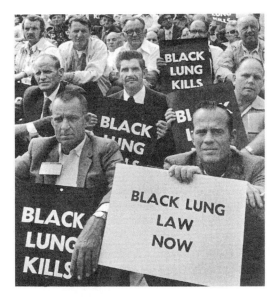

FIGURE 34-1 ● Protest by union members that was part of the movement that led to the passage of the black lung legislation (Coal Mine Safety and Health Act) in 1969. (Photograph by Earl Dotter.)

BENEFITS OF UNIONIZATION

Workers belong to unions for a variety of reasons. Two important reasons are to have input about their working conditions and to have representation ensuring that they will be treated fairly at the workplace. Unionized workers generally fare much better in terms of salary and benefits than their non-unionized counterparts. Union workers in the United States earn approximately one-third more than non-union workers. The wage difference is even greater for minorities and women. Union workers also are more likely than non-union workers to receive health care, retirement, and short-term disability benefits (Fig. 34-1).[3]

About 42 million workers in the United States would choose to have union representation if they could.[4] The U.S. labor movement has been trying to address this need by developing innovative strategies to bring unionization to workers in new and expanding sectors of the economy. In addition to providing professional representation and other services to existing members, unions are seeking to involve workers (organized or unorganized) in actively finding solutions to the issues that affect them.

Promoting active worker involvement both attracts and retains members.

Many labor leaders have discovered that, in addition to protecting their members, health and safety advocacy can be a dynamic and powerful issue in building the union. Hundreds of thousands of workers go to work each day in pain. Workers navigate through their work shifts anxious about their unsafe working conditions. For many, health and safety is a matter of basic human dignity and respect. In a recent poll, a safe and healthy workplace was ranked "essential" or "very important" by 98 percent of workers who responded; to be treated with respect by the employer was ranked high by 94 percent, a living wage by 87 percent, and health benefits by 75 percent.[5]

New Approaches for a Changing Workforce

The U.S. workforce of the early 21st century is increasingly made up of women, people of color, and recent immigrants. These groups, often lacking power and an organized voice, are typically channeled into the lowest paid, most dangerous, and highly stressful jobs.

Labor is seeking ways to reach out to these workers and to address their special concerns (Fig. 34-2). Unions are taking the lead in advocating for equal access to health and safety training and

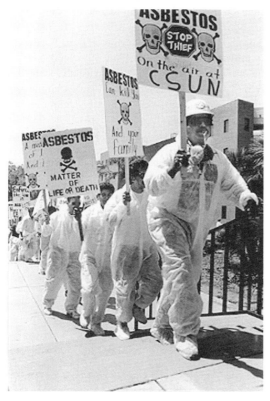

FIGURE 34-2 • Immigrant workers who strip asbestos insulation from older buildings march through the Northridge, Los Angeles, campus of California State University, protesting (a) efforts by contractors to keep them from organizing a union and (b) dangerous conditions on the job. (Photograph by David Bacon.)

OSHA services. For example, they argue that training, literature, and complaint processes should take into account workers' own languages and cultures. Unions have also pushed for new protections against hazards of particular concern to low-wage workers, such as workplace violence, ergonomic hazards, and pesticide exposure. Some unions are now establishing alliances with community organizations that serve immigrant and low-wage workers. For example, unions have joined forces with community groups in campaigns to demand a "living wage" rather than just a minimum wage in local communities.

Some unions have also helped launch alternative *workers' centers* to reach out to those who are not yet ready to join a union or who find union recognition a difficult and lengthy battle. For example, the Teamsters sponsor a community-based immigrant and workers' rights center in California's Salinas Valley called the Citizenship Project. It offers an array of immigration and naturalization services and other rights-related assistance to agricultural and other workers.

In recent years, some community groups and/or faith-based organizations have created their own workers' centers independent of unions. Those centers sometimes take the initiative to address worker health and safety through advocacy, support, and education in the community. For example, the Workplace Project, a center in Long Island, New York, grew out of the struggles of Latino immigrants to respond to nonpayment or underpayment of wages, high rates of workplace injuries, job displacement, and other workplace issues. The center has created worker committees for factory workers, day laborers, women working in child care and housecleaning, and maintenance workers. It also offers classes in labor history, health and safety, workers' compensation, organizing, and immigrant and worker rights.

A UNION APPROACH TO OCCUPATIONAL HEALTH AND SAFETY

In 1911, a fire broke out at the Triangle Shirtwaist Company on New York's Lower East Side. About 150 employees, almost all of them young immigrant women and girls, perished when the fire swept through the upper floors of the loft building in which they worked. Many burned to death; others jumped and died. The safety exits on the burning floors had been securely locked, allegedly to prevent "loss of goods." The International Ladies Garment Workers Union (ILGWU), along with the rest of organized labor in New York City and around the country, led an outraged response to the tragedy. A state factory investigation committee was formed and paved the way for many long-needed reforms in industrial safety, fire prevention, and child labor protection.[6,6a]

Since the time of the Triangle Shirtwaist Factory fire, U.S. unions have continued to promote worker health and safety through a combination of political action, collective bargaining, technical assistance, and worker education.

Political Action

Unions lobbied throughout the 20th century for national health and safety standards. By the 1960s, increased interest in occupational safety and health was supported by two parallel political movements.

The environmental movement began to question the long-term effects of chemicals on health. The civil rights movement made individuals more aware of their rights. These movements created a climate of reform, which encouraged others, including unions and workers, to advocate for new health and safety laws. (See Chapter 35.)

In 1968, labor leaders worked with President Lyndon Johnson's office to propose a government agency to develop and enforce comprehensive national workplace health and safety rules. A major national disaster that year gave impetus to these efforts—78 miners died in Farmington, West Virginia. As a result of this tragedy, and at the urging of the United Mine Workers union, the Federal Coal Mine Safety and Health Act (MSHAct) was passed. In 1970, the Occupational Safety and Health Act (OSHAct) was also enacted, extending health and safety rights to nearly all U.S. workers.[7]

Unions today carry on their advocacy for laws and regulations that affect wages, hours, and working conditions, including health and safety. International unions have petitioned for several re-cent OSHA rules, covering essential issues, such as blood-borne pathogen exposure on the job, ergonomic hazards, and fall protection. A new or improved OSHA standard is always subjected to intense debate, and when adopted usually is the direct result of concerted union advocacy countered by rigorous opposition from industry. Unions mobilize their members to lobby and provide testimony at hearings on proposed OSHA standards and generally give voice to both organized and unorganized workers' concerns.

Collective Bargaining/ Representation

Unions bargain directly with employers for comprehensive agreements aimed at improving working conditions, including health and safety (Box 34-3). This can include (a) health and safety committees or representatives, (b) the right to refuse unsafe work, (c) improvements in the workplace environment, (d) protective equipment, and (e) special safety grievance procedures. Some unions also

---

BOX 34-3

Sample Health and Safety Contract Language

General Duty to Protect

The Company is committed to providing a safe and healthy work environment and encourages the active involvement and support of all employees. To achieve this end, the Company will:

- establish responsibilities of all levels of management and hold them accountable for implementing programs and procedures,
- ensure through proper support and training that all employees are aware of hazards and accept responsibility for working safely...
- ensure that all operations conduct business in compliance with applicable safety and health laws and regulations.

(UAW and Navistar, 1995)

Committees

The Parties shall maintain occupational safety and health committees at the national, regional, and establishment levels ... Written minutes of each meeting will be maintained and distributed to each committee member and made available to employees upon request.

(AFGE and U.S. General Services Administration, 1990)

Research/Studies

Joint Studies: At either party's request, a study may be initiated to review work stations, ergonomics of the jobs, and other health and safety issues in a particular department. Such a study shall be jointly designed by the parties and conducted by a mutually agreeable expert(s) in the area of occupational health issues. The cost for such a study shall either be equally borne by the parties or funded by other sources, such as foundations or other grants. All implementation issues and recommendations resulting from said study shall be resolved only by mutual agreement of the parties.

(Local 2 and San Francisco Multi-employer Hotel Group, 1999–2004)

(continued)

BOX 34-3

Sample Health and Safety Contract Language *(Continued)*

Training

Violence in the Workplace procedures shall be published and distributed. The District and the AFT shall be responsible for providing an education and training program. Clerical/Technical unit employees shall attend the initial

training and shall receive appropriate release time for this and subsequent training. The AFT and the District shall develop procedures for training new employees. . .
(AFT Local 1521 and Los Angeles Community College District, 1998)

Source: *Collective bargaining for health and safety—A handbook for unions. Berkeley, CA: Labor Occupational Health Program, 2000.*

---

negotiate for the right of access to employer facilities to investigate hazards and for the right to accompany government or company personnel when they conduct safety inspections, surveys, and monitoring. When health and safety clauses are included in the contract, unions have a tool for addressing workplace hazards immediately through existing means of contract enforcement, rather than depending on OSHA. The collective bargaining agreement also can address hazards not yet covered by OSHA standards or fill in the gaps where current standards are inadequate.

Unions also have negotiated for a greater role in occupational health research. An example is the Hotel Employees and Restaurant Employees Union in San Francisco, which incorporated language about joint labor–management health studies into its contract with the Hotel Multi-Employer Group. The language allows either party to request a study to assess the work stations, workloads, ergonomic issues, and other health and safety problems. It calls for joint design of such studies, shared costs, and mutual agreement on researchers and recommendations. Similarly, many of the most important studies of hazards in the auto industry have been conducted as a result of contract language negotiated by the United Auto Workers (UAW).

Effective enforcement of the union contract is just as important as contract language. Unions and their members need to monitor workplaces and to see whether health and safety agreements are being kept. Typically, a worker or union can file a grievance if there is a perceived violation of the contract. By including in the union contract a "general duty clause" regarding health and safety in the workplace, a grievance can be filed about nearly any

unsafe practice or condition. Such a clause states that the employer has a duty to keep the workplace safe.

Besides contract bargaining and enforcement, unions represent members' health and safety concerns in a number of other ways. These can include filing complaints with OSHA or other agencies, organizing direct actions, and mobilizing public support through the media.

Education and Assistance

Unions conduct numerous training programs for their members. Many unions have developed training manuals, videos, and factsheets on a wide range of health and safety topics. Some have received funding from federal agencies, such as OSHA or the National Institute of Environmental Health Sciences (NIEHS), to train members about specific issues, such as noise, radiation, construction safety, ergonomics, hazardous waste, and health care hazards.

Worker training is required under many federal and state health and safety regulations. Normally this is the employer's responsibility. However, some union contracts make clear what training the employer must provide, what training the union will give, and how training is to be delivered. For example, several Canadian Auto Workers contracts specify that union members will deliver all education and training for employees. These members attend 2-week instructor training programs provided by the Canadian Workers Health and Safety Center to prepare them to assume this training role.[8]

Unions also provide technical assistance to members facing hazards. Some international unions and larger regional bodies have health and safety departments with professional staff, such as industrial hygienists or nurses. Many local unions also work with committees on occupational safety and health (COSH groups). These are local coalitions of union members, occupational health professionals, lawyers, and students located throughout the United States. They provide advice, training, support, and sometimes materials and equipment. University programs, government agencies, and occupational health clinics also provide technical support to unions and their members, as well as to unorganized workers.

Applying Union Principles to Health and Safety

Whether through political action, collective bargaining, other forms of representation, or educational programs, unions are guided in their health and safety efforts by several basic principles that are the cornerstone of the labor movement. The most fundamental is a commitment to preserving, expanding, and defending workers' rights. These principles are listed below.

The Right to Protection

Unions advocate for safety programs that identify and effectively control hazards. They generally oppose the type of program that blames workers for injuries and illnesses. Instead of emphasizing unsafe acts, unions demand safe working conditions. They insist on recognition of the fundamental principle of the OSHAct—that employers are responsible for providing a safe and healthful workplace. This principle means that workers have a right to be protected from hazards.

Similarly, unions advocate for the most protective solutions to problems. These usually eliminate hazards at their source, rather than relying on personal protective equipment used by individual workers. For example, eliminating the use of toxic chemicals or installing effective ventilation is preferable, where possible, to relying on the individual use of respirators that are hot, uncomfortable, and fallible.

The right to protection also means that that workplaces must institute effective injury and illness prevention programs, including such elements as (a) systems to identify and control hazards in a timely manner; (b) training of all workers on the potential hazards they face and skills needed to participate actively in health and safety; and (c) mechanisms that allow workers to report symptoms, injuries, and potential hazards without fear of reprisal. When prevention efforts fail and workers are injured, unions advocate for timely medical care, compensation for any lost wages, and appropriate return to work policies.

The Right to Participate and Act

Unions advocate for the right of workers to participate fully in all aspects of workplace health and safety programs. They also support worker participation in the development and implementation of local, state, and national policies. Worker and union participation takes many forms, including joint labor–management health and safety committees in which unions have equal membership, equal control of the agenda, and an equal leadership role; opportunities for input on new equipment and technology; and a role in setting research agendas and in reviewing and analyzing resulting data.[7] To ensure their ability to participate fully in health and safety activities, workers need an environment in which they can voice concerns and advocate for change without fear of reprisals. To this end, unions have pushed for strong antidiscrimination provisions and strict "whistleblower" protections both in laws and in collective bargaining agreements. Finally, unions have fought for the right of workers to refuse hazardous work and have battled to protect from discrimination and defend workers who exercise this right.

The Right to Know

In order to participate on a full and equal footing with management, workers need access to all relevant information about the hazards they face on the job. Unions successfully fought for an OSHA Hazard Communication, or *right to know*, standard that gives workers access to material safety data sheets (MSDSs) that provide information on specific chemicals, chemical labels, records of exposure or medical monitoring, logs of workplace injuries and illnesses, and training about various types of hazards.

Some unions have gone further to demand that workers have the right to understand the information they are given. This right to understand means that information and training must be presented in ways that are accessible to all workers and that methods and materials must be adapted to take into account differences in language, literacy, culture, and technical expertise. [9] This right is particularly critical given the growing numbers of non-English-speaking workers in the United States, many of whom work in the most dangerous jobs.

A UNION APPROACH TO ENVIRONMENTAL HEALTH

In October 1948, an industrial suburb of Pittsburgh, Pennsylvania, was enveloped in a "killer smog." Stagnant air conditions trapped emissions from a local zinc works and a steel mill in the town of Donora. Over a 5-day period, more than 20 people died and thousands more became ill as a direct result of the sulfur dioxide, zinc, cadmium, and other contaminants in the thick smog. It was the worst recorded industrial air pollution accident in U.S. history. The United Steelworkers, who represented workers from the mill, joined in the demand that employers be held accountable for poisoning their members and others in the community. [10]

This incident marked the beginning of the U.S. labor movement's involvement in environmental advocacy in the post–World War II period, well before the rise of the popular environmentalist movement of the 1960s and 1970s.[1] Unions became involved not only in antipollution efforts for clean air and water but also in conservationist issues, such as preservation of wilderness areas for the enjoyment of a working class with growing leisure time. Despite its early adoption of environmental principles, labor has a mixed history in working for environmental health.

Labor Pioneers in Environmental Health

By fighting for the elimination or reduction of hazardous chemicals in the workplace, unions contribute to the protection of the surrounding environment. Workers want a safe, clean environment not just in the workplace but also where they live, play, and send their children to school. As a result, unions have put their political clout behind some important battles for environmental protection. For example, in 1972, just 2 years after labor finally won the fight for passage of the OSHAct, it also helped win passage of the Clean Water Act amendments.

Walter Reuther, president of the UAW, was an early advocate for the environment. Under his leadership, the union created a Department of Conservation and Resource Development in 1967, predating the first Earth Day in 1970. The UAW lobbied on behalf of numerous bills to control disposal of toxic waste, promote recycling, and pass a National Environmental Policy Act.

Tony Mazzocchi, a leader of the Oil, Chemical, and Atomic Workers (OCAW), like Mr. Reuther, was a leading labor advocate for environmental protection. The OCAW argued for regulatory protection of the environment although its members were among the most vulnerable to job displacement due to new environmental restrictions. He led his union to take a visionary role in recognizing the potential catastrophe of leaving environmental pollution unchecked.

Another early leader in labor's advocacy for environmental health was Cesar Chavez of the United Farm Workers Union (UFW). The UFW led campaigns beginning in the 1960s to raise awareness of the hazards of pesticides used on food crops. It built a successful alliance to fight for pesticide protection for both consumers and workers.

Jobs versus the Environment

As the post–World War II years of economic growth and security gave way to the economic decline of the 1980s, tensions between labor and the environmental movement grew. More and more, fights for environmental protection were perceived by labor as a threat to union jobs, which already were declining at an alarming rate. In some cases, union jobs actually were lost as older, environmentally damaging industries closed down, with little or no concern for the displaced workforce. But in other cases, the threat of plant closures was used as a tool by industry to enlist labor support in a fight against environmental control. Claims that regulation would cost jobs were exaggerated or false.[11,12]

These tensions reached their peak in the "timber wars" in the Pacific Northwest, especially following the listing of the spotted owl under the Endangered Species Act, which restricted logging. Timber workers actively fought environmental activists, labeled by some as "tree huggers," who appeared to care more about owls than about humans who were losing their only livelihood.

As a result of these well-publicized conflicts, the labor movement developed a reputation for being anti-environmentalist. Similarly, many workers came to view the environmental movement as anti-labor and uncaring about workers. Public opinion generally held that labor would always side with the employers against environmental protection and in favor of jobs. However, even in these years, the labor movement was never monolithic on the question of the environment. Those sectors of the labor movement that did feel directly threatened by job loss soon came to find that they were losing jobs to international competition anyway. Thus, a renewed era of labor–environmental collaboration began to develop.

New Alliances

By the dawn of the 21st century, strife between environmentalists and labor started to fade. One survey found that 64 percent of union leaders reported their relationships with environmentalists as "good" or "very good." Only 10 percent identified their relationships as "poor" or "very bad." The worst relations were found in regions where the timber industry is a dominant employer. Other than in these places, labor leaders expressed considerable commitment to common concerns with the environmental movement, including restricting use of toxic chemicals, protecting air and water quality, and incorporating environmental standards into international trade agreements.[13]

Important new alliances have been built on the premise of a "just transition" from polluting industries to environmentally friendly jobs. Beginning in 1996, a coalition of environmental and economic justice organizations and the OCAW came together to promote dialogue between communities of color affected by polluting industries and workers who rely on those industries for their jobs. This exchange of concerns led to the establishment of a Just Transition Alliance, which promotes policies in local communities to address conflicts between jobs and a clean environment.

Just transition principles hold that the costs of achieving sustainable development, a healthy economy, and a clean environment should not be borne by workers or by the community. They call for compensation and other reparations, including re-education and training, for both workers and community members affected by polluting industries or by their closing.[14]

More blue-green alliances are taking shape, many of them joining in the call for "just transition." These alliances often call for placing equal emphasis on policies that will:

- protect worker health;
- protect community health;
- promote sustainable, environmentally friendly employment; and
- preserve union representation, maintenance of living standards, safety, and decent working conditions in newly created jobs that replace jobs in polluting industries.

These new alliances have sprouted among labor and environmental advocates in a variety of fields, including urban development, land use, energy policy, and international trade agreements. Construction unions and environmentalists have found common ground by fighting for smart growth rather than no-growth policies. By jointly advocating for development in already urbanized areas, they promote both union construction jobs and control of the health hazards associated with urban sprawl. Similarly, the Apollo Alliance has put forward a national sustainable energy policy that would create new high-wage, high-skilled jobs promoting environmental health. In developing this policy, a coalition of top leaders of the labor and environmental movements joined forces to call for investment in energy-efficient buildings and technologies, such as hybrid cars and solar–powered buildings, and to decrease dependence on oil for a more sustainable future.

Perhaps the most publicized coalitions of labor and environmentalists have been in the area of international trade agreements. Unions and environmentalists have jointly advocated for the inclusion and enforcement of trade sanctions in such agreements to ensure that global competitors in developing nations maintain adequate standards to protect workers and the environment. The news media labeled the protests in Seattle at the 1999 meeting of the World Trade Organization (WTO) as a coalition of "teamsters and turtles." Environmentalists showed up in turtle costumes to protest the WTO ruling against the U.S. Sea Turtle Conservation Act, marching side-by-side with large labor contingents, including the Teamsters union.[15]

One premise of these alliances is that environmental health advocates who wish to make common cause with the labor movement need to address the issue of jobs. At the same time, labor needs to be more consistent in opposing "job blackmail" (or "job fear") that can undermine its defense of environmental health. Unions must be committed to countering employers who threaten to move jobs because of environmental regulation. Not only does labor benefit by finding important allies in the environmental movement for workers' rights, but it also helps create both sustainable jobs and cleaner, safer community environments for its members.

TEN TIPS FOR WORKING WITH UNIONS

The first steps toward working effectively with labor unions are understanding the basic functions and structure of union and knowing some of the history of labor's involvement with occupational and environmental health. It is also useful to learn from the experience of other professionals who have worked in collaboration with unions. The following are tips, based on advice from practicing public health professionals and others.[7,16]

1. *Involve the union in your work in as many ways as possible.* Unions can be important allies in your efforts to improve health and safety in the workplace and the community. You will avoid difficulties, and gain substantial insight, by working with the union from the start.

   "Hearing from the unions gives me a complete, more balanced view of the reality of the workplace. Just hearing from management won't give you the whole picture. You need to hear from the shop floor. It allows me to propose interventions that are likely to work in the real world" [*a NIOSH researcher*].

2. *Don't be surprised when the union takes an adversarial stance.* It is the job of the union to advocate for its members.

   "Sometimes I can be frustrated when the union takes a very tough stand. But I have to remind myself that without their support we would have no health and safety regulations, we would have no health and safety programs. We would have no jobs in this field" [*an industrial hygienist*].

3. *Educate yourself about labor.* Find out which unions represent the workforce you interact with. Learn about the union structure. Who are the elected officials, paid staff, executive board members, and shop stewards? Does the union have a designated safety representative? Does it have a community services department? Find out with whom you should communicate. In addition to your local union contacts, many labor unions have staff at the national level who spe-

cialize in safety and health. Get to know your union contacts and find out what their concerns are. Be proactive.

   "It can be complicated working with unions, knowing who to go to for what. You have to get to know the players. When do you need to talk to elected leaders? When do you want staff and when do you want the steward? When is it a good idea to talk with the international union and when would it be stepping on toes? If I'm not sure, I ask" [*a community organizer*].

4. *Show respect for union leadership.* Unions have hierarchies just like other institutions. Go through proper channels. Although you may have good informal contacts with individual union members, be sure to make official requests through the elected leadership.

   "Despite all of the stereotypes about 'big business and big unions,' unions are actually one of the few democratic institutions around. Local leaders are elected by the grass roots. It is important to respect these elected leaders" [*a union health and safety director*].

5. *Get to know the rank–and–file membership of the union.* Although it is important to get the buy-in of the union leadership, it is also important to hear directly from the workers. Ask questions and listen carefully.

   "Sometimes I can't understand a position the union is taking. But if I get out and see for myself and talk with folks, I might understand it better. And sometimes I might get my own point of view across. Someone is always more open to your point of view if you show you are listening, too" [*an environmental activist*].

6. *Visit the workplace.* Tour the workplace with a union guide. Arrange to "shadow" a worker through the workday. There is no substitute for seeing working conditions firsthand.

   "You think you know what the hazards are in a particular industry, but I guarantee that the reality will blow you away" [*a public health student*].

7. *Get to know the collective bargaining agreement at the workplace.* Find out what the provisions are for health and safety. Does the contract call for joint labor–management health and safety committees? How are safety and health grievances handled? Are there training or other requirements that go above and beyond what OSHA requires?

"One piece of advice? Read the union contract. Work with it—it is just as important as what is spelled out in the OSHA regulations" [*a company safety director*].

8. *Share information with the union.* Keep the union fully informed about the results of all occupational and environmental health investigations. Arrange for union participation in research projects and work with the union to notify workers of the results.

"We did a cancer study of our workforce. We had an advisory committee of experts, but even more importantly we involved the union. They played a critical role all the way through the process, from designing the study to keeping the workers informed" [*an occupational medicine physician*].

9. *Understand that unions have competing priorities.* Health and safety may be important, but so are organizing, negotiating the union contract, representing members, mobilizing politically around local and national elections, and holding union elections. The union may not always be able to work with you on your timetable. Be flexible.

"I have learned to expect the unexpected. Just because we have a deadline for our research doesn't mean the union can get to our agenda on our timetable. Most people who work for unions are working long and hard hours, under enormous pressure. If there is a strike, an election, a crisis, then we have to be prepared to wait" [*a university researcher*].

10. *Establish your credibility.* If you are an outsider or newcomer, you may be viewed with suspicion until you are known to be a steadfast, ethical advocate for health and safety. Never compromise your integrity.

"Make sure the union knows you as a credible professional who is open to hearing concerns, will follow through, and will speak out honestly for health and safety.

Go out on a limb. Be a real advocate for health and safety. Establish your track record" [*an occupational health nurse*].

ACKNOWLEDGMENTS

The authors wish to thank Debra Chaplan, Eugene Darling, Pam Tau Lee, Diane Stein, and Jenice View for their thoughtful comments. We also thank Frank Mirer and Michael Silverstein for their excellent chapter in the fourth edition of this book, which inspired us.

REFERENCES

1. Dewey S. Working for the environment: Organized labor and the origins of environmentalism in the United States, 1948–1970. Environmental History 1998;3:45–63.
2. Lerner S. An immodest proposal: A new architecture for the house of labor. New Labor Forum 2003;12:9–30.
3. Bureau of Labor Statistics. Labor force statistics from the current population survey: Union members summary. Washington, DC: Bureau of Labor Statistics, 2000.
4. Freeman R, Rogers J. A proposal to American labor. The Nation, June 2004.
5. AFL-CIO. The union difference. 2004. Available at <http://www.aflcio.org/aboutunions/joinunions/whyjoin/uniondifference/>.
6. Berman D. Death on the Job. New York: Monthly Review Press, 1978.
6a. Von Drehle D. Triangle: The fire that changed America. New York: Grove Press, 2003.
7. Silverstein M, Mirer F. Labor unions and occupational health. In: Levy BS, Wegman DH, eds. Occupational health: Recognizing and preventing work-related disease and injury. 4th ed. Philadelphia: Lippincott Williams & Wilkins, 2000, pp. 715–27.
8. Labor Occupational Health Program. Collective bargaining for health and safety. Berkeley, CA: Labor Occupational Health Program, Center for Occupational and Environmental Health, University of California at Berkeley, 2000.
9. Labor Occupational Health Program. The right to understand. Berkeley, CA: Labor Occupational Health Program, Center for Occupational and Environmental Health, University of California at Berkeley, 2000.
10. Pennsylvania Department of Environmental Protection. Donora Smog kills 20. 1948. Available at <http://www.dep.state.pa.us/dep/rachel_carson/donora.htm>.
11. Freudenberg W, Wilson L, O'Leary D. Forty years of spotted owls? A longitudinal analysis of logging industry job losses. Sociol Perspect 1998;41:1–26.
12. Kazis R, Grossman R. Fear at work. Philadelphia: New Society, 1991.
13. Obach B. Labor-environmental relations: An analysis of the relationship between labor unions and environmentalists. Soc Sci Q 2002;83.
14. The Just Transition Alliance Website 2004. Available at <http://www.jtalliance.org>.
15. Kohn RE. A Heckscher-Ohlin-Samuelson interpretation of the labor-environmental coalition in Seattle. Atl Econ J 2002;30:26–33.
16. Baker R, Szudy B, Guerriero J. Working with labor unions: What occupational health nurses need to know. AAOHN J 2000;48:563–70.

BIBLIOGRAPHY

Delp L, Ottman-Kramer M, Schurman S, et al. Teaching for change: Popular education and the labor movement. Los Angeles: UCLA Center for Labor Research and Education and George Meany Center for Labor Studies/The National Labor College, 2002.

A collection of articles about the role of popular education. Includes several examples of creative union activities in occupational and environmental health, including participatory research with hotel room cleaners, using theater for worker health and safety, Just Transition efforts, and others.

Labor Occupational Health Program. Tools of the trade: A health and safety handbook for activists. Berkeley: Labor Occupational Health Program. University of California at Berkeley, 2005.

A practical "how to" resource guide for unions and community groups advocating for worker protection. Contains multiple "real life" examples of union approaches to health and safety.

<www.aflcio.org>

Web site with useful information about the U.S. labor movement and the AFL-CIO's advocacy for health and safety.

<www.cpwr.com>

Web site of the research and training arm of the Building and Construction Trades Department of the AFL-CIO. Useful information about the building trades union and their work for health and safety. Also provides links to the Center to Protect Workers' Rights electronic library of information on construction hazards (eLCOSH).

<www.jtalliance.org>

Web site of the Just Transition Alliance, addressing collaborative efforts of labor and environmental justice advocates.

<www.njwec.org>

Web site of the New Jersey Work Environment Council, pioneers in organizing grassroots campaigns to help labor and environmental movements speak with a unified voice.

<www.nycosh.org>

Web site of the New York Committee on Occupational Safety and Health. In addition to news on developments in New York State, the site provides useful nationwide resources on a wide range of health and safety topics. Links available to all of the other COSH groups in the United States.

CHAPTER 35

The Role of Nongovernmental Organizations in Environmental Health

Stephanie Pollack

Long before there was an environmental movement in the United States, the country faced serious environmental problems—polluted air, sewage-choked rivers, and the growing use and dispersion of toxic substances. Until the modern environmental movement was born in roughly 1970, these problems were addressed not as "environmental" issues but as public health concerns. As the environmental movement grew and acquired its legal, regulatory, and bureaucratic framework during the 1970s, environmental issues were frequently severed from their origins in the field of public health, while at the same time public health practitioners struggled to adapt to the new environmental protection paradigm with mixed success. The fields of both public health and environmental protection have suffered as a result of their often-artificial separation. Over time, public health practitioners have increasingly focused on the need to play an active role in addressing those public health concerns whose origins lie at least in part in environmental factors. The environmental movement, for its part, has increasingly focused on the connections among the environment, environmental pollution, and human health. Both the environmental movement and public health profession have come to acknowledge the importance of reintegrating the issues of environmental protection and public health. Both have moved into the 21st century with sights firmly fixed on working together to address an increasingly complicated set of local, national, and global environmental health challenges.

PUBLIC HEALTH ISSUES AND THE ENVIRONMENTAL MOVEMENT

There are thousands of local, state, and national environmental nongovernmental (or nonprofit) organizations (NGOs) in the United States that together comprise the environmental movement (Figs. 35-1 and 35-2). The broad and diverse environmental movement encompasses a collection of very different organizations and even other movements that have evolved over more than 100 years. During that time, new issues were added to the collection of environmental concerns that originally had focused more on the natural environment than on people and their health. Many of the different strands that comprise the environmental movement in the United States are involved with the relationship between people's environment and their health.

Natural Resources Protection

Perhaps the greatest number of organizations that characterize themselves as "environmental groups" focus their efforts on issues related to land and natural resources issues, such as wildlife, wilderness, biodiversity, and land protection. This strand of the environmental movement traces its origins to the "preservation" and "conservation" movements that arose at the end of the 19th century and beginning of the 20th century, when the American frontier closed and people became concerned about the unfettered exploitation of natural resources. Both movements were concerned largely with issues of natural

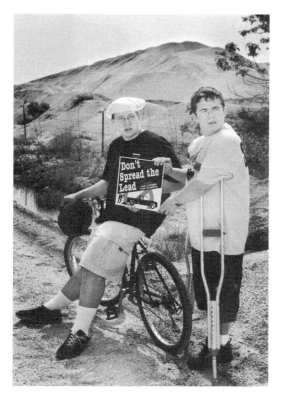

FIGURE 35-1 ● Community-based lead poisoning prevention program. (Photograph by Earl Dotter.)

resources rather than public health. The *preservation movement* focused on preserving wilderness for its spiritual, aesthetic, and recreational benefits. The *conservation movement* focused on ensuring the wise use of natural resources, such as forests, water, and rangeland, to ensure that they would be available for the benefit of future generations.

From their early days, NGOs were a critical part of the conservation and preservation movements. Indeed, many of today's environmental organizations trace their roots to those movements, including the Sierra Club (founded in 1892), the National Audubon Society (founded in 1905), the National Parks Conservation Association (founded in 1919), the Wilderness Society (founded in 1935), and the National Wildlife Federation (founded in 1936).[1]

Many organizations in this part of the environmental movement focus little of their attention on issues of public health or even human beings, rejecting an anthropocentric approach to issues of wildlife and wilderness in favor of one that values the natural environment for its own sake. Others, however, have embraced an approach that embraces those public health issues at the intersection of the human and natural environments. The Sierra Club, for example, now has as its very human-focused motto "Explore, enjoy and protect the planet." It was an early and important participant in battles

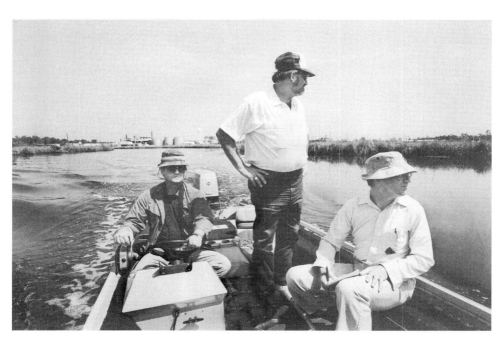

FIGURE 35-2 ● Community group assesses water pollution. (Photograph by Earl Dotter.)

over health-related environmental issues, such as air pollution. The Trust for Public Land was founded in 1951 explicitly to focus on the protection of land—"To improve the health and quality of life of American communities." This organization and others like it frequently cite public health benefits for land protection and open space, including the role green space plays in mitigating air and water pollution and providing opportunities for recreation to combat Americans' increasingly sedentary and unhealthy lifestyles.

Antipollution Organizations

While the conservation and preservation movements were worrying about the health and sustainability of America's natural resources, other Americans had begun to focus on the kinds of air and water pollution issues that would later be categorized as environmental issues. The air and water pollution that were to become major issues for the environmental movement in the 1970s had actually been on the public health agenda for nearly a century before that, categorized as public health "nuisances" and considered the responsibility of local and state public health authorities rather than the federal government. For as the Industrial Revolution and urban migration of the late 19th century evolved into the dirty, overcrowded cities and polluted air and water of the early 20th century, the U.S. public health movement turned its attention from the issues of quarantine and sanitation to the issues of food and water contamination and industrial wastes.[2]

Perhaps the first health-related environmental movement in the United States was the *anti-smoke* movement that arose during the late 1800s. *Smoke* was the term used for air pollution from industrial sources as well as from coal used for domestic heating. Anti-smoke campaigns were launched in large U.S. cities during the late 1800s and early 1900s, often by women's organizations that felt they had a role to play in protecting their homes and families from air, water, noise, and garbage pollution. Groups, such as the Women's Organization for Smoke Abatement in St. Louis and an anti-smoke league in Chicago, succeeded in passing smoke ordinances at the city level and spurring "smoke inspectors," who were part of the public health apparatus of most large American cities by 1912, to locate and fine the worst polluters.[1]

Pollution of water supplies was another "environmental" issue that gained attention at the be-

ginning of the 20th century, a time when bays, rivers, and lakes were used as dumps for untreated sewage from growing cities and industrial discharges from mills and factories. By the 1880s, public health authorities and, later, water boards began building systems for providing clean water supplies and treating sewage.[1] But raw sewage and industrial wastes continued to pollute many water bodies and, by the turn of the century, organized efforts began to address water pollution. This time, the moving force was sportsmen concerned about the destruction of fishing streams by industrial pollution and raw sewage. Their target was not local public health authorities but the federal government. In 1922, a group of sportsmen brought together many smaller organizations concerned about water pollution and founded the Izaak Walton League—an NGO still active today. The "Ikes" successfully convinced President Calvin Coolidge to conduct the first national water pollution inventory in 1927 and later lobbied successfully for one of the first federal antipollution laws, the Water Pollution Control Act of 1948.[3] In a pattern that would be repeated throughout the history of the environmental movement, the initial impetus for action was natural resources protection, rather than public health; the resulting efforts, however, would lay the groundwork for reducing the adverse impacts of polluted water on human health.

The Modern Environmental Movement

The birth of the modern environmental movement is often traced to the 1962 publication of Rachel Carson's book *Silent Spring*, which chronicled the effect of the pesticide DDT on bird and animal populations. Suddenly, the ecosystem and human health effects of pesticides, previously known only to a small group of scientists, were brought to the public's attention. And, at a time when the civil rights and antiwar movements of the 1960s were already causing many Americans to question the status quo, the issue of environmental quality quickly moved into the forefront of public concern.[1] The environmental movement gained steam rapidly with the first Earth Day in 1970, which attracted 20 million Americans to participate in rallies, teach-ins, and other activities around the country. That same year, President Richard Nixon signed a reorganization plan that combined parts of 15 different federal agencies, including a number of health-related functions, into the nation's first environmental regulatory agency, the Environmental Protection Agency (EPA). Statutory responsibilities for protecting the nation's air and water soon followed with the passage of the Clean Air Act of 1970 and the federal Water Pollution Control Act of 1972. For the first time, the United States had a regulatory agency charged with setting health-based standards to limit the pollution of the country's air and water.

A new generation of environmental NGOs played a critical role in spurring the enactment and enforcement of these new environmental protection laws. Some, such as Friends of the Earth (founded in 1969) and Greenpeace (founded in 1971), were "grassroots" organizations that depended on a large membership to generate public pressure for environmental protection. But the passage of federal environmental protection laws also spawned a new kind of environmental NGO—the environmental law organization, staffed by lawyers (and often scientists and others) whose mission was to bring polluters as well as recalcitrant government regulators to court. The Environmental Defense Fund (whose name was later shortened to Environmental Defense, or ED) was founded in 1967 by four scientists and a lawyer who sued to halt the use of the pesticide DDT. The Natural Resources Defense Council (NRDC) was founded in 1970 to secure passage and enforcement of environmental protection laws and quickly helped to win congressional approval of the Clean Water Act. A group of lawyers who had brought the Sierra Club's first lawsuit in 1969 formed a separate group called the Sierra Club Legal Defense Fund in 1971 in order to provide legal representation to the growing environmental movement; Earthjustice, as it has been called since 1997, has since represented more than 600 local, state, and national environmental groups in lawsuits. All of these environmental law organizations eventually became involved in important environmental health battles, including those over lead poisoning and air pollution.

The Antitoxics Movement

By the end of the "Environmental Decade" of the 1970s, a new environmental bureaucracy and movement had grown up around a series of federal environmental protection laws that were generally divided according to the "media" or pathway of environmental exposure. The Clean Air Act addressed pollutants in the air, the Clean Water Act and Safe Drinking Water Act addressed water pollution, and the Resource Conservation and Recovery Act and Toxic Substances Control Act addressed exposure to and disposal of toxic materials and hazardous industrial wastes. Each of these statutes and their implementing regulations were designed to improve public health by providing for health-based standards to limit environmental exposures to hazardous pollutants. But during a decade of regulatory and judicial battles over the appropriate process and legal standards for administering these new laws, the increasingly legally oriented and Washington, DC–based environmental movement sometimes seemed to lose sight of the big picture—the public's concern that people were getting sick and dying as a result of environmental pollution.

During the late 1970s and early 1980s, the environmental movement "came home," refocusing on core public health concerns in communities throughout the United States. Like the anti-smoke movement a century earlier, this movement was driven in part by women seeking to protect the health of their children and families. This *antitoxics* movement was born in the Niagara Falls suburb of Love Canal, New York; the woman who gave birth to it was Lois Gibbs, a housewife whose son and daughter had both suffered from serious health problems that she believed were related to a nearby waste disposal site where the Hooker Chemical Company had dumped 20,000 tons of toxic chemicals. In 1978, a total of 833 families had to be moved out of Love Canal—a pattern that would be repeated later in the dioxin-laced community of Times Beach, Missouri. Residents of communities across the United States became alarmed about the pollution of their air, drinking water, and neighborhoods by a myriad of toxic substances. Their activism focused both on demanding the clean-up of existing sources of toxics pollution and on preventing the siting of additional facilities to handle or dispose of toxic wastes.

The antitoxics movement gave rise to a new set of environmental NGOs, including hundreds of community-based groups focused on local environmental health issues. This grassroots antitoxics movement was supported by a number of national "umbrella" organizations providing technical, legal, and strategic support; the two largest such groups are the National Toxics Campaign and the Center for Health, Environment and Justice (which started out in 1981 as Lois Gibbs' Citizens

Clearinghouse for Hazardous Waste).[1] Antitoxics organizations have frequently been derided, sometimes even by medical and public health practitioners, as "not in my backyard" (NIMBY) groups because of their opposition to the siting of a wide variety of waste-processing facilities. The antitoxics movement, however, must be credited with catalyzing important changes in the public health paradigm underlying environmental protection efforts. The media-based environmental protection laws of the early 1970s had focused on controlling pollution at the "end of the pipeline" through a complicated system of "command-and-control" regulations. Antitoxics activists, however, wanted environmental regulation to focus on preventing pollution in the first place by changing industrial production and waste-disposal practices. Another key demand of the antitoxics movement was the *right to know* about toxic exposures in the community.[4] In 1986, responding to this new strain of environmentalism, Congress passed a new kind of environmental law that was not based on the principles of command-and-control. The Emergency Planning and Community Right to Know Act required companies to publicly report their annual emissions of toxic substances into air, land, and water. The resulting Toxics Release Inventory (TRI) revealed the enormous extent of toxics use in the United States. Indeed, even a decade later, in 1997, the TRI identified 2.58 billion pounds of toxic substances released into air and water in the United States—a staggering figure that nonetheless represented a 43 percent decline from the first TRI due to a combination of community pressure and voluntary industry changes in use and disposal of toxic materials.[1]

The Environmental Justice Movement

Whereas the antitoxics branch of the environmental movement focuses on reducing exposure to toxic substances in all communities, the environmental justice movement, born in the 1980s, focuses on the environmental and health threats that disproportionately impact low-income and tribal communities and communities of color (see also Chapter 31). One key impetus for this environmental movement has been public health data documenting serious disparities in the ways in which people of color, tribal people, and those living in low-income communities are affected by exposure to lead-based paint hazards, air pollution, drinking water con-

tamination, proximity to hazardous facilities, and unequal enforcement of environmental laws. The birth of the environmental justice movement is often traced to a 1987 report by the Commission for Racial Justice of the United Church of Christ, entitled *Toxic Waste and Race in the United States*. In response to this and other evidence of disproportionate exposure to environmental hazards, the First National People of Color Environmental Leadership Summit was held in 1991. Then, in 1992, EPA established an Office of Environmental Justice. As explained by Charles Lee, author of the 1987 report and director of the EPA office, "[I]n little over a decade, what was a loose alliance of community-based activists, church-based civil rights leaders, and academic researchers has transformed into a vibrant social movement that sought to systematically examine and develop proactive strategies to address issues of environmental degradation in people of color, tribal and poor communities."[5]

By 2000, a directory of environmental justice groups identified more than 400 organizations in 45 states, including groups such as Mothers of East Los Angeles (which successfully blocked construction of a hazardous waste incinerator) and West Harlem Environmental Action in New York City (which works on issues ranging from lead poisoning to asthma to odors from a nearby sewage treatment plant). These organizations have been represented in court by, and worked in partnership with, mainstream environmental groups such as Earthjustice and the Natural Resources Defense Council. Like the antitoxics movement of the 1980s, the environmental justice movement of the 1990s helped to refocus the larger environmental movement in the United States back toward the issues of public health that drive the environmental concerns of many Americans.

THE ENVIRONMENTAL MOVEMENT AND PUBLIC HEALTH: THE CASE OF ENVIRONMENTAL LEAD EXPOSURE

One issue that clearly illustrates the benefits of the involvement of the environmental movement in public health matters has been the century-long effort to prevent childhood lead poisoning by reducing or eliminating environmental lead exposure. Lead poisoning prevention provides a particularly intriguing case study because the early battles over both leaded gasoline and lead-based paint took place in the first part of the 20th century and were characterized as public health issues; in contrast, subsequent rounds occurred during the past three decades, after the birth of the environmental movement and the creation of the EPA. In both cases, the public health goal of primary prevention was achieved only by addressing the population-wide effects of lead exposure through the environmental paradigm of pollution control and prevention.

Leaded Gasoline

The Ethyl Corporation was created in 1923 by three major oil companies in order to produce tetraethyl lead as a gasoline additive. Almost immediately public health flags were raised when workers at production plants began suffering from acute lead poisoning. But, at the time, there was no federal agency, such as EPA, with the ability and authority to determine whether lead could safely be added to gasoline. In response to pressure from state health officials, who suspended sales of ethyl gasoline in New Jersey and Pennsylvania, the Ethyl Corporation withdrew its product from the market and asked the Surgeon General to set up an expert panel to make recommendations.

The Surgeon General convened a one-day conference at which industry representatives and public and occupational health practitioners sparred over the safety of leaded gasoline. The expert panel subsequently concluded that "there are at present no good grounds for prohibiting the use of ethyl gasoline." Although the panel did call for further public safety studies, these were never conducted. As a result of this decision to allow leaded gasoline to be introduced widely throughout the United States, an estimated 7 million tons of lead were burned in gasoline in the United States during the 20th century.

The problem, of course, was that the burden of proof was on public health advocates to show that tetraethyl lead would cause harm, rather than on the industry to demonstrate its safety. But that paradigm changed with the advent of environmental regulation. With its well-documented adverse health impacts, especially on children, lead was a frequent candidate for regulatory attention. During the period between 1978 and 1995, the Consumer Product Safety Commission limited the allowable amount of lead in paint; the Food and Drug Administration banned the use of lead-based solder in food cans; EPA banned the use of lead in plumbing, fixtures,

fittings, and solder used in water supply systems; and, most importantly, EPA phased out the use of lead in gasoline, starting in 1973 and concluding in 1995.[6]

The result was a major public health victory: the proportion of children with elevated blood lead levels plummeted. In the late 1970s, among children aged 1 to 5, 88 percent had elevated blood lead levels; by the late 1990s, this proportion had dropped to less than 5 percent. Most of this decline was attributable to the reduction, and ultimately elimination, of lead in gasoline. Because elevated blood lead levels cause learning and attentional deficits and decrease IQs, this decline in population blood lead levels means that millions of American children are healthier and will be more productive citizens. One study calculated that the gain in earning power that each generation of newborn children experience as a result of not being exposed to the same level of lead as their counterparts a generation earlier amounts to over $200 billion.[7]

The environmental-era battle to remove lead from gasoline was just as frustrating and even lengthier than the earlier efforts to prevent the introduction of lead into gasoline. The phase-out began in 1973 and was not complete until 1995, but the result was far superior from a public health perspective. The Clean Air Act of 1970 required EPA to set standards on the lead content of gasoline in order to ensure that lead did not poison the catalyst used in the catalytic converters then being installed on automobiles to reduce air pollution. But EPA went beyond the statutory requirements and proposed the complete phase-out of lead in gasoline, citing evidence that lead harmed the brains of young children. Environmental groups, such as the Environmental Defense Fund and Natural Resources Defense Council, supported this approach in both the regulatory proceedings and later in court, because the Ethyl Corporation challenged the EPA action in a lawsuit. The company claimed that the agency had failed to establish that lead "will endanger" public health and "present a significant risk of harm," as required by the Clean Air Act. The Ethyl Corporation won the first round of litigation before a three-judge panel, with Judge J. Skelly Wright dissenting on the grounds that EPA had the authority and obligation to act to protect health, even when scientific evidence is incomplete. On appeal, the full court agreed with the dissent and upheld the EPA phase-out of lead in gasoline, given "the special judicial interest in favor of protection of the health and welfare of people, even in areas where certainty does not exist."[8] In other words, enactment of the Clean Air Act had reversed the public health paradigm of the 1920s, in which the burden was on advocates to establish adverse health effects. In its place, the Clean Air Act established a new environmental paradigm that allowed regulators to protect public health even in the face of uncertainty as to the causal relationship between an environmental exposure and adverse health effects.

Lead-Based Paint Hazards

The health hazards of childhood exposure to lead-based paint were, like the adverse effects of adding tetraethyl lead to gasoline, well-known to public health researchers and authorities in the first half of the 20th century. Physicians documented cases of lead poisoning caused by children ingesting lead paint from toys and cribs as early as 1910, yet lead pigment manufacturers and their trade association continued to promote the use of lead-based paint as healthful.[9] No federal regulatory agency had the authority to regulate the addition of lead pigment to paint. A handful of communities, including Baltimore, banned the use of lead-based paint in housing, but most took no action.

As with leaded gasoline, the regulation of lead-based paint hazards did not occur in earnest until the environmental protection paradigm took hold in the 1970s. In 1971, Congress enacted the first Lead-Based Paint Poisoning Prevention Act to address lead-based paint hazards in public housing and then, in 1978, the Consumer Product Safety Commission limited the allowable amount of lead in paint, ensuring that most housing built after that date would not contain lead-based paint hazards. But banning the use of new lead paint could not, like banning the addition of lead in gasoline, eradicate the public health threat because millions of housing units already contained lead-based paint hazards. And so, even as population blood lead levels were declining in the 1980s and 1990s due to the phase-out of lead in gasoline, significant populations of young children remained at risk of lead poisoning caused by deteriorating paint and lead dust hazards, especially in older, low-income housing. While local and state health departments, supported by the Centers for Disease Control and Prevention (CDC), were working to screen, identify, and treat

lead-poisoned children, "the public health response was confined almost entirely to belatedly reacting to already poisoned children."[10] What was needed was the implementation of an environmental model of primary prevention—reducing children's exposure to lead-based paint hazards before they become lead poisoned. Public health researchers have found that the benefits of intervention after children are poisoned are small; trying to control lead-contaminated dust without addressing the underlying paint hazards has also had limited success. The most effective primary prevention strategy is the adoption and enforcement of lead poisoning prevention statutes focused on removing the environmental exposure from lead-based paint hazards rather than on treating lead-poisoned children after the fact.[11]

Although the full story of addressing lead-based paint hazards has yet to be completed, the shift to an environmental exposure/primary prevention paradigm has begun to yield results. In 1992, a new federal lead law was adopted that enlisted the regulatory powers of both EPA and the U.S. Department of Housing and Urban Development (HUD) to set health-based standards for lead dust and other lead-based paint hazards in older housing. Drawing on the experience of the antitoxics movement, the federal law (Title X) gives renters and homebuyers a right to know about lead hazards in older housing. Citing data that low-income children are at 8 times higher risk and African-American children at 5 times higher risk than other children, lead poisoning prevention advocates have also enlisted the environmental justice movement in their work to eradicate childhood lead poisoning.[10] Children's blood lead levels have continued to drop; the remaining challenge, perhaps the most difficult of all, is to focus on the highest risk environmental exposures found primarily in distressed housing in low-income communities.[6]

COMING FULL CIRCLE: THE CHANGING RELATIONSHIP BETWEEN THE ENVIRONMENTAL AND PUBLIC HEALTH MOVEMENTS

Many state environmental protection departments were created by removing existing personnel, functions, and resources from public health agencies. The reorganization that created EPA, for example, included removing the air pollution control bureau from the Department of Health, Education, and Welfare. Local public health agencies, too, had their environmental protection functions stripped away from them during the 1970s.

This artificial bifurcation of public health and environmental protection has had unfortunate consequences for the efficacy of both movements. Thankfully, the pendulum is swinging back toward a more integrated approach. The environmental movement is contributing to this reintegration by focusing on the *precautionary principle*, which elegantly combines the imperatives of public health and environmental protection. More broadly, numerous environmental organizations have begun to recognize and act on the connection between public health and some of the most pressing environmental health challenges of the 21st century, including childhood asthma, sprawl, and global climate change.

Separating Environmental Protection from Public Health

The artificial bifurcation of the fields of public health and environmental protection in the 1970s, when federal and state environmental departments were first created, has undermined the efficacy of both the public health response to environmental pollution and the environmental response to public health problems. When environmental health and protection activities were moved out of local and state public health agencies, the word "health" was conspicuously omitted from the titles of the newly created environmental departments. Once environmental protection was severed from public health protection, it was sometimes too easy for environmental regulators to focus on the process and minutiae of standard-setting and regulatory enforcement and lose sight of the public health basis for their regulatory authority. At the same time, public health agencies, shorn of environmental responsibilities, risked becoming isolated from their counterparts in the environmental agencies. Communication has often been poor, with public health practitioners neglecting to convey important information to environmental regulators and environmental regulators failing to make use of available public health resources.[12]

Thankfully, the unfortunate consequences of this balkanized approach to environmental health have become evident and efforts are now underway to reintegrate public health and environmental protection. A pivotal event was a workshop in 2000 sponsored by the Institute of Medicine on "Rebuilding the Unity of Health and the Environment: A New Vision of Environmental Health for the 21st Century."[13] The workshop participants sought to identify strategies that could be merged to produce an integrated approach to protecting both the environment and health. The issue of fragmentation among environmental and public health agencies and organizations has since been addressed by the Pew Environmental Health Commission, the CDC, and the Agency for Toxic Substances and Disease Registry, which are working to develop a "shared vision" for federal environmental public health activities.

It is far too late to structurally recombine environmental and public health functions into single agencies at the federal or state level. But it is not too late to ensure better and more strategic collaboration, cooperation, and communication. Historically, public health agencies first assumed and later gave up important "environmental" responsibilities. As Duffy has explained in his history of public health in the United States, a "fundamental role of public health departments has always been to recognize community and individual health problems, find a way to solve them, and then, when feasible, turn the problem over to some other agency or body."[2] The problem is not that environmental protection was transferred from public health to environmental agencies, but that both sides failed to understand the importance of continuing to work together to tackle complicated and daunting environmental health challenges.

Reintegrating Environment and Public Health: The Precautionary Principle

One opportunity to bring the relationship between the environmental movement and public health full-circle back to an integrated approach is the increasing interest in basing environmental health policy on the precautionary principle. Stated simply, the *precautionary principle* holds that protective action should be taken by environmental regulators when there is evidence that not to do so would cause harm to public health or the environment.[14] The broadly based movement working to incorporate the precautionary principle into local, state, federal, and even international environmental protection efforts evolved as the environmental movement evolved. B. Mayer and colleagues note that the modern environmental movement initially focused its efforts on command-and-control, end-of-pipe technological fixes for pollution. The antitoxics movement rejected this approach and pushed for pollution prevention and toxics use reduction, more "upstream" approaches designed to address the dispersion of toxic substances before they contaminate homes and communities. But even these approaches often failed to address public health concerns, as the desired end was the reduction in the use of toxic substances rather than the elimination of adverse health effects that could be caused even by the remaining uses.[4]

The precautionary principle represents the next step in moving environmental control to a new paradigm, one in which environmental and public health regulators are expected to act to protect health and the environment even in the face of uncertainty. Applying the precautionary principle requires examining all possible alternatives before allowing a potentially harmful activity. And environmental and public health proponents of the precautionary principle embrace the role of an informed citizenry in evaluating alternatives, categorizing potential harm, and deciding how best to protect public health and the environment.[14]

CONCLUSION

The environmental health challenges of the 21st century are even more complicated and daunting than those that led to the creation of the environmental movement nearly 35 years ago. Urban sprawl is not only destroying the countryside and causing air and water pollution, but it is also contributing to a sedentary lifestyle, which is a critical factor in the nation's obesity epidemic. Childhood asthma rates are rising. Both outdoor and indoor air quality issues will need to be addressed to ensure that environmental pollution does not exacerbate the health problems of the increasing number of children and adults with respiratory illnesses. In addition to its ecosystem impacts, global climate change presents public health impacts associated with disease and death related directly to temperature increases, increased incidence of severe weather events, and changes in patterns of water- and vector-borne diseases.

History teaches us that public health practitioners are more likely to achieve their goal of primary prevention of disease when they work with environmental organizations to implement strong regulatory systems. Similarly, environmental activists and organizations have been far more successful when they have been able to enlist public health research and public health practitioners in support of their efforts. Tackling the complicated and critical environmental health challenges of the 21st century will require the coordinated, combined efforts of an energized public health movement and a powerful environmental movement. Together, environmentalists and public health practitioners can and will accomplish far more than either can alone.

Collaborating with Environmental NGOs

The environmental movement of the 21st century includes hundreds of nongovernmental organizations working at the local, state, national, and international levels (for a list of the major environmental organizations, see the Appendix to this chapter). These organizations, as described at the beginning of the chapter, address a broad range of issues, only some of which involve the environment and its relation to public health.

These organizations use a variety of tools, including education and information dissemination, advocacy, and technical assistance and consultation. Some of these organizations focus on one issue or a closely related set of issues; others focus on a broad range of environmental health issues.

Health professionals may find it useful to contact local, state, or national organizations in order to obtain technical information and to become more knowledgeable about current issues related to environmental health. Some groups can also help connect experts and local community organizations, which can benefit from collaboration with public health practitioners. Health professionals play a vital role in many environmental NGOs by serving as resources, technical advisors, and members of their boards and committees.

REFERENCES

1. Merchant C. The Columbia guide to American environmental history. New York: Columbia University Press, 2002.
2. Duffy J. The sanitarians: A history of American public health. Chicago: University of Illinois Press, 1990.

3. History of the Izaak Walton League: Water. <www. iwla.org/history>.

4. Mayer B, Brown P, Linder M. Moving further upstream: From toxics reduction to the precautionary principle. Public Health Reports 2002;117:574–86.

5. Lee C. Environmental justice: Building a unified vision of health and the environment. Environ Health Perspect 2002;110(Supp 2):141–4.

6. Goldman L. Linking research and policy to ensure children's environmental health. Environ Health Perspect 1998;106(Supp. 3):857–62.

7. Grosse SD, Matte TD, Schwartz J, et al. Economic gains resulting from the reduction in children's exposure to lead in the United States. Environ Health Perspect 2002;110:563–9.

8. Ethyl Corp. *v.* EPA, 541 F.2d 1, D.C. Circuit Court of Appeals, 1976, cert. denied 426 U.S. 941 (1976).

9. Rosner D, Markowitz G. Industry challenges to the principle of prevention in public health: The precautionary principle in historical perspective. Public Health Reports 2002;117:501–12.

10. Ryan D, Levy B, Pollack S, et al. Protecting children from lead poisoning and building healthy communities. Am J Public Health 1999;89:822–44.

11. Brown MJ, Gardner J, Sargent J, et al. The effectiveness of housing policies in reducing children's lead exposure. Am J Public Health 2001;91:621–4.

12. Kotchian S. Perspectives on the place of environmental health and protection in public health and public health agencies. Annu Rev Public Health 1997;18:245–259 at 249.

13. Institute of Medicine. Rebuilding the unity of health and the environment: A new vision of environmental health for the 21st century. Washington, DC: National Academies Press, 2001.

14. Kurland J. The heart of the precautionary principle in democracy. Public Health Reports 2002;117:498–500.

APPENDIX

ENVIRONMENTAL ORGANIZATIONS

The American Council for an Energy-Efficient Economy (ACEEE) is dedicated to advancing energy efficiency as a means of promoting both economic prosperity and environmental protection.

1001 Connecticut Avenue, NW, Suite 801
Washington, DC 20036
202-429-8873
<www.aceee.org>

The Center for Health, Environment and Justice provides technical information and training to grassroots community environmental activists about how to organize and about the rights of local communities.

P.O. Box 6806
Falls Church, VA 22043
703-237-2249

The Center for a Livable Future promotes policies to protect health, the environment and sustainable living.

Johns Hopkins University
615 North Wolfe Street
Baltimore, MD 21205
410-955-5000
<www.jhsph.edu/Environment>

Clean Water Network is an alliance of more than 1,000 organizations working to protect our nation's water resources.

1200 New York Avenue, NW Suite 400
Washington, DC 20005
202-289-2395
<www.cwn.org/cwn/>

Center for Renewable Energy and Sustainable Technology (CREST) provides information about energy efficiency, renewable energy, and sustainable technology information and connections.

Renewable Energy Policy Project
1612 K Street, NW, Suite 202
Washington, DC 20006
202-293-2898
<www.crest.org/index.html>

The Earth Island Institute provides organizational support in developing projects to protect the global environment.

300 Broadway, Suite 28
San Francisco, CA 94133-3312
415-788-3666

Earthjustice is a non-profit public interest law firm that defends the right of all people to a healthy environment.

426 17th Street, 6th Floor
Oakland, CA 94612-2820
510-550-6700
<www.earthjustice.org>

Earthwatch sponsors scientific field research to improve understanding of the planet and its inhabitants.

3 Clock Tower Place, Suite 100
Box 75
Maynard, MA 01754
800-776-0188

The Energy & Environmental Research Center (EERC) performs multidisciplinary research and development of innovative energy and environmental technologies for the protection of air, water, and soil.

University of North Dakota
P.O. Box 9018
15 North 23rd Street
Grand Forks, ND 58202-9018
701-777-5000
<www.undeerc.org>

Environmental Defense combines science, economics, and law to find economically sustainable solutions to environmental problems.

257 Park Avenue South
New York, NY 10010
212-505-2100
<www.environmentaldefense.org>

The Environmental Literacy Council offers links to environmental resources on the Web.

1625 K Street, NW, Suite 1020
Washington, DC 20006-3868
202-296-0390

The Environmental Working Group provides the public with locally relevant information on the environment.

1436 U Street, NW, Suite 100
Washington, DC 20009
202-667-6982
<www.ewg.org>

Friends of the Earth USA focuses on the underlying social and economic causes of environmental problems.

1717 Massachusetts Avenue, NW, 600
Washington, DC 20036-2002
877-843-8687
<www.foe.org>

Greenpeace uses nonviolent, creative confrontation to expose global environmental problems and force solutions.

702 H Street, NW, Suite 300
Washington, DC 20001
202-462-1177
<www.greenpeace.org>

The League of Conservation Voters is a bipartisan group working to educate voters and win elections on behalf of the environment.

1920 L Street, NW, Suite 800
Washington, DC, 20036
202-785-8683,
<www.lcv.org>

The National Environmental Trust is a nonpartisan organization dedicated to educating the American public on contemporary environmental issues.

1200 18th Street, NW, Fifth Floor
Washington, D.C. 20036
<www.environet.policy.net>

The Natural Resources Defense Council protects the environment and human health through advocacy, litigation, research, and education.

40 West 20th Street
New York, NY 10011
212-727-2700
<www.nrdc.org>

The Public Interest Research Group (PIRG) is an association of watchdog organizations dedicated to safeguarding the public interest and protecting the environment.

U.S. PIRG Education Fund
218 D Street, SE
Washington, DC 20003
202-546-9707
<www.pirg.org>

The Sierra Club is a grassroots environmental organization that works to protect communities and the planet.

85 Second Street, 2nd Floor
San Francisco, CA 94105
415-977-5500
<www.sierraclub.org>

The Trust for Public Land helps conserve land for recreation and spiritual nourishment and to improve the health and quality of life of communities.

116 New Montgomery Street, 4th Floor
San Francisco, CA 94105
415-495-4014

The Union of Concerned Scientists is dedicated to advancing responsible public policies in areas where science and technology play a critical role.

2 Brattle Square
Cambridge, MA 02238-9105
617-547-5552
<www.ucsusa.org>

The Woods Hole Research Center addresses global environmental issues through scientific research and education.

P.O. Box 296
Woods Hole, MA 02543-0296
508-540-9900
<www.whrc.org>

World Resources Institute helps governments and private organizations cope with environmental, resource, and development challenges of global significance.

10 G Street, NE, Suite 800
Washington, DC 20002
202-729-7600
<www.wri.org>

Acknowledgment

Portions of this list were adapted from the National Resources Defense Council Web site.

CHAPTER 36

Responding to Community Environmental Health Concerns

Henry A. Anderson and Henry Nehls-Lowe

Improved health owes less to advances in medical science than to changes in external environment, and to a favorable trend in the standard of living. We are healthier than our ancestors not because of what happens when we become ill but because we do not become ill: and we do not become ill not because of specific protective therapy but because we live in a healthier environment.
—*Rene Dubos,* Man Adapting, *1969 Pulitzer Prize.*

Over the past three decades, communities have seen unprecedented advances as well as challenges in environmental public health. Many of the specific hazards of particular interest and relevance to communities are discussed in other chapters of this book. From the community and community resident perspective, two advances stand out as especially valuable in informing and maintaining community awareness of environmental health issues.

The first is the *community right-to-know movement* that continues to identify environmental health disparities and empower communities by providing easy access to information. It allows communities to become more knowledgeable about their environment, sources of exposure, and proposals that might adversely impact their health and quality of life. The implementation of this conceptual framework has been especially valuable to low-income and minority communities, which are often disproportionally affected by current and past environmental decisions. While highlighting disparities, the right-to-know concept benefits all. Community members are now mailed results of water quality testing done by their municipal water authorities. They are familiar with the new Environmental Protection Agency (EPA) index of air quality (IAQ) that most weather pages and programs report daily along with wind-chill and heat indices. They can go to their local libraries to review data repositories for Superfund site investigations in their communities. A major strength of the Agency for Toxic Substances and Disease Registry (ATSDR), created by the Superfund law (see Chapter 3), is its community outreach and support function. Community right-to-know precepts facilitate greater involvement in crafting community-based solutions. Communities can receive grants to hire their own experts and support their community-based organizations. In the occupational health sector, workers have a comparable right to know that has been codified in regulation and has led to the availability of material safety data sheets (MSDSs). The right-to-know principles have also been incorporated into epidemiologic research strategies described as community-based participatory research.

The second advance that has been critical to support right-to-know is the World Wide Web. Data and information that was previously almost exclusively in the domain of scientists and environmental health professionals are now available to all. Search engines can locate thousands of sources of information. For example, a recent Internet search on polychlorinated biphenyls (PCBs) identified more than 103,000 sources of information. A community can use the Internet to locate contacts in other communities with similar challenges. The Internet has also provided a means for governments to provide data for community use. Web access to the EPA's Toxics Release Inventory (TRI) has been a staple for community understanding of sources of potential exposure in its area. However, while unfettered access to raw data and a plethora of differing interpretations of that data is the hallmark of the Internet, seldom is there a consensus of opinion upon which a citizen can rely and act. Thus, the individual searching for answers on the Internet often comes away with more questions than answers. If questions remain after such a search or the conclusion is that action is needed, communities often turn to local or state governments for help.

Communities find that the greatest challenge is converting the information they now have into action. Obtaining information used to be the bottleneck, now more than ever the bottleneck is finding someone to respond. More than 40 states have followed the federal example and split environmental law enforcement from public health. Communities often start with the regulatory agencies before contacting public health. The public health system remains the primary resource to assist communities to respond to their identified health concerns, especially when enforcement of environmental laws seems unable to help.[1] (See Chapter 35.)

In most states, public health service delivery is a tiered system, usually organized around geopolitical boundaries—city, county, region, and state.[2] Typically, a county or large city health department provides primary services. More specialized services are most often provided by a secondary system at the regional or state level. In some instances, the state health department may provide direct services when the local resources cannot. Environmental public health at the local level is provided by public health sanitarians, environmental health specialists, and public health nurses with generalist skills. Core local activities include investigating infectious disease outbreaks, indoor air complaints, private well or septic system concerns, and factory emissions. Larger county, city, and state health departments usually are able to employ staff with more specialized skills and training and to deploy more sophisticated equipment and laboratory support. The community and local health care practitioners turn to this interrelated system when they have environmental heath concerns that require action.

Responding to community environmental health concerns is labor- and resource-intensive, not just to conduct the studies but also to effectively interpret and communicate the results and risks so they are understandable to the public. The funding and staffing of environmental public health has not kept pace with the exponentially expanding access to information on the World Wide Web and awareness of environmental threats to health. When the local resources are insufficient, state personnel and resources augment response efforts. If both are overextended, as can happen when responding to a natural disaster such as a flood, tornado, or hurricane, the state can request assistance from the federal government, specifically the Centers for Disease Control and Prevention (CDC), which can rapidly deploy field epidemiologists to support state and local efforts.

Community concern may begin with (a) a newly identified exposure and fear that adverse health effects may result; or (b) the perception that some disease may be occurring more frequently than expected because of a suspected exposure. The latter situation may lead to an investigation of a disease cluster.[3] Regardless of whether the initial request for assistance begins as an exposure or a disease concern, when the community suspects the cause is environmental, the environmental public health program often leads the investigation.

A fundamental principle of public health is the prevention of disease by avoiding exposures to harmful levels of toxic exposures in the environment. Despite a preventive approach, environmental health agencies typically respond to a case when chemical exposure is discovered. Sometimes, environmental health agencies address the emergency response situation of a chemical spill or accident, which results in actual or potential acute chemical exposures to the public. Environmental agencies also frequently address long-term exposure of the public to contaminants that are discovered in well water or surface soils.

EXPOSURE EVALUATION

When the public is known or suspected to be exposed to chemical contamination, environmental health agencies must determine the level of any exposures. Exposure evaluations rely on either environmental screening or sampling data. If a chemical spill occurs, the first responders arriving at the scene are typically firefighters or hazardous-waste management teams with professional judgment and field-chemical screening equipment, and they determine the level of existing hazards and actions needed to control them. When environmental health agencies learn that a neighborhood has chemical contamination that originates from an old dumpsite, laboratory analysis of environmental media, such as drinking water, soils, sediments, indoor air, or even fish tissue, reveals the levels of contaminants. Unfortunately, high costs of laboratory analysis do not allow environmental samples to be randomly collected everywhere but forces environmental investigations to focus only on places where contamination is suspected. Even when contamination is discovered in environmental media, an evaluation is needed to determine whether people are actually being exposed and the frequency, duration, and degree of their exposure. An exposure evaluation must examine each possible exposure pathway.

RISK ASSESSMENT

When people are exposed to contaminated soil or drinking water, a risk assessment must be performed to determine whether the exposure represents an unacceptable health risk and an intervention is needed (Fig. 36-1). A risk assessment examines the exposure, empirical toxicological data of the contaminants of concern, and potentially sensitive populations who may be exposed. For some media, such as ground water, risk assessments are fairly straightforward because state and federal agencies have established drinking-water

standards for many chemicals. These standards take into account children and other sensitive people and assume that people daily ingest 2 L of contaminated water for a lifetime. However, for contaminated soil there is no similar standard but rather a range of guidelines. These guidelines require investigators to first establish (a) how often the public comes in contact with affected soils, (b) whether the area is residential or industrial, and (c) if children are visiting this area. For ambient or indoor air, occupational guidelines are suitable for a work setting. Yet, occupational guidelines are not appropriate for a residential or a commercial setting where occupational safety practices are not being implemented. The contaminant of concern is often a substance that does not have an exposure guideline for drinking water, residential soil, or workplace air—making the conduct of a risk assessment even more challenging.

EXPOSURE PREVENTION AND INTERVENTION

Once it is evident that the public is either likely to have or has a high risk of being exposed to an unacceptable level of chemical contaminants, actions are needed to prevent or halt the exposure. Interim actions, such as providing bottled water or fencing a contaminated abandoned property, may be sufficient to halt exposures. But bottled water may not be adequate if there are high concentrations of a solvent in tap water that can be released to indoor air by washing dishes or, showering, and residents

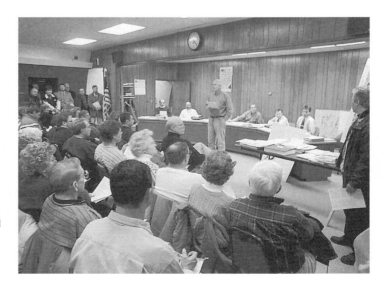

FIGURE 36-1 ● Holding public meetings with environmental and public health experts is essential to answering the community's questions and concerns. (Courtesy of Wisconsin Division of Public Health.)

are exposed by breathing affected indoor air. Each exposure intervention must consider and rule out all potential exposure pathways that may exist.

EVACUATION

If a highly contaminated area is discovered in a residential area or a chemical spill is spreading a toxic vapor cloud, the only appropriate action is the relocation or evacuation of the residents or workers. Evacuation or relocation is costly and stressful for both evacuees and responders. Although decisions to evacuate are carefully and thoughtfully made, this is often a time-critical decision made under duress by the responders. Evacuation decisions incorporate a buffer zone that is protective of public safety for those beyond the affected area. This zone area can be expanded in case the incident worsens and there is an increased risk of an explosion or the spreading of chemical contamination. Sometimes, if an airborne chemical plume is quickly dispersing, people may receive a significant exposure when evacuating, and "in-place" sheltering is the best action.

REENTRY

Once an incident is controlled and a clean-up is being planned, decisions are needed about what conditions are safe to allow the public to return to their homes and businesses. The reentry decisions take into account a risk assessment of the acceptable threshold of contaminant because total removal of all residuals is not usually feasible. In addition, air deposition of burning by-products onto adjacent properties during an industrial fire may affect reentry decisions.

PUBLIC INFORMATION AND RISK COMMUNICATION

As soon as environmental health agencies become involved with a chemical spill or discovery of environmental contamination, they must immediately prepare for and respond to community health questions and concerns about the situation. The risk communication skills of health agencies are a pivotal function in conveying health information to the public throughout the incident (Fig. 36-2).

FOLLOW-UP ACTIONS: HEALTH STUDIES, BIOLOGICAL MONITORING, AND DISEASE TRACKING

If the public is exposed to contaminants at a level that poses an unacceptable health risk, environmental health agencies decide what additional actions should be taken. For certain chemicals, immediate biological monitoring can give insight or even determine if people had a significant exposure. For some substances, medical monitoring may determine if those exposed to contaminants developed a specific illness or symptoms. Such medical monitoring could be part of a longer health study that tracks whether the rates of certain illnesses

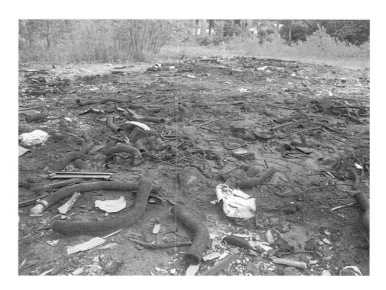

FIGURE 36-2 ● This waste site contains the remains from automobile wrecks and potentially contaminates the soil with heavy metals and other contaminants. (Courtesy of Wisconsin Division of Public Health.)

or symptoms increase over time or are higher than those of a comparison population.[4] Conducting these follow-up actions can be very expensive and time-consuming, especially if they continue for a long time. Although these findings may be informative and useful, they may also be inconclusive.

The following are examples of responses. A particular benefit of the Internet is the ability for state and local governments to make these reports available, or at least provide an inventory of such reports so they are available, to a broader audience.

The first example is a response to an acute exposure to mercury. Unfortunately, such spills have become common and create a cross-contamination issue greater than most consider. Unusual in this example is the availability of portable direct-read laboratory equipment that allowed rapid exposure assessment and resolution of community concerns. A critical activity involved communicating with all affected groups—from managers to students.

The second example is more typical of site-specific community concerns and reflects the problems that can develop from evolving land use in communities. This type of response is typical of the investigations performed by states that are supported by the Agency for Toxic Substance and Disease Registry (ATSDR) site-investigation funding. Biomonitoring, a new investigative tool of state and local health departments, was used to demonstrate that exposures were occurring at levels atypical for the general population. This finding helped to determine that the cause of the exposure was off-site.

The third and last example is a complex "outbreak" investigation involving multiple state and local agencies. The availability of federal support allowed for a more comprehensive study than would otherwise have been possible. While effective and open communication was important, it may also have contributed to expanding and prolonging the "outbreak."

Example 1: Mercury Spill at a High School

At 1:15 p.m. on January 30, 2004, elemental metallic mercury was spilled from an open-ended glass manometer at the back of a high-school chemistry classroom. A student reportedly attached one end of a rubber hose to the manometer and the other end to a pressurized air port. The student then reportedly opened the air port, which forced air into the

manometer and blew most of the mercury from the manometer. An estimated 4 tablespoons (60 cc) of mercury spilled onto nearby tables and counters and onto the floor. Mercury particles were also observed attached to the ceiling tiles directly above where the manometer was located. Shortly after this spill occurred, it was discovered by school personnel, who quickly reported it to school administrators, who implemented the school district's emergency procedure plan.

Responding to a request by school district officials, teams of firefighters and hazardous materials workers arrived at the school. After consulting with emergency response officials, the school district retained a hazardous waste clean-up contractor. Also responding to the incident were the Wisconsin Department of Natural Resources, the Wisconsin Department of Health and Family Services (DHFS), and the County Department of Human Services (DCHS).

Immediately after the spill was discovered, the high school science wing was cleared of students, faculty, and staff, and then secured. Soon after, the entire school was locked down and, to prevent the potential spread of mercury contamination, all students, faculty, and staff were not allowed to leave the building until they were screened for mercury contamination. The 70 students who were in chemistry class during or immediately after the spill were sent to locker rooms, where they removed their clothing and shoes and placed them in plastic bags, showered, and dressed in chemically resistant suits. These students were then transported to another school, where they were picked up by their parents and taken home. Their bagged clothes were transported to the community center. On Saturday, students and their parents were allowed to pick up their clothes and shoes if it was determined that their bags were free of mercury—with the use of a mercury analyzer that DHFS had recently procured. But seven had sufficiently high mercury vapor levels to retain and properly dispose of the clothing and shoes.

Students, faculty, and staff who had not gone in or near the chemistry classroom where the spill occurred were only required to have their shoes screened for mercury before they were allowed to leave the building, in order to ensure that mercury was not being tracked or carried around the school. Only one person, a science teacher who was in the chemistry classroom when the spill occurred, had elevated mercury vapors coming from her shoes, which were collected and properly disposed. Repeated screening of her clothes did not detect elevated mercury vapors.

The hazardous waste contractors used mercury field-screening meters to screen all indoor areas of the school for elemental mercury vapors. They observed beads of elemental mercury in the chemistry classroom where the mercury had been spilled. They also found elevated mercury vapors in this classroom and in the adjacent hallway and science office. Mercury vapor concentrations at the classroom doorway ranged between 2 and 3 $\mu g/m^3$ and where the spill had occurred between 14 to 22 $\mu g/m^3$. All areas of the school were double-checked to confirm that mercury was elevated only inside of and very near the chemistry classroom. The contractors then collected and removed all visible mercury from the classroom and used clean-up methods to appropriately remove mercury residues from the classroom, the adjacent hallway, and selected nearby rooms. They also thoroughly ventilated the classroom and science wing. As a precautionary measure, they also wet-mopped flooring throughout the school with a special amalgamating solution to ensure the removal of any mercury residues that may have previously escaped detection. The clean-up staff worked through the night and completed the clean-up by 3:00 p.m. on the day after the spill.

Application of Existing Public Health Guidelines and Protocols

The ATSDR chronic inhalation minimal risk level (MRL) for mercury vapor in air is 0.2 $\mu g/m^3$. ATSDR defines an MRL as an "estimate of daily human exposure to a hazardous substance at or below which that substance is unlikely to pose a measurable risk of harmful (adverse), noncancerous effects." (The inhalation of elemental mercury vapors has not been found to cause cancer in humans.)

Students, faculty, and staff who had been in the chemistry classroom at the time of the spill had breathed mercury vapors only for a short time. Taking into consideration the levels of mercury they had breathed, it was not likely that this exposure caused any harmful health effects and, as a result, it was thought that this exposure posed no apparent human health hazard.

The *Suggested Action Levels for Indoor Mercury Vapors in Homes or Businesses with Indoor Gas Regulators* of ATSDR were the clean-up goals used. ATSDR recommends that after a spill, mercury va-

por levels in the breathing zone of a home not exceed 1.0 $\mu g/m^3$ and that at or below this level is acceptable for reoccupancy of any structure. Exceeding the action level of 1 $\mu g/m^3$ prompts the need for clean-up or other remedial actions to reduce exposures, and exceeding 10 $\mu g/m^3$ prompts isolation of residents from exposure and actions taken to remediate the spill. ATSDR also recommends an action level of 10 $\mu g/m^3$ when testing the air from a plastic bag in which mercury-contaminated clothing has been placed, indicating that it is to be obtained from the owner.

Biomonitoring Recommendations and Results

As a further precautionary measure, DHFS and DCHS offered urine laboratory screening for mercury. A total of 42 urine samples were brought to the emergency department at the local hospital by Tuesday, February 3, and then submitted to the Wisconsin State Laboratory of Hygiene for testing. Only one of the 41 urine samples had a mercury level above the detection limit—at 6 $\mu g/L$, within the acceptable range. DCHS mailed the results and explanatory letters directly to the students' parents on Thursday, February 5.

Air Sampling Before Reentry

As a follow-up activity, air samples were collected from selected locations to provide a final, confirmatory evaluation. A third-party contractor had collected air samples in the high school, on January 31, by drawing air through glass tubes filled with appropriate sampling media. Tests of these samples did not detect any mercury vapors.

DHFS provided these data to school district officials on the afternoon of February 1. It had concluded that the data demonstrated that the clean-up had effectively removed all of the elemental mercury that had been spilled. School district officials then decided to reopen the high school the following day.

Risk Communication Employed

Communication among all involved parties was critically important throughout the response to the spill. DHFS staff members used their expertise in risk communication to assist school administrators in developing and communicating appropriate health messages that were effective. They also assisted the school superintendent and the county health officer in drafting written communications and preparing for a Friday evening press conference to share with parents and media representatives information concerning the situation and prudent actions being taken to address it. They wrote to the superintendent on Sunday to interpret air sampling results and to state that the school was ready to open on Monday. They also wrote letters to students' parents on Tuesday, informing them why mercury spills are of concern and explaining that low background levels of mercury vapor found in all bags of clothes that were returned to the students meant there was no further health concern. They assisted the DCHS health officer in writing letters to parents that interpreted mercury levels in their children's urine specimens. At the school board meeting on Monday night, they presented the public health implications of the incident and answered questions from board members and the public. Because the school board meeting was televised, they used the opportunity to promote the proper removal and disposal of mercury sources, such as oral thermometers and thermostats, from homes and businesses.

Representatives of the school district, the responding public health agencies—DHFS and DCHS—the hospital emergency department, and the Wisconsin Poison Center all collaborated in the response to the incident. During the course of the response, the poison center received approximately 50 telephone calls from concerned parents about the spill. No callers described adverse health effects associated with acute or chronic mercury exposure. School officials and DCHS personnel informed parents that they should seek medical care for their children from their physicians or the emergency department if their children experienced neurologic or other symptoms related to mercury exposure. The emergency department received several inquiries but no known or suspected mercury-related adverse health effects.

Example 2: Health Concern at a Hazardous-Waste Remediation Site[5]

Site History: How the Problem Began and Progressed

In the summer of 1997, some people residing at the former Northwestern Barrel Company in South Milwaukee complained about odors coming from on-site soil treatment activities. Some reported experiencing symptoms when odors were strong. Residents requested that DHFS conduct a public health assessment of site conditions in order to quantify exposure to any contaminants being released and to evaluate possible adverse health impacts.

When the company operated from 1940 to 1964, waste materials—mostly paint-related—were disposed into multiple pits located near the edge of a bluff overlooking Lake Michigan. Leachate from the pits stained the bluff edge and drained to the beach. The site was identified for detailed investigation and remediation.

By 1996, condominiums, apartments, and single-family homes had been built over the property. Three apartment complexes and two condominium complexes—with about 195 residences—were within 100 yards of the property. Another four-condominium complex—with 80 units built in 1968—was on the southwestern corner of the property. Two of these condominium buildings had been built very close to the foundation of one of the previous industrial buildings. A 1952 aerial photograph indicated the 80-unit complex was located where drums were once stored. Yet another 8-unit condominium, built in 1982, was located north of these condominiums. Finally, a 24-unit apartment complex, built in 1991, was on the northwest corner of the property. In addition to the 195 apartments adjacent to the property, approximately 210 single-family dwellings were within 300 yards of the property. DHFS estimated that altogether about 1,000 people lived within 300 yards of the property.

Chemical analysis from 1995 of subsurface soil samples revealed the presence of elevated levels of inorganic chemicals, volatile organic compounds (VOCs), and semivolatile organic compounds (SVOCs). The highest lead level detected was 45,700 mg/kg. In one sample, total VOCs comprised more than 7 percent of soil by weight. The highest level of xylenes found was 36,000 mg/kg.

During November and December 1996, as part of the remediation plan, soils were excavated from these disposal pits, placed on a prepared clay pad, covered with plastic sheeting, and stockpiled on the property. In May 1997, EPA approved a request for the on-site treatment/stabilization of the soil by adding Portland cement to minimize the leaching of lead and to facilitate disposal of the soil as non-hazardous waste.

Soil treatment/stabilization and removal activities were initiated in June 1997 and were scheduled to last about 3 weeks. A canvas tent was erected to house the soil-mixing equipment and minimize release of fugitive dust and VOCs. Soil piles were

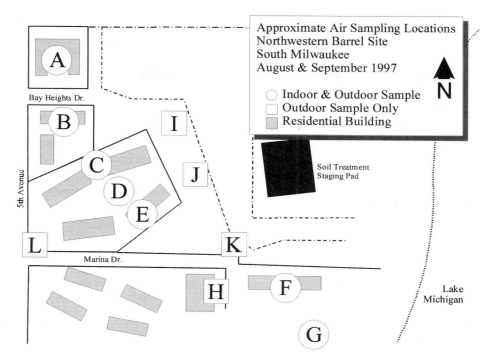

FIGURE 36-3 ● Approximate air-sampling locations at the Northwestern Barrel site, South Milwaukee, 1997. (Courtesy of Wisconsin Division of Public Health.)

uncovered and transferred with heavy equipment to a screening device (located outside the mixing tent), which sifted debris from the soil. Soil piles were covered when operations ceased. However, a high water content was found in stockpiled soils, along with much debris, considerably slowing the soil-mixing operation. These and other logistical issues resulted in extending of treatment/stabilization activities for 3 more months beyond the planned completion date, until September 1997.

Organic vapors from the property were released into the air by on-site soil treatment/stabilization and removal activities. Two environmental consultants used direct-readout instruments to regularly monitor air quality at and near the treatment area fence (Fig. 36-3). The air monitoring equipment that they used provided information on levels of airborne particulates and total VOCs, oxygen percentage in the air, and proximity to the lower explosive limit. An organic vapor monitor (OVM) was primarily used to make direct readings of the VOC concentration in air. During soil-treatment activities, OVM readings were reported as high as 352 ppm within the canvas tent, although these values often ranged between 30 and 150 ppm. The highest outdoor VOC

level of 147 ppm was observed immediately outside the tent. On June 23, total VOCs were measured inside the tent at 157 ppm. Later that day, contractors used compound-specific, hand-held, colormetric Draeger tubes to test air inside the tent and found benzene at 6 ppm (TLV = 0.5 ppm), styrene at 15 ppm, and toluene at 125 ppm (TLV = 50 ppm). On-site workers used appropriate personal protective equipment that permitted working in the presence of these vapors. Along the fence line, total VOCs were usually not measurable with the OVM.

These direct readings indicated that fence-line air concentrations of VOCs and particulates were not at acutely hazardous levels. Direct readout meters, such as organic vapor meters (OVMs), are useful tools when field screening for VOCs. However, there are limitations to such air monitoring instrumentation:

- OVM instruments are not compound-specific.
- They may not accurately measure airborne VOCs at concentrations less than 1 ppm.
- OVM use at the property required daily calibration, in accordance with the manufacturer's guidelines.

- Evidence of OVM calibration was to be written on the daily fugitive air emissions monitoring logs, but calibration notations were missing on 31 daily monitoring logs for site activities between June 5 and September 24, 1997.
- Air was monitored only by the environmental consultants during weekdays, but not during evenings or weekends, when there was no work being done at the property.

Listening to and Communicating with the Affected Community

On certain days between June and September 1997, a number of residents complained about bad odors coming from the soil treatment area at the property, initially on June 29. On that day, the Wisconsin Department of Natural Resources (DNR) observed that air was stagnant and issued an ozone alert for southeastern Wisconsin. Complaints from nearby residents were also noted in the site air-emissions monitoring log on July 24, July 31, and September 15. Typically, residents complained about air quality when there were light winds from the east or northeast, which carried vapors from the treatment area toward condominiums and apartments located less than 100 yards to the west.

DHFS responded to citizen air-quality complaints by visiting the property several times. During a July 11 visit, a light easterly breeze was blowing from Lake Michigan, across the treatment area, and toward several of the nearby apartment and condominium buildings. Residents again complained about a paint-like odor, which was evident to DHFS personnel as they walked around the apartment and condominium areas. VOCs were detected inside and immediately outside the treatment tent, but not on the perimeter of the treatment area.

Some residents reported adverse health effects, particularly when they noticed strong odors coming from the treatment area, including headache, sore throat, lethargy, and burning eyes. One resident recalled that he smelled similar odors and experienced similar symptoms when the two pit areas were excavated in 1996. In October 1997, one resident informed DHFS that she had developed a respiratory problem shortly after moving into a nearby apartment in mid-June that was diagnosed as asthma. She reported that the severity of her asthma symptoms was temporally associated with odors coming from the treatment

area. She was hospitalized twice for asthma during July. She reported that her asthma improved when odors subsided and after on-site soil treatment ended in September.

Responding to Concerns: Investigating Exposure

As a result of reported symptoms, DHFS initiated an exposure investigation, evaluating the VOC levels in blood of residents who complained of both poor air quality and symptoms. Before selecting survey participants, residents were asked questions to identify other possible VOC exposures that might confound interpretation of their blood VOC levels. DHFS then conducted VOC analysis of air samples collected in and around selected residents' homes, between their homes and the treatment area, and along the perimeter of the treatment area. DHFS offered blood VOC testing to approximately 20 people who lived near the property and had complained about odors coming from the property, three of whom agreed to provide blood samples.

Responding to Concerns: Selecting Study Subjects

DHFS contacted residents who had air-quality complaints about the property in order to identify those who experienced health effects associated with airborne contaminants from the property. Participants were informed that blood samples would be collected when wind conditions carried VOC vapors from the treatment area toward their residences. Nearby residents who provided blood samples were selected because (a) they planned to be at home for the duration of the day, and (b) they did not report a possible alternative confounding exposure to solvents (such as pumping gasoline, smoking cigarettes, or using household solvents).

Blood samples were collected on two separate days approximately 1 week apart. Subjects were interviewed when their blood samples were collected. On August 28, two of the three participating individuals reported they smelled odors coming from the soil treatment area: one said it smelled like paint thinner, and the other, like sweet perfume, with a burnt characteristic. Both individuals characterized the odors as weaker than usual. While neither of these individuals said they had an odor-related illness on August 28, one said he often had headaches on the afternoons of days when he

TABLE 36-1

Residential Blood Volatile Organic Compound (VOC) Sampling (All Blood Concentrations in μg/L)

| | Observed Average Blood VOC Concentration | | NHANES III Blood VOC Concentrations | | | |
| | | | Nonsmokers Only | | Smokers and Nonsmokers | |
Subject and Chemical	August 28	September 3	50th Percentile (Median)	95th Percentile	50th Percentile (Median)	95th Percentile
Subject 1: Sample location C						
Benzene	0.04	0.03	0.05	0.09	0.06	0.48
Ethylbenzene	0.04	0.03	0.05	0.23	0.06	0.25
Styrene	0.03	0.01	0.03	0.08	0.04	0.18
Toluene	0.08	0.27	0.21	1.00	0.28	1.50
Xylene (total)	0.19	0.12	0.25	0.97	0.30	1.08
Subject 2: Sample location C						
Benzene	*0.04*		*0.05*	*0.09*	*0.06*	*0.48*
Ethylbenzene	*0.01*		*0.05*	*0.23*	*0.06*	*0.25*
Styrene	*0.01*		*0.03*	*0.08*	*0.04*	*0.18*
Toluene	*0.05*		*0.21*	*1.00*	*0.28*	*1.50*
Xylene (total)	*0.09*		*0.25*	*0.97*	*0.30*	*1.08*
Subject 3: Sample location F						
Benzene	*0.03*	*0.03*	*0.05*	*0.09*	*0.06*	*0.48*
Ethylbenzene	*0.12*	*0.29**	*0.05*	*0.23*	*0.06*	*0.25*
Styrene	*0.05*	*0.13**	*0.03*	*0.08*	*0.04*	*0.18*
Toluene	*0.10*	*0.17*	*0.21*	*1.00*	*0.28*	*1.50*
Xylene (total)	*0.61*	*1.68**	*0.25*	*0.97*	*0.30*	*1.08*

Data in boldface exceed NHANES III 95th percentile for nonsmoking subjects only. Outlined blood VOC concentrations exceed NHANES III 95th percentile for all subjects.

noticed odors coming from the treatment area all day long. The third subject reported often having sore throats, which she attributed to air coming from the treatment area.

On September 3, a second set of samples was collected from two of these individuals when one reported an odor coming from the soil treatment area. This person described the odor as a paint thinner, although weaker than usual. These people did not report any odor-related symptoms on September 3. All of these individuals stated that they were nonsmokers. No subjects reported using any products or materials containing VOCs on the days that samples were obtained. Blood results from these three residents were compared with VOC blood concentrations of non–occupationally exposed participants of the Third National Health and Nutrition Examination Survey (NHANES III) (Table 36-1).

Eliciting Broader Community Health Concerns

As a follow-up, DHFS, in November 1997, sent letters and surveys to approximately 240 nearby households, asking residents about their health concerns related to the 1997 soil clean-up at the property; of the 59 households (25 percent) that responded, 16 reported illness or symptoms perceived as possibly related to contaminants at the site. Generally, people reported combinations of 12 respiratory symptoms, including nose and throat irritation, asthma, nosebleed, increased respiratory infections, wheezing, and coughing. Eight people reported severe or frequent headaches. All respondents reported at least one of the following symptoms: skin rash, lightheadedness, loss of appetite, weight gain, nausea, loss of energy, arthritis, muscle aches, weight loss, and discomfort. Most people who felt ill believed their symptoms were caused by exposure to airborne chemicals. To a lesser extent, people were concerned about soil contact while they were gardening or walking their dogs or their children were playing in soil and water. Twenty people reported outdoor air-quality conditions associated with the property that they believed increased their sensitivity to chemicals. They reported chronic illnesses affecting their lungs, liver, sinuses, eyes, circulatory system, and kidneys. Two women were concerned about respiratory exposures they had had during pregnancy.

Communication of Public Health Conclusions

Ethylbenzene and xylene levels were higher in the September 3 air samples from Location F (about 100 yards from the soil treatment area) and the fenceline than the August 28 samples. Both fenceline samples were south of the treatment area and in between Location F and the treatment area.

Indoor and outdoor air samples taken from residences next to the treatment area showed the presence of relatively low concentrations of site-related VOCs and SVOCs. None of these substances were found in air at concentrations known to cause illness with short- or intermediate-term exposures. The VOCs with the highest offsite concentrations were ethylbenzene (40 ppbv), styrene (85 ppbv), toluene (46 ppbv), and total xylenes (179 ppv). None of these aromatic VOCs were found at a concentration that exceeds an ATSDR acute or intermediate minimal risk level.

Nearby residents were exposed to slightly elevated levels of several airborne VOCs during soil treatment at the property. Analysis of blood samples collected from three residents showed that one in Location F on September 3 had high blood concentrations of ethylbenzene, styrene, and xylene; between August 28 and September 3, his blood concentrations of ethylbenzene and xylene seemed to correlate with indoor and outdoor air concentrations of these substances at Location F.

Example 3: 1995 Outbreak of Unexplained Symptoms

Setting the Stage

One of the mandated pollutant control activities under the Clean Air Act Amendments of 1990 was requiring that only reformulated gasoline (RFG) be sold in many major metropolitan areas in the United States, starting in January 1995. By November 1994, RFG containing at least 2.0 percent oxygen by weight was to be sold in ozone-nonattainment areas. (*Nonattainment* was defined as having exceeded the federal ambient ozone standard at least once a year. Nonattainment areas included metropolitan Chicago, Milwaukee, Los Angeles, San Diego, Baltimore, Houston, New York, Philadelphia, and Hartford.)

The oxygen content of RFG has been increased by supplementation with ethanol or ether-based compounds, such as methyl *tert*-butyl ether (MTBE), ethyl *tert*-butyl ether (ETBE), and tertiary amyl methyl ether (TAME), at concentrations of up to 11 percent by weight. The use of such chemicals in automobile fuel is not new. MTBE has been used to enhance octane in U.S. gasoline since 1979, with concentrations of up to 7 percent by weight in premium grades. Oxygenated gasoline was first used in Denver in 1988 to reduce ambient carbon monoxide levels. Local government agencies did not register any unusual public reactions to the change in gasoline at that time.

In November 1992, oxygenated gasoline was introduced in several carbon monoxide nonattainment areas, including Stamford, Connecticut, and Anchorage and Fairbanks, Alaska. Soon after, the Alaska Department of Public Health began receiving numerous health complaints attributed to the use of oxygenated gasoline. Consequently, after less than 2 months of implementation, the program was discontinued. During the period when oxygenated gasoline was used and 6 weeks after it was discontinued, the Alaska Department of Public Health had conducted a study comparing self-reported health effects among occupationally exposed groups (drivers, mechanics, and service-station operators). The rate of self-reported symptoms decreased after the program was terminated.[6]

RFG Introduction in Milwaukee

Approximately 6 weeks after the November 1994 introduction of RFG in Milwaukee, government agencies began to receive the first of more than 3,500 telephone calls from people reporting various symptoms they attributed to RFG use. An interagency response was organized, which included establishment of well-publicized telephone hotlines for the public to register concerns, a standard system of complaint-reporting for hotline operators, public meetings, and distribution of information to the health care providers and general public. In February 1995, the Governor of Wisconsin requested that the state Bureau of Public Health (BPH) and Department of Natural Resources (DNR) investigate these symptoms and determine if RFG use was causing them.[7,8]

Outbreak Investigation

Random-Digit-Dial Survey

The Wisconsin Survey Research Laboratory conducted a random-digit-dial (RDD), computer-assisted telephone interview (CATI) survey between February 24 and March 19. The survey included questions on demographic information, health status, awareness of the Clean Air Act, use of RFG, and activities related to purchasing gasoline and driving. All respondents were asked: "Since November 1, 1994, have you experienced any unusual health symptoms unrelated to cold or flu or any other chronic health problem you may have?" Those responding positively were asked if they had noted headache, nausea, eye irritation, dizziness, diarrhea, rashes, muscle aches, throat irritation, difficulty breathing, back pain, fever, "spaciness" or lightheadedness, sinus congestion, "funny smells," or other symptoms. They were also asked when symptoms began and if symptoms were noted while driving, sitting in an idling vehicle, pumping gasoline, on the job, or during other specific activities. Analysis units consisted of the six-county Milwaukee ozone nonattainment area ("Milwaukee"); the six-county Chicago ozone nonattainment area ("Chicago"); and all of Wisconsin, except for the ozone nonattainment area ("Wisconsin"). The sample design specified 500 adults in each of these three areas.

People exposed to RFG were defined as living in either Chicago or Milwaukee—the two study areas where RFG use was required. Those exposed to specific RFG components were further defined in separate analyses as car owners in Chicago or Milwaukee who reported (a) usually buying brands and grades of gasoline containing MTBE; and/or

(b) usually or occasionally buying gasoline from pumps not displaying the label ethanol.

Air Monitoring

Ambient air monitoring was conducted twice by the DNR staff at three service stations, three roadway locations, and one parking garage in the Milwaukee area between February 21 and March 9. Service stations, with and without stage 2 vapor recovery (a system by which gasoline vapors are drawn back into the gasoline storage tank), were chosen. Specific areas were chosen for sampling based on the number of complaints received from people living or working in the area. Air samples were also collected from one service station and two urban roadway locations outside of the area where RFG use was mandated.

Standard EPA air-sampling methods were used to determine target gasoline components in ambient air. Air samples collected over 1 to 3 hours were analyzed for benzene, toluene, ethylbenzene, xylene, MTBE, ETBE, ethanol, and methanol. Personal breathing zone monitoring equipment was worn by DNR personnel for 15 minutes during automotive refueling. Air concentrations of gasoline components were also measured at one permanent air-monitoring station located in a residential area of Milwaukee. Sample concentrations were determined for 24-hour periods every sixth day during the study period. Eleven samples were collected.

Study Results

RDD Survey

The overall response rate was 59 percent, with regional response rates ranging from 41 percent in Chicago to 71 percent in Wisconsin. Demographic and health status characteristics of the sampled populations closely matched those in the general population in each area. Milwaukee respondents, however, were much more likely to be aware of issues related to RFG and specific oxygenates than respondents from the other two areas.

The prevalence of each unexplained symptom was higher in Milwaukee than in Chicago or Wisconsin. The most common unexplained symptoms reported among all three populations were headache, throat irritation, and sinus congestion. Prevalence of unexplained back pain and fever—symptoms not previously associated with solvent exposure—was also higher in Milwaukee than the other two areas. Differences in unexplained

TABLE 36-2

Variables Included in Analysis

Demographic Information	Health Status	RFG Exposure	RFG Knowledge
Ages 33–45	Cigarette smoker	Car owner	Live in an area where RFG is required
Ages 46–57	Physician-diagnosed asthma	Commute >1 h/day	Heard of MTBE
Ages 58+	Cold/flu since November 1		
Nonwhite race			
Female gender			

RFG, reformulated gasoline.

symptom prevalence between Chicago and Wisconsin were not statistically significant.

Half of the Milwaukee respondents and 10 percent of Chicago respondents reported purchasing RFG since November 1, 1994. Milwaukee respondents who reported purchasing RFG were significantly more likely to report symptoms and attribute them to RFG than the rest of the Milwaukee respondents. Similar, but not statistically significant, patterns were seen among Chicago and Wisconsin respondents.

Forty-three (64 percent) of Milwaukee respondents and six (46 percent) of Chicago respondents reporting unexplained headaches since November 1, associated their headaches with pumping gasoline, and 51 (76 percent) of Milwaukee respondents and 8 (61 percent) of Chicago respondents associated their headache with driving or idling. A similar pattern of attribution was seen among the other symptoms. Approximately half of the respondents reported symptom onset after January 1.

Risk ratios were determined in a multiple logistic regression model for the entire study population based on area of residence and cold or flu history status. Milwaukee residents were between 3 and 35 times more likely to report each individual symptom than residents of either Chicago or Wisconsin. Individuals reporting a cold since November 1 were between 2 and 12 times more likely to report each unexplained symptom, except rashes, muscle aches, and back pain.

To determine predictors of symptoms within each region, risk ratios were determined for respondents in each of the three areas separately. A

multiple logistic regression model was created so that individual risk factors related to demographic characteristics, health status, or potential exposure to gasoline could be analyzed simultaneously. Table 36-2 shows the variables included in this analysis.

In the analysis, none of the risk factors included in the model were associated with symptom prevalence in Chicago or Wisconsin. In Milwaukee, only cold status, hearing about MTBE, and knowledge of living in an area where RFG is required predicted symptoms. None of the demographic or RFG exposure risk factors included predicted the other symptoms.

Few people were able to recall specific information about the gasoline they purchased. In all areas studied, approximately one-third of survey respondents indicated the brand and grade of gasoline usually purchased, and one-fourth reported whether they remembered whether the pump dispensing that gasoline was labeled ethanol. Among these few responders, neither of these exposure definitions was predictive of any symptom, suggesting that symptoms were not predominantly associated with one type of RFG.

Air Monitoring

At all roadside locations, toluene and benzene were gasoline components detected at the highest concentrations. MTBE and ETBE were detected at all roadside, service station, and parking ramp locations in the Milwaukee metropolitan area but not in every sample collected. MTBE was also detected at a service station, but not at roadside locations, outside the area where RFG is required. This finding may result from premium grades of nonreformulated gasoline containing up to 7 percent MTBE. The highest gasoline-related hydrocarbon concentrations were found in the personal breathing zone of people refueling at a self-service pump and were approximately 1,000 times those measured in ambient air samples.

Interpreting and Communicating the Results: Trying to Make Public Health Sense from the Outbreak

The introduction of RFG in November 1994 was temporally associated with an outbreak of unusual health symptoms among Milwaukee residents. Whether the outbreak was caused by an acute toxic reaction to RFG remained elusive, and other explanations appeared more plausible.

In designing the investigation, it was hypothesized that if the observed excess in unusual symptom prevalence in Milwaukee represented a toxic response to RFG use, symptom prevalence in Chicago should have been similar to Milwaukee. Chicago was the best available "positive exposure" control. Correspondence from, and discussions with, oil industry representatives indicated that Milwaukee and Chicago service stations received RFG gasoline from the same distributors and through the same pipelines. Compliance sampling by EPA in February 1995 reported comparable use of MTBE as the oxygenate in gasoline in Milwaukee and Chicago. Unfortunately, it was not possible to conduct air monitoring in Chicago during the outbreak period, which could have provided comparability of validated ambient air concentrations. Geographic proximity and shared weather conditions, which influence air pollutant concentration and distribution, provide qualitative support for the assumption that ambient air concentrations of RFG components in Chicago would be comparable to those in Milwaukee. Field monitoring studies documented that stage II vapor recovery systems at gasoline stations significantly reduced exposure to gasoline vapors to operators filling their gasoline tanks. A March 1995 survey of 884 service stations in the six-county Milwaukee area found 35 percent of stations had such equipment. The proportion of such stations in Chicago was unknown; however, the significance of any differences is probably small. Of individuals experiencing unusual symptoms in each city, the proportion experiencing them while pumping gasoline was not significantly different.

The markedly higher prevalence of self-reported unusual symptoms in Milwaukee—approximately four times that in Chicago—could not be explained by potential RFG exposure differences in the two cities. Symptom prevalence in Wisconsin outside of Milwaukee, a control area where RFG was not sold during the study period, was identical to that in Chicago, supporting the conclusion that the excess seen in Milwaukee was unlikely a toxic response but rather initiated by factors other than exposure to RFG vapors.

Concentrations of RFG components during fueling were frequently 1,000 times higher than ambient concentrations. If an acute toxic response were contributing to the occurrence of unusual symptoms, a dose–response relationship should exist and would predict a higher prevalence of symptoms experienced during refueling than while driving or idling in traffic. The finding that a similar proportion of symptomatic individuals reported experiencing their symptoms while fueling as while driving or idling argues against a toxic response. Time spent commuting, a surrogate measure for "nonrefueling" exposure, was also unrelated to symptom occurrence. Finally, the unusual symptoms began for 50 percent of the symptomatic respondents over 2 months after initiation of the RFG program. This delay in symptom onset is inconsistent with a toxic exposure–acute response relationship and is quite different from the immediate symptom response seen when the oxygenated fuels program was initiated in Alaska.

It had also been hypothesized that different RFG formulations might elicit different symptom responses and, thus, analyses attempted to identify subgroups with predominant use of a single RFG formulation. MTBE received the most attention, perhaps due to its sharp odor at low concentrations, having been the oxygenate present in the Alaska oxygenated fuel-associated outbreak, and concern over its carcinogenicity. MTBE air concentrations found in this study were elevated but within the range of those found in previous studies. Thus, Milwaukee exposure conditions were not unusual. Unusual symptoms were not associated with different RFG formulations. Milwaukee residents reporting usually purchasing gasoline containing MTBE were no more likely to report symptoms than those purchasing gasoline containing ethanol—although the strength of this conclusion is limited by the comparatively small number of individuals who consistently purchased gas from one station. Previously published clinical studies support a conclusion that the MTBE concentrations measured in this study would be unlikely to cause acute, short-term health problems.[9]

Knowledge of RFG, defined as reporting purchasing RFG since November 1, 1994, was five times greater among Milwaukee residents than among residents of the other two study areas. Knowledge of RFG issues was also high among Wisconsin residents, perhaps because Milwaukee newspapers are distributed throughout the state. In the Alaska study, symptom prevalence markedly decreased after termination of the oxygenated fuels program. In the Milwaukee study, knowledge of RFG and awareness of RFG issues were major factors in this outbreak of unusual symptoms.

Anecdotal evidence suggests that Milwaukee was unique in the United States regarding media attention to RFG. In late January 1995, a national television "news magazine" broadcast a story about the health complaints in Alaska related to the introduction of oxygenated gasoline. In Milwaukee, the story was immediately followed by a 1-week local television series and radio talk show programs devoted to the subject. Newspaper and television stories erroneously listed January 1, 1995, as the date on which the RFG program began; on that date, gasoline prices in the Milwaukee area had risen by approximately 16 cents per gallon. This price increase did not occur in Chicago and was later found to be unjustified in Milwaukee, based on the wholesale cost of gasoline.

A computer search of newspaper stories appearing in the *Milwaukee Journal* and *Milwaukee Sentinel*, newspapers read throughout Wisconsin, found that between February 10 and March 17, 63 stories (nearly two per day) about RFG appeared in these newspapers, often on the front page. Media attention was limited in the rest of the region, with only three related articles published in the *Chicago Tribune* during this period, one of which discussed the concerns of Milwaukee residents and questioned the lack of such concerns in Chicago, highlighting the Milwaukee television stories and the lack of media attention in other areas. Although RFG had been used in the area since November 1994, the symptom outbreak coincided with media attention to the RFG issue in mid-January 1995.

Beginning January 26, 1995, public response to the introduction of RFG was facilitated by the establishment of a toll-free complaint hotline at the Region V office of the EPA and by television and radio stations broadcasting local telephone numbers of relevant government agencies. Whereas more than 5,000 Wisconsin residents called, only 10 Illinois residents called (6 of whom worked in Wisconsin), and no one from other states. In February and March 1995, the Wisconsin Bureau of Public Health sent a brief survey to all state health departments and received 20 responses, indicating that 4 states used RFG and 10 used oxygenated gasoline. Between November 1994 and February 1995, no other state health department reported more than 10 health-related complaints related to gasoline exposure.

Analyses support a conclusion that public knowledge of the RFG program and heightened awareness of negative RFG issues, associated with a gasoline price increase and subsequent media attention, may have led a disproportionate number of Milwaukee residents to consider "unusual" symptoms they were experiencing from colds, flu, or other diseases and attribute them to RFG exposure. Such responses are not unusual. For example, in 1980, after publicity about the relative risk of toxic shock syndrome (TSS) among users of Rely tampons, the proportion of women with toxic shock who thought they had used Rely tampons was significantly higher after publicity than before.

Perhaps more than others, Milwaukee residents have a healthy respect for the consequences of environmental exposures. Such concern in Milwaukee was not unfounded, because an outbreak of gastrointestinal symptoms, which affected an estimated 400,000 people in the city less than 2 years earlier, was later attributed to the presence of *Cryptosporidium* in the public water supply.[10]

Final Public Health Message

All gasoline, whether RFG or more traditional formulations, contains toxic components known to cause adverse health effects among significantly exposed humans, and exposure should be avoided. DHFS concluded that the outbreak of unusual symptoms in the general Milwaukee population in early 1995, while roughly coinciding with the mandatory introduction of RFG, was unlikely to have represented a widespread, general public toxic response to exposure to RFG vapors or combustion products. The data collected and analyses performed supported more plausible alternative sociologic explanations. The relevance of these explanations was supported by:

- the localization of the outbreak to Milwaukee;
- the uniquely high news and media attention in Milwaukee;
- anger over the marked rise in gasoline prices;
- the increased prevalence and attribution of all types of symptoms as "unusual";
- the strong association between health symptoms and knowledge of RFG surrogate variables;
- the occurrence of a previous cold or the flu with unusual symptom prevalence;
- the lack of a dose–response relationship; and
- the appreciation in Milwaukee, as a consequence of the cryptosporidiosis outbreak, that environmental exposures can cause widespread illness.

Mandatory RFG sale continued in Milwaukee during and after the "outbreak." During the following winter of 1995–1996, no gasoline-related health complaints were received by local Wisconsin government agencies.

Although some people in Milwaukee may have had an acute toxic response, they could not be separated from the more complex interplay of contributing factors. To assist those individuals, the study concluded that stage 2 vapor recovery systems markedly reduced exposure to all gasoline vapors while fueling. People concerned about potential adverse health effects were advised to patronize service stations with such equipment.

REFERENCES

1. Anderson H, Sieger T. Environmental health in Wisconsin – Challenges for the 21st century. Wisconsin Medical Journal 2000;99:10–14.
2. National Association of County and City Health Officials. Community revitalization and public health: Issues, roles, and relationships for local health agencies. Washington, DC: NACCHO, 2000.
3. Fiore BJ, Hanrahan LP, Anderson, HA. State health department response to disease cluster reports: A protocol for investigation. Am J Epidemiol 1990;132:S14–S22.
4. Thacker SB, Stroup DF, Parrish RG, et al. Surveillance in environmental public health: Issues, systems, and sources. Am J Public Health 1996;86:633–8.
5. Agency for Toxic Substances and Disease Registry. Former Northwestern Barrel Company (Marina Cliffs): Public Health Assessment and Ambient Air Exposure Investigation: Public Comment Release. Atlanta, GA: ATSDR, 2002.
6. Moolenaar RL, Hefflin BJ, Ashley DL, et al. Methyl tertiary butyl ether in human blood after exposure to oxygenated fuel in Fairbanks, Alaska. Arch Env Health 1994;49:402–9.
7. Anderson HA, Hanrahan LH, Goldring J, et al. An investigation of health concerns attributed to reformulated gasoline use in southeastern Wisconsin: Phase 1—Final report. Madison, WI: Department of Health and Social Services, Wisconsin, Division of Health, Bureau of Public Health, 1995.
8. Anderson HA, Hanrahan LH, Goldring J, et al. An investigation of health concerns attributed to reformulated gasoline use in southeastern Wisconsin: Phase 2, telephone registered health concerns—Final report. Madison, WI: Wisconsin DHSS, DOH, BPH, 1995.
9. White MC, Johnson CA, Ashley DL, et al. Exposure to methyl tertiary-butyl ether from oxygenated gasoline in Stamford, Connecticut. Arch Env Health 1995;50: 183–9.
10. MacKenzie WR, Hoxie NJ, Proctor ME, et al. A massive outbreak in Milwaukee of cryptosporidium infection transmitted through the public water supply. N Eng J Med 1994;331:161–7.

BIBLIOGRAPHY

ATSDR Public Health Assessment Tutorial. Available at: <http://www.atsdr.cdc.gov/training/public-health-assessment-overview/html/>
Provides an overview of the health assessment approach used by states and the federal Agency for Toxic Substances and Disease Registry when addressing known or suspected environmental contamination that the public may be exposed to.

U.S. EPA Exposure Assessment Guidance Overview. Available at <http://www.epa.gov/opptintr/exposure/docs/exposurep.htm>.
A systematic approach to evaluating when people are exposed to chemical contamination.

Morgan MT. Environmental health. 3rd ed. Belmont, CA: Wadsworth/Thompson Learning, 2003.
A comprehensive summary of the practices used in protecting the public from environmental health hazards.

Burke R. Hazardous materials chemistry for emergency responders: Street chemistry. Boca Raton, FL: CRC Press, 1997.
Useful chemical information and case studies of hazardous material events.

CHAPTER 37

Regulations in Practice: Assessing and Enforcing Compliance with Health and Safety Regulations

Michael Silverstein and Michelle T. Watters

The important features that distinguish regulatory and enforcement agencies from the rest of government are [that] the core of their mission involves the imposition of duties. They deliver obligations, rather than services. Society entrusts regulatory and enforcement agencies with awesome powers. They can impose economic penalties, place liens upon or seize property, limit business practices, suspend professional licenses, destroy livelihoods....How regulatory and enforcement agencies use these powers fundamentally affects the nature and quality of life in a democracy.[1]

There is little debate that generally accepted norms, standards, or codes of behavior and commerce are essential for people to live and work together successfully in groups as simple as families or athletic teams or as complex as entire communities. Some such norms ensure predictability and facilitate interaction, such as weights and measures. Others are necessary for protection and safety, such as rules of the road. In other cases, the purpose of such norms is to protect fairness and equity by ensuring a "level playing field," such as measures to ensure competitiveness, prevent discrimination, or discourage cheating. Still other societal standards are essentially moral or ethical, such as "acceptable" styles or amounts of clothing.

There is also little disagreement that some standards are so important they should be mandatory and codified into enforceable statutes, rules, and regulations. Few would argue against ethical pro-

hibitions against murder being written into criminal laws and enforced vigorously. However, consensus is rarely reached so easily. There is considerable debate about when our behavior should be governed by enforceable rules and regulations rather than voluntary standards. Even when there is general agreement that enforceable rules are needed, there are substantial differences about exactly what these rules should say and how they should be enforced. There is broad consensus that legal speed limits are necessary on public thoroughfares but less agreement about what these limits should be, and even less about vehicle-related safety matters, such as seatbelt or motorcycle-helmet use.

There have been few fields in which the debate about the role of government regulation versus voluntary self-control has been more pronounced than that of occupational and environmental health. Over the past 35 years since our laws protecting worker and environmental health were substantially strengthened, their implementation has repeatedly become the stage for clashes between advocates for personal (or corporate) freedom versus public responsibility, private property versus public stewardship, and economic control versus equal opportunity. As these conflicts have worked themselves through the three branches of government, the requirements for occupational and environmental protections have been more sharply defined, and a complex infrastructure of regulatory agencies and related institutions has evolved to ensure compliance with them.

Achieving this compliance has proved to be a more challenging strategic undertaking than simply establishing the laws and rules and then deputizing law officers to enforce them. Hybrid strategies have been proposed that combine traditional coercive methods like inspections, citations, and litigation with tools of encouragement, education, and persuasion that use market and other economic incentives.

The resulting programs, policies, and procedures have become something of a maze for the uninitiated. Nonetheless, students and practitioners of public health need to understand and appreciate the roles, responsibilities, rights, and relationships that have emerged from these regulatory maneuvers if they are to apply their professional skills effectively.

For example, if patients are fearful that their health is threatened by workplace chemical exposures, what avenues are open to their physicians for ensuring that all legal obligations for identifying and controlling hazards have been met? The purpose of this chapter is to provide a review of the way that the environmental and occupational health regulatory structure affects public health practice and to provide some basic tools for working within it (see also Chapter 3).

WORKPLACE SAFETY AND HEALTH REGULATION: RIGHTS, ROLES, AND RESPONSIBILITIES UNDER THE OCCUPATIONAL SAFETY AND HEALTH ACT

The Occupational Safety and Health Act of 1970 (OSHAct) was simple, yet profound, in its declaration of a national "purpose and policy . . . to assure so far as possible every working man and woman in the Nation safe and healthful working conditions." It established the Occupational Safety and Health Administration (OSHA) as the principal regulatory and enforcement agency to achieve this purpose. However, jurisdiction is vested elsewhere in several situations:

- *Mines*: The Mine Safety and Health Administration and the Mine Safety and Health Act cover approximately 3,500 coal mines and 12,450 metal and other mines.
- *Industries regulated by other federal agencies*: The OSHAct permits other federal regulatory agencies to assume safety and health responsibil-

ity for certain industries. For example, the Federal Aviation Administration has claimed jurisdiction for hazards faced by airplane crews and the U.S. Department of Energy (DOE) has jurisdiction for workplace hazards at its weapons manufacturing facilities.
- *State and local government employers and employees*: In 24 states and two territories (see below), local and state government employers and employees are covered by the state safety and health agencies. In all other states and territories, these public employees and employers are not covered at all by OSHA regulations and are not subjected to OSHA enforcement.
- *Federal government employees*: No federal agency employees are covered by OSHA regulations or are subjected to OSHA enforcement. Instead, the OSHAct directs each federal agency head to maintain an effective and comprehensive occupational safety and health program that is consistent with OSHA standards. However, OSHA must perform various services for the federal agencies, including consultation, training, record keeping, inspections, and evaluations. But, compliance with these directives is voluntary, and there are no sanctions or penalties for violating them.
- *Motor vehicle and driver safety*: Jurisdiction in this area is split, with some requirements under the control of OSHA and some under the U.S. Department of Transportation (DOT). For example, DOT is responsible for commercial driver medical certification, including alcohol and controlled substances testing. Although there are no OSHA general industry standards concerning workplace motor vehicle safety, there are some limited OSHA rules for motor vehicle use, such as for marine terminals, construction vehicles, and agricultural tractors.
- *Ionizing radiation protection*: Although OSHA has some limited rules covering workplace exposure to ionizing radiation, DOE and the Nuclear Regulatory Commission (NRC) both have more extensive radiation standards that reflect technological and safety advances since the OSHA rules were adopted in 1974.

The OSHAct has a simple statement of roles and responsibilities:

- OSHA is established within the U.S. Department of Labor and is authorized "to set mandatory occupational safety and health standards applicable to businesses" and to provide "an effective enforcement program."

- Each employer "shall comply with occupational safety and health standards." In addition, where there are no specific standards, each employer still has a general duty to "furnish to each of his employees employment and a place of employment which are free from recognized hazards that are causing or are likely to cause death or serious physical harm."
- Each employee "shall comply with occupational safety and health standards and all rules, regulations, and orders issued . . . which are applicable to his own actions and conduct."

The OSHAct provided the opportunity for individual states to assume responsibility for regulation and enforcement as long as the state program would be at least as effective as federal OSHA. Twenty-one states (and Puerto Rico) have assumed safety and health coverage for both private and public sectors and an additional three states (and the Virgin Islands) have assumed coverage for public sector workplaces only. Federal OSHA has jurisdiction in 29 states and the District of Columbia for private sector workplaces only. It is a glaring omission of the OSHAct that public sector employees do not have the rights and protections of the law except in those states that have assumed jurisdiction. And even in these states, federal employees are not protected. (A listing of state plan programs, including contact information, is available at <www.osha.gov/fso/osp/index.html>.)

Regardless of whether the safety and health laws are administered by federal OSHA or a state program, the basic regulatory and enforcement structure is the same:

- Employers must comply with two types of specific regulations. First, there are safety rules covering safety hazards, such as those associated with machinery and tools, working at heights, electrical energy, stairs and ladders, compressed gases, conveyors, cranes and hoists, and flammables and combustibles. Second, there are health rules for hazards involving chemicals and biological agents, such as asbestos, benzene, lead, and several hundred other specific chemicals; entry into confined spaces; blood-borne pathogens; ventilation; and respiratory protection. (These

rules may be found at <www.osha.gov/comp-links.html>.)
- Employers must also protect employees from exposure to any other recognized hazards for which there are no specific standards. For example, although there is no OSHA ergonomics standard for hazards causing work-related musculoskeletal disorders, employers still have a "general duty" to reduce exposure to highly repetitive motions, heavy and awkward lifting, awkward postures, high hand force, and vibration. When OSHA seeks to enforce these "general duty" requirements, it must be able to prove that the hazards are in fact "recognized" by the employer or the industry and that there are feasible means of reducing the exposures.
- Employers in some states, but not those covered by federal OSHA, have additional requirements such as those for joint employer–employee safety committees or for written safety and health programs.
- OSHA and its state counterparts are authorized to inspect workplaces and to issue citations and penalties when rules have been violated. Two types of inspections are conducted. First, employees and former employees have a right to file written complaints, which must be investigated, usually with an on-site inspection. Second, OSHA may send an inspector to a workplace without having first received a complaint, for example as part of a program to focus attention on a particularly high-risk industry. (Information about filing complaints may be found at <www.osha.gov/as/opa/worker/html>.)
- Employers—but not employees—may request a consultation visit from a state agency authorized by OSHA to provide such visits. These visits are free and carry no risk of penalty, although there is a requirement that any violations of OSHA regulations identified be corrected in a timely manner. (Information about consultation services may be found at <www.osha.gov/dcsp/smallbusiness/consult.html>.)
- Employers have a right to appeal the results of an OSHA inspection. (Employees can only appeal the time given for the employer to abate the violation.) The independent Occupational Safety and Health Review Commission or a comparable state appeals board hears these appeals. Further appeals are available through state or federal courts.

- Employers are prohibited from discriminating against an employee who has filed a complaint or otherwise exercised any rights under the OSHAct. OSHA and its state counterparts investigate discrimination complaints.

The federal and state OSHA laws cover approximately 8 million workplaces. In 2003, there were approximately 2,100 federal and state inspectors to enforce the OSHA law. In federal fiscal year 2002, these inspectors conducted 97,437 inspections (almost 40 percent by federal inspectors and the remainder by state inspectors). At current levels of funding and staffing, it would take federal OSHA about 115 years to inspect every workplace in its jurisdiction once. The state plans would take about 60 years to visit every workplace in their jurisdictions. Consultation visits are provided substantially less frequently than inspections. Only 34,404 were conducted in federal fiscal year 2003.

OSHA's enforcement presence is also limited by restrictions on the way that the agency can spend money in its budget. For many years, Congress has adopted riders to annual appropriations bills for OSHA that prohibit the agency from inspecting certain workplaces. For example, in 2003, OSHA was not permitted to do any inspections, including in response to complaints or after fatalities, on farms with 10 or fewer employees (unless the farm has an active temporary labor camp). At non-farm workplaces with 10 or fewer employees in selected low-hazard industries, OSHA was permitted to conduct inspections only in limited circumstances, such as in response to complaints and after fatalities.

Penalties for violations of the safety and health laws are relatively low compared to penalties for violation of many environmental regulations. The maximum penalty for a serious violation—one that poses a substantial probability of death or serious physical harm—is $7,000. If the violation is willful or repeated, the penalty may increase to $70,000. In federal fiscal year 2002, the penalties for serious violations averaged $867 for federal OSHA and $902 for state plans. The OSHAct also establishes a criminal penalty of up to $10,000 and 6 months imprisonment for employers whose willful violation of an OSHA standard caused the death of an employee. However, criminal charges have rarely been pursued. There have been less than 100 criminal convictions and less than 20 imprisonments since OSHA was established more than 30 years ago.

HOW TO USE OSHA

How to Request an OSHA Inspection

- *File a complaint*: Anyone can file an OSHA complaint with an OSHA office by phone, fax, e-mail, or in writing. (Complaint instructions and forms may be found at <www.osha.gov/as/opa/worker/complain.html>.)
- *If you are not an employee or a union representative, try to have an employee designate you in writing as his or her representative*: Because the OSHAct specifically directs OSHA to investigate when it receives a complaint from an employee or representative of employees, these complaints get the most serious and timely consideration. OSHA will look into all other complaints, but will consider them "referrals," and there is less certainty that they will actually do a workplace inspection after a referral than a complaint.
- *File the complaint in writing and sign it*: OSHA considers signed, written complaints to be "formal complaints." OSHA will look into all other complaints but will consider them "informal," and there is less certainty that they will actually perform a workplace inspection after an informal complaint than a formal one. OSHA is required to keep names confidential upon request.
- *Provide as much specific information about the issues of concern as possible*: The OSHAct requires unannounced, on-site inspections only when there are reasonable grounds to believe that there is an imminent danger at a workplace or that a violation of an OSHA rule threatens physical harm.
- *Call the OSHA area office and talk to an inspector or supervisor*: Although this is not required, it will increase the likelihood that OSHA will respond quickly and seriously.

How to Request an Onsite Consultation

- Determine what agency provides free safety and health consultation services in your state. OSHA consultation services are funded primarily by federal OSHA but delivered by the 50 state governments, most commonly through a state labor department or university. (The list of consultation programs can be found at <www.osha.gov/dcsp/smallbusiness/consult_directory.html>.)

- OSHA will not conduct a consultation visit without an invitation from the employer. If you are not an employer but feel that an employer might benefit from an OSHA consultation, you might talk with the employer to try to convince the employer to seek assistance. Or you might contact the state consultation program office and suggest that a consultant call the employer. The consultation program will contact an employer and offer its services, but a consultant will only enter the workplace if the employer responds positively and invites a consultant in.

How to File a Discrimination Complaint

- The OSHAct prohibits an employer from discriminating against any employee for having filed a complaint or exercising any rights afforded by the act. Some examples of discrimination are firing, demotion, transfer, layoff, losing opportunity for overtime or promotion, assignment to an undesirable shift, denial of benefits such as sick leave, blacklisting with other employers, and reducing pay or hours.
- Employees believing they have been discharged or otherwise discriminated against may file a complaint with OSHA or a state counterpart agency within 30 days of the alleged discrimination. Complaints can be telephoned, faxed, or mailed. OSHA conducts an interview with each complainant to determine the need for an investigation. OSHA or the state must then complete an investigation within 90 days of the complaint. If evidence supports the worker's claim, OSHA will ask the employer to restore the worker's job, earnings, and benefits. If the employer objects, OSHA may take the employer to court to seek relief for the worker.

How to Find OSHA Standards

First, determine whether the workplace in which you are interested is in a state covered by federal OSHA or by a state agency. (You can find this out on the OSHA Web site: <www.osha.gov/fso/osp/index.html>.) OSHA rules and related documents can be found at <www.osha.gov/comp-links.html>. OSHA also has developed a decision logic that helps employers determine which specific rules apply to their workplaces. (This can be found at <www.osha.gov/dcsp/compliance_

assistance/quickstarts/index.html>.) States may adopt safety and health rules that differ from OSHA rules as long as they are "at least as effective as" the federal rules. Each of the state OSHA programs has its own Web site with links to its specific rules.

ENVIRONMENTAL HEALTH REGULATION

Federal Framework of Environmental Legislation and Regulation

Paralleling the increase in awareness and concern for occupational safety and health that occurred in the 1960s was recognition of the degradation of the environmental quality and the concomitant negative impact on health and well-being. Publication of Rachel Carson's *Silent Spring* in 1962 provided a treatise on the harm that had been done to the environment from pesticide use, while media coverage of the oil spill off the coast of Santa Barbara, California, and the fire on Cleveland's Cuyahoga River in 1969 provided a visual reminder of the paucity of environmental regulations and enforcement. These events intensified the impetus for the passage of major environmental legislation in the 1970s (Table 37-1).

Historically, environmental legislation, including federal laws such as the Clean Air Act of 1963, emphasized state, regional, or local control. Some laws involved conservation measures, while others were media-based and provided for technical, rather than regulatory, oversight by federal agencies. Local public health environmental regulations were often sanitation-based. Through zoning and local ordinances, restrictions were placed on the location of dumps, burning of garbage, and disposal of garbage. The intent of these sanitation laws was to not so much to improve environmental quality as to address local public health issues, such as the prevention of disease transmission by rodent control, and to address nuisance-related issues, such as unsightliness and odor.

The National Environmental Policy Act of 1969 (NEPA) made protection of the environment a national charter. Its lofty goals were

- "To declare a national policy which will encourage productive and enjoyable harmony between man and his environment."
- "To promote efforts which will prevent or eliminate damage to the environment and biosphere and stimulate the health and welfare of man."

TABLE 37-1

Major U.S. Environmental Laws

Statute	Year Enacted	Scope
National Environmental Policy Act (NEPA)	1970	Established a national environmental charter, required environmental impact statements of federal projects, created the CEQ
Clean Air Act (CAA)	1970	Standards to improve air quality by reduction of air emissions from mobile and stationary sources
Clean Water Act (CWA)	1972	Standards for protecting the nation's surface waters
Federal Insecticide, Fungicide and Rodenticide Act (FIFRA)	1972	Registration and testing of herbicides and pesticides
Endangered Species Act (ESA)	1973	Identification and protection of endangered and threatened species and their habitat
Safe Drinking Water Act (SWDA)	1974	Standards for public water drinking systems and protection of aquifers
Toxic Substance Control Act (TSCA)	1976	Regulation of chemicals by testing and reporting requirements; regulations on PCBs and asbestos
Resource Conservation and Recovery Act (RCRA)	1976	Regulation of the treatment, storage, and disposal of hazardous and nonhazardous waste from active and future facilities; "cradle to grave" management
Comprehensive Environmental Response, Compensation, and Liability Act (CERCLA) (Superfund)	1980	Funding and enforcement for clean-up of abandoned or historical hazardous waste sites and emergency spills; created ATSDR
Superfund Amendments and Reauthorization Act (SARA)	1986	Expanded the scope of CERCLA, increased the focus on human health problems from hazardous waste sites
Emergency Planning and Community Right to Know Act (EPCRA)	1986	Provision of SARA that required reporting of releases and inventories of regulated chemicals and plans for emergency response to releases
Pollution Prevention Act (PPA)	1990	Provided pollution prevention goals with an emphasis on source reduction
Oil Pollution Act (OPA)	1990	Strengthened EPA's ability to respond to catastrophic oil spills

- "To enrich our understanding of the ecological systems and natural resources important to the Nation."

NEPA required an environmental impact statement be prepared by federal agencies for all significant federal projects. Citizens were given a voice in the decision process for these projects through public meetings and public review periods for documents. The act also established the Center for Environmental Quality (CEQ) to advise the executive branch on environmental matters and to review all environmental impact statements.

In ushering in the new decade of environmental advocacy, it became apparent that the piecemeal approach of having multiple departments and agencies addressing specific environmental issues would not adequately fulfill the charter for national environmental protection. Concern about the bias and objectivity that may occur from giving the primary mission of environmental protection to an existing agency encouraged the move toward the creation of an independent agency. In 1970, President Richard Nixon announced the reorganization of the government that would involve the creation of an independent agency, the Environmental Protection Agency

(EPA), to establish and enforce environmental standards. EPA would also conduct research, provide assistance to other agencies and states in combating environmental pollution, and assist the CEQ in recommending to the president new policies for environmental protection.

The organizational structure for EPA was derived from the old Federal Water Pollution Control Agency. Thus, there was a smooth transition to enforcement of the 1972 Clean Water Act (CWA). The major goals of the CWA, last amended in 1987, are to eliminate pollutant discharges into the nation's lakes, rivers, and streams and to make these waters safe for fishing and recreation. The 1963 Clean Air Act was amended, and EPA was also mandated to oversee the improved 1970 Clean Air Act (CAA). The CAA, last amended in 1990, targeted improvement of air quality by reduction of air emissions from mobile and stationary sources.

Other major environmental statutes enacted during the 1970s for which EPA had primary responsibility addressed pesticides (Federal Insecticide, Fungicide, and Rodenticide Act), drinking water (Safe Drinking Water Act), industrial chemicals (Toxic Substance Control Act), and hazardous and nonhazardous waste (Resource Conservation and Recovery Act). Although these acts covered current and future releases to the land, air, and water, they did not address the numerous abandoned or historical hazardous waste sites in the United States. The Comprehensive Environmental Response, Compensation, and Liability Act (CERCLA), commonly known as Superfund, was enacted in 1980 to provide funding for the clean-up of abandoned facilities and authority to respond to emergency releases.

Environmental legislation during the 1980s was marked by amendments to many of the acts that broadened the scope of the statutes and expanded EPA's ability for enforcement. A notable addition to these statutes was provisions for including more direct community involvement in sites. The Superfund Amendments and Reauthorization Act (SARA) encouraged greater citizen participation in decisions on how sites should be cleaned up. Prior to SARA, citizens had been included in most environmental statutes by provisions that allowed them to sue the owner or operator of a pollutant source or to sue EPA or the state that had not enforced the act.

A separate provision of SARA was the Emergency Preparedness and Community Right to Know Act (EPCRA). EPCRA required that facilities with potentially hazardous substances notify state and local authorities for the purpose of emergency planning. The act also required the preparation of material safety data sheets (MSDSs) that are provided to local authorities and the workplace in accordance with OSHA regulations. The Toxic Release Inventory (TRI), established by EPCRA, required that certain manufacturers report the release and inventories of listed chemicals. (The TRI, information on permitted facilities for land, air, and water releases, location of National Priorities List [NPL] and other hazardous waste sites, and report cards on drinking water and recreational beaches are available on the Internet.)

EPA, which regulates pesticides, has a role in provisions involving pesticides in food under the Food Quality Protection Act and the Federal Food, Drug and Cosmetic Act, although the Food and Drug Administration (FDA) is the primary agency for enforcing these laws. Under FIFRA, decisions to ban pesticide use are based in part on adverse effects to species listed under the Endangered Species Act (ESA). This law, which is administered by the U.S. Fish and Wildlife Service (USFWS), is a powerful piece of legislation for environmental protection, as evidenced by (a) relocation or reconsideration of dams and airport and roadway construction to prevent habitat destruction, and (b) the heated debates on logging in old forests on the West Coast that endanger the spotted owl.

The Freedom of Information Act (FOIA), which became law in 1966, provides a strong mechanism for the public in researching environmental contamination problems in the community. FOIA allows citizens to make requests for government information to any branch of the federal government. Citizens do not have to give their identity or state why they are requesting the information. Some restrictions on FOIA include early draft documents, some confidential enforcement information, and national security information. Some medical or personnel records will require a consent form from the person whose records are requested.

Federal agencies have offices that deal with FOIA requests, and their Internet sites describe procedures for making these requests. The agency's Internet sites also contain public domain material that would not be subject to FOIA. In making the request, the search can be most effective if the request is as specific as possible, so learning what type of information each agency collects due to the reporting requirements under the various pieces of legislation will make the search more successful. Payment for photocopying and time may be required, although a fee waiver may be requested. Many states have a comparable version of the FOIA.

Agencies Involved in Legislation

For most of the environmental legislation, EPA has the lead responsibility. At its inception in 1970, about 4,000 employees were reassigned from several government agencies that had administered some media-specific environmental legislation. For example, EPA incorporated the National Air Pollution Control Administration from the Department of Health, Education and Welfare (HEW) and took over the function of pesticide registration from the Department of Agriculture (USDA). By 2003, EPA had expanded to include more than 17,600 workers. EPA maintains ten regional offices to carry out programs mandated by federal statutes.

EPA works with many other agencies in responding to emergencies, enforcing regulation, and providing technical assistance, including the U.S. Coast Guard (USCG), the FDA, the NRC, USDA, and OSHA. Much of the compliance and enforcement aspects of the environmental legislation remain under the purview of the state environmental protection or natural resources departments. EPA enters into agreements with states with an approved program for implementing environmental protection programs; each agreement specifies when EPA will step in and take enforcement action in an approved state program. States may enact their own environmental protection laws, as long as they are at least as stringent as the federal laws.

To assist in evaluating public health impacts involving hazardous waste sites, the Agency for Toxic Substances and Disease Registry (ATSDR) was created by the CERCLA legislation in 1980. ATSDR does not have a regulatory role; it makes public health recommendations to EPA concerning all NPL sites and other hazardous waste sites as well as emergency responses. ATSDR also receives requests from other federal, state, and local agencies and from citizens to investigate public health concerns from hazardous releases and to provide health education. Toxicological profiles are compiled about hazardous chemicals. ATSDR has cooperative agreements with 22 states that provide funding so that state public health departments can provide health consultations and public health im-

pact evaluations for hazardous sites within their own boundaries.

The National Center for Environmental Health (NCEH), which is part of the Centers for Disease Control and Prevention (CDC), is another federal agency involved in health research and policy. One of the programs at NCEH is environmental public health tracking, which attempts to link hazards, exposures. and health effects. In 2003, the NCEH was joined administratively to ATSDR. The National Institute of Environmental Health Science (NIEHS), one of the institutes of the National Institutes of Health (NIH), performs and supports research on how environmental factors and human susceptibility interact in human health and disease.

Nongovernmental organizations, such as the Sierra Club, the Natural Resources Defense Council, and Environmental Defense, promote environmental programs and policies on the national level (see Chapter 35). Regional air pollution control authorities, watershed protection associations, and local and county health or environmental departments also fulfill advocacy, enforcement, and programmatic functions—providing opportunities for direct local-citizen involvement and input on environmental decisions.

PUTTING ENVIRONMENTAL REGULATIONS TO WORK

Despite all of the environmental regulations that are in place, hazardous releases to the environment occur and some facilities either unwittingly or knowingly disobey the laws. Citizens may also become concerned by what they perceive is an elevated level of disease in their community. Confronted by these environmental impacts, citizens may be unsure of what recourse is available for addressing these issues. One of the first distinctions to make is ascertaining whether there is an immediate threat to the public's health.

An environmental violation involves noncompliance with an environmental regulation that does not pose an immediate threat to the public's health. Examples include tampering with emission control devices, unpermitted dredging of wetlands, falsifying records, and improper treatment or disposal of wastes. Reporting of possible environmental violations can often be made at the state or local level. Some complaints such as for odor, noise, or garbage are more likely addressed by city or county government agencies. State environmental agencies are responsible for many of the permit and reporting requirements of the federally mandated programs for pollution control. The ten regional offices of EPA also can assist in addressing the violations to federal regulations.

An accidental or intentional release of hazardous material involving a chemical, oil, or radioactive release into the air, water, or land that poses an immediate threat to the public's health or to the environment constitutes an environmental emergency. There are numerous small releases that occur around industrial facilities or roadways and may cause little disruption to the community. In an average year, about 12,000 transportation accidents involving hazardous materials occur. Local emergency responders may clean up these smaller spills or, in the case of on-site releases, the operator of the facility may assist in the clean-up. Other releases are more serious and require action by the National Response Center (NRC), which is the primary federal hazardous substances communications center. People should report oil or hazardous waste spills, illegal dumping, transportation emergencies, or chemical accidents by calling the NRC at (800) 424-8802. The U.S. Coast Guard staffs the NRC 24 hours a day. After receiving a report, the NRC notifies the federal on-scene coordinator (OSC) that is assigned to the geographic area where the incident occurred. The Coast Guard manages incidents occurring in tidal or coastal areas, while EPA handles releases to inland waterways or land spills. The Department of Defense and DOE have jurisdiction over releases on their respective federal properties.

EPA's on-scene coordinators are part of the Superfund Emergency Response and Removal Program. After notification of a release, an OSC evaluates the site to determine if federal response is necessary. The OSC coordinates with local and state responders and other federal agencies to protect the public and to remove the threat. The OSC also interacts with members of the community to inform them of the situation and to ensure that their concerns are considered. The Coast Guard's National Strike Force, EPA's Environmental Response Team, and the National Oceanic and Atmospheric Administration (NOAA) scientific support coordinators provide technical assistance to the OSCs on-site evaluation and clean-up technologies. ATSDR also has an Emergency Response Section to provide consultation on public health-related issues where there is a hazardous release.

Once a site is brought to the attention of the OSC, actions to clean up or stabilize immediate threats to the environment and public health are initiated. This may involve disposal or treatment of the hazardous substance and methods to prevent the spread of the contaminant. ATSDR may issue a public health advisory that provides recommendations to EPA about activities to implement that will reduce adverse health effects. As part of the response, community residents may be provided with an alternative drinking water supply, fences may be installed to prevent access and direct contact, and residents may even be temporarily relocated. Once the emergency response actions are completed, long-term clean-up actions may be required at the site. The Superfund Emergency Response and Removal Program also conducts long-term clean-up projects at other sites that are not commonly considered "emergencies," such as the discovery of abandoned waste sites. EPA may stabilize a site and identify responsible parties to recover expended costs and pay for any long-term remedial actions.

An important component to the emergency response actions is community involvement. Community-involvement staff at EPA work with the public, media, and local officials to provide information about the response. A written record of response actions is maintained that is available to the public. EPA also considers the community a valuable resource for knowledge of site history and activities. Community input on clean-up plans increases the likelihood of community acceptance of proposed responses. At some sites, community advisory groups are established to act as a liaison between the community and EPA. Under SARA, technical assistance grants from EPA are available to communities to allow them to hire technical experts to assist them in understanding hazardous-waste problems.

In the event of a sudden release, the risk to health from an environmental contaminant is fairly apparent. For some of the historic and abandoned waste sites, environmental releases may be more insidious. Groundwater contamination may have been occurring gradually over time at fairly low levels. Community members may first be alerted to the possibility of a contaminant in their environment by the suspicion that an increase rate of disease is occurring in their neighborhood. One source of information on disease rates is the state or local health department. Many states contain registries on new cancer cases and birth outcomes.

Death certificate data may also be available for the community.

Statistical information on adverse health outcomes other than cancer is very limited. Even with registry data, very few clusters of disease are found from environmental contamination. It is difficult to identify a cluster from an environmental source for several reasons: Cancer is a common disease. The latency of most cancers is greater than 10 years. It is difficult to quantify exposure over time. And migration of people in and out of a community may be high. In addition, the levels of a contaminant to which community members are exposed may be very low, so concern may focus on the added risk of disease that arises from exposure to the hazardous chemical.

Citizens or community groups can request that ATSDR address their health concerns about an environmental contaminant from a release site by petitioning the agency in writing. Petition letters should include:

- Contact information, including the name of the group, if any;
- Name, location, and description of the facility or release; and
- Information about human exposure to a hazardous substance, including how many people might be exposed.

Any exposure or health data or additional information about the site is also helpful to include. Petition letters should be sent to: Assistant Administrator, ATSDR, 1600 Clifton Road, NE (E28), Atlanta, GA 30329-4027.

Once the petition letter is received by ATSDR, an acknowledgment letter is sent to the petitioner within 10 days and contact is made by the petition coordinator with the regional office to obtain a history of involvement at the site by EPA and state and local agencies. Basic information is gathered about the site. Within 30 days, the ATSDR holds a preliminary petition meeting with agency staff to review the information. Three Phase 1 criteria are applied and must be met for the petition to continue to the next phase:

- "Has ATSDR prepared, or is ATSDR preparing, a public health assessment or equivalent document that addresses the health concerns in the petition?"
- "Has a hazardous substance been released into the environment?"

- "Is an ATSDR public health assessment or other ATSDR program activity an appropriate response to the petition?"

If Phase 1 criteria are not met, the petitioner is sent a written response with explanation.

Within the next 1 to 3 months, a site team is assembled that includes environmental scientists, physicians, toxicologists, epidemiologists, and other appropriate staff members. The team gathers environmental and exposure data available from the site and identifies public health issues and the petitioner's concerns. A scoping visit may be made to the site to meet with the petitioner and other community members and to gather additional data. A postscoping debriefing session is held to determine if the following three Phase 2 criteria are all met.

- "Are the location, concentration, and toxicity of the hazardous substances related to the petition, site or release possibly of public health concern?"
- "Is there an exposed or potentially exposed population as indicated in the petition and as determined by evaluating human exposure pathways for the hazardous substance release(s)?"
- "Is there a plausible relationship between possible human exposure to a release of hazardous substances and community health concerns, adverse health concerns, or adverse health outcomes?"

If a consensus is reached that all three Phase 2 criteria are met, then a decision is made as to which of the following public health responses is most appropriate: a public health assessment, a health consult, a public health advisory, or community health education.

Between the 46th and 180th day from receipt of the petition letter, the petitioner is sent a letter explaining whether further action will be taken and in what form. If the complaint is accepted for investigation, a site plan is developed, and the public health activity is undertaken. ATSDR or a state public health agency with a cooperative agreement with ATSDR may take the lead for the site.

A public health assessment (PHA) or health consultation is a written, comprehensive evaluation about the hazardous substance released at a site and the likelihood that exposure by inhalation, ingestion, or direct contact can occur or has occurred—and if the level of exposure could result in harm. As part of the evaluation, environmental and health data are reviewed and community concerns are addressed. Depending on the complexity of the site, community advisory panels may be formed to act as a liaison with ATSDR and the community to facilitate information exchange. If a public health hazard is determined to be present at the site, recommendations are made for reducing or eliminating the exposure. ATSDR works with EPA and state and local environmental and health agencies to ensure that the recommendations can be implemented. Before the PHA becomes final, there is a public release of the document for community review and comment. A public meeting may also be held to discuss the findings and public health action plan (see Box 37-1 for an example of an ATSDR evaluation).

BOX 37-1

Hydrogen Sulfide Exposure

The rainfall in fall 2001 and spring 2002 was much greater than usual in Warren Township, Ohio. That was about the time the residents began to find that the odors coming from the adjacent landfill were becoming worse (Fig. 37-1). Not only was the rotten egg-like smell foul, but residents living near the landfill complained of headaches and nausea and also had health concerns of exacerbation of asthma, difficulty breathing, and eye irritation. The odor would cause schoolchildren attending classes at the elementary and high schools located within a half-mile of the landfill boundaries to come home with headache and nausea. Although there were other sources of hydrogen sulfide in the community, the Warren Recycling, Incorporated, (WRI) landfill was identified as the primary source of the hydrogen sulfide gas.

The WRI landfill is located in an area of mixed commercial and residential use; around the periphery of the property, residential yards abut the fence line. The 200-acre property, which was purchased by WRI in 1994, is used as a construction and demolition debris (C&DD) landfill. Two of the phased landfills on the property are filled and covered, while the third phased landfill is currently active.

A major component of C&DD landfills is gypsum drywall. Because gypsum is composed of calcium sulfate, the C&DD landfills tend to produce more hydrogen sulfide and less methane gas as compared to municipal solid waste landfills. Four tons of gypsum drywall can produce about 1 ton of hydrogen sulfide. The bacterial decomposition is greatest and accelerated when there is little oxygen and when there is water infiltration.

Acute exposure to 5 to 10 parts per million (ppm) hydrogen sulfide can cause shortness of breath. Chronic exposures to lower levels of hydrogen sulfide has been reported to cause eye, throat, and lung irritation; nausea; headache; sleeping difficulties; weight loss; chest pain; and asthma attacks in communities with 0.3 to 4 ppm hydrogen sulfide in ambient air. Eye irritation is also found with low-level acute exposure.

Residents called the City of Warren Health Department to complain about the odors. The city sent inspectors out who confirmed the odors. The Ohio EPA also received complaints and sent inspectors to the site. In February 2002, Warren Township held a public meeting to discuss problems with the WRI landfill. Residents were reassured that the problem was now being addressed by the recent construction of new wells to vent the gas. The citizens were also told that the city had portable detection monitors that could be brought to homes to take readings when there were odor concerns.

Odor problems persisted. Our Lives Count (OLC), a citizen's group, was formed in early 2002 to "deal with an unpleasant 'rotten egg' smell in Warren Township area that is affecting our health, homes and our community." The OLC ensured that regulators were kept aware of continuing odor problems in their community emanating from the landfill. A special local school board meeting to address air-quality concerns was held in March 2002. It was proposed that WRI pay for an independent lab to sample air quality. Attendees were told that WRI was spraying neutralizing agents at the site to reduce the odor.

In late April 2002, after continued odor and health complaints, the LaBrae School District

(continued)

<hr>

BOX 37-1

Hydrogen Sulfide Exposure (Continued)

and the Warren Township Board of Trustees petitioned the Agency for Toxic Substances and Disease Registry (ATSDR) to evaluate whether the hydrogen sulfide in ambient air posed a health risk to the community. In May 2002, a consultant selected by the school district and township conducted continuous air monitoring at five locations in the community, including the elementary and high schools. Air monitoring results showed hydrogen sulfide at levels up to 13 ppm. Hydrogen sulfide levels consistently exceeded the ATSDR intermediate environmental evaluation guide of 0.03 ppm.

ATSDR, OEPA, and the Ohio Department of Health (ODH) held a community meeting in August 2002. More than 160 people were interviewed about their health concerns and exposure history. Based on the site visit and the available data, ATSDR wrote a health consult that was issued in September 2002. Because the consultant's data had incomplete quality assurance data, ATSDR concluded "hydrogen sulfide in air currently presents a public health hazard to area residents and school children." Recommendations included:

- Schools in the area should install hydrogen sulfide alarms and evacuation plans for the schools should be established;
- Residential indoor and ambient air should be monitored for at least a season;
- Private wells should be sampled to ensure that hydrogen sulfide was not present at levels of concern; and
- Groundwater monitoring wells should be installed to evaluate whether leachate was affecting drinking water aquifers.

Implementation of the recommendations was a collaborative effort among ATSDR, EPA, ODH, OEPA, the regional air pollution control agency, the local fire and police departments, the hazmat coordinator for Trumball County, and the LeBrae School District. ATSDR also agreed

to perform an exposure investigation (EI) to further characterize the site. Paired hydrogen sulfide monitors, one to collect indoor and the other for outdoor samples, were installed at six residences for a 4-month period starting in mid-November 2002. The high school air was also monitored for a 5-week period, starting in January 2003. The maximum peak outside hydrogen sulfide concentration was 6.1 ppm, which lasted 15 minutes; the maximum peak indoor concentration was 0.038 ppm, which lasted 120 minutes.

The conclusion of the EI was that an urgent public health hazard existed at the site and that "People with pre-existing cardiopulmonary disease or respiratory problems are at risk from the levels of hydrogen sulfide present in outdoor air in residential areas." The potential for fire or explosion at the landfill vents and the unrestricted access to the landfill also posed a threat to the community. A public meeting was held in June 2003 to present the sampling results and conclusion; a document summarizing the exposure investigation results was issued in November 2003. One of the recommendations of the EI was to conduct a health study.

The OEPA signed a Consent Order with WRI in July 2003 that required engineering controls, emission characterization, groundwater monitoring, leachate collection, and a gas collection system at the site. In January 2004, the OEPA denied WRI a new air permit for the landfill that would have allowed the landfill to accept more waste. The decision was based in part on the ATSDR classification of the facility as an urgent public health hazard and letters by the ODH and EPA recommending against issuing the license. Another major contributing factor to this decision was the more than 800 odor complaints by the citizens that were logged by the OEPA since February 2002 regarding hydrogen sulfide coming from the site.

EFFECTIVENESS OF REGULATIONS

There are three basic premises underlying the regulatory framework: Once rules are in place, those affected will comply with them—-either voluntar-

ily or when faced with enforcement action:

- Compliance with the rules will result in decreased exposure to hazards; and
- Decreased exposure will result in improved health and well-being.

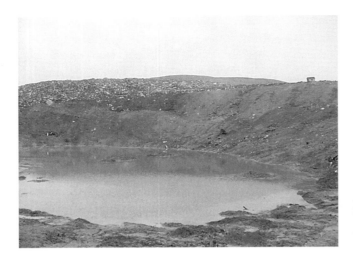

FIGURE 37-1 ● Exposed waste surrounds a pool of leachate emitting hydrogen sulfide gas at a CERCLA (Superfund) remediation site in Warren, Ohio. (Photograph by Michelle Waters.)

While there have been only a few empirical tests of this logic and the evidence is mixed, it does appear that adoption and enforcement of some occupational and environmental rules has had a positive impact (Fig. 37-2.)

Effectiveness of Occupational Health Legislation

Many workplaces are not fully compliant with OSHA rules. Approximately 70 percent of OSHA inspections result in at least one violation being cited. In 1993, 51 percent of OSHA inspections of large construction contractors—and 69 percent of other contractors—found at least one OSHA violation. Among 2,060 large national construction contractors, 76 percent of whom had at least one OSHA inspection during the 1987–1993 period, there was only a 6 percent increase in the likelihood of compliance being found at a second inspection.[2]

What we know about the match between hazards cited in OSHA inspections and the causes of workplace fatalities and injuries is disappointing.[2] For example, in 1994 in the construction industry,

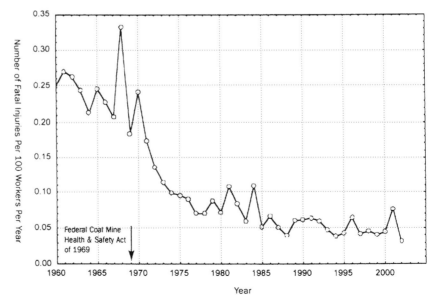

FIGURE 37-2 ● Rate of fatal injuries in underground coal mines, 1960–2002. (Source: Occupational Safety and Health Administration.)

42 percent of OSHA citations were for fall-protection violations, but only 19 percent of the injuries were from falls. In contrast, 31 percent of injuries were from being struck by objects at work, but only 4 percent of the OSHA citations were for violations directly related to these hazards. An even more striking discrepancy is that 30 percent of all workers' compensation claims are for work-related musculoskeletal disorders, yet there are no OSHA standards for ergonomics, except in California. These data suggest that increased compliance with the rules that have been adopted will be, at best, only partially effective in reducing hazards and preventing injuries.

There have been only a few recent analytic studies examining whether safety and health rules and their enforcement have resulted in reductions in workplace injuries and illnesses. These studies have examined two questions: Do rules make a difference in the specific workplaces where they are enforced? Do rules have a broader deterrent impact in workplaces beyond those with specific enforcement interventions?

A direct, positive impact of OSHA enforcement in workplaces where inspections have taken place has been found in several studies. A study of injury rates for the 1979–1985 period in a large group of manufacturing facilities after OSHA inspections found that there was a 15 to 22 percent decline in lost-workday injury rates in the 3 years after inspections where penalties had been imposed, compared with no decline in workplaces with inspections but no penalties.[3,4] However, a subsequent study for the 1987–1991 and 1991–1998 periods found substantially smaller effects.[5]

Another group of studies has examined the impact of inspections on specific workplaces in the State of Washington. Workers' compensation claims rates declined 22 to 27 percent for employers at fixed-site workplaces in the year after a safety and health inspection, compared with a 5 to 7 percent decline in comparable workplaces without inspections.[6,7] Similar effects after consultation visits could not be demonstrated. In addition to these general industry effects, a more specific enforcement effect was found after enforcement of the fall-protection rule of the State of Washington in the construction industry. Workers' compensation claims for fall injuries were 2.3 times as likely to decrease among workplaces that were inspected and cited for violations of the rule than control workplaces.[8]

One recent study has reported evidence for a general deterrent impact on falls among carpenters in the construction industry after adoption of the new fall-protection rule in the State of Washington.[9] However, other evidence that inspections in some workplaces result in decreased injuries in other, uninspected workplaces has been mixed; a series of studies in the 1970s and 1980s found very small positive effects or none at all.

A provocative summary of regulatory effectiveness in 1978 is still worth our attention: "Expectancies of being cited for initial safety and health violations, and the fine levels if cited, are so low under OSHA that they are of little value in preventing violations of the Act. Those employers who obey the law would do so regardless of the penalties. Employers at whom the sanctions are aimed—those who will correct violations only if it is economically profitable for them to do so—are not being affected. Thus the current sanctions antagonize employers who attempt to obey the law, while having little impact on those employers who will obey the law only if it is economically profitable."[10]

Effectiveness of Environmental Health Enforcement

Since the "burning" of the Cuyahoga River in 1969, much progress has been made toward its restoration. Once considered a "dead" river, the fish populations are recovering and standard exceedances of heavy metals and fecal coliform bacteria are dropping. The Cuyahoga River Remedial Action Plan is an aggressive and comprehensive plan targeting environmental, socioeconomic, recreational, and human health issues. Although much work remains, the Clean Water Act and the Great Lakes Water Quality Agreement have resulted in significant improvements to this designated "American Heritage River."

The nation has also shown significant improvement in air quality during the past 35 years. Nationally, from the passage of the Clean Air Act in 1970 to 1997, there was a 75 percent decrease in particulate matter emissions, a 32 percent decrease in carbon monoxide emissions, and a 98 percent reduction in lead emissions[11] (Fig. 37-3). The reduction of primary pollutants was achieved by controls on industrial sources and motor vehicles and the banning of leaded gasoline. The estimated health benefit for children predicted to occur by 2010 because of the CAA is $1 to $2 billion from 10,000

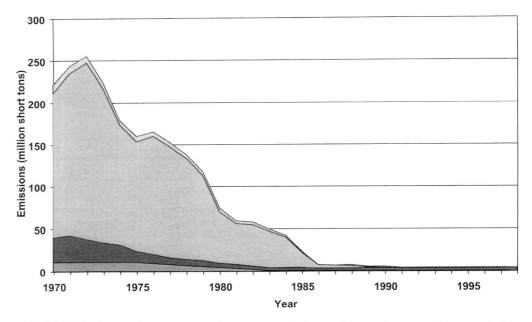

FIGURE 37-3 ● Lead emissions, United States, 1970–1998. From bottom, the sources shown are: fuel, combustion, industrial processing, on-road (transportation), and non-road. Since lead was removed from gasoline, these levels have sharply decreased. (Source: U.S. Environmental Protection Agency.)

fewer asthma hospitalizations, 40,000 fewer emergency department visits, 20 million fewer school absences, and 10,000 fewer infants of low birthweight.[12]

Since the passage of Superfund and the creation of the Emergency Response and Removal Program, EPA has responded to more than 6,000 hazardous substance and oil emergencies. Between 1980 and 1997, the program has contained or treated more than 7 million cubic yards of contaminated soil or debris and 981 million gallons of contaminated liquids.[13] At the long-term remedial Superfund sites, EPA has completed clean-ups at nearly 900 sites and is proceeding on the almost 1,300 sites on the National Priorities List. In early 2004, the Love Canal site in Niagara Falls, New York, was proposed for de-listing from the NPL.

One key to the success of the environmental legislation is that EPA is an enforcement agency and will initiate criminal and civil prosecution for violating federal environmental laws. The use of administrative or judicial responses can force compliance, remedy the violation, require penalties, impose prison sentences, or result in contractor listing on EPA's List of Violating Facilities. In contrast to OSHA, which limits the amount of fines that can be imposed for violations, EPA can impose fines

as well as recover clean-up costs from responsible parties, which can cost millions of dollars. In fiscal year 2002, EPA's enforcement settlements resulted in $4 billion in injunctive relief to correct violations and restore the environment and $26 million in administrative penalties. Also in fiscal year 2002, 674 criminal cases were initiated, criminal violators paid in excess of $62 million in criminal penalties, and convicted environmental criminals were sentenced to 215 years of prison time.

Although the improvements made to the environment since the 1970s through clean-ups and deterring polluters are noteworthy, challenges remain. The problems with the use of DDT that Rachel Carson wrote of in *Silent Spring* have been replaced by concern over brominated flame retardants and perfluorooctanoates (PFOAs and C-8s). In 2000, at least 2.1 million tons of electronic waste (e-waste), which often contains toxic metals, were generated in the United States. With improved analytical methodologies and lower detection limits, pharmaceuticals and personal care products are recognized as emerging water pollutants.

Ironically, some environmental problems result from environmental laws. For example, the amendments to the Clean Air Act in 1990 required some areas to use oxygenated fuels to reduce tailpipe emissions. Methyl *tert*-butyl ether (MTBE) was one of the additives used for this fuel. From leaks and spillage, MTBE is now detected in about 2 percent of more than 2,200 water systems tested in California.

EPA's approach to legislation, which focuses on distinct media such as air and water, is in part at fault. For enforcement and compliance issues, this format works well for structuring divisions within EPA. In practice, however, pollution control is more encompassing. For example, installation of air pollution control technology will reduce the amount of air emissions, but will increase the waste streams for other media that will require treatment or disposal. Wet collectors create additional wastewater, while electrostatic precipitators and fabric filtration result in solid or hazardous waste. For addressing regional impacts of pollutants on the environment, especially in site clean-ups, a more comprehensive approach is desirable. A hazardous waste spill that has contaminated soil becomes a groundwater problem when the liquid waste percolates into the aquifer and becomes an air problem when vapors off-gas or migrate into homes.

Despite the overall effectiveness of environmental legislation, there has been some erosion of EPA's ability for enforcement in recent years. Concerns about the nation's economic well-being and terrorism have resulted in a sharp decline in antipollution regulations.[14] One method of cutting programs back is by reducing funding, which affects both the number of personnel for implementing programs and the remedial activities at sites. In early 2004, EPA's inspector general announced that clean-up of 11 of the country's worst hazardous waste sites had not started because of lack of funding and that other waste sites were on hold or activities were spread out over longer periods. In the mid to late 1990s, EPA completed about 75 clean-ups a year; in the early 2000s, the number of clean-ups completed each year was between 40 and 50. The trading of air-pollution credits to allow businesses more flexibility in pollution reduction goals may reduce the nation's ability to achieve air quality goals because of the widespread dispersal of pollutants. (This issue is relevant to the debate on easing regulations on mercury emissions.) Reinterpretation of the Clean Water Act concerning wetlands will exclude many acres of these valuable ecosystems from protection. For reasons of security, information available as a result of community right-to-know laws and the

FOIA process has been restricted. In order to ensure continued effectiveness of environmental laws and regulations, our nation will need to balance competing priorities between environmental protection and business and economic development, as well as competing priorities among various environmental protection needs.

REFERENCES

1. Sparrow M. The regulatory craft. Washington, DC: Brookings Institution Press, 2000:2.
2. Weil D. Assessing OSHA performance: New evidence from the construction industry. Journal of Policy Analysis and Management 2001;20:651–74.
3. Scholz J, Gray W. OSHA enforcement and workplace injuries: A behavioral approach to risk assessment. Journal of Risk and Uncertainty 1990;3:283–305.
4. Gray W, Scholz J. Does regulatory enforcement work? A panel analysis of OSHA enforcement. Law Soc Rev 1993;27:177–213.
5. Gray W, Mendeloff J. The declining effects of OSHA inspections on manufacturing injuries, 1979–1998: National Bureau of Economic Research Working Paper 9119, Cambridge, MA: National Bureau of Economic Research, 2002.
6. Baggs J, Silverstein B, Foley M. Workplace health and safety regulations: Impact of enforcement and consultation on workers' compensation claims rates in Washington State. Am J Ind Med 2004;43:483–94.
7. Fan J, Foley M, Silverstein B. Impact of WISHA activities on compensable claims rates in Washington State, 2001–2002. Olympia, WA: Washington State Department of Industries SHARP Technical Report 70-3-2003.
8. Nelson NA, Kaufman J, Kalata J, et al. Falls in constructive injury rates for OSHA-inspected employers before and after citation for violating the Washington State Fall Protection Standards. Am J Ind Med 1997;31:296–302.
9. Lipscomb H, Leiming L, Dement J. Work related falls among union carpenters in Washington State before and after the vertical fall arrest standard. Am J Ind Med 2003;44:157–65.
10. Gleason J, Barnum D. Effectiveness of OSHA sanctions in influencing employer behavior: Single and multi-period decision models. Accident Analysis & Prevention 1978;10:35–49.
11. U.S. Environmental Protection Agency. EPA Region 5–30 years of environmental progress. EPA-905-R-00-002. Washington, DC: USEPA, 2000.
12. Wong EY, Gohlke J, Griffith WC, et al. Assessing the health benefits of air pollution reduction for children. Environ Health Perspect 2004;112:226–32.
13. U.S. Environmental Protection Agency. The EPA emergency response and removal program. Over two decades of protecting human health and the environment. EPA 540-K-00-002. Washington, DC: USEPA, 2000.
14. Greenberg M. Is public support for environmental protection decreasing? An analysis of U.S. and New Jersey data. Environ Health Perspect 2004;112:121–5.

BIBLIOGRAPHY

Sparrow M. The regulatory craft. Washington, DC: Brookings Institution Press, 2000.

This is a thoughtful and probing examination of the strategies that government agencies use to ensure compliance with regulations. Based on his own experience with community oriented policing, he argues for a "problem solving" approach that uses enforcement authority firmly but creatively. His conceptual discussion is sound and his numerous examples are compelling.

Baggs J, Silverstein B, Foley M. Workplace health and safety regulations: Impact of enforcement and consultation on workers' compensation claims rates in Washington State. Am J Ind Med 2003;43:483–94.
There have been relatively few systematic evaluations of the effectiveness of government enforcement policies and programs. This article provides evidence from a state OSHA program for the impact of workplace safety and health enforcement on injury and illness rates. <http://www.osha.gov/>

This is the main Web site for OSHA. It has links to sources covering many of the subjects addressed in this chapter. <http://www.epa.gov>
This is the main Web site for EPA. It has links to sources covering many of the subjects addressed in this chapter. <http://www.atsdr.cdc.gov>
This is the main Web site for ATSDR. It has links to sources covering many of the subjects addressed in this chapter.

The findings and conclusions in this chapter are those of the authors and do not necessarily represent the views of the Centers for Disease Control and Prevention.

Index

Note: Numbers followed by f indicate figures; those followed by t indicate tables.